# Management of Small Animal Distal Limb Injuries



Steven F. Swaim, DVM, MS
Janet Welch, DVM, DACVS
Robert L. Gillette, DVM, MSE

TETON NEWMEDIA
INNOVATIVE PUBLISHING OF VETERINARY & HUMAN MEDICINE

Executive Editor: Carroll C. Cann
Design and Production: www.fiftysixforty.com

Teton NewMedia
P.O. Box 4833
Jackson, WY 83001
1-888-770-3165
www.tetonnm.com



PRINTED IN THE UNITED STATES OF AMERICA

ISBN # 978-1-893441-27-9

Print number 5 4 3 2 1

Library of Congress Cataloging-in-Publication Data on file.

# Preface

Distal limb injuries in dogs and cats are a common occurrence, to include injuries of this area in sporting and working dogs. Such injuries may involve soft tissues, hard tissues, or both, and they present the practitioner with a challenge in management to achieve a functional limb for the animal. In some cases treatment is aimed at preventing limb amputation.

The general purpose of this book is to provide the practitioner with treatment options that are available for reconstruction and salvage following distal limb injury. Effort was made to make the book practitioner-friendly by presenting each topic from the standpoint of Definition and Indications, Technique, Aftercare, and Advantages and Disadvantages.

The materials and methods described in the book are for the most part those that the authors have used and found practical and effective although other materials and methods are available.

# Acknowledgements

The authors are grateful for the contribution of several people in the production of this book. The editorial work of Carroll Cann and material processing of Mike Albiniak are greatly appreciated. Thanks go to Barbara Webster for her work in doing the word processing of the soft tissue injury section of the book. Kudos go to Amanda Stahl for the fine medical illustrations she supplied. Drs. Jennifer Pendergraft and Julia Albright covered the topic of acral lick dermatitis very effectively. The information from Drs. Dawn Boothe and Bonnie Campbell on the use of systemic antibiotics in Chapter 1 is appreciated.

# Dedication

This book is dedicated to the veterinarians, residents, interns, veterinary students, veterinary technicians, and especially the animals that will benefit from its use.

# Contributors

**Albright, M.A., D.V.M.**
Diplomat America College of Veterinary Behaviorists
Assistant Professor of Veterinary Behavior
PetSafe Chair of Small Animal Behavioral Research
College of Veterinary Medicine
University of Tennessee
Knoxville, TN 37996

**Robert L. Gillette, D.V.M., M.S.E.**
Head - Sports Medicine and Rehabilitation Department
Center for Integrative Medicine
Red Bank Veterinary Hospital
210 Newman Springs Road
Red Bank, NJ 07701

**Jennifer Pendergraft, D.V.M., M.S.**
Diplomat American College of Veterinary Dermatology
and Otology
Assistant Professor
James L. Voss Veterinary Teaching Hospital
Colorado State University
Fort Collins, CO 80523

**Steven F. Swaim, D.V.M.,M.S.**
Professor Emeritus
Scott-Ritchey Research Center and Department of
Clinical Sciences
College of Veterinary Medicine
Auburn University
Auburn, Alabama 36849

**Janet A. Welch, D.V.M.,**
Diplomat American College of Veterinary Surgeons
Specialty Services Surgeon
VCA Boston Road Animal Hospital
1235 Boston Road
Springfield, MA 01119

*Medical Illustrator*
**Amanda Stahl McKay, B.F.A., M.S. M. I.**
637 Huntington Road
#E6
Athens, GA 30606

# Table of Contents


## Part One: Soft Tissue Injuries

**Chapter 1:** Initial Management of Contaminated and Infected Wounds

- Preliminary Procedures ... 2
- Debridement and Lavage ... 11
- Wound Closure Assessment ... 17
- Topical Lavage Agents ... 19
- Antibiotics and Antibacteriels ... 24
- Enzymes ... 28
- Wound Healing Stimulants ... 29
- Other Topical Agents ... 32

**Chapter 2**: Bandages, Splints and Slings

- Primary Bandage Layer ... 38
- Adhesive Tape Stirrups ... 46
- Secondary Bandage Layer ... 48
- Tertiary Bandage Layer ... 50
- Padding Materials ... 55
- Specialty Appliances ... 60
- Carpal Flexion Splint ... 63
- Carpal Sling ... 65
- Velpeau Sling ... 66
- 90/90 Sling ... 67

**Chapter 3:** Carpal-Metacarpal/Tarsal-Metatarsal Wounds

- Primary Wound Closure ... 72
- Delayed Primary Closure ... 73
- Secondary Wound Closure ... 74
- Peripheral Nerve Injury and Repair ... 76
- Wound Drainage ... 79
- Wounds With Apposable Edges - No Tension ... 86
- Wounds With Apposable Edges - Tension ... 95
- Various Shaped Wounds ... 105
- Wounds Over the Carpus and Tarsus - Apposable Edges ... 113
- Wounds with Nonapposable Edges - Potential for Apposition and Relief of Tension - Related Scars ... 118
- Wounds Over the Carpus and Tarsus - Nonapposable Edges ... 136
- Wounds With Nonapposable Edges - No Potential for Apposition ... 139
- Wounds With Exposed Bones and Joints ... 163

**Chapter 4:** Paw Wounds

- Hemostasis ... 168
- Dorsal Digital Wounds ... 168
- Palmar/Plantar Pad Wounds - Pad Surface Wounds ... 169
- Deep Abrasion, Partial Avulsions and Deep Burns ... 171
- Pad Punctures ... 173
- Pad Lacerations ... 175
- Metacarpal/Metatarsal Pad Loss ... 179
- Deep Pad Ulceration - Bandaging ... 179
- Pad Replacement: Phalangeal Fillet ... 181
- Pad Replacement: Pouch Flap (Cats) ... 186
- Pad Replacement: Tubed Pedicle Flaps (Cats) ... 188
- Pad Replacement: Pad Grafts ... 190
- Pad Replacement: Mesh Grafts (Cats) ... 193
- Interdigital Wounds ... 194
- Interdigital Pododermatitis ... 194
- Superficial Interdigital (Web) Lacerations ... 204
- Deep Interdigital Lacerations ... 205
- Digit Orthopedic Wounds and Soft Tissue Salvage ... 206
- Digit Space Filling: Phalangeal Fillet ... 209

**Chapter 5:** Specific Wounds - Snakebite and Acral Lick Dermatoses

- Snake Bite Wounds ... 212
- Acral Lick Dermatitis ... 216

**Chapter 6:** Onychectomy, Deep Digital, Flexor Tenectomy and Digit Amputation

- Onychectomy ... 228
- Deep Digital Flexor Tenectomy (Cats) ... 233
- Dewclaw Amputation ... 234
- Digit Amputation ... 236

## Part Two: Orthopedic Injuries

**Chapter 7:** Orthopedic Injuries of the Tarsal Area

- Anatomy of the Distal Hind Limb ... 246
- Ligament and Tendon Injuries ... 250
- Sprain Injury ... 251
- Tarsal Shearing Wounds Treated by Open Wound Healing, Prosthetic Imbrication and External Fixation ... 261
- Severe Tarsal Shearing Wounds Treated by Early Arthrodesis Using External Fixation ... 264
- Severe Tarsal Shearing Wounds Treated by Delayed Arthrodesis Using Bone Plating ... 267
- Plantar Intertarsal Subluxation and Luxation ... 271
- Dorsal Intertarsal Subluxation ... 275
- Luxation of the Base of the Talus ... 278
- Tarsometatarsal Joint Subluxation ... 279
- Talocalcaneal Luxation ... 281
- Strain Injury ... 282
- Injury to the Common Calcaneal Tendon ... 286
- Rupture or Laceration of the Common Calcaneal Tendon ... 287
- Avulsion of the Gastrocnemius Tendon Insertion ... 289
- Chronic Calcaneal Tendonitis ... 295
- Gastrocnemius Tears at the Musculotendinous Junction ... 296
- Rupture of the Gastrocnemius Muscle ... 297

Luxation of the Superficial Digital
Flexor Tendon ... 298
Transarticular External Fixation of the Tarsus ... 299
Malleolar Fractures ... 305
Distal Tibial Physeal Fractures ... 307
Fractures of the Tarsal Bones ... 307
Fractures of the Calcaneus ... 308
Talus Fractures ... 312
Central Tarsal Fractures ... 316
Central Tarsal Bone Fracture - Luxation ... 320
Fractures of the Numbered Tarsal Bones ... 321

**Chapter 8:** Orthopedic Injuries of the Carpal Area
Anatomy of the Distal Forelimb ... 324
Hyperextension Injury ... 327
Collateral Ligament Instability of the
Antebrachiocarpal Joint ... 331
Luxation of the Antebrachiocarpal
(Radiocarpal) Joint ... 335
Middle Carpal Subluxation ... 336
Distal Fractures of the Radius and Ulna ... 337
Distal Radial and Ulnar Fractures: Noncominuted
and Closed ... 341
Distal Radial and Ulnar Fractures:
Cominuted or Open ... 344
Angular Limb Deformity ... 345
Radial Carpal Bone Fractures ... 352
Radial Carpal Bone Luxation ... 354
Accessory Carpal Bone Fractures ... 355
Soft Tissue Injury Related to the
Accessory Carpal Bone ... 357

**Chapter 9:** Orthopedic Injuries to the Metatarsal,
Metacarpal and Phalangeal Areas
Anatomy of the Metatarsal, Metacarpal
and Phalangeal Areas ... 360
Metacarpal and Metatarsal Fractures ... 362
Phalangeal Fractures ... 367
Ligamentous Injuries of the Phalanges ... 369
Sesamoid Fragmentation ... 371

**Part Three: Atheletic and Working Dog Injuries**

**Chapter 10:** Athletic and Working Dog Injuries
General Information ... 378
Skin Injuries ... 379
Cracked Nails ... 379
Bruised Nails ... 380
Avulsed Nails ... 380
Pad Injuries ... 381
Muscle Injuries ... 382
Interosseous Myositis or Muscle Strain ... 382
Interosseous Muscle Tears or Ruptures ... 383
Synovial Injuries ... 384
Acute Carpal Synovitis ... 384
Chronic Carpal Synovitis ... 384
Acute Sesamoidal Synovitis ... 385
Chronic Sesamoidal Synovitis ... 386
Toe Dislocations ... 386
Tendon Injuries ... 388
Palmar or Plantar Lacerations ... 390

**Index** ... 393

# Part One:
# Soft Tissue Injuries

# Chapter 1

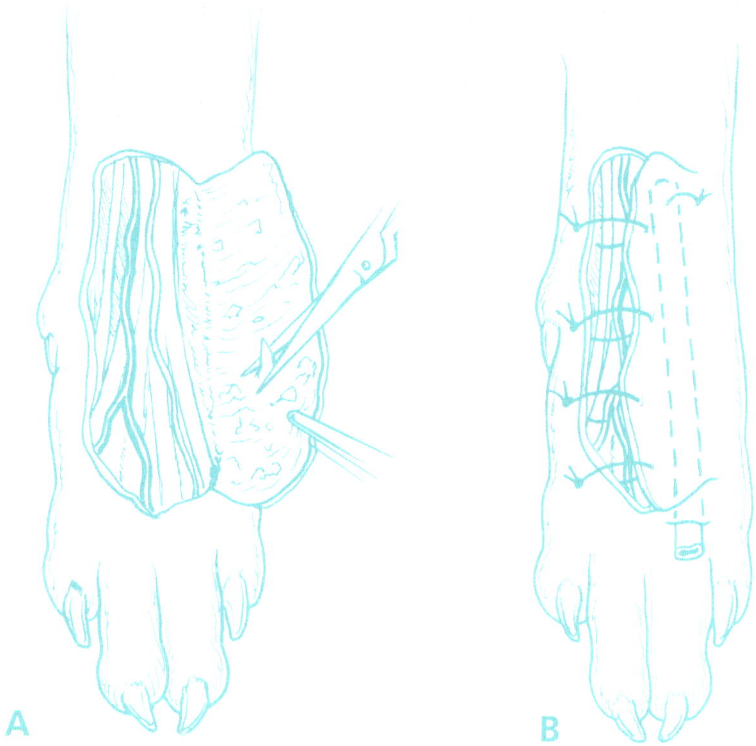


## Initial Wound Management of Contaminated and Infected Wounds

Steven F. Swaim, D.V.M., M.S.

# Contaminated and Infected Wounds-Preliminary Procedures

## Definition and Indications

When there has been a short time lapse since wound infliction the wound is considered to be contaminated. Tissues have been traumatized and inoculated with microorganisms; however, they have not started to propagate in devitalized tissue or invade viable wound tissues. When microorganisms adhere to the tissues and replicate but do not cause host injury, the wound is colonized, and healing is delayed. The wound is infected when microorganisms are replicating in the wound and causing host injury. This also affects healing. Infected wounds show signs of inflammation and may have exudates associated with them. A neutrophilia may also be present in the late stages of infection.

Numerous factors govern the time at which a wound progresses from a contaminated to an infected wound (Table 1-1).

**Table 1-1. Factors Governing Progression From a Contaminated to an Infected Wound**

| |
|---|
| 1. Blood supply to wound tissues |
| 2. Amount and type of traumatized tissue |
| 3. Number and pathogenicity of inoculated microorganisms |
| 4. Amount and type of foreign debris |
| 5. Animal's age |
| 6. Animal's immunocompetence |

Six preliminary procedures are indicated in the initial management of contaminated or infected distal limb wounds prior to surgical intervention: 1) preparation for transport to veterinary facilities, 2) initial patient evaluation, 3) microbial evaluation and therapy, 4) protection of the wound during periwound preparation, 5) periwound preparation, and 6) anesthesia and analgesia.

## Techniques

### Preparation for Transport to Veterinary Facilities

When a wound has been recently inflicted and there are no fractures or luxations present, a dry gauze or improvised bandage of clean linen should be held firmly in place to protect the wound, prevent additional contamination and help control hemorrhage. In the presence of open fractures or shearing injuries with loss of collateral ligamentous support of joints, especially the intracarpal or intratarsal joints, a splint of some type should be incorporated in the bandage. A magazine wrapped around the limb can serve this purpose.

### Initial Evaluation of the Patient

At the time of presentation to veterinary facilities, a thorough history should be taken. This should include health and medical factors that could have a bearing on wound management. A note should be made of circumstances causing the wound and any emergency therapy that has been administered. An "ABC" (airway, breathing, consciousness) survey should be performed, followed by assessment of the animal's state of consciousness. With a critically wounded animal, resuscitation and stabilization should be performed prior to caring for superficial wounds.

A detailed physical examination, as well as hematologic, biochemical, radiographic, ultrasonographic and electrocardiographic examinations are performed as indicated after the animal has been stabilized.

A sterile supportive bandage composed of a gauze pad primary dressing, absorbent secondary wrap and outer tertiary tape should be applied to the distal limb injury while other life-saving procedures and patient assessment procedures are being performed. If culture and sensitivity tests are to be performed, samples should be taken before bandaging. The primary dressing can contain a topical antimicrobial agent (Kerlix AMD, Super Sponges, Covidien Tyco/ HealthCare /Kendall, Mansfield, MA). These contain 0.2% polyhexamethylene biguanide. Sterile gauze pads coated with a water-miscible antibiotic ointment or a saline-moistened gauze containing an antibiotic or nonirritating antiseptic solution can also be used. A 0.05% chlorhexidine diacetate (Nolvasan solution, Ft. Dodge Animal Health, Ft. Dodge, IA) or chlorhexidine gluconate (ChloxheriDerm Disinfectant, Dermatologics in Veterinary Medicine Pharmaceuticals, Inc., Miami, FL) solution may be used as an antiseptic dressing. (See Topical Agents in this Chapter)

When the distal limb injury is evaluated, sterile gloves should be worn. The vascular and neural integrity of the distal limb should be evaluated, as should the orthopedic structures (bones, ligaments, and tendons). During the examination the degree of contamination or infection should be considered. The potential for the limb to become functional again and the surgical techniques that might be necessary for repair should be considered along with the anticipated time and expense to the owner.

It is human nature to look at the obvious damage and assess it and to overlook damage that may not be easily seen. For instance, neurologic damage will not be as readily observed as a distal radial and ulnar fracture. Neurologic assessment should be an important part of the examination. There is no sense in doing extensive and expensive soft tissue and orthopedic reconstruction on a forelimb that has radial/brachial avulsion injury.

## Microbial Evaluation and Therapy

Evaluation of the wound flora is usually not performed on recent wounds. However, if a recent wound is potentially serious a swab of the wound should be taken prior to wound lavage for aerobic and anaerobic bacterial culture and sensitivity testing. Alternatively, tissues from the wound can be submitted for culture and sensitivity testing.

If a wound has been present for a few days and is infected or in chronic nonhealing wounds (e.g. acral lick dermatitis wounds) wound tissue should be collected for microbial evaluation. For chronic wounds, this includes fungal evaluation. The surface of these wounds should be thoroughly cleansed to help rid it of surface contaminants before taking the biopsy. Proper collection vials should be used. Personnel of a microbiology laboratory can be consulted about collection and handling techniques, especially when dealing with chronic wounds that may be infected with fungal or unusual organisms.

The use of systemic antimicrobials should be approached rationally and judiciously, with clinical signs playing an important role in decisions on their use. Superficial wounds with little tissue damage and minimal to moderate contamination in a healthy animal can be properly lavaged and debrided and may not require topical or systemic antibiotic therapy. Conversely, systemic antibiotic therapy is indicated when there has been severe tissue damage, to include bone and/or joint trauma, there is questionable tissue remaining after debridement, the animal is severely immune-compromised, the wound tissues show signs of infection and inflammation, and/or there are signs of systemic infection. In such cases, parenteral antibiotic administration may be indicated until the animal's general health allows continuation of antibiotic therapy in oral form.

In addition to bacteria being sensitive to the antibiotic used, it is also important to make sure the dose, dose interval, and tissue penetration are such that effective antibiotic levels are reached in the wound.

Often, initial antibiotic therapy in wound management is done empirically based on clinical judgment. If this is the case, the antibiotic selected should be effective against the bacteria that are expected to be in the wound which are likely to cause postoperative wound infection. There is some information about systemic antibiotics that can be of clinical importance in wound therapy. Drugs with long half – lives are preferred to drugs with short half – lives (e.g. amoxicillin with or without clavulanic acid). Routine use of drugs with residual effects (e.g. cefovecin) should be avoided and based on susceptibility data. In the presence of marked inflammatory debris, drugs which accumulate in phagocytic white blood cells should be considered (e.g. fluorinated quinolones, macrolides, clindamycin). While first tier drugs (e.g. amoxicillin – clavulanic acid, cephalexin) are encouraged when appropriate, such drugs are commonly underdosed. While fluorinated quinolones are characterized by excellent distribution, if resistance occurs it will be high – level, multidrug resistance, and in the case of *Staphyloccoccus* may include methicillin – resistance.

*Staphylococcus* and *Streptococcus* spp. Are usually present in recent wounds, and the first generation cephalosporins [e.g. cephalexin (Keflex, Dista Products Co., Division of Eli Lilly & Co., Indianapolis, IN), or cefadroxil (Cefa-Drops or Cefa-Tabs, Ft. Dodge Animal Health, Ft. Dodge, IN)] can be used for prophylaxis. The Cephalosporins can be given intravenously at anesthesia induction and may be repeated every 90 minutes during surgery. This is followed by oral administration postoperatively. A combination trimethoprim and sulfadiazine (Tribrissen tablets, Schering-Plough Animal Health Corp., Union, NJ) can be used for wound therapy, as can amoxicillin (Amoxi-inject, Amoxi-Tabs, Pfizer animal Health Group). A combination of amoxicillin-trihydrate and clavulanate potassium (Clavamox tablets or drops, Pfizer Animal Health Group) can be used to treat more aggressive wounds. Aminoglycosides could be considered for wounds that have a heavy gram-negative bacterial flora. Cephoxitin and potentiated sulfonamides are also commonly effective against gram negative aerobes. For broader spectrum coverage with one antibotic, the fluoroquinolones [e.g. enrofloxacin (Baytril, Bayer Corp., Agriculture Corp., animal Health, Shawnee Mission, KS)] can be used.

In the presence of contaminated distal limb wounds with orthopedic instability, intravenous antibiotics, such as the first generation cephalosporin, cefazolin (Cephazolin for injection, Westward Pharmaceutical Corp., Eatontown, NJ), are in order when gram positive organisms are present. Enrofloxacin or aminoglycocides can be used if gram negative organisms are present.

If anaerobes are present, ampicillin (Ampicillin injectable, American Pharmaceutical Partners, Schaumburg, IL, or ampicillin capsules, Teva, Sellersville, PA), clindamycin (Antirobe, Pharmica and Upjohn Co., Kalamazoo, MI), metronidazole (Metronidazole tablets, Teva, Sellersville, PA) are effective. These three antibiotics are also available for intravenous injection, Azithromycin (Zythromax, Pfizer, New York, NY) is also effective against anaerobes, as is the second generation cephalosporin cefoxitin (Mefoxin, ESI Lederle, Philadelphia, PA) If a wound has bone involvement, extensive soft tissue injury, or is grossly contaminated or infected, a second generation cephalosporin such as cefoxitin or a combination of drugs that provide broad spectrum coverage (including anaerobes) may be considered.

The effectiveness of systemic antibiotic therapy can be evaluated by repeating culture examination 3 or 4 days following initial culture and sensitivity tests. If there is no growth, the initial therapy can be continued. However, a change in antibiotic therapy should be considered when 1) another antibiotic is indicated by culture and sensitivity tests, 2) there has been little improvement in the wound's appearance after 2 to 3 days of the initial therapy, or 3) the animal's general condition has worsened with signs of septicemia.

When systemic antibiotics are used, they should be administered as soon as possible following wound infliction. Administration of antibiotics within the first 3 hours helps ensure adequate levels in the wound fluids to contact bacteria before they are surrounded by thick tenacious coagulum. When wounds are badly contaminated or infected, a combination of systemic and topical antibiotics is indicated. Systemic antibiotics are usually administered for 5 to 7 days unless extensive antibiotic therapy is indicated. Once an open soft tissue wound has entered a repair stage of healing and has a healthy bed of granulation tissue, systemic and topical antibiotics are generally not needed. However, if there is bone infection, systemic antibiotic therapy is prolonged, possibly as long as 6 to 8 weeks.

## Protection of the Wound During Periwound Preparation

To effectively protect the wound while the area around it is prepared, the wound is covered with a water-soluble lubricating gel (K-Y Jelly, Johnson & Johnson, New Brunswick, NJ) or a water-soluble lubricating gel that contains chlorhexidine gluconate (Surgilube, Savage Laboratories, Melville, NY). The gel often tends to gravitate from the wound due to the limb's elevated position while the wound is being treated. Thus, a thin coat of the gel may be applied as an adhesive to hold a sterile dry gauze sponge over the wound. Once applied, the edges of the gauze may be trimmed with scissors so the gauze more accurately fits the wound and preparation of skin near the wound edge is easier.

After the area around the wound has been clipped, the original protective gauze sponge is replaced with a fresh sponge and gel. The skin around the wound is prepared for aseptic surgery, using care not to get preparation detergents or solutions in the wound even though it is covered with the sponge and gel. The sponge and gel are removed just prior to injecting local analgesic if this is to be used.

## Periwound Preparation

The paw is an area of high contamination, and this combined with the multiple intertriginous areas and hair provide an ideal area for bacterial growth when exudate, serum, and blood-producing wounds are present. Thus, for all wound management and surgical techniques performed on the palmar/plantar paw surface, the paw should be properly prepared for aseptic surgery.

For thorough preparation of a paw, towel forceps can be placed through the ends of the nails on the third and fourth digits. Gauze is tied through the rings of the forceps, then a length of gauze is used to suspend the limb while hair is clipped and the paw is scrubbed (Figure 1-1).

All hair should be clipped from the paw. Standard clippers (Oster Clippers, Oster Professional Products, McMinnville, TN) with a No. 40 blade can be used to clip the majority of the hair from the paw. However, to adequately clip the hair in the interdigital and interpad areas, a small pair of clippers with a one-inch wide head (Oster Finisher, Oster Professional Products, McMinnville, TN) (Figure 1-2) should be used.

The nails should be clipped, including those of the third and fourth digits being used for limb suspension after scrubbing and antiseptic application. If any groove remains on the palmar/plantar surface of the nails after clipping, it is cleaned with the point of an 18-gauge needle.

Because of their residual antimicrobial action, especially in the presence of organic material (i.e. blood and exudate), the author prefers to use chlorhexidine-containing products for preparing the paws for surgery.

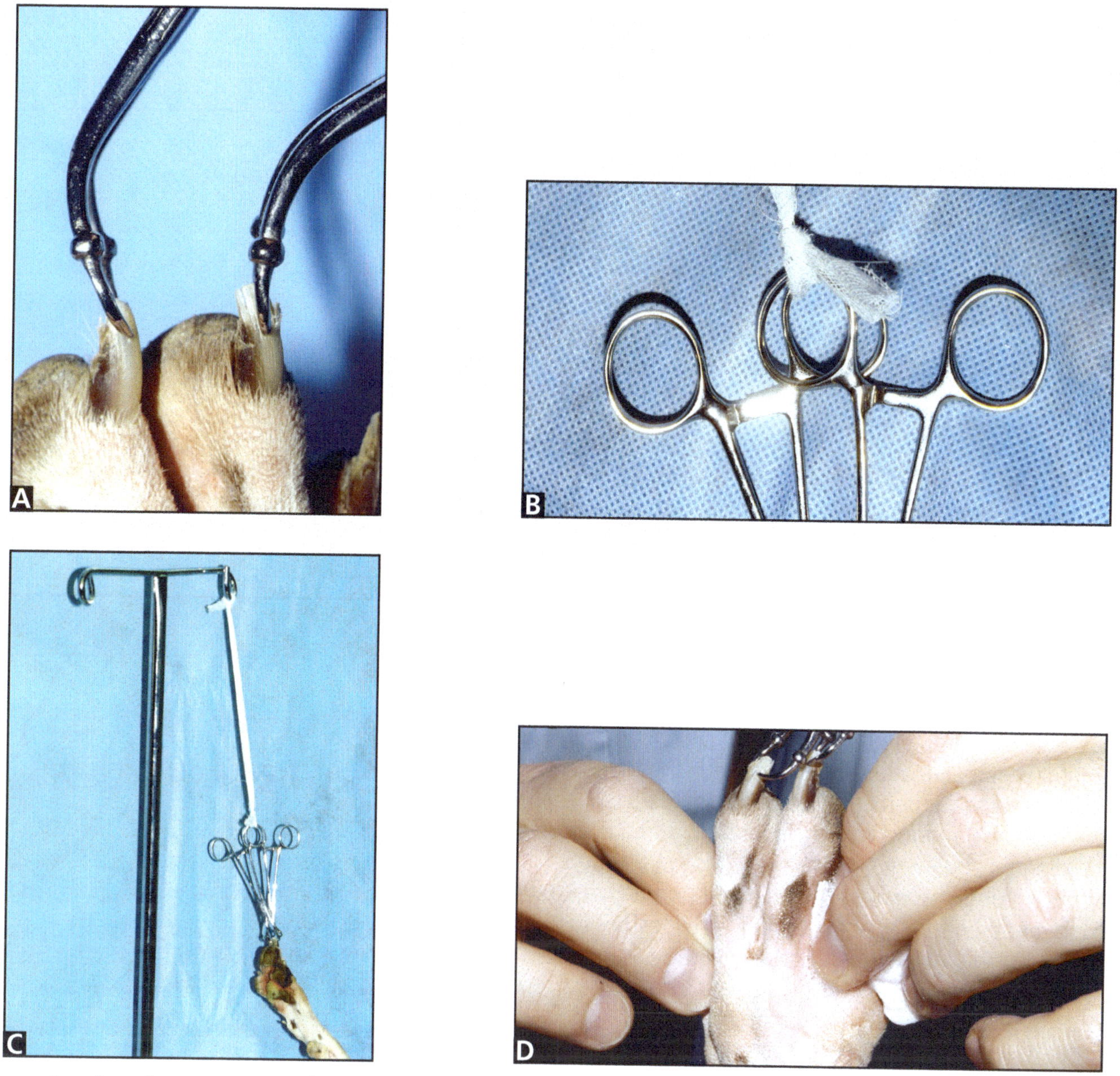

**Figure 1-1.** Preparation of paw for surgery. **A.** Towel forceps placed through the distal ends of the nails on digits 3 and 4. **B.** Gauze through the rings on the forceps. **C.** Limb suspended by gauze and towel forceps. **D.** Interdigital and interpad areas are open for surgical preparation (From Swaim SF, Henderson RA: Small Animal Wound Management, 2nd ed. : Baltimore: Williams & Wilkins, 1997, 333.)

These are chlorhexidine diacetate (Nolvasan Surgical Scrub and Nolvasan Solution, Ft. Dodge Animal Health, Ft. Dodge, IA) or chlorhexidine gluconate (ChlorhexiDerm Scrub and ChlorhexiDerm Disinfectant, Dermatologics in Veterinary Medicine Pharmaceuticals, Inc., Miami, FL). The paw is scrubbed 3 times with the scrub solution with a tap water rinse between scrubs. If there is still debris coming off the palmar/plantar surface of the paw, additional scrubs are done. After scrubbing the paw, 3 applications of chlorhexidine solution are applied to the paw.

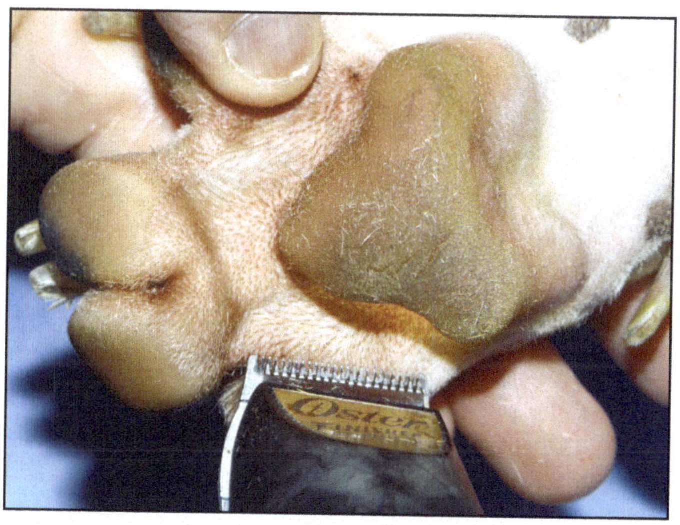

**Figure 1-2.** Small finishing clippers with a one inch wide head for clipping hair in the intedigital and interpad areas of the paw.

To protect the paw while transporting the animal to the surgery room, sterile aluminum foil can be removed from an autoclaved roll and wrapped around the distal limb (Figure 1-3). This provides a sterile, water-impervious covering and no towel forceps or

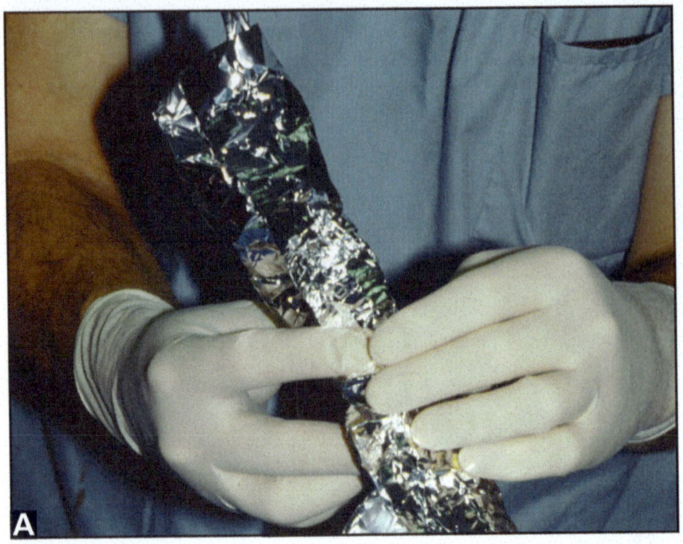

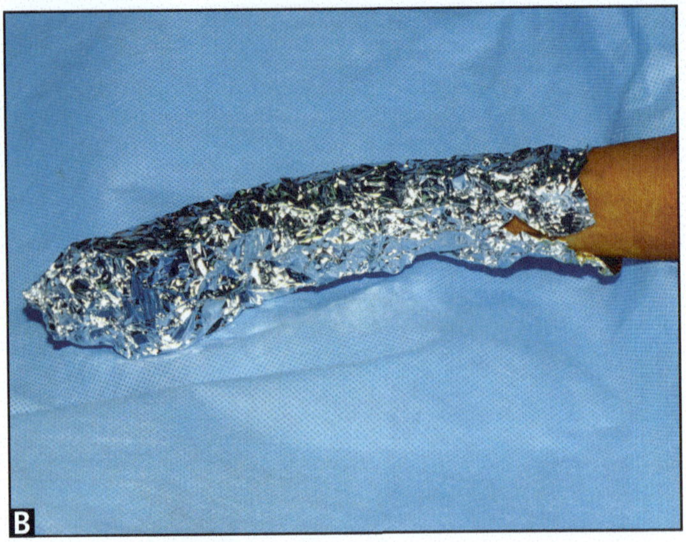


**Figure 1-3.** Aluminum foil for draping of a surgically prepared paw and distal limb. **A.** Sterile aluminum foil removed from an autoclaved roll/box being wrapped around a limb. **B.** Aluminum foil wrapping completed. (From Swaim SF, Henderson RA: Small Animal Wound Management, 2nd ed.: Baltimore: Williams & Wilkins, 1997, 334.)

gauze ties are needed to hold it in place (Janssens L., Antwerp, Belgium. Personal Communication, 1990).

## Anesthesia and Analgesia

General anesthesia, local or regional anesthesia, and/or regional analgesia may be used for wound management. General anesthesia is the first choice if the animal is in good physical condition and a good candidate for general anesthesia. If a compromised physical condition makes the animal a poor candidate for general anesthesia local or regional anesthesia combined with a neuroleptanalgesic drug are in order.

Prior to wound irrigation and manipulation to remove foreign debris from its surface, a surgical sponge can be placed on the wound and saturated with warm 2% lidocaine, without epinephrine. When left in place for 2 to 3 minutes it appears to make wound surface lavage and manipulation more comfortable for the animal (Figure 1-4A).

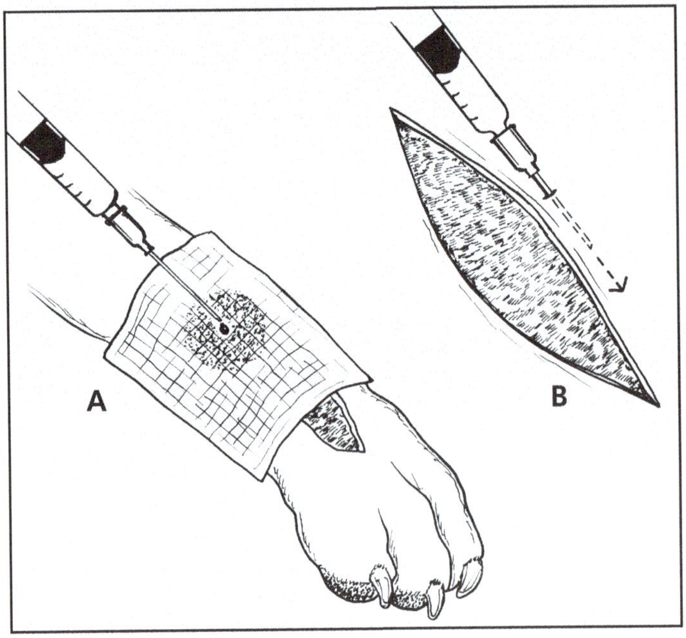


**Figure 1-4.** Local anesthesia. **A.** Topical anesthesia: warm 2% lidocaine applied to surgical sponges. **B.** Local anesthesia: warm 1% or 2% lidocaine without epinephrine or bupivicaine injected through intact skin parallel to wound edge.

Neuroleptanalgesia combined with local anesthesia are commonly used before wound lavage and debridement. The tranquilizer sedates the animal and the analgesic helps control pain. Lidocaine, 1% or 2% without epinephrine, or bupivicaine is injected through intact skin parallel to the wound edge using a 23 or 25 gauge needle (Figure 1-4B). Lidocaine has a relatively rapid onset of action and short duration of effect, 5 to 10 minutes and 1 to 2 hours, respectively. Whereas, bupivacaine has a relatively longer onset of action and longer duration of effect, 20 minutes and 4 to 6 hours, respectively. The toxicity levels of the drugs when given intravenously should be borne in mind when administering them locally or regionally. In dogs, toxic effects of lidocaine are seen at approximately 10 mg/kg, and 3 to 5 mg/kg with bupivacaine. In cats total doses should not exceed 2.5 mg/kg of lidocaine and 1.0 mg/kg of bupivacaine. The total dose of bupivacaine should not exceed 2 mg/kg in dogs. If desired, lidocaine and bupivacaine can be combined at a maximum of 1.5 mg/kg each.

To help prevent the initial pain of analgesic injection, 0.1 ml of injectable sodium bicarbonate can be added for each ml of lidocaine. Other measures to increase the comfort of local anesthesia injection are 1) warming the anesthetic agent if it has been refrigerated; although, refrigeration of such agents is not necessary, 2) slow injection, 3) pinching the skin up at the point of needle insertion, and 4) injection into subcutaneous tissue.

Regional analgesia in conjunction with neuroleptanalgesia can also be used for distal limb and paw surgery. One form of regional analgesia is a ring block of the limb with the analgesic drug. Using a 23 to 25 gauge needle, analgesic drug is injected from the skin to the bone circumferentially proximal to the wound. Ring block with bupivacaine has been described for onychectomy pain (Figure 1-5).

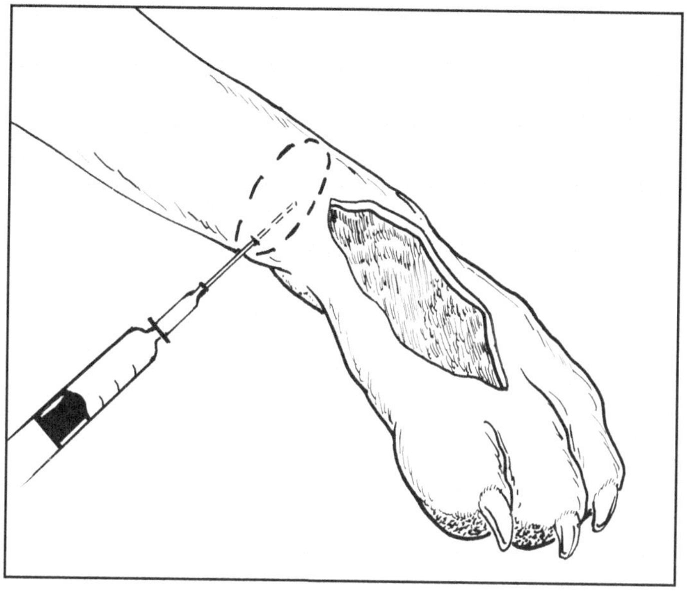

**Figure 1-5.** Regional anesthesia of forelimb. Ring block from skin to bone circumferentially proximal to the wound.

On the distal forelimb/paw a regional nerve block can be performed on the superficial radial, dorsal cutaneous and palmar branches of the ulnar nerve for the forelimb, and the median nerve for procedures on the paw (Figure 1-6). As an example, injection of 0.1 to 0.2 ml of 0.5% bupivacaine per site (not to exceed a total dose of 5mg/kg) is useful in providing analgesia for onychectomy in cats. This provides analgesia for 4-6 hours. The paw can also be blocked by inserting the needle just distal to the carpus on the proximal-medial aspect of the metacarpus and injecting a small amount of local anesthetic to produce a small bleb. Repeated small injections are made continuing across the dorsum of the metacarpus to the lateral aspect. The block is completed by inserting the needle in the depression just distal to the accessory carpal pad, aspirating and injecting a small amount of local anesthetic, ensuring a continuous infiltration from the medial aspect to the lateral aspect. For the distal pelvic limb, a regional nerve block can be performed on the superficial and deep peroneal nerves and the tibial nerve. The superficial peroneal nerve is located subcutaneously where it crosses the dorsal surface of the hock, slightly on the medial side. The deep peroneal nerve is located parallel to the cranial tibial artery (this becomes the dorsal pedal artery as it descends distal to the tarsus). The tibial nerve is palpated beneath the skin between the gastrocnemius tendon and the tibia just proximal to the hock. Injection for this nerve should be immediately dorsal to the hock as the nerve receives a branch from the caudal cutaneous sural nerve proximal to that level.

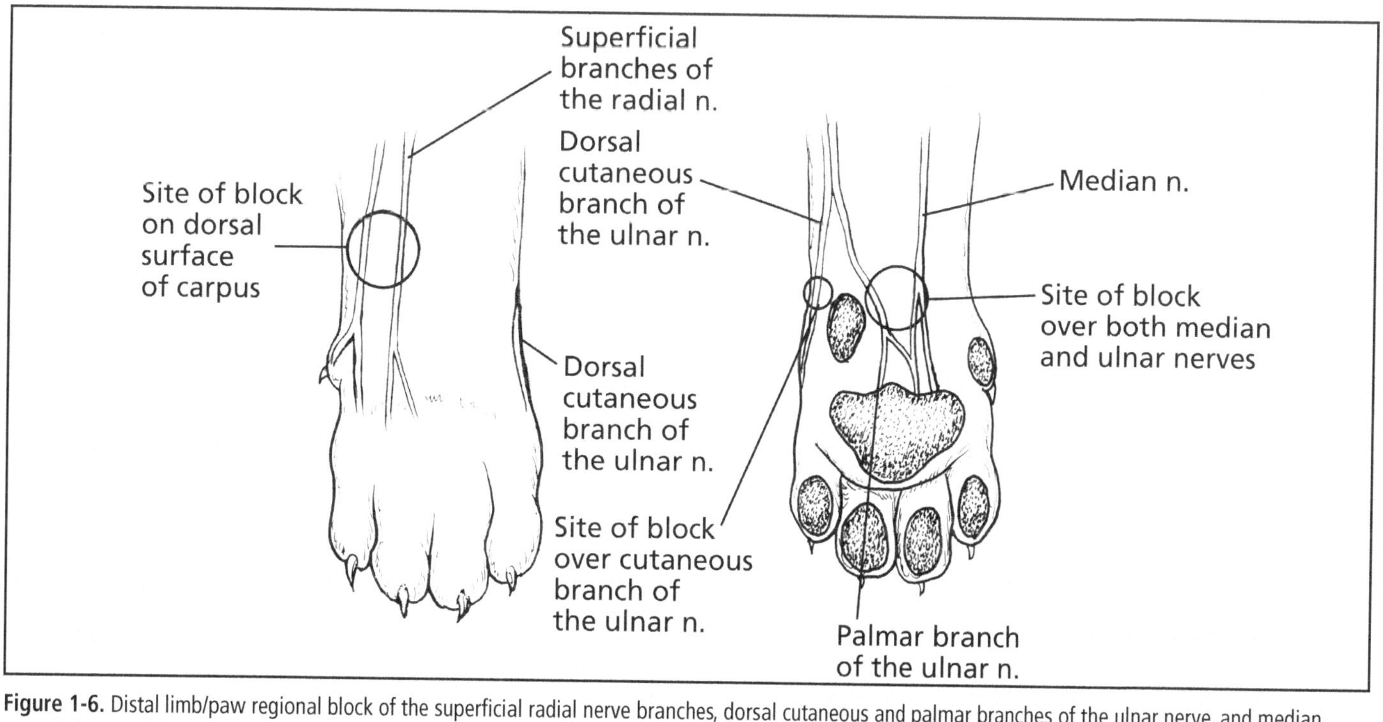


**Figure 1-6.** Distal limb/paw regional block of the superficial radial nerve branches, dorsal cutaneous and palmar branches of the ulnar nerve, and median nerve (often used for feline onychectomy). (Afer Pascoe P: Local and regional anesthesia and analgesia. Semin. Vet Med and Surg (Small Animal) 12:94, 1997.)

Digital regional blocks can be accomplished by inserting a fine needle subcutaneously on each side of a digit and injecting 0.5 to 1.0 ml of local anesthetic agent on each side to block the dorsal and palmar/plantar branches of the digital nerves (Figure 1-7). As an alternative, the common dorsal and palmar/plantar digital nerves can be blocked by injections dorsally and ventrally at the distal end(s) of the metacarpal/metatarsal space(s).

For distal forelimb wounds, a brachial plexus block can be considered as a regional block. A 22 gauge, 3.75 to 7.5 cm needle is used depending on the animal's size. For cats, a 1.5 inch needle is used. After preparing the cranial scapulohumeral area aseptically, the needle is inserted medial to the shoulder joint toward the costochondral junction of the first palpable rib, lateral to the thoracic wall, and parallel to the vertebral column (Figure 1-8). Aspiration is performed to assure that a large vessel has not been penetrated. The local anesthetic agent is injected as the needle is withdrawn. An alternative is to inject local anesthetic while withdrawing the needle 75% of the distance inserted. The needle is then withdrawn and inserted 2 more times, approximately 30 degrees dorsal and 30 degrees ventral with aspiration for blood at each insertion. Anesthetic is injected while withdrawing the needle. Local anesthetic dose can be as high as 1.5 mg/kg of lidocaine or bupivacaine.

Epidural blocks could be considered for management of pain associated with distal limb and paw surgery. It can be used for intraoperative pain management

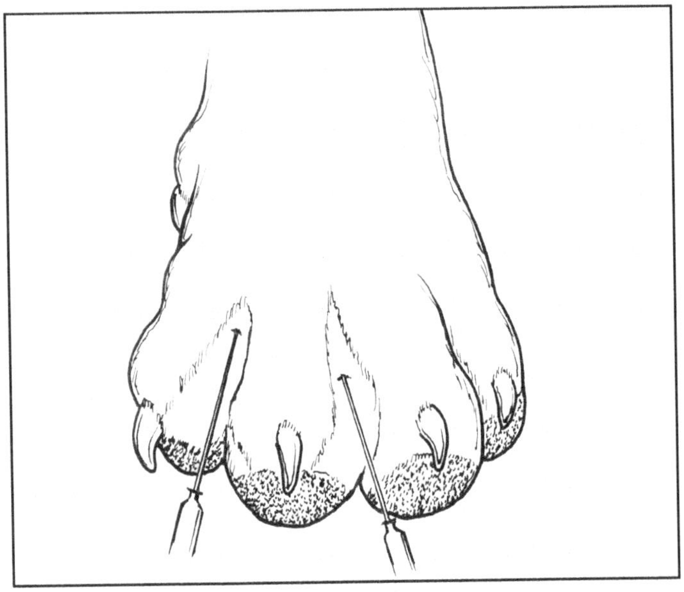

**Figure 1-7.** Digital nerve block with subcutaneous injection on each side of the digit to block the dorsal and palmar/plantar branches of the digital nerves. (After Hall LW, Clarke KW, Trim CM: Veterinary Anesthesia, 10th ed.: Philadelphia: WB Saunders, 2001, 385.)

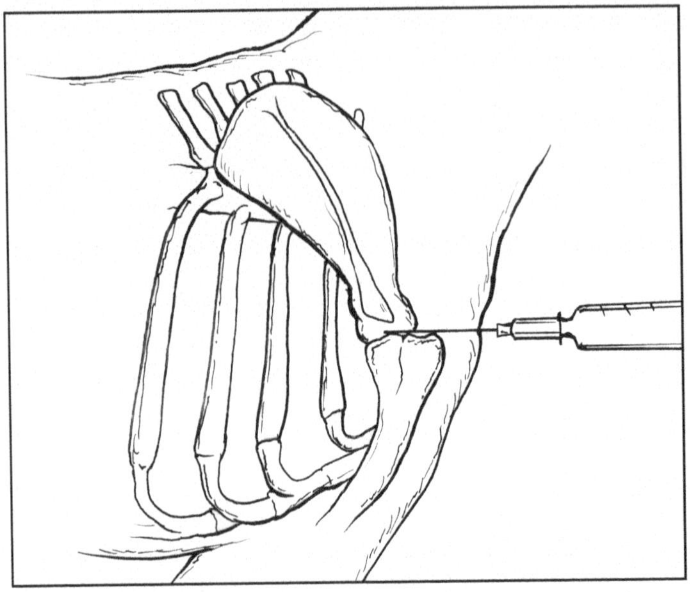

**Figure 1-8.** Brachial plexus block. The needle is placed medial to the scapulohumeral joint toward the costochondral junction, lateral to the thoracic wall and parallel to the vertebral column. (After Carroll GL: Perioperative multimodal analgesic therapy. In Fossum TW, et al: Small Animal Surgery, 3rd ed.: St. Louis: Mosby, 2007, 130.)

in high-risk patients as well as for postoperative pain management. For pelvic limb orthopedic procedures, both local anesthetic agents and opioid analgesic agents can be used. With forelimb orthopedic procedures only opiod analgesics can be used. The technique is contraindicated in the presence of coagulation abnormalities, pyoderma and sepsis. Epidural administration of local anesthetics, but not opioids is contraindicated with hypolipemia. The dose of local anesthetic should be reduced for geriatric, pregnant and obese patients as well as with space occupying lesions or conditions in which venous engorgement is expected. Local anesthetic dose should also be reduced to 25 to 50% of the normal dose if cerebrospinal fluid (CSF) is encountered when performing the epidural tap. Epidural blocks can be performed on dogs under neuroleptanalgesia; however, general anesthesia is usually required for safe administration in cats.

After aseptic preparation of the skin from just cranial to the wings of the ilium to the second sacral vertebra and as wide as the ilium wing, an eye drape is placed over the area. The skin and subcutaneous tissue over the lumbosacral space is injected with lidocaine in the conscious animal. The animal may be placed in sternal or lateral recumbency; however, sternal recumbency may be precluded if the animal has upper pelvic limb trauma. If the animal is in sternal recumbency the pelvic limbs are flexed and pulled cranially. The right and left iliac crests are palpated with the thumb and middle finger of one hand. The dorsal spine of $L_7$ and the median sacral crest are palpated with the index finger. The dorsal spine of $L_6$ may be easier to palpate with the dorsal spine of $L_7$ just caudal to it. The spinal needle size depends on the animal's size (<10 kg - 1.5 inch x 22 G, 10 to 45 kg - 2.5 inch x 22 G, >45 kg - 3.5 inch x 20G). With the needle in the opposite hand, it is inserted through the skin with the bevel directed cranially, with continued insertion on the dorsal midline perpendicular to the skin and centered at the $L_7$ and $S_1$ interarcual space. Alternatively, the needle is inserted on the dorsal midline immediately behind and parallel to the spinous process of $L_7$ to the dorsal arch of $L_7$. The needle point is advanced through the tissues to the interarcual space between $L_7$ and $S_1$. The needle then penetrates the ligamentum flavum into the epidural space (Figure 1-9). In dogs, but not cats, a change in resistance to needle advancement is felt as the needle penetrates the ligamentum flavum. The "hanging drop" technique can be used to check proper placement of the needle. With a drop of sterile saline in the hub of the needle, it will disappear into the epidural space when the needle penetrates it. If the needle strikes bone during advancement, the caudal aspect of the dorsal arch of $L_7$ or the cranial aspect of $S_1$ may have been encountered. The needle should be withdrawn slightly, and the angle of penetration should be changed slightly cranial or caudal (dependent on position of the needle relative to $L_7$ or $S_1$). The needle is then advanced off the edge of the bone into the interarcual space. With unsuccessful needle placement, it should be withdrawn, the landmarks repalpated, and the needle reinserted. Needle placement is checked by removing the stylet and checking for CSF or blood in the needle. No CSF should be present. Gentle aspiration may be performed. If CSF is encountered, the local anesthetic dose is reduced to 50% of the normal dose. If blood appears in the needle, it should be withdrawn and repositioned. Injection of 0.5 ml to 1.0 ml of air with a glass syringe should meet no resistance, and air should not bubble back along the needle to distend the skin at the injection site or result in crepitus. If the syringe plunger is pushed back by air, it indicates the needle is not in the desired location. In cats 0.1 to 0.2 ml of air should be used. In dogs and cats, 2% lidocaine is injected at 3 to 5 mg/kg or 0.5% bupivicaine at 1.5 to 2.5 mg/kg with the dose depending on the level and extent of block required. Following injection of the anesthetic or analgesic drug, the needle stylet is replaced and the needle is removed. The animal is then positioned with the affected side (operative site) down for 20 minutes. Elevation of the animal's head for the first 10 minutes should be done to avoid excess cranial advancement of the block.

## Aftercare

After the preliminary procedures of wound management have been accomplished, the wound itself is ready for debridement and lavage, placement of topical medication and application of a bandage/splint. If a wound is considered to be sufficiently prepared after debridement and lavage, the appropriate technique for closure is performed.

## Advantages and Disadvantages

Packing a wound with gauze or clean linen under

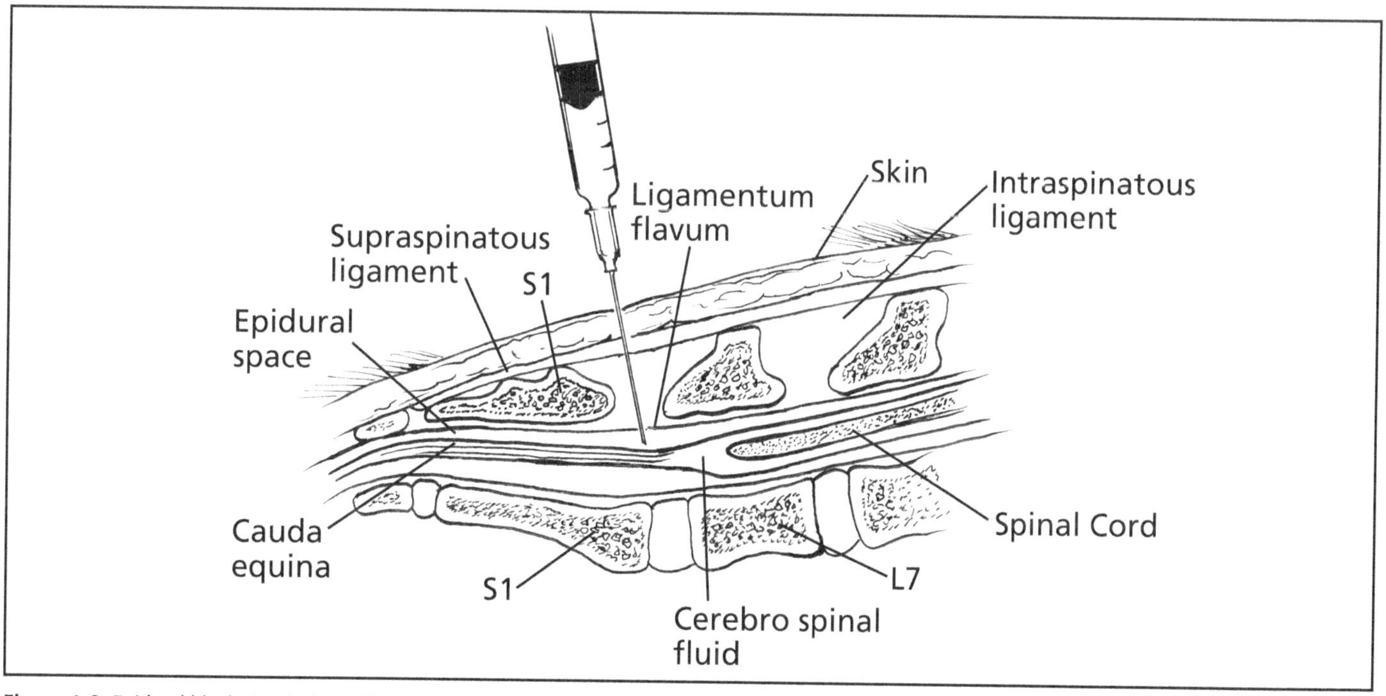


**Figure 1-9.** Epidural block. A spinal needle is inserted into the epidural space through the ligamentum flavum at the intrarcual space between L7 and S1. (After Carroll GL: Perioperative multimodal analgesic therapy. In Fossum TW, et al: Small Animal Surgery, 3rd ed: St. Louis: Mosby, 2007, 130.)

pressure is safer than tourniquet application. A tourniquet applied too loosely does not provide sufficient hemostasis; whereas, one applied too tightly may cause neurovascular damage to underlying tissue.

Although it may involve more expense, a culture and sensitivity test from a potentially serious wound may assure that antimicrobial therapy is accurate. Cultures of wound tissue, rather than surface swabs, on chronic wounds helps assure accurate microbial analysis of causative organisms rather than surface contaminants.

Use of sterile water soluble lubricating gels and gauze sponges to protect the wound while preparing the area around the wound is simpler than temporary wound closure with sutures, staples or towel clamps.

An advantage to the use of neuroleptanalgesia is that the narcotic portion of the drug can be counteracted with an antagonist if the animal develops problems while under the effects of the drugs. A surgical sponge soaked with 2% lidocaine and initially placed over the wound makes preliminary procedures more comfortable for the animal; however, no surgical debridement can be performed. When using local anesthesia good analgesia is possible.

A brachial plexus block can provide good intraoperative and postoperative analgesia. However, it can be less reliable than an epidural block because it is a relatively blind technique without using a nerve locator. Other disadvantages have been described for brachial plexus blocks. A large hematoma may result if brachial plexus vessels are punctured. If the needle enters the thorax air can enter the pleural cavity. The brachial plexus can be damaged resulting in neuritis or permanent paralysis. Infection can result if aseptic technique is not used in doing the block.

Epidural anesthesia can provide hours of relative comfort for an animal. However, if aseptic techniques is not used for injection, septic meningitis or myelitis can result. If the anesthetic agent is injected in the subarachnoid space, there may be more cranial advancement of the drug. Excess cranial advancement of the drug can interfere with intercostal efferent nerves to cause respiratory difficulty. A gross overdose may cause phrenic nerve paralysis and respiratory arrest.

The toxic effects of lidocaine and bupivacaine should be borne in mind when using these drugs. These include restlessness, muscle tremors, seizures, cardiopulmonary depression, coma and death.

# Suggested Readings


1. Aaron DN: Management of open musculoskeletal injuries. Semin Vet. Med Surg (Small Anim) 3: 290, 1988.
2. Anderson D: Wound management in small animal practice. In Practice 18: 115, 1996.
3. Anderson D: Management of open wounds. In Williams J, Moores A, eds.: BSAVA Manual of Canine and Feline Wound Management and Reconstruction, 2nd ed.: Glouster (UK): BSAVA, 2009, 37.
4. Brainard BM, Hofmeister EH: Anesthesia monitoring. In Tobias KM, Johnston SA, eds.: Veterinary Surgery, Small Animal, Vol 1: St. Louis: Elsevier-Saunders, 2012, 248.
5. Bright RM, Probst CW: Management of superficial skin wounds. In Slatter DH, ed.: Textbook of Small Animal Surgery. Philadelphia: WB Saunders, 1985, 431.
6. Carroll GL: Treatment of perioperative pain. In Fossum TW, ed.: Small Animal Surgery, 2nd ed: St. Louis: Mosby, 2002, 93.
7. Carroll GL: Treatment of perioperative multimodal pain. In Fossum TW, ed.: Small Animal Surgery, 3rd ed: St. Louis: Mosby, 2007, 130.
8. Dernell WS: Initial wound management. Vet Clin No Am Small Anim Pract. 36: 713, 2006.
9. Fahie MA: Primary wound closure. In Tobias KM, Johnston SA, eds.: Veterinary Surgery, Small Animal, Vol 2: St. Louis: Elsevier-Saunders, 2012, 1197.
10. Gaynor JS, Mama KR: Local and regional anesthetic techniques for alleviation of perioperative pain. In Gaynor JS, Muir WW, eds.: Handbook of Veterinary Pain Management, 2nd ed.: Philadelphia: Elsevier, 2009, 277.
11. Hall LW, Clarke KW, Trim CM: Veterinary Anesthesia, 10th ed.: Philadelphia: WB Saunders, 2001, 225, 385.
12. Heath MM: Surgical preparation: Part I, Preoperative preparation of the patient. Vet Tech 7:253, 1985.
13. Hosgood G: Open wounds. In Tobias KM, Johnston SA, eds.: Veterinary Surgery, Small Animal, Vol. 2: St. Louis: Elsevier-Saunders, 2012, 1210.
14. Johnston DE: Care of accidental wounds. Vet. Clin No Amer Small Anim Pract 20: 27, 1990.
15. Knapp DW: Management of the open wound. In Birchard SJ, Sherding RG, eds.: Saunders Manual of Small Animal Practice, 2nd ed.: Philadelphia: WB Saunders, 2000, 399.
16. Knapp DW: Management of the open wound. In Birchard SJ, Sherding RG, eds.: Saunders Manual of Small Animal Practice, 3rd ed.: St. Louis: Saunders-Elsevier, 2006, 549.
17. Krahwinkel DJ, Boothe HW: Topical and systemic medications for wounds. Vet Clin No Am Small Anim Pract 36: 739, 2006.
18. Lamont LA: Perioperative pain management. In Harari J, ed.: Small Animal Surgery Secrets, 2nd ed.: Philadelphia: Hanley and Belfus, 2004, 20.
19. Liptak JM: An overview of topical management of wounds. Australian Veterinarian 75: 408, 1997.
20. Lozier SM: Topical Wound Therapy. In Harari, J ed.: Surgical Complications and Wound Healing in Small Animal Practice. Philadelphia: WB Saunders, 1993, 63.
21. Muir WW: Anesthetic techniques. In Slatter DH, ed.: Textbook of Small Animal Surgery, 2nd ed.: Philadelphia: WB Saunders, 1993, 2245.
22. Pascoe P: Local and regional anesthesia and analgesia. Semin Vet Med and Surg (Small Anim) 12: 94, 1997.
23. Pavletic MM: Atlas of Small Animal Reconstructive Surgery, 2nd ed.: Philadelphia: WB Saunders, 1999, 21.
24. Pavletic MM: Atlas of Small Animal Wound Management and Reconstructive Surgery, 3rd ed.: Ames, IA: Wiley-Blackwell, 2010, 31.
25. Quandt JE, Rawlings CR: Reducing postoperative pain in dogs: Local anesthetic and analgesic techniques. Compend Contin Educ (Small Anim) 18: 101, 1996.

26. Rochat MC: Preventing and treating osteomyelitis. Vet Med 96: 678, 2001.
27. Swaim SF, Pope ER: Limb degloving injuries: pathophysiology and management. Semin Vet Med Surg (Small Anim).
28. Swaim SF, Riddell KP, Geiger DL, et.al: Evaluation of surgical scrub and antiseptic solutions for surgical preparation of canine paws. J Am Vet Med Assoc 198: 1941, 1991.
29. Swaim SF, Henderson RA: Small Animal Wound Management, 2nd ed.: Baltimore: Williams and Wilkins, 1997, 13.
30. Swaim SF: Acute superficial soft tissue injuries. In Bistner SI, Ford RB, Raffe MR, eds.: Handbook of Veterinary Procedures and Emergency Treatments, 7th ed.: Philadelphia: WB Saunders, 2000, 257.
31. Swaim SF, Bohling MW: Current concepts in small animal superficial open wound management. Medecien Veterinaire Du Quebec 33: 99, 2003.
32. Swaim SF, Renberg WC, Shike KM: Small Animal Bandaging, Casting, and Splinting Techinques. Ames, IA: Wiley-Blackwell, 2011, 43.
33. Usatine RP, Moy BL: Anesthesia. In Usatine RP, Moy RL, Tobinick EL, Siegel DM, eds.: Skin Surgery: A Practical Guide. St. Louis: Mosby, 1998, 20.
34. Waldron DR, Trevor P: Management of superficial skin wounds. In Slatter DH, ed.: Textbook of Small Animal Surgery, 2nd ed.: Philadelphia: WB Saunders, 1993, 269.
35. Waldron DR, Zimmerman-Pope N: Superficial skin wounds. In Slatter DH, ed.: Textbook of Small Animal Surgery. 3rd ed.: Philadelphia: WB Saunders, 2003, 259.
36. Williams JM, Fowler D: Wound management and reconstruction. In Fowler D, Williams JM, eds.: Manual of Canine and Feline Wound Management and Reconstruction. Cheltenham (UK): BSAVA, 1999, 1.

# Debridement and Lavage

## Definition and Indications

"The germ is nothing; it is the terrain in which it grows, which is everything." - Pasteur. The goal of debridement is to free wounds of material that would support bacterial growth and thus provide a terrain conducive to uncomplicated wound healing. In addition, it removes tissue that physically blocks ingrowth of fibroblasts and endothelial cells. It makes the wound easier to assess and shortens the inflammatory stage of healing as reflected by decreased exudate production. Debridement is the single most important factor in management of contaminated wounds.

Surgical wound debridement on the distal limb and paws is a form of layered debridement involving the removal of devitalized tissue and foreign debris from acute and chronic wounds. More specifically, it is selective wound debridement in removing these materials. Wound lavage is done simultaneously with surgical debridement by delivering copious quantities of lavage solution to the wound to aid in the removal of devitalized tissue and foreign debris.

Foreign debris within a wound can be hair, plant material including wood, various forms of soil, and gunshot missiles. In general, the more organic the debris is, the greater is the tissue reaction to it if it is left in the wound. Soil can compromise tissues markedly. Small, highly charged soil particles, infection-potentiating fractions (IPF's) in soil can inhibit antibiotics, leukocytes, antibodies, and bactericidal serum activity. Soils rich in organic matter or clay have high IPF concentrations. Sand has lower IPF concentrations. It may be possible to pick and lavage some debris from a wound. However, some debris may be so firmly imbedded in the tissue that it will be necessary to surgically debride the wound.

Nonsurgical debridement involves the use of enzymes or bandages for debridement. Nonsurgical debridement can be considered when 1) surgical debridement could jeopardize vital structures, 2) the animal is a poor anesthetic risk, or 3) when the wound must be cleaned of small amounts of foreign debris and necrotic tissue, e.g. after surgical debridement.

## Techniques

Five factors require attention during debridement: 1) devitalized, contaminated and infected tissue removal; 2) foreign debris removal; 3) attaining adequate hemostasis; 4) delivering adequate lavage solution; and 5) drainage of dead space.

Surgical gloves, cap, and mask should be worn by the surgeon during debridement. For practical purposes, cold sterilization of instruments can be used with periodic placing of the instruments in the solution. This helps prevent placing contaminated instruments back into the wound as the wound becomes cleaner with progression of the procedure. Ideally, instruments should be rinsed with saline and/or be wiped free of cold sterilization solution before replacement in the wound. Toothed forceps and sharp scissors or a scalpel blade are the primary instruments used in debridement.

It has been stated that decreasing amounts of tissue should be excised in the order of - subcutis, skin, fascia and muscle, blood vessels and tendons. However, it should be remembered that regardless of the tissue type, if it is definitely not viable, it should be removed.

*Tissue color and attachment serve as good indicators of tissue viability. Tissues that are very dark or very white are usually nonviable. If these tissues have been present for any length of time, they may have begun to separate from underlying viable tissues.* It is not necessary to have tissues bleed to have adequate debridement. This is especially true when debridement is performed early following trauma. At this time some vessels on the wound surface or at the skin edges may be in a state of temporary spasm, which will subside with time. Thus, based on capillary hemorrhage, a conservative approach should be used. If capillary hemorrhage is encountered at debridement, it may be controlled by temporary pressure on the area or by the topical application of polysaccharide hemostatic beads (HemaBlock, Abbott Animal Health, North Chicago, IL). Fine-point electrocoagulation may also be considered for hemostasis, using care not to leave large pieces of charred tissue in the wound. If vessels are encountered that require ligation, 4-0 synthetic absorbable material is preferred. Guidelines for debriding tissues that are present on the distal limb are given in Table 1-2.

*Because tissue for reconstruction of distal limb and paw wounds is at a premium, staged debridement is very important in wound management. Obviously nonviable tissue is removed at the time of debridement, leaving any tissue that is viable or questionable. The wound is bandaged. At subsequent bandage changes tissue that has changed from questionable to obviously nonviable is removed. The wound is rebandaged and the process is repeated until the wound has viable tissue. At this time, reconstructive options are considered.*

When a partial degloving wound results in a skin flap with a broad base of attachment, the skin should be maintained for reconstruction if possible. The tissue on the dermal surface of such flaps often contains debris and nonviable tissue. During debridement, as much tissue as possible should be retained on this surface of the flap to help ensure that the blood supply to the flap is retained. Because debridement is limited, a ¼ inch diameter Penrose drain is placed under the flap and the flap is replaced over the wound. If the flap's edge cannot be reapposed to the opposite side of the wound, the edge of the flap may be tacked down with sutures (Figure 1-10). This keeps the flap from retracting until future reconstructive procedures can be performed. An alternative is to place an adjustable horizontal mattress suture which can be used over time to gradually stretch the skin for eventual wound edge apposition.

For nonsurgical debridement, an enzymatic debriding agent is placed on a wide-mesh gauze primary bandage which is placed on the wound. Adherent bandages in the form of dry-to-dry or wet-to-dry dressings can also be considered for nonsurgical debridement. Moist wound healing is another effective option for nonsurgical debridement. It supports autolytic selective debridement of white blood cells. Moist wound healing is achieved with moisture retentive dressings. (See

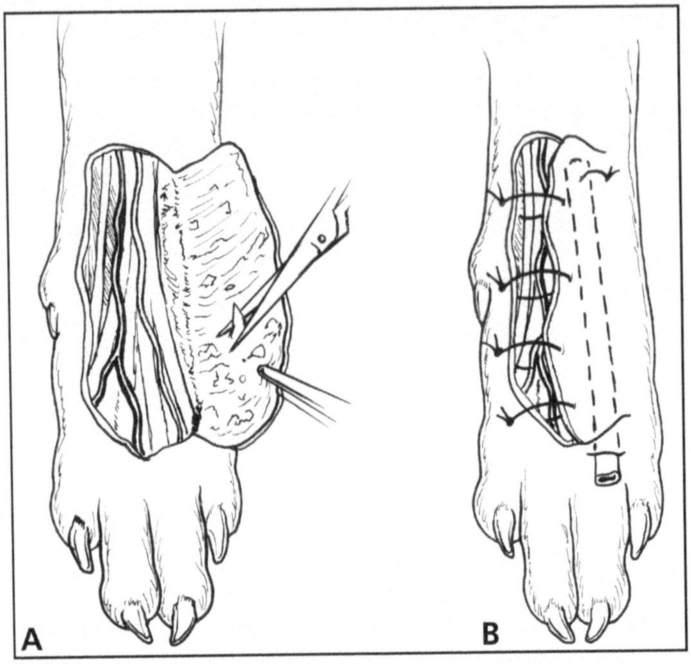


**Figure 1-10.** Wound management of a partial degloving wound with a flap that has a broad base of attachment and partial loss of skin. **A.** Conservative debridement of the flap's dermal surface to retain blood supply. **B.** A ¼ inch diameter Penrose drain placed under the flap and flap tacked into position with sutures.

the Enzymes section in this Chapter, and Chapter II, Bandages, Pads, Splints and Slings - Primary Bandage Layer - Gauze Pad Dressing, Polyurethane Foam Sponge, and Hydrogels.) Although the author (SFS) has not utilized it yet, biological debridement in the form of maggots is gaining favor as a means of nonsurgical debridement.

Wounds should be lavaged with copious quantities of warm lavage solution during debridement. Various solutions have been described for wound lavage, to include tap water, physiologic saline, and balanced electrolyte solutions (lactated Ringer's or Ringer's solutions). The goal of lavage is to reduce bacterial numbers mechanically by loosening and flushing them away along with devitalized tissue and foreign debris. In an effort to help reduce bacterial numbers in wounds, antibiotics, antiseptics (chlorhexidine or povidone iodine), and soaps have been added to lavage solution. A commonly used antiseptic solution is a 0.05% chlorhexidine diacetate (Nolvasan Solution, Ft. Dodge Animal Health, Ft. Dodge, IA) or gluconate (ChlorhexiDerm Disinfectant, Dermatologics in Veterinary Medicine Pharmaceuticals, Inc., Miami, FL) solution made by adding 1 part of the chlorhexidine solution to 40 parts of sterile water. The use of castile soap (50 ml in 3 L of saline) has been described for lavaging cortical bone.

Several techniques are available to deliver lavage solutions to wounds. A bulb syringe has been used to

**Table 1-2. Specific Tissue Debridement**

| Tissue | Appearance | Technique and Comments |
|---|---|---|
| Skin | 1. Skin with normal appearance near area of trauma.<br><br>2. Damaged skin edges<br>A. Sharp laceration<br>B. Ragged; grey, white or black color<br><br>3. Dark or pale flaps<br>A. Turgid dark flap with sharp demarcation line between normal and darker tissue (poor prognosis for darker tissue).<br>B. Turgid dark flap with no line of demarcation between normal and darker tissue (better prognosis for darker tissue).<br>C. Definite dark (leathery) or pale (shiny soft white) flap.<br><br>4. Large thick flaps that are not contused and have a very tenuous pedicle of attachment.<br><br>5. Abraded skin<br><br>6. Contused skin | 1. Observe for possible future signs of impaired circulation.<br><br>2.<br>A. Little if any debridement needed.<br>B. Excise cleanly (caution: excision back to active bleeding could lead to excision of viable skin due to temporary vessel occlusion by vasospasm, edema, or flap position.<br><br>3.<br>A. Observe for 48-72 hours. Trim definitely devitalized tissue.<br>B. Same as A.<br>C. Excise flap.<br><br>4. Excise flap, remove all subcutaneous tissue, mesh it, and place it as a graft.<br><br>5. Clean, retain, and observe. Debride later if necessary.<br><br>6. Observe. Debride later if necessary. |
| Fascia | 1. Loose ragged fragments | 1. Excise with a thin border of normal fascia. |
| Blood vessels | 1. Severed<br><br>2. Intact in an area of pathologic tissue and/or debris. | 1. Ligate and depend upon collateral circulation.<br><br>2. Cleanse gently and cover. Localized enzymatic debridement. |
| Nerves | 1. Exposed intact<br><br>2. Cleanly severed without trauma, ends are identifiable and apposable.<br><br>3. Severed with trauma and contamination, ends are identifiable and apposable. | 1. Cleanse gently and cover. Localized enzymatic debridement.<br><br>2. Anastomose<br><br>3. Perform temporary anastomosis to prevent retraction. Defer definitive anastomosis until healthy wound tissue is present (21 days). |
| Muscle | 1. Friable, no hemorrhage, no contraction with stimulation, imbedded dirt, darker or paler than normal.<br><br>2. Cat muscle normally appears pale. | 1. Remember the 4 "C's" of muscle debridement - color, capacity to bleed, contractility, and consistency. Excise muscle until remaining muscle bleeds, and contracts normally (color may be deceptive unless obviously darker or lighter). Remember vessels may be in spasm in viable tissue early following injury.<br>*Use staged debridement, removing nonvital tissue as it becomes evident.* |

Table 2-1 Continued

| Tissue | Appearance | Technique and Comments |
|---|---|---|
| | | 2. Debride cautiously. Use staged debridement removing nonvital tissue as it becomes evident |
| Tendons | 1. Contaminated and denuded of paratenon.<br><br>2. Cleanly severed without trauma, ends are identifiable.<br><br>3. Severed with trauma and contamination, identifiable ends.<br><br>4. Severed and frayed ends not identifiable, with large gaps in tendon. | 1. Provide coverage.<br><br>2. Anastomose<br><br>3. Perform temporary anastomosis to prevent retraction. Defer definitive anastomosis until healthy wound tissue is present (21 days).<br><br>4. Debride frayed ends, no anastomosis (flexor tendon loss in paws and distal limbs leads to greater abnormalities than extensor tendon loss). |
| Joints | 1. Debris or clots<br><br>2. Cartilage and/or bone fragments.<br><br>3. Torn joint capsule and ligaments.<br><br>4. Gunshot wounds.<br><br>5. Skin and subcutaneous wound over joint.<br><br>6. Unstable joint. | 1. Lavage thoroughly.<br><br>2. Discard small pieces of bone and cartilage, replace large pieces and smooth sharp bone edges.<br><br>3. Suture partially or totally when possible.<br><br>4. Remove bullets/pellets or fragments.<br><br>5. Usually left open for delayed primary closure.<br><br>6. Immobilize joint. |
| Bone | 1. Periosteal covering present.<br><br>2. Dirt imbedded in bone.<br><br>3. Dirt in broken end.<br><br>4. Fragments | 1. Needs bandage or tissue coverage.<br><br>2. Massage gently during lavage. Use Castile soap lavage solution. Remove with a brush, currette, or rongeur. (Up to 3 hours from injury - low pressure lavage. Six or more hours postinjury - high pressure lavage.)<br><br>3. Remove with currette or cut off bone end. Lavage the area with low pressure (bulb syringe or syringe with no needle).<br><br>4. Retain fragments with soft tissue attachments. Remove sequestra that do not have soft tissue attachments. Use clinical judgement - bone can be removed later, but it is hard to replace. Immobilize fractures. |

flush wounds with open fractures. A syringe without a needle can also be used for this purpose. These provide lavage at very low pressure. For more, pressure, lavage solution can be delivered to a wound through a 30 ml syringe with an 18 gauge needle. An intravenous administration set can be placed in a bag of lavage solution. A three-way stopcock valve is attached to the other end of the administration set, and the syringe and needle are attached to the three-way stopcock (Figure 1-11). The wound can be lavaged by turning the valve on the stopcock to alternately fill and empty the syringe. A plastic squeeze bottle with a small aperture for fluid delivery can be used for wound lavage (Figure 1-12A). Squeezing the bottle supplies fluid under pressure. A plastic bottle with a trigger-type delivery mechanism can also be used for wound lavage. The delivery mechanism is adjusted to deliver a stream rather than a spray of fluid (Figure 1-12B). A one-L bag of lavage solution placed in a pressurized cuff inflated to 300 mm Hg and delivered through a 16-18 gauge needle has also been used for lavage. Another type of lavage apparatus can be made by using an 18 gauge needle to make holes in the top of a plastic bottle of physiologic saline solution. Inverting the bottle and squeezing it delivers a series of streams of fluid to the wound. For lavage of distal limb wounds, making one or two holes in the top allows more direct lavage of the smaller wounds, rather than the shower effect of many holes. These delivery mechanisms deliver fluid at varying pressures. However, a one-L bag of lavage solution placed in a pressure cuff pressurized to 300 mm Hg and delivered through a 16 or 18 gauge needle provides about 7 psi of pressure. This is within the 7-8 psi range recommended for wound lavage. Other commercially available wound lavage equipment is available. These generally deliver fluids at a higher pressure and are capable of pulsatile delivery of fluids.

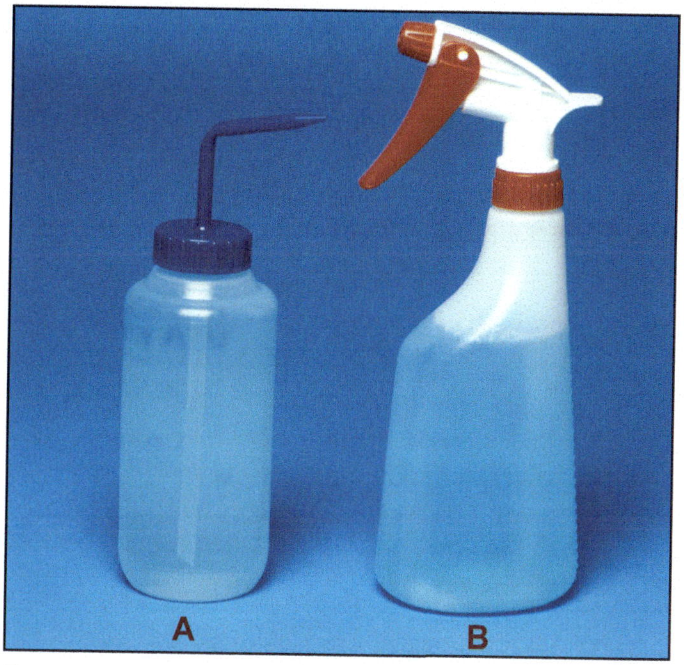


**Figure 1-12.** Wound lavage apparatus. **A.** Plastic squeeze bottle with a small aperture for fluid delivery. **B.** Plastic bottle with a trigger – type delivery apparatus that is adjusted to deliver a stream of fluid. (From Swaim SF, Henderson RA: Small Animal Wound Management, 2nd ed.: Baltimore: Williams & Wilkins, 1997, 25.)

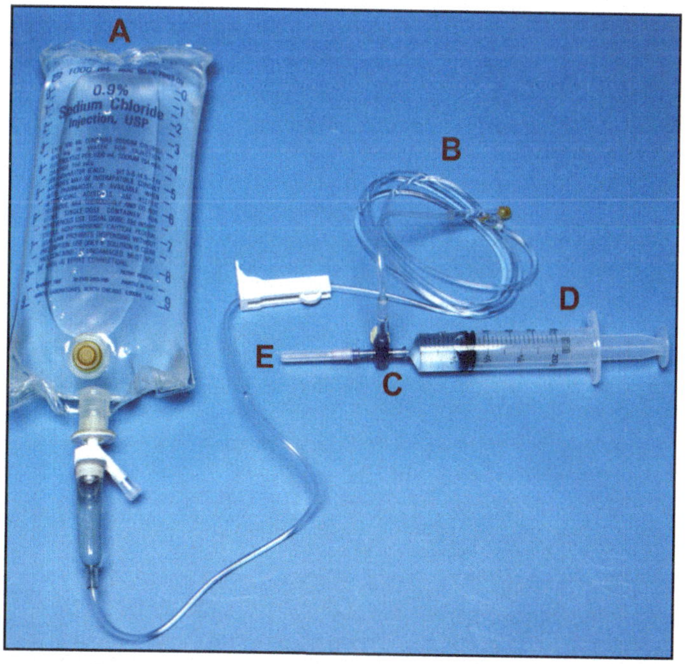


**Figure 1-11.** Wound lavage apparatus. *(A)* Container of lavage solution. *(B)* Intravenous administration set. *(C)* Three – way stopcock valve. *(D)* 30 ml syringe. *(E)* 18 guage needle. (From Swaim SF, Henderson RA: Small Animal Wound Management, 2nd ed.: Baltimore: Williams & Wilkins, 1997, 24.)

## Aftercare

If a wound can be classified as clean or clean contaminated after debridement and lavage, the appropriate technique for wound closure can be performed. If debridement has been extensive, or when it is believed that contaminated or infected tissue remains in the wounds, a drain should be placed as part of the closure procedure. Some wounds should be allowed to heal as open wounds until the tissues are healthy enough to allow closure.

## Advantages and Disadvantages

Selective debridement, especially when used in a staged fashion, on the distal limb allows accurate tissue evaluation and conservation which is important when considering wound closure on the distal limb where skin is at a premium. Sharp debridement is also the most rapid method of debridement. A disadvantage of surgical debridement is the possibility of removing viable tissue that could be used later for reconstruction.

When using nonsurgical debridement, it should be remembered that delicate vessels, nerves, and tendons could be damaged at the time of bandage removal when an adherent bandage is used. Thus, enzymatic debridement around these delicate structures should be considered. Although enzymatic debridement is a painless technique to debride without damaging viable tissues, it is a slower form of debridement.

An advantage to adding antibiotics to a lavage solution is that tissues that appear normal may have circulatory compromise. The antibiotic in the lavage solution supplies antibiotic to the areas of inadequate systemic delivery. In addition, although mechanical action removes most bacteria, an antibiotic or antiseptic in the lavage may also be helpful in reducing bacteria in a wound.

When looking at the effect of lavage pressure on soft tissues, it can have the advantage of reducing bacterial numbers and removing foreign debris and necrotic tissue. However, it may have the disadvantage of driving bacteria and debris into the loose tissue planes, damaging underlying tissue, and reducing the resistance to infection. This is often a factor with high pressure lavage. In addition, pressure of 50 psi or higher has been found to inhibit new bone formation. Another disadvantage of lavage is that it is less effective when used by itself on chronic wounds. With such wounds, it should be used in combination with surgical debridement and topical antimicrobials.

With exposed bone, as is often seen in distal limb wounds, the lavage solution and lavage pressures have advantages and disadvantages. Castile soap lavage solution has been found effective in removing bacteria from cortical bone - more so than antibiotic lavage solution. Soap has also been found to be less damaging to bone than chlorhexidine or povidone iodine. There are also indications that castile soap irrigation may reduce *Pseudomonas aeruginosa* in wounds. Although it is not generally thought to deliver sufficient pressure for effective lavage, a bulb syringe can be beneficial in lavaging in the area of open fractures. It could possibly help prevent seeding of the medullary canal with bacteria. A syringe without a needle can serve the same purpose.

Low pressure lavage is effective in removing bacteria from bone if used within 3 hours of inoculation of the bone, but not at 6 hours. Low pressure does not cause damage to the bone. High pressure lavage (70 psi), is effective at removing bacteria from bone at both 3 and 6 hours after inoculation; however, it causes more macroscopic bone damage. In the presence of fractures (i.e. intraarticular), high pressure pulsatile lavage has the disadvantage of being detrimental to early new bone formation which could increase the risk of nonunion. In addition, high pressure pulsatile lavage in a contaminated fracture can result in bacterial seeding into the medullary canal and damage to the architecture of the bone. Based on the fact that both soft tissue and bone can be involved in distal limb wounds and the fact that high pressure lavage can be detrimental to both soft tissue and bone, early lavage at a low pressure would appear to be the best scenario in wound management.

## Suggested Readings

1. Aaron DN: Management of open musculoskeletal injuries. Semin Vet Med Surg (Small Anim) 3: 290, 1988.
2. Anderson D: Wound management in small animal practice. In Practice 18: 115, 1996.
3. Anderson D: Management of open wounds. In Williams J, Moores A, eds.: BSAVA Manual of Canine and Feline Wound Management and Reconstruction, 2nd ed.: Glouster (UK): BSAVA, 2009, 37.
4. Anglen JO, Apostles S, Christensen G, et al: The efficacy of various irrigation solutions in removing slime-producing *Staphylococcus.* J Orthop Trauma 8: 390, 1994.
5. Anglen JO, Apostles S, Christensen G, et al: Removal of surface bacteria by irrigation. J Orthop Rsch 14: 251, 1996.
6. Anglen JO, Wound irrigation in musculoskeletal injury. J Am Acad Orthop Surg 9: 219, 2001.
7. Bhandri M, Adili A, Lachowski RJ: High pressure pulsatile lavage of contaminated human tibiae: An *in vitro* study. J Orthop Trauma 12: 479, 1998.
8. Bhandri M, Schemitsch EH, Adili A, et al: High and low pulsatile lavage of contaminated tibial fractures: An *in vitro* study of bacterial adherence and bone damage. J Orthop Trauma 13: 256, 1999.
9. Bhandri M, Adili A, Schemitsch EH: The efficacy of low-pressure lavage with different irrigating solutions to remove adherent bacteria from bone. J Bone and Joint Surg 83: 412, 2001.
10. Bowler PG, Duerden BI, Armstrong DG: Wound microbiology and associated approaches to wound management. Clin Microbiol Rev 14: 244, 2001.
11. Conroy BP, Anglen JO, Simpson WA, et al: Comparison of castile soap, benzalkonium chloride, and bacitracin as irrigation solutions for complex contaminated orthopaedic wounds. J Orthop Trauma 13: 332, 1999.
12. Dernell WS: Initial wound management. Vet Clin No Am Small Anim Pract 36: 713, 2006.
13. Dirschl DR, Duff GP, Dahners LE, et al: High pressure pulsatile lavage irrigation of intraarticular fractures: Effects on fracture healing. J Orthop Trauma 12: 460, 1998.
14. Doughty D: Dressings and more: Guidelines for topical wound management. Nurs Clin No Am 40: 217, 2005.
15. Esterhai JL, Queenan J: Management of soft tissue wounds associated with type III open fractures. Orthop Clin No Am. 22: 427, 1991.
16. Gall TT, Monnet E: Evaluation of fluid pressures of common wound-flushing techniques. Am J Vet Res 71: 1384, 2010.
17. Hassinger SM, Harding G, Wongworawat MD, et al: High-pressure pulsatile lavage propogates bacteria in soft tissue. Clin Orthop and Rel Res 439: 27, 2005.
18. Hedlund CS: Surgery of the integumentary system. In Fossum TW, ed: Small Animal Surgery, 2nd ed.: St. Louis: Mosby, 2002, 134.

19. Hedlund CS: Surgery of the integumentary system. In Fossum TW, ed: Small Animal Surgery, 2nd ed.: St. Louis: Mosby, 2007, 159.
20. Hosgood G: Open wounds. In Tobias KM, Johnston SA, eds.: Veterinary Surgery, Small Animal, Vol. 2: St. Louis: Elsevier-Saunders, 2012, 1210.
21. Johnston DE: Care of accidental wounds. Vet Clin No Am Small Anim Pract 20: 27, 1990.
22. Jones G, Wall R: Maggot therapy in veterinary medicine. Rsch Vet Sci 85: 394, 2008.
23. Karuppasamy K, Hutton MJ, Lef MJ: A novel system for irrigation of open fractures. Injury 35: 980, 2004.
24. Knapp D: Management of the open wound. In Birchard SJ, Sherding RG, eds.: Saunders Manual of Small Animal Practice, 2nd ed.: Philadelphia: WB Saunders, 2009, 399.
25. Knapp D: Management of the open wound. In Birchard SJ, Sherding RG, eds.: Saunders Manual of Small Animal Practice, 3rd ed.: St. Louis: Saunders, Elsevier, 2006, 549.
26. Koeveker G: Surgical debridement of wounds. In Falanga V, ed.: Cutaneous Wound Healing. London: Martin Dunitz, 2001, 233.
27. Krahwinkel DJ, Boothe HW: Topical and systemic medications for wounds. Vet Clin No Am Small Anim Pract 36: 739, 2006.
28. Lam DG, Rastomjee D, Dyan Y: Wound irrigation: A simple reproducible device. Ann Roy Coll Surg Engl 82: 346, 2000.
29. Lees MJ, Fretz PB, Bailey JV, et al: Factors influencing wound healing: Lessons from military wound management. Compend Contin Educ Equine 11: 850, 1989.
30. Liptak JM: An overview of topical management of wounds. Australian Veterinarian 75: 408, 1997.
31. Lozier S, Pope E, Berg J: Effects of four preparations of 0.05% chlorhexidine diacetate on wound healing in dogs. Vet Surg 21: 107, 1992.
32. Mason LK: Treatment of contaminated wounds of the abdomen and thorax. In Harari J, ed.: Surgical Complications and Wound Healing in Small Animal Practice. Philadelphia: WB Saunders, 1993, 33.
33. McPhail CM: Surgery of the integumentary system. In Fossum TW, ed: Small Animal Surgery, 4th ed.: St. Louis: Mosby, 2013, 190.
34. Ndikuwera J, Winstanley EW: High pressure pulsatile lavage and high pressure syringe lavage in treatment of contaminated wounds in dogs. J Small Anim Pract 26: 3, 1985.
35. Pavletic MM: Atlas of Small Animal Reconstructive Surgery, 2nd ed.: Philadelphia: WB Saunders, 1999, 21.
36. Pavletic MM. Atlas of Small Animal Wound Management and Reconstructive Surgery, 3rd ed.: Ames, IA: Wiley-Blackwell, 2010, 31.
37. Pope ER: Lavage of open wounds: Chlorhexidine recommended. Vet Med Rep 2: 185, 1990.
38. Probst CW: Lavage of open wounds: Successful management without topical antiseptics. Vet Med Rep 2: 184, 1990.
39. Rodeheaver GT: Wound cleansing, wound irrigation, wound disinfection. In Krasner DL, Rodeheaver GT, Sibbald RG, eds.: Chronic Wound Care, 3rd ed.: Wayne, PA: HMP Communications, 2001, 369.
40. Seligson D, Henry SL: Treatment of compound fractures. Am J Surg 161: 693, 1991.
41. Sherman RA: Maggot versus conservative debridement therapy for the treatment of pressure ulcers. Wound Rep Reg 10: 208, 2002.
42. Sherman RA, Hall MJR, Thomas S: Medicinal maggots: An ancient remedy for some contemporary afflictions. Annu Rev Entomol 45: 55, 2000.
43. Svboda SJ, Bice TG, Gooden HA, et al: Comparison of bulb syringe and pulsed lavage irrigation with use of a bioluminescent musculoskeletal wound model. J Bone and Joint Surg 88: 2167, 2006.
44. Swaim SF, Pope ER: Early management of limb degloving injuries. Semin Vet Med Surg (Small Animal) 3: 274, 1988.
45. Swaim Sf, Henderson RA: Small Animal Wound Management, 2nd ed.: Baltimore: Williams and Wilkins, 1997, 13.
46. Swaim SF: Acute superficial soft tissue injuries. In Bistner SI, Ford RB, Raffe MR, eds.: Handbook of Veterinary Procedures and Emergency Treatments, 7th ed.: Philadelphia: WB Saunders, 2000, 257.
47. Swaim SF, Bohling MW: Current concepts in small animal open wound management. Medecin Veterinaire Du Quebec. 33: 99, 2003.
48. Waldron DR, Zimmerman-Pope N: Superficial skin wounds, In Slatter DH, ed.: Textbook of Small Animal Surgery. 3rd ed.: Philadelphia: WB Saunders, 2003, 259.
49. Williams JM: Open wound management. In Fowler D, Williams JM, eds.: Manual of Canine and Feline Wound Management and Reconstruction. Cheltenham (UK): BSAVA, 1999, 3

# Wound Closure Assessment

## Definition and Indications

Wound closure assessment first requires evaluation of the wound from the standpoint of health of the tissues and second from the standpoint of tissue available for wound closure. Because some wounds have extensive tissue damage and are badly contaminated or infected, they are allowed to heal completely by contraction and epithelialization (second intention). Other wounds will have tissue that is healthy enough following initial wound management to allow immediate closure (primary closure). Still other wounds will require open wound management for a period to provide tissue healthy enough for closure (delayed primary and secondary closure).

The wound size and availability of tissue for wound closure also govern the type of closure to be used. Skin may be readily available for closure without tension or with use of appropriate relaxing or stretching procedures skin edges can be apposed. In other instances, the extent of skin loss may be so great that a skin graft or flap will be necessary for reconstruction.

## Technique

Assessment of tissue viability and health requires clinical judgment at the time of initial management and at subsequent bandage changes when staged debridement is being performed. The severity of wound contamination, tissue damage, and circulatory compromise are the major factors governing tissue health and viability. (See Debridement and Lavage and Table 1-2 - Specific Tissue Debridement.)

To assess the amount of skin present for wound closure, the fingers can be used to attempt apposition of the wound edges, or skin edges can be grasped with atraumatic forceps and gentle traction can be used in an attempt to appose the edges. Wound edge apposition should be attempted before the wound has entered the inflammatory stage of healing. The edema and enlargement of underlying tissue during this stage will impair moving the skin over the wound.

## Aftercare

After assessing the health of the wound tissues and the availability of skin for wound closure, the next step is to proceed with the appropriate wound management techniques. If it is decided to allow a wound to heal as an open wound due to the condition of the tissues, the appropriate topical medications as well as bandages and splints should be used to support healing. These wounds have exposed and damaged muscles, tendons, ligaments, nerves, blood vessels, bones and joints. However, they will cover with granulation tissue and the wound will heal by contraction if the defect is not too large.

When the condition of the tissues qualifies it as a clean wound, primary closure may be performed with placement of a drain to control dead space as needed. Primary closure may also be performed on mildly contaminated wounds that have minimal debris and necrotic tissue. These wounds should receive thorough debridement and lavage as well as some type of drainage. Such wounds should be watched closely for postoperative complications. Delayed primary closure may be more appropriate for these wounds. Moderate and heavily contaminated wounds are candidates for longer delays with open wound treatment before closure. When the condition of the tissues warrants treatment of the wounds until healthy tissue is present to be followed by wound closure, topical medications with bandages and splints are needed in early aftercare. Later aftercare would consist of using the appropriate surgical repair of the wounds.

When wound edges appose easily, the appropriate suture pattern can be used for closure. Wound edges that cannot be apposed initially, but which in the judgment of the surgeon will eventually appose if the wound is allowed to heal by second intention, may lend themselves to use of a skin stretching or relaxing procedure for closure. Finally, for wound edges that obviously will not appose, a skin graft or flap technique will be needed. Some wounds may fall into a "grey area" making it difficult to decide if a stretching or relaxing procedure would provide closure or whether a skin graft or flap is needed. In such instances, the stretching or relaxing techniques should be considered first. If they do not result in complete closure, the remaining wound may heal as an open wound or a smaller graft will be necessary for final closure.

If it is necessary to flex a joint (i.e. carpal or tarsal area) to obtain wound edge apposition, it is best to consider a graft or flap for reconstruction. The greater the need for flexion for skin edge apposition, the greater is the indication for a graft or flap.

## Advantages and Disadvantages

The advantages and disadvantages of wound closure assessment are related to the procedures and techniques used in the aftercare. If the health of the tissue is not assessed properly and a wound is closed too soon, complications may ensue. When second intention healing is used for treatment of the wound, it allows staged debridement as well as maximal wound drainage. However, the wounds may require longer to heal with the added expense of hospital visits, bandages and medications. Some wounds will not heal completely by contraction and epithelialization or will cover with fragile epithelium that is easily damaged. If bandages and/or restraint devices are not used to prevent an animal from molesting the wound, the result may be a chronic nonhealing wound (See Chapter 5). On dogs, granulation tissue may occasionally proliferate above the wound edge to impair contraction and epithelialization.

When allowed to heal by second intention, large wounds over the flexion surface of joints (i.e. carpal and tarsal areas) may develop a contractual deformity of a webbed scar or area of tight scar tissue across the joint. These limit joint extension and require reconstructive surgery to correct the deformity (Figure 1-13).

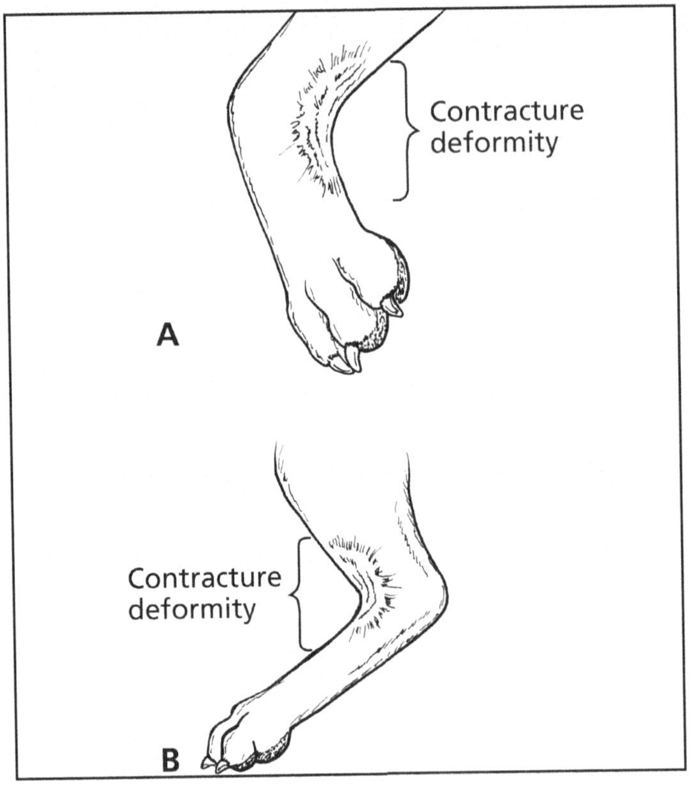


**Figure 1-13.** Contractural deformity. **A.** Contractural deformity resulting from a large open wound healing on the carpal flexion surface. **B.** Contractural deformity resulting from a large open wound healing on the tarsal flexion surface. Joint extension is limited.

Large wounds on the paws that heal by second intention are subject to contraction that pulls pads out of their normal position. This results in ulceration when weight is borne on skin not designed for weight-bearing (Figure 1-14).

The advantages and disadvantages of the various techniques for closing wounds are stated with information about each technique within the text.

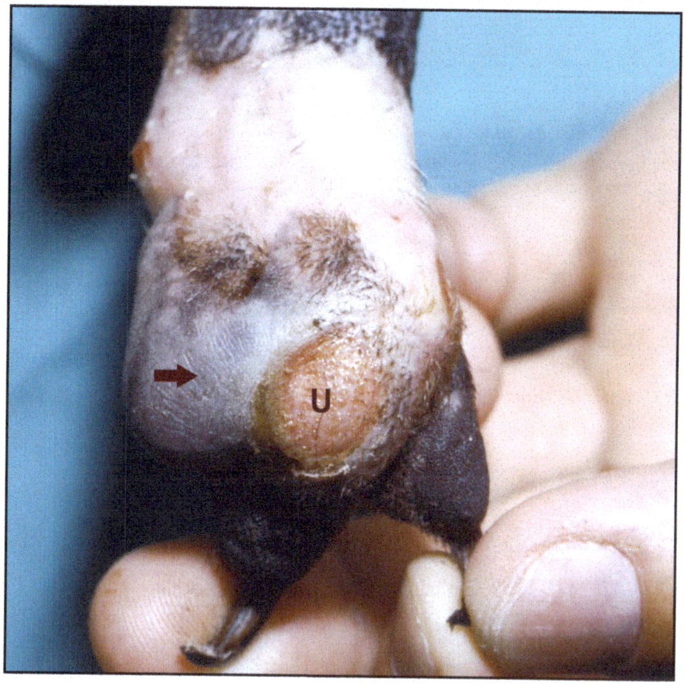


**Figure 1-14.** Result of a large paw wound that healed by second intention. Contracture has pulled the metatarsal pad *(arrow)* out of line, resulting in an ulcer *(U)* in adjacent skin. (From Swaim SF: Foot salvage techniques in dogs and cats: options, "do's" and "don'ts". J Amer Hosp Assoc 21:511, 1985.)

# Suggested Readings


1. Dernell WS: Initial wound management. Vet Clin No Am Small Anim Pract 36: 713, 2006.
2. Hosgood G: Open wounds. In Tobias KM, Johnston SA, eds.: Veterinary Surgery, Small Animal, Vol. 2: St. Louis. Elsevier Saunders, 2012, 1210.
3. Pavletic MM: Atlas of Small Animal Reconstructive Surgery, 2nd ed.: Philadelphia: WB Saunders, 1999, 21.
4. Pavletic MM: Atlas of Small Animal Wound Management and Reconstructive Surgery, 3rd ed.: Ames, IA: Wiley-Blackwell, 2010, 31.
5. Swaim SF, Henderson RA: Small Animal Wound Management, 2nd ed.: Baltimore: Williams and Wilkins, 1997, 13.


# Topical Lavage Agents

This section does not present an extensive coverage of topical wound care agents. It presents information on some of the vulnerary agents used by the authors in wound management.

# Tap Water

## Definition and Indications

Tap water is that which comes from the water faucets of the veterinary medical establishment. Boiled and cooled water as well as distilled water can be used for wound lavage. Water is indicated in the initial management of wounds to lavage wounds that are heavily contaminated with debris.

## Technique

A hose with a spray nozzle which is located near a commercial sink is the most effective way to deliver tap water to a heavily contaminated wound. Such hose and nozzle fixtures are components of commercial surgical preparation tables (Figure 1-15A). The nozzle is used to deliver warm water to the wound. With the animal lying on the grate of the surgical preparation table, the water is drained away from the animal and the wound as it is used. If a commercial surgical preparation table is not available, a wound lavage area can be improvised by placing a removable cage door over a bath tub. The tap water supply of the tub is used to lavage the wound, with the cage door serving as the grate (Figure 1-15B).

## Aftercare

Ideally, physiologic saline or lactated Ringer's or Ringer's solution should be used to lavage the wound after tap water lavage. However, because of the limited contact time between the wound and water, it is not essential that the solution be isotonic.

## Advantages and Disadvantages

Tap water provides an inexpensive means of delivering a large quantity of lavage solution to a wound for removing gross debris. A degree of comfort can be provided to the animal by adjusting the temperature at the tap. The multijet delivery of water by the nozzle does not force irrigating fluid into tissues as much as a single orifice irrigating apparatus.

Tap water is not isotonic and has the potential to cause cellular damage, e.g. fibroblast damage. The advantage of removing gross debris and bacteria from a wound, which could cause significant tissue damage and infection, overrides the relatively small detrimental effect of lack of isotonicity. Studies have indicated that there is either no difference between saline and tap water in lavaging wounds or that tap water may be superior to sterile saline in cleaning soft tissue wounds.

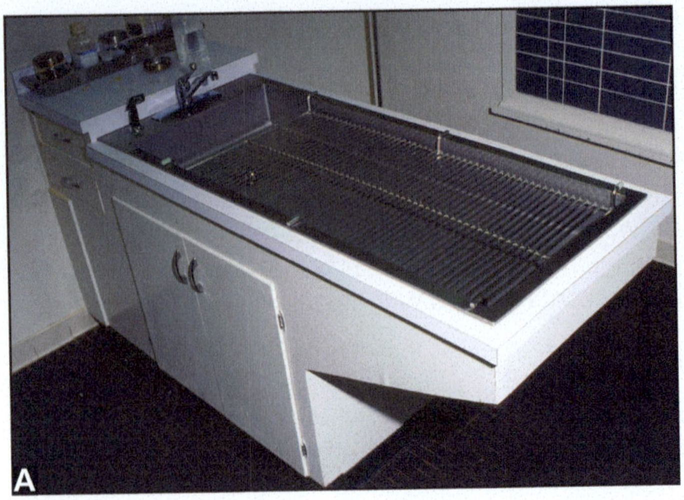

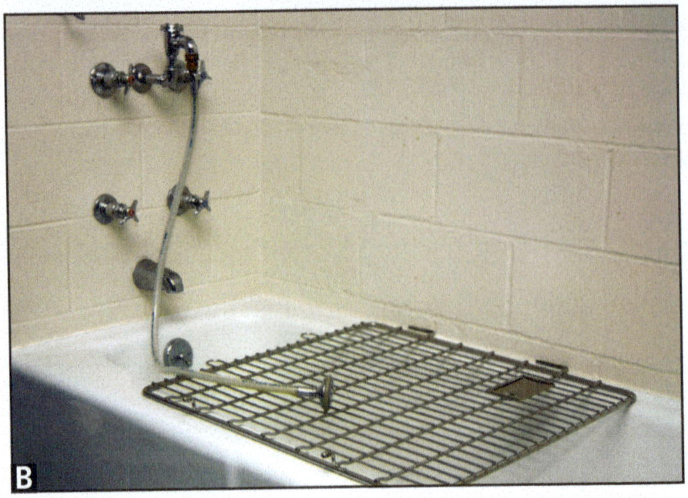

**Figure 1-15.** Equipment for lavaging wounds with tap water. **A.** Commercial surgical preparation table with grate and a hose/nozzle to deliver tap water. **B.** A cage door laid over a bathtub as a grate and a hose nozzle to deliver tap water. (From Swaim SF, Henderson RA: Small Animal Wound Management, 2nd ed.: Baltimore: Williams & Wilkins, 1997, 72.)

## Suggested Readings


1. Angeras MH, Brandberg A, Falk A, et al: Comparison between sterile saline and tap water for the cleaning of traumatic soft tissue wounds. Eur J Surg 158: 347, 1992.
2. Bansal BC, Wiebe RA, Perkins SD, et al: Tap water for irrigation of lacerations. Am J Emerg Med 20: 469, 2002.
3. Buffa EA, Lubbe AM, Verstraete FJM, et al: The effects of wound lavage solutions on canine fibroblasts: An in vitro study. Vet Surg 26: 460, 1997.
4. Dernell WS: Initial wound management. Vet Clin No Am Small Anim Pract 36: 713, 2006.
5. Fernandez RS, Griffiths R, Ussia C: Water for wound cleansing. Intern J Evid-Based Healthcare 5: 305, 2007.
6. Fernandez RS, Griffiths R: Water for wound cleansing (Review) Cochrane Collab. Wiley and Sons, Ltd. 2010, 1.
7. Hosgood G: Open wounds. In Tobias KM, Johnston SA, eds.: Veterinary Surgery, Small Animal, Vol. 2: St. Louis: Elsevier Saunders, 2012, 1210.
8. Johnston DE: Care of accidental wounds. Vet Clin No Am Small Anima Pract 20: 27, 1990.
9. Mason LK: Treatment of contaminated wounds of the abdomen and thorax. In Harari J, ed.: Surgical Complications and Wound Healing in Small Animal Practice. Philadelphia: WB Saunders, 1993, 33.
10. Moscati RM, Reardon RF, Lerner EB, et al: Wound irrigation with tap water. Acad Emerg Med 5: 1076, 1998.
11. Moscati RM, Mayrose J, Fincher L, et al: Comparison of normal saline with tap water for wound irrigation. Am J Emerg Med 16: 379, 1998.
12. Moscati RM, Mayrose J, Reardon RF, et al: A multicenter comparison of tap water versus sterile saline for wound irrigation. Acad Emerg Med 14: 404, 2007.
13. Probst CW: Lavage of open wounds: Successful management without topical antiseptics. Vet Med Rep 2: 184, 1990.
14. Rodeheaver GT: Wound cleansing, wound irrigation, wound disinfection. In Krasner DL, Rodeheaver GT, Sibbald RG, eds.: Chronic Wound Care, 3rd ed.: Wayne, PA: HMP Communications, 2001, 369.
15. Salami AA, Imosemi IO, Owoeye OO: A comparison of the effects of chlorhexidine, tap water, and normal saline on healing wounds. Int J Morphol 24: 673, 2006.
16. Svboda SJ, Owens BD, Gooden HA, et al: Irrigation with potable water versus normal saline in a contaminated musculoskeletal wound model. J Trauma – Inj Infec Crit Care 64: 1357, 2008.
17. Swaim DF, Henderson RA: Small Animal Wound Management, 2nd ed.: Baltimore: Williams and Wilkins, 1997, 53.
18. Waldron DR, Zimmerman-Pope N: Superficial skin wounds. In Slatter DH, ed.: Textbook of Small Animal Surgery, 3rd ed.: Philadelphia: WB Saunders, 2003, 259.


## Isotonic Saline, Lactated Ringer's, or Ringer's Solutions

### Definition and Indications

Contaminated and infected wounds may be lavaged with isotonic saline solution, lactated Ringer's solution, or Ringer's solution to remove debris and reduce the amount of bacteria in a wound by means of their washing action. For home care, an acceptable saline solution can be made by adding 2 teaspoons of salt to one liter of boiling water followed by cooling before use.

### Technique

The reader is referred to the section on Debridement and Lavage in this chapter for information on techniques to deliver lavage solutions to wounds.

### Aftercare

No special aftercare is required following wound lavage with isotonic saline, lactated Ringer's solution or Ringer's solution.

### Advantages and Disadvantages

Because these solutions are isotonic, iso-osmotic, and sterile, they are physiologic and should cause no tissue damage. When used in large quantities, there may be some tissue retention of these fluids to give an edematous appearance. Because these solutions do not have any antibacterial properties, their efficacy in wound lavage is based on the mechanical process of solution delivery to rid the wound of debris and bacteria. Studies have indicated that there is either no difference between saline and tap water in lavaging wounds or that tap water may be superior to saline in cleaning soft tissue wounds.

## Suggested Readings


1. Angeras MH, Brandberg A, Falk A, et al: Comparison between sterile saline and tap water for the cleaning of acute traumatic soft tissue wounds. Eur J Surg 158: 347, 1992.
2. Aaron DN: Management of musculoskeletal injuries. Semin Vet Med Surg 3: 290, 1988.
3. Buffa EA, Lubbe AM, Verstraete TJM, et al: The effects of wound lavage solutions on canine fibroblasts: An in vitro study. Vet Surg 26: 460, 1997.
4. Dernell WS: Initial wound management. Vet Clin No Am Small Anim Pract 36: 713, 2006.
5. Daly WR: Wound infections. In Slatter DH, ed.: Textbook of Small Animal Surgery: Philadelphia: WB Saunders, 1985, 37.
6. Johnston DE: Care of accidental wounds. Vet Clin No Am Small Animal Pract 20: 27, 1990.
7. Mason LK: Treatment of contaminated wounds of the abdomen and thorax. In Harari J, ed.: Surgical Complications and Wound Healing in Small Animal Practice. Philadelphia: WB Saunders, 1993, 33.
8. Moscati RM, Mayrose J, Fincher L, et al: Comparison of normal saline and tap water for wound irrigation. Am J Emerg Med 16: 379, 1998.
9. Moscati RM, Mayrose J, Reardon RF, et al: A multicenter comparison of water versus sterile saline for wound irrigation. Acad Emerg Med 14: 404, 2007.
10. Owen BD, White DW, Wenke JC: Comparison of irrigation solutions and devices in a contaminated musculoskeletal wound survival model. J Bone and Joint Surg 91: 92, 2009.
11. Pavletic MM: Atlas of Reconstructive Surgery, 2nd ed.: Philadelphia. WB Saunders, 1999, 21.
12. Pavletic MM: Atlas of Small Animal Wound Management and Reconstructive Surgery, 3rd ed.: Ames, IA: Wiley-Blackwell, 2010, 31.
13. Probst CW: Lavage of open wounds: Successful management without topical antiseptics. Vet Med Rep 2: 184, 1990.
14. Rodeheaver GT: Wound cleansing, wound irrigation, wound disinfection. In Krasner DL, Rodeheaver GT, Sibbald RG, eds.: Chronic Wound Care, 3rd ed.: Wayne, PA: HMP Communications, 2001, 369.
15. Salami AA, Imosemi IO, Owoeye OO: A comparison of the effects of chlorhexidine, tap water and normal saline on healing wounds. Int J Morphol 24: 673, 2006.
16. Svboda SJ, Owens BD, Gooden HA, et al: Irrigation with potable water versus normal saline in contaminated musculoskeletal wound model. J Trauma – Inj Infec Crit Care 64: 1357, 2008.
17. Swaim SF, Henderson RA: Small Animal Wound Management, 2nd ed.: Baltimore: Williams and Wilkins, 1997, 53.
18. Waldron DR, Zimmerman-Pope N: Superficial skin wounds. In Slatter DH, ed.: Textbook of Small Animal Surgery, 3rd ed.: Philadelphia: WB Saunders, 2003, 259.


# Chlorhexidine

### Definition and Indications

Chlorhexidine is a bisbiguanide compound effective against gram-positive and gram- negative bacteria molds, yeasts, and viruses. It is more effective against gram-positive than gram-negative bacteria and has less activity against fungi. It is inactive against spores. Chlorhexidine diacetate (Nolvasan solution, Ft. Dodge Animal Health, Ft. Dodge, IA) or gluconate (ChlorhexiDerm Disinfectant, Dermatologics in Veterinary Medicine Pharmaceuticals, Inc., Miami, FL) may be used for wound lavage. A 0.05% solution is indicated for lavage of contaminated or infected wounds to reduce bacterial numbers and expose remaining bacteria to its antimicrobial activity.

### Technique

The reader is referred to the section on Debridement and Lavage for information on techniques to deliver lavage solutions to wounds. A 0.05% solution is prepared by diluting one part of 2% stock solution with 40 parts of sterile water.

### Aftercare

No special aftercare is required after wound lavage with chlorhexidine solution.

### Advantages and Disadvantages

Chlorhexidine has a broad spectrum of antimicrobial activity that results in an immediate and reliable reduction in bacterial counts as well as a sustained residual activity. It also has the advantages of not being inactivated by organic matter, blood, and other lavage fluids. Chlorhexidine does not seem to have the disadvantages of systemic absorption, causing hypersensitivity, or toxicosis.

Inflammation of synovial membranes exposed to 0.05% chlorhexidine solution has been reported. However, synovial fluid changes and lameness were no different from joints flushed with lactated Ringer's solution. Joint lavage with 0.05% chlorhexidine diacetate was not recommended.

If physiologic saline or lactated Ringer's solution are used to dilute chlorhexidine diacetate, a precipitate forms. However, this does not seem to affect its antibacterial effects against *Staphylococcus intermedius in vitro*. Neither does this precipitate have a negative effect on wound contraction or epithelialization *in vivo*.

Some gram-negative bacteria may be resistant to chlorhexidine.

# Suggested Readings


1. Amber EI, Henderson RA, Swaim SF, Gray BW: A comparison of antimicrobial efficiency and tissue reaction of four antiseptics on canine wounds. Vet Surg 12:63, 1983.
2. Anderson MA, Payne JT, Kreager JM, et al: Effects of intra-articular chlorhexidine diacetate lavage on the stifle in healthy dogs. Am J Vet Res 54:1784, 1993.
3. Atiyeh BS, Dibo SA, Hayek SN: Wound cleansing, topical antiseptics and wound healing. Int Wound J 6: 420, 2009.
4. Dernell WS: Initial wound management. Vet Clin No Am Small Animal Pract 36: 713, 2006.
5. Drosou A, Falabella A, Kirsner RS: Antiseptics and wounds: An area of controversy. Wounds 15: 149, 2003.
6. Fahie MA, Shettko D: Evidence-based wound management: A systemic view of therapeutic agents to enhance granulation and epithelialization. Vet Clin No Am Small Animal Pract 37: 559, 2007.
7. Hedlund CS: Surgery of the integumentary system. In Fossum TW, ed.: Small Animal Surgery, 3rd ed.: St. Louis: Mosby, 2007, 159.
8. Krahwinkel DJ, Boothe HW: Topical and systemic medication for wounds. Vet Clin No Am Small Animal Pract 36: 739, 2006.
9. Lee AH, Swaim SF, McGuire JA, Hughes KS: The effects of chlorhexidine diacetate, povidone iodine, and polyhydroxydine on wound healing in dogs. J Am Anim Hosp Assoc 24:77, 1988.
10. Lemarié RJ, Hosgood G: Antiseptics and disinfectants in small animal practice. Compend Contin Educ Pract Vet 17:1339,1995.
11. Lozier SM, Pope ER, Berg J: Effects of four preparations of 0.05% chlorhexidine diacetate on wound healing in dogs. Vet Surg 21:107, 1992.
12. Main RC: Should chlorhexidine be used in wound cleansing. J Wound Care 17: 112, 2008.
13. MacPhail CM: Surgery of the integumentary system. In Fossum TW, ed.: Small Animal Surgery, 4th ed.: St. Louis: Mosby, 2013, 190.
14. Pavletic MM: Atlas of Small Animal Wound Management and Reconstructive Surgery. 3rd ed.: Ames IA: Wiley-Blackwell, 2010: 31, 51.
15. Platt J, Bucknall RA: An experimental evaluation of antiseptic wound irrigation. J Hosp Infec 5:181,1984.
16. Pope ER: Lavage of open wounds: chlorhexidine solution is recommended. Vet Med Rep 2:185, 1990.
17. Prince HN, Nonemaker WS, Norgard RC, Prince DL: Drug resistance studies with topical antiseptics. J Pharm Sci 67:1629,1978.
18. Rosenberg A, Alatary SB, Peterson AF: Safety and efficiency of the antiseptic chlorhexidine gluconate. Surg Gynecol Obstet 143:789,1976.
19. Russell AD: Chlorhexidine: Antibacterial action and bacterial resistance. Infection 14:212, 1986.
20. Salami AA, Inosemi IO, Owoeye OO: A comparison of the effects of chlorhexidine, tap water, and normal saline on healing wounds. Int J Morphol 24: 673, 2006.
21. Sanchez IR, Swaim SF, Nusbaum KE, et al: Effects of chlorhexidine diacetate and povidone-iodine on wound healing in dogs. Vet Surg 17:291, 1988.
22. Sebben JE: Surgical antiseptics. J Am Acad Dermatol 9:759, 1983.
23. Swaim SF: Bandages and topical agents. Vet Clin North Am Small Animal Pract 20:47, 1990.
24. Swaim SF, Henderson RA: Small Animal Wound Management, 2nd ed.: Baltimore: Williams and Wilkins, 1997, 53.
25. Waldron DR, Zimmerman-Pope N: Superficial skin wounds. *In* Slatter DH, ed.: Textbook of Small Animal Surgery, 3rd ed.: Philadelphia: WB Saunders, 2003, 259.


# Povidone Iodine

## Definition and Indications

Iodine has a broad spectrum of antimicrobial activity against gram-positive and gram-negative bacteria, fungi, viruses, protozoa and yeasts. Povidone iodine is a complex of iodine with polyvinylpyrrolidone. It is a form of "tamed iodine". Iodine is slowly released from the complex as "free iodine", which is responsible for the antimicrobial activity. *In vitro*, dilute solutions have been shown to have more bactericidal activity than full-strength solutions. This is attributed to more free iodine in the dilute solutions. Povidone iodine is indicated as a lavage for contaminated and infected wounds to reduce the bacterial flora and to expose remaining bacteria to its antimicrobial activity.

## Technique

The reader is referred to the section on Debridement and Lavage for information on techniques to deliver lavage solutions to wounds. Diluting one part of 10% stock solution with 9 parts of sterile water or electrolyte solution provides a 1% solution for wound lavage. Because blood, exudate and other organic material inactivate povidone iodine, wounds should be thoroughly lavaged with water, isotonic saline, lactated Ringer's solution, or Ringer's solution before applying povidone iodine.

## Aftercare

If povidone iodine is to be the only topical medication applied, it should be applied relatively often during the day because its bactericidal activity only lasts 4 to 8 hours.

## Advantages and Disadvantages

Povidone iodine provides a broad spectrum of antimicrobial activity with small amounts of free iodine being constantly released. However, several disadvantages are associated with it. It has a broad antimicrobial spectrum, but reduced bacteriocidal activity caused by the complexing of iodine with polyvinylpyrrolidone. Its short residual activity is associated with its inactivation by organic materials such as red and white blood cells, necrotic tissues, exudate, fat, hemoglobin and the cornstarch used to pack surgical gloves. Its residual activity is 4 to 6 hours and this is reduced in the presence of organic matter. Povidone iodine is toxic to the cells essential to wound healing, and the higher the concentration of the solution, the more toxic it is; thus, having an adverse effect on healing. A 1% solution is advocated for wound lavage. Some bacteria develop a resistance to povidone iodine.

Povidone iodine is absorbed from tissues and has potential to cause renal failure, metabolic acidosis due to its acidic nature, and thyroid malfunction. These factors would be of relatively more concern with use on larger wounds on the body than on the smaller wounds of the distal limb. However, they should be considered when using povidone iodine as a wound lavage.

The detergent form of povidone iodine has been found to be detrimental to wound healing, and *in vitro* studies have suggested that povidone iodine solution and scrub may have deleterious effects on exposed bone, a factor often encountered in distal limb wounds.

## Suggested Readings


1. Amber EI, Henderson RA, Swaim SF, Gray BW: A comparison of antimicrobial efficacy and tissue reaction of four antiseptics on canine wounds. Vet Surg 12:63, 1983.
2. Atiyeh BS, Dibo SA, Hayek SN: Wound cleansing, topical antiseptics and wound healing. Intnat Wound J 6: 420, 2009.
3. Balogh D, Bauer M, Riccabona G: The influence of povidone iodine treatment on thyroid hormones in severe burns. J Hosp Infec 6 (Suppl.):147, 1985.
4. Berkelman RL, Holland BW,Anderson RL: Increased bactericidal activity of dilute preparations of povidone-iodine solutions. J Clin Microbiol 15:635,1982.
5. Bolton L, Oleniacz W, Constantine B, et al: Repair and antibacterial effects of topical antiseptic agents *in vivo*. Mod Dermatol 2:145,1985.
6. Dernell WS: Initial wound management. Vet Clin No Am Small Animal Pract 36: 713, 2006.
7. Drosou A, Falabella A, Kirsner RS: Antiseptics on wounds: An area of controversy. Wounds 15: 149, 2003.
8. Durani P, Leaper D: Povidone-iodine: Use in hand disinfection, skin preparation and antiseptic irrigation. Internat Wound J 5: 376, 2008.
9. Flynn J: Povidone-iodine as a topical antiseptic for treating and preventing wound infection: a literature review. Br J Community Nurs 8: 536, 2003.
10. Georgiade NG, Harris WA: Open and closed treatment of wounds with povidone-iodine. Plast Reconstr Surg 52:640,1973.
11. Hedlund CS: Surgery of the integumentary system. In Fossum TW, ed.: Small Animal Surgery, 3rd ed.: St. Louis: Mosby, 2007, 159.
12. Kaysinger KK, Nicholson NC, Ramp WK, Kellam JF: Toxic effects of wound irrigation solutions on clutured tibiae and osteoblasts. J Orthop Trauma 9:303,1995.
13. Krahwinkel DJ, Boothe HW: Topical and systemic medications for wounds. Vet Clin No Am Small Animal Pract 36: 739, 2006.
14. Kramer SA: Effects of povidone-iodine on wound healing: A review. J Vascular Nurs 17:17, 1999.
15. Lee AH, Swaim SF, McGuire JA, Hughes KS: The effects of chlorhexidine diacetate, povidone iodine, and polyhydroxydine on wound healing in dogs. J Am Anim Hosp Assoc 24:77, 1988.
16. Lemarié RJ, Hosgood G: Antiseptics and disinfectants in small animal practice. Compend Contin Educ Pract Vet 17:1339,1995.
17. MacPhail CM: Surgery of the integumentary system. In Fossum TW, ed.: Small Animal Surgery, 4th ed.: St. Louis: Mosby, 2013, 190.
18. Pavletic MM: Atlas of Small Animal Wound Management and Reconstructive Surgery, 3rd ed.: Ames, IA: Wiley-Blackwell, 2010, 51.
19. Pietsch J, Meakins JL: Complications of povidone-iodine absorption in topically treated burn patients. Lancet 1:280,1976.
20. Reimerk K, Wichelhaus TA, Schafer, et al: Antimicrobial effectiveness of povidone-iodine and consequences of new application areas. Dermatology 204: 114, 2002.
21. Rodeheaver G, Bellamy W, Kody EM, et al: Bactericidal activity and toxicity of iodine-containing solutions in wounds. Arch Surg 117:181,1982.
22. Rodeheaver GT: Wound cleansing, wound irrigation, wound disinfection. *In* Krasner DL, Rodeheaver GT, Sibbald RG, eds.: Chronic Wound Care, 3rd ed.: Wayne PA: HMP Communications, 2001, 369.
23. Sanchez IR, Swaim SF, Nusbaum KE, et al: Effects of chlorhexidine diacetate and povidone-iodine on wound healing in dogs. Vet Surg 17:291, 1988.
24. Schneider W, Ahuja S, Klebe I: Clinical and bacteriological studies of the polyvinyl pyrrolidone-iodine complex. *In* World Congress on Antisepsis. New York: P. H. Publishing Co., 1976, 100.
25. Sebben JE: Surgical antiseptics. J Am Acad Dermatol 9:759, 1983.
26. Selvaggi G, Monstrey S, Van Landuy K: The role of iodine in antisepsis and wound management: A reappraisal. Acta Chir Belg 103: 241, 2003.
27. Silva JE: Effects of iodine and iodine containing compounds on thyroid function. Med Clin North Am 69:881, 1985.
28. Swaim SF: Bandages and topical agents. Vet Clin North Am Small Anim Pract 20:47, 1990.
29. Swaim SF, Henderson RA: Small Animal Wound Management, 2nd ed.: Baltimore: Williams and Wilkins, 1997, 53.
30. Waldron DR, Zimmerman-Pope N: Superficial skin wounds. *In* Slatter DH, ed.: Textbook of Small Animal Surgery, 3rd ed.: Philadelphia: WB Saunders, 2003, 259.
31. Zamora JL: Povidone-iodine and wound infection. Surgery 95:121, 1984.
32. Zamora JL: Chemical and microbiologic characteristics and toxicity of povidone-iodine solutions. Am J Surg 151:400,1986.
33. Zamora JL, Price MD, Chuang P,Gentry LO: Inhibition of povidone-iodine's bactricidal activity by common organic substances: A experimental study. Surgery 98:25, 1985.


# Hydrogen Peroxide

## Definition and Indications

Hydrogen peroxide is frequently used to lavage wounds. Upon contact tissue catalases convert it to a foam of water and oxygen. It has a brief period of broad spectrum, antimicrobial activity which does not penetrate tissues. It is more effective against gram-positive bacteria. It is indicated as an initial one time lavage for wounds that are badly contaminated with debris and/or that have a high potential for anaerobic organism contamination.

### Technique

Unlike other lavage solutions Hydrogen peroxide should not be delivered to wounds under pressure.

### Aftercare

Wounds lavaged with hydrogen peroxide do not require any special aftercare.

## Advantages and Disadvantages

When hydrogen peroxide is used as an initial wound lavage, it may be beneficial in removing dirt and debris from deep wounds by its effervescent action. However, most distal limb wounds are not deep wounds as compared to some wounds on other parts of the body. Because of its minimal bactericidal potency hydrogen peroxide has minimal antiseptic action. It has more effect as a sporicidal agent. If it is delivered under pressure or if its drainage is restricted, its foaming action can result in forcing the agent and debris between tissue planes. This can result in wound enlargement and tissue emphysema. When applied to wounds that are in the repair stage of healing with new epithelium visible, it can be detrimental to the tissues. *In vitro* studies have indicated that hydrogen peroxide may have deleterious effects on exposed bone, a factor often encountered in distal limb injuries. The available 3% solution and lower concentrations injure cells. When using hydrogen peroxide to remove debris from a wound, the benefit from this should be weighed against the potential for tissue damage that may result.

# Suggested Readings


1. Baldry MGC: The bactericidal, fungicidal and sporicidal properties of hydrogen peroxide and peracetic acid. J Appl Bacteriol 54:417,1983.
2. Bolton L. Oleniacz W, Constantine B, et al: Repair and antibacterial effects of topical antiseptic agents *in vivo*. Mod Dermatol 2:145,1985.
3. Brown CD, Zitelli JA: A review of topical agents for wounds and method of wounding. Guidelines for wound management. J Dermatol Surg Oncol 19:732, 1993.
4. Drosou A, Falabella A, Kirsner RS: Antiseptics on wounds: An area of controversy. Wounds 15: 149, 2003.
5. Gruber RP, Vistnes L, Pardoe R: The effects of commonly used antiseptics on wound healing. Plast Reconst Surg 55:472,1975.
6. Kaysinger KK, Nicholson NC, Ramp WK, Kellam F: Toxic effects of wound irrigation solutions on cultured tibiae and osteoblasts. J Orthop Trauma 9:303,1995.
7. Lau WY, Wong SH: Randomized prospective trial of topical hydrogen peroxide in appendectomy wound infection. Am J Surg 142:393,1981.
8. Lemarié RJ, Hosgood G: Antiseptics and disinfectants in small animal practice. Compend Contin Educ Pract Vet 17:1339,1995.
9. Lineweaver W, McMorris S, Soucy D, Howard R: Cellular and bacterial toxicities of topical antimicrobials. Plast Reconst Surg 75:394,1985.
10. Lineweaver W, Howard R, Soucy D, et al: Topical antimicrobial toxicity. Arch Surg 120:267,1985.
11. Lineweaver W, McMorris S, Howard R: Effects of topical disinfectants and antibiotics on human fibroblasts. Surg Forum 33:37,1982.
12. Reybrouck G: The bactericidal activity of aqueous disinfectants applied on living tissues. Pharm Weekbl (Sci) 7:100, 1985.
13. Rodeheaver GT: Wound cleansing, wound irrigation, wound disinfection. *In* Krasner DL, Rodeheaver GT, Sibbald RG, eds.: Chronic Wound Care, 3rd ed.: Wayne PA, HMP Communications, 2001, 369.
14. Sleigh JW, Linter SP: Hazards of hydrogen peroxide. Br Med J (Clin Res Ed) 291: 1706, 1985.
15. Stringer MD, Lawrence JC, Lilly HA: Antiseptics and the casualty wound. J Hosp Infect 4:410, 1983.
16. Swaim SF: Bandages and topical agents. Vet Clin North Am Small Anim Pract 20:47, 1990.
17. Swaim SF, Henderson RA: Small Animal Wound Management, 2nd ed.: Baltimore: Williams and Wilkins, 1997, 53.


# Antibiotics and Antibacterials Bacitracin, Neomycin, Polymixin

## Definition and Indications

Bacitracin, neomycin, and polymixin are three bactericidal antibiotics that are combined as a topical triple antibiotic ointment for wound treatment. There are numerous manufacturers of the ointment. The medication is primarily indicated for small wounds in the early stages of wound management.

## Technique

Because these antibiotics are poorly absorbed by wound tissues, they should be used early in the wound management process before organisms have invaded the wound tissues. Thus, the three antibiotics should be considered as more effective in preventing than in treating infections. The triple antibiotic ointment can be placed on a piece of surgical gauze to provide a nonadherent semiocclusive primary bandage layer, or it can be placed on a commercial nonadherent dressing pad. This form of antibiotic therapy is generally indicated for smaller wounds, which would include wounds on the distal limbs and paws.

## Aftercare

Bandages should be changed as needed depending upon how much the wound is draining. In general, bandages are changed more frequently in the early stages of wound healing when there is more drainage. The antibacterial activity lasts about 12 hours. At the time of bandage change, the skin around the wound should be observed for signs of allergic reaction to the drugs, especially neomycin. However, allergic reactions are uncommon. Once the wound is epithelialized, this medication is of limited benefit.

## Advantages and Disadvantages

The triple antibiotic medication has a wide spectrum of bactericidal activity, with all 3 antibiotics having a synergistic effect against organisms. These antibiotics are effective against the most common disease causing pathogens found in wounds. Bacitracin is particularly effective against *Streptococcus pyogenes* and neomycin against *Staphylococcus aureus*. Polymixin B has been found effective against methacillin-resistant *Staphylococcus aureus*. A combination of bacitracin and polymixin B sulfate may be effective against both gram-positive and gram-negative organisms, and neomycin and polymixin provide coverage against some gram-negative bacteria.

The limited tissue absorption of these antibiotics by wound tissues can be considered both an advantage and disadvantage. High concentrations of these antibiotics can be applied to wounds with little concern about systemic absorption and toxicity (nephrotoxicity, ototoxicity, neurotoxicity). However, with this limited absorption they are not as effective on infected wounds. Application of large quantities of the antibiotics could possibly result in systemic absorption with side effects such as nephrotoxicity, ototoxicity, and neurotoxicity. There is more potential for allergic sensitization to neomycin than to the other topical antibiotics. The enhanced re-epithelialization of wounds has been associated with the zinc bacitracin component of these antibiotics.

A disadvantage of the three antibiotics is their ineffectiveness against *Pseudomonas* species. Another disadvantage is the inactivation of bacitracin and polymixin B by purulent exudates. Although zinc bacitracin enhances epithelialization, it can retard wound contraction.

## Suggested Readings

1. Bolton L, Oleniacz W, Constantine B, et al: Repair and antibacterial effects of topical antiseptic agents *in vivo*. Mod Dermatol 2:145,1985.
2. Bono RA, Van Zile PS, Li Q, et al: Topical triple antibiotic as a novel therapeutic choice in wound management and infection prevention: A practical perspective. Expert Rev Anti-infect Ther 5: 773, 2007.
3. Booth JH, Benrimoj SI, Nimo GR: *In vitro* interactions of neomycin sulfate, bacitracin, and polymixin B sulfate. Int J Dermatol 33:517,1994.
4. Brown CD, Zitelli JA: A review of topical agents for wounds and methods for wounding: guidelines for wound management. J Dermatol Surg Oncol 19:732,1993.
5. Diehr S, Hamp A, Jamison B: Do topical antibiotics improve wound healing? J Fam Pract 56: 140, 2007.
6. Dire DJ, Coppola M, Dwyer DA, et al: Prospective evaluation of topical antibiotics for preventing infections in uncomplicated soft tissue wounds repaired in the ED. Acad Emerg Med 2:4, 1995.
7. Eaglstein WH, Mertz P, Alvarez OM: Effects of topically applied agents on healing wounds. Clin Dermatol 2:112,1984.
8. Fahie MA, Shettko D: Evidence-based wound management: A systematic review of therapeutic agents to enhance granulation and epithelialization. Vet Clin No Am Small Animal Pract 37: 559, 2007.
9. Glotzer DJ, Goodman WS, Geronimus LH: Topical antibiotic prophylaxis in contaminated wounds. Arch Surg 100:589, 1970.
10. Hedlund CS: Surgery of the integumentary system. *In* Fossom TW, ed.: Small Animal Surgery, 2nd ed.: St. Louis: Mosby, 2002, 134.
11. Hedlund CS: Surgery of the integumentary system. In Fossum TW, ed.: Small Animal Surgery, 3rd ed.: St. Louis: Mosby, 2007, 159.
12. Hosgood G: Open wounds. In Tobias KM, Johnston SA, eds.: Veterinary Surgery, Small Animal, Vol 2: St. Louis: Elsevier-Saunders, 2012, 1210.
13. Kaye ET: Topical antibacterial agents. Infect Dis Clin No Am: 14: 321, 2000.
14. Krahwinkel DJ, Boothe HW: Topical and systemic medications for wounds. Vet Clin No Am Small Animal Pract 36: 739, 2006.
15. Langford JH, Artemi P, Benrimoj SI: Topical antimicrobial prophylaxis in minor wounds. Ann Pharmacother 31:559, 1997.
16. Leyden JJ, Sulzberger MB: Topical antibiotics in minor skin trauma. Am Fam Pnysician 23:121, 1982.
17. Lio PA, Kaye ET: Topical antibacterial agents. Infec Dis Clin No Am 23: 945, 2009.
18. Lionelli GT, Lawrence WT: Wound Dressings. Surg Clin No Am 83: 2003.
19. MacPhail CM: Surgery of the integumentary system. In Fossum TW, ed.: Small Animal Surgery, 4th ed.: St. Louis: Mosby, 2013, 190.
20. Noyes HE, Chi NH, Linh LT, et al: Delayed topical antimicrobials as adjuncts to systemic antibiotic therapy in war wounds. Bacteriologic Studies. Mil Med 132, 1967.
21. Pavletic MM: Atlas of Small Animal Wound Management and Reconstructive Surgery, 3rd ed.: Ames IA: Wiley-Blackwell, 2010, 51.
22. Rudolph R: Nonsurgical maintenance of the chronic problem wound. *In* Rudolph R, Noe JM, eds.: Chronic Problem Wounds. Boston: Little, Brown, 1983, 29.
23. Scott DW, Miller WH, Griffin CE: Muller and Kirk's Small Animal Dermatology, 6th ed.: Philadelphia: WB Saunders, 2001, 274.
24. Swaim SF: Bandages and topical agents. Vet Clin North Am Small Anim Pract 20:47, 1990.
25. Swaim SF, Henderson RA: Small Animal Wound Management, 2nd ed.: Baltimore: Williams and Wilkins, 1997, 53.
26. Watcher M, Wheeler R: The role of topical antibiotics in the healing of full-thickness wounds. J Dermatol Surg Oncol 15:1188,1989.
27. Yoshida T, Hiramatsu K: Potent *in vitro* bactericidal activity of polymixin B against methicillin-resistant *Staphylococcus aureus* (MRSA). Microbiol Immunol 37:853,1993.

# Silver Sulfadiazine

## Definition and Indications

Silver sulfadiazine 1% is a water-miscible cream made by several manufacturers. It has a wide spectrum of antimicrobial activity and is indicated in the treatment of burn and other necrotic wounds. It is especially effective against *Pseudomonas spp.* The medication may be indicated when treating wounds where it is desirable to inhibit wound contraction, i.e. over a flexion surface to help prevent wound contracture or when it is desirable to enhance wound epithelialization.

New silver dressings are available in the form of nanoparticle slow release impregnated dressings and ionic silver-impregnated dressings. These are available in various forms – waterproof foam, alginate, permeable polyester mesh, and carboxymethylcellulose fiber dressings. They have a wide spectrum of antimicrobial activity to include aerobic and anaerobic bacteria as well as yeasts and filamentous fungi.

## Technique

Silver sulfadiazine is applied to a wound by placing it on the contact layer of the bandage. The drug is often used as an antimicrobial when preparing a distal limb wound for a skin graft. The medication is usually discontinued approximately 24 hours prior to the skin grafting procedure at which time topical gentamicin sulfate is used.

## Aftercare

No special aftercare is required with the topical use of silver sulfadiazine. Bandages are changed as necessary depending upon the amount of wound drainage. Bandage changes are generally more frequent in the early stages of wound management.

## Advantages and Disadvantages

Silver sulfadiazine has the advantage of having a wide spectrum of antimicrobial activity against gram-positive and gram-negative bacteria as well as most fungi. It has been shown that combining 1% chlorhexidine gluconate with 1% silver sulfadiazine increases the antibacterial activity of the silver sulfadiazine. It is painless upon application, nonstaining, nonsensitizing, and is relatively nontoxic. It has also been found to stimulate re-epithelialization of wounds. The ability of its antimicrobial activity to penetrate necrotic tissue and eschar is a significant advantage of the medication.

There may be delayed separation of eschar from burn wounds with silver sulfadiazine use. There is also the possibility of absorption with depressed bone marrow activity and lymphocyte proliferation with silver sulfadiazine. Additionally, there may be deposits in the liver, kidney and other organs. These would probably be more of a factor with large body wounds than distal limb wounds. However, it should be borne in mind especially if it is used over a period of time on a distal limb wound. Silver sulfadiazine has a negative effect on fibroblasts. Thus, it can slow wound contraction. This could be considered an advantage if it is indicated to slow wound contraction over a flexion surface (i.e. caudal carpal area or cranial tarsal area) to help prevent flexion contracture deformity.

# Suggested Readings


1. Atiyeh BS, Costagliola M, Hayek SN, et al: Effect of silver on burn wound infection control and healing: Review of the literature. Burns 33: 139, 2006.
2. Bolton L, Oleniacz W, Constantine B, et al: Repair and antibacterial effects of topical antiseptic agents in vivo. Mod Dermatol 2:145,1985.
3. Brown CD, Zitelli JA: A review of topical agents for wounds and methods for wounding: guidelines for wound management. J Dermatol Surg Oncol 19:732, 1993.
4. Demling RH, DeSanti L: Effect of silver on wound management. Wounds 13 (Suppl A): 1, 2001.
5. Eaglstein WH, Mertz PM: Effects of topical medicaments on the rate of repair of superficial wounds. *In* Dineen P, Hildick-Smith G, eds.: The Surgical Wound. Philadelphia: Lea & Febiger, 1981, 150.
6. Eaglstein WH, Mertz PM, Alvarez OM: Effect of topically applied agents on healing wounds. Clin Dermatol 2:112,1984.
7. Gamelli RL, Paxton TP, O'Reilly: Bone marrow toxicity of sulfadiazine. Surg Gynecol Obstet 117:115,1993.
8. Hedlund CS: Surgery of the integumentary system. *In* Fossum TW, ed.: Small Animal Surgery, 2nd ed.: St. Louis: Mosby, 2002, 134.
9. Hedlund CS: Surgery of the integumentary system. In Fossum TW, ed.: Small Animal Surgery, 3rd ed.: St. Louis: Mosby, 2007, 159.
10. Hosgood G: Open wounds. In Tobias KM, Johnston SA, eds.: Veterinary Surgery: Small Animal, Vol. 2: St. Louis: Elsevier-Saunders, 2012, 1210.
11. Krahwinkel DJ, Boothe HW: Topical and systemic medications for wounds. Vet Clin No Am Small Animal Pract 36: 739, 2006.
12. Lunsdown AB, Williams A: How safe is silver in wound care? J Wound Care 13: 131, 2004.
13. Lee ARC, Moon HK: Effect of topically applied silver sulfadiazine on fibroblast cell proliferation and biomechanical properties of the wound. Arch Pharma Rsch 26: 855, 2003.
14. Leitch IO, Kucukcelebi A, Robson MC: Inhibition of wound contraction by topical antimicrobials. Aust NZ J Surg 63:289,1993.
15. Lionelli GT, Lawrence WT: Wound dressings. Surg Clin No Am 83: 2003.
16. MacPhail CM: Surgery of the integumentary system. In Fossum TW, ed.: Small Animal Surgery, 4th ed.: St. Louis: Mosby, 2013, 190.
17. Muller MJ, Hollyoak MA, Moavani Z, et al: Retardation of wound healing by silver sulfadiazine reversed by aloe vera and nystatin. Burns. 29: 834, 2003.
18. Pavletic MM: Atlas of Small Animal Wound Management and Reconstructive Surgery, 3rd ed.: Ames IA: Wiley-Blackwell, 2010, 51.
19. Snelling CF, Roberts FJ: Comparison of 1% silver sulfadiazine with and without 1% chlorhexidine digluconate for topical antibacterial effect in the burnt infected rat. J Burn Care Rehab 9:35, 1988.
20. Stefanides MM, Copeland CE, Kominos SD, Yee RB: *In vitro* penetration of topical antiseptics through eschar of burn patients. Ann Surg 183:358,1976.
21. Swaim SF: Bandages and topical agents. Vet Clin North Am Small Anim Pract 20:47, 1990.
22. Swaim SF, Henderson RA: Small Animal Wound Management, 2nd ed.: Baltimore: Williams and Wilkins, 1997, 53.
23. Watcher M, Wheeland R: The role of topical antibiotics in the healing of full-thickness wounds. J Dermatol Surg Oncol 15:1188,1989.
24. Wright JB, Lam K, Burrell RE: Wound management in an era of increasing bacterial antibiotic resistance: A role for topical silver treatment. Am J Infec Control 26:572, 1998.
25. Wright JB, Lam K, Hansen D, Burrell RE: Efficacy of topical silver against fungal burn wound pathogens. Am J Infec Control 27:344, 1999.
26. Zapata-Sirvent RL, Hansborough JF: Cytotoxicity to human leukocytes by topical antimicrobial agents used for burn care. J Burn Care Rehab 14:132,1993.


# Nitrofurazone

## Definition and Indications

Nitrofurazone is available as a 0.2% topical antimicrobial medication in a water soluble polyethylene glycol base. It has a broad gram positive spectrum but has little effect on *Pseudomonas spp*. It is indicated for treating wounds, burns, and cutaneous ulcers in dogs and cats.

### Technique

The medication is placed on a fine-mesh gauze sponge as a contact bandage layer. The medication is often used as an antimicrobial when preparing a distal limb wound for a skin graft. Its application is usually discontinued approximately 24 hours before the graft is placed. At that time, topical gentamicin sulfate is used.

### Aftercare

No special aftercare is necessary with nitrofurazone wound treatment. The frequency of bandage changes is dependent on the amount of wound drainage, with bandage changes being more frequent in the early stages of wound healing when drainage is more copious.

### Advantages and Disadvantages

The polyethylene glycol base of nitrofurazone dressings makes the gauze to which it is applied nonadherent. This can be advantageous in the repair stage of healing. The hydrophilic nature of polyethylene glycol has the advantage of drawing homeostatic fluids up through wound tissues to dilute tenacious exudates so they can be more readily absorbed into bandages. In addition, if the animal is on a systemic antibiotic, wound tissues are bathed with antibiotic-laden fluids as they are drawn up through the wound. The hydrophilic nature of the medication increases the capillarity of the primary bandage layer; thus, wound fluid is moved from the primary layer into the intermediate layer more effectively. However, because it is water soluble, the nitrofurazone is washed out of the primary layer as wound fluid moves up through the bandage. The slowing of epithelialization by nitrofurazone that has been reported by others has not been the experience of the author.

*In vitro*, blood and serum have been shown to result in a slight reduction of antibacterial activity of nitrofurazone soluble dressing. If the medication leeches through to the outer bandage layer, its yellow coloring may be mistaken for urine soilage of the bandage.

## Suggested Readings

1. Bolton L, Oleniacz W, Constantine B, et al: Repair and antibacterial effects of topical antiseptic agents *in vivo*. Mod Dermatol 2:145,1985.
2. Coffey RP, Rice TL, Thomason PD: Effects of blood and serum on *in vitro* antibacterial activity of nitrofurazone. Am J Hosp Pharm 48:1496, 1991.
3. Doughty D: Dressings and more: Guidelines for topical wound management. Nurs Clin No Am 40: 217, 2005.
4. Eaglstein WH, Mertz PM: Effects of topical medicaments on the rate of repair of superficial wounds. *In* Dineen P, Hildick-Smith G, eds.: The Surgical Wound. Philadelphia: Lea & Febiger, 1981, 150.
5. Eaglstein WH, Mertz PM, Alvarez OM: Effect of topically applied agents on healing wounds. Clin Dermatol 2:112,1984.
6. Hedlund CS: Surgery of the integumentary system. *In* Fossum TW, ed.: Small Animal Surgery, 2nd ed.: St. Louis: Mosby, 2002, 134.
7. Hedlund CS: Surgery of the integumentary system. In Fossum TW, ed.: Small Animal Surgery, 3rd ed.: St. Louis: Mosby, 2007, 159.
8. Krahwinkel DJ, Boothe HW: Topical and systemic medications for wounds. Vet Clin No Am Small Animal Pract 36: 739, 2006.
9. Lee AH, Swaim SF, Yang SL, Wilken LO, et al: The effects of petrolatum, polyethylene glycol, nitrofurazone, and a hydroactive dressing on open wound healing. J Am Anim Hosp Assoc 22:443, 1986.
10. Noe JM, Kalish S: The mechanism of capillarity in surgical dressings. Surg Gynecol Obstet 143:454,1976.
11. Noe JM, Kalish S: The problem of adherence in dressed wounds. Surg Gynecol Obstet 147:185,1978.
12. Noe JM, Kalish S: Dressing materials and their selection. *In* Rudolph R, Noe JM, eds.: Chronic Problem Wounds. Boston: Little, Brown, 1983, 37.
13. MacPhail CM: Surgery of the integumentary system. In Fossum TW, ed.: Small Animal Surgery, 4th ed.: St. Louis: Mosby, 2013, 190.
14. Pavletic MM: Atlas of Small Animal Wound Management and Reconstructive Surgery, 3rd ed.: Ames, IA: Wiley-Blackwell: 2010, 51.
15. Swaim SF: Bandages and topical agents. Vet Clin North Am Small Anim Pract 20:47, 1990.
16. Swaim SF, Henderson RA: Small Animal Wound Management, 2nd ed.: Baltimore: Williams and Wilkins, 1997, 53.

## Gentamicin Sulfate

### Definition and Indications

Gentamicin sulfate is available as a 0.1% wide-spectrum antibiotic ointment. It is used for topical treatment of bacterial wound infections. It is particularly effective against some gram-negative organisms found in wounds, i.e. *Pseudomonas aeruginosa, Escherichia coli, Proteus vulgaris*. The medication has been found to be particularly effective in preparing distal limb wounds for application of skin grafts and for postoperative bacterial control following grafting. Collagen-gentamicin implants/sponges have been used to treat wound infections in people, to include treating foot ulcers that have a high bacterial load.

### Technique

The medication in the form of an ointment, not cream, can be placed on a fine-mesh gauze sponge or a nonadherent dressing pad for placement on a wound or a graft. When placing it on a graft, the coating should be applied in a very thin coating to a nonadherent dressing pad. Thus, it does not interfere with fluid absorption of the pad. When the medication is used to prepare a wound for grafting, it is applied approximately 24 hours prior to grafting, replacing either silver sulfadiazine or nitrofurazone that has been used previously.

### Aftercare
No special aftercare is needed when using gentamicin sulfate topically. The frequency of bandage changes is dependent on the amount of wound drainage with changes being more frequent in the early stages of wound management when there is more fluid production.

### Advantages and Disadvantages
When bacitracin-neomycin-polymixin therapy is not effective in controlling gram-negative bacteria in a wound, especially *Pseudomonas* spp., gentamicin sulfate ointment has been found to be effective by the authors.

## Suggested Readings

1. Fahie MA, Shettko D: Evidence-based wound management: A systemic review of therapeutic agents to enhance granulation and epithelialization. Vet Clin No Am Small Anim Pract 37: 559, 2007.
2. Friberg O, Svedjeholm R, Soderquist: Treating sternal wound infections after cardiac surgery with implantable gentamicin-collagen sponge. J Am Med Assoc 304: 2123, 2010.
3. Griffis CD, Metcalfe S, Bowling FL, et al: The use of gentamicin-impregnated foam in the management of diabetic foot infections: A promising delivery system. Expert Opin Drug Deliv 6: 639, 2009.
4. Guerro EB, Ferguson TB, Lin M, et al: Effect of an implantable gentamicin-collagen sponge on sternal wound infections following cardiac surgery: A randomized trial. J Am Med Assoc 304: 755, 2010.
5. Hedlund CS: Surgery of the integumentary system. *In* Fossum TW, ed.: Small Animal Surgery, 2nd ed.: St. Louis: Mosby, 2002, 134.
6. Hedlund CS: Surgery of the integumentary system. In Fossum TW, ed.: Small Animal Surgery, 3rd ed.: St. Louis: Mosby, 2007, 159.
7. Krahwinkel DJ, Boothe HW: Topical and systemic medications for wounds. Vet Clin No Am Small Anim Pract 36: 739, 2006.
8. Lee AH, Swaim SF, Yang ST, et al: Effects of gentamicin solution and cream on the healing of open wounds. Am J Vet Res 45: 1487, 1984.
9. Lio PA, Kaye ET: Topical antibacterial agents. Infec Dis Clin No Am 23: 945, 2009.
10. MacPhail CM: Surgery of the integumentary system. In Fossum TW, ed.: Small Animal Surgery, 4th ed.: St. Louis: Mosby, 2013, 190.
11. Pavletic MM: Atlas of Small Animal Wound Management and Reconstructive Surgery, 3rd ed.: Ames, IA: Wiley-Blackwell, 2010, 51.
12. Swaim SF: Bandages and topical agents. Vet Clin North Am Small Anim Pract 20:47, 1990.
13. Swaim SF, Henderson RA: Small Animal Wound Management, 2nd ed.: Baltimore: Williams and Wilkins, 1997, 53.
14. Yetrim I, Ozkan OV, Dervisoglu A, et al: Effect of local gentamicin application on healing and wound infection in patients with modified radical mastectomy: A prospective randomized study. J Internat Med Rsch 38: 1442, 2010.


## Enzymes
## Trypsin-Balsam of Peru-Castor Oil
### Definition and Indications
The particular enzymatic agent used by the author contains trypsin, balsam of Peru and castor oil (Granulex-V, Bertek Pharmaceuticals, Sugarland, TX). The trypsin clears the wound of debris. The balsam of Peru acts to stimulate angiogenesis, i.e. granulation tissue in the wound. Epithelialization is enhanced in the wound by the castor oil as it provides a moist environment and reduces premature epithelial drying and cornification. It also serves as an analgesic.

Enzymatic debridement is indicated in patients that are poor anesthetic risks and as an adjunct to conservative surgical debridement. Enzymatic debriding agents work synergistically with endogenous enzymes. Trypsin liquefies coagulum and crusts. It also dissolves blood clots and breaks down necrotic tissue without harming viable tissue. Thus, bacteria in these substances are better exposed to cellular and humoral immune factors as well as any antimicrobial agents that are present. This form of debridement is particularly useful in treating wounds on the distal limbs to help assure that only nonviable tissue is removed, retaining tissue that can be used for reconstruction. When used following conservative surgical debridement to remove definitely nonviable tissue, the enzyme degrades remaining questionable tissue that is actually nonviable so that it is either absorbed into the bandage and removed at the next bandage change or it is more defined as nonviable and easily removed at the next debridement of the staged surgical debridement procedure.

### Technique
Following conservative surgical debridement to remove definitely nonviable tissue, the compound is sprayed on the wound and covered with a wide-mesh surgical gauze sponge primary bandage layer.

### Aftercare
No special aftercare is needed when using this compound. Bandages are changed daily.

### Advantages and Disadvantages
A general advantage of enzymatic debridement is that it allows postponement of surgical debridement until the animal has been stabilized and is a better anesthesia candidate. As the enzymes are used as an adjunct to conservative surgical debridement they have

the advantage of defining viable from nonviable tissue, thus providing a more accurate debridement.

In addition to debriding a wound, enzymes such as trypsin have been found to decrease the bacterial flora of wounds. The debriding action of the compound aids in the removal of coagulum, exudate and necrotic debris which would support bacterial growth. The enzymatic liquefaction of coagulum allows systemic and/or topical antibiotics to contact bacteria that have been surrounded by the coagulum. Coagulum liquefaction also enhances its absorption into the bandage which further aids in lowering the bacterial flora of the wound. A specific advantage of the combination of trypsin, balsam of Peru and castor oil compound is the stimulation of granulation tissue and support of epithelialization provided by the latter 2 components of the compound, respectfully.

Local inflammation, a pyogenic reaction, and a stinging sensation have been reported with topical application of trypsin. However, this has not been noted in our experience. Burned skin and necrotic bone do not lend themselves to enzymatic debridement.

## Suggested Readings


1. Beitz JM: Wound debridement: Therapeutic options and care considerations. Nurs Clin No Am 40: 233, 2005.
2. Hedlund CS: Surgery of the integumentary system. *In* Fossum TW, ed.: Small Animal Surgery, 2nd ed.: St. Louis: Mosby, 2002, 134.
3. Hedlund CS: Surgery of the integumentary system. In Fossum TW, ed.: Small Animal Surgery, 3rd ed.: St. Louis: Mosby, 2007, 159.
4. Hosgood G: Open wounds. In Tobias KM, Johnston SA, eds.: Veterinary Surgery: Small Animal, Vol 2: St. Louis: Elsevier-Saunders, 2012, 1210.
5. Krahwinkel DJ, Boothe HW: Topical and systemic medications for wounds. Vet Clin No Am Small Animal Pract 36: 739, 2006.
6. Lozier SM: Topical wound therapy. *In* Harari J, ed.: Surgical Complications and Wound Healing in Small Animal Practice. Philadelphia: WB Saunders, 1993, 63.
7. MacPahil CM: Surgery of the integumentary system. In Fossum TW, ed.: Small Animal Surgery, 4th ed.: St. Louis: Mosby, 2013, 190.
8. Pavletic MM: Atlas of Small Animal Wound Management and Reconstructive Surgery, 3rd ed.: Ames, IA: Wiley-Blackwell, 2010, 51.
9. Riser HG, Patton R, Roetting LC: Tryptic debridement of necrotic tissue. Arch Surg 63:568,1951.
10. Schultz GS, Sibbald RG, Falanga V, et al: Wound bed preparation: A systematic approach to wound management. Wound Repair and Regeneration 11 (2 Suppl): 1, 2003.
11. Shelby RW, Taylor LE, Garnes AL, Prigot A: Enzymatic debridement with activated whole pancreas. Am J Surg 96:545,1958.
12. Sherry S, Fletcher A: Proteolytic enzymes: A therapeutic evaluation. Clin Pharmacol Ther 1:202, 1960.
13. Swaim SF: Management and bandaging of soft tissue injuries of dog and cat feet. J Am Anim Hosp Assoc 21:329, 1985.
14. Swaim SF: Bandages and topical agents. Vet Clin North Am Small Anim Pract 20:47, 1990.
15. Swaim SF, Henderson RA: Small Animal Wound Management, 2nd ed.: Baltimore: Williams and Wilkins, 1997, 53.


# Wound Healing Stimulants

## Acemannan

### Defintion and Indications

Acemannan is a beta (1, 4)-linked acetylated mannan. It is available as a topical hydrogel wound dressing (CarraVet Acemannan Wound Gel, CarraVet, Inc., Newnan, GA). Acemannan modulates the production of interleukin-1 (IL-1) and tumor necrosis factor-alpha (TNF-a) by wound macrophages in the inflammatory stage of healing. These cytokines are present at levels that enhance the early stages of healing. They result in enhanced fibroblast proliferation, neovascularization, epidermal growth and motility, and collagen deposition. They also bind growth factors involved in wound healing to stabilize them, thus prolonging their stimulating effects on granulation tissue formation.

The medication is indicated in the early inflammatory stage of healing and can be continued into the repair stage of healing. It can be used for treating superficial and deep partial-thickness burns, lacerations, dermal ulcers and abrasions on horses, dogs and cats.

### Technique

The wound should first be debrided and lavaged. The hydrogel should be applied over the entire wound and its borders and then be covered by a gauze sponge or a nonadherent primary bandage pad. An absorbent secondary bandage wrap is placed over this, followed by the outer bandage layer. The bandage is changed daily.

Because the medication has been noted to have its greatest effect in the first seven days of its use, it has been used in a 7-day sequential therapy regimen. The medication is used sequentially with one of the other wound healing stimulants (see sequential 7 day therapy)

### Aftercare

No special aftercare is needed.

### Advantages and Disadvantages

The primary advantage of acemannan is stimulation of the wound healing process. It can be used to stimulate earlier healing of severe traumatic wounds, to include wounds with exposed bone such as would be seen in distal limb wounds.

## Suggested Readings


1. Hedlund CS: Surgery of the integumentary system. *In* Fossum TW, ed.: Small Animal Surgery, 2nd ed.: St. Louis: Mosby, 2002, 134.
2. Hedlund CS: Surgery of the integumentary system. In Fossum TW, ed.: Small Animal Surgery, 3rd ed.: St. Louis: Mosby, 2007, 159.

3. Krahwinkel DJ, Boothe HW: Topical and systemic medications for wounds. Vet Clin No Am Small Animal Pract 36: 739, 2006.
4. MacPhail MC: Surgery of the integumentary system. In Fossum TW, ed.: Small Animal Surgery, 4th ed.: St. Louis: Mosby, 2013, 190.
5. Pavletic MM: Atlas of Small Animal Wound Management and Reconstructive Surgery, 3rd ed.: Ames, IA: Wiley-Blackwell, 2010, 51.
6. Swaim SF, Riddell KP,McGuire JA: The effects of topical medications on the healing of open pad wounds in dogs. J Am Anim Hosp Assoc 28:499, 1992.
7. Swaim SF, Vaughn DM, Kincaid SA, et al: Effects of locally injected medications on the healing of pad wounds in dogs. Am J Vet Res 57:394, 1996.
8. Swaim SF, Henderson RA: Small Animal Wound Management, 2nd ed.: Baltimore: Williams and Wilkins, 1997, 53.
9. Swaim SF, Gillette RL: An update on wound medications and dressings. Compend Contin Educ 20:1133,1998.
10. Tizzard IR, Carpenter RH, McAnalley BH, Kemp MC: The biologic activities of mannans and related complex carbohydrates. Mol Biother 1:290, 1989.
11. Tizzard IR, Busbee D, Maxwell B, et al: Effects of acemannan, a complex carbohydrate, on wound healing in young and aged rats. Wounds 6:201,1994.

# Tripeptide Copper Complex

## Definition and Indications

The tripeptide copper complex medication is a hydrogel containing glycyl-L-histidyl-L-lysine tripeptide complexed with copper (lamin Hydrating Gel Wound Dressing, Folica, Dayton, NJ). It is a chemo-attractant for mast cells and monocytes/macrophages in wounds. Macrophages produce growth factors which are important in the progression of wound healing. Mast cells play an important role in neovascularization of wounds. The medication enhances various aspects of wound healing to include neovascularization, reepithelialization, collagen deposition, and wound contraction.

The medication is indicated to enhance the healing of acute wounds. It is indicated for use in the late inflammatory and early repair stages of healing on into the late repair stage of healing. The medication could also be used to stimulate slow or nonhealing wounds into an active state of healing.

Empirically, the author has found it to be effective in stimulating chronic wounds into active healing in cats, barring the presence of underlying complications.

## Technique

The wound should be debrided and lavaged, followed by application of the hydrogel over the entire wound. The wound should then be covered with a gauze sponge or nonadherent primary bandage pad. This is followed by an absorbent secondary bandage wrap and an outer bandage layer. The bandage is changed daily.

This medication has been noted to have its greatest effect in the first seven days of its use. Thus, it has been used in a 7-day sequential therapy regimen. (See Sequential 7-day Therapy). It is used sequentially with one of the other wound healing stimulants. It has a tendency to cause over-production of granulation tissue above the wound edges. Thus, it should be used judiciously as wound healing progresses - i.e. every-other day.

## Aftercare

Wounds treated with topical tripeptide copper complex do not require any special aftercare. However, on the second or third day of treatment the surface of the wound will have an exudate on its surface which may have a blue tint to it. The color is related to the blue color of the gel. Under the exudate is healthy granulation tissue. The exudate should be lavaged from the wound surface before applying more of the hydrogel.

## Advantages and Disadvantages

The advantage of tripeptide copper complex tropical hydrogel is its stimulation of the wound healing process. The medication may stimulate over-production of granulation tissue above the wound edges which could mechanically slow wound contraction.

# Suggested Readings

1. Canapp SO, Farese JP, Schultz GS, et al: The effects of topical tripeptide-copper-complex on healing of ischemic open wounds. Vet Surg 32:515, 2003.
2. Cangul IT, Gul NY, Topal A, et al: Evaluation of the effects of topical tripeptide-copper complex and zinc oxide on open wound healing in rabbits. Vet Derm 17: 417, 2006.
3. Downey D, Larrabee F, Voci V, Pickart L: Acceleration of wound healing using glycyl-histidyl-lysine-Cu2+. Surg Forum 48:573, 1985.
4. Fahie MA, Shettko D: Evidence-based wound management: A systematic review of therapeutic agents to enhance granulation tissue and epithelialization. Vet Clin No Am Small Animal Pract 37: 559, 2007.
5. Fish FS, Katz I, Hien NT, et al: Evaluation of glycyl-L-histidyl-L-lysine copper complex in acute wound healing: Effect in post Moh's surgery wounds. Wounds 3:171, 1991.
6. Gul NY, Topal A, Cangul IT, et al: The effects of topical tripeptide copper complex and helium-neon laser on wound healing in rabbits. Vet Derm 19: 7, 2008.
7. Hedlund CS: Surgery of the integumentary system. *In* Fossum TW, ed.: Small Animal Surgery, 2nd ed.: St. Louis: Mosby, 2002, 134.
8. Hedlund CS: Surgery of the integumentary system. In Fossum TW, ed.: Small Animal Surgery, 3rd ed.: St. Louis: Mosby, 2007, 159.
9. Krahwinkel DJ, Boothe HW: Topical and systemic medications for wounds. Vet Clin No Am Small Animal Pract 36: 739, 2006.
10. MacPhail MM: Surgery of the integumentary system. In Fossum TW, ed.: Small Animal Surgery, 4th ed.: St. Louis: Mosby, 2013, 190.
11. Maquart FX, Bellon G, Chaquor B, et al: In vivo stimulation of connective tissue accumulation by the tripeptide-copper complex glycyl-L-histidyl-L-lysine-Cu2+ in rat experimental wounds. J Clin Invest 92:2368, 1993.
12. Maquart FX, Pickart L: Stimulation of collagen synthesis in

fibroblast cultures by the tripeptide-copper complex glycyl-L-histidyl-L-lysine-Cu2+. FEBS Lett 238:34, 1998.
13. Palvetic MM: Atlas of Small Animal Wound Management and Reconstructive Surgery, 3rd ed.: Ames, IA: Wiley-Blackwell, 2010, 51.
14. Pickart L: lamin. A human factor with multiple healing properties. In Sorenson JRJ, ed.: Biology of Copper Complexes: Clinton NJ: Humana Press, Inc., 1987, 273.
15. Swaim SF, Bradley DM, Spano JS, et al: Evaluation of multipeptide-copper complex medications on open wound healing in dogs. J Am Anim Hosp Assoc 29:519, 1993.
16. Swaim SF, Vaughn DM, Kincaid SA, et al: Effects of locally injected medications on the healing of pad wounds in dogs. Am J Vet Res 57:394, 1996.
17. Swaim SF, Gillette RL: An update on wound medications and dressings. Compend Contin Educ 20:1133, 1998.
18. Zetter BR, Rasmussen N, Brown L: Methods in laboratory investigation: An *in vivo* assay of chemoattractant activity. Lab Investig 53:362, 1985.

# Maltodextrin N.F. (D-Glucose Polysaccharide)

## Definition and Indications

Maltodextrin N.F., a D-glucose polysaccharide, is a hydrophilic, soluble powder or gel (Intracell-Mcleod Pharmaceuticals, Ft. Collins, CO) that may be used to cleanse and promote healing of contaminated and infected wounds. Maltodextrin may yield available glucose from polysaccharide hydrolysis to provide energy for cell metabolism to enhance healing. In addition, the medication has been reported to cause chemotaxis of polymorphonuclear cells, lymphocytes and macrophages into wounds. These then increase the level of growth factors necessary for healing.

It is indicated in treating acute wounds from the early inflammatory through the repair stages of healing. The medication may also be used to treat chronic wounds and ulcers to stimulate them into an active state of healing. Because of its hydrophilic nature, the powder form of the drug could be used in treating wounds where reduction of edema in the wound area is desired in the inflammatory stage of healing. The powder form of the drug is indicated for exudating wounds and the gel for drier wounds.

## Technique

After the wound is debrided and lavaged, the medication is applied over the wound at a depth of about ¼ inch. This is covered with a gauze sponge or non-adherent primary bandage pad followed by an absorbent secondary bandage wrap and an outer tertiary layer. The bandage is changed at least daily and possibly more often with a highly productive wound. The frequency of bandage change can decrease as fluid production by the wound decreases.

Maltodextrin has been used in a 7-day sequential therapy regimen. (See Sequential 7-day Therapy). It is used sequentially with one of the other wound healing stimulants.

## Aftercare

No special aftercare is needed when treating a wound with the Maltodextrin N.F. If a non-adherent bandage pad becomes dry and adheres to the wound, saline should be placed on the pad to help ensure that the wound healing process will not be disturbed at bandage change.

## Advantages and Disadvantages

Advantages of the medication include softening of necrotic tissue, rapid penetration of wound irregularities, nontoxicity, no systemic absorption, and effectiveness in infected and noninfected wounds. In addition, a reduction of wound odor, exudate, and infection are advantages. The hydrophilic nature of the medication; whereby, the body's own homeostatic fluids are drawn up through the wound tissues to bathe them from the inside is an advantage. If the animal is on systemic antibiotics, these fluids will be laden with antibiotics. The fluids dilute exudates for better absorption into the bandage. Maltodextrin has also been reported to have antibacterial and bacteriostatic properties.

# Suggested Readings

1. Fahie MA, Shettko D: Evidence-based wound management: A systematic review of therapeutic agents to enhance granulation and epithelialization. Vet Clin No Am Small Animal Pract 37: 559, 2007.
2. Hedlund CS: Surgery of the integumentary system. In Fossum TW, ed.: Small Animal Surgery, 3rd ed.: St. Louis: Mosby, 2007, 159.
3. Krahwinkel DJ, Boothe HW: Topical and systemic medications for wounds. Vet Clin No Am Small Animal Pract 36: 739, 2006.
4. MacPhail CM: Surgery of the integumentary system. In Fossum TW, ed.: Small Animal Surgery, 4th ed.: St. Louis: Mosby, 2013, 190.
5. McFadden EA: Multidex gel for use in wound care. J Pediatric Nurs 12:125,1997.
6. Pavletic MM: Atlas of Small Animal Wound Management and Reconstructive Surgery, 3rd ed.: Ames, IA: Wiley-Blackwell, 2010, 51.
7. Silvetti AN: An effective method of treating long enduring wounds and ulcers by topical applications of solutions and nutrients. J Dermatol Surg Oncol 7:501,1981.
8. Silvetti AN: The antimicrobial effect of maltodextrin N.F. in the healing of chronic wounds and ulcers including pressure ulcers. Proc Symp Adv Wound Care and Med Res Forum Wound Repair, 1994, 70.
9. Swaim SF, Henderson RA: Small Animal Wound Management, 2nd ed.: Baltimore: Williams and Wilkins, 1997, 53.
10. Swaim SF, Gillette RL: An update on wound medications and dressings. Compend Contin Educ 20:1133,1998.
11. White GW: Maltodextran NF powder: A new concept in equine wound healing. J Equi Vet Sci 15:296,1995.

# Sequential 7-day Therapy

### Definition and Indications

This regimen of therapy is used based on the author's (SFS) observation that medications tend to have their greatest effect during the first seven days of use. The three wound healing stimulants are used in a sequential fashion to stimulate healing in large and/or deep wounds. On distal limb wounds the use is primarily to enhance healing of large wounds whether they are to be allowed to heal by second intention or to have a reconstructive procedure performed.

### Technique

During the first week acemannan is applied to the wound as described for that medication. During the second week maltodextrin N.F. (D-glucose polysaccharide) is applied to the wound as described for that medication, and tripeptide copper complex is applied as described for that medication during the third week.

### Aftercare

The aftercare stated for each of the medications should be kept in mind when that medication is being used. If at some point in therapy the granulation tissue appears to be exuberant, which could mechanically interfere with contraction and epithelialization, use of the medication should be decreased or discontinued based on clinical judgment.

### Advantages and Disadvantages

The advantages and disadvantages of the sequential 7-day therapy are those that have been stated for each of the wound healing stimulants.

Based on one author's imperical observation an advantage of the sequential 7-day regimen is that it gets the healing process underway quickly with acemannan resulting in early appearance of granulation tissue. This is followed by continued stimulation of the process by the action of the other 2 medications.

# Suggested Readings

(See Suggested Readings for Acemannan, maltodextrin N.F. (D-glucose polysaccharide), and tripeptide copper complex.

# Other Topical Agents

## Sugar

### Definition and Indications

Granulated sugar is sucrose in the form of table sugar. It is indicated to cleanse and promote the healing of open contaminated or infected wounds. Sugar may provide a local source of cellular energy as well as be a chemo-attractant for macrophages which play a vital role in wound healing. It also accelerates sloughing of devitalized tissue and promotes the formation of a protective protein layer on the wound.

Sugar is indicated to treat acute wounds from the early inflammatory stage until they have reached the repair stage of healing. It could also be used to treat chronic wounds and ulcers to stimulate them into an active stage of healing with a healthy bed of granulation tissue.

Sugar is hydrophilic in nature. Its high osmolarity results in body fluids and nutrients being drawn through regenerating tissues. This can result in reduced inflammatory edema of the area. In addition, as sugar draws fluid from the wound, it creates an environment of low water activity in the wound. This inhibits bacterial growth. It has also been stated that high concentrations of sugar alter wound pH which produces a toxic environment for invading microorganisms. There is also speculation that sugar undergoes fermentation within a wound to create alcohols that act as antiseptics. It has been reported to be effective in wounds infected with *Staphylococcus, Streptococcus, Enterobacter, E.coli, Klebsiella, Pseudomonas,* and *Serratia.*

### Technique

Following wound debridement, lavage, and patting the wound almost dry, sugar is placed in a thick coat on the wound (1 cm thick). The wound is covered by a gauze sponge or non-adherent primary bandage pad followed by an absorbent secondary bandage wrap and an outer tertiary wrap. Initially, bandages are changed twice daily when the wound is highly productive. Strike through is a definite indication for bandage change. The frequency of bandage change can become less as fluid production by the wound decreases, e.g. when there is still undissolved sugar on the wound at bandage change. Sugar therapy can be discontinued once granulation tissue is present.

### Aftercare

No special aftercare is needed when treating a wound with sugar.

### Advantages and Disadvantages

Sugar is reported to have a rapid antibacterial and deodorizing action. It enhances granulation tissue formation and epithelialization in accelerating wound healing. Sugar is readily available and inexpensive. Hyperglycemia does not result from its topical application. The potential for causing fluid, electrolyte and protein imbalances due to the hydrophilic nature of sugar drawing large quantities of these through the tissues is less with distal limb wounds than it would be with large body wounds. Sugar is not sterile, and it may contain additives such as corn starch or one percent tricalcium to prevent clumping. It is unknown how these additives impact wound healing.

## Suggested Readings


1. Anderson D: Management of open wounds. In Williams J, Moores A, eds.: BSAVA Manual of Canine and Feline Wound Management and Reconstruction, 2nd ed.: Glouster (UK): BSAVA, 2009, 37.
2. Chirife J, Scarmato GA, Herszage L: Scientific basis for use of granulated sugar in treatment of infected wounds. Lancet 1:560,1982.
3. Chirife J, Herszage L, Joseph A, Kohn ES: *In vitro* study of bacterial growth inhibition in concentrated sugar solutions: Microbiological basis for the use of sugar in treating infected wounds. Antimicrob Agents Chemother 23:766,1983.
4. Dawson J: The role of sugar in wound healing: A comparative trial of the healing of infected wounds using traditional gauze/antiseptic packing and granulated sugar. Ann Royal Coll Surg Engl 78:82,1996.
5. Fahie MA, Shettko D: Evidence-based wound management: A systemic review of therapeutic agents to enhance granulation and epithelialization. Vet Clin No Am Small Animal Pract 37: 559, 2007.
6. Hedlund CS: Surgery of the integumentary system. In Fossum TW, ed.: Small Animal Surgery, 3rd ed.: St. Louis: Mosby, 2007, 159.
7. Hosgood G: Open wounds. In Tobias KM, Johnston SA, eds.: Veterinary Surgery, Small Animal, Vol 2: St. Louis: Elsevier-Saunders, 2012, 1210.
8. Kamat N: Use of sugar in infected wounds. Trop Doct 23:185,1993.
9. Krahwinkel DJ, Boothe HW: Topical and systemic medications for wound. Vet Clin No Am Small Animal Pract 36: 739, 2006.
10. MacPhail CM: Surgery of the integumentary system. In Fossum ed.: Small Animal Surgery, 4th ed.: St. Louis: Mosby, 2013, 190.
11. Mathews KA, Binnington AG: Wound management using sugar. Compend Contin Educ 24:41, 2002.
12. Molan PC, Cooper RA: Honey and sugar as a dressing for wounds and ulcers. Trop Doct 30:249,2000.
13. Pavletic MM: Atlas of Small Animal Wound Management and Reconstructive Surgery, 3rd ed.: Ames, IA: Wiley-Blackwell, 2010, 51.
14. Podrasky DL, Flynn KT: Topical sugar for healing: Kitchen magic or science? Ost Wound Manag 18:24, 1988.
15. Rund C: Alternative topical therapies for wound care. *In* Krasner DL, Rodeheaver GT, Sibbald RG, eds.: Chronic Wound Care, 3rd ed.: Wayne, PA: HMP Communications, 2001, 329.


# Honey

## Definition and Indications

Honey is a natural product produced by bees. It is composed of 40% glucose, 40% fructose, and 20% water, vitamins, trace elements and amino acids. Honey has several properties that make it beneficial in wound management. It decreases inflammatory edema, attracts macrophages that are essential in wound healing, accelerates sloughing/debridement of devitalized tissue, provides local cell energy, protects wound tissues from free oxygen radicals with its antioxidants, and reduces periwound maceration. It also increases wound collagen content and collagen maturation. Honey has been reported to lower wound prostaglandin levels and elevate nitric oxide end products which may explain its therapeutic properties in healing.

Honey also has antimicrobial properties. It contains inhibine, an enzyme from the pharyngeal glands of the bees. Inhibine breaks down into hydrogen peroxide and gluconolactone. Unlike commercially available 3% hydrogen peroxide, which can damage mammalian cells and slow healing, the concentration of hydrogen peroxide generated from honey is much lower, and this low level harms bacteria but not mammalian cells. The hydrogen peroxide is a mild disinfectant and gluconolactone equates to gluconic acid, a mild antibiotic. Honey also contains propolis, a substance gathered from plant buds to repair cracks in a hive. The active ingredient of propolis is galangine, a food preservative. Honey has a low pH (3.6 to 3.7) which increases its antibacterial effects. Like sugar, the high osmolarity of honey results in low water activity in the wound and an antibacterial effect. Honey has also been found to inhibit the growth of some fungi. Thus, honey has a mild disinfectant, a mild antibiotic, a low pH, a high osmolarity and food preservative qualities to give it natural antimicrobial properties. It has been reported to be effective against a wide variety of gram positive and gram negative bacteria, including *E.coli, Proteus mirabilis, Pseudomonas aeruginosa, Salmonella typhimurium, Serratia marcescens, Staphylococcus aureus, Streptococcus pyogenes,* and *Candida albicans.* Manuka honey contains higher levels of antimicrobial phytochemicals.

Honey is indicated to treat acute wounds from the early inflammatory stage into the repair stage of healing. Chronic wounds and ulcers could also be treated with honey to stimulate them into an active state of healing with a bed of healthy granulation tissue.

### Technique

Wounds should be debrided and lavaged. Grossly contaminated wounds should be lavaged with body temperature tap water delivered by a spray nozzle. After lavage, wounds should be patted dry. The honey used to treat wounds must be unpasteurized and ideally should not have been heated above 37° C. Honey can be poured into the wound then covered with a gauze, applied on gauzes, which are then placed on the wound, or be applied by gauzes that have been saturated in honey. The absorbent secondary wrap and tertiary bandage layer are then applied. The frequency of bandage change can be from one to three times daily depending on how rapidly the honey is diluted by exudates. At bandage changes, the wound should be lavaged before a new application of honey. Honey application can be discontinued when healthy granulation tissue is present and epithelialization has started.

### Aftercare

No special aftercare is needed when treating a wound with honey.

### Advantages and Disadvantages

Honey is a cost-effective wound treatment and is effective against the growth of bacteria and in deodorizing wounds. It also serves as a viscous barrier to wound invasion by bacteria. Honey enhances wound healing by stimulating the formation of granulation tissue and epithelialization of wounds. It has been reported to be less painful than sugar when applied.

There are issues to be considered when using honey. Raw unprocessed honey is not sterile, and may be contaminated with pesticides and other chemicals which bees may carry. A known reaction to bees by an animal should be considered before using honey. The potential for causing fluid, electrolyte, and protein imbalances due to the hydrophilic nature of honey drawing large quantities of these through the tissues is less with distal limb wounds than it would be with a large body wound.

## Suggested Readings


1. Al-Wai N, Salom K, Al-Ghamdi AA: Honey for wound healing, ulcers, and burns: data supporting its use in clinical practice. Sci Word J 11: 766, 2011.
2. Anderson D: Management of open wounds. In Williams J, Moores A, eds.: BSAVA Manual of Canine and Feline Wound Management and Reconstruction, 2nd ed.: Glouster (UK): BSAVA, 2009, 37.
3. Bergmann A, Yani J, Weiss J, et al: Acceleration of wound healing by topical application of honey: An animal model. Am J Surg 145:374,1983.
4. Cooper RA, Molan PC: Honey in wound care. J Wound Care 8:340, 1999.
5. Cooper RA, Molan PC,Harding KG: Antibacterial activity of honey against strains of *Staphylococcus aureus* from infected wounds. J Royal Soc Med 92:283, 1999.
6. Efem SE, Udoh KT, Iwara CI: The antimicrobial spectrum of honey and its clinical significance. Infection 20:227, 1992.
7. Efem SE: Clinical observations on the wound healing properties of honey. Br J Surg 75:679,1998.
8. Fahie MA, Shettko D: Evidence-based wound management: A systemic review of therapeutic agents to enhance granulation and epithelialization. Vet Clin No Am Small Animal Pract 37: 559, 2007.
9. Frankel S, Robinson GE, Berenbaum MR: Antioxidant capacity and correlated characteristics of 14 unifloral honeys. J Apic Res 37:27,1998.
10. Harris S: Honey for the treatment of superficial wounds: A case report and review. Primary Intention Nov18, 1994.
11. Hedlund CS: Surgery of the integumentary system. In Fossum TW, ed.: Small Animal Surgery, 3rd ed.: St. Louis: Mosby, 2007, 159.
12. Hosgood G: Open Wounds. In Tobias KM, Johnston SA, eds.: Veterinary Surgery, Small Animal, Vol. 2: St. Louis: Elsevier-Saunders, 2012, 1210.
13. Ingle R, Levin J, Polinder K: Wound healing with honey: A randomized controlled trial. South Afric Med J 96: 831, 2006.
14. Krahwinkel DJ, Boothe HW: Topical and systemic medications for wounds. Vet Clin No Am Small Anim Pract 36: 739, 2006.
15. Langemo DK, Hanson D, Anderson J, et al: Use of honey for wound healing. Advan Skin Wound Care 22: 113, 2009.
16. Lee DS, Sinno S, Khachemoune A: Honey and wound healing: An overview. Am J Clin Derm 12: 181, 2011.
17. MacPhail CM: Surgery of the integumentary system. In Fossum TW, ed.: Small Animal Surgery, 4th ed.: St. Louis: Mosby, 2013, 190.
18. Mathews KA, Binnington AG: Wound management using honey. Compend Contin Educ 24:53, 2002.
19. Molan PC: The antibacterial activity of honey. 1: The nature of the antibacterial activity. Bee World 73:15,1992.
20. Molan PC: The role of honey in managing wounds. J Wound Care 8:415, 1999.
21. Molan PC, Cooper RA: Honey and sugar as a dressing for wounds and ulcers. Trop Doct 30:249,2000.
22. Mphande AN, Killowe C, Phalira S, et al: Effects of honey and sugar dressings on wound healing. J Wound Care 16: 317, 2007.
23. Pavletic MM: Atlas of Small Animal Wound Management and Reconstructive Surgery, 3rd ed.: Ames, IA: Wiley-Blackwell, 2010, 51.
24. Rund C: Alternative topical therapies for wound care. In Krasner DL, Rodeheaver GT, Sibbald RG, eds.: Chronic Wound Care, 3rd ed.: Wayne, PA: HMP Communications, 2001, 329.
25. White JW, Stubers MH, Shepartz AI: The identification of inhibine, the antibacterial factor in honey, as hydrogen peroxide and its origin in a honey glucose-oxidase system. Biochem Biophys Acta 73:57,1963.
26. White JW: Inhibine and glucose oxidase in honey: A review. Amer Bee J 106:214, 1966.


## Collagen Products
## Activated Bovine Collagen
### Definition and Indications

An activated bovine collagen dressing is available in powder form (Cellerate RX, Wound Care Innovations, Ft. Lauderdale, FL). It effectively absorbs wound drainage. Following studies with this form of medication, it is believed the hydrophilic action could be utilized in cleansing contaminated and infected wounds, as well as reducing edema in the wound area in the inflammatory stage of healing.

The medication is indicated for treating acute wounds from the early inflammatory through the repair stage of healing.

### Technique

The wound is debrided and lavaged followed by application of the activated bovine collagen powder to the wound surface at about a ¼ inch depth. Alternatively, a gel or spray is applied to the wound surface. A gauze pad or nonadherent primary bandage pad is placed over the medication followed by an absorbent secondary bandage wrap and an outer tertiary wrap. The bandage is changed at least daily and possibly more often in the early inflammatory stages on a highly productive wound. The frequency of bandage change can decrease as fluid production decreases.

### Aftercare

No special aftercare is needed when treating a wound with the bovine collagen powder.

### Advantages and Disadvantages

Because of its hydrophilic nature, activated bovine collagen powder is useful in reducing wound odor, exudate and infection. If the animal is on systemic antibiotics, the fluids drawn up through the wound bathe the wound with antibiotic-laden fluids. These fluids dilute exudates for better absorption into the bandage. The moist wound environment created by the medication has been found to enhance wound epithelialization. Research has shown the powder form of collagen does not induce a histologic inflammatory reaction in the wound tissues.[6]

## Suggested Readings


1. Fahie MA, Shettko D: Evidence-based wound management: A systematic review of therapeutic agents to enhance granulation and epithelialization. Vet Clin No Amer Small Animal Pract 37: 559, 2007.
2. Hedlund CS: Surgery of the integumentary system. In Fossum TW, ed.: Small Animal Surgery, 3rd ed.: St. Louis: Mosby, 2007, 159.
3. Krahwinkel DJ, Boothe HW: Topical and systemic medications for wounds. Vet Clin No Am Small Animal Pract 36: 739, 2006.
4. MacPhail CM: Surgery of the integumentary system. In Fossum TW, ed.: Small Animal Surgery, 4th ed.: St. Louis: Mosby, 2013, 190.
5. Pavletic MM: Atlas of Small Animal Wound Management and Reconstructive Surgery, 3rd ed.: Ames, IA: Wiley-Blackwell, 2010, 51.
6. Swaim SF, Gillette RL, Sartin EA, et al: Effects of a hydrolyzed collagen dressing on the healing of open wounds in dogs. Am J Vet Res 61:1574, 2000.

# Chapter 2

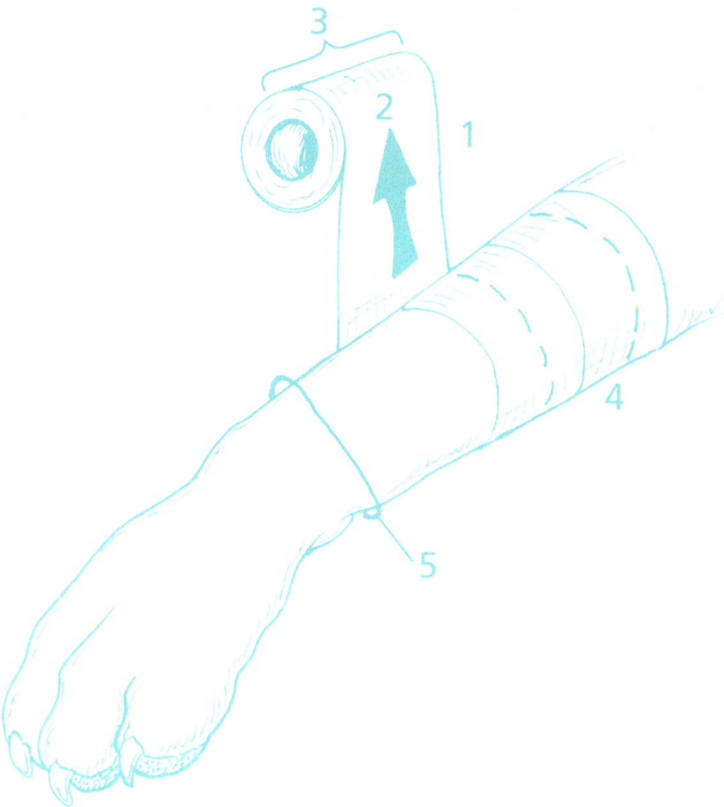


## Bandages, Pads, Splints, and Slings

Steven F. Swaim, D.V.M., M.S.

# General Information

This section will present information on the various materials that can be used in bandaging, padding, splinting and placing slings on the distal limb and paw areas. The presentation is not an extensive coverage of products used for these procedures. The materials presented are those primarily used by the authors. Information on the techniques for applying the different bandage, splint and sling configurations is also presented throughout the text in the *Technique* and *Aftercare* sections of the various procedures and conditions.

# Primary Bandage Layer: Gauze Pad Dressings

## Definition and Indications

The gauze pad dressings used in bandaging have a wide mesh that does not have cotton filler. It is one of the older forms of dressing, but it is still useful. When used over a closed wound, they absorb the small amount of fluid that drains between the wound edges. When used on open wounds exudate is absorbed by the gauze and dries by evaporation, attaching the dressing to the scab that forms. In addition, the open mesh entraps foreign bodies and loose necrotic tissue which are removed at bandage change. An antimicrobial gauze pad is available (Kerlix AMD, Super Sponges, Covidien,Tyco/HealthCare/Kendall, Mansfield, MA). It is impregnated with 0.2% polyhexamethylene biguanide.

Gauze pad dressings are indicated over closed wounds to absorb the small amount of exudate that drains from the suture line to keep the area dry. When used on open wounds, gauze pad dressings are indicated as adherent dressing to help debride the wound of necrotic tissue and debris. When used in this manner, they can be used as dry-to-dry or wet-to-dry dressings. When there is a copious amount of low-viscosity exudate a dry-to-dry dressing is indicated; however, a wet-to-dry dressing is indicated for wounds with a viscous exudate (coagulum). The antimicrobial gauze pads are indicated for wound debridement of infected wounds.

## Techniques

### Dry-to-dry dressing

The dressing pad is applied to the wound followed by absorbent secondary wrap and a porous outer layer. The bandage remains in place until the primary and secondary materials have absorbed fluid and debris from the wound and the fluid has evaporated, leaving a dry primary layer. At bandage removal the gauze-entrapped necrotic tissue and foreign debris is removed. The antimicrobial gauzes are used as a dry-to-dry dressing.

### Wet-to-dry dressing

A gauze wet with warm sterile saline, lactated ringers solution or 1:40 dilution (0.05%) of chlorhexidine diacetate (Nolvasan solution, Ft. Dodge Animal Health, Ft. Dodge, IA) or gluconate (Chlorhexiderm solution, Dermatologics in Veterinary Medicine Pharmaceuticals, Miami, FL) in water is placed on the wound. Alternatively, a sterile gauze can be placed on the wound followed by wetting with the solution from a sterile spray bottle, pour bottle, or syringe. Bandage application is more comfortable for the animal if the wetting solution has been warmed in a microwave oven. An absorbent secondary wrap and porous tertiary layer are applied over the gauze. The wetting solution dilutes the viscous exudate for better absorption into the bandage. After the bandage dries by evaporation, fibrin, foreign debris and necrotic tissue adhered to the gauze are removed from the wound at bandage change.

## Aftercare

The frequency of bandage change is dependent upon the fluid productivity of the wound. For closed wounds without a drain, bandage change may be done every 2 to 3 days. For open or drained distal limb and paw wounds, daily bandage change is usually sufficient. However, if the bandage over an open wound is saturated with exudate and is not adhered to the wound, more frequent bandage change is indicated. Generally, the frequency of bandage change decreases as the wound progresses from the inflammatory/debridement stage to the repair stage.

When removing an adherent gauze from dogs and cats it can be soaked with warm saline to make removal more comfortable for the animal. Alternatively, in dogs the outer gauze layers can be removed down to the last 2-3 layers over the wound. These layers are moistened with warm 2% lidocaine – sodium bicarbonate solution. The lidocaine should not contain epinephrine. The two medications are mixed in a 9:1 ratio by volume. This prevents the stinging sensation of the lidocaine. The final layers are removed after 2 to 3 minutes. Occasionally, sedation is needed for bandage removal.

Adherent bandage debridement is used in conjunction with staged debridement. The wound is usually cleared of necrotic tissue and debris by 3 to 5 days. At this time the application of medications, i.e. antibiotics/antibacterials and wound healing stimulants can be considered. Once the wound has entered the later inflammatory or early repair healing stage, another form of dressing should be selected that will favor progression of wound healing, For example, a moisture retentive dressing.

## Advantages and Disadvantages

Adherent gauze pads provide a cost effective way of removing large amounts of exudates from wounds in the early stages of healing. They also provide a means of completing wound debridement when used in conjunction with staged surgical debridement. In addition to wound debridement, antimicrobial gauze pads have the advantage of providing antimicrobial treatment of infected wounds without the effort of placing medications on the pads. When saline is used to wet a gauze there is a hydrophilic principle involved. Water evaporates from the saline solution making the gauze hypertonic. Thus, water is drawn from the wound into the dressing. As the dressing becomes isotonic, the cycle is repeated.

These adherent bandages have several disadvantages. The primary disadvantage of adherent gauze pads is pain and damage to viable cells at bandage removal. The dry wound environment of these bandages does not support the function of proteases and cells involved in wound repair cleanup. Dry guaze disperses more bacteria into the air during bandage change; thus, contaminating the area and increasing the possibility of cross – contamination between wounds. Fiber from adhered bandages may remain attached to the wound surface resulting in an inflammatory reaction. Frequent removal of wound fluid with these types of bandages reduces the availability of growth factors and cytokines essential for healing. If wet-to-dry bandages are too wet, tissues may macerate, and if fluid reaches the outer bandage layer, bacteria may move centrally toward the wound. At the other extreme, if bandages become too dry, the tissues may dessicate. On the distal limb, dessication of exposed bones, tendons, ligaments, nerves and blood vessels could have serious consequences. With a heavy Pseudomonas infection, a 0.05% chlorhexidine wetting solution in a wet-to-dry bandage may not be sufficient to control infection. Solutions of 0.1% or 0.5% may control infection; however, at these increased strengths these tend to slow granulation tissue formation.

# Suggested Readings


1. Anderson D: Management of open wounds. In Williams J, Moores A, eds.: BSAVA Manual of Canine and Feline Wound Management and Reconstruction, 2nd ed.: Glouster (UK): BSAVA, 2009, 37.
2. Bohling MW, Campbell BG, Swaim SF: Open wound care. Clinician's Brief Jan 19, 2007.
3. Bohling MW, Swaim SF: Bandaging and drainage techniques. In Bojrab MJ, ed.: Current Techniques in Small Animal Surgery, 5th ed.: Jackson, WY: Teton NewMedia, 2014, 13.
4. Bolton LL, Monte K, Pirone LA: Moisture and healing: Beyond the jargon. Ostomy Wound Manage S6 (Suppl): 515, 2000.
5. Campbell BG: Dressings, bandages and splints for wound management in dogs and cats.Vet Clin No Am Small Anim Pract 36: 759, 2006.
6. Campbell BG: Bandages and drains. In Tobias KM, Johnston SA, eds.: Veterinary Surgery, Small Animal, Vol 1: St. Louis: Elsevier – Saunders, 2012, 221.
7. Compton – Johnson S, Wilson J: Infected wound management: Advanced technologies, moisture retentive dressings and die – hard methods. Crit Care Nurs Q 24: 64, 2001.
8. Cutting KF: Wound exudates: Composition and functions. Br J Community Nurs 8 (Suppl): S4, 2003.
9. Hedlund CS: Surgery of the integumentary system. In Fossum TW, ed.: Small Animal Surgery, 2nd ed.: St. Louis: Mosby, 2002, 134.
10. Hedlund CS: Surgery of the integumentary system. *In* Fossum TW, ed.: Small Animal Surgery, 3rd ed.: St. Louis: Mosby, 2007, 159
11. Hosgood G: Open wound. In Tobias KM, Johnston SA, eds.: Veterinary Surgery, Small Animal, Vol. 2: St. Louis: Elsevier – Saunders, 2012, 1210.
12. Lee AH, Swaim SF, McGuire JA, Hughes KS: Effects of chlorhexidine diacetate, povidone iodine, and polyhydroxydine on wound healing in dogs. J Am Anim Hosp Assoc 24:77, 1988.
13. Lee WR, Tobias KM, Bemis DA, Rohrback BW: In vitro efficacy of a polyhexamethylene biguanide-impregnated gauze dressing against bacteria found in veterinary patients. Vet Surg 33:404, 2004.
14. Lim JK, Saliba L, Smith LJ, et al: Normal saline wound dressing - is it really normal? Br J Plast Surg 53:42, 2000.
15. Lozier SM: Topical wound therapy. *In* Harari J, ed.: Surgical Complications and Wound Healing in the Small Animal Practice. Philadelphia: WB Saunders, 1993, 63.
16. MacPhail CM: Surgery of the integumentary system. In Fossum TW, ed.: Small Animal Surgery, 4th ed.: St. Louis: Mosby, 2013, 190.
17. Mertz P, Cazzaniga A, Serralta V, et al: The effect of an antimicrobial gauze dressing impregnated with 0.2% polyhexamethylene biguanide as a barrier to prevent *Pseudomonas aeruginosa* wound invasion. Mansfield, MA: Kendall, Wound Care Research and Development, 2001.
18. Miller CW: Bandages and drains. *In* Slatter DH, ed.: Textbook of Small Animal Surgery. 3rd ed.: Philadelphia: WB Saunders, 2003, 244.
19. Noe JM, Kalish S: The problem of adherence in dressed wounds. Surg Gynecol Obstet 147:185, 1978.
20. Pavletic MM: Atlas of Small Animal Reconstructive Surgery, 2nd ed.: Philadelphia: WB Saunders, 1999, 107.
21. Pavletic MM: Atlas of Small Animal Wound Management and Reconstructive Surgery, 3rd ed.: Ames IA: Wiley – Blackwell, 2010, 81.
22. Popovich DM, Alexander D, Rihman M, et al: Strike – through contamination in sterile dressings: A clinical analysis. Clins Nurs Res 4: 195, 1995.
23. Rogers AA, Walmsley RS, Rippon MG, Bowler PG: Absorption of serum-derived proteins by primary dressings: Implications for dressing adhesion to wounds. J Wound Care 8:403, 1999.
24. Reitsma AM, Rodeheaver GT: Effectiveness of a new antimicrobial gauze dressing as a bacterial barrier. Mansfield, MA: Kendall Co., 2001.
25. Swaim SF: The effects of dressings and bandages on wound healing. Sem Vet Med Surg (Sm Anim) 4:274, 1989.
26. Swaim SF: Bandages and topical agents. Vet Clin North Am Small Anim Pract 20:47, 1990.
27. Swaim SF, Wilhalf D: The physics, physiology, and chemistry of bandaging open wounds. Compend Contin Educ Pract Vet 7:146, 1985.

28. Swaim SF, Henderson RA: Small Animal Wound Management, 2nd ed.: Baltimore: Williams and Wilkins, 1997, 53.
29. Swaim SF, Renberg WC, Shike KM: Small Animal Bandaging, Casting and Splinting Techniques. Ames IA: Wiley – Blackwell, 2011, 3.
30. Williams JM: Open wound management. *In* Fowler D, Williams JM, eds.: Manual of Canine and Feline Wound Management and Reconstruction. Cheltenham, England: BSAVA, 1999, 37.

# Polyurethane Foam Sponge

## Definition and Indications

Polyurethane foam sponge material (Hydrasorb Foam Sponge, Covidien, Tyco/Health Care/Kendall, Mansfield, OH) is a highly absorbent, conformable, permeable nonadherent dressing (Figure 2-1A & B). It is classified as a moisture retentive dressing. It maintains a moist wound surface while absorbing excess fluid. Thus, it supports autolytic debridement. It also stimulates a healthy granulation tissue bed. The sponge can be used over wounds that are producing large quantities of fluid in the inflammatory stage of healing. The dressing can also be used on wounds that are in the repair stage of healing because it does not adhere to the wound surface and disrupt healing tissue at bandage changes.

## Technique

After wound debridement and lavage, the semiocclusive foam sponge is cut to the appropriate shape and size for the wound. It is placed over the wound followed by an absorbent secondary bandage wrap and a porous tertiary wrap. When indicated, topical medications can be placed on the sponge.

## Aftercare

When used on highly productive wounds in the inflammatory stage of healing, bandages are changed at least daily. Due to the storage capacity of the sponges, the bandages can be changed less frequently as healing progresses and fluid production decreases. The sponges can be used effectively with staged debridement, with the sponges absorbing wound exudate and surgical debridement removing necrotic tissue and foreign debris.

## Advantages and Disadvantages

Polyurethane foam sponges have many of the attributes of the ideal wound dressing. In the early stages of healing, polyurethane sponges provide an effective means of removing large amounts of fluid from wounds while stimulating granulation tissue formation. They maintain a moist wound environment to support healing, but prevent tissue maceration. The sponges provide cushioning and thermal insulation for wounds, and they promote epithelialization. They can be used as the primary dressing layer throughout the wound healing process.

In the later stages of healing as wounds produce less fluid, a dry sponge may adhere at the wound edge.

# Suggested Readings

1. Anderson D: Management of open wounds. In Williams J, Moores, A eds.: BSAVA Manual of Canine and Feline Wound Management, 2nd ed.: Glouster (UK): BSAVA, 2009, 37.
2. Bohling MW, Campbell BG, Swaim SF: Open wound care. Clinician's Brief, Jan.: 19, 2007.
3. Bohling MW, Swaim SF: Bandaging and drainage techniques. In Bojrab MJ, ed.: Current Techniques in Small Animal Surgery, 5th ed.: Jackson, WY: Teton NewMedia, 2014, 13.
4. Campbell BG: Dressings, bandages, and splints for wound management in dogs and cats. Vet Clin No Am Small Anim Pract. 36: 759, 2006.
5. Campbell BG: Bandages and drains. In Tobias KM, Johnston SA, eds.: Veterinary Surgery, Small Animal, Vol. 1: St. Louis: Elsevier – Saunders, 2012, 221.
6. Casey G: Modern wound dressings. Nurs Stand 15: 47, 2000.

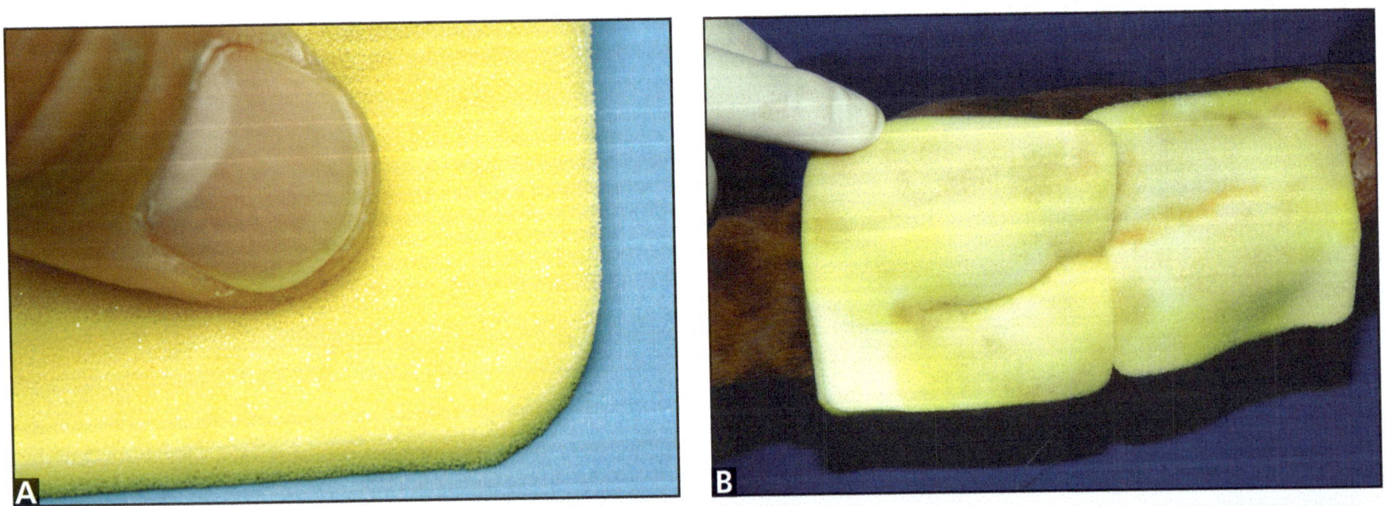


**Figure 2-1.** Polyurethane foam sponge primary bandage. **A.** Dressing Pad. **B.** Dressing pad conforming to a concavity on a limb wound surface (crease in dressing).

7. Compton – Johnston S, Wilson J: Infected wound management: Advanced technologies, moisture retentive dressings, and die – hard methods. Crit Care Nurs Q 24: 64, 2001.
8. Hedlund CS: Surgery of the integumentary system. In Fossum TW, ed.: Small Animal Surgery, 3rd ed.: St. Louis: Mosby, 2007: 159.
9. MacPhail CM: Surgery of the integumentary system. In Fossum TW, ed.: Small Animal Surgery, 4th ed.: St. Louis: Mosby, 2013, 190.
10. Miller CW: Bandages and drains. *In* Slatter DH, ed.: Textbook of Small Animal Surgery. 3rd ed.: Philadelphia: WB Saunders, 2003, 244.
11. Pavletic MM: Atlas of Small Animal Wound Management and Reconstructive surgery, 3rd ed.: Ames IA: Wiley – Blackwell, 2010, 81.
12. Seaman S: Dressing selection in chronic wound management. J Am Pediatr Med Aassoc 92:24, 2002.
13. Swaim SF, Henderson RA: Small Animal Wound Management, 2nd ed.: Baltimore: Williams and Wilkins, 1997, 53.
14. Swaim SF, Gillette RL: An update on wound medications and dressings. Compend Contin Educ Pract Vet 20:1133, 1998.
15. Swaim SF, Renberg WC, Shike KM: Small Animal Bandaging, Casting and Splinting Techniques. Ames, IA: Wiley – Blackwell, 2011, 3.
16. Turner TD: Interactive dressings used in the management of human soft tissue injuries and their potential in veterinary practice. Vet Derm 8:235, 1997.
17. Williams JM: Open wound management. In Fowler D, Williams JM, eds.: Manual of Canine and Feline Wound Management and Reconstruction. Cheltenham, England: BSAVA, 1999, 7.

# Hydrogels

## Definition and Indications

A hydrogel dressing used in veterinary medicine is a thin, semitransparent, nonadherent, occlusive, conformable sheet composed of a water - rich hydrophilic polyethylene oxide polymer between two thin synthetic sheets (CarraVet Clear Hydrogel Sheet, CarraVet, Inc. Newman, GA). Other hydrogel dressings are available that contain or are used as a vehicle for antibiotics, antimicrobials, or other dressing agents. The occlusive nature of polyethylene oxide dressing enhances the wound healing process. Angiogenesis is promoted, and with the new blood supply there is delivery of oxygen and antibacterial systems to the wound, to include systemic antibiotics. The moist environment provided by this moisture retentive dressing is especially effective in stimulating reepithelialization of wounds.

Because hydrogels have only a weak tendency to absorb fluid and biological components such as proteins and cells, i.e. exudate, these dressings are primarily indicated for wounds in the repair stage of healing when the exudate is decreased and of a serous nature. These would be considered clean open wounds with minimal to moderate drainage that are usually in their second week of management. Since they are capable of donating large amounts of moisture to wounds. They can also be used to rehydrate a dry wound bed and facilitate autolytic debridement and removal of dry eschar. These dressings could also be used on partial – thickness wounds, i.e. abraision wounds, to enhance epitheliazation. The sheets are well suited for moderate sized limb wounds due to their conformability by which they wrap around a limb and adhere to surrounding skin.

## Technique

Prior to dressing application, the skin around the wound should be cleaned and dried along with wiping the wound surface with an antiseptic solution. The dressing is then cut to the appropriate size for the wound and the blue synthetic sheet is peeled off one surface of the dressing leaving the clear synthetic sheet in place. The hydrogel surface is placed on the wound (Figure 2-2A-C). This is followed by a secondary bandage wrap and tertiary bandage layer. The dressing may be left in place for 2 days.

## Aftercare

After removing the dressing the wound surface and surrounding skin should be cleared of residual gel before placing a new dressing. As healing occurs and fluid production decreases, the time between bandage changes can increase. However, if a hydrogel containing an antibiotic or antimicrobial is being used, daily change may be indicated to maintain their activity in the wound. Use of the occlusive dressing should be discontinued after the wound is epithelialized. If the wound and surrounding tissue begin to appear macerated due to the moist environment under the dressing, the dressing should be discontinued. The polyurethane foam sponge dressing provides the desired wound environment at this point.

## Advantages and Disadvantages

The gel nature of hydrogel dressings enhances epithelialization and provides wound comfort while the semitransparent nature allows wound observation. The occlusive nature of the dressings can limit contamination of the wound. Conversely, any bacteria under the bandage are in a favorable environment for proliferation. It has been reported that the dressings are compatible with other topical agents. Because they are used in the repair stage of healing, fewer bandage changes are necessary with these dressings. Although hydrogel dressings have a tendency to cause exuberant granulation tissue, they reportedly stimulate contraction of forelimb wounds in dogs.

# Suggested Readings

1. Anderson D: Management of open wounds. In Williams J, Moores A, eds.: BASAVA Manual of Canine and Feline Wound Management and Reconstruction, 2nd ed.: Glouster (UK): BSAVA, 2009, 37.

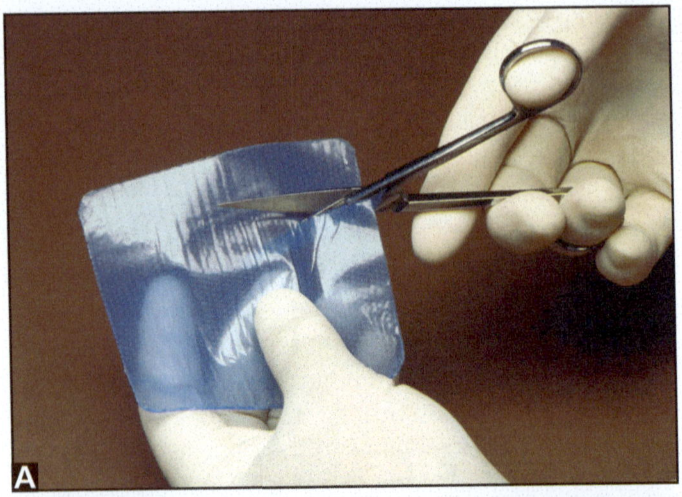

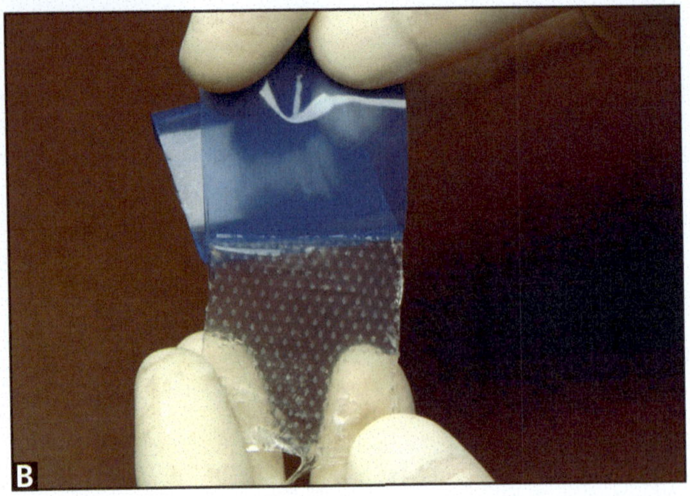

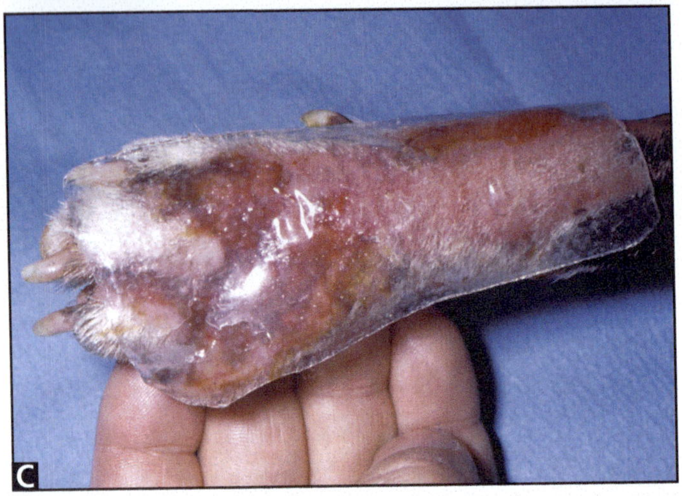

**Figure 2-2.** Hydrogel primary dressing. **A.** Cutting dressing to the size and shape needed. **B.** One synthetic sheet being peeled from one surface of the dressing. **C.** The hydrogel surface placed on the wound. (From Swaim SF, Henderson RA: Small Animal Wound Management, 2nd ed.: Baltimore: Williams & Wilkins, 1997, 63 & 64.)


2. Bohling MW, Campbell BG, Swaim SF: Open wound care. Clinician's Brief Jan., 19: 2007.
3. Bohling MW, Swaim SF: Bandage and drainage techniques. In Bojrab MJ, ed.: Current Techniques in Small Animal Surgery, 5th ed.: Jackson, WY: Teton NewMedia, 2014, 13.
4. Campbell BG: Dressings, bandages and splints for wound management in dogs and cats. Vet Clin No Small Animal Pract 36: 759, 2006.
5. Campbell BG: Bandages and drains. In Tobias KM, Johnston SA, eds.: Veterinary Surgery, Small Animal, Vol. 1: St. Louis: Elsevier – Saunders, 2012, 221.
6. Compton – Johnson S, Wilson J: Infected wound management: Advanced technologies, moisture retentive dressings, and die – hard methods. Crit Care Nurs Q 24:64, 2001.
7. Eaglstein WH: Moist wound healing with occlusive dressings: A clinical focus. Dermatol Surg 27:175, 2001.
8. Eaglstein WH, Mertz PM, Falanga V: Occlusive dressings. Amer Fam Pract 35:211, 1987.
9. Hedlund CS: Surgery of the integumentary system. In Fossum TW, ed.: Small Animal Surgery, 3rd ed.: St. Louis, Mosby, 2007, 159.
10. Hutchinson JJ: Infection under occlusion. Ostomy/Wound Management 4:28, 1994.
11. Krahwinkel DJ, Boothe HW: Topical and systemic medications for wounds. Vet Clin No Am Small Animal Pract 36: 739, 2006.
12. MacPhail CM: Surgery of the integumentary system. In Fossum TW, ed.: Small Animal Surgery, 4th ed.: St. Louis: Mosby, 2013, 190.
13. Miller CW: Bandages and drains. In Slatter DH, ed.: Textbook of Small Animal Surgery. 3rd ed.: Philadelphia: WB Saunders, 2003, 244.
14. Morgan PW, Binnington AG, Miller CW, et al: The effects of occlusive and semiocclusive dressings on the healing of acute full-thickness wounds on the forelimbs of dogs. Vet Surg 23:494, 1994.
15. Pavletic MM: Atlas of Small Animal Reconstructive Surgery, 2nd ed.: Philadelphia: WB Saunders, 1999, 107.
16. Pavletic MM: Atlas of Small Animal Wound Management and Reconstructive Surgery, 3rd ed.: Ames, IA: Wiley – Blackwell, 2010, 81.
17. Ramsey DT, Pope ER, Wagner-Mann C, et al: Effects of three occlusive dressing materials on healing of full-thickness wounds in dogs. Am J Vet Res 56:941, 1995.
18. Seaman S: Dressing selection in chronic wound management. J Pediatr Med Association 92:24, 2002.
19. Swaim SF: The effects of dressings and bandages on wound healing. Sem Vet Med Surg (Sm Anim) 4:274, 1989.
20. Swaim SF, Henderson RA: Small Animal Wound Management, 2nd ed.: Baltimore: Williams and Wilkins, 1997, 53.
21. Swaim SF, Gillette RL: An update on wound medications and dressings. Compend Contin Educ Pract Vet 20:1133, 1998.
22. Swaim SF, Renberg WC, Shike KM: Small Animal Bandaging, Casting and Splinting Techniques. Ames, IA: Wiley – Blackwell, 2011, 3.
23. Turner TD: Interactive dressings used in the management of human soft tissue injuries and their potential in veterinary practice. Vet Derm 8:235, 1997.
24. Williams JM: Open wound management. In Fowler D, Williams JM, eds.: Manual of Canine and Feline Wound Management and Reconstruction. Cheltenham, England: BSAVA, 1999, 37.

# Extracellular Matrix Scaffolds

## Definition and Indications

A porcine-derived small intestinal submucosa product (Vet BioSISt, Global Veterinary Products, New Buffalo, MI) is available for use as a primary layer in wound management (Figure 2-3). It is an extracellular matrix scaffold (EMS) dressing that is an acellular biodegradable sheet with a three – dimensional ultra-structure. The dressing is reportedly composed of small intestinal stratum compactum and submucosa, containing collagen (types I, III, IV, V, VI, and VIII), fibronectin, hyaluronic acid, chondroitin suflate A, heparin, and heparin sulfate. It has also been reported to contain fibroblast growth factor 2, a transforming growth factor beta-like compound, and vascular endothelial growth factors. The dressing acts as a matrix that host stem cells use to invade the wound to deposit a site – specific matrix. Thus, the dressing is gradually replaced by host tissue with characteristics of the normal adjacent tissue.

The material has been evaluated for its effect on healing of full-thickness cutaneous wounds in rodents and dogs as well as on distal limb wounds with exposed bone in dogs.

Another EMS dressing is derived from porcine urinary bladder submucosa matrix.

## Technique

The wound is debrided and lavaged to eliminate infection. If there will be drainage from the wound, the dressing should be fenestrated. A 1.5 mm diameter biopsy punch can be used to make small round holes that allow adequate wound drainage. The dressing is applied to the wound with the rough side against the wound. No topical medications, cleaning agents or exudates should be present on the wound. Ideally, the dressing should be placed under the skin at the wound edge. However, it can be placed on top of the skin, which makes application easier. The dressing can be rehydrated with saline prior to application, but working with it in the lyophilized form may be easier. If tissue fluids have not hydrated the dressing by the time application is completed, saline may be used to hydrate it. The collagen sheet is sutured or stapled to the wound edges (Figure 2-4). A semipermeable nonadherent bandage pad is placed over the EMS dressing followed by an absorbent secondary wrap and tertiary bandage layer.

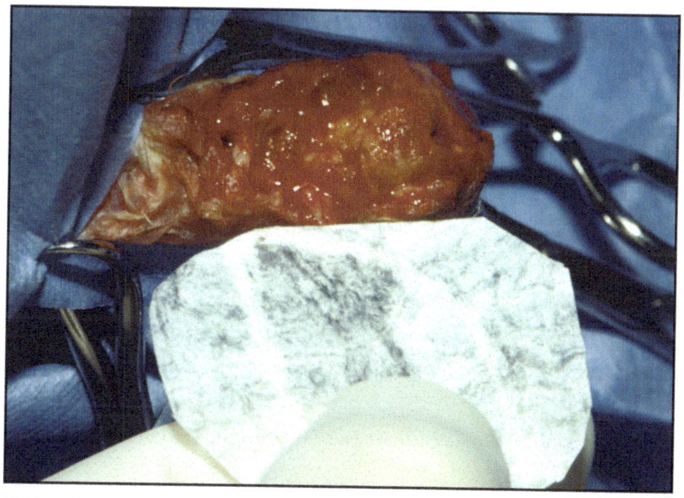

**Figure 2-3.** Extracellular matrix scaffold, porcine – derived, small intestinal submucosa primary dressing.

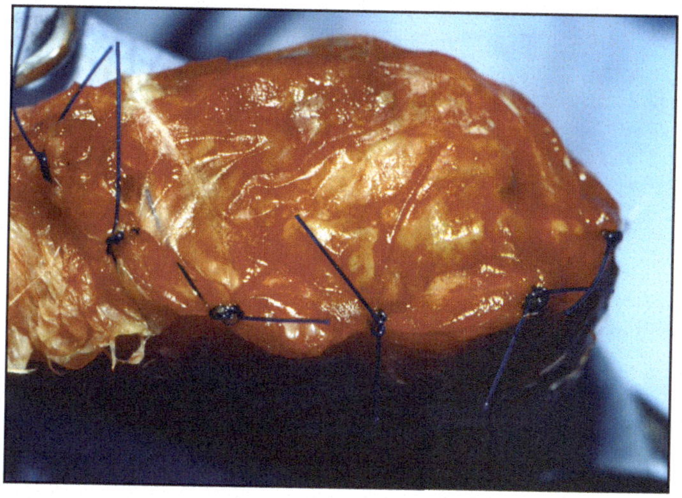

**Figure 2-4.** Extracellular matrix scaffold porcine derived, small intestinal submucosa primary dressing sutured over a wound.

## Aftercare

The outer portions of the bandage are changed in three to four days; however, the EMS dressing is left in place. As the center of the dressing degenerates, an additional sheet of dressing is placed over the wound without removing the peripheral portions of the original dressing. The additional dressing is not sutured or stapled in place. If the added dressing tends to slip off the wound surface, tape can be used to hold it in position. Usually, drainage from the wound has decreased by this time and tape is adequate to hold the dressing in place. The outer bandage is replaced and left in place four to seven days. After two to three applications in this manner no further applications of the EMS dressing are required. Wound management continues with appropriate bandaging for a granulating wound.

## Advantages and Disadvantages

The EMS dressing product provides a unique method for enhancing wound healing by acting as a matrix that host stem cells use to invade a wound in the healing process. Although it is of porcine origin, it does not tend to incite a specific or marked inflammatory response.

It may enhance the appearance of granulation tissue in a wound, but it either has no effect or a negative effect on wound contraction. When it is not sutured over a wound, the collagen matrix has a tendency to migrate. This may be more of a problem as the wound progresses in healing and additional sheets of the product are placed over the wound.

# Suggested Readings


1. Badylak SF, Park K, Peppas N, et. al.: Marrow – derived cells populate scaffolds composed of xenogeneic extracellular matrix. Exp Hematol 29: 1310, 2001.
2. Badylak SF: The extracellular matrix as a scafforld for tissue reconstruction. Semin Cell Dev Biol 13: 377, 2002.
3. Badylak SF, Xenogeneic extracellular matrix as a scaffold for tissue reconstruction. Transpl Immunol 12: 367, 2004.
4. Badylak SF, Freytes DO, Gilbert TW: Extracellular matrix as a biological scaffold material: Structure and function. Acta Biomat 5: 1, 2009.
5. Bibbo C: The porcine small intestinal submucosa (SIS) patch in foot and ankle reconstruction. J Foot Ankle Surg. 49: 123, 2010.
6. Bohling MW, Swaim SF: Bandage and drainage techniques. In Bojrab MJ, ed.: Current Techniques in Small Animal Surgery, 5th ed.: Jackson, WY: Teton NewMedia, 2014, 13.
7. Brennan EP, Reing J, Chew D, et. al.: Antibacterial activity within degradation products of biological scaffolds composed of extracellular matrix. Tiss Engin 12: 2949, 2006.
8. Campbell BG: Dressings, bandages and splints for wound management in dogs and cats. Vet Clin No Am Small Animal Practice 36:759, 2006.
9. Doillon CJ, Whyne CF, Berg RA, et al: Fibroblast – collagen sponge interactions and the spatial deposition of newly synthesized collagen fibers *in vitro* and *in vivo*. Scan Electron Micros 3: 1313, 1984.
10. Fahie MA, Shettko D: Evidence – based wound management: A systematic review of therapeutic agents to enhance granulation and epithelialization. Vet Clin No Am Small Animal Pract 37: 559, 2007.
11. Hedlund CS: Surgery of the integumentary system. In Fossum TW, ed.: Small Animal Surgery, 3rd ed.: St. Louis, Mosby, 2007, 159.
12. Hosgood G: Open wound. In Tobias KM, Johnston SA, eds.: Veterinary Surgery, Small Animal, Vol 2.: St. Louis: Elsevier – Saunders, 2012, 1210.
13. Krahwinkel DJ, Boothe HW: Topical and systemic medications for wounds. Vet Clin No Am Small Animal Pract 36: 739, 2006.
14. MacPhail CM: Surgery of the integumentary system. In Fossum TW, ed.: Small Animal Surgery, 4th ed.: St. Louis: Mosby, 2013, 190.
15. Norsworthy GD: Closure of difficult surgical defects using an extracellular matrix bioscaffold. Vet Forum 22:35, 2005.
16. Pavletic MM: Atlas of Small Animal Wound Management and Reconstructive Surgery, 3rd ed.: Ames IA: Wiley – Blackwell, 2010, 81.
17. Prevel CD, Eppley BL, Summerlin DJ, et al: Small intestinal submucosa: Utilization as a wound dressing in full-thickness rodent wounds. Ann Plast Surg 35:381,1995.
18. Schallberger SP, Stanley BJ, Hauptman JG, et al: Effects of porcine small intestinal submucosa on acute full – thickness wounds in dogs. Vet Surg 37: 515, 2008.
19. Swaim SF, Renberg WC, Shike KM: Small Animal Bandaging, Casting and Splinting Techniques. Ames, IA: Wiley – Blackwell, 2011, 3.
20. Voytik-Harbin SL, Brightman AO, Kraine MR, et al: Identification of extractable growth factors from small intestinal submucosa. J Cell Biochem 67:478, 1997.
21. Winkler JT, Swaim SF, Sartin EA, et al: The effect of a porcine-derived small intestinal submucosa product on wounds with exposed bone in dogs. Vet Surg 31:541, 2002.


# Nonadherent Semiocclusive Pads

## Definition and Indications

Commercially available nonadherent semiocclusive pads ( Telfa "Ouchless" Adhesive Pads, Covidien, Tyco/ HealthCare/ Kendall, Mansfield, MA) absorb fluid from a wound that will be absorbed by the secondary layer. Thus, they prevent tissue maceration; however, they retain sufficient moisture over a wound to prevent tissue dehydration while enhancing reepithelialization of the wound. Another commercially available nonadherent dressing (Adaptic, Johnson & Johnson, New Brunswick, NJ) is coated with petrolatum to give it nonadherency.

Gauze pads can be prepared to provide a nonadherent semiocclusive dressing by coating them with a nitrofurazone/polyethylene glycol combination topical medication or a petrolatum-based antibiotic ointment. (See Chapter 1, Antibiotics and Antibacterials). Autoclaving gauze pads with petrolatum also produces a nonadherent dressing.

Nonadherent semiocclusive pads are indicated for full-thickness wounds that are in the repair stage of healing, with a healthy granulation tissue bed, serosanguinous exudate and epithelialization starting from the wound edges. They are also indicated for sutured wounds and partial-thickness wounds that will heal by reepithelialization. Strips of these pads can be used for wounds in the interdigital spaces. The nonadherent property of the dressings avoids damage to newly formed tissue at dressing changes.

### Technique

Nonadherent semiocclusive pads are placed on the wound followed by an absorbent secondary wrap and a porous tertiary bandage layer. For interdigital wounds, appropriate-sized strips are cut from pads and placed between the digits (Figure 2-5). For wounds on the dorsum of the digits or on the pads of a medium sized dog a nonadherent semiocclusive pad with adhesive edges may be used to "diaper" bandage the paw. Triangular portions are cut from either side of the pad at its midpoint along the adhesive edges of the pad (Figure 2-6A). The pad is placed on the palmar/ plantar surface of the paw and adhered to the medial and lateral aspects of the paw (Figure 2-6B). The pad is then folded to cover the dorsum of the paw, and the remaining adherent strips are adhered to the edges of the bandage already in place (Figure 2-6C & D). Notching the bandage allows smooth folding and a good fit. Depending on the amount of drainage from the wound, bandages are changed every 1 to 2 days.

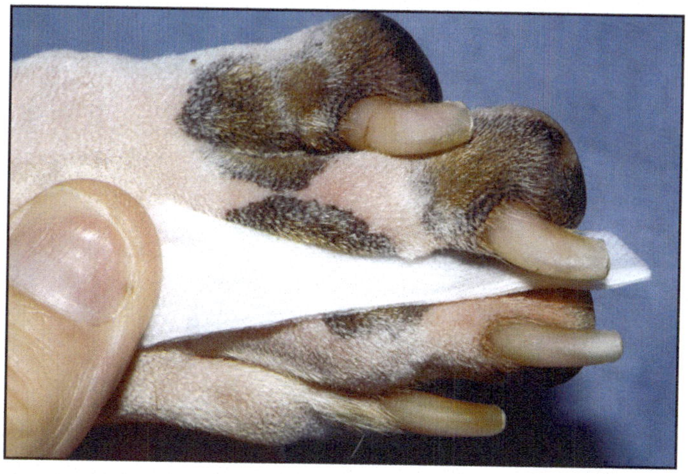

**Figure 2-5.** Strip of nonadherent semiocclusive pad placed between digits for interdigital wound.

To prepare petrolatum - impregnated gauzes, the gauze pads are placed in an autoclaveable container and petrolatum is placed on top of them. After covering the container it is autoclaved. The petrolatum is melted by the heat of autoclaving, and it is pulled down through the gauzes by gravity to coat them.

When bandages are changed, the lid is removed from the container, a gauze is removed from the top of the stack and placed on the wound. If this form of petrolatum gauze or the commercial form is used in the early repair stage of healing, it should be discontinued when new epithelium begins to appear at the wound edge. At this time a nonadherent dressing that does not contain petrolatum should be used.

A semiocclusive nonadherent petrolatum-base antibiotic ointment gauze or nitrofurazone/polyethylene glycol gauze can be prepared by spreading a thin layer of medication on the gauze using a tongue depressor just prior to putting it on the wound.

## Aftercare

Depending on the amount of drainage from the wound, bandages are changed every 1 to 2 days. If petrolatum impregnated gauze is used, it should be discontinued when epithelialization begins. One of the commercially available nonadherent semiocclusive pads should then be used.

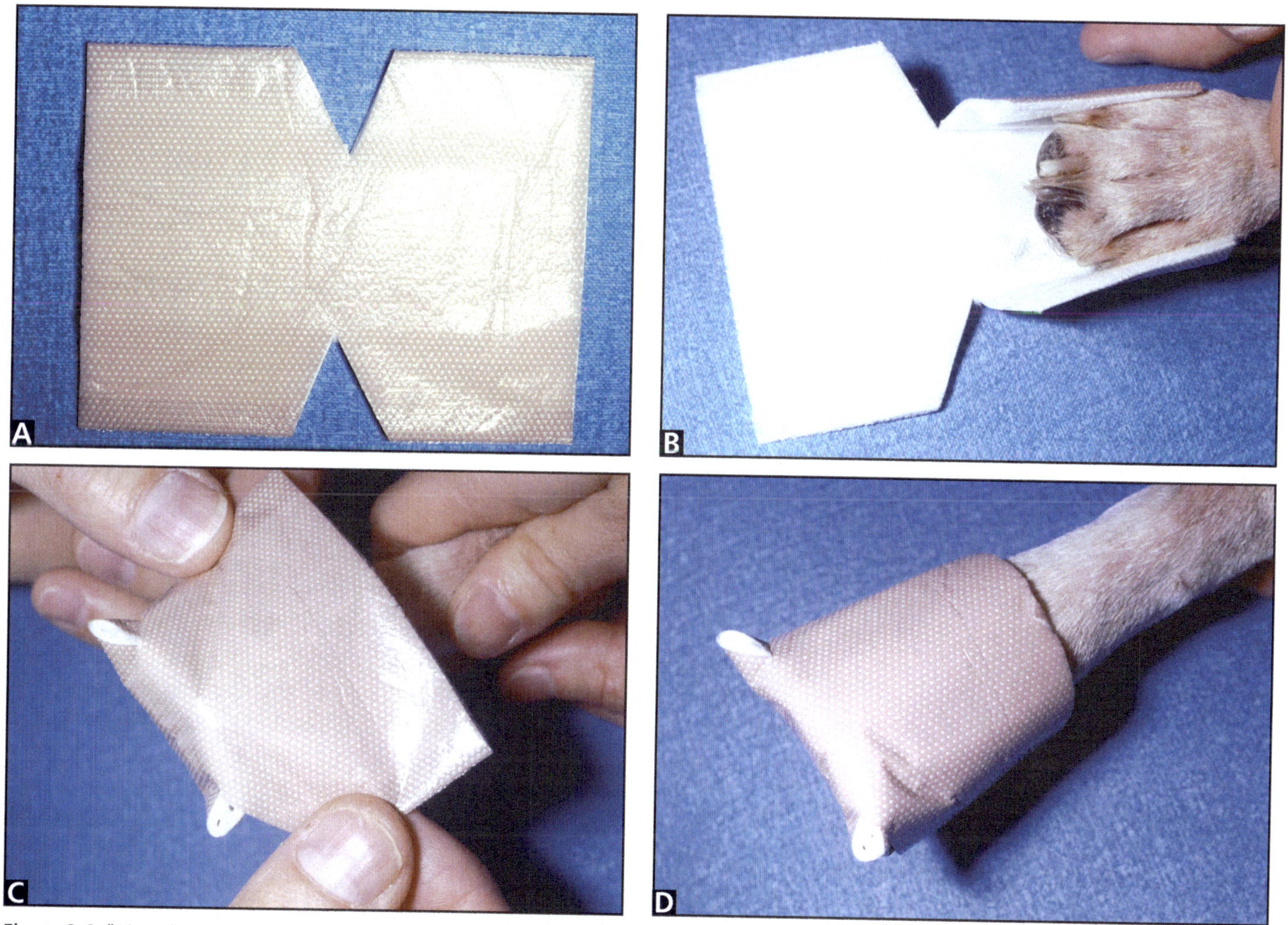


**Figure 2-6.** "Diaper" paw bandage. **A.** Triangular notches are cut at the midpoint of either side of the adhesive edge of a nonadherent pad. **B.** One half of the pad is applied to the palmar/plantar surface of the paw and adhered to the medial and lateral aspects of the paw. **C.** and **D.** The other half of the pad is folded over the paw's dorsal surface, and the remaining adherent strips are adhered to the first half of the pad. (From Swaim SF, Henderson RA: Small Animal Wound Management, 2nd ed.: Baltimore: Williams & Wilkins, 1997, 339.)

## Advantages and Disadvantages

Nonadherent semiocclusive pads provide a moist environment conducive to healing, especially epithelialization. Removal of such bandages does not disturb the healing process. In addition to being antibacterial, nitrofurazone/ polyethylene glycol gauzes are also hydrophilic. With the hydrophilic property, homeostatic fluid is drawn through wound tissues to bathe them and dilute wound coagulum for better absorption into the bandage. Petrolatum-based antibiotic ointment gauzes provide antibacterial activity as well as nonadherence.

A disadvantage of the hydrophilics of nitrofurazone/ polyethylene glycol gauzes is the wound fluid drawn through the bandage can leach out or dilute the polyethylene glycol, thus necessitating more frequent bandage changes. Nonadherent semiocclusive pads that contain petrolatum have the disadvantage of delaying epithelialization of wounds. In addition, petrolatum-impregnated gauzes prepared by autoclaving gauzes with petrolatum are inconsistent in their content of petrolatum. Gauzes at the top of the stack are lightly coated; whereas, those at the bottom of the stack are heavily coated to the point of creating an occlusive bandage. Thus, in addition to delaying epithelialization, the fluid retention may lead to tissue maceration.

When gauze is used as the nonadherent semiocclusive pad, the mesh size of the gauze has advantages and disadvantages. A wide-mesh gauze allows more wound fluid absorption into the secondary bandage layer. However, granulation tissue and possibly epithelium grows into the interstices of the mesh more readily to result in adherence of the bandage. Frequent bandage changes may help prevent this. With fine-mesh gauze there is less tendency for the bandage to adhere to the wound, but the gauze interstices tend to occlude easily, especially if the gauze is coated with medication. Thus, fluid absorption into the secondary bandage layer is restricted.

# Suggested Readings

1. Anderson D: Management of open wounds. In Williams J, Moores A, eds.: BSAVA Manuual of Canine and Feline Wound Management and Reconstruction, 2nd ed.: Glouster (UK): BSAVA, 2009, 37.
2. Bohling MW, Swaim SF: Bandage and drainage techniques. In Bojrab MJ, ed.: Current Techniques in Small Animal Surgery, 5th ed.: Jackson, WY: Teton NewMedia 2014, 13.
3. Campbell BG: Dressings, bandages and splints for wound management in dogs and cats. Vet Clin No Am Small Animal Pract 36: 759, 2006.
4. Campbell BG: Bandages and drains. In Tobias KM, Johnston SA, eds.: Veterinary Surgery, Small Animal, Vol. 1: St. Louis: Elsevier – Saunders, 2012, 221.
5. Eaglstein WH, Mertz PM: Inert vehicles do affect wound healing. J Invest Dermatol 74:90, 1980.
6. Eaglstein WH, Mertz PM: Effect of topical medicaments on the rate of repair of superficial wounds. *In* Dineen P, Hildick-Smith G, eds.: The Surgical Wound. Philadelphia: Lea and Febiger, 1981, 150.
7. Hedlund CS: Surgery of the integumentary system. *In* Fossum TW, ed.: Small Animal Surgery, 2nd ed.: St. Louis: Mosby, 2002, 134.
8. Hedlund CS: Surgery of the integumentary system. In Fossum TW, ed.: Small Animal Surgery, 3rd ed.: St. Louis: Mosby, 2007, 159.
9. Lee AH, Swaim SF, McGuire JA, Hughs KS: Effects of nonadherent dressing materials on the healing of open wounds in dogs. J Am Vet Med Assoc 190:416, 1987.
10. Lee AH, Swaim SF, Yang ST, et al: The effects of petrolatum, polyethylene glycol, nitrofurazone and a hydroactive dressing on open wound healing. J Am Anim Hosp Assoc 22:443, 1986.
11. Lozier SM: Topical wound therapy. *In* Harari J, ed.: Surgical Complications and Wound Healing in Small Animal Practice. Philadelphia: WB Saunders, 1993, 63.
12. MacPhail CM: Surgery of the integumentary system. In Fossum TW, ed.: Small Animal Surgery, 4th ed.: St. Louis: Mosby, 2013, 190.
13. Miller CW: Bandages and drains. *In* Slatter DH, ed.: Textbook of Small Animal Surgery, 3rd ed.: Philadelphia: WB Saunders, 2003, 244.
14. Noe JM, Kalish S: The mechanism of capillarity in surgical dressings. Surg Gynecol Obstet 143:454, 1976.
15. Noe JM, Kalish S: The problem of adherence in dressing wounds. Surg Gynecol Obstet 147:185, 1978.
16. Noe JM, Kalish S: Dressing materials and their selection. *In* Rudolph R, Noe JM, eds.: Chronic Problem Wounds. Boston: Little, Brown, 1983, 37.
17. Pavletic MM: Atlas of Small Animal Wound Management and Reconstructive Surgery, 3rd ed.: Ames, IA: Wiley – Blackwell, 2010, 81,
18. Swaim SF, Wilhalf D: The physics, physiology, and chemistry of bandaging open wounds. Compend Contin Educ Pract Vet 7:146, 1985.
19. Swaim SF: The effects of dressing and bandages on wound healing. Semin Vet Med Surg (Small Anim) 4:274, 1989.
20. Swaim SF: Bandages and topical agents. Vet Clin North Am Small Anim Pract 20:47, 1990.
21. Swaim SF, Henderson RA: Small Animal Wound Management, 2nd ed.: Baltimore: Williams and Wilkins, 1997, 53.
22. Swaim SF, Renberg WC, Shike KM: Small Animal Bandaging, Casting and Splinting Techniques. Ames, IA: Wiley – Blackwell, 2011, 3.
23. Williams JM: Open wound management. *In* Fowler D, Williams JM, eds.: Manual of Canine and Feline Wound Management and Reconstruction. Cheltenham, England: British Small Animal Association, 1999, 37.

# Adhesive Tape Stirrups

## Definition and Indications

Adhesive tape "stirrups" can be placed in distal limb and paw bandages as part of the primary bandage layer. They serve to secure bandages on the limb. They are 2 strips of adhesive tape, usually one inch wide, that are placed on opposite sides of the limb, i.e. dorsal and volar or medial and lateral. The strips extend beyond the end of the paw and are folded back for incorporation in the secondary bandage layer to secure the bandage.

## Technique

Before placing adhesive tape stirrups, pieces of cotton can be placed between the digits on the dorsal paw surface and between the digital and metacarpal/metatarsal pads on the volar surface (Figure 2-18A & B).

Two strips of 1-inch wide adhesive tape are adhered to the skin of the limb parallel to the long axis of the limb. The strips are on opposite sides of the limb (dorsal and volar or medial and lateral) (Figure 2-7A & B). The strips should be paced to avoid open wounds, and if they are placed over suture lines, they should be placed over a primary bandage covering.

After placing the secondary bandage wrap, the strips are folded back over the surface of the secondary wrap in one of 2 ways. The adhesive surfaces of the strips can be adhered together beyond the paw for a length from 3 to 8 inches, depending on the length of the bandage/leg. This single strip is then folded back onto the secondary bandage surface (Figure 2-8). With the second technique, each strip is twisted 180 degrees and folded back onto the secondary bandage layer. Thus, the adhesive surface of each strip is adhered to the secondary layer (Figure 2-9). The tertiary bandage layer is applied to secure the stirrups in the bandage.

## Aftercare

At bandage changes, it may be possible to remove the bandage and leave the stirrups in place to be incorporated in the subsequent bandage. Otherwise, new stirrups may need to be placed at bandage changes. In the presence of wounds with drainage, the stirrup portions on the skin may become saturated with exudate necessitating their change at each bandage change. On some wounds it will not be possible to use stirrups, e.g. circumferential mesh skin graft over the metacarpal/metatarsal area. In such cases, bandage security comes from proximal fixation (taping) of the bandage.

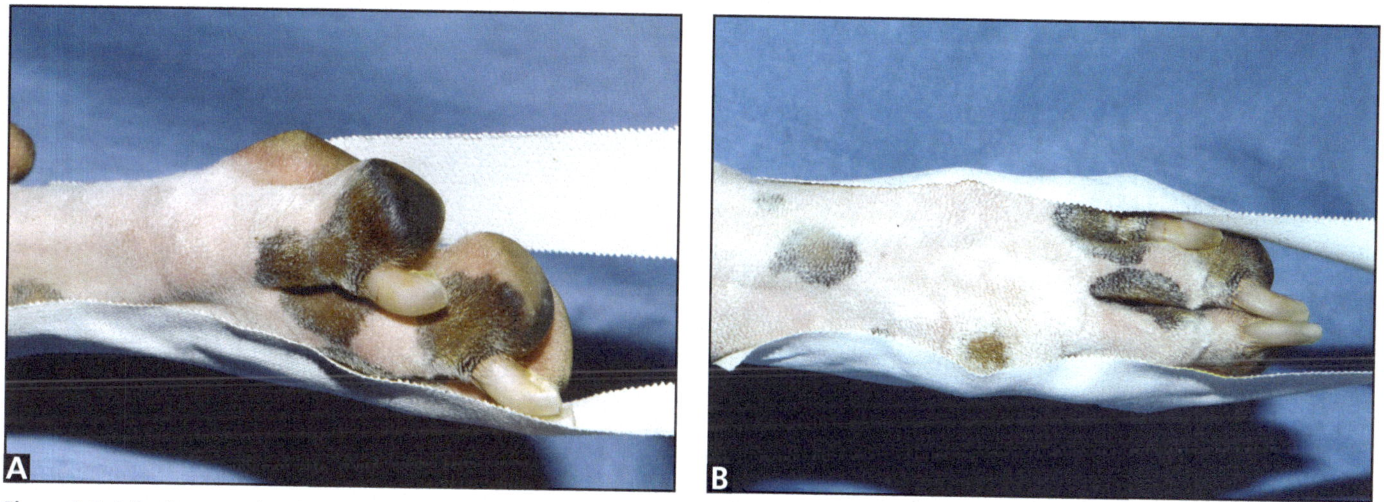


**Figure 2-7.** Adhesive tape stirrups. **A.** Tape strips on the dorsal and volar aspects of the distal limb and paw. **B.** Tape strips on the medial and lateral aspects of the distal limb and paw.

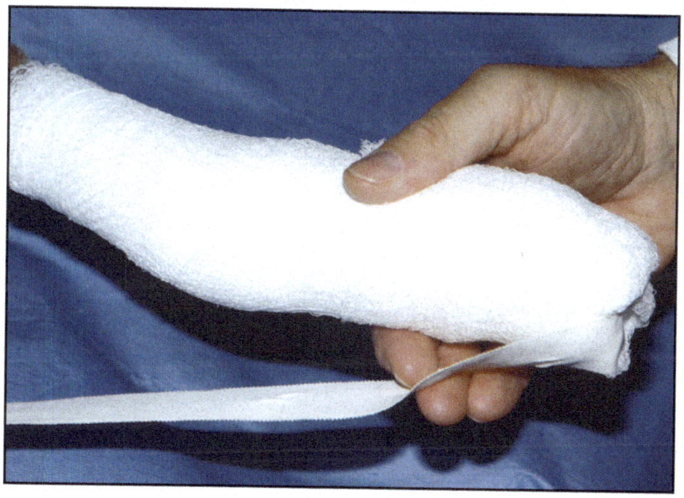

**Figure 2-8.** Adhesive tape strips of stirrup adhered together, being folded back onto the surface of the secondary bandage layer.

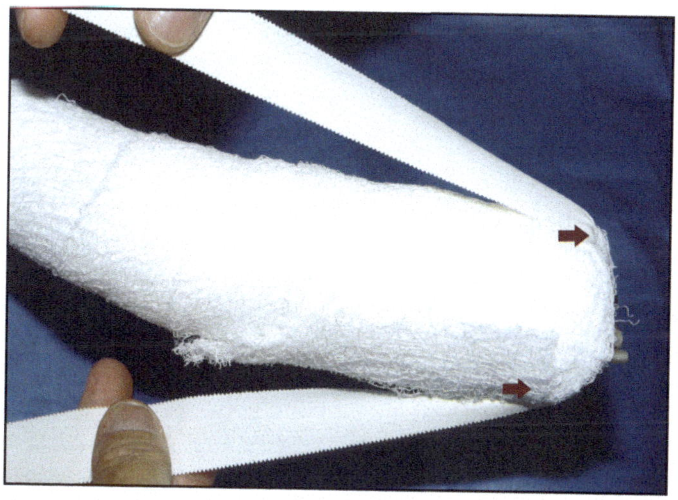

**Figure 2-9.** Adhesive strips of stirrup twisted *(arrows)* and being folded back onto the surface of the secondary bandage layer.

## Advantages and Disadvantages

The primary advantage of tape stirrups is the security they provide in keeping a bandage and splint in place. A disadvantage of stirrups is the difficulty of placement in the presence of open wounds or suture lines on the distal limb and paw.

# Suggested Readings


1. Campbell BG: Dressings, bandages and splints for wound management in dogs and cats. Vet Clin No Am Small Animal Pract 36: 759, 2006.
2. Campbell BG: Bandages and drains. In Tobias KM, Johnston SA, eds.: Veterinary Surgery, Small Animal, Vol. 1: St. Louis: Elsevier – Saunders, 2012, 221.
3. Hedlund CS: Surgery of the integumentary system. *In* Fossum TW, ed.: Small Animal Surgery, 2nd ed.: St. Louis: Mosby, 2002, 134.
4. Hedlund CS: Surgery of the integumentary system. In Fossum TW, ed.: Small Animal Surgery, 3rd, ed.: St. Louis: Mosby, 2007, 159.
5. MacPhail CM: Surgery of the integumentary system. In Fossum TW, ed.: Small Animal Surgery, 4th ed.: St. Louis: Mosby, 2013, 190.
6. Pavletic MM: Atlas of Small Animal Wound Management and Reconstructive Surgery, 3rd ed.: Ames, IA: Wiley – Blackwell, 2010, 81.
7. Swaim SF, Renberg WC, Shike KM: Small Animal Bandaging, Casting and Splinting Techniques, Ames, IA: Wiley – Blackwell, 2011, 43.


# Secondary Bandage Layer: Roll Dressings

## Definition and Indications

The secondary bandage layer is placed over the primary bandage layer. It serves to absorb blood, serum, exudate, bacteria, enzymes and debris as capillary action moves them through the primary layer. One form of the dressing is a thick absorptive gauze roll (Kerlix Roll, Covidien, Tyco HealthCare/Kendall, Mansfield, MA). A secondary gauze roll impregnated with the antimicrobial 0.2% polyhexamethylene biguanide is available (Kerlix® AMD Roll, Covidien, Tyco HealthCare/Kendall, Mansfield, MA). Absorbent cotton and a cast padding material (Specialist Cast Padding, BSN Medical, Rutherford College, NC) have also been used as a secondary layer. The primary function of the dressing is to absorb exudate, and thus bacteria, away from the wound. In addition, the dressing provides padding against trauma, splinting to limit movement, and packing to obliterate dead space and prevent edema. It also serves as filling to equalize the circumference of a limb bandage for secure fitting of a splint to be incorporated in the bandage (Figure 2-10A & B).

## Technique

To assure maximum absorption of exudate from a wound the secondary layer should be wrapped on the limb such that contact between the secondary layer, primary layer and wound surface are assured. However, excess pressure should not be applied when wrapping the limb. The amount of pressure governs the amount of fluid absorbed from the wound by this layer; thus, excessive pressure can decrease the absorptive capacity of the bandage and could lead to tissue maceration. The secondary bandage layer should be placed evenly along the limb. Application is from distal to proximal with 50% overlap with each wrap. The practice of twisting the bandage material 180 degrees to get a narrow portion to pull underlying bandage into an uneven area should be avoided. Such a twist increases pressure under this twist. The number of layers of secondary wrap may be governed by the amount of wound drainage. A thicker wrap would be indicated for a more productive wound.

At the distal end of a distal limb/paw bandage, the roll dressing is turned at a right angle in preparation

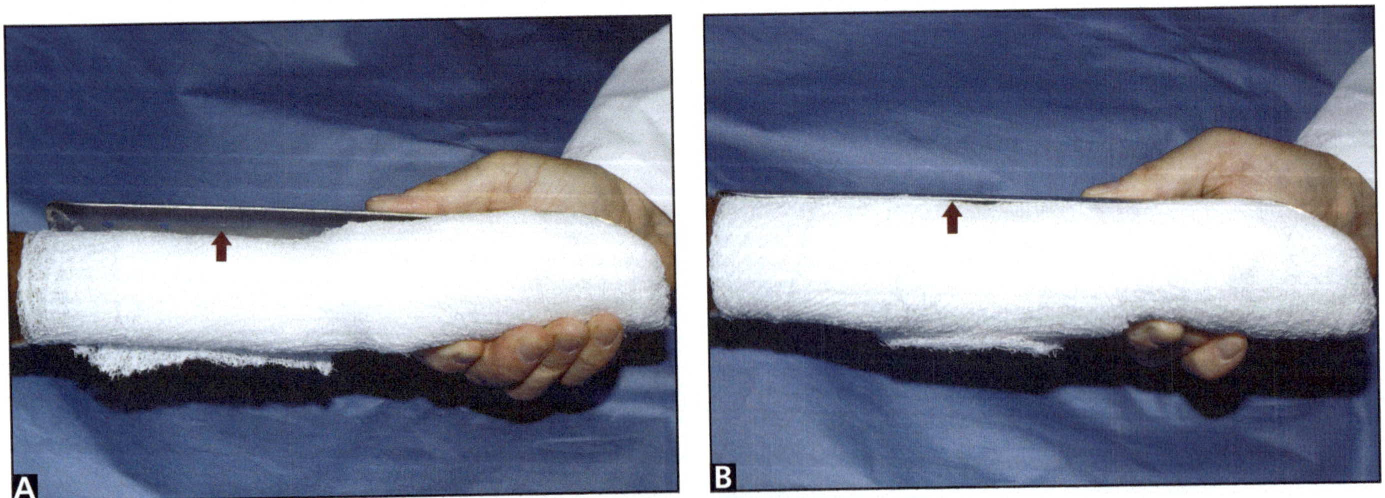


**Figure 2-10.** Equalizing the circumference of a limb bandage for even fit of a splint. **A.** Space between the limb and splint before applying secondary bandage wrap proximal to the paw *(arrow)*. **B.** Circumference of bandage equalized with secondary bandage wrap proximal to the paw and splint fitting smoothly against the bandage *(arrow)*.

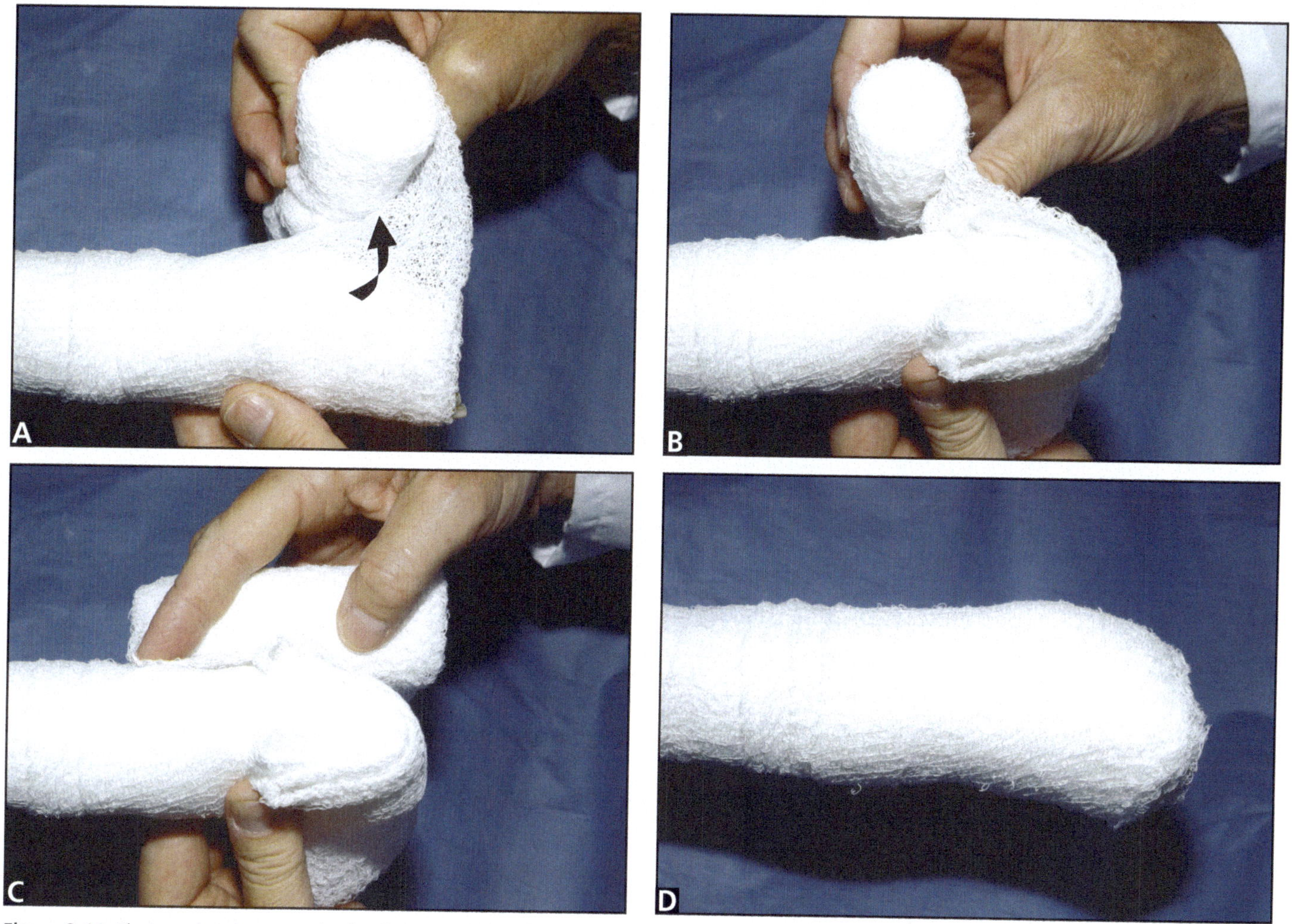


**Figure 2-11.** Placing a bandage over the distal end of the paw. **A.** Secondary bandage roll is turned 90 degrees *(arrow)* in preparation for placing layers over end of paw. **B.** Secondary bandage folded back – and – forth several times over end of paw. **C.** Secondary bandage roll is turned 90 degrees again for circumferential wrap to pull in the protruding edges. **D.** Completed paw bandage.

for placing layers over the end of the bandage (Figure 2-11A). Bandage material is folded back and forth over the end of the paw several times (Figure 2-11B). It is then turned at a right angle again and wrapped circumferentially around the paw area, pulling in the protruding edges of the folds (Figure 2-11C). This gives a smooth bandage enclosing the paw (Figure 2-11D), which is preferred by the author. It would be especially necessary to use this technique in the presence of wounds involving the digits. An alternative technique is to wrap the paw starting at the level of the second and fifth digits and wrap obliquely so the third and fourth digits are not covered by the bandage but remain exposed to allow evaluation of bandage tightness (Figure 2-12).

When absorbent roll cotton is used as a secondary layer, care should be taken that it does not contact the wound surface, where it will be difficult to remove. Likewise, cast padding can have considerable lint associated with it which should be kept out of wounds.

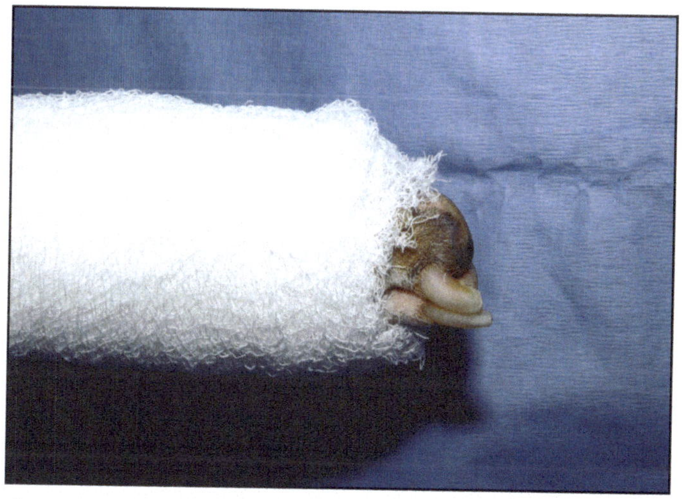

**Figure 2-12.** Paw bandage with secondary bandage wrap applied so that the 3rd and 4th digits remain exposed.

## Aftercare

The frequency of bandage change is dependent upon the amount of exudate being produced. At the minimum, daily bandage changes should be done early in wound management. Bandages should be changed before exudate has reached the tertiary bandage layer, especially if the tertiary layer is porous. If this layer becomes wet, exogenous bacteria can contaminate the wound. As healing progresses and less exudate is produced by the wound, bandage changes may be less frequent. At bandage change, the tertiary layer should be incised longitudinally and cut away from the secondary layer, and the secondary layer should be unwrapped from the limb rather than cutting through it. Cutting through the entire thickness of the secondary bandage layer can be difficult and painful for the animal, especially if it is wet with exudate.

## Advantages and Disadvantages

The primary advantage of the secondary bandage layer is its property of absorbing exudate and its associated bacteria away from a wound. With a porous tertiary bandage layer, fluid can evaporate from the exudate. This helps inhibit bacterial growth. With the 0.2% polyhexamethylene biguanide impregnated secondary dressing (Kerlix AMD, Tyco HealthCare Kendall, Mansfield, MA) there is the advantage of inhibiting wound bacteria as well as exogenous bacteria that may be in the secondary layer.

An advantage of cast padding as a secondary layer wrap is that it is difficult to wrap too tightly because it will tear if too much tension is placed on it while wrapping. When cast padding is used as the secondary layer under an elastic adhesive tape, it provides relatively more protection from pressure.

In a highly productive wound, absorption may be faster than evaporation, and exogenous bacteria or bacteria in the wound may proliferate in the culture media provided by the bandage. In addition to limiting the amount of exudate absorbed from a wound, tight application of the secondary bandage layer, especially gauze-type material, along with tight application of the tertiary bandage layer can splint the wound edges so that wound contraction is impeded. If cotton or cast padding contact the wound, they become wet with wound fluid and may be difficult to see for complete removal. Thus, small amounts remain and can act as foreign bodies.

# Suggested Readings


1. Anderson D: Management of open wounds. In Williams J, Moores A, eds.: BSAVA Manual of Canine and Feline Wound Management and Reconstruction, 2nd ed.: Glouster (UK): BSAVA, 2009, 37.
2. Baxter H, Ballard K: Bandaging: A vital skill, Nurs Times, 97: 57, 2001.
3. Bohling MW, Swaim SF: Bandages and drainage techniques. In Bojrab MJ, ed.: Current Techniques in Small Animal Surgery, 5th ed.: Jackson, WY: Teton NewMedia, 2014, 13.
4. Campbell BG: Dressings, bandages and splints for wound management in dogs and cats. Vet Clin No Am Small Animal Pract 36: 759, 2006.
5. Campbell BG: Bandages and drains. In Tobias KM, Johnston SA, eds.: Veterinary Surgery, Small Animal, Vol. 1: St. Louis: Elsevier – Saunders, 2012, 221.
6. Hedlund CS: Surgery of the integumentary system. *In* Fossum TW, ed.: Small Animal Surgery, 2nd ed.: St. Louis: Mosby, 2002, 134.
7. Hedlund CS: Surgery of the integumentary system. In Fossum TW, ed.: Small Animal Surgery, 3rd ed.: St. Louis: Mosby, 2007, 159.
8. MacPhail CM: Surgery of the integumentary system. In Fossum TW, ed.: Small Animal Surgery, 4th ed.: St. Louis: Mosby, 2013, 190.
9. Malimson PD: On twisting bandages: An experimental study. Br J Plast Surg 37:626, 1984.
10. Miller CW: Bandages and drains. *In* Slatter DH, ed.: Textbook of Small Animal Surgery, 3rd ed.: Philadelphia: WB Saunders, 2003, 244.
11. Noe JM, Kalish S: The mechanism of capillarity in surgical dressings. Surg Gynecol Obstet 143:454, 1976.
12. Noe JM, Kalish S: Dressing materials and their selection. *In* Rudolph R, Noe JM, eds.: Chronic Problem Wounds. Boston: Little, Brown, 1983, 37.
13. Pavletic MM: Atlas of Small Animal Reconstructive Surgery. 2nd ed.: Philadelphia: WB Saunders, 1999, 107.
14. Pavletic MM: Atlas of Small Animal Wound Management and Reconstructive Surgery, 3rd ed.: Ames, IA: Wiley – Blackwell, 2010, 81.
15. Simpson AM, Beale BS, Radlinsky M: Bandaging in dogs and cats: Basic principles. Comp Cont Educ 23: 12, 2001.
16. Swaim SF: The effects of dressings and bandages on wound healing. Semin Vet Med Surg (Small Anim) 4:274, 1989.
17. Swaim SF: Bandages and topical agents. Vet Clin North Am Small Anim Pract 20:47, 1990.
18. Swaim SF, Wilhalf D: The physics, physiology, and chemistry of bandaging open wounds. Compend Contin Educ Pract Vet 7:146, 1985.
19. Swaim SF, Henderson RA: Small Animal Wound Management, 2nd ed.: Baltimore: Williams and Wilkins, 1997, 53.
20. Swaim SF, Renberg WC, Shike KM: Small Animal Bandaging, Casting, and Splinting Techniques. Ames, IA: Wiley – Blackwellm 2011, 3.
21. Williams JM: Open wound management. In Fowler D, Williams JM, eds.: Manual of Canine and Feline Wound Management and Reconstruction. Cheltenham, England: BSAVA, 1999, 37.


# Tertiary Bandage Layer: Porous Adhesive Tape

## Definition and Indications

The tertiary bandage layer secures the other bandage layers in place. In addition, it helps immobilize the bandaged distal limb, especially when the tape fixes a splint in the bandage. Porous adhesive tape (Zonas Porous Tape, Johnson & Johnson, Arlington, TX or Curity Standard Porous Tape, Covidien, Tyco Healthcare/Kendall, Mansfield, MA) allows fluid evaporation from the bandage. It is indicated for exudative or transudative wounds; whereby, the evaporation helps provide a partially dry wound atmosphere as a means of inhibiting bacterial growth.

## Technique

When using porous adhesive tape, strips of tape can be pretorn before applying them over underlying bandage materials (Figure 2-13A). Alternatively, the tape can be rolled off the roll as it is applied to the bandage. However, with this technique, it is necessary to secure the tape near the bandage with one hand while pulling additional tape from the roll (Figure 2-13B). In this way the danger of applying tape too tightly is reduced. Mild but not constrictive pressure should be applied when placing the tape in overlapping fashion.

At the proximal end of the bandage half the width of the last strip of tape should be on the next-to-last piece of tape applied. The remaining half width should be on the hair/skin above the bandage. For more security, additional wraps can be taken to incorporate more hair on the limb, thus helping prevent slippage. To help ensure that the tape adheres to the hair, a hand can be pressed against the tape over the hair for approximately a minute. The heat of the animal's body and the hand help make the adhesive material of the tape adhere to the hair. Another technique to help ensure tape adhesion to the skin is to spray some polymeric solution of hexamethyldisiloxane acrylate (Cavilon No Sting Barrier Film, 3M Health Care, St. Paul, MN) on the skin adjacent to the top of the bandage. After it dries it leaves a clear film to which the tape sticks better than to skin alone. In addition, when the tape is removed the film helps prevent epidermal stripping when the tape is removed.

At the distal end of distal limb-paw bandage, 2 strips of 2-inch wide adhesive tape are placed at right angles to each other over the end of the bandage. A final circumferential tape wrap is wrapped around these to secure them in place (Figure 2-14A & B).

## Aftercare

The bandage should be changed at least daily on heavily exudative wounds to remove absorbed exudate. As wounds enter the repair stage, bandages may be changed less frequently. With porous adhesive tape, if bandages are not changed often enough absorbed wound fluid may reach the bandage surface and predispose the bandage to exogenous bacterial contamination.

When porous adhesive tape has been used for a distal limb-paw bandage, a plastic bag/sack (e.g. bread sack) can be placed over the bandage when the animal is in a wet or potentially contaminating environment, such as outdoors for urinary and bowel functions in wet grass. Rubber bands should not be used to affix the plastic sack on the leg. Tape should be used to secure it to the hair on the limb above the bandage. This helps prevent the possibility of a rubber band slipping off of the bag and going unnoticed under the hair until it is causing circumferential limb damage.

To provide comfort for the animal the bandage should be removed in layers. Using a razor blade or scalpel blade, *only* the tertiary layer is incised carefully along the bandage length. At the proximal end of the bandage where tape of the tertiary layer may be adhered to the skin and hair for security, bandage scissors and digital manipulation are used to release

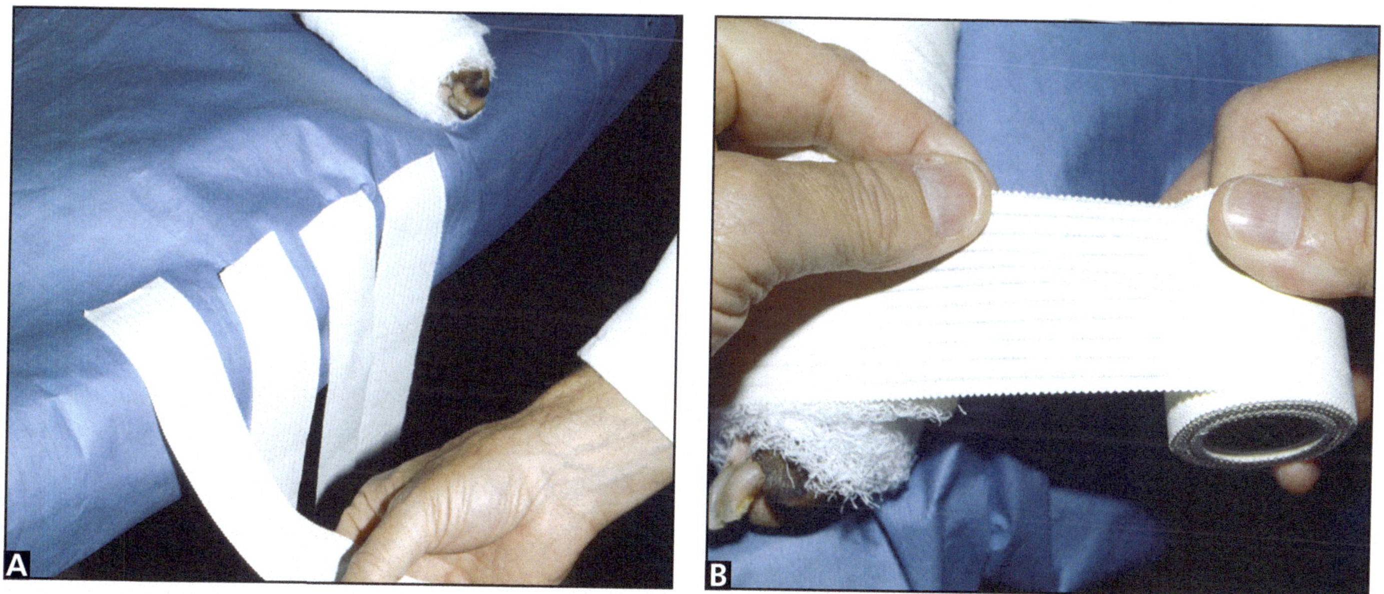


**Figure 2-13.** Applying outer bandage layer. **A.** Pretearing adhesive tape strips before applying them to bandage. **B.** Applying tape from a roll. Tape is held near the bandage with one hand while pulling another length of tape from the roll.

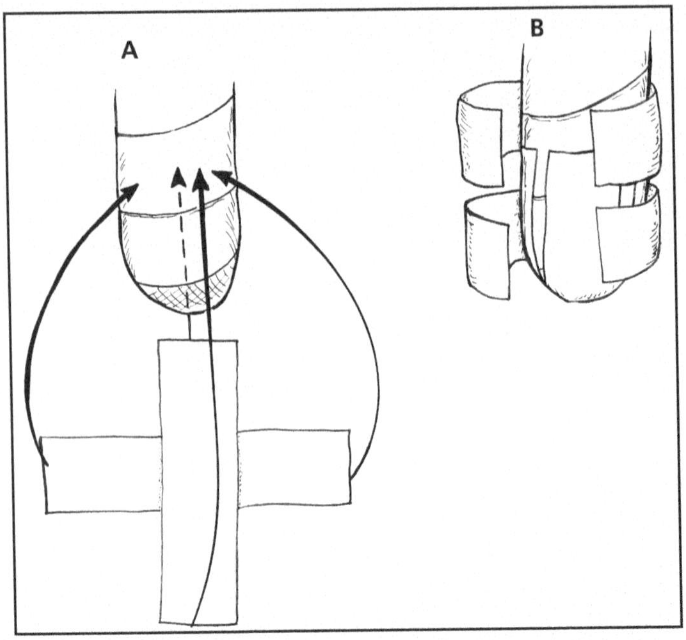


**Figure 2-14.** Taping the distal end of a paw bandage. **A.** Two tape strips are applied at right angles to each other. **B.** Circumferential tape strips are applied after the right angle strips are applied.

the tape attachment. The tertiary layer is then removed by peeling it away from the secondary layer. If there is some attachment between the two layers bandage scissors are used to snip the attachment. An end of the secondary layer is located or created and this layer is unwrapped from the limb.

## Advantages and Disadvantages

The primary advantage of porous adhesive tape is the evaporation of fluid which it provides. It's adhesive property which helps affix it to the skin and hair of the limb to prevent bandage slippage are also advantageous.

The porosity of the tape can also be a disadvantage in that it allows the ingress of exogenous contamination which in turn can lead to secondary wound contamination. Conversely, wound fluid reaching the surface of the bandage can contaminate the environment. The pain and irritation that accompany epidermal stripping when adhesive tape is removed is a disadvantage. However, placing the polymeric solution of hexamethyldisiloxane acrylate on the skin prior to placing the tape helps prevent this.

If adhesive tape is applied under too much pressure, the underlying bandage components are compressed, limiting the bandage's capacity to absorb exudate. Tight application can also constrict blood supply to underlying tissues which can lead to avascular necrosis.

# Suggested Readings


1. Anderson D: Management of open wounds. In Williams J, Moores A, eds.: BSAVA Manual of Canine and Feline Wound Management and Reconstruction, 2nd ed.: Glouster (UK): BSAVA, 2009, 37.
2. Bohling MW, Swaim SF: Bandage and drain techniques. In Bojrab MJ, ed.: Current Techniques in Small Animal Surgery, 5th ed.: Jackson, WY: Teton NewMedia, 2014, 13.
3. Campbell BG: Dressings, bandages and splints for wound management in dogs and cats. Vet Clin No Am Small Animal Pract 36: 759, 2006.
4. Campbell BG: Bandages and drains. In Tobias KM, Johnston SA, eds.: Veterinary Surgery, Small Animal, Vol. 1: St. Louis: Elsevier – Saunders, 2012, 221.
5. Hedlund CS: Surgery of the integumentary system. *In* Fossum TW, ed.: Small Animal Surgery, 2nd ed.: St. Louis: Mosby, 2002, 134.
6. Hedlund CS: Surgery of the integumentary system. In Fossum TW, ed.: Small Animal Surgery, 3rd ed.: St. Louis: Mosby, 2007, 159.
7. MacPhail CM: Surgery of the integumentary system. In Fossum TW, ed.: Small Animal Surgery, 4th ed.: St. Louis: Mosby, 2013, 190.
8. Miller CW: Bandages and drains. *In* Slatter DH, ed.: Textbook of Small Animal Surgery, 3rd ed.: Philadelphia: WB Saunders, 2003, 244.
9. Pavletic MM: Atlas of Small Animal Reconstructive Surgery. 2nd ed.: Philadelphia: WB Saunders, 1999, 107.
10. Pavletic MM: Atlas of Small Animal Wound Management and Reconstructive Surgery, 3rd ed.: Ames, IA: Wiley – Blackwell, 2010, 81.
11. Simpson AM, Beale BS, Radlinsky M: Bandaging in dogs and cats: Basic principles. Comp Cont Educ 23: 12, 2001.
12. Swaim SF: The effects of dressings and bandages on wound healing. Semin Vet Med Surg (Small Anim) 4:274, 1989.
13. Swaim SF: Bandages and topical agents. Vet Clin North Am Small Anim Pract 20:47, 1990.
14. Swaim SF, Wilhalf D: The physics, physiology, and chemistry of bandaging open wounds. Compend Contin Educ Pract Vet 7:146, 1985.
15. Swaim SF, Henderson RA: Small Animal Wound Management, 2nd ed.: Baltimore: Williams and Wilkins, 1997, 53.
16. Swaim SF, Renberg WC, Shike KM: Small Animal Bandaging, Casting and Splinting Techniques. Ames, IA: Wiley – Blackwell, 2011, 3.
17. Williams JM: Open wound management. In Fowler D, Williams JM, eds.: Manual of Canine and Feline Wound Management and Reconstructive Surgery. Cheltenham, England: BSAVA, 1999, 37.


# Waterproof Adhesive Tape

## Definition and Indications

Nonporous waterproof adhesive tape provides an occlusive bandage that can protect a wound from exogenous contamination. This tape is indicated as the outer bandage layer on bandages that are subject to such contamination, i.e. paw bandages. The author has found the application of a commercial waterproof tape (Duck Brand Tape, Shur Tech Bands, Avon, OH) over the tertiary bandage layer to be effective for waterproofing a paw bandage.

## Technique

The techniques for applying waterproof adhesive tape are the same as for applying porous adhesive tape. (See

Porous Adhesive Tape in this chapter.) However, the author uses it over the tertiary bandage layer, i.e. porous adhesive tape. Contact with the skin and hair of the limb are avoided. Security of the bandage to these is assured with medical grade porous adhesive tapes and the polymeric solution of hexamethyldisiloxane acrylate.

### Aftercare

Paw bandages should be changed frequently due to the location of the wound and physiology of the area. Not only does waterproof tape keep exogenous fluid out of a bandage, but it also retains endogenous fluid that is in the bandage. Thus, exudate from a wound combined with the normal sweat from a dog's pads can lead to considerable moisture in a bandage. This can result in tissue maceration and/or exacerbation of any infection present.

### Advantages and Disadvantages

The main advantage of waterproof tape is its occlusive nature in helping protect the wound from exogenous contamination. In addition, the strong slick surface of the tape makes it difficult for an animal to damage the bandage by licking and chewing.

A disadvantage of waterproof adhesive tape is the potential for tissue maceration and exacerbation of infection from retained fluid. It should be remembered that if an animal is in an area where exogenous fluid contamination is highly possible and the bandage is not completely occlusive, any moisture that gets into the bandage will be retained.

## Suggested Readings


1. Bohling MW, Swaim SF: Bandage and drain techniques. In Bojrab MJ, ed.: Current Techniques in Small Animal Surgery, 5th ed.: Jackson, WY: Teton NewMedia, 2014, 13.
2. Campbell BG: Dressings, bandages and splints for wound management in dogs and cats. Vet Clin No Am Small Animal Pract 36: 759, 2006.
3. Campbell BG: Bandages and drains. In Tobias KM, Johnston SA, eds.: Veterinary Surgery, Small Animal, Vol. 1: St. Louis: Elseveir – Saunders, 2012, 221.
4. Hedlund CS: Surgery of the integumentary system. *In* Fossum TW, ed.: Small Animal Surgery, 2nd ed.: St. Louis: Mosby, 2002, 134.
5. Hedlund CS: Surgery of the integumentary system. In Fossum TW, ed.: Small Animal Surgery, 3rd ed.: St. Louis: Mosby, 2007, 159.
6. MacPhail CM: Surgery of the integumentary system. In Fossum TW, ed.: Small Animal Surgery, 4th ed.: St. Louis: Mosby, 2013, 190.
7. Pavletic MM: Atlas of Small Animal Reconstructive Surgery. 2nd ed.: Philadelphia: WB Saunders, 1999, 107.
8. Pavletic MM: Atlas of Small Animal Wound Management and Reconstructive Surgery, 3rd ed.: Ames, IA: Wiley – Blackwell, 2010, 81.
9. Swaim SF: Bandages and topical agents. Vet Clin North Am Small Anim Pract 20:47, 1990.
10. Swaim SF, Wilhalf D: The physics, physiology, and chemistry of bandaging open wounds. Compend Contin Educ Pract Vet 7:146, 1985.
11. Swaim SF, Henderson RA: Small Animal Wound Management, 2nd ed.: Baltimore: Williams and Wilkins, 1997, 53.
12. Swaim SF, Renberg WC, Shike KM: Small Animal Bandaging, Casting and Splinting Techniques. Ames, IA : Wiley – Blackwell, 2011, 3.


## Elastic Adhesive Tape-Pressure Bandage

### Definition and Indications

Elastic adhesive tape is compliant and it provides dynamic continuous pressure to a wound as the animal moves. These bandages are used to help control minor hemorrhage. They may also be used to help prevent periwound edema, especially transudative passive edema. Pressure adhesive tape is also indicated to immobilize limb fractures prior to definitive surgery, prevent exuberant granulation tissue, and help obliterate dead space.

### Technique

An elastic adhesive tape (Vetrap, 3M Animal Care Products, St. Paul, MN) and other elastic tapes should be carefully wrapped over underlying bandage materials to provide even but not excessive pressure. Adequate secondary bandage wrap should be evenly placed on the limb prior to placing the elastic adhesive tape. Using cast padding as the secondary bandage wrap can provide relatively more protection from pressure of an elastic adhesive tape tertiary layer.

Five factors govern the amount of pressure caused by elastic adhesive tape. These need to be considered when applying elastic adhesive tape.

1. The elasticity of the material used. Higher elasticity equates to more pressure.
2. The amount of tension placed on the tape as it is applied.
3. The width of the tape. The narrower the tape, the greater the local (tourniquet-type) pressure.
4. The number and overlap of layers applied. Pressure is additive with these.
5. The circumference of the bandaged limb. The smaller the circumference, the greater the possible pressure (Figure 2-15).

When applying the tape, the same principles should be followed that are used in applying porous adhesive tape off of the roll. Unrolling and rerolling elastic bandage material before applying it off the roll makes it easier to apply in a relaxed, nonstretched manner. Another technique is to hold the tape near the bandage with one hand while pulling the next length of tape off of

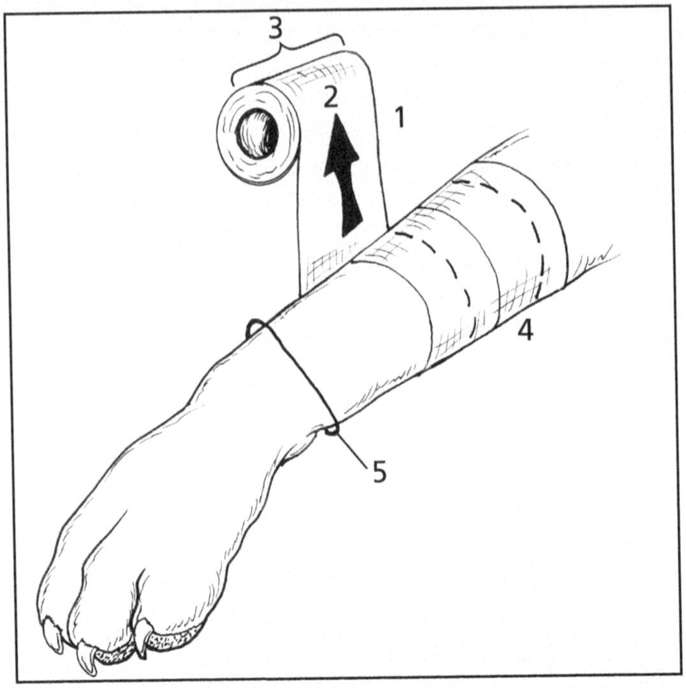


**Figure 2-15.** Five factors governing the pressure caused by elastic adhesive tape. *(1)* Elasticity of the tape, *(2)* Amount of tension used in application, *(3)* Width of tape, *(4)* Number and overlp of layers, and *(5)* Circumference of the bandaged limb.

the roll for application on the bandage (See Figure 2-13B). This aslo helps prevent placing the tape under too much tension. There should be one-third to one-half overlap of wraps. Another guideline for applying the tape is to apply it so that the textured pattern of the material is slightly distorted but visible.

When elastic adhesive tape is applied to a limb, it should be placed with even distribution of pressure. However, care should be used when progressing from an area of smaller circumference to one of larger circumference, i.e. from distal to proximal. Less tension should be used when applying the distal portion of the bandage to avoid excessive bandage constriction on this area of smaller circumference. Adding padding in areas of smaller circumference could be considered to increase effective limb radius to avoid pressure.

It should be remembered that on some animals there may be certain areas that are narrower than more distal areas, i.e. immediately proximal to the carpus and tarsus and proximal to the digits in some dogs. Tight application in these areas could result in a tourniquet effect.

If elastic adhesive tape is used to temporarily immobilize a limb, i.e. prior to definitive fracture repair, a more substantial secondary wrap is needed.

If elastic adhesive tape is used to bandage over a very convex surface (i.e. the point of the hock or point of the elbow), care should be used to avoid too much pressure. Bandages over these areas normally produce pressure; thus, elastic tape has the potential for causing excess pressure over the areas. Placing additional padding over the areas increases rather than decreases the pressure; therefore, it is best to pad around these points with a "donut"-type pad (see Padding Material, Cast Padding in this Chapter) (Figure 2-16).

To help assess the pressure of a distal limb bandage applied with elastic adhesive tape, the bandage can be applied leaving the third and fourth digits exposed enough so they can be used to monitor sensation and circulation several times daily.

## Aftercare

When considering the relationship of pressure to the circumference of the bandaged part, pressure bandages should be used carefully on the distal limb and paw to avoid circulatory compromise and potential tissue loss. If pressure bandages are used to control minor hemorrhage, they should be left in place a relatively short time. They should be checked within 24 hours. If the third and fourth digits are left exposed to monitor circulation, they should be observed for loss of sensation, cyanosis (of pink nails), swelling, and hypothermia as indicators that the bandage may

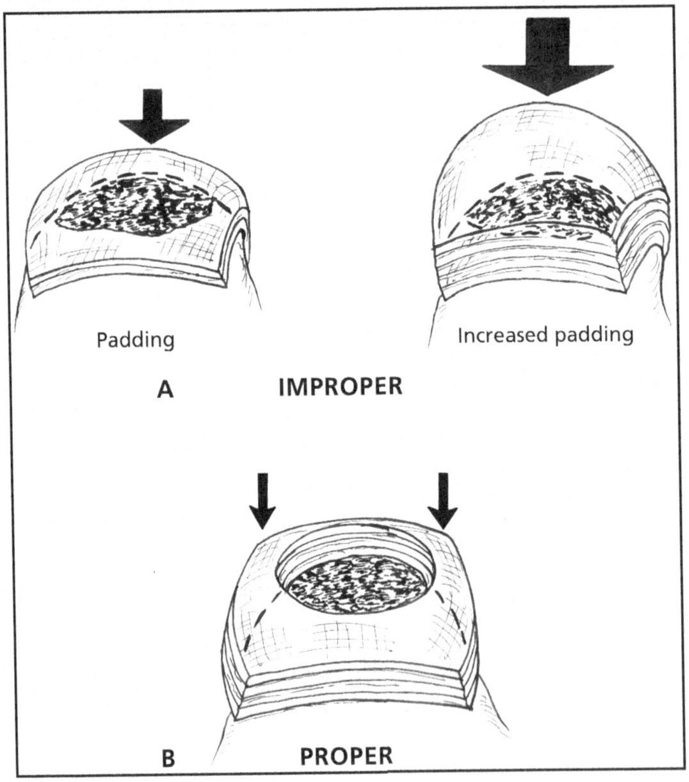


**Figure 2-16.** Improper and proper padding over convex surfaces (i.e. point of the hock and point of the elbow). **A.** Improper – Additional padding over a convex surface increases pressure when outer bandage layers are applied *(increased size of arrow)*. **B.** A "donut" – type cast padding pad distributes pressure around the convex surface *(small arrows)*.

be too tight. If the animal licks or chews at a pressure bandage it may be an indication that the bandage is too tight. If the animal is released to the owner's care after pressure bandage application, written instructions should be given to them related to bandage complications. If any of the above signs are noticed, the entire bandage should be removed and the limb examined. If pressure bandages are removed and the paws become markedly edematous within a matter of hours, it is a sign of reperfusion injury. The increased vascular permeability with resulting edema leads to increased tissue pressure on vessels in deep tissues. This in turn causes tissue ischemia and avascular necrosis. The occurrence of paw edema after bandage removal has a guarded to poor prognosis. The usual result is loss of paw tissue, especially in cats following bandage removal after onychectomy.

### Advantages and Disadvantages

The advantages of pressure bandages are related to their indications. Elastic bandage materials provide good conformation of the bandage to the limb. Because the elastic tapes adhere to themselves, minimal external taping is needed to secure the bandage in place. The tape does not adhere to the skin; thus, there is no discomfort with bandage removal. However, because the tape adheres to itself, wraps of the bandage are unable to move relative to each other, and joint flexion or extension can result in increased pressure at focal points around joints.

The main disadvantages of pressure bandages are their tendency to cause circulatory compromise and pressure induced neuropathies if they are applied too tightly. Pressure injury can be the result of local skin compression, especially over a bony prominence or it may be the result of a local tourniquet effect with deeper tissue ischemic necrosis which can include the secondary ischemia caused by the edema of reperfusion injury. Tissue loss from pressure bandages includes loss of full-thickness skin, underlying tissues, to include digital tendons; digits, metacarpal and metatarsal pads; or the entire limb. As a result, surgical procedures to correct or salvage such losses are necessary.

## Suggested Readings


1. Anderson DM, White RAS: Ischemic bandage injuries: A case series and review of the literature. Vet Surg 29:488, 2000.
2. Anderson D: Management of open wounds. In Williams J, Moores A, eds.: BSAVA Manual of Canine and Feline Wound Management and Reconstruction, 2nd ed.: Glouster (UK): BSAVA, 2009, 37.
3. Campbell BG: Dressings, bandages and splints for wound management in dogs and cats. Vet Clin No Small Animal Pract 36: 759, 2006.
4. Campbell BG: Bandages and drains. In Tobias KM, Johnston SA, eds.: Veterinary Surgery, Small Animal, Vol. 1: St. Louis: Elsevier – Saunders 2012, 221.
5. Hedlund CS: Surgery of the integumentary system. In Fossum TW, ed.: Small Animal Surgery, 3rd ed.: St. Louis: Mosby, 2007, 159.
6. MacPhail CM: Surgery of the integumentary system. In Fossum TW, ed.: Small Animal Surgery, 4th ed.: St. Louis: Mosby, 2013, 190.
7. Miller CW: Bandages and drains. *In* Slatter DH, ed.: Textbook of Small Animal Surgery, 3rd ed.: Philadelphia: WB Saunders, 2003, 244.
8. Noe JM, Kalish S: Dressing materials and their selection. *In* Rudolph R, Noe JM, eds.: Chronic Problem Wounds. Boston: Little, Brown, 1983, 37.
9. Pavletic MM: Atlas of Small Animal Wound Management and Reconstructive Surgery, 3rd ed.: Ames, IA: Wiley – Blackwell, 2010, 81.
10. Swaim SF: The effects of dressings and bandages on wound healing. Semin Vet Med Surg (Small Anim) 4:274, 1989.
11. Swaim SF: Bandages and topical agents. Vet Clin North Am Small Anim Pract 20:47, 1990.
12. Swaim SF, Wilhalf D: The physics, physiology, and chemistry of bandaging open wounds. Compend Contin Educ Pract Vet 7:146, 1985.
13. Swaim SF, Renberg WC, Shike KM: Small Animal Bandaging and Casting Techniques. Ames, IA: Wiley – Blackwell, 2011, 43.
14. Thomas S, Dawes C, Hay P: A critical evaluation of some extensible bandages in current use. Nursing Times 76:1123, 1980.


## Padding Materials: Cast Padding

### Definition and Indications

Cast padding material (Specialist Cast Padding, (BSN Medical, Rutherford College, NC) can be used to create a "donut"-type pad to be placed over convex prominences where skin could be injured by cast or splint pressure. The 2 most common areas of use on the distal limb are, 1) over the carpal pad, and 2) over the calcaneal process of the calcaneus tarsal bone.

When the cast padding is used as a "donut"-type pad, the principle involved is to place the hole of the "donut" over the prominence so the surrounding padding absorbs the pressure and there is no pressure on the skin over the prominence.

A second use for the material is as the secondary layer of bandages. It serves to absorb, pad, splint, pack, and contour the bandage. (See Secondary Bandage Layer, Roll Dressings in this chapter.)

A third use of the padding is as padding in the interdigital and interpad areas of the paw. It serves to pad these areas and absorb moisture.

### Technique

To make a "donut"-type pad several layers of cast padding are folded on each other to make a pad approximately 3 inches x 3 inches (Figure 2-17A). The pad is then folded over on itself, and bandage scissors are used to cut a slit in the pad's center (Figure 2-17B). After unfolding the pad, digital tension is used on the edges of the slit to enlarge it to a nearly round opening ("donut" hole) Figure 2-17C). The pad is then placed over the prominence with the opening over the prominence (Figure 2-17D). The secondary bandage layer is then wrapped around the limb to hold the pad in place, followed by application of the outer bandage layer.

When used as the secondary bandage layer, cast padding is applied as described under Secondary Bandage Layer, Roll Dressings.

For interdigital padding, small pieces are torn from the cast padding and placed in the interdigital areas and the interpad area on the palmar/plantar paw surface (Figure 2-18). The secondary bandage layer holds these in place.

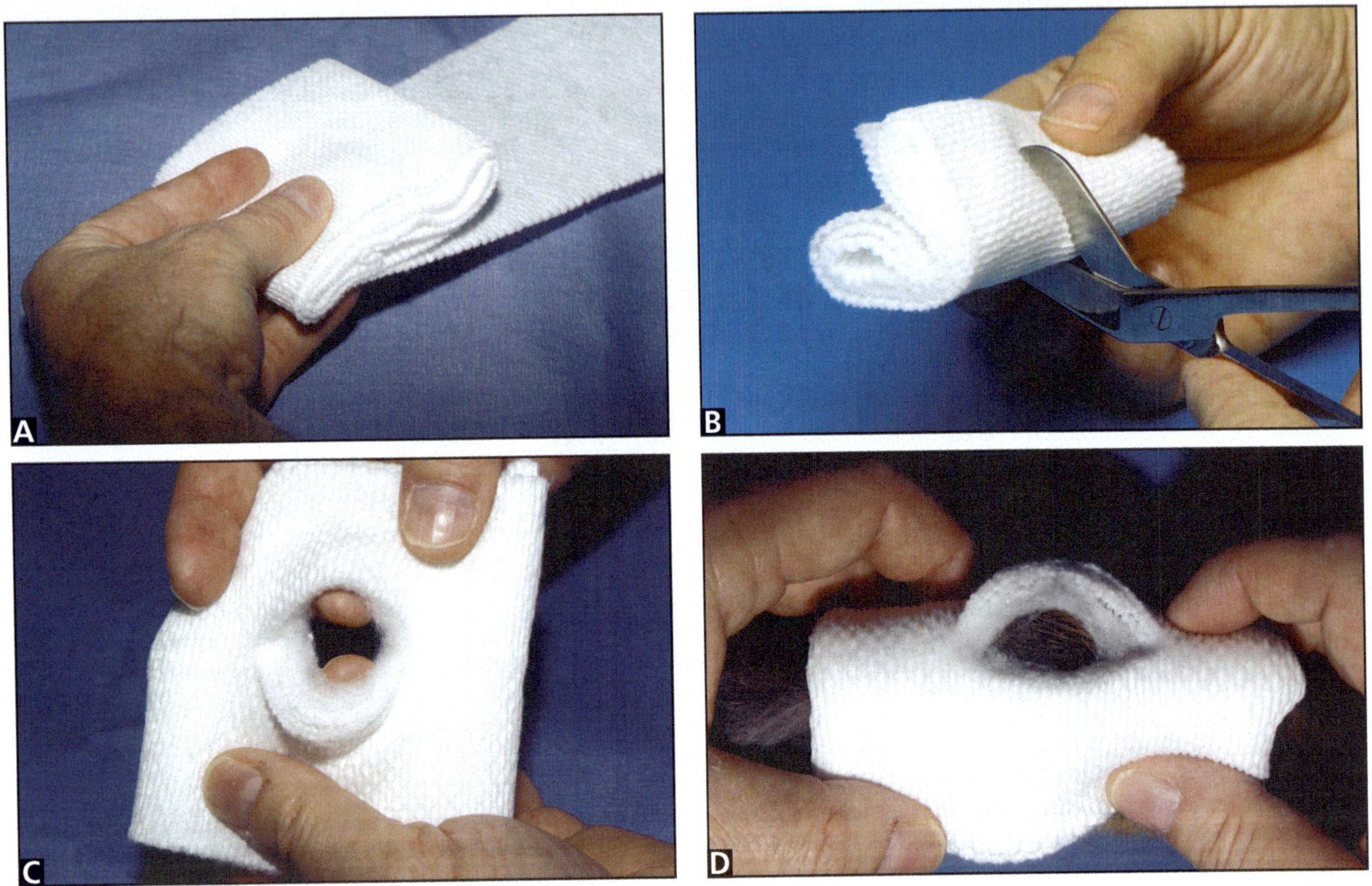


**Figure 2-17.** "Donut" – type pad for convex surfaces. **A.** Several layers of cast padding are folded together to make a 3 inch x 3 inch pad. **B.** The pad is folded on itself and a slit is cut in its center. **C.** Digital tension is used to form the slit into a round hole. **D.** Pad is placed with the hole over a convex surface (calcaneal tuber). (From Swaim SF, Henderson RA: Small Animal Wound Management, 2nd ed.: Baltimore, Williams & Wilkins, 1997, 132.)

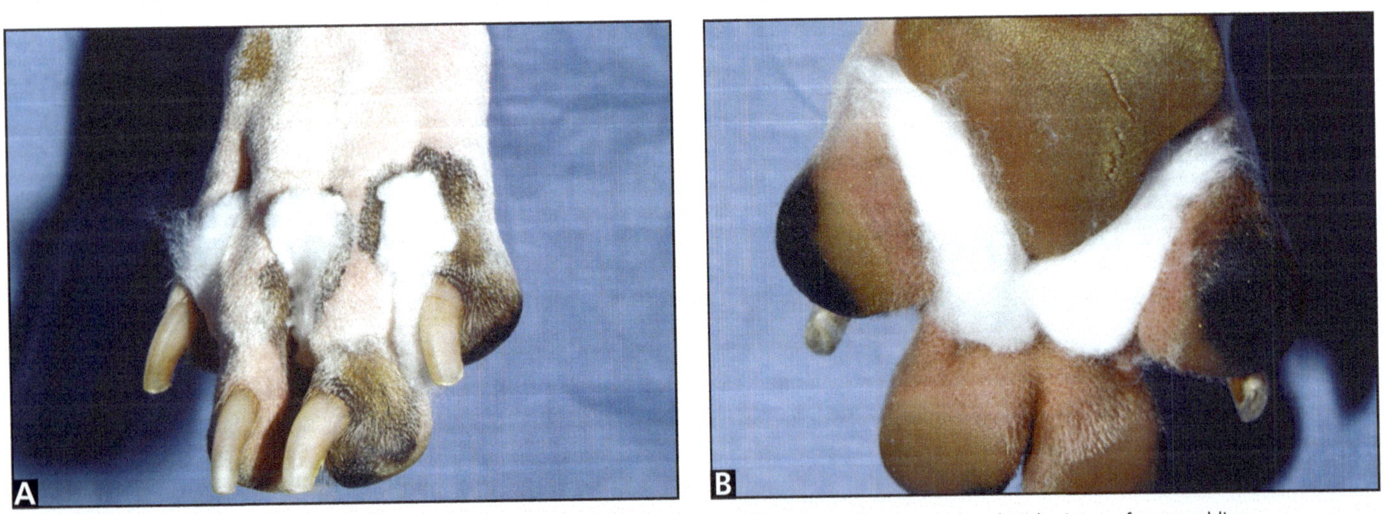


**Figure 2-18. A.** Padding the interdigital spaces and **B.** space between the digital and metacarpal/metatarsal pad with pieces of cast padding.

## Aftercare

When bandages are changed, the "donut"-type pad can be saved and reused 2 to 3 times if it has not become wet or soiled. After 2 to 3 uses, it should be discarded because it will have compressed to the point where it is not functional for pressure relief.

Aftercare when cast padding is used as the secondary bandage layer is as described for Secondary Bandage Layer, Roll Dressings.

Generally, interdigital and interpad pieces of cast padding are replaced at each bandage change.

## Advantages and Disadvantages

The main advantage of cast padding is that it is inexpensive and one roll will provide numerous "donut"-type pads and interdigital pads. Advantages and disadvantages of cast padding as a secondary bandage layer are as described for Secondary Bandage Layer, Roll Dressings in this chapter.

# Suggested Readings


1. Bohling MW, Swaim SF: Bandage and drainage techniques. In Bojrab MJ, ed.: Current Techniques in Small Animal Surgery, 5th, ed.: Jackson, WY: Teton NewMedia, 2014, 13.
2. Campbell BG: Dressings, bandages and splints for wound management in dogs and cats. Vet Clin No Am Small Animal Pract 36: 759, 2006.
3. Campbell BG: Bandages and drains. In Tobias KM, Johnston SA, eds.: Veterinary Surgery, Small Animal, Vol. 1.: St. Louis: Elsevier – Saunders, 2012, 221.
4. Hedlund CS: Surgery of the integumentary system. *In* Fossum TW, ed.: Small Animal Surgery, 2nd ed.: St. Louis: Mosby, 2002, 134.
5. Hedlund CS: Surgery of the integumentary system. In Fossum TW, ed.: Small Animal Surgery, 3rd ed.: St. Louis: Mosby, 2007, 159.
6. Miller CW: Bandages and drains. *In* Slatter DH, ed.: Textbook of Small Animal Surgery, 3rd ed.: Philadelphia: WB Saunders, 2003, 244.
7. Pavletic MM: Atlas of Small Animal Wound Management and Reconstructive Surgery, 3rd ed.: Ames, IA: Wiley – Blackwell, 2010, 81.
8. Swaim SF, Henderson RA: Small Animal Wound Management, 2nd ed.: Baltimore: Williams and Wilkins, 1997, 53 and 87.
9. Swaim SF, Renberg WC, Shike KM: Small Animal Bandaging, Casting and Splinting Techniques: Ames, IA : Wiley – Blackwell: 2011, 3 & 43.


# Foam Sponge Padding

## Definition and Indications

Foam sponge padding (Comfor™ Foam, HiTech Foam, Lincoln, NE) is available for inclusion in the secondary layer of paw bandages. The padding of medium compressibility (blue color) is the padding of choice. The padding is used to relieve pressure on pads to assist in the wound healing process on pads. Pressure on pads tends to spread pad tissue, thus interfering with open wound healing and leading to wound disruption of sutured wounds. The foam sponge padding can be used to off load the metacarpal/metatarsal pad or the digital pads. This form of pad pressure relief is indicated for small to medium sized dogs that have moderate pad wounds.

## Technique

For pressure relief on the metacarpal/metatarsal pad, a piece of foam sponge is cut to the size and basic shape of the palmar/plantar surface of the paw. The foam sponge pad thickness is split in half using a number 10 scalpel blade or razor blade to provide a pad approximately 1.25 cm. thick. The blade is also used to cut a hole in the foam sponge in the area that will lie over the metacarpal/metatarsal pad wound, providing a "donut"-type pad. The pad is then incorporated on the palmar/plantar surface of the paw bandage in the secondary wrap (Figure 2-19A). For better pressure

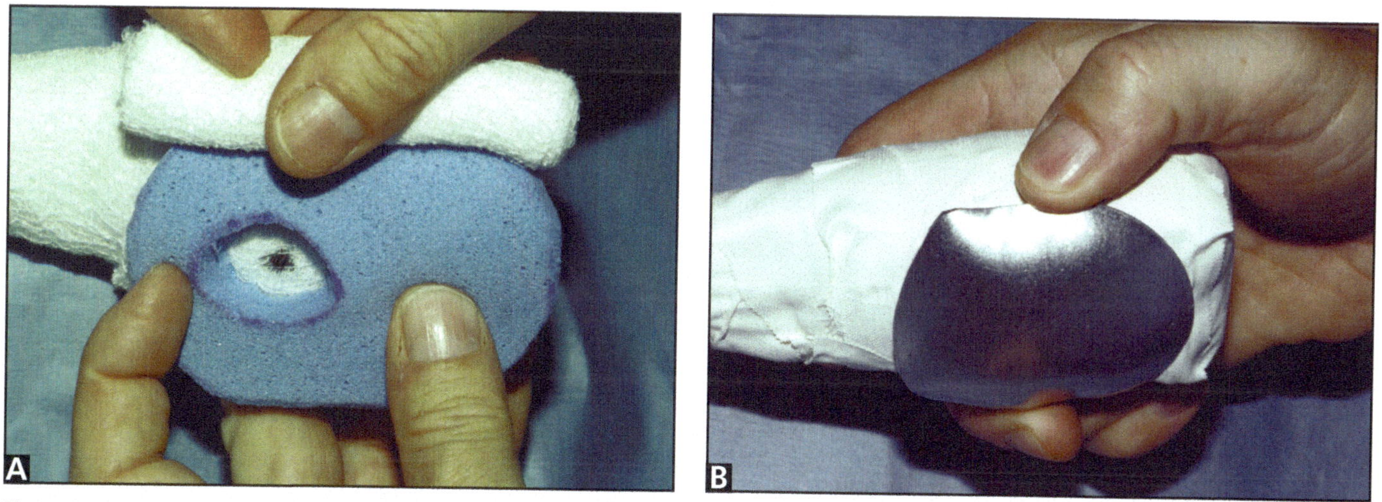


**Figure 2-19.** Pressure relief on the metacarpal/metatarsal pad. **A.** "Donut" – type foam sponge pad being incorporated in secondary bandage wrap on the palmar surface of the paw. **B.** Cup portion of a metal splint incorporated in the bandage under a "donut" – type sponge pad. (From Swaim SF, Marghitu DB, Rumph PF. Et al: Effects of bandage configuration on paw pad pressure in dogs: A preliminary study. J Am Anim Hosp Assoc 39: 212, 2003.)

relief, the cup portion of a Mason metasplint can also be incorporated in the bandage underlying the foam sponge pad (Figure 2-19B).

For pressure relief on the digital pad surfaces for either soft tissue or orthopedic injuries, padding is not placed under the digit but under the metacarpal/metatarsal pad to direct pressure away from the digital pad surfaces. To accomplish this a foam sponge is cut in a triangular shape approximately the size of the metacarpal/metatarsal pad. The thickness of the foam sponge pad is split in half to approximately 1.25 cm. thickness with a number 10 scalpel blade or razor blade. The pad is then incorporated on the palmar/plantar surface of the paw bandage over the metacarpal/metatarsal pad in the secondary wrap (Figure 2-20A). For better pressure relief, the cup portion of a Mason metasplint can also be incorporated in the bandage underlying the foam sponge pad (Figure 2-20B).

## Aftercare

At the time of bandage change all portions of the bandage are changed and the foam sponge pad is saved to be incorporated in the next bandage. For draining wounds, it may be necessary to have 2 pads. Thus, if one pad becomes soiled with drainage it can be rinsed with antiseptic solution and allowed to dry for incorporation at the next bandage change.

## Advantages and Disadvantages

The main advantage of foam sponge pads is the pressure relief they provide in the area of a wound. For the metacarpal/metatarsal "donut"-type pad the off loading principle is that of distributing pressure on tissues around the wound rather than on the wound (Figure 2-21A). With the metacarpal/metatarsal triangle pad the off loading principle is that of elevating the digits by placing padding under the metacarpal/metatarsal pad (Figure 2-21B). Another advantage of the sponge foam is that ingenuity on the part of the clinician could provide other types of padding that could be used in practice.

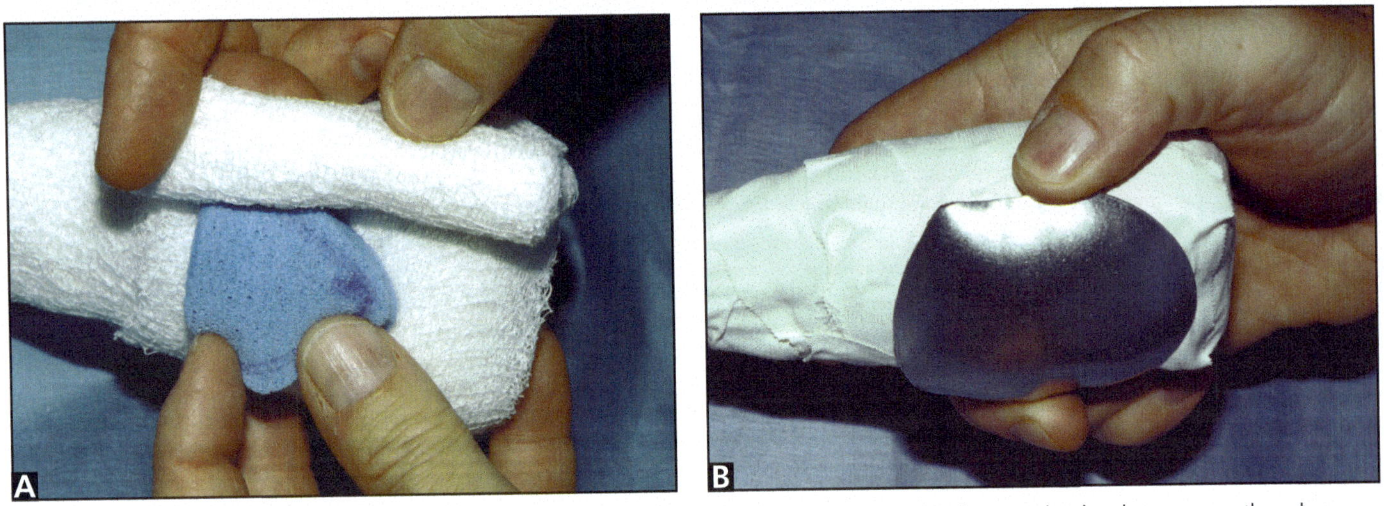


**Figure 2-20.** Pressure relief on the digital pads. **A.** A triangular – shaped foam sponge pad incorporated in the secondary bandage wrap on the palmar surface of the metacarpal pad. **B.** Cup portion of a metal splint incorporated in the bandage under a triangular sponge pad. (From Swaim SF, Marghitu DB, Rumph PF, et al: Effects of bandage configuration on paw pad pressure in dogs: A preliminary study. J Am Anim Hosp Assoc 39: 211, 2003.)

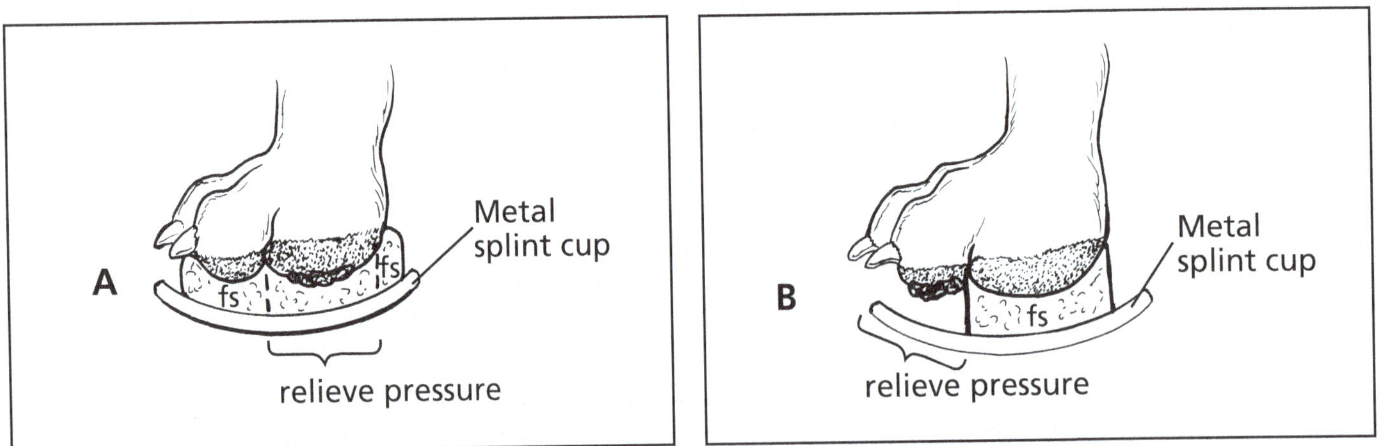


**Figure 2-21.** Side view of the off loading principle for pad pressure relief. **A.** Foam sponge *(fs)* with hole in its center (broken line) used with a metal splint cup to relieve pressure on the metacarpal/metatarsal pad. **B.** Foam sponge *(fs)* used with a metal splint cup to relieve pressure on digital pads.

# Suggested Readings


1. Bohling MW, Swaim SF: Bandage and drainage techniques. In Bojrab MJ, ed.: Current Techniques in Small Animal Surgery, 5th ed.: Jackson, WY: Teton NewMedia 2014, 13.
2. Campbell BG: Dressings, bandages and splints for wound management in dogs and cats. Vet Clin No Am Small Animal Pract 36: 759, 2006.
3. Campbell BG: Bandages and drains. In Tobias KM, Johnston SA, eds.: Veterinary Surgery, Small Animal, Vol. 1: St. Louis: Elsevier – Saunders, 2012, 221.
4. Hedlund CS: Surgery of the integumentary system. In Fossum TW, ed.: Small Animal Surgery, 3rd ed.: St. Louis: Mosby, 2007, 159.
5. MacPhail CM: Surgery of the integumentary system. In Fossum TW, ed.: Small Animal Surgery, 4th ed.: St. Louis: Mosby, 2013, 190.
6. Pavletic MM: Atlas of Small Animal Wound Management and Reconstructive Surgery, 3rd ed.: Ames, IA: Wiley – Blackwell, 2010, 81.
7. Swaim SF, Marghitu DB, Rumph PF, et al: Effects of bandage configuration on paw pad pressure in dogs: A preliminary study. J Am Anim Hosp Assoc 39:209, 2003.
8. Swaim SF: Management of bandaging of soft tissue injuries of dog and cat feet. J Am Anim Hosp Assoc 21:329, 1985.
9. Swaim SF, Henderson RA: Small Animal Wound Management, 2nd ed.: Baltimore, Williams and Wilkins, 1997, 295.
10. Swaim SF, Renberg WC, Shike KM: Small Animal Bandaging, Casting and Splinting Techniques. Ames, IA: Wiley – Blackwell: 2011, 43.


# Stockinette Padding

## Definition and Indications

Cotton Stockinette or synthetic orthopedic stockinette that is used to line casts can be used to provide inexpensive temporary padding and coverage for the paws of small dogs and cats. The covering is indicated for abrasive and pressure-type lesions that result from abnormal placement of the paw due to a temporary peripheral nerve lesion that has the potential for recovery in time, i.e. a neuropraxic lesion (Figure 2-22A).

## Technique

A length of 2 inch diameter stockinette is placed on the distal limb extending from the proximal metacarpal/metatarsal level to the end of the digits. The stockinette is cut one to two inches beyond the digits (Figure 2-22B). The distal end of the stockinette is folded back onto the paw. If the lesion is on the dorsal aspect of the paw, the stockinette is folded dorsally. Conversely, if the lesion is on the palmar/plantar paw surface the stockinette is folded to this surface (Figure 2-22C). The distal end of the stockinette is then taped in place with a circumferential wrap of 1-inch wide adhesive tape, and the proximal end of the stockinette is also taped

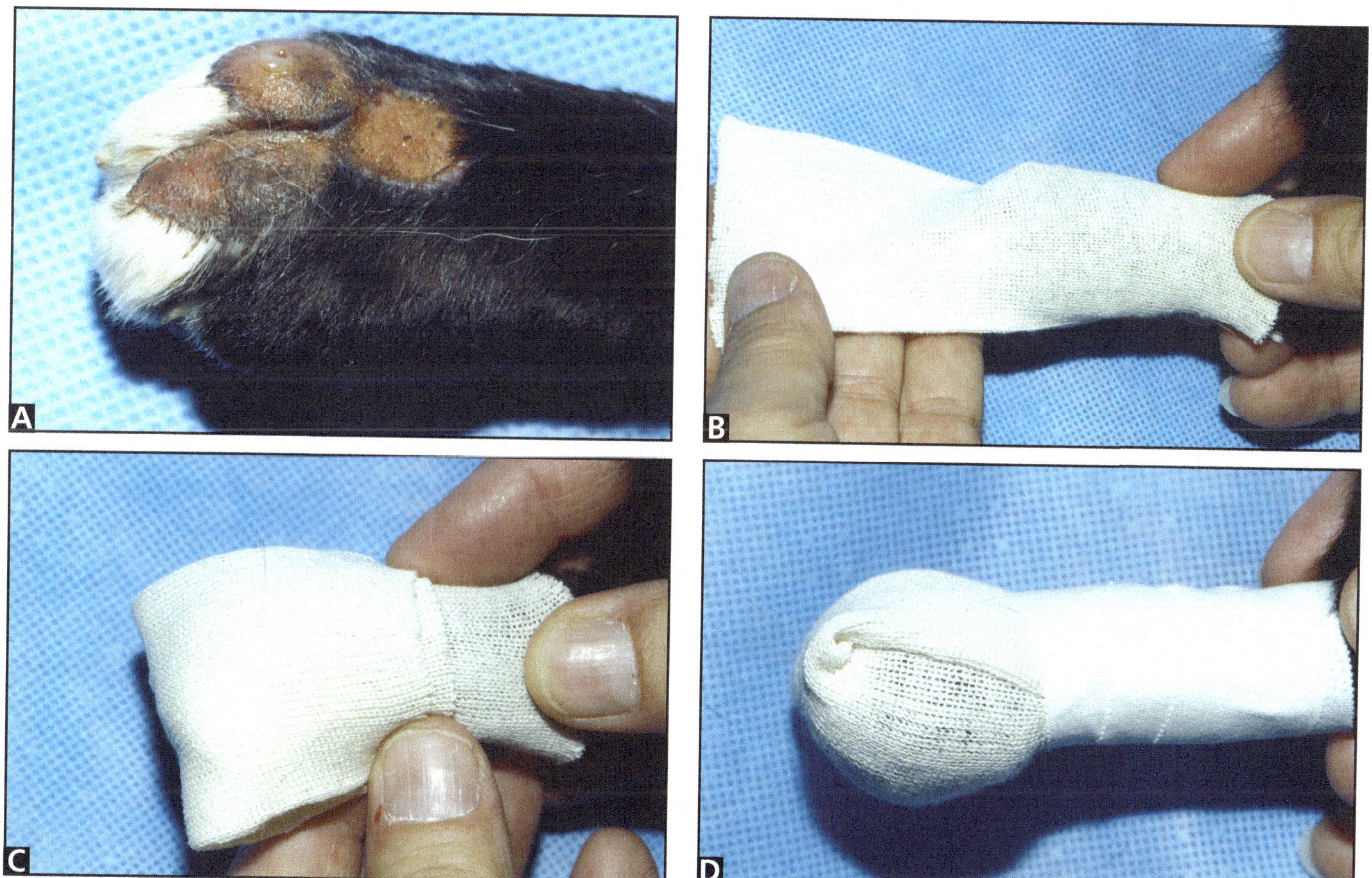

**Figure 2-22.** Stockinette padding bandage. **A.** Abrasion lesion on the dorsum of a cat's paw resulting from neurologically induced abnormal gait. **B.** Length of 2 – inch diameter stockinette on the metatarsal area, extending 2 inches beyond digits. **C.** Distal end of stockinette folded back on dorsum of paw. **D.** Distal and proximal ends of stockinette taped in place with strips of 1 – inch wide adhesive tape. The tape strips overlap. A triple thickness of stockinette is over the lesion.

in place with a strip of 1-inch wide adhesive tape that is placed circumferentially with half its width on the stockinette and half on the hair of the limb. This strip may overlap the first strip (Figure 2-22D).

## Aftercare

The animal's exercise should be limited and preferably confined to soft surfaces. The stockinette should be observed over the area of the abrasion/pressure lesion periodically to determine when the stockinette should be changed due to wear. Keeping the stockinette dry is also important. Placing a piece of waterproof tape over the area of stockinette that receives the most pressure/wear will help prolong the usefulness of the stockinette cover and avoid frequent changes.

## Advantages and Disadvantages

The 3 layers of stockinette covering the lesion provide protection on paws of small dogs and cats until the animal can position the paw normally after nerve regeneration occurs (See Figure 2-22D). The covering is inexpensive. However, it would not be sufficient for larger dogs because of the wear the dog would place on the stockinette. Some form of bootie would be a better choice in such instances.

# Suggested Readings

1. Swaim SF, Renberg WC, Shike KM: Small Animal Bandaging, Casting and Splinting Techniques. Ames, IA.: Wiley – Blackwell: 2011, 43.

# Specialty Appliances

Specialty appliances are bandages, splints, and slings used to protect distal limb and paw soft tissue and orthopedic wounds from the deleterious effects of movement and pressure. The appliances covered are those primarily used by the author. These include various uses of metal splints, a carpal flexion splint, a carpal sling,the Velpeau sling and the 90/90 sling. Other types of splints may be necessary on occasion. These will be covered in sections of the text where they are applicable.

# Metal Splints

## Definition and Indications

The metal splints used on distal limbs and paws are those of the aluminum Mason metasplint design (Mason Metasplints, Jorgensen Labs, Inc., Loveland, CO). These have a paw cup and straight portion to the splint and come in different sizes (Figure 2-23). The splints are used in varying ways in combination with limb bandages to treat distal limb and paw wounds.

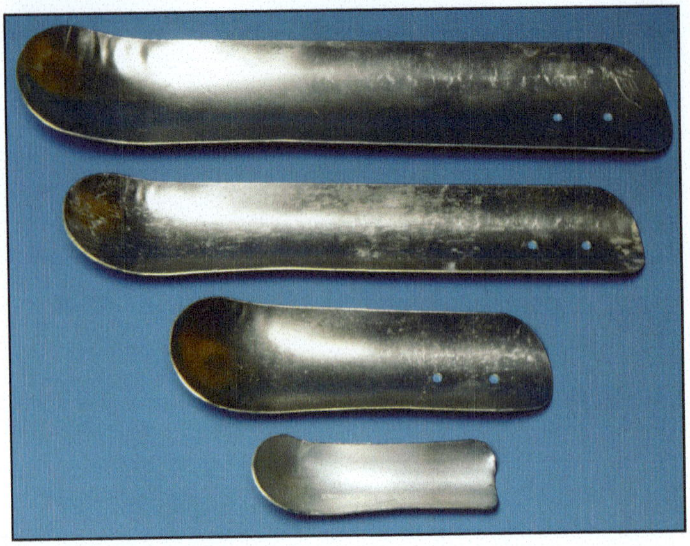

**Figure 2-23.** Mason metasplints of various sizes.

### Paw Cup

The cup portion of a metal splint can be cut from the splint with metal cutting shears or cast cutting shears with serrated blades. The cup is then placed in the palmar/plantar surface of the bandage. It can be placed alone to confine spreading of the metacarpal/metatarsal pad as the animal bears weight. It can also be used in combination with a foam sponge pad to off load the digital pads on the metacarpal/metatarsal pad. (See Padding Materials, Foam Sponge Padding in this chapter.)

### Full Splints

Full metal splints can be incorporated in forelimb bandages to immobilize orthopedic injuries from the digits to the carpal area and soft tissue injuries from the digits to the midantebrachial area. They can be incorporated in hind limb bandages to immobilize orthopedic wounds of the digits and soft tissue wounds of the paw and metatarsal area.

### "Clam Shell" Splint

Two full metal splints are applied over a forelimb bandage to immobilize orthopedic injuries from the digits to the carpal area and soft tissue injuries from the digits to the midantebrachium. They are incorporated in hind limb bandages to immobilize orthopedic wounds of the digits and soft tissue wounds of the paw and metatarsal area.

"Clam shell" splints are indicated when major reconstructive or salvage surgery has been done on the paw, and it is necessary to off load the paw maximally. They are quite useful in large dogs where considerable pressure could be placed on such surgical repairs.

### One-Half "Clam Shell" Splint

One metal splint is applied to the plantar surface of a hind limb bandage to immobilize orthopedic wounds of the digits and soft tissue wounds of the paw and metatarsal area.

One-half "clam shell" splint is indicated when major reconstructive or salvage surgery has been done on the paw and it is necessary to off load the paw maximally. However, the front portion of a whole "clam shell" splint causes pressure irritation of the skin on the dorsal aspect of the tarsal area.

## Techniques

### Paw Cup

As the last layer of the secondary wrap is applied to a paw bandage, the paw cup portion of a metal Mason metasplint is incorporated on the palmar/plantar surface of the bandage. The tertiary portion of the bandage is then applied.

The paw cup may be used with a foam sponge "donut"-type pad for relief of metacarpal/ metatarsal pad pressure, or a foam sponge triangle pad for relief of digital pad pressure. The cup is incorporated in the bandage under the sponge pad in these instances (See Figure 2-19A & B).

### Full Splints

A paw bandage is applied, usually with adhesive tape stirrups for security. Additional secondary wrap is applied to the level of the elbow or hock to make the surface of the bandage circumferentially equal along its length. The appropriate size of metal splint is placed on the volar surface of the bandage and taped in place with or to the tertiary bandage layer (Figure 2-24A & B). It is important to have a cast padding "donut"-type pad over the carpal pad of the forelimb and over the point of the hock of the hind limb.

### "Clam Shell" Splint

A paw bandage is applied with adhesive tape stirrups for security. Additional secondary wrap is applied to the level of the elbow or hock to make the surface of the bandage circumferentially equal along its length. The tertiary bandage layer of adhesive tape is placed. Two metal splints of the appropriate size are placed on opposite sides of the bandage. On the forelimb the splints should extend to near the elbow and to near the hock on the hind limb. The splints are usually placed on the cranial and volar/plantar bandage surfaces but may be applied on the medial and lateral surfaces. They are placed with the paw cups facing each other and extending approximately 1 to 1½ inches beyond the end of the paw (Figure 2-25A). Strips of 2-inch wide adhesive tape are used to tape the splints in place (Figure 2-25B). It is important to use adhesive tape for the tertiary bandage layer and to tape the splints in place. The adhesion of the tape of these 2 layers between the splints gives security to the splints so they do not slip dorsally with weight bearing. A gauze sponge should be taped over the sharp ends of the paw cups to protect them from abrasion and the clients' floors and carpets from damage (Figure 2-25C).

### One-Half "Clam Shell" Splint

The technique for applying the one-half "clam shell" splint is like that for applying the "clam shell" splint; however, the cranial portion of the splint is not applied to the hind limb (See "Clam Shell" Splint). The length of splint extending beyond the end of the bandage should be shortened for stability (Figure 2-26).

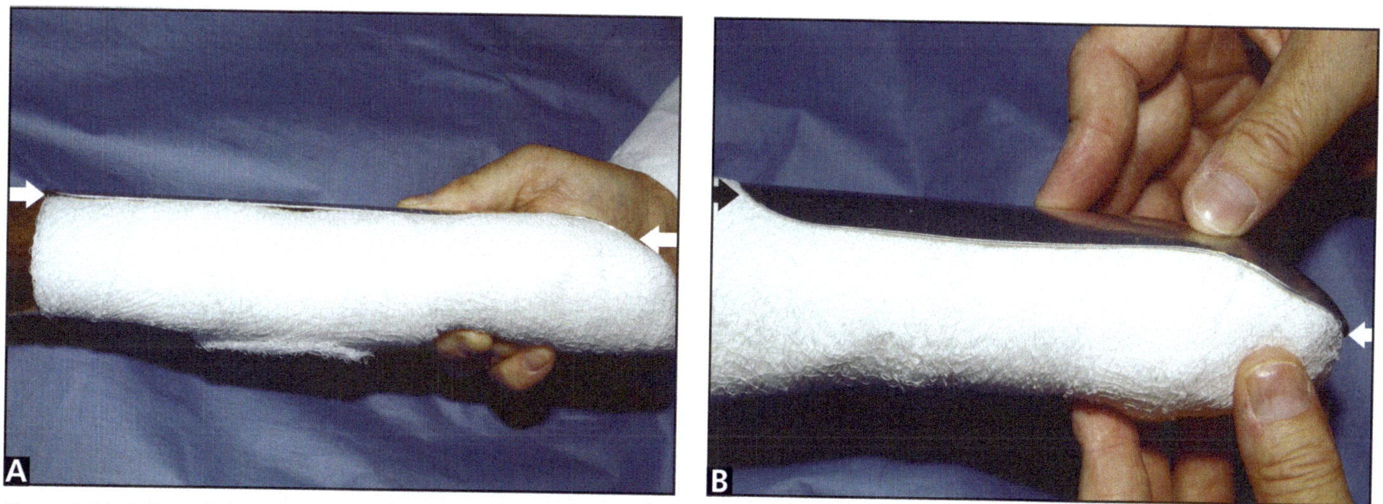


**Figure 2-24.** Full metal splint. A full metal splint held over the caudal surface of a **A.** forelimb bandage (between arrows), **B.** a pelvic limb bandage (between arrows).

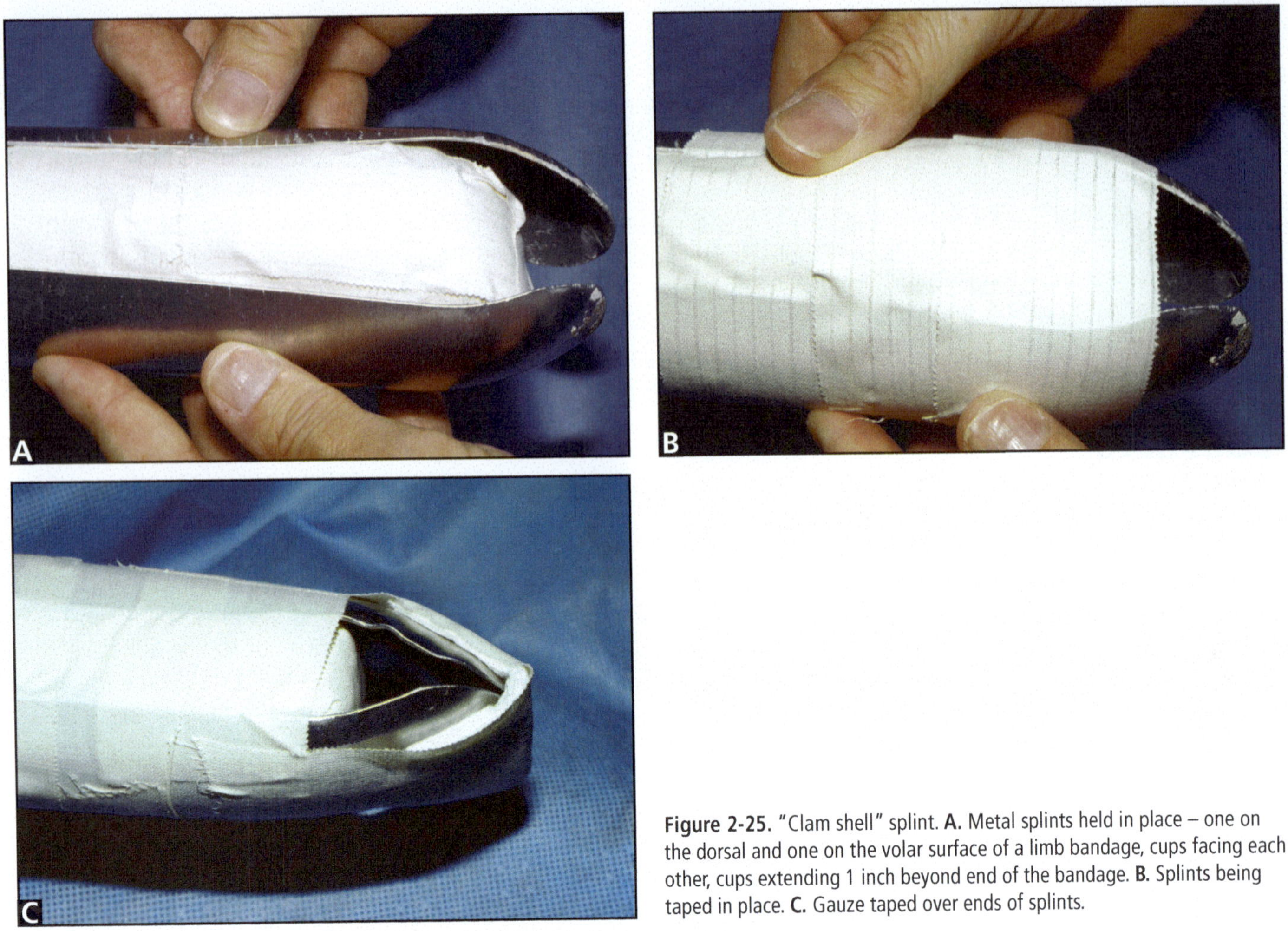


Figure 2-25. "Clam shell" splint. A. Metal splints held in place – one on the dorsal and one on the volar surface of a limb bandage, cups facing each other, cups extending 1 inch beyond end of the bandage. B. Splints being taped in place. C. Gauze taped over ends of splints.

## Aftercare

### Paw Cup

No special aftercare is necessary when using paw cups in bandages. If foam sponge padding is used in conjunction with the paw cups it is advisable to have 2 pads in case one gets soiled. It can be cleaned with antiseptic while the second one is in use.

### Full Splints

When changing a bandage that has a full splint in it, the status of the carpal pad should be noted. If it shows signs of pressure injury, the cast padding "donut"-type pad should be made thicker to help alleviate the pressure on it. If the splint is being used to immobilize a skin grafted area, i.e. over a joint, care should be used at bandage change that the joint is not moved while the bandage is being changed.

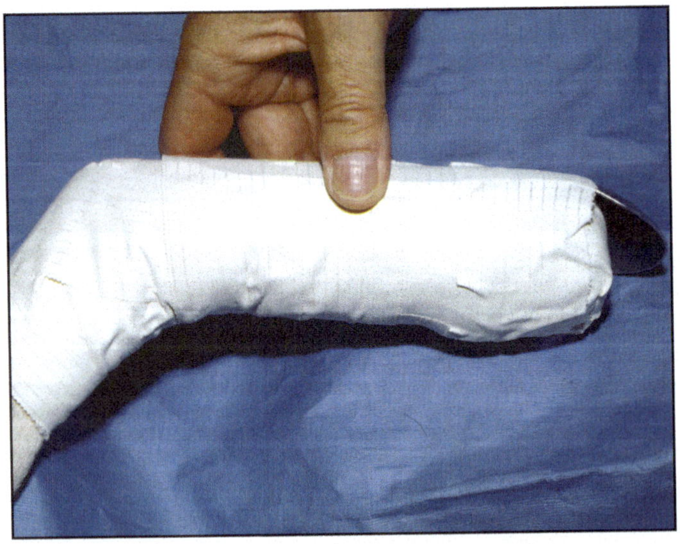

Figure 2-26. One – half "clam shell" splint on a pelvic limb.

### "Clam Shell" Splint

The same precaution regarding pressure injury to the carpal pad by a full splint should be used with "clam shell" splints. When using "clam shell" splints on the hind limb, the cranial surface of the tarsal area should be observed for evidence of pressure irritation by the dorsal edge of the dorsal splint, caused by the animal bearing weight on the splints. If this is noticed the cranial splint can be omitted if the clinical judgement indicates a one-half "clam shell" splint will still be effective. If it is believed full "clam shell" support is needed, the splints may be placed on the medial and lateral sides of the limb.

### One-Half "Clam Shell" Splint

If a one-half "clam shell" splint does not appear to be providing the support or protection desired, a "clam shell" splint with splints on the medial and lateral aspects of the limb should be considered.

## Advantages and Disadvantages

### Paw Cup

When a paw cup is used without sponge foam padding, it confines the metacarpal/metatarsal pad so it does not spread; thus, helping prevent this factor that can impair healing. When used with a foam sponge "donut"-type pad it provides more reduction of metacarpal/metatarsal pad pressure than a pad alone. The same is true of the use of the foam sponge triangle with the cup to off load the digits (See Figure 2-21A & B).

### Full Splints

The advantage and a full splint in treating soft tissue injuries is that it immobilizes joints to enhance wound healing over them. A disadvantage is the potential pressure injury they can cause on the carpal pad if a cast padding "donut"-type pad is not used with them.

### "Clam Shell" Splint

These splints serve as a local crutch to place the paw in a "toe dancing" position and provide maximum relief of pressure on paw reconstructive and salvage procedures to enhance healing. They are particularly advantageous for large dogs where their weight could cause significant pressure on repair procedures if not abated by the splints. As with full splints, the splints have the potential of causing pressure injury to the carpal pad if it is not adequately padded with a cast padding "donut"-type pad.

### One-Half "Clam Shell" Splint

This splint has the same advantages as the "clam shell" splint. It prevents the pressure irritation that can occur over the cranial tarsal surface. It may not provide as much support as the "clam shell" splint. Reducing the length of the splint extending beyond the end of the paw can help compensate for this.

## Suggested Readings


1. Bohling MW, Swaim SF: Bandage and drainage techniques. In Bojrab MJ, ed.: Current Techniques in Small Animal Surgery, 5th ed.: Jackson, WY: Teton NewMedia 2014, 13.
2. Bradley DM, Scardino MS, Swaim SF: Construction of a weight-bearing surface on a dog's distal pelvic limb. J Am Anim Hosp Assoc 34:387, 1998.
3. Campbell BG: Dressings, bandages and splints for wound management in dogs and cats. Vet Clin No Am Small Animal Pract 36: 759, 2006.
4. Campbell BG: Bandages and drains. In Tobias KM, Johnston SA, eds.: Veterinary Surgery, Small Animal, Vol. 1: St. Louis: Elsevier – Saunders, 2012, 221.
5. Hedlund CS: Surgery of the integumentary system. In Fossum TW, ed.; Small Animal Surgery, 3rd ed.: St. Louis: Mosby: 2007, 159.
6. MacPhail CM: Surgery of the integumentary system. In Fossum TW, ed.: Small Animal Surgery, 4th ed.: St. Louis: Mosby, 2013, 190.
7. Pavletic MM: Atlas of Small Animal Wound Management and Reconstructive Surgery, 3rd. ed.: Ames, IA: Wiley – Blackwell, 2010, 81.
8. Swaim SF: Management of bandaging of soft tissue injuries of dog and cat feet. J Am Anim Hosp Assoc 21:329, 1985.
9. Swaim SF: Bandaging and splinting techniques. In Kirk RB, Bistner SI, Raffe MR, eds.: Handbook of Veterinary Procedures and Emergency Treatment, 7th ed.: Philadelphia: WB Saunders, 2000, 549.
10. Swaim SF, Henderson RA: Small Animal Wound Management, 2nd ed.: Baltimore, Williams and Wilkins, 1997, 295.
11. Swaim SF, Marghitu DB, Rumph PF, et al: Effects of bandage configuration on paw pad pressure in dogs: A preliminary study. J Am Anim Hosp Assoc 39:209, 2003.
12. Swaim SF, Renberg WC, Shike KM: Small Animal Bandaging, Casting and Splinting Techniques. Ames, IA: Wiley – Blackwell: 2011, 43.


# Carpal Flexion Splint

## Definition and Indications

The carpal flexion splint is indicated for preventing weight-bearing on the forelimb. It is used following procedures such as orthopedic repairs on the carpus and below, digital flexor tendon repair, and major paw reconstruction and salvage procedures.

## Technique

Adhesive tape stirrups are applied to the dorsal and caudal aspect of the distal limb with the carpus in slight flexion (Figure 2-27A). A length of 2-inch diameter orthopedic stockinette is applied to the limb. This is followed by wrapping the lower limb with cast padding material (Specialist Cast Padding, BSN Medical, Rutherford College, NC). To conform the cast padding to the structures of the lower limb, it is next wrapped with an elastic gauze roll (Kling, Johnson and Johnson, Arlington, TX) (Figure 2-27B). Two-inch wide fiberglass casting tape ( Vecast Plus, Veterinary Casting Tape, 3M St. Paul, MN) is used to construct a splint for the dorsal and volar surfaces of the bandage. The elastic gauze is used to wrap the splints in place (Figure 2-27C). The stirrups are then folded back

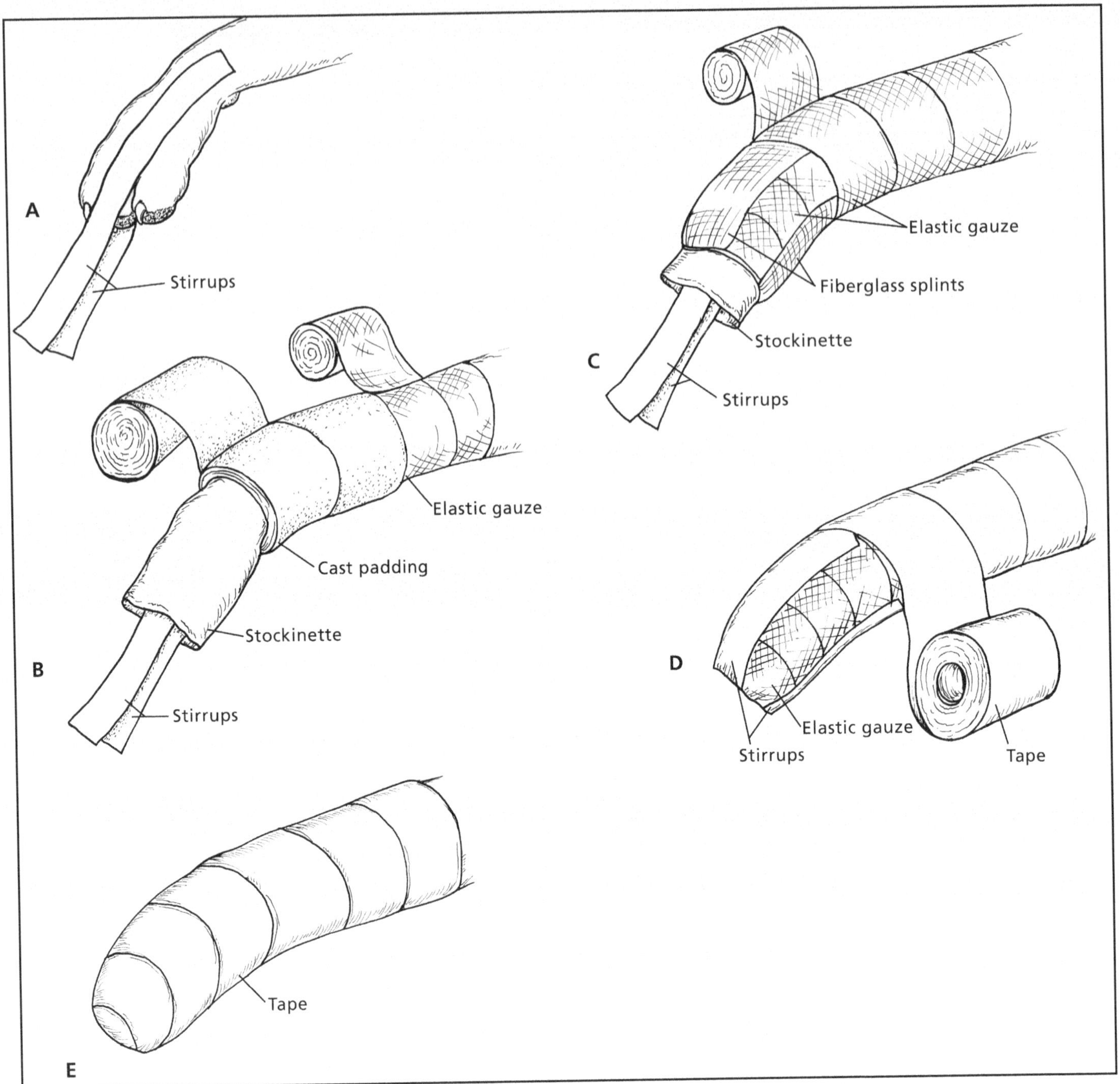


**Figure 2-27.** Carpal flexion splint. **A.** Forelimb flexed slightly with tape stirrups in place. **B.** Stockinette in place; cast padding and elastic gauze roll being applied. **C.** Fiberglass splints being wrapped in place. **D.** Stirrups folded back and being taped. **E.** Completed splint.

over the outside of the bandage splint (Figure 2-27D) and are taped in place to complete the splint (Figure 2-27E).

## Aftercare

The splint is observed and changed as indicated depending upon the condition being treated. Likewise, the length of time the splint is left in place is dependent on the condition being treated. With generalized soft tissue injury in the area of the carpus, prolonged flexion immobilization can result in adhesions that interfere with carpal extension. To help prevent contracture deformities, limited extension should be returned within 3 to 4 weeks.

## Advantages and Disadvantages

Carpal flexion provides good protection for flexor tendon repairs. It can also provide a nonweight-bearing environment for healing of paw reconstructive and salvage procedures. The potential for carpal contractural complications is a disadvantage of the technique.

# Suggested Readings

1. Canapp SO Campana DH: Orthopedic coaptation devices and small animal prosthetics. In Tobias KM, Johnson SA, eds.: Veterinary Surgery, Small Animal, Vol. 1: St. Louis: Elsevier – Saunders, 2012, 628.

2. DeCamp CE: External coaptation. *In* Slatter DH, ed.: Textbook of Small Animal Surgery, 3rd ed.: Philadelphia: WB Saunders, 2003, 1835.
3. Swaim SF, Renberg WC, Shike KM: Small Animal Bandaging, Casting and Splinting Techniques. Ames, IA: Wiley – Blackwell: 2011, 43.

# Carpal Sling

## Definition and Indications

The carpal sling is indicated for preventing weight – bearing on the forelimb without having to immobilize the entire limb. It can be used when it is important that the dog not bear weight for a short period of time, e.g. for such procedures as orthopedic repair on the carpus and below when the repair is not sufficiently strong to withstand immediate walking forces. The sling would also be indicated for paw reconstructive surgery or wound management on a paw pad,

## Technique

With the dog in lateral recumbency with the affected limb up, the carpus is palpated to insure the flexion is comfortable (Figure 2-28A).The carpus is flexed but not beyond 90 degrees. The paw and distal

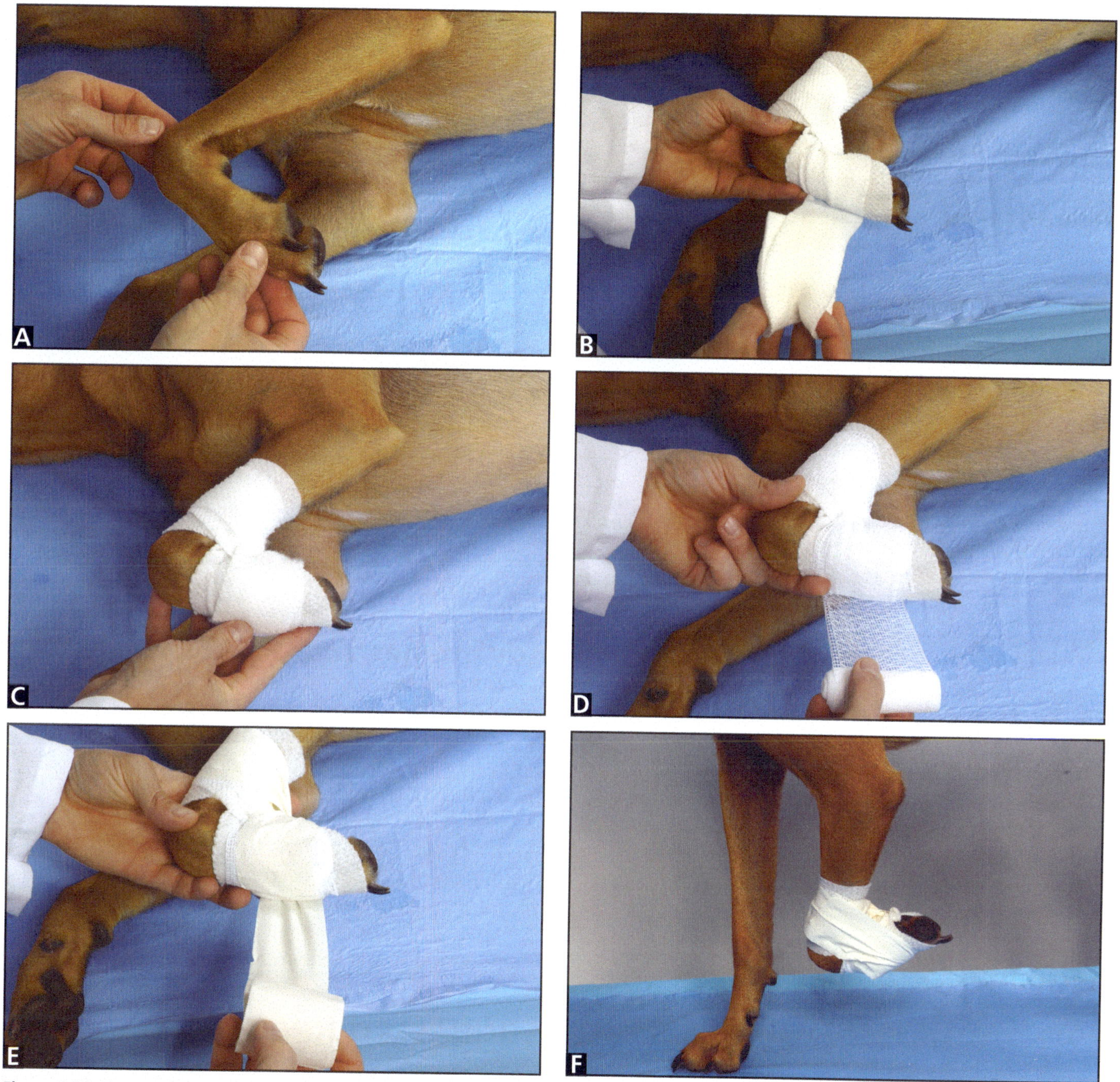


**Figure 2-28.** The Carpal Sling. **A.** Palpating the carpus to assure comfort with flexion. **B. & C.** Carpus is flexed and the paw and distal antibrachium are wrapped with cast padding in a figure-of-eight pattern. **D.** Elastic gauze roll placed over the cast padding. **E.** Two – inch wide porous adhesive tape placed in a figure-of-eight pattern without tension. **F.** Entire bandage is wrapped with two – inch wide porous adhesive tape. Dog standing comfortably with carpus in flexion. (From Swaim SF, Renberg WC, Shike KM: Small Animal Bandaging, Casting and Splinting Techniques. Ames, IA: Wiley – Blackwell: 2011, 76-8)

antibrachium are wrapped with cast padding in a figure – of – eight pattern Figure 2-28B & C). A layer of elastic gauze roll is applied over the cast padding (Figure 2-28D). Two – inch wide porous adhesive tape is applied in a figure – of – eight pattern without tension (Figure 2-28E) and a final wrap of the entire bandage is made with two – inch wide porous adhesive tape Figure 2-28F). The dog should be able to stand comfortably without the sling slipping.

### Aftercare

The dog is observed carefully twice a day to assure that the digits are not swelling and the sling is not slipping. The sling should not be used for longer than two weeks. If the sling is being used to treat paw pad injuries, it may be necessary to remove it periodically to allow wound treatment if the pads are not readily accessable in the sling.

### Advantages and Disadvantages

Movement is important for joint health. This sling allows movement of the shoulder and elbow joint, and thus has an advantage over the Velpeau sling which immobilizes these joints. However, the sling will result in some temporary carpal stiffness after it is removed. A disadvantage of the sling is that the dog may slip the sling off cranially.

## Suggested Readings

1. Swaim SF, Renberg WC, Shike KM: Small Animal Bandaging, Casting and Splinting Techniques. Ames, IA: Wiley – Blackwell: 2011, 43.
2. Canapp SO, Campana DM: Orthopedic coaptation devices and small animal prosthetics. In Tobias KM, Johnston SA, eds.: Veterinary Surgery, Small Animal, Vol. 1: St. Louis: Elsevier – Saunders, 2012, 628.

## Velpeau Sling

### Definition and Indications

The Velpeau sling prevents weight bearing on the forelimb by holding the carpus, elbow and shoulder joint in flexion. The sling can thus be used as an adjunct in the healing of orthopedic and soft tissue injuries of the distal limb and paw.

### Technique

The animal should be awake and in a standing position, being supported by an assistant as it stands on 3 limbs. With the carpus and paw in moderate flexion, cast padding is wrapped around the carpus and paw. This padding should prevent hyperflexion of the paw. Cast padding is then wrapped around the trunk of the dog to cover the flexed forelimb completely. For adequate security the cast padding is alternately wrapped cranial and caudal to the opposite forelimb. The bandage is then wrapped with elastic gauze followed by elastic tape or porous adhesive tape (Figure 2-29). A window can be cut in the lateral surface of the bandage for daily assessment of the digits and paw.

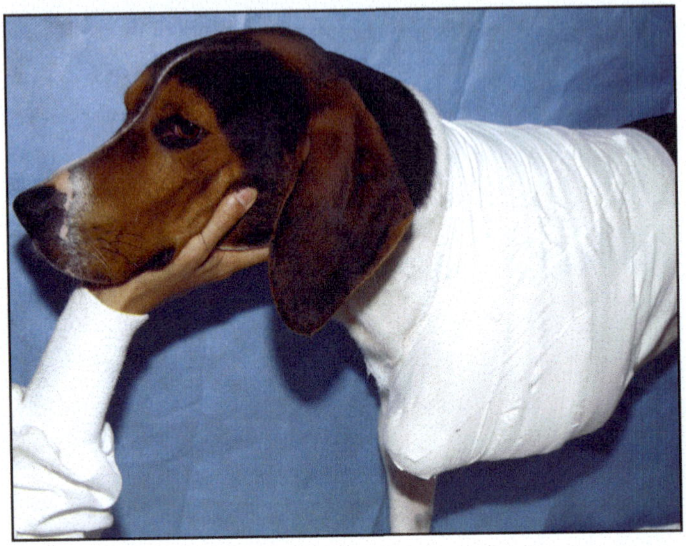

**Figure 2-29.** Velpeau sling in place.

### Aftercare

The sling is observed daily. If the wounds on the distal limb and paw lend themselves to it, it may be possible to treat them through the window cut in the lateral side of the bandage. The animal should be strictly confined while wearing the sling. The owners should be made aware that if the bandage loosens or slips it could cause serious vascular impairment that could result in tissue loss.

### Advantages and Disadvantages

The sling provides a comfortable bandage with few complications. However, abrasions may develop in the opposite axilla if the bandage rubs as the dog walks. It may be necessary to remove some bandage material in the area if this occurs. If the flexed carpus and paw are compressed by elastic gauze or tape, if the sling loosens or slips, or if there is a preexisting vascular obstruction of the paw, necrosis of the skin and underlying structures may result. If the sling is used for more than 2 weeks, joint contracture can occur due to the severe flexion of the forelimb joints.

## Suggested Readings

1. Anderson DA, White RAS: Ischemic bandage injuries: A case series and review of the literature. Vet Surg 29:488, 2000.
2. Canapp SO, Campana DH: Orthopedic coaptation devices and small animal prosthetics. In Tobias KM, Johnston SA, eds.: Veterinary Surgery, Small Animal, Vol. 1: St. Louis: Elsevier – Saunders, 2012, 628.

3. DeCamp CE: External coaptation. *In* Slatter DH, ed.: Textbook of Small Animal Surgery, 3rd ed.: Philadelphia: WB Saunders, 2003, 1835.
4. Johnson AL: Fundamentals of orthopedic surgery and fracture management. In Fossum TW, ed.: Small Animal Surgery, 4th ed.: St. Louis: Mosby, 2013, 1033.
5. Lange DN, Bartels KE: Splinting techniques. *In* Bojrab MJ, ed.: Current Techniques in Small Animal Surgery, 4th ed.: Baltimore: Williams and Wilkins, 1998, 1304.
6. Swaim SF, Renberg WC, Shike KM: Small Animal Bandaging, Casting and Splinting Techniques. Ames, IA: Wiley – Blackwell, 2011, 43.

# 90/90 Sling

## Definition and Indications

The 90/90 sling prevents weight – bearing on the pelvic limb and achieves flexion of the hock and stifle joints. It is indicated for treating orthopedic conditions where these qualities are needed. It could be considered for preventing weight – bearing on a hind paw after significant surgery had been performed on the pads.

## Technique

The dog is placed in lateral recumbency with the affected limb up, and a long length of 2 – inch wide porous adhesive tape is laid along the femoral area as a reserve piece of tape. It is folded so its remaining length lies along the dog's body. The length of tape along the femoral area has the adhesive side up. After folding the tape, the remaining length is adhesive side against the body (Figure 2-30A). This reserve length of tape will be used later in the procedure.

Several layers of cast padding are wrapped around the metatarsal area (Figure 2-30B). Two – inch wide porous adhesive tape is placed on the metatarsal area by placing it on the caudal surface with the adhesive side against the initial wrap (Figure 2-30C). The tape is brought cranially such that the adhesive sides meet cranially and the tape does not completely encircle the metatarsal area (Figure 2-30D). This helps guard against placing the tape too tightly around the metatarsal area.

The hock and stifle are flexed and the tape that was placed around the metatarsal area is brought up the lateral aspect of the femoral area and around the cranial femoral area with the adhesive side against the dog. The tape should cross over the reserve piece of tape lying along the length of the femoral area at a 90 degree angle. The reserve piece should extend four to six inches ventrally past the crossing piece (Figure 2-30E).

The tape coming from the metatarsal area is then taken down the medial aspect of the femoral area and taken around the caudal aspect of the metatarsal area. This passage is repeated to provide two layers (Figure 2-30F).

The ventral end of the reserve piece of tape is folded over to secure its attachment to the tape that started on the metatarsal area (Figure 2-30G). The remaining length of the reserve piece of tape is twisted so the adhesive side is against the dog. It is brought up the femoral area for passage around the dorsum of the dog (Figure 2-30H). The tape is taken down the other side of the dog and around the abdomen (Figure 2-30I). Care is taken in male dogs that the tape does not interfere with the prepuce. The final result is that the dog can stand with the hock and stifle flexed with no weight – bearing on the paw (Figure 2-30J).

## Aftercare

There is an increased chance of causing bandage – related wounds with the 90/90 sling than with other bandages because the skin is thin where it is applied in the caudal abdominal area and tape is applied directly to the skin. Close observation is necessary to watch for slipping of the sling with development of bandage – related wounds. A particular area to observe for pressure wounds is the caudal aspect of the metatarsal area. The sling should be modified immediately or removed if any wounds develop.

Recheck visits to the veterinarian are advised, and the sling should not be left in place longer than 10 to 14 days. Removal may be uncomfortable for the dog because the tape was placed directly on the skin. There are commercial products available to help in the removal of adhesive tape bandages.

After removing the sling, the dog may not use the limb for one or two days due to stiffness of the joints.

## Advantages and Disadvantages

The 90/90 sling is a good means of preventing weight – bearing on a pelvic limb. However, it does not allow range of motion exercises, and it may be prone to causing bandage – related wounds.

# Suggested Readings

1. Swaim SF, Renberg WC, Shike KM: Small Animal Bandaging, Casting and Splinting Techniques. Ames, IA: Wiley – Blackwell: 2011, 43.

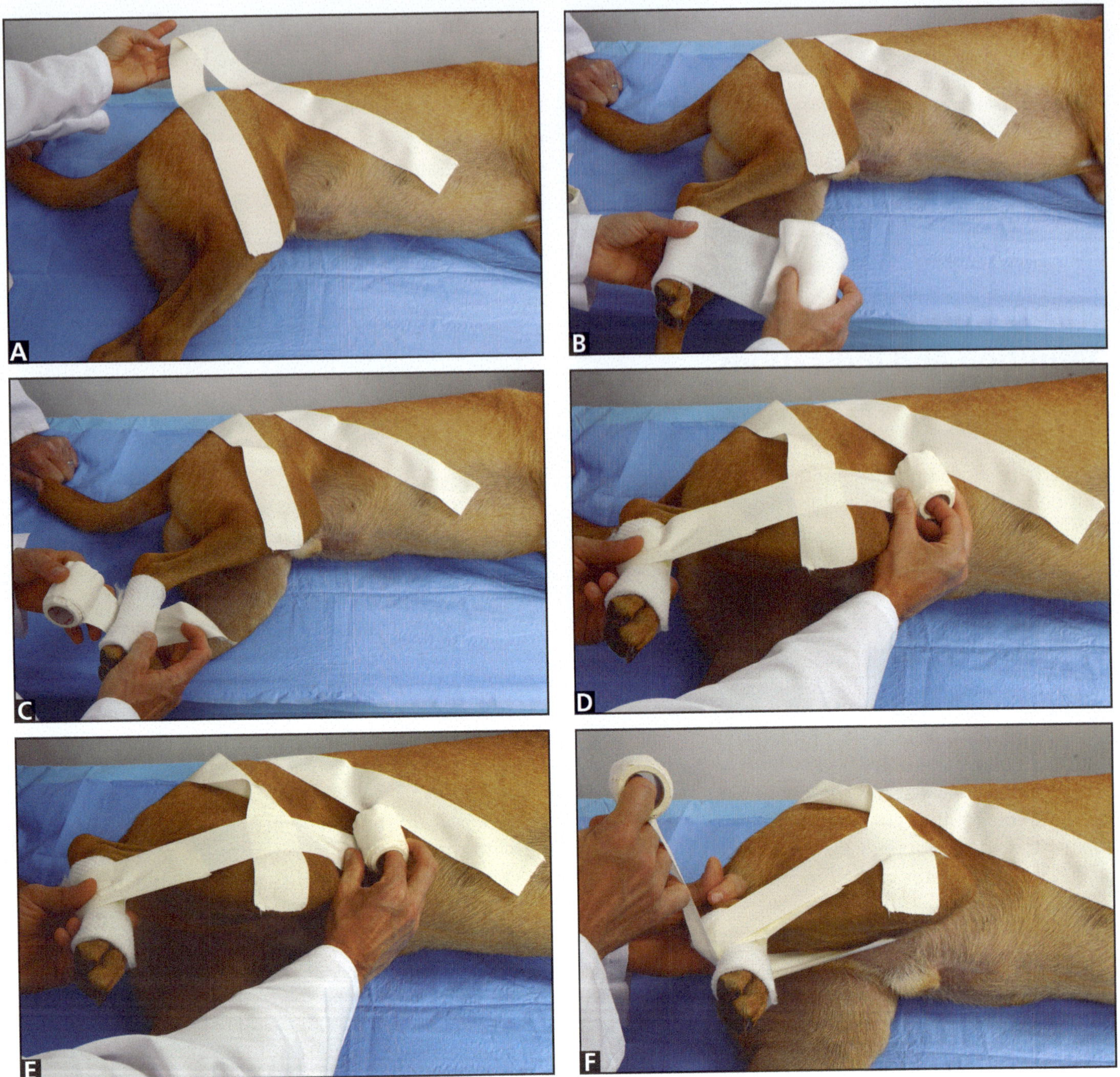

**Figure 2-30.** The 90/90 Sling. **A.** A dog in lateral recumbency with affected limb up. The reserve piece of tape in position – segment adhesive side up along femoral area, segment adhesive side down along body. **B.** Several layers of cast padding are placed around metatarsal area. **C.** Two – inch wide porous adhesive tape being placed on the metatarsal area. The adhesive side is against the caudal metatarsal area. **D.** Tape is brought cranially so adhesive sides meet cranially. **E.** Hock and stifle flexed with tape brought up the lateral aspect of the femoral area. It passes over the reserve piece of tape at a 90 degree angle and around the cranial aspect of the femoral area with adhesive side against the dog. **F.** Tape is brought down the medial side of the femoral area and returned around the caudal metatarsal area. This passage is repeated to give 2 layers.

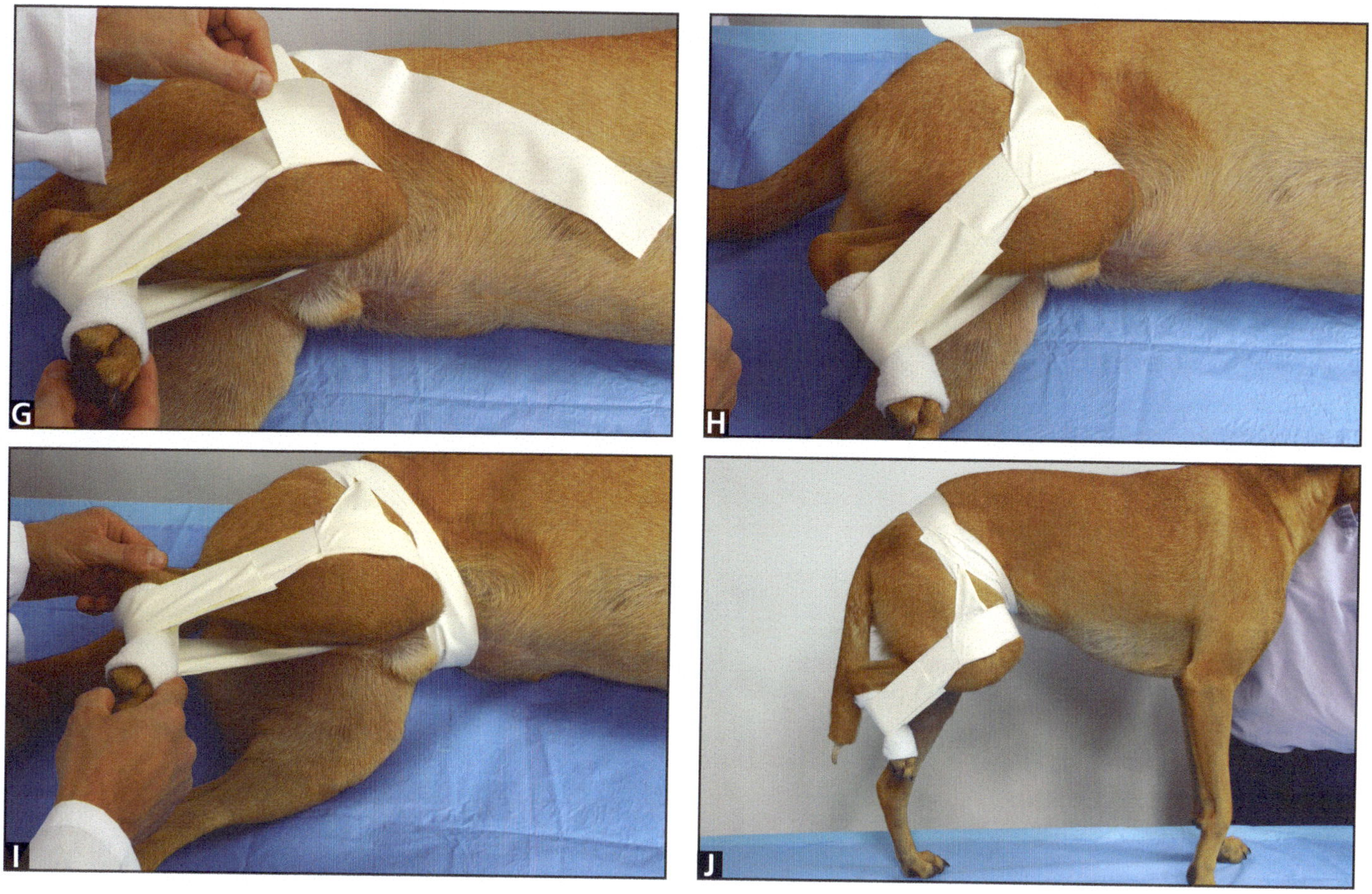

**Figure 2-30.** (continued) **G.** The ventral end of the reserve piece of tape is folded over to secure its attachment to the tape that started on the metatarsal area. **H.** The remaining end of the reserve piece of tape is twisted so the adhesive side is against the dog. It goes up the femoral area and over the dorsum of the dog. **I.** The tape goes down the other side and around the abdomen. **J.** Dog standing with hock and stifle flexed with no weight bearing on the paw. (From Swaim SF, Renberg WC, Shike KM: Small Animal Bandaging, Casting and Splinting Techniques. Ames, IA: Wiley – Blackwell: 2011, 105).

# Chapter 3

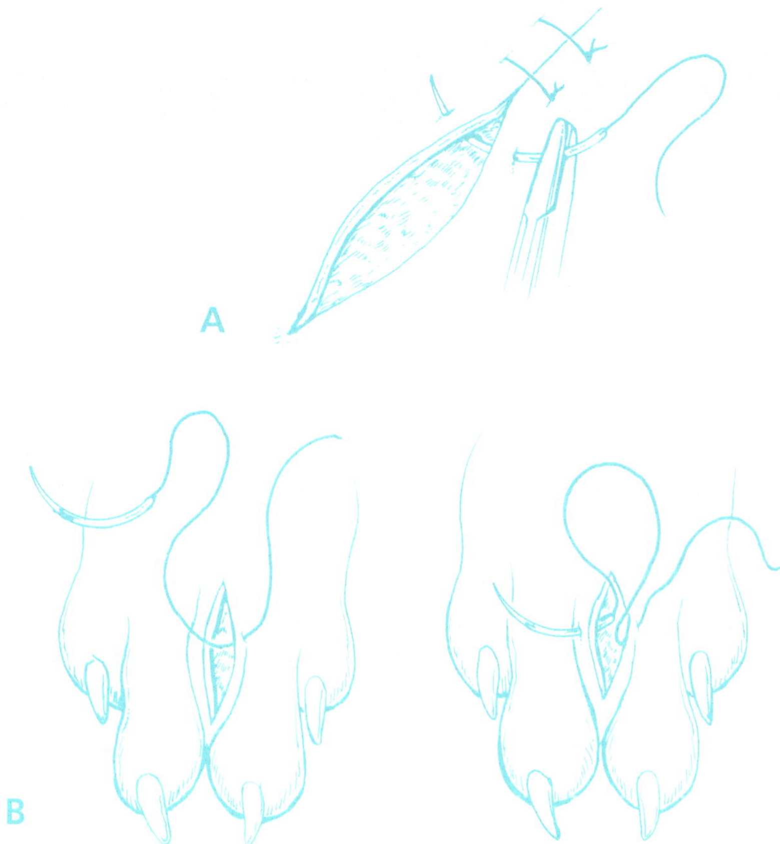


# Carpal-Metacarpal/Tarsal-Metatarsal Wounds

Steven F. Swaim, D.V.M., M.S.

# Primary Wound Closure

## Definition and Indications

Primary wound closure is performed relatively soon after the wound has been inflicted. These wounds are considered clean or clean contaminated wounds. Closure could be within the first 6 hours after infliction. It should be performed when the animal and the wound tissues are in good condition. There should be a minimal amount of contamination and tissue trauma or thorough debridement and lavage should result in tissue suitable for wound closure and the surgeon believes healing will progress uneventfully. Good hemostasis, lack of dead space and closure without tension are other qualities indicating primary closure. A surgical wound created under aseptic conditions is an example of the ideal for primary closure.

### Technique

Thorough lavage, debridement, and when indicated, antimicrobial prophylaxis are part of wound management. Drainage is also indicated when there has been considerable trauma and there is considerable foreign material in the tissues, as often occurs with degloving and crushing degloving wounds on the distal limb (See Drains in this chapter).

Transected tendons can be anastomosed in clean wounds. Large motor nerves that are sharply transected can also be primarily apposed. Usually there is a little subcutaneous tissue present on the distal limb, and buried sutures in this area are generally intradermal. However, depending on the breed and size of the animal, there may be sufficient subcutaneous tissue to allow closure and thus provide support to the wound closure if tension is a factor. Usually, absorbable 3-0 to 4-0 monofilament or multifilament suture material is used. Depending upon the nature of the wound, an interrupted or continuous suture pattern can be used. Care should be used to avoid incorporation of any major vessels, nerves, or tendons in placing sutures. The fewest number of the smallest diameter suture material should be used. The suture material should have minimal adverse effects on the healing process, to include not having the potential for converting a contaminated wound to one that is infected.

Skin closure may be with 2-0 to 4-0 nonabsorbable suture material using one of several suture patterns or skin staples.

### Aftercare

Primarily closed wounds should be observed for 7 to 10 days after closure. When a drain has been used in a primarily closed wound, bandages should be used to protect the wound and drain. The amount and nature of drainage will govern the frequency of bandage change, and these should be assessed at each bandage change. The drain should be removed when the amount of drainage observed in the bandage has decreased to a minimal amount.

## Advantages and Disadvantages

With proper evaluation and management, primarily closed wounds should heal uneventfully within 7 to 10 days. However, hematoma, seroma, and/or infection may result if evaluation, management, and closure have not been properly accomplished. The result is prolonged wound management. Adhesions sometimes form between subcutaneous sutures and underlying tissues, e.g. tendons. This can result in lameness, especially in performance dogs.

If a wound is closed under too much tension, it is possible to create a "biologic tourniquet", whereby the tight skin interferes with circulation. If the limb becomes edematous distal to the closure site, the paw feels hypothermic, and/or the base of the nails appears cyanotic on dogs with light colored nails it indicates a "biologic tourniquet". Suture removal should be considered followed by use of one of the skin stretching techniques, relaxing incisions, or a flap or graft.

# Suggested Readings


1. Bellah JR, Williams JM: Wound closure options and decision making. *In* Fowler D, Williams JM, eds.: BSAVA Manual of Canine and Feline Wound Management and Reconstruction. Shurdington, Cheltenham, UK: BSAVA, 1999, 25.
2. Bohling MW, Swaim SF: Management of the traumatic wound by primary closure. Birchard SJ, Sherding RG, eds.: Saunders Manual of Small Animal Practice, 3rd ed.: St. Louis: Saunders, Elsevier, 2006, 541.
3. Dernell WS: Initial wound management. Vet Clin No Am Small Animal Pract 36: 2006, 713.
4. Hedlund CS: Surgery of the integumentary system. *In* Fossum TW, ed.: Small Animal Surgery, 2nd ed.: St. Louis: Mosby, 2002, 134.
5. Hedlund CS: Surgery of the integumentary system. In Fossum TW, ed.: Small Animal Surgery, 3rd ed.: St. Louis: Mosby, 2007, 159.
6. Hosgood G: Open wounds. In Tobias KM, Johnston SA, eds.: Veterinary Surgery, Small Animal, Vol. 2: St. Louis: Elsevier – Saunders, 2012, 1210.
7. Johnston DE: Care of accidental wounds. Vet Clin North Am, Small Anim Pract 20:27, 1990.
8. MacPhail CM: Surgery of the integumentary system. In Fossum TW, ed.: Small Animal Surgery, 4th ed.: St. Louis: Mosby, 2013, 190.
9. Mason LK: The treatment of contaminated wounds including wounds of the abdomen and thorax. *In* Harari J, ed. Surgical Complications and Wound Healing in the Small Animal Practice. Philadelphia: WB Saunders, 1993, 33.
10. Pavletic MM: Atlas of Small Animal Reconstructive Surgery, 2nd ed.: Phialdelphia: WB Saunders, 1999, 21.

11. Pavletic MM: Atlas of Small Animal Wound Management and Reconstructive Surgery, 3rd ed.: Ames, IA: Wiley – Blackwell, 2010, 31.
12. Swaim SF: Acute superficial soft tissue injuries. *In* Bistner SI, Ford RB, Raffe MR, eds.: Kirk and Bistner's Handbook of Veterinary Procedures and Emergency Treatment, 7th ed.: Philadelphia: WB Saunders, 2000, 257.
13. Swaim SF: Management of the traumatic wound by primary closure. *In* Birchard SJ, Sherding RG, eds.: Saunders Manual of Small Animal Practice, 2nd ed.: Philadelphia: WB Saunders, 2000, 392.
14. Swaim SF, Henderson RA: Small Animal Wound Management, 2nd ed.: Baltimore: Williams and Wilkins, 1997, 13.
15. Waldron DR, Zimmerman-Pope N: Superficial skin wounds.. *In* Slatter DH, ed.: Textbook of Small Animal Surgery, 3rd ed: Philadelphia: WB Saunders, 2003, 259.
16. Williams J: Decision – making in wound closure. In Williams J, Moores A, eds.: BSAVA Manual of Canine and Feline Wound Management and Reconstruction, 2nd ed.: Glouster (UK): BSAVA, 2009, 25.

# Delayed Primary Closure

## Definition and Indications

Delayed primary closure is wound closure between 3 and 5 days after the wound occurs, before granulation tissue forms. These wounds may have heavy contamination, purulent exudates, residual necrotic or questionable tissue, edema, erythema, lymphangitis and skin tension. Thus, they require surgical and medical management to improve the possibility of uncomplicated healing.

## Technique

Wounds as described above should be managed with staged debridement, lavage, topical and/or systemic antibiotics and appropriate bandages. When bandages are changed each day, staged debridement and lavage should be performed to remove obviously devitalized tissue. Questionable tissue is left and evaluated the following day. Topical and systemic medication can be administered. When delayed primary closure is performed, the materials and methods are the same as those used for primary wound closure. A drain should be placed in the wound if there is any concern about the status of the wound tissue at the time of closure.

With wounds of several days duration that are clean, sharp, and uninfected with no devitalized or questionable tissue the wound surface should be cleansed, drains should be placed as needed, and the wound should be closed.

## Aftercare

(See Primary Closure)

## Advantages and Disadvantages

Delayed primary closure allows observation of contused, contaminated or infected tissue and the progression of the early healing process. Staged wound debridement and maximal wound drainage are also advantages of this type of closure. Delayed primary closure of wounds provides better mechanical strength than primary closure, and if it is properly performed, healing is usually complete within 7 to 10 days. However, if procedures are not performed properly, wound infection and disruption may occur resulting in the need for extended wound management.

If closure is too tight a "biologic tourniquet" may result; whereby, the tight skin interferes with circulation. This should be evaluated and managed as described for primary closure.

# Suggested Readings

1. Bellah JR, Williams JM: Wound closure options and decision making. *In* Fowler D, Williams JM, eds.: BSAVA Manual of Canine and Feline Wound Management and Reconstruction. Shurdington, Cheltenham, UK: BSAVA, 1999, 25.
2. Bohling MW, Swaim SF: Management of the traumatic wound by primary closure. In Birchard SJ, Sherding RG, eds.: Saunders Manual of Small Animal Practice, 3rd ed.: St. Louis: Saunders, Elsevier, 2006, 541.
3. Dernell WS: Initial wound management. Vet Clin No Small Animal Pract 36: 2006, 713.
4. Hedlund CS: Surgery of the integumentary system. *In* Fossum TW, ed.: Small Animal Surgery, 2nd ed.: St. Louis: Mosby, 2002, 134.
5. Hedlund CS: Surgery of the integumentary system. In Fossum TW, ed.: Small Animal Surgery, 3rd ed.: St. Louis: Mosby, 2007, 159.
6. Hosgood G: Open wounds. In Tobias KM, Johnston SA, eds.: Veterinary Surgery, Small Animal, Vol. 2: St. Louis: Elsevier – Saunders, 2012, 1210.
7. Johnston, DE: Care of accidental wounds. Vet Clin North Am Small Anim Pract 20:27, 1990.
8. MacPhail CM: Surgery of the integumentary system. In Fossum TW, ed.: Small Animal Surgery, 4th ed.: St. Louis: Mosby, 2013, 190.
9. Mason LK: The treatment of contaminated wounds, including wounds of the abdomen and thorax. *In*: Harari, J. ed.: Surgical Complications and Wound Healing in the Small Animal Practice. Philadelphia: WB Saunders, 1993, 33.
10. Pavletic MM: Atals of Small Animal Reconstructive Surgery, 2nd ed.: Philadelphia: WB Saunders, 1999, 21.
11. Pavletic MM: Atlas of Small Animal Wound Management and Reconstructive Surgery, 3rd ed.: Ames, IA: Wiley – Blackwell, 2010, 31.
12. Shepard GH. The healing of wounds after delayed primary closure: an experimental study. Plast Reconst Surg 48:358, 1971.
13. Swaim SF: Acute superficial soft tissue injuries. *In* Bistner SI, Ford RB, Raffe MR, eds: Kirk and Bistner's Handbook of Veterinary Procedures and Emergency Treatment, 7th ed.: Philadelphia: WB Saunders, 2000, 257.
14. Swaim SF: Management of traumatic wounds by primary closure. *In* Birchard SJ, Sherding RG, eds: Saunders Manual of Small Animal Practice, 2nd ed.: Philadelphia: WB Saunders, 2000, 392.
15. Swaim, SF, Henderson RA: Small Animal Wound Management, 2nd ed.: Baltimore: Williams and Wilkins, 1997, 13.
16. Waldron DR, Zimmerman-Pope N: Superficial skin wounds. *In* Slatter DH, ed.: Textbook of Small Animal Surgery, 3rd ed: Philadelphia: WB Saunders, 2003, 259.
17. Williams J: Decision – making in wound closure. In Williams J, Moores A, eds.: BSAVA Manual of Canine and Feline Wound Management and Reconstruction, 2nd ed.: Glouster (UK): BSAVA, 2009, 25.

# Secondary Wound Closure

## Definition and Indications

Secondary closure of a wound is closure 5 days or longer following wound infliction, when a bed of healthy granulation tissue is starting to form. This type of closure is indicated when it is necessary to leave a wound open longer than 5 days to accomplish adequate management to provide tissue that is suitable for wound closure. Closure of a wound that is well into the repair stage of healing with a well developed bed of granulation tissue is also secondary closure as is closure of a disrupted wound in which granulation tissue has formed.

With the relative sparsity of excess skin on the distal limbs, as granulation tissue develops and matures, movement of adjacent skin for wound closure becomes more difficult than such closure on other areas of the body.

## Technique

Prior to secondary closure, a wound should be managed as an open wound, with staged debridement and lavage at each daily bandage change. Topical and systemic medication can be administered. Beyond the fourth or fifth day following injury, granulation tissue continues to form, the skin edges become increasingly adherent to the underlying tissue, the wound tissue becomes less compliant, and epithelium begins to advance over the granulation surface.

It may be possible to appose and suture the wound edges if there is sufficient skin around the wound to allow closure, the wound is small, and the wound has not progressed too far into the proliferative stage of healing. For such closure, the wound surface should be gently cleansed with a surgical sponge and antiseptic solution or sterile physiologic saline before the wound edges are sutured. Closure should be done before epithelial tissue has begun to advance over the granulation tissue (Figure 3-1).

Wounds on the distal limb that are in the later repair stage of healing should be assessed as to whether secondary closure is the best option for wound closure. If there is sufficient skin surrounding the wound,

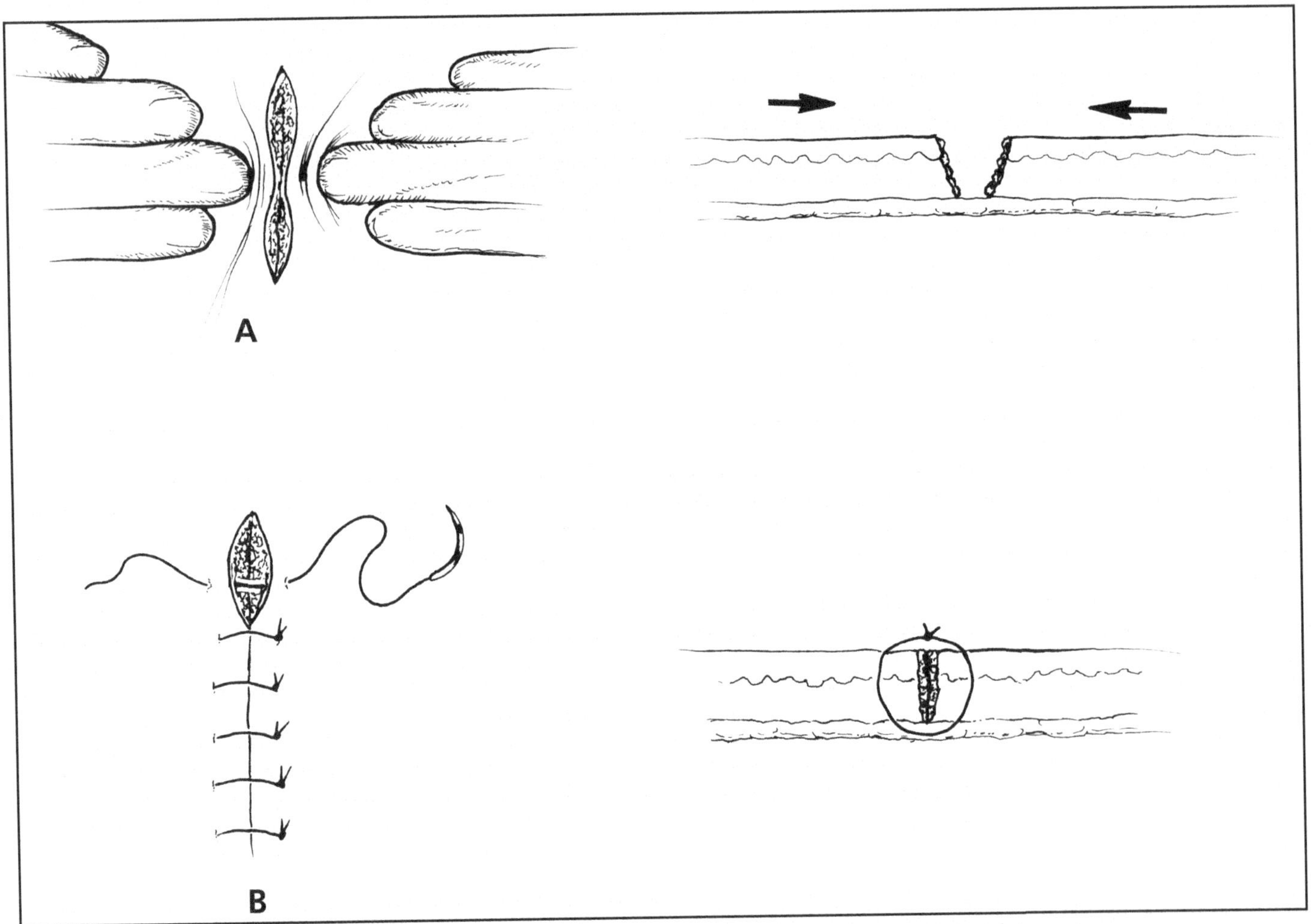


**Figure 3-1.** Secondary closure of a wound. **A.** Manipulation of wound edges to determine if they can be apposed. **B.** Suturing wound edges together with a thin covering of granulation tissue. (After Lee AH, Swaim SF: Granulation tissue: How to take advantage of it in management of open wounds. Compend Contin Educ Pract Vet 10: 166, 1988.)

to allow closure, then secondary closure should be performed. However, if the amount of skin is relatively sparse, but it appears that it could eventually be stretched to cover the wound, skin expanding procedures should be considered for closure.

When a wound is in the later repair stage of healing, the surface should be gently cleansed with an antiseptic solution or physiologic saline on a surgical sponge. An incision is made around the wound at the junction of epithelial tissue with haired skin and the junction of epithelium with granulation tissue. The epithelial tissue at the wound edge is then removed. The skin around the wound is undermined, and the wound edges are advanced and sutured over the granulation tissue (Figures 3-2A-C). If tension is a factor, a continuous intra-dermal suture may be used to help appose the wound edges prior to placement of the skin sutures.

Another technique to close wounds that have a bed of granulation tissue and epithelium at the wound edge is to excise both of these completely. The resulting wound is then closed (Figure 3-2D-E). Wound

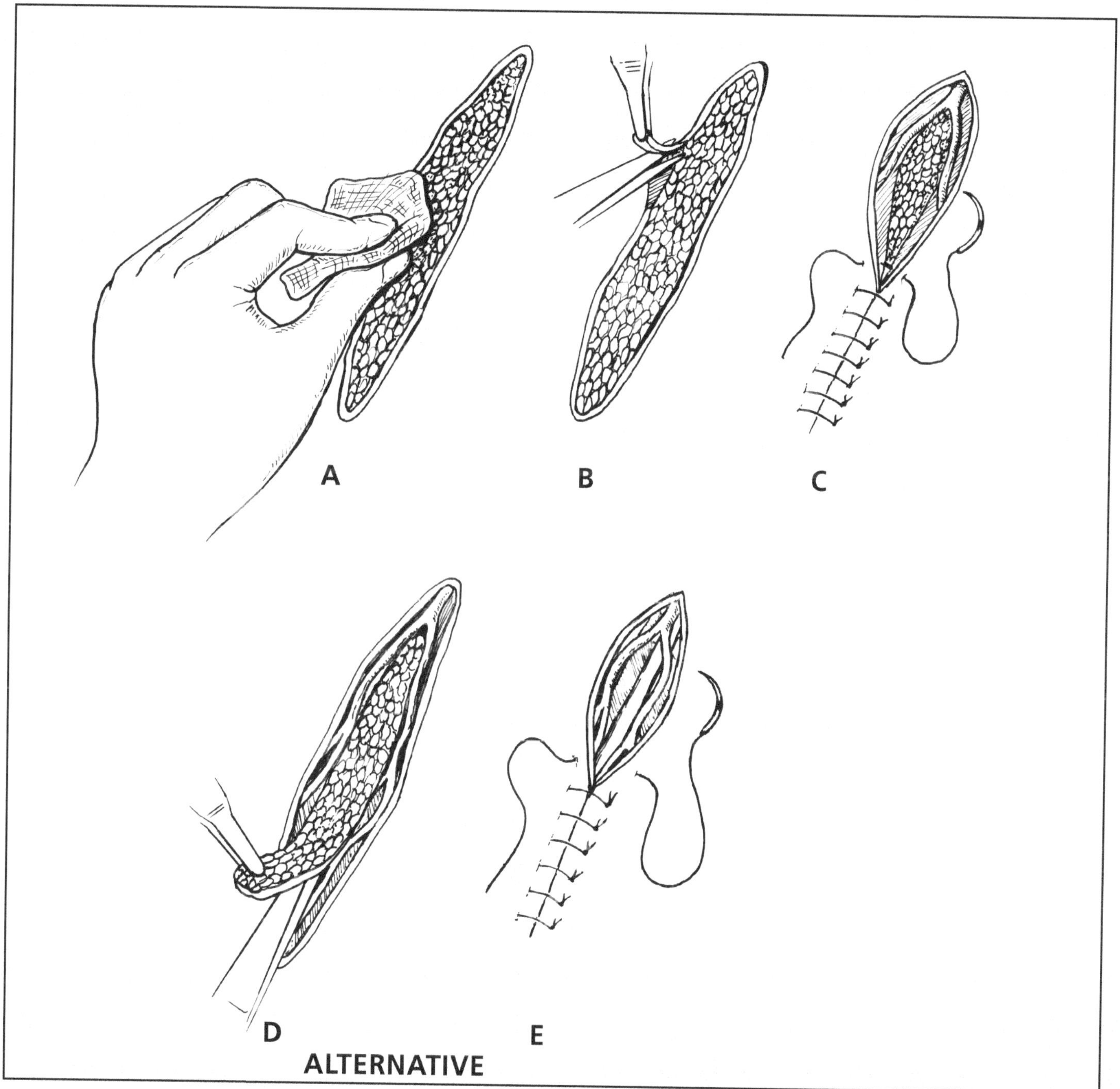


**Figure 3-2.** Closure of a wound in the later repair stage of healing with considerable granulation tissue. **A.** Cleansing the wound surface. **B.** Removing epithelium at the wound edge. **C.** Wound edges being sutured over the granulation tissue. Alternative technique: **D.** Remove epithelium and granulation tissue. **E.** Wound closure after epithelium and granulation tissue removal.

assessment should be performed before performing this kind of closure on the distal limb. The procedure may have some advantages and disadvantages.

A third option for secondary wound closure is use of some type of reconstructive surgical procedure such as a graft or flap. These are used when tension is a factor in wound closure.

When a sutured wound has disrupted, but has already formed a bed of granulation tissue, it may be possible to resuture the wound without disrupting the granulation tissue, provided the granulation tissue is healthy. As with the other forms of secondary closure, the surgeon should assess the condition and availability of tissue in and around the wound before performing the procedure. If the wound is to be resutured, the underlying cause of disruption should be corrected first. These causes include undue tension on the skin edges, use of improper suture material, improper knot tying, poor suturing technique, tissue ischemia and necrosis, hematomas, infection, poor nutritional status of the animal, and retention of foreign material in the wound.

### Aftercare

(See Primary Closure)

### Advantages and Disadvantages

When wound closure is delayed, it helps ensure that all necrotic tissue and infections have been removed and the wound is in the reparative stage. The presence of granulation tissue helps control infection in the wound, and it fills tissue defects. Once closed, healing can then progress without complication, and the gain in tensile strength will occur faster than with primary closure since the wound is already in the reparative stage of healing.

Wound closure in the presence of granulation tissue may be more difficult because the tissue is not as pliable. This is especially so on the distal limbs where skin is also relatively sparse.

Removing the entire granulation tissue bed prior to wound closure can debulk the area, reduce limb diameter and make wound closure easier. However, the presence of underlying vessels, nerves, and tendons could be damaged during dissection. A skin graft or flap would probably be a better option for wound closure.

Suturing the granulating wound edges of a disrupted wound may not be as cosmetic as a primarily closed wound; however, the tensile strength of the wound is attained sooner. With time and maturation, the appearance of the area improves.

If closure is too tight a " biologic tourniquet" may result; whereby, the tight skin interferes with circulation. This should be evaluated and managed as described for primary closure.

## Suggested Readings

1. Bellah JR, Williams JM: Wound closure options and decision making. *In* Fowler D, Williams JM, eds.: BSAVA Manual of Canine and Feline Wound Management and Reconstruction. Shurdington, Cheltenham, UK: BSAVA, 1999, 25.
2. Bohling MW, Swaim SF: Management of the traumatic wound by primary closure. In Birchard SJ, Sherding RG, eds.: Saunders Manual of Small Animal Practice, 3rd ed.: St. Louis: Saunders, Elsevier, 2006, 541.
3. Dernell WS: Initial wound management. Vet Clin No Am Small Animal Pract 36: 2006, 713.
4. Hedlund CS: Surgery of the integumentary system. In Fossum TW, ed.: Small Animal Surgery, 2nd ed.: St. Louis: Mosby, 2002, 134.
5. Hedlund CS: Surgery of the integumentary system. *In* Fossum TW, ed.: Small Animal Surgery, 3rd ed.: St. Louis: Mosby, 2007, 159.
6. Hosgood G: Open wounds. In Tobias KM, Johnston SA, eds.: Veterinary Surgery, Small Animal, Vol. 2: St. Louis: Elsevier – Saunders, 2012, 1210.
7. Johnston DE: Care of accidental wounds. Vet Clin No Small Animal Pract 20: 27, 1990.
8. Lee AH, Swaim SF: Granulation tissue: How to take advantage of it in management of open wounds. Compend Contin Edu Pract Vet 10:163, 1987.
9. MacPhail CM: Surgery of the integumentary system. In Fossum TW, ed.: Small Animal Surgery, 4th ed.: St. Louis: Mosby, 2013, 190.
10. Mason LK: The treatment of contaminated wounds, including wounds of the abdomen and thorax. *In* Harari J, ed.: Surgical Complications and Wound Healing in the Small Animal Practice. Philadelphia: WB Saunders, 1993, 33.
11. Pavletic MM: Atlas of Small Animal Reconstructive Surgery, 2nd ed.: Philadelphia: W B Saunders, 1999, 21.
12. Pavletic MM: Atlas of Small Animal Wound Management and Reconstructive Surgery, 3rd ed.: Ames, IA: Wiley – Blackwell, 2010, 31.
13. Swaim SF, Henderson RA: Small Animal Wound Management, 2nd ed.: Baltimore: Williams and Wilkins, 1997, 13.
14. Waldron DR, Zimmerman-Pope N: Superficial skin wounds.. *In* Slatter DH, ed.: Textbook of Small Animal Surgery, 3rd ed: Philadelphia: WB Saunders, 2003, 259.
15. Williams J: Decision – making in wound closure. In Williams J, Moores A, eds.: BSAVA Manual of Canine and Feline Wound Management and Reconstruction, 2nd ed.: Glouster (UK): BSAVA, 2009, 25.

## Peripheral Nerve Injury and Repair

### Nerve Injury

Peripheral nerve injuries may result from compression, crushing, stretching, laceration or complete transection. These injuries are usually secondary to traumatic events to include motor vehicle accidents, fractures, gunshot wounds, bite wounds, leg-hold trap injuries, lacerations, and occasionally iatrogenic causes (e.g. accidental severance during a surgical procedure). With severe trauma to the distal limb, such as a degloving injury, large sections of nerves may be missing, and it is not possible to identify nerves for repair. In such cases, it should be remembered that studies have shown that collateral innervation grows into areas from adjacent nerves.[5]

## Suggested Readings

1. Diamond J, Foerter A: Recovery of sensory function in skin deprived of its inneration by lesion of the peripheral nerve. Exp Neurol 115:100, 1992.
2. Rodkey WG, Sharp NJH: Surgery of the peripheral nervous system. *In* Slatter DH, ed.: Textbook of Small Animal Surgery, 3rd ed.: Philadelphia: WB Saunders, 2003, 1218.
3. Seim HB: Surgery of the peripheral nerves. *In* Fossum TW, ed.: Small Animal Surgery, 2nd ed.: St. Louis: Mosby, 2002, 1346.
4. Shores A: Peripheral nerve injury and repair. *In* Bojrab MJ, ed.: Current Techniques in Small Animal Surgery, 4th ed.: Baltimore: Williams and Wilkins, 1998, 73.
5. Swaim SF, Bradley DM, Steiss JE, et al: Free segmental paw pad grafts in dogs. Am J Vet Res 54:2161, 1993.

# Nerve Repair

## Definition and Indications

Neurorrhaphy is described in veterinary the literature. However, it is performed infrequently, and with even less frequency in the distal limb areas due to the small diameter of nerves in the area. An example of an instance requiring neurorrhaphy would be damage to a large diameter nerve in the carpal or tarsal area, (i.e. superficial radial nerve or the superficial peroneal or tibial nerve) in a large dog. Identifiable nerve ends and some magnification would be indicated for the procedure.

### Primary Repair

Epineural neurorrhaphy is the anastomosis of the severed nerve ends by placing fine sutures in the epineural connective tissue of the nerve.

### Delayed Repair

Epineural neurorrhaphy is performed on the separated nerve ends just as with primary repair. However, the condition of the nerve and surrounding tissues indicates a delay in performing the neurorrhaphy.

When there has been stretching of a nerve or nerve injury is associated with crushing or is openly contaminated, neurorrhaphy should be delayed until soft tissue infection or contamination has been adequately treated and there is healthy tissue in the area. In addition, the delay allows time for the traumatized nerve to degenerate such that nonviable nerve is demarcated from viable nerve and can be removed prior to neurorrhaphy.

## Techniques

### Primary Repair

Nerves that have been cleanly and sharply severed need minimal debridement and length can be preserved. Magnifying loupes with twofold to sixfold magnification facilitate the surgical procedures because the nerves are small. Microsurgical instruments facilitate accurate neurorrhaphy. These include microsurgical scissors, microneedle holder, fine tipped jewelers forceps, and tissue forceps with microfine teeth.

To debride the nerve, it is carefully wrapped in a soft material such as a Penrose drain, wide umbilical tape, plastic surgical drape, or moistened paper. The wrapping material is held snugly around the nerve with forceps or a surgical clamp, using care not to crush the nerve. This makes the nerve segment to be debrided firm and easily stabilized. The nerve end is placed on a tongue depressor. Transverse cuts are made evenly and accurately across the nerve end with a scalpel or razor blade beginning at the end of the nerve. Each cut is perpendicular to the long axis of the nerve. Accurate debridement is revealed by noting the characteristic fascicular pattern of the nerve (Figure 3-3A). This helps assure that debrided nerve ends make accurate contact at anastomosis. Lint-free neurosurgical sponges or gentle suction are used to remove blood from the nerve ends.

An attempt should be made to appose the transected debrided nerve ends. If there is longitudinal tension, dissection is performed proximally and distally along the nerve to reduce tension. If tension is still present, positioning the distal limb (i.e. flexion or extension) should be attempted to try and relieve tension on the anastomotic site.

The wrapping material is removed from the nerve ends and they are placed on a light-colored soft material (i.e. Penrose drain) to enhance visualization for suturing. The nerve ends are positioned in anatomic contact such that each fascicle in one nerve end aligns with each fascicle in the apposing nerve end. Alignment of longitudinal epineural blood vessels will help in correct fascicle alignment (Figure 3-3B). Neurorrhaphy is performed with 8-0 to 10-0 monofilament, nonabsorbable suture material on a swaged-on fine taper point microsurgical needle. With the nerve ends aligned and apposed, the needle is placed through the epineurium of one nerve end, avoiding inclusion of underlying neural elements. The needle is then passed in like manner in the apposing nerve end and it is tied. A second suture is placed 180° from the first (Figure 3-3C). Long ends are left on these 2 sutures to be used to gently manipulate the nerve for placement of 2 additional sutures 90 degrees to the previous 2 sutures (Figure 3-3D). The suture line is then evaluated for anatomic alignment and security. Additional sutures can be placed if necessary; however, the minimum number of sutures, usually 4 or 5 are used for neurorrhaphy. Any blood clots in the area are removed with moistened lint-free neurosurgical sponges and hemostasis is ensured. Any remaining long suture ends are cut, and the area is lavaged with sterile saline.

### Delayed Repair

When the condition of the wound warrants delayed repair, the wound should be debrided and the severed nerve located. A simple interrupted suture of bright-colored, 5-0 or 6-0 monofilament, nonabsorbable suture material should be placed epineurally between the severed nerve ends to loosely approximate them. The suture should be cut leaving long tags. This prevents retraction of the nerve ends and provide easy identification when definitive repair is done. After early

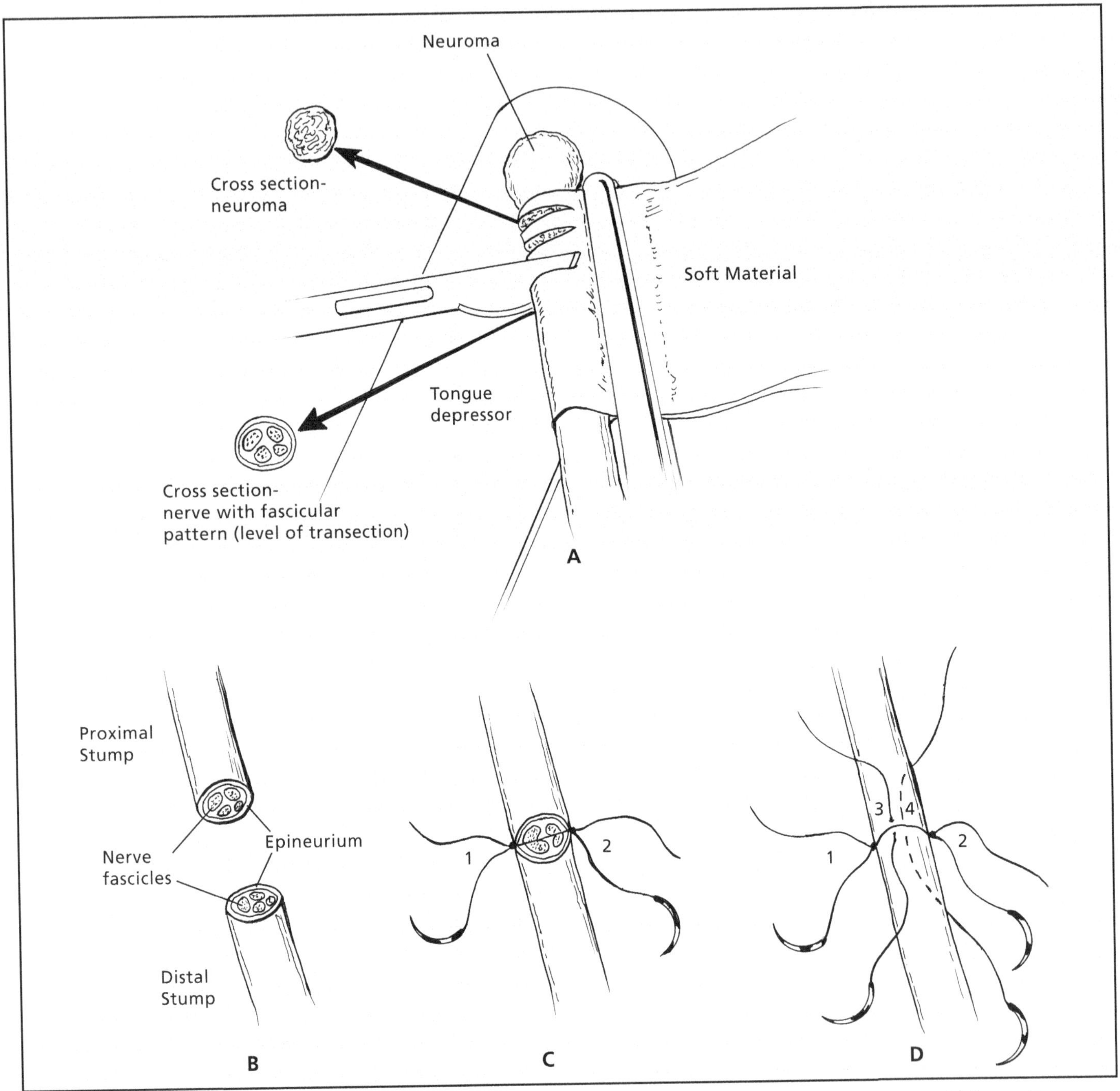


**Figure 3-3.** Epineural neurorrhaphy. **A.** Each nerve end is wrapped with soft material which is carefully secured around the nerve with forceps. The nerve end is placed on a tongue depressor and transverse cuts are made evenly and accurately across the nerve segment. When the characteristic fascicular pattern is noted, the nerve is completely transected. **B.** The nerve ends are laid on a light colored soft material (Penrose drain) with accurate alignment of the fasciles and epineural blood vessels. **C.** Neruorrhaphy is begun with 2, 8-0 to 10-0 monofilament nonabsorbable sutures placed 180 degrees from each other. **D.** The ends of these sutures are left long to manipulate the nerve for placement of the final 2 sutures, 90 degrees from these first 2 sutures. (After Seim HB: Surgery of the peripheral nerves. In Fossum TW, ed.: Small Animal Surgery, 2nd ed.: St. Louis: Mosby, 2002, 1348).

wound management is complete and there is a bed of healthy tissue, the bright-colored suture is used to locate the nerve. Scar tissue is carefully dissected from around the temporary neurorrhaphy site to isolate the nerve and mobilize it. The bright-colored suture is removed and the nerve ends are debrided as described in Primary Repair. Debridement may need to be more extensive than with a clean acute focal neurotmesis because there is a greater chance that the 2 nerve ends may have to be freed by undermining or the limb will have to be positioned by coaptation postoperatively to prevent tension on the neurorrhaphy site.

## Aftercare

### Primary Repair

A padded bandage that provides moderate immobilization should be applied for 1 to 2 weeks in a tensionless neurorrhaphy. However, if there is any tension on the neurorrhaphy or if it was necessary to position the limb to attain a tensionless neurorrhaphy the limb should be rigidly immobilized in a cast for 3 weeks. The cast can be bivalved at the end of the third week. Bandaging should be continued for 2 to 3 more weeks, using half of the bivalved cast for immobilization. During this period of coaptation, exercise should be strictly limited. Following this, the limb is gradually allowed to return to a neutral position. After all bandages are discontinued, a gradual return to normal exercise over 2 to 3 weeks takes place. Physical therapy of affected muscles, tendons, and joints is recommended until signs of reinnervation occur. Therapy includes heat application, muscle massage, tendon stretching and passive range of motion exercises.

It is imperative that the insensitive portion of the lower limb be protected from self-mutilation during the healing time.

### Delayed Repair

(See Primary Repair)

## Advantages and Disadvantages

### Primary Repair

With clean, sharp lacerations healing is generally better than with injuries involving avulsion, crushing, and open chronic wounds. Thus, early neurorrhaphy has the advantages of better healing, reinnervation, and normal end-organ function. Young animals have a much more rapid and complete regeneration of injured nerves than older animals. The best chance of functional nerve regeneration is when regeneration will be within a distance of 10 to 15 cm. Distal limb injuries would fall within this range.

If there is failure of a coaptation device or lack of owner compliance postoperatively disruption of the neurorrhaphy can occur. There can be a neuroma formation at the nerve end, and it may be painful or cause signs of parasthesia, i.e. dog continually licking at the area resulting in a lick granuloma-type lesion. Failure of reinnervation or reinnervation with inadequate function of the end-organ can result.

### Delayed Repair

(See Primary Repair)

## Suggested Readings

1. Platt SR, de Costa RC: Cervical spine. In Tobias KM, Johnston SA, eds.: Veterinary Surgery, Small Animal, Vol.1: St. Louis; Elsevier – Saunders, 2012, 410.
2. Rodkey WG, Sharp NJH: Surgery of the peripheral nervous system. *In* Slatter DH, ed.: Textbook of Small Animal Surgery, 3rd ed.: Philadelphia: WB Saunders, 2003, 1218.
3. Seim HB: Surgery of the peripheral nerves. *In* Fossum TW, ed.: Small Animal Surgery, 2nd ed.: St. Louis: Mosby, 2002, 1346.
4. Shores A: Peripheral nerve injury and repair. *In* Bojrab MJ, ed.: Current Techniques in Small Animal Surgery, 4th ed.: Baltimore: Williams and Wilkins, 1998, 73.

# Wound Drainage

## Open Drainage

### Definition and Indications

There is an adage - the best drain for a wound is an open wound. Open drainage provides maximum drainage from a wound. Such drainage should be a part of open wound management, either prior to wound closure or as part of second intention healing. It is indicated for wounds that are heavily contaminated or infected and/or wounds that are associated with considerable tissue contusion. Many of the wounds on the distal limbs of small animals lend themselves to open drainage.

### Technique

(See Chapter 1)

Wound lavage, debridement, and application of topical medications and bandages are associated with open wound drainage. Drainage can be enhanced by using topical medications and dressings that have a hydrophilic nature or that are highly absorbent, e.g. sugar, honey, Maltodextrin N.F.-D-glucose polysaccharide (Intracell, Macleod Pharmaceuticals, Ft. Collins, CO), hydrolyzed bovine collagen (Cellerate RX, Wound Care Innovations, Ft. Lauderdale, FL), or polyurethane foam dressing (Hydrasorb, Foam Sponge, Covidien, Tyco/ Health Care/ Kendall, Mansfield, MA). These medications and dressings with hydrophilic properties tend to draw fluids up through wound tissues bathing the wound from the inside with the body's homeostatic fluids. Because the wound is open, these fluids are then absorbed into overlying bandage material.

### Aftercare

Periodic bandage change should be done when using open wound drainage. In the inflammation and debridement stages, when fluid production is copious, bandage changes should be at least daily. At the time of bandage change, staged debridement and wound lavage are performed. As healing progresses and fluid production decreases, bandage changes become less frequent. If open drainage is being used in conjunction with delayed primary or secondary closure, these procedures are performed when the surgeon believes the tissues are healthy enough for closure.

### Advantages and Disadvantages

The primary advantage of open drainage is the maximal drainage of wound fluids from the contaminated or infected wound. This helps assure that no pockets of infection develop. Open drainage also assists in the rapid progression of the wound into the repair stage of healing. When hydrophilic dressings or medications are being used in conjunction with systemic antibiotics, the fluid being drawn up through wound tissues is antibiotic laden. A potential disadvantage of open drainage could be secondary contamination of the wound if an animal removes a bandage and the wound becomes heavily contaminated, e.g. fecal contamination.

## Suggested Readings

(See suggested readings for Polyurethane Foam Sponges, Maltodextrin N.F., (D – glucose polysaccharide), Sugar, Honey and Collagen Products).

## Passive Drains

### Definition and Indications

Passive drains function by utilizing the principles of pressure differentials, overflow, and gravity. Tissue movement and pressure bandages also assist in the function of passive drains. Such drains provide an egress path of least resistance to the surface of a wound as the majority of fluid drains along the outer surface of the drain. On the distal limb, they are used in the treatment of bite wounds, lacerations, skin avulsions or separations, seromas, or abscesses. An absorbent bandage is usually placed over the exterior portion of such drains to absorb drained fluids. The most applicable passive drain for small animal distal limbs is the soft, thin, radiopaque, cylindrical latex rubber drain (Penrose drain). The most applicable drain size for distal limb wounds is the ¼-inch diameter drain. For small wounds or wounds on the distal limbs of small dogs and cats, a strip of rubber can be cut lengthwise from a ¼-inch diameter Penrose drain to place in the wound (Figure 3-4).

Wound drainage is indicated 1) when there is an abscess or other established area of fluid accumulation; 2) when foreign material or tissue of questionable viability cannot be excised; 3) when massive wound contamination is inevitable; and 4) when it is necessary to prevent the accumulation of blood, exudate, serum or air in a dead space or potential dead space. A common indication for drainage on the distal limb is the degloving injury where a flap of skin has been reflected off of the underlying tissue (Figure 3-5, & See Figure 1-10). Vigorous debridement of debris from the dermal side of the flap is not feasible since blood supply to this flap of skin is located in the subcutaneous tissue. Therefore, a drain is used under the flap.

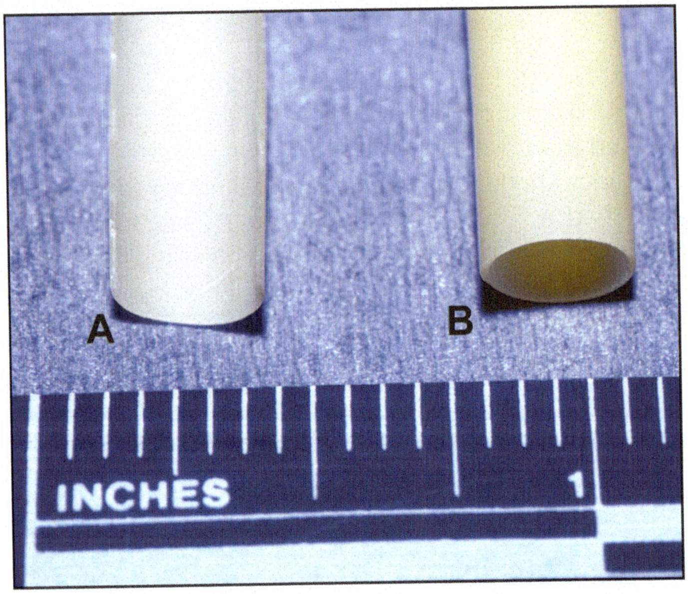


**Figure 3-4.** Passive drains for distal limb wounds. **A.** Strip drain made by cutting one side out of a ¼-inch diameter Penrose drain. **B.** One quarter inch diameter Penrose drain.

### Techniques

#### Single-exit drain

Fenestrations are not usually cut in flat (Penrose) drains. Fenestrations do not improve their drainage capacity, and they could weaken the drain making it subject to tearing. The fewest number and smallest diameter of drains should be used and the fewest number of gravitationally dependent exit holes should be made in the skin.

The entire distal limb should be clipped and prepared

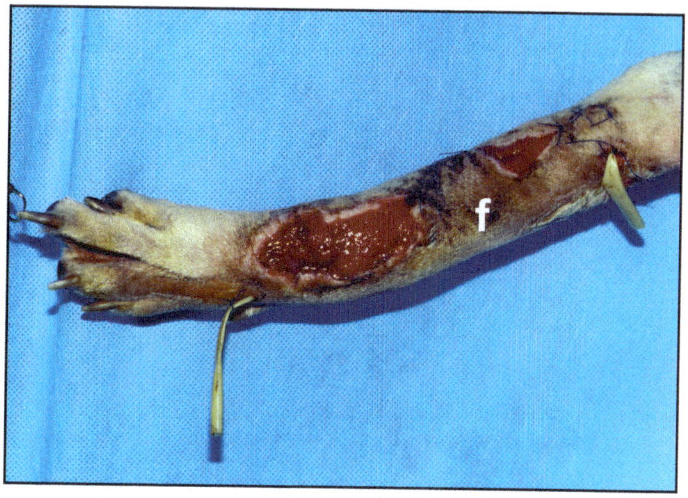


**Figure 3-5.** A Penrose drain placed under a skin flap *(f)* after the flap had been replaced in position.

aseptically to avoid accumulation of any drainage fluid in the hair. This especially includes all interdigital and palmar/plantar interpad areas.

The length of the drain placed in the wound should be noted in the animal's record. This can be compared with the length of drain that is removed to ensure that the entire length has been removed. Drains should be secured in a wound so that they cannot be prematurely removed or cannot retract into the wound.

With an open wound, the proximal end of the drain is placed in the most proximal area of the wound and, if possible off to one side so that it does not lie directly under the suture line. A simple interrupted suture of 3-0 nonabsorbable monofilament suture material is passed through the skin, through the drain's proximal end, and back through the skin. As the suture is tied, it anchors the proximal end of the drain in place. Long tags can be left on this suture to identify it as the drain-anchor suture. When the drain is removed, the suture is cut to free the proximal end of the drain (Figure 3-6).

Drains should be placed parallel to the long axis of the limb, i.e. vertically, to obtain maximum flow by gravity.

At the distal end of the wound, drains should exit through a stab incision at least 1 cm from the primary incision to prevent incisional dehiscence. Curved hemostatic forceps are used to make a tunnel between the distal aspect of the wound and a point just under the skin approximately 1 cm distal to the distal aspect of the wound. With the tips of the forceps directed outward and slightly separated, a scalpel blade is used to incise the skin between the forcep's blades. The incision should be large enough to allow the drain to exit with sufficient opening around the drain to allow wound drainage. The distal end of the drain is pulled through this opening and is sutured to the edge of the opening with a simple interrupted nonabsorbable suture. The wound is then sutured (Figure 3-7). Contact between the drain and the skin suture line should be avoided; thus, when a drain is placed, it may be directed to one side of the wound so it does not lie directly under the suture line. Subcutaneous tissue, if present, can be sutured over the drain to separate it from the skin suture line. Because of the small diameter of the distal limb and sparsity of subcutaneous tissue, these maneuvers to avoid contact of the drain with the suture line may be difficult, and a combination of the two may be helpful in accomplishing the task. When subcutaneous and skin sutures are placed, care should be taken that they do not incorporate the drains. If suture(s) incorporate a drain, drain removal is not possible until the sutures are removed.

If there is sufficient subcutaneous tissue present on the distal limb to allow its closure over a drain, the following technique can be used to prevent drain incorporation in the suture line. The drain is placed in the wound via the distal drain hole. The proximal end of the drain is placed at the desired level in the wound,

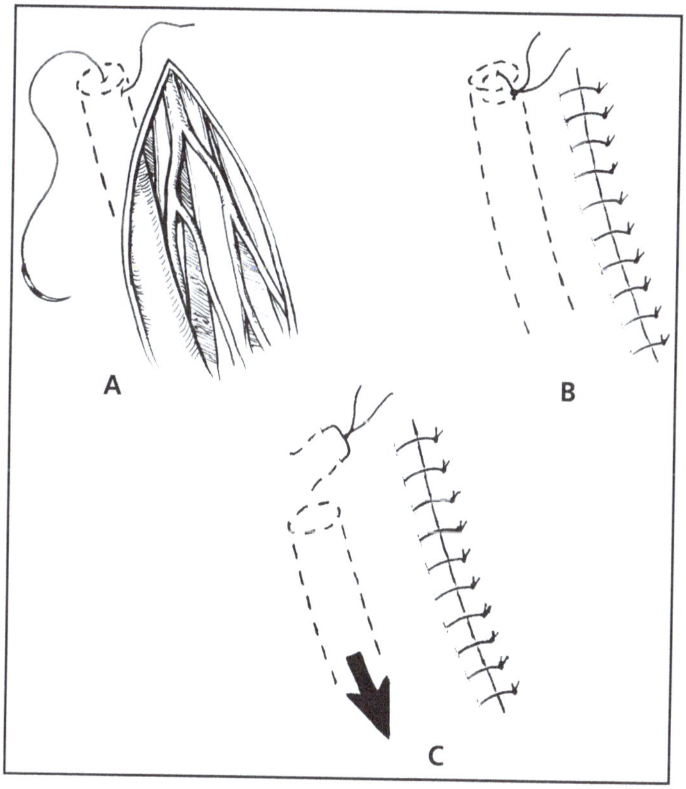


**Figure 3-6.** Anchoring the end of a drain in the proximal end of a wound. **A.** One end of the drain is placed in the proximal end of the wound and off to one side. A nonabsorbable simple interrupted anchor suture is placed through the skin, the end of the tube, and back through the skin. **B.** The anchor suture is tied, leaving long tags and the wound is closed. **C.** At the time of drain removal, the anchor suture is cut and the drain is removed *(arrow)*. (After Bohling MW, Swaim SF: Bandaging and drainage techniques. In Bojrab MJ, ed.: Current Techniques in Small Animal Surgery, 5th ed.: Jackson, WY: Teton NewMedia, (in press).

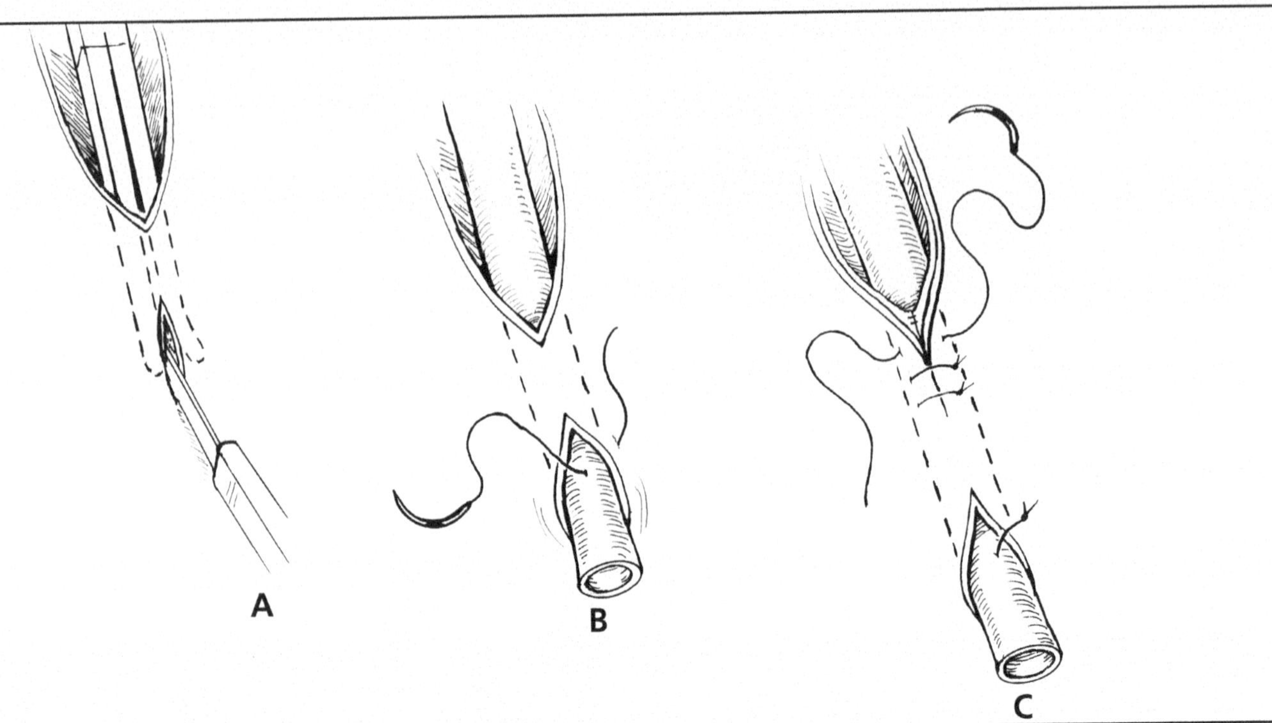


**Figure 3-7.** Placing the distal end of a drain. **A.** Hemostats are tunneled subcutaneously near the distal end of the wound and an incision is made over their tips. **B.** The distal end of the drain is pulled through the incision. It is anchored with a simple interrupted suture. **C.** Wound closure with closure of subcutaneous tissue over the drain if possible. (After Bohling MW, Swaim SF: Bandaging and drainage techniques. In Bojrab MJ, ed.: Current Techniques in Small Animal Surgery, 5th ed.: Jackson, WY : Teton NewMedia, (In press).

and the point where the drain exits the distal drain hole is marked on the drain. The drain is then pulled out the proximal end of the wound. As a result the mark on the drain at the distal drain hole is pulled into the wound. The subcutaneous tissue is then sutured. After every 2 to 3 suture bites, both ends of the drain are grasped, and the drain is pulled back and forth to ascertain if any suture bite has incorporated the drain. If the drain does not move freely it indicates suture incorporation, and the previous 2 to 3 sutures can be removed and replaced. Once all sutures are placed and the drain moves back and forth freely in the wound, traction is placed on the distal end of the drain to pull the proximal end within the wound and replace the previously placed mark on the drain at the level of the distal drain hole. The skin can then be closed without danger of incorporating the drain since it is protected by subcutaneous tissue. At the level of the proximal end of the drain, a deep simple interrupted skin suture can be placed in such a manner as to incorporate the end of the drain. When it is tied, it anchors the drain in the proximal end of the wound. Long tags are left on this suture to identify it as the anchoring suture. The distal drain anchoring suture can then be placed (Figure 3-8). The same technique can be used when only the skin is being sutured; however, it may not be necessary since the skin edges may be observed more closely in relation to the drain as sutures are placed.

A retrieval suture can be placed in the proximal end of a drain to help assure removal of the proximal end of a drain as it is pulled from a wound. A nonabsorbable suture with a swaged needle is passed through one end of a Penrose drain. A knot is tied in the suture against the drain such that the end of the suture without the needle ("tail" of the suture) is approximately 2 to 3 cm longer than the length of drain to be placed in the wound (Figure 3-9A). The end of the drain with the attached retrieval suture is placed at the proximal end of the wound. The needle on the retrieval suture is passed through the skin at this area, and the suture with the attached proximal end of the drain is pulled up under the dermal surface of the skin. A simple interrupted suture of nonabsorbable material is placed in the skin near the emergence point of the retrieval suture. The retrieval suture is tied to one of the tags on this suture, and the segment of suture with the needle is removed (Figure 3-9B). The drain and "tail" of the retrieval suture are placed within the wound and out through the exit hole distal to the distal end of the wound (Figure 3-9C). The wound is closed and the distal end of the drain is anchored as previously described. At the time of drain removal, the simple interrupted proximal anchor suture is removed as is the distal anchor suture. The distal end of the drain and retrieval suture are pulled distally for drain removal (Figure 3-9D).

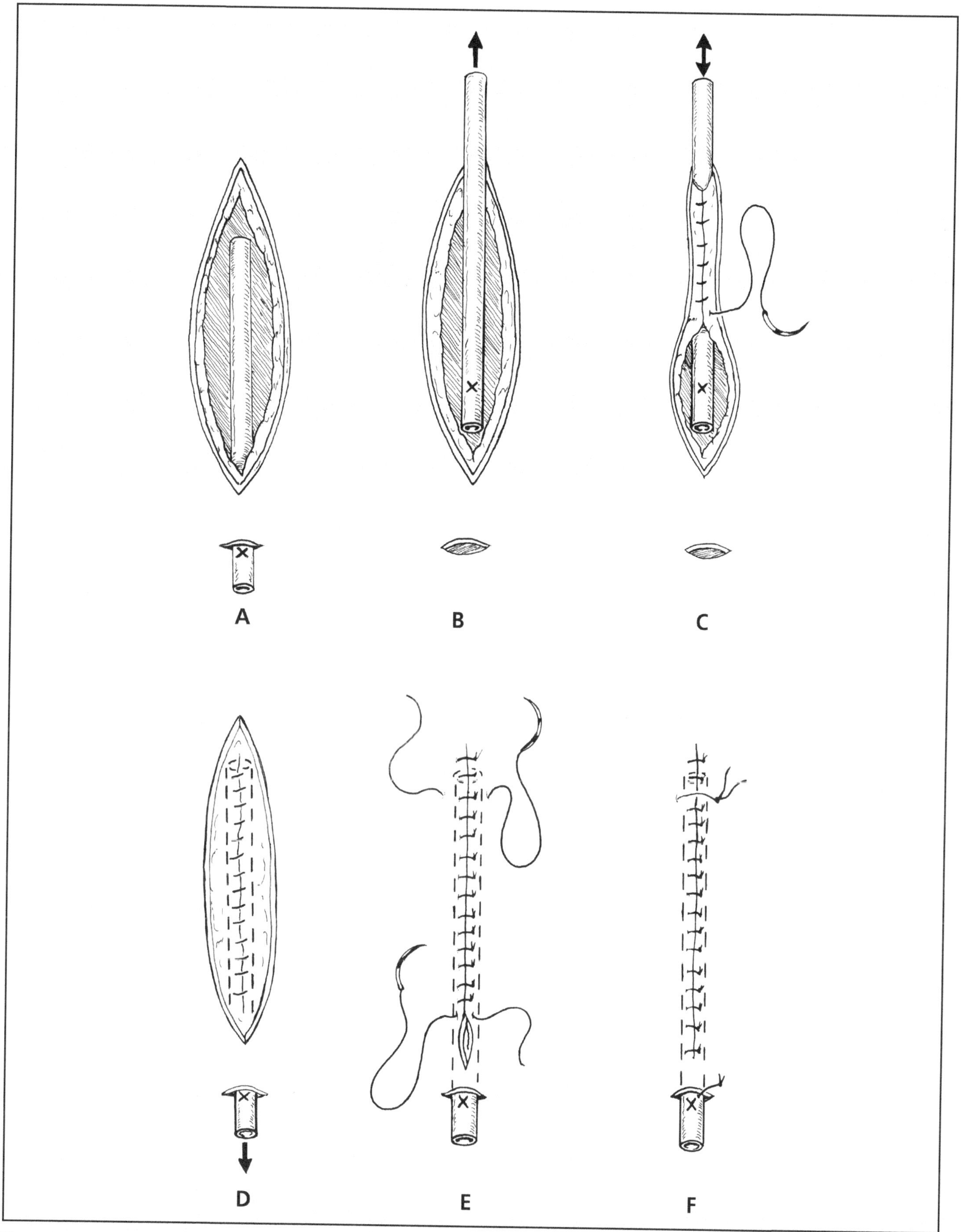


**Figure 3-8.** Prevention of drain incorporation in the suture line. **A.** Drain placed in wound via distal drain hole, with the proximal end of the drain at the desired level in the wound. Point of exit is marked on distal drain end "x". **B.** Drain is pulled out the proximal end of the wound. **C.** Subcutaneous tissue is sutured with periodic movement of the drain to assure no suture is through the drain. **D.** Subcutaneous tissue is closed and the distal drain end is pulled out drain hole to the "x". **E & F.** Skin closure and suture placement to anchor the proximal and distal ends of the drain.

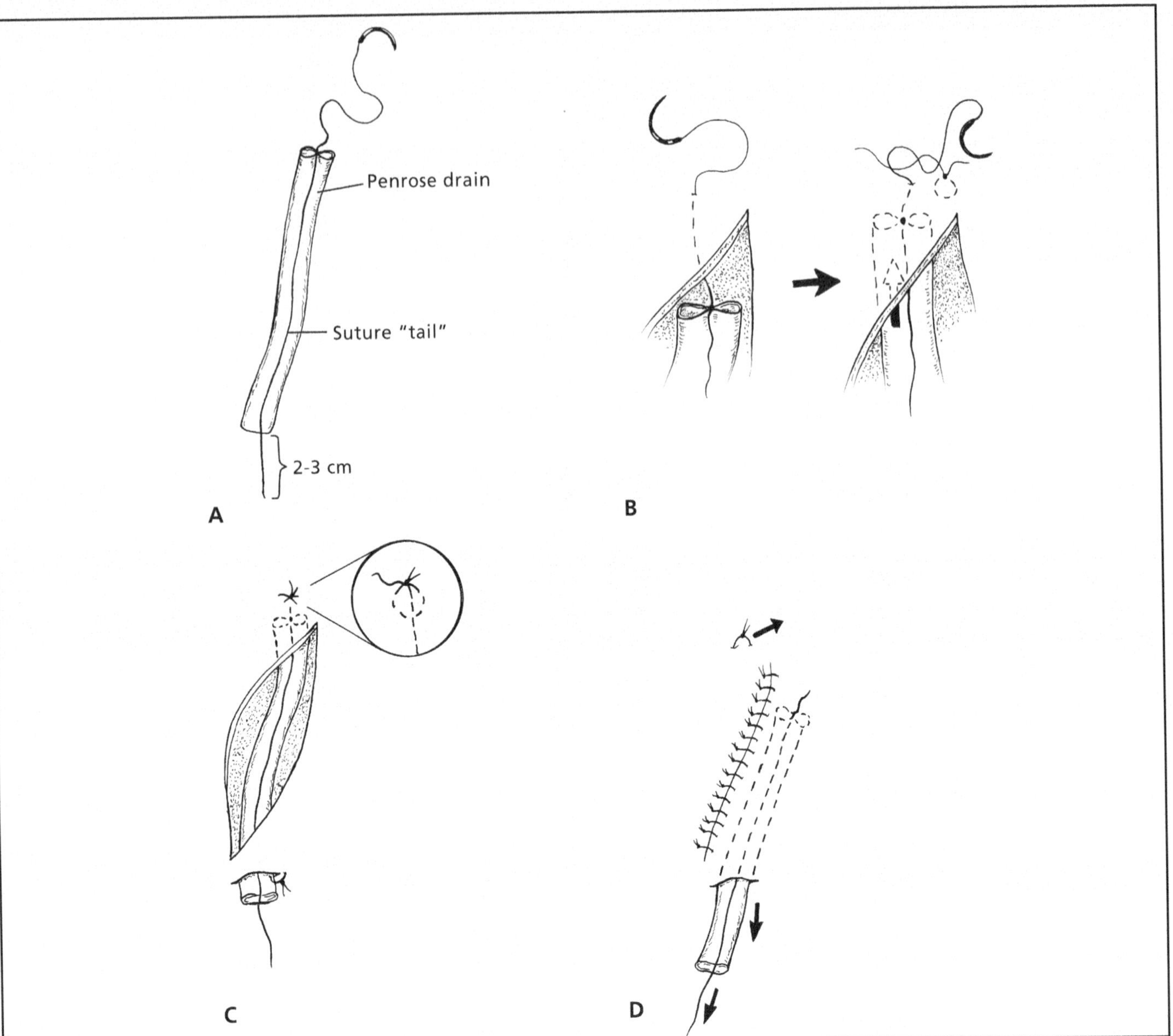


**Figure 3-9.** Placing a retrieval drain. **A.** A nonabsorbable suture is placed in the end of a Penrose drain. A length of suture is left on the unneedled end of the suture (*"tail"*) which is 2-3 cm longer than the drain to go in the wound. **B.** The needled end of the suture is passed through the skin adjacent to the proximal wound end and tied to one tag of a simple interrupted anchor suture in the area. **C.** Proximal end of the drain is fixed in place. On the skin surface is a suture knot with 3 tags. (2 with anchor suture and one with retrieval suture.) Distal end of drain and suture *"tail"* emerge at opening distal to distal wound end. **D.** Drain is removed by distal traction on drain and retrieval suture *"tail"* (*arrows*) after the anchoring suture is cut.

## Double-exit drain

Ports of exit are made near both the proximal and distal ends of the wound. To prevent suture incorporation of a drain, a similar technique to that described for a single exit drain can be used. However, the drain is pulled back and forth at its point of emergence from the proximal and distal drain holes.

# Aftercare

An antibiotic ointment is placed over the drain exit ports. However, it should not be sufficient in amount to obstruct the drain exit hole. This is followed by placing sterile wide-mesh absorbent gauzes over the end of the drain. The capillary action of the gauze supplements the action of the drain. An absorbent secondary bandage wrap is placed over the gauzes, followed by a porous adhesive tape or elastic outer wrap. The wound and drain are protected from molestation by the bandage, and at removal the amount and nature of the drainage can be assessed by examining the bandage. A wire basket muzzle or an Elizabethan collar may be needed for further protection from molestation.

The bandage should be changed at least daily, and the area around the drain exit should be cleansed with an antibacterial solution. The amount and nature of drainage fluid will determine when the drain should be removed. When infection is present, the discharge will be exudative at first, and become transudative serosanguinous in nature with the amount decreasing as healing progresses. The drain can be removed when the drainage has decreased to a small amount, and it remains about the same in amount and consistency from one bandage change to the next.

To remove a drain, all skin-drain tacking sutures are removed. For double-exit drains, the proximal end of the drain protruding beyond the exit hole is cut off flush with the skin. Thus, as traction is placed on the distal end of the drain and the drain is pulled through the drain tract, the possibility of contaminating the tract is reduced. Once removed, the drain should be examined to confirm that all of it has been removed. To remove a drain with a retrieval suture, the proximal end of the retrieval suture is cut where it emerges through the skin. The simple interrupted suture it is tied to is removed. The distal anchoring suture in the drain is cut, and traction is placed on the distal end of the drain and the "tail" of the retrieval suture to remove it from the wound. The "tail" of the retrieval suture helps assure that the proximal end of the drain is removed from the wound.

Double-exit drains are usually used in highly contaminated or infected wounds. Antibiotics or antiseptics can be used to lavage the wound from the proximal tube emergence site. However, caution should be taken not to flush the drain with a large amount of fluid over a long time. This could interfere with the wound healing process.

## Advantages and Disadvantages

Penrose drains are easily sterilized, and they are readily available. They are malleable and do not exert pressure on adjacent blood vessels or other structures, which is an advantage on the distal limb where there is an abundance of vessels, nerves, tendons and ligaments closely subjacent to the skin.

Lavaging a wound from the proximal tube emergence site of a double-exit drain exposes the length of the wound tract to the lavage solution. However, if the solution only follows the path of least resistance, the drain tract, it will not reach the branching crevices of the wound.

Bacterial ascension along a drain and decreasing resistance to bacterial colonization are potential disadvantages of all drains. The proximal incision for a double exit drain has been stated to provide a portal for retrograde contamination.

If an animal molests a drain, it may be removed before it has accomplished its purpose, or it may tear off leaving part of the drain in the wound. If a drain tears at the time of removal, the length of the removed section can be compared to the original drain length to determine how much is retained. Radiography can be used to ascertain whether any of a radiopaque Penrose drain is still in a wound. Surgical intervention is required to remove any remaining parts of a torn drain.

# Suggested Readings


1. Baines SJ: Surgical drains. *In* Fowler D, Williams JM, eds.: BSAVA Manual of Canine and Feline Wound Management and Reconstruction. Shurdington, Cheltenham, UK: BSAVA, 1999, 47.
2. Bohling MW, Swaim SF: Bandage and drainage techniques. In Bojrab MJ, ed.: Current Techniques in Small Animal Surgery, 5th ed.: Jackson, WY: Teton NewMedia 2014, 13.
3. Campbell BG: Bandages and drains. In Tobias, KM, Johnston SA, eds.: Veterinary Surgery, Small Animal, Vol. 1: St. Louis: Elsevier – Saunders, 2012, 221.
4. Dernell WS: Initial wound management. Vet Clin No Am Small Animal Pract 36: 2006, 713.
5. Fox JW, Golden GT: The use of drains in subcutaneous surgical procedures. Am J Surg 132:673, 1976.
6. Golousky D, Conolly WB: Observations on wound drainage with a review of the literature. Med J Aust 1:289, 1976.
7. Hak DJ: Retained broken wound drains: A preventable complication. J Orthop Trauma 14:212, 2000.
8. Hampel NL: Surgical drains. *In* Harari J, ed.: Surgical Complications and Wound Healing in the Small Animal Practice. Philadelphia: WB Saunders, 1993, 319.
9. Hampel NL, Johnson RG: Principles of surgical drains and drainage. J Am Animal Hosp Assoc 21:21, 1985.
10. Hedlund CS: Surgery of the integumentary system. *In* Fossum TW, ed.: Small Animal Surgery, 2nd ed.: St. Louis: Mosby, 2002, 134.
11. Hedlund CS: Surgery of the integumentary system. In Fossum TW, ed.: Small Animal Surgery, 3rd ed.: St. Louis: Mosby, 2007, 159.
12. Hosgood G: The history of surgical drainage. J Am Vet Med Assoc 196:42, 1990.
13. Ladlow J: Surgical drains in wound management and reconstructive surgery. In Williams J, Moores A, eds.: BSAVA Manual of Canine and Feline Wound Management and Reconstruction, 2nd ed.: Glouster (UK): BSAVA, 2009, 54.
14. Lee AH, Swaim SF, Henderson RA: Surgical drainage. Compend Contin Educ Pract Vet 8:94, 1986.
15. MacPhail CM: Surgery of the integumentary system. In Fossum TW, ed.: Small Animal Surgery, 4th ed.: St. Louis: Mosby, 2013, 190.
16. Miller CW: Bandages and drains. *In* Slatter DH, ed.: Textbook of Small Animal Surgery, 3rd ed. Philadelphia: WB Saunders, 2003, 244.
17. Morrow LL: No more lost drain tubes. Vet Forum 19:28, 2002.
18. Pavletic MM: Atlas of Small Animal Reconstructive Surgery, 2nd ed.: Philadelphia, WB Saunders, 1999, 21.
19. Pavletic MM: Atlas of Small Animal Wound Management and Reconstructive Surgery, 3rd ed.: Ames, IA: Wiley – Blackwell, 2010, 51.
20. Roush JK: Use and misuse of drains in surgical practice. Probs in Vet Med. 2:482, 1990.
21. Scardino MS, Swaim SF: Wound drainage techniques. *In* Bojrab MJ, ed.: Current Techniques in Small Animal Surgery, 4th ed.: Baltimore: Williams and Wilkins, 1998, 34.
22. Swaim SF: Acute soft tissue injuries. *In* Bistner SI, Ford RB, Raffe MR, eds.: Kirk and Bistner's Handbook of Veterinary Procedures and Emergency Treatment, 7th ed.: Philadelphia: WB Saunders, 2000, 257.
23. Swaim SF, Henderson RA: Small Animal Wound Management, 2nd ed.: Baltimore: Williams and Wilkins, 1997, 13.

# Wounds with Apposable Edges - No Tension

## Planning Wound Closure on the Distal Limbs

### General Information

The patient's skin, surgeon's hands and imagination as well as instruments can be used to plan the closure of an existing wound (e.g. traumatic wound) or a proposed wound (e.g. the wound resulting after removal of a tumor, localized infection or granulomatous lesion). Planning wound closure is indicated so the proper technique(s) can be decided upon.

Planning should be done with the animal unsedated; however, if the lesion is painful, it may be necessary to sedate or anesthetize the animal.

With intact skin, the thumb and fingers can be used to pinch the skin together on either side of the lesion, elevating the lesion, and thus determine if it will be possible to appose the skin on either side of the defect after lesion removal (Figure 3-10). When dealing with skin tumors they should be palpated gently and cytologically inspected before surgery.

If an open wound is present, the wound edges may be pushed together to determine whether there is enough skin for closure. Towel forceps or staples may be used to appose wound edges in an anesthetized animal. This may include converting an irregular shaped wound into a multiarmed closure, using the towel forceps or staples to determine which points can be pulled together easiest to result in closure with the least wound tension (Figure 3-11).

The development of "dog ears" should be considered when planning wound closure on the distal limbs. Because skin is sparse on the distal limbs, the surgeon should take advantage of all the remaining skin in closure. Thus, if a planned closure results in large "dog ear" formation, the surgeon may want to consider another type of closure that does not require removing "dog ear" skin, especially if the planned closure had tension associated with it. A closure technique that takes advantage of "dog ear" skin should be considered if possible.

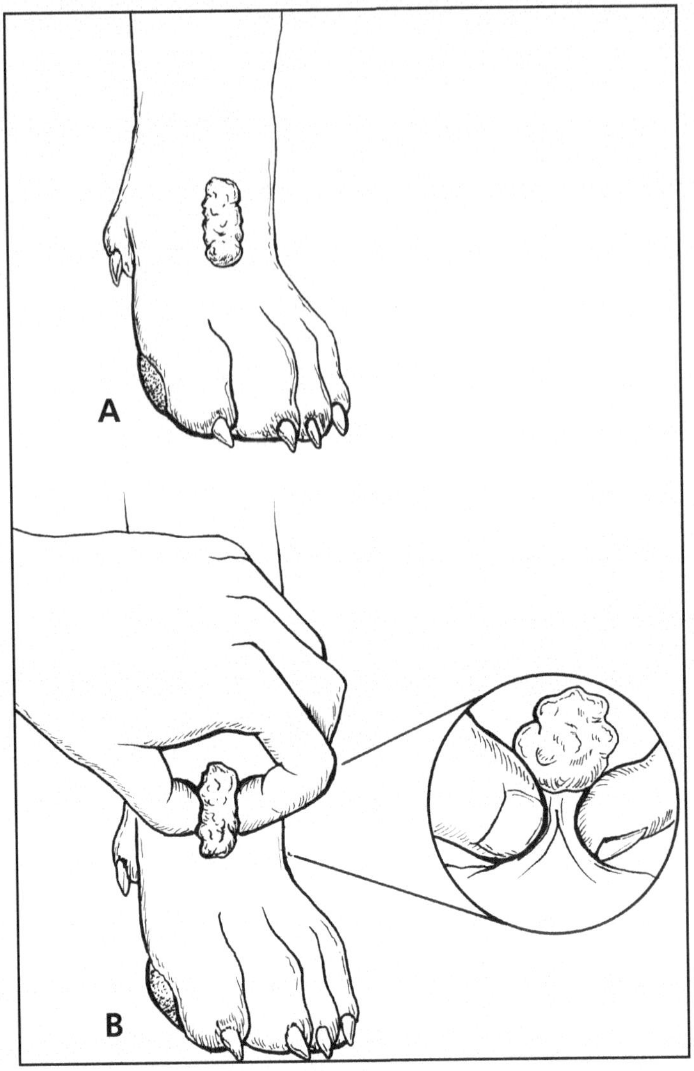


**Figure 3-10.** Pinching the skin together on either side of a lesion to determine if primary skin edge apposition will be possible after lesion removal. **A.** Lesion on the distal limb. **B.** Pinching skin under the lesion.

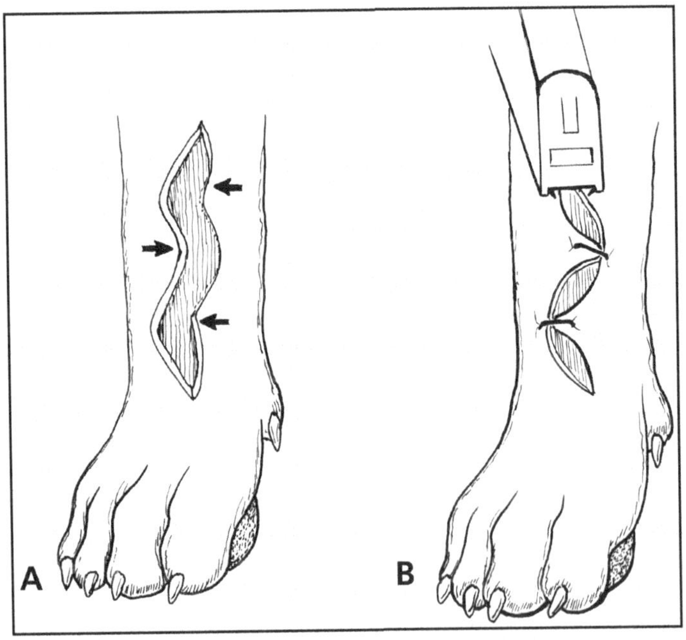


**Figure 3-11.** Planning closure of an irregularly shaped wound. **A.** Potential movement of skin points for closure *(arrows)*. **B.** Staples used to approximate wound edges at points to provide a multiarmed wound for closure.

# Closure - Skin Sutures/Staples Intradermal Closure

## Definition and Indications

Intradermal sutures should be continuous sutures within the dermis. When placed in this area, they serve to appose the wound edges and they can also act as tension sutures. As apposition sutures, they appose the skin edges with little or no suture material exposed on the surface of the wound. They also help control capillary hemorrhage from the skin edges.

As a tension suture they help prevent wound disruption and scar widening. If skin tension is not excessive they can be used in conjunction with skin apposition sutures. They can also be used with other forms of tension sutures if tension is more significant.

Because there is little subcutaneous tissue in the distal limb area, these sutures would be the ones used to help appose wound edges rather than subcutaneous sutures. Because of the thinness of the skin on the distal limb of cats and some dogs, (e.g. Greyhounds), these sutures could be difficult to use and could be contraindicated in these animals. Continuous intradermal sutures are primarily indicated for distal limb wounds due to the sparsity of subcutaneous tissue that would help protect underlying vessels, tendons, and nerves from the irritation and scar tissue that might result from knots on interrupted intradermal sutures.

## Techniques

For use on distal limb wounds, a 4-0 to 3-0 absorbable suture material is used. Reverse cutting needles should be used to decrease the possibility of sutures cutting through the dermis. Although taper-point needles are more difficult to pass through the dermis, they make a circular hole that is more resistant to the suture cutting through the dermis.

A continuous 4-0 to 3-0 monofilament nonabsorbable suture can be placed such that it can be removed at a later time. A simple interrupted suture is placed just beyond one end of the wound, and the needle is passed from this point through the commissure of the wound (Figure 3-12A). The suture is continued by passing the needle on alternating sides of the wound horizontally in the dermis. Passage of the suture between bites in the dermis should be truly perpendicular to the wound edge. The bites are the size of the arc of the needle. Since the suture is to be removed, suture removal is easier on long wounds if the suture is passed through the skin to the outside at 5 to 8 cm lengths along the wound (Figure 3-12B).

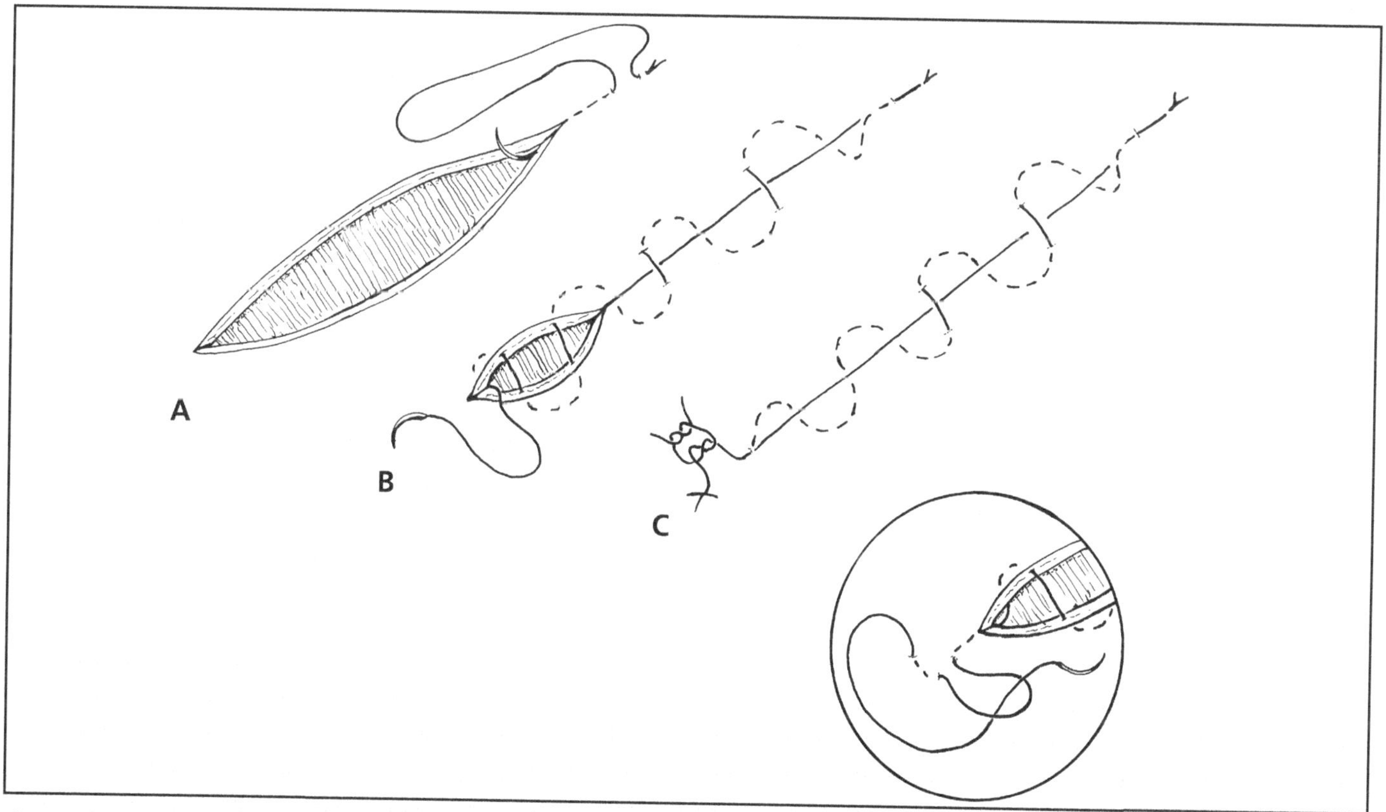


**Figure 3-12.** Placing a continuous intradermal suture (nonabsorbable). **A.** Simple interrupted suture beyond one end of the wound with needle passed through wound commisure. **B.** Suture placement with occasional exteriorized loop. **C.** Ending suture by passing needle through other wound commisure and cutting a long tag which is tied to one tag of a simple interrupted suture. *(Inset)* Alternative suture ending. Needle is passed out through the commisure. A bite is taken in adjacent skin. The resulting loop is tied to the free suture end.

When the suture is removed, these areas of external suture material are cut. This provides suture ends that can be grasped for suture removal by segments. This procedure is used on long wounds. For wounds 2.5 to 5 cm long, it is not necessary to externalize segments of the suture. To end the suture, the needle is passed out through the other wound commisure. The suture is cut and a simple interrupted suture is placed in line with the wound. The cut end of the running suture is tied to it (Figure 3-12C). Alternatively, after the suture is passed out the commissure of the wound, a bite is taken through the skin from the outside. The resulting loop is then tied to the free end of the suture (Figure 3-12C, inset).

An absorbable monofilament 4-0 to 3-0 continuous intradermal suture may be left in place. The beginning knot is buried by placing the first 2 bites from deep-to-superficial and superficial-to-deep, respectively (Figure 3-13A & B). Intradermal suturing is continued along the length of the wound (Figure 3-13C & D). To end the suture with a swaged needle, a four step technique can be used to secure the suture with a buried knot. First, the needle passes from superficial-to-deep near the commisure of the wound and a 2 cm loop of suture material is drawn from the wound (Figure 3-13E1). Second, the needle is passed from deep-to-superficial on the opposite side of the wound (Figure 3-13E2). Third, the needle is taken back across the wound and inserted from superficial-to-deep toward the base of the loop (Figure 3-13E3). Fourth, the free suture strand and loop are tied together to pull the remaining wound edges together and bury the knot (Figure 3-13E4).

## Aftercare

A continuous nonabsorbable intradermal suture is usually removed 10 to 14 days postoperatively. For removal, it is cut at the ends and at any loops that were left exposed. The suture segments are then gently removed.

## Advantages and Disadvantages

Intradermal tension sutures are less prone to molestation by the animal than other types of exposed tension sutures. These sutures help prevent scar widening following the removal of skin apposition sutures. If the knots are large on absorbable intradermal sutures or if the knots are not sufficiently buried, they may result in pressure and local skin necrosis. Any scar tissue that might form as a result of buried knots could cause adhesions to underlying tissues, e.g. tendons. This could result in lameness, especially in performance dogs. Removal of a nonabsorbable continuous intradermal suture may be uncomfortable for the animal as the suture is pulled through the skin. This is especially so if segments of the suture have not been exteriorized along the suture line, which can be cut at suture removal for removal of shorter segments. Compared to skin sutures that penetrate the full-thickness of the skin, continuous intradermal sutures may not be as strong.

# Suggested Readings

1. Bellenger CR: Sutures. Part II: the use of sutures and alternative methods of closure. Compend Contin Edu Pract Vet 4:587, 1982.
2. Bohling MW, Swaim SF: Management of the traumatic wound by primary closure. In Birchard SJ, Sherding RG, eds.: Saunders Manual of Small Animal Practice, 3rd ed.: St. Louis; Saunders – Elsevier, 2006, 541.
3. Bennett RG: Fundamentals of Cutaneous Surgery, St. Louis: CV Mosby, 1988, 355.
4. Boothe HW: Instrument and tissue handling, In Tobias KM, Johnston SA, eds.: Veterinary Surgery, Small Animal, Vol. 2: St. Louis: Elsevier – Saunders, 2012, 201.
5. Fahie MA: Primary wound closure. In Tobias KM, Johnston SA, eds.: Veterinary Surgery, Small Animal, Vol. 2: St. Louis: Elsevier – Saunders, 2012, 1197.
6. Jankauskas S, Cohen IK, Grabb WC: Basic technique of plastic surgery. *In* Smith JW, Aston SJ, eds.: Plastic Surgery, 4th ed.: Boston: Little, Brown, 1991, 3.
7. Knecht CD, Allen AR, Williams DJ, et al: Fundamental Techniques in Veterinary Surgery, 3rd ed.: Philadelphia: WB Saunders, 1987, 54.
8. MacPhail CM: Biomaterial, suturing, and hemostasis. In Fossum TW, ed.: Small Animal Surgery, 4th ed.: St. Louis: Mosby, 2013, 64.
9. Pavletic MM: Atlas of Small Animal Reconstructive Surgery, 2nd ed.: Philadelphia: WB Saunders, 1999, 131.
10. Pavletic MM: Atlas of Small Animal Wound Management and Reconstructive Surgery, 3rd ed.: Ames, IA: Wiley – Blackwell, 2010, 241.
11. Scardino MS, Swaim SF, Henderson RA, Wilson ER: Enhancing wound closure on the limbs, Compend Contin Educ Pract Vet 18:919, 1996.
12. Smeak DD. Buried continuous intradermal suture closure. Compend Contin Educ Pract Vet 14:907, 1992.
13. Stanley BJ: Tension relieving techniques: In Tobias KM, Johnston SA, eds.: Veterinary Surgery, Small Animal, Vol. 2: St. Louis: Elsevier – Saunders, 2012, 1221.
14. Swaim SF: Management of skin tension in dermal surgery. Compend Contin Educ Pract Vet 2:758, 1980.
15. Swaim SF: Management of the traumatic wound by primary closure. *In* Birchard SJ, Sherding RG, eds.: Saunders Manual of Small Animal Practice, 2nd ed.: Philadelphia: WB Saunders, 2000, 392.
16. Swaim SF, Henderson RA: Small Animal Wound Management, 2nd ed.: Baltimore: Williams and Wilkins, 1997, 143.
17. Trout NJ: Principles of plastic and reconstructive surgery. *In* Slatter DH, ed.: Textbook of Small Animal Surgery, 3rd ed.: Philadelphia: WB Saunders, 2003, 274.
18. Williams J: Decision – making in wound closure. In Williams J, Moores A, eds.: BSAVA Manual of Canine and Feline Wound Management and Reconstruction, 2nd ed.: Glouster (UK): BSAVA, 2009, 25.

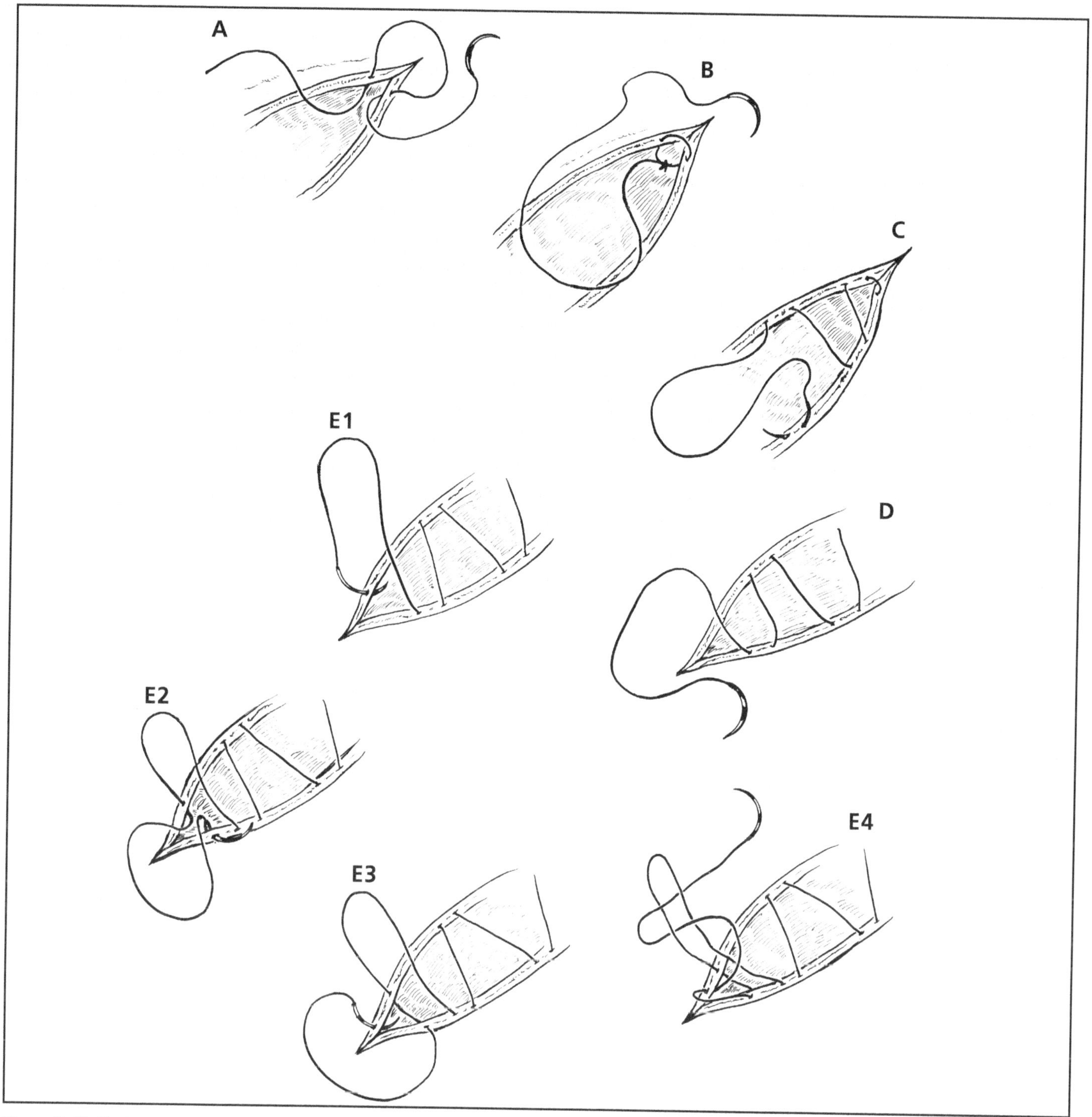


**Figure 3-13.** Placing a continuous intradermal suture ( absorbable – swaged needle). Beginning the suture. **A.** Needle is passed from deep – to – superficial on one side of the wound and superficial – to – deep on the opposite side of the wound. **B.** Suture is tied burying the knot. **C.** & **D.** Suturing continued along the wound. Ending the suture after the majority of the wound has been closed by pulling on the suture. **E1.** Needle is passed from superficial – to – deep and a loop of suture material is lifted from the wound. **E2.** The needle is inserted from deep – to – superficial on the opposite side of the wound. **E3.** Needle is taken back across the wound and inserted superficial – to – deep toward the base of the loop. **E4.** The free end of the suture is tied to the loop for a buried knot.

# Simple Interrupted Skin Sutures

## Definition and Indications

Each suture is a segment of suture material that is passed perpendicular to the plane of the tissue/wound edge. The ends of the suture emerge from the tissue on opposite sides of the wounds an equal distance from the wound edges on each side (Figure 3-14). These sutures are indicated for apposition of wound edges when there is no tension on the wound edges. They may also be used in conjunction with tension sutures to attain final cosmetic wound edge apposition.

## Technique

For wound closure on the distal limbs, 3-0 to 2-0

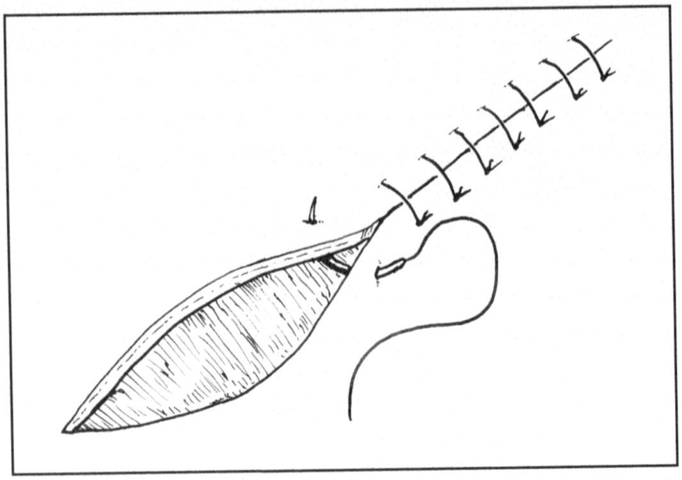

**Figure 3-14.** Simple interrupted skin sutures. Each suture is passed perpendicular to the plane of the wound, equidistant from each edge of the wound.

monofilament synthetic sutures material (i.e. polypropylene or nylon) swaged on a curved, cutting needle is used. Sutures are placed such that equal amounts of tissue are included in the suture from each side of the wound. The needle is inserted and emerges about 2 to 3 mm from the wound edge. Because the needle is curved in shape, a twisting or rolling motion of the surgeon's wrist should be used when passing the needle through the skin. This passes the needle in a curving fashion to match its curved shape. This manner of passing the needle can result in a slight angle of placement so that a slightly greater amount of the deeper part of the dermis is taken. As the needle passes through the opposite side of the wound, the curved pattern of passage can again result in slightly more deep dermis being included in the suture (Figure 3-15). The suture is tied with a square knot or a surgeon's knot with the suture ends held relaxed and untwisted. The knot should be offset so it does not rest on the incision. Equal tension is placed on the suture strands for a secure symmetrical knot.

The needle may be passed through both sides of the wound in one motion if the wound edges are closely apposed and the location of the wound (e.g. on a relatively flat surface) allows such passage (Figure 3-16A). However, if there is some separation of the wound edges or the location of the wound would make such simultaneous passage awkward (e.g. an interdigital wound), the needle may be passed completely through one skin edge and withdrawn from the wound before passing it through the opposite edge (Figure 3-16B).

Sufficient sutures should be placed close enough together to adequately coapt the skin edges without a gap between the edges. Fewer sutures are needed to appose the edges of thick skin and edges of wounds that are parallel to tension lines.

Occasionally it is necessary to suture wound edges that are not on the same plane. When the skin is thick enough to allow it, placing the suture at the same depth in the dermis from the skin surface on both wound edges is effective in evening the wound edges (Figure 3-17).

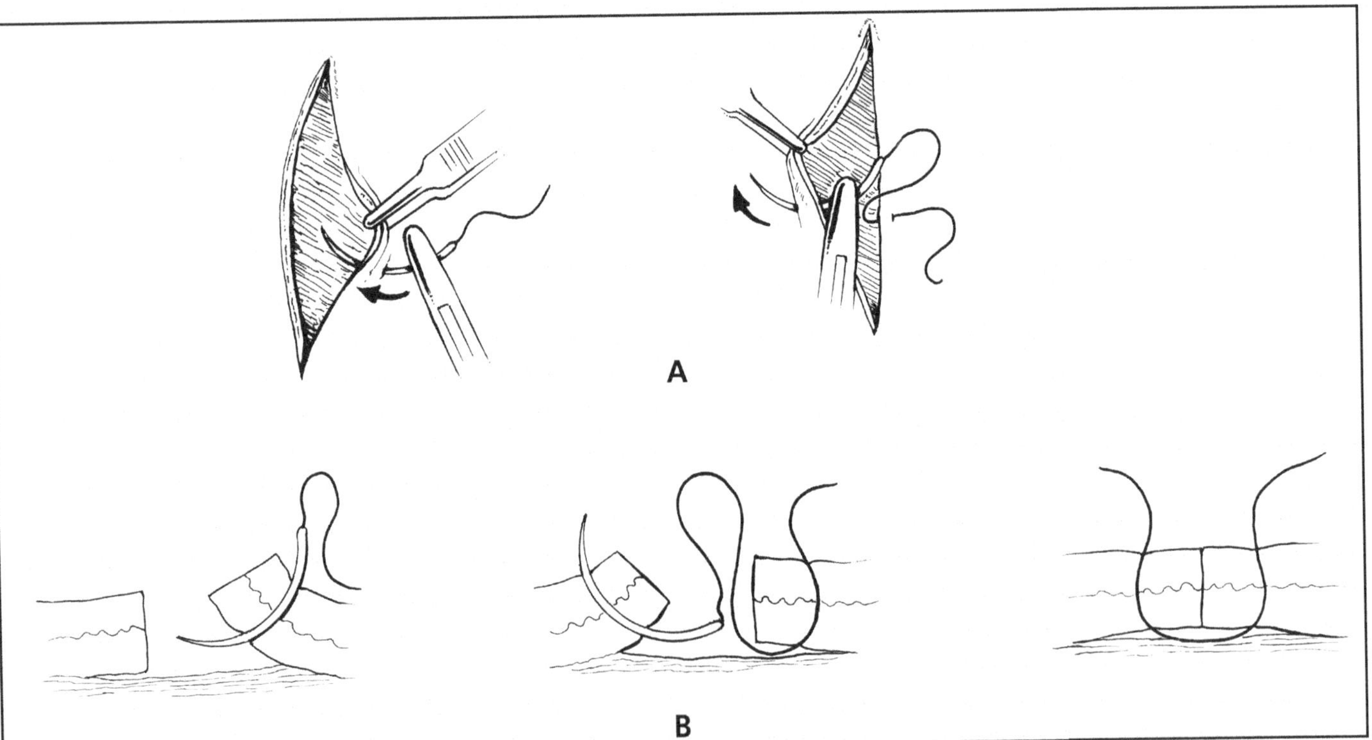


**Figure 3-15.** Placing simple interrupted skin sutures. **A.** A twisting or rolling motion of the surgeon's wrist to pass a curved needle through the skin facilitates needle passage *(arrow)*. **B.** Such passage results in a slight angle of placement with slightly greater amount of deeper dermis in the suture.

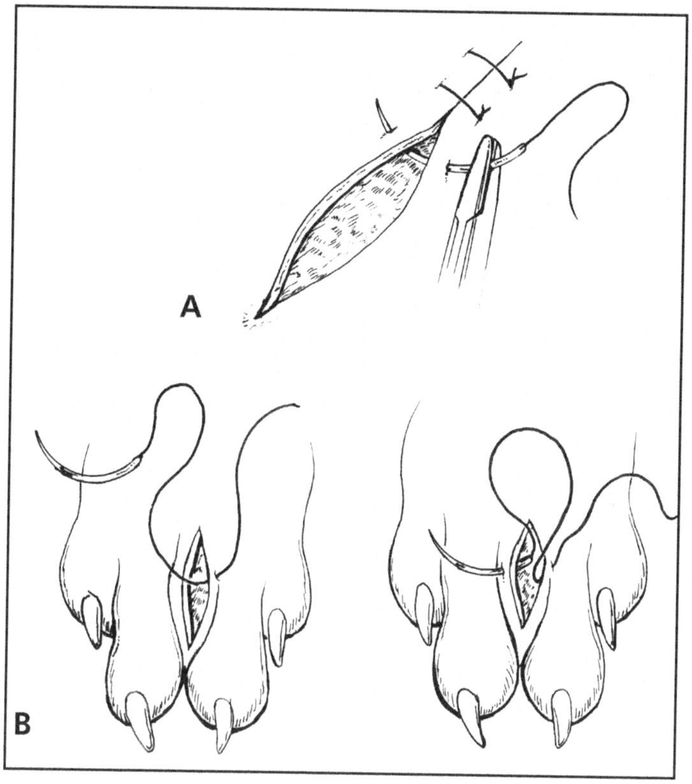


**Figure 3-16.** Needle passage. **A.** Simultaneous needle passage through both sides of the wound. **B.** Complete passage of the needle through one side of the wound before passage through the opposite side of the wound. Used when wound is in an awkward location or edges are widely separated.

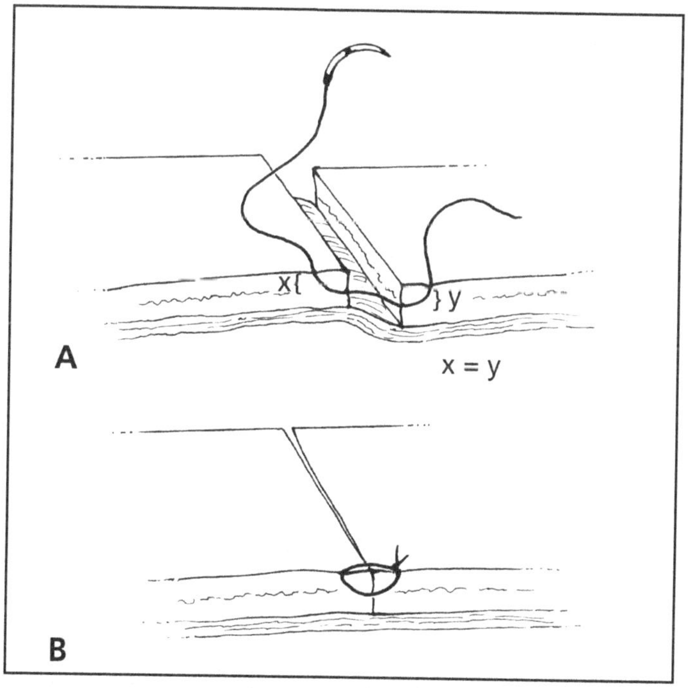


**Figure 3-17.** Suturing wound edges on slightly different planes. **A.** Placing sutures at the same depth in the dermis from the skin surface on both wound edges. **B.** Wound edges are leveled when the suture is tied. (After Trout NJ: Principles of plastic and reconstructive surgery. In Slatter DH, ed.: Textbook of Small Animal Surgery, 3rd ed.: Philadelphia: WB Saunders, 2003, 275.)

If there is a tangential cut in the skin, the edges can be sutured with unequal suture placement. On the "acute" side of the wound the needle is passed far from the wound edge (wide bite) and it is passed near to the wound edge (narrow bite) on the "obtuse" side of the wound (Figure 3-18).

When suturing a horizontal wound, a right-handed person should suture from right to left; whereas, a left-handed person should suture from left to right. When suturing a vertically oriented wound, suturing should begin at the most distal end of the wound.

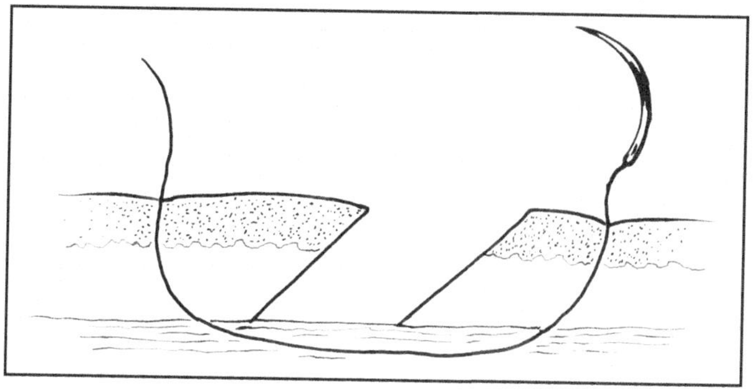

**Figure 3-18.** Suturing a tangential cut. The fist bite on the "acute" side of the wound is placed far from the wound edge (wide bite). On the "obtuse" side of the wound the suture is placed near to the wound edge (narrow bite). (After Knowles RP: Injuries to the skin muscle and tendon, In Some Techniques and Procedures in Small Animal Surgery. Bonner Springs Kansas: Veterinary Publishing Co., Inc., 1963, 141.)

## Aftercare

In general sutures are removed 7 to 10 days after surgery.

## Advantages and Disadvantages

Simple interrupted sutures have the advantage of being quickly and easily placed. They also maintain good tissue apposition with mobility between sutures. They cause minimal alteration in blood supply to the wound edges, and if one suture fails, the others remain intact. Additionally, the surgeon can adjust the tension of each suture along the wound as the spreading forces dictate. If there is a small amount of subcutaneous dead space beneath and between the wound edges, it can be obliterated by taking a small bite in the subcutaneous tissue as the suture is placed. The bite must be small so that a large amount of subcutaneous tissue is not pulled up and interposed between the skin edges, which might interfere with wound healing.

Simple interrupted sutures have the disadvantage of using a greater amount of suture material, and it takes a relatively longer time to place this suture pattern than continuous suture patterns. If they are tied with too much tension, they cause skin inversion which is undesirable. Also, tight placement can result in sutures cutting into the skin, especially if postoperative swelling occurs.

## Suggested Readings


1. Bellah JR, Williams JM: Wound closure options and decisions. In Fowler D, Williams JM: BSAVA Manual of Canine and Feline Wound Management and Reconstruction. Shurdington, Cheltenham, UK: BSAVA, 1999, 25.
2. Bellenger CR: Sutures: Part II. The use of sutures and alternative methods of closure. Compend Contin Educ Pract Vet 4: 587, 1982.
3. Bennett RG: Fundamentals of Cutaneous Surgery, St. Louis: CV Mosby, 1988, p 355.
4. Fahie MA: Primary wound closure. In Tobias KM, Johnston SA, eds.: Veterinary Surgery, Small Animal, Vol. 2: St. Louis: Elsevier – Saunders, 2012, 1197.
5. Fossum TW: Biomaterials, suturing, and hemostasis. *In* Fossum TW, et al: Small Animal Surgery, 2nd ed.: St. Louis: Mosby, 2002, 43.
6. Fossum TW: Biomaterials, suturing and hemostasis. In Fossum TW, ed.: Small Animal Surgery, 3rd ed.: St. Louis: Mosby, 2007, 57.
7. Jankauskas S, Cohen IK, Grabb WC: Basic technique of plastic surgery. *In* Smith JW, Aston SJ, eds.: Plastic Surgery, 4th ed.: Boston: Little, Brown, 1991, 3.
8. Knecht CD, Allen AR, Williams DJ, et al: Fundamental Techniques in Veterinary Surgery, 3rd ed.: Philadelphia: WB Saunders, 1987, 54.
9. MacPhail CM: Biomaterial, suturing, and hemostasis. In Fossum TW, ed.: Small Animal Surgery, 4th ed.: St. Louis: Mosby, 2013, 64.
10. McGregor IA: Fundamental Techniques of Plastic Surgery, 8th ed.: Edinburgh: Churchill Livingston, 1989, 3.
11. Pavletic MM: Atlas of Small Animal Wound Management and Reconstructive Surgery, 3rd ed.: Ames, IA: Wiley – Blackwell, 2010, 241.
12. Stashak TS: Equine Wound Management, Philadelphia: Lea & Febiger, 1991, 52.
13. Swaim SF, Henderson RA: Small Animal Wound Management, 2nd ed.: Baltimore: Williams and Wilkins, 1997, 13.
14. Trout NJ: Principles of plastic and reconstructive surgery. *In* Slatter DH, ed.: Textbook of Small Animal Surgery, 3rd ed.: Philadelphia: WB Saunders, 2003, 274.
15. Williams J: Decision – making in wound closure. In Williams J, Moores A, eds.: BSAVA Manual of Canine and Feline Wound Management and Reconstruction, 2nd ed.: Glouster (UK): BSAVA, 2009, 25.


# X-Matress (Cruciate) Sutures

### Defintion and Indications

X-mattress sutures are interrupted sutures placed in the pattern their name implies. They are particularly useful in suturing the skin after digital amputations.

### Technique

The needle is inserted 3 to 4 mm from the wound edge on one side of the wound. It is passed to the opposite side of the wound the same as for the placement of a simple interrupted suture (Figure 3-19A). The needle is advanced 5 mm and crosses the wound. At this point, the needle is passed through the skin a second time parallel to the first passage (Figure 3-19B). The suture ends are now on opposite sides of the wound; they are tied to form an "x" on the wound surface (Figure 3-19C & D). The sutures can be also be placed as a continuous suture.

### Aftercare

Sutures are removed 7 to 10 days after surgery.

### Advantages and Disadvantages

These sutures provide a stronger closure than simple interrupted sutures. They also resist tension such as might occur when weight is borne on nearby tissue, i.e. adjacent digits (Figure 3-9E). These sutures prevent eversion of the wound edges. If they are tied under tension, they do not obstruct the vasculature at the wound edge. Because they are interrupted, they provide wound edge security. However, they require more suture material and time for placement. If they are tied under too much tension, they may cause skin edge inversion at the point where the suture crosses over the incision/wound.

## Suggested Readings


1. Boothe HW: Instrument and tissue handling techniques. In Tobias KM, Johnston SA, eds.: Veterinary Surgery, Small Animal, Vol. 2: St. Louis: Elsevier – Saunders, 2012, 201.
2. Fahie MA: Primary wound closure. In Tobias KM, Johnston SA, eds.: Veterinary Surgery, Small Animal, Vol. 2: St. Louis: Elsevier – Saunders, 2012, 1197.
3. Fossum TW: Biomaterials, suturing, and hemostasis. In Fossum TW, ed.: Small Animal Surgery, 3rd ed.: St. Louis: Mosby, 2007, 57.
4. Knecht CD, Allen AR, Williams DJ, et al: Fundamental Techniques in Veterinary Surgery, 3rd ed.: Philadelphia: WB Saunders, 1987, 54.
5. McPhail CM: Biomaterials, suturing, and hemostasis. In Fossum TW, ed.: Small Animal Surgery, 4th ed.: St. Louis: Mosby, 2013, 64.
6. Pavletic MM: Atlas of Small Animal Wound Management and Reconstructive Surgery, 3rd ed.: Ames IA: Wiley – Blackwell, 2010.
7. Swaim SF, Henderson RA: Small Animal Wound Management, 2nd ed.: Baltimore: Williams and Wilkins, 1997, 13.
8. Trout NJ: Principles of plastic and reconstructive surgery. *In* Slatter DH, ed.: Textbook of Small Animal Surgery, 3rd ed.: Philadelphia: WB Saunders, 2003, 274.


# Staples

### Definition and Indications

Staples are wires available as regular width (4.8 to 6.1 mm) and wide width (6.5 to 7.0 mm). When applied, they form rectangles that appose and secure wound edges together. Each staple is composed of a cross-member that passes over the top of the closed wound perpendicular to it, two legs that penetrate into the skin, and two pointed tips that lie beneath the skin parallel to the cross-member. There is a gap between the cross member and the incision to accommodate swelling. Some staples are arcuate or

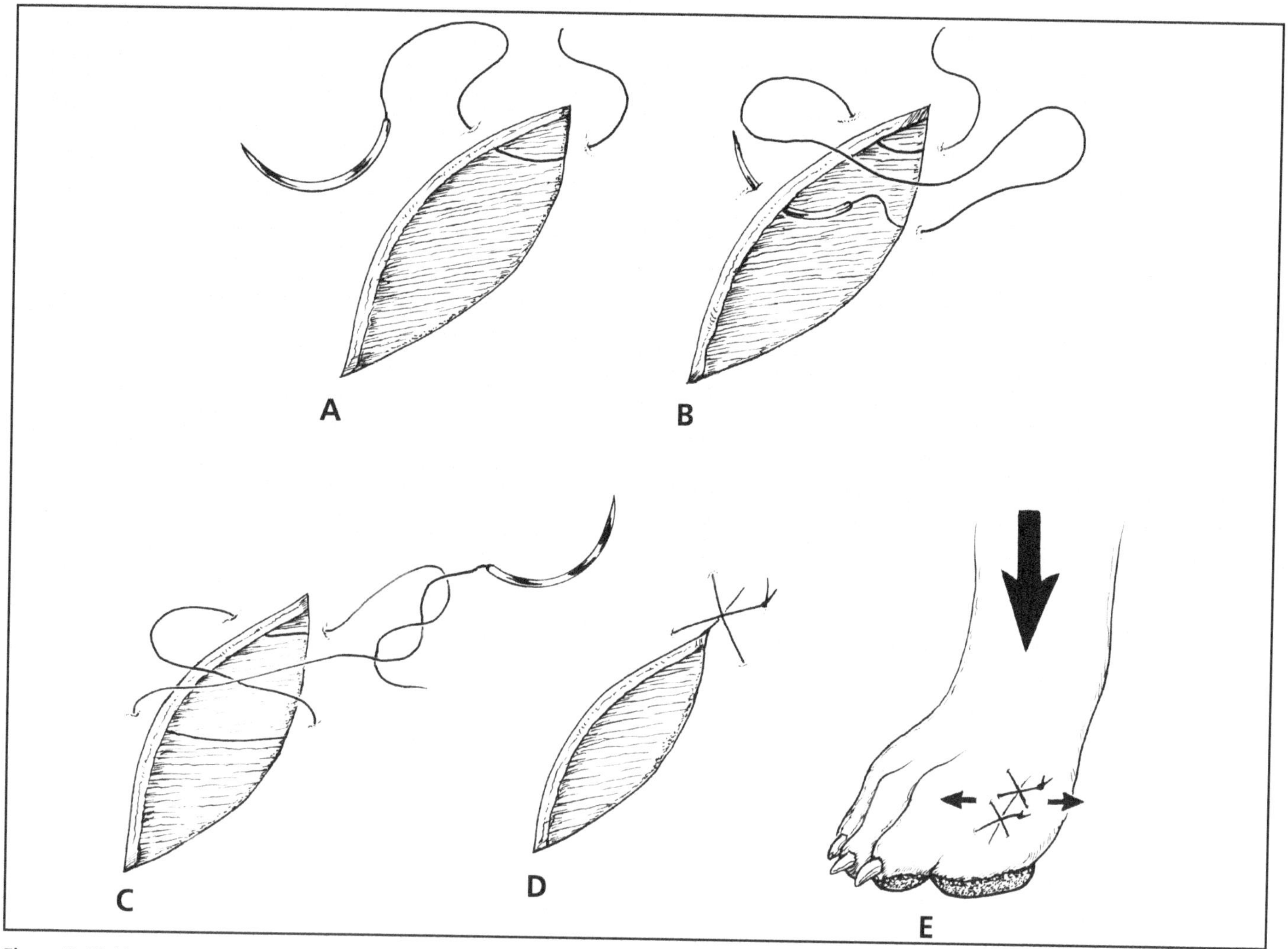


**Figure 3-19.** X-mattress suture. **A.** First suture passage is the same as a simple interrupted suture. **B.** Needle is advanced across the wound and passed parallel to the first passage. **C.** Tying the suture. **D.** Tied suture forms an "X" over the wound. **E.** Sutures resist tension *(small arrows)* when weight is borne *(large arrows)* on nearby tissue. (A-D After Swaim SF, Henderson RA: Small Animal Wound Management, 2nd ed.: Baltimore: Williams & Wilkins, 1997, 34.)

triangular in shape. An absorbable polymer subcuticular staple (Insorb, Incisive Surgical, Inc., Plymouth, MN) is available. Staples are contained and dispensed from a self-contained, light-weight plastic unit. Some staple units apply staples by a palm grip while others apply the staples with a finger pinch-type grip. Staples are indicated when speed is an important factor in wound closure. The primary indication for skin staples on distal limb injuries is the rapid application of mesh skin grafts. Staples can also be used to secure drapes or stockinette to the skin, secure dressings over skin grafts, and move skin flaps into place when used as modified skin hooks.

## Technique

To appose wound edges for staple placement, traction can be placed on either end of the wound using towel clamps or stay sutures, or forceps may be used for edge apposition. When skin tension is a factor in wound closure, intradermal sutures are usually placed before staples are inserted. To apply the staples, the dispensing part of the applicator is placed at a 90° angle to the wound with the indicator arrow over the center of the apposed wound edges (Figure 3-20A). As the delivery mechanism of the applicator is compressed, a staple is inserted and bent into the skin, with one-half of the staple being on each side of the apposed wound edge (Figure 3-20B & C). Disengagement of the staple from the applicator may require either forward or backward movement of the instrument.

Staples can be used to quickly appose points of an unusually shaped wound. The resulting arms of the wound can then be sutured or stapled for final closure.

## Aftercare

Staples are usually removed 7 to 10 days after surgery using a special staple removing instrument (Figure 3-20D-F).

## Advantages and Disadvantages

Staples provide a rapid everted and accurate means of closing skin wounds. Speed and simplicity of closure are the primary advantages of staple closure. Staples are inert and cause little inflammation. They resist infection and result in minimal iatrogenic trauma when they are applied. Skin staples may be removed faster than sutures. They also cause minimal interference with the skin edge vasculature. Skin staples have been reported to be cost effective and more economical than sutures. The absorbable subcuticular polymer staples have been reported to resist infection.

There may be skin edge overlap if staples are applied at an oblique angle rather than perpendicular to the wound. Overlap of wound edges may also occur if the staple is shifted to the right or left over the suture line so it gathers more skin from one side. Obvious "cross marks" over the closed wound may be caused if the cross-member is in contact with the skin and becomes imbedded in the skin. Occasionally, staples rotate in the skin, and they must be manipulated into the proper position for application of the removal instrument (Figure 3-20G). This may cause some discomfort to the animal. When placed under a cast or splint, the rigid staple apposed against the cast of splint could cause pressure necrosis. There have been reports in humans of increased infection problems with staple – closed wounds compared to suture closed wounds, following orthopedic procedures.

## Suggested Readings


1. Bellenger CR: Sutures: Part II. The use of sutures and alternative methods of closure. Compend Contin Educ Pract Vet 4:587, 1982.
2. Bennett RG: Fundamentals of Cutaneous Surgery, St. Louis: CV Mosby, 1988, 445.
3. Brickman KR, Lambert RW: Evaluation of skin stapling for skin closure in the emergency department. Ann Emerg Med 18:1122, 1989.
4. Dernell W, Harari J: Surgical devices and wound healing. *In* Harari J, ed.: Surgical Complications and Wound Healing in Small Animal Practice, Philadelphia: WB Saunders, 1993, 349.
5. Fahie MA: Primary wound closure. In Tobias KM, Johnston SA, eds.: Veterinary Surgery, Small Animal, Vol. 2: St. Louis: Elsevier – Saunders, 2012, 1197.
6. Fernandez AP, Solopek LS, Rodheaver PF, et. al.: A revolutionary advance in skin closure compared to current methods. J Long – Term Eff Med Impl. 16:19, 2006.
7. Fossum TW: Biomaterials, suturing, and hemostasis. In Fossum


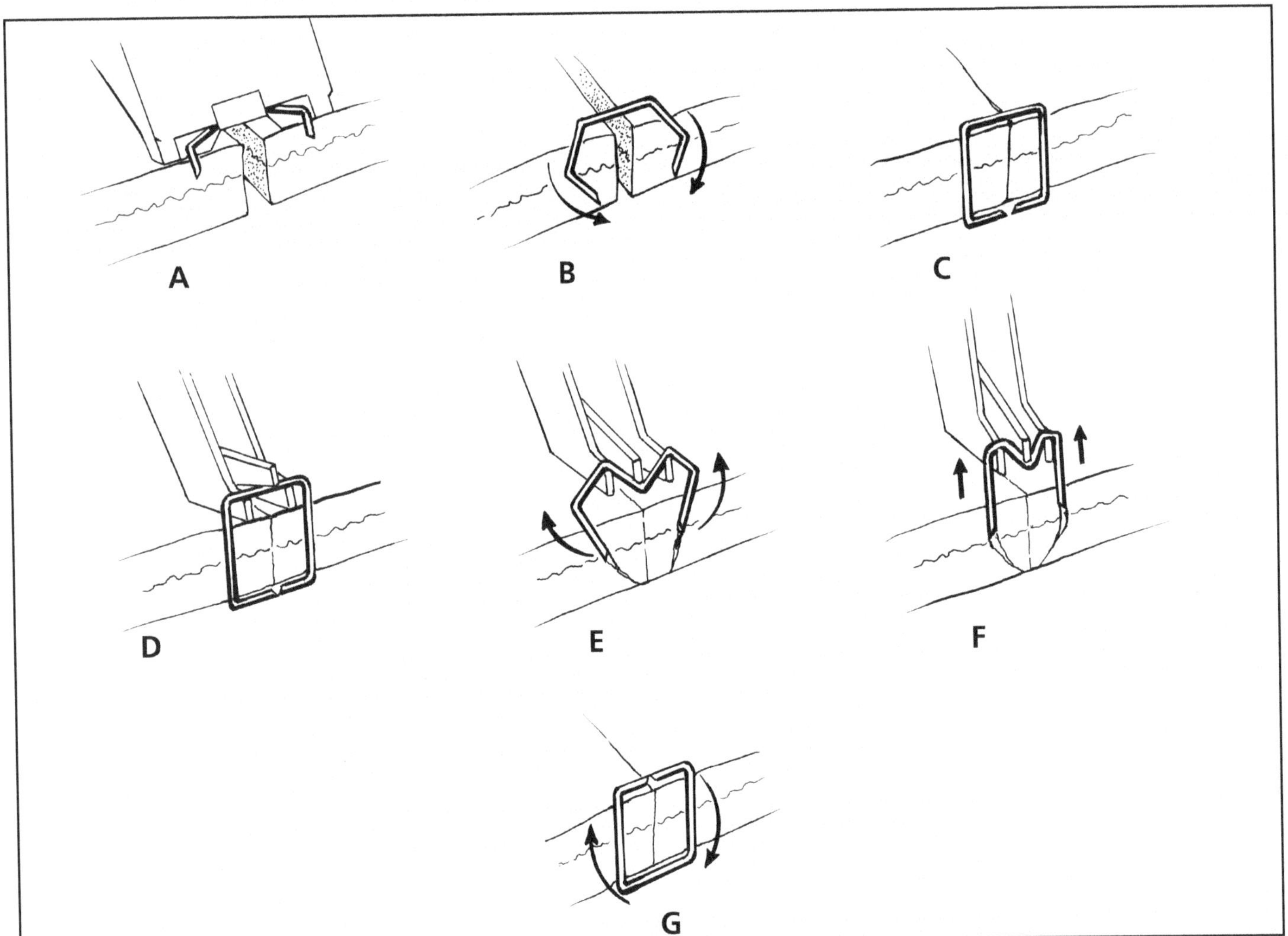


**Figure 3-20.** Skin staples. **A.** Staple dispensing port centered over almost – apposed skin edges. **B.** Dynamics of staple inserting. **C.** Staple in place apposing skin edges. **D.** Staple remover in place. **E.** Staple being opened. **F.** Staple open and ready for removal. **G.** Staples can rotate during the healing process. (After Swaim SF, Henderson RA: Small Animal Wound Management, 2nd ed.: Baltimore : Williams & Wilkins, 1997, 39.)

TW, ed.: Small Animal Surgery, 3rd ed.: St. Louis: Mosby, 2007, 57.
8. Hammer DL: The use of skin staples in small animal surgery. Vet Rep, Solvay 3:9, 1990.
9. Hess JL, De Young DW, Riley MGI, et al: Comparison of stainless steel staple and synthetic suture material on skin wound healing. J Am Anim Hosp Assoc. 15:569, 1979.
10. Jankauskas S, Cohen IK, Grabb WC: Basic technique of plastic surgery. *In* Smith JW, Aston SJ, eds.: Plastic Surgery, 4th ed.: Boston: Little, Brown, 1991, 3.
11. Johnson A, Rodeheaver GT, Durand LS, et al: Automatic disposable stapling devices for wound closure. Ann Emerg Med 10:631, 1981.
12. Kanegaye JT, Vance CW, Chan L: Comparison of skin stapling devices and standard sutures for pediatric scalp lacerations: A randomized study of cost and time benefits. J Pediat 130:808, 1997.
13. Lefreniere R, Kefchan AS: The use of the skin stapler for drape fixation during operations. Surg Gynecol Obstet 162:73, 1986.
14. MacPhail CM: Surgery of the integumentary system. In Fossum TW, ed.: Small Animal Surgery, 4th ed.: St. Louis: Mosby, 2013, 190.
15. Pavletic MM: Atlas of Small Animal Wound Management and Reconstructive Surgery, 3rd ed.: Ames, IA: Wiley – Blackwell, 2010.
16. Porter DB: A clinical evaluation of the Proximate stapling system for closing skin incisions. Vet Med Sm Anim Clin 76:320, 1981.
17. Smith TO, Sexton D, Mann C, Donell S: Sutures versus staples for skin closure in orthopeaedic surgery: meta – analysis. Br Med J 340: 1199, 2010.
18. Stillman RM, Marino CA, Seligman SJ: Skin staples in potentially contaminated wounds. Arch Surg 119:821, 1984.
19. Swaim SF, Henderson RA: Small Animal Wound Management, 2nd ed.: Baltimore: Williams and Wilkins, 1997, 13.
20. Syed KA, Gandhi R, Davey JR, et al: Risk of wound infection is greater after skin closure with staples than with sutures in orthopaedic surgery. J Bone Joint Surg Am 92:2732, 2010.
21. Tobias KM: Surgicel stapling devices in veterinary medicine: A review. Vet Surg 36:341, 2007.
22. Trout NJ: Principles of plastic and reconstructive surgery. *In* Slatter DH, ed.: Textbook of Small Animal Surgery, 3rd ed.: Philadelphia: WB Saunders, 2003, 274.
23. Waldron DR: Skin and fascia staple closure. Vet Clin North Am Small Anim Pract 24:413, 1994.
24. Williams J: Decision – making in wound closure. In Williams J, Moores A, eds.: BASAVA Manual of Canine and Feline Wound Management and Reconstruction, 2nd ed.: Glouster (UK): BSAVA, 2009, 25.

# Wounds with Apposable Edges - Tension

## Wound Tension on the Distal Limbs

### General Information

In general, skin is less abundant on the limbs than on the trunk of dogs and cats, with the abundance varying with the breed of animal. A blood hound has relatively more skin on its limbs that can be used for wound closure than a greyhound (Figure 3-21). The quantity of extra skin decreases progressively as you move distally on the limbs. Although skin is not abundant on the limbs, it is possible to move skin cranially and caudally on the limbs for wound closure. The amount of tension on wound closure will depend upon how much skin is available. However, wounds on the limbs that are closed under too much tension can constrict the tissues, resulting in a "biologic tourniquet" with distal limb circulatory insufficiency (Figure 3-22).

Wounds over or near the extensor surface of the carpal and tarsal joints tend to disrupt with joint flexion since flexion places tension on wound edges to separate them. Whether the reconstruction is by simple appositional suturing, special tension suturing, or use of skin grafts, joint flexion tends to disrupt healing.

Another form of tension that results in poor healing over the carpal and tarsal joints is contractural tension on the flexor surfaces of the carpal or tarsal areas. Large wounds that are allowed to heal as open wounds in these areas may be pulled into flexion deformity as wound contraction ends in wound contracture (Figure 3-23 and See Figure 1-13).

The following material will provide information about relieving tension on skin where it is possible to appose the wound edges. This will include information on

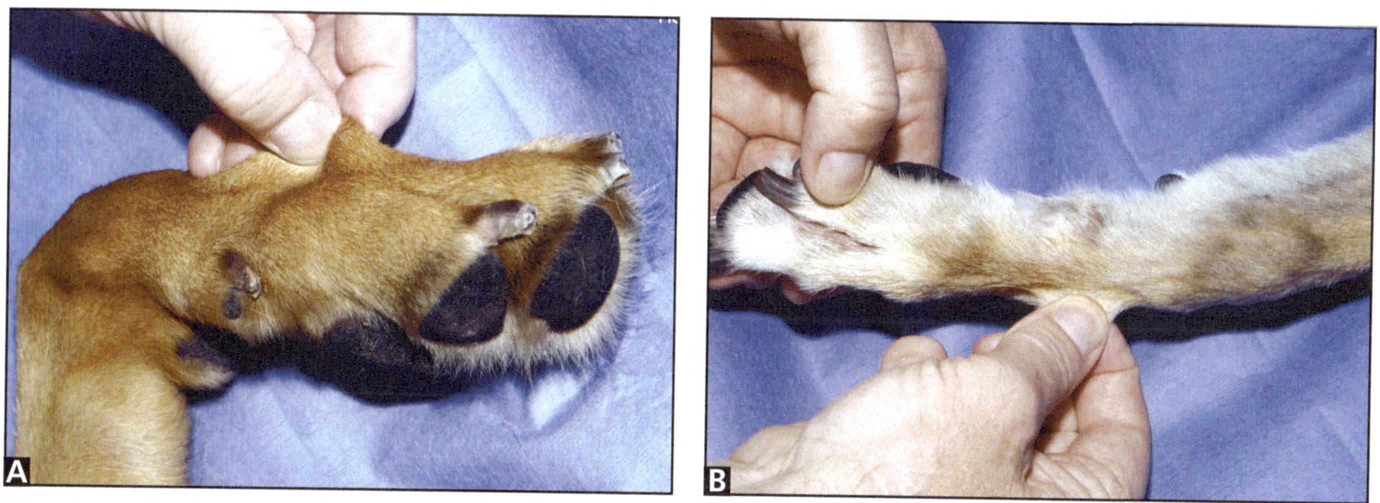


**Figure 3-21.** Difference in the amount of skin on the distal limbs of different breeds of dogs. **A.** Bloodhound – more. **B.** Greyhound – less.

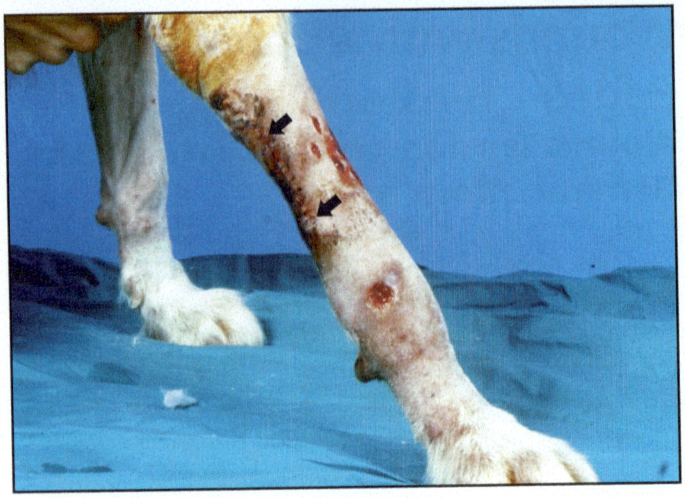

**Figure 3-22.** "Biologic tourniquet" resulting from skin being closed under too much tension (between arrows) with swelling distal to the "tourniquet".

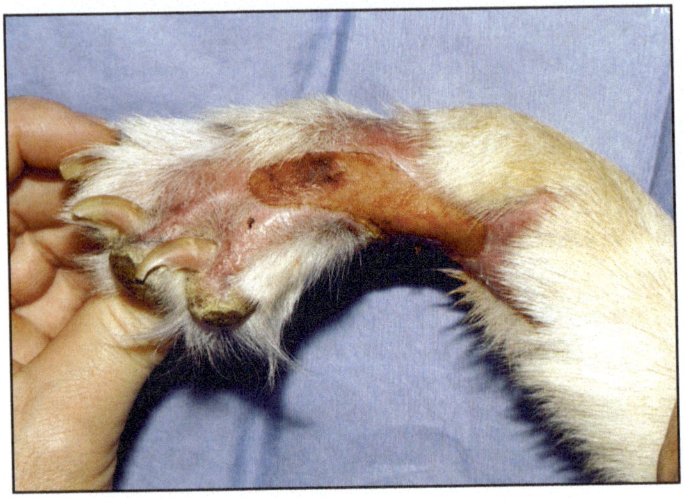

**Figure 3-23.** Contractual flexion of the carpus resulting from tension caused by second intention healing of a large open wound on the flexion surface or the carpus. (From Swaim SF, Hinkle SH, Bradley DM: Wound Contraction: Basic and clinical factors. Compend Contin Edu Vet Pract 23: 29, 2001.)

techniques which the author has found beneficial in dealing with such wounds. It will include the topics of 1) undermining, 2) various tension sutures, 3) closure of various shaped wounds that may commonly be encountered on the distal limbs where tension may be a factor, and 4) management of wounds over the carpus and tarsus.

# Undermining

## Definition and Indications

Undermining of skin on the distal limb is done using scissors or a scalpel to separate the skin from underlying structures. The full elastic potential of the skin can then be utilized to stretch it in wound closure endeavors.

Undermining is indicated to relieve skin tension prior to apposing wound edges, to isolate vessels and nerves within a wound, and to release the skin from underlying dense scar tissue at the edge of chronic wounds.

## Techniques

Skin is undermined parallel to the anticipated direction of skin advancement. Blunt undermining may be performed by advancing closed scissor blades beneath the skin to the depth of undermining and then opening them (Figure 3-24A). The scissors are withdrawn from under the skin with the blades still open. For undermining on the distal limb, curved blunt-blunt scissors (i.e. Metzenbaum scissors) are effective. The curve of the scissors is placed against the curve of the limb for most effective use. Because a relatively small area will be undermined, the points of the scissors will primarily be used in the procedure. The blunt end of a scalpel handle may also be inserted under the skin and moved back and forth as a means of blunt dissection (Figure 3-24B). Undermining should be done in the loose areolar fascia deep to the dermis to preserve blood supply to the skin. If skin has been recently traumatized it should be undermined gently because the additional insult to the skin vasculature could result in slough. When the status of the skin vasculature is questionable, delayed primary closure is indicated after resolution of contusions, edema and infection.

Sharp-sharp scissors can be used for fine dissection around specific structures such as vessels and nerves. The need for such dissection is more prevalent on the distal limb where such structures are abundant. The scissor points delicately engage the connective tissue around such structures with minimal pressure. When the blades are opened they separate the tissue atraumatically. The surgeon should be careful not to close the scissors until the points are well retracted from the wound to help assure that no vessels or nerves are inadvertently cut.

Sharp undermining may be performed by carefully snipping dense fascial attachments with scissor blades (Figure 3-24C). The procedure is often combined with blunt scissor undermining. This type of undermining on the distal limb would most likely be used in the presence of dense scar tissue under the skin. Small amounts of tissue would be snipped at a time, using care not to damage nerves or vessels in the area. Sharp undermining of skin adherent to underlying fascia by dense scar tissue may also be performed using a scalpel blade to cut the dense connective tissue parallel to the undersurface of the skin (Figure 3-24D). Again, care must be used on the distal limb not to damage vessels and nerves. Care must also be used not to undermine too shallow when cutting through dense scar tissue at

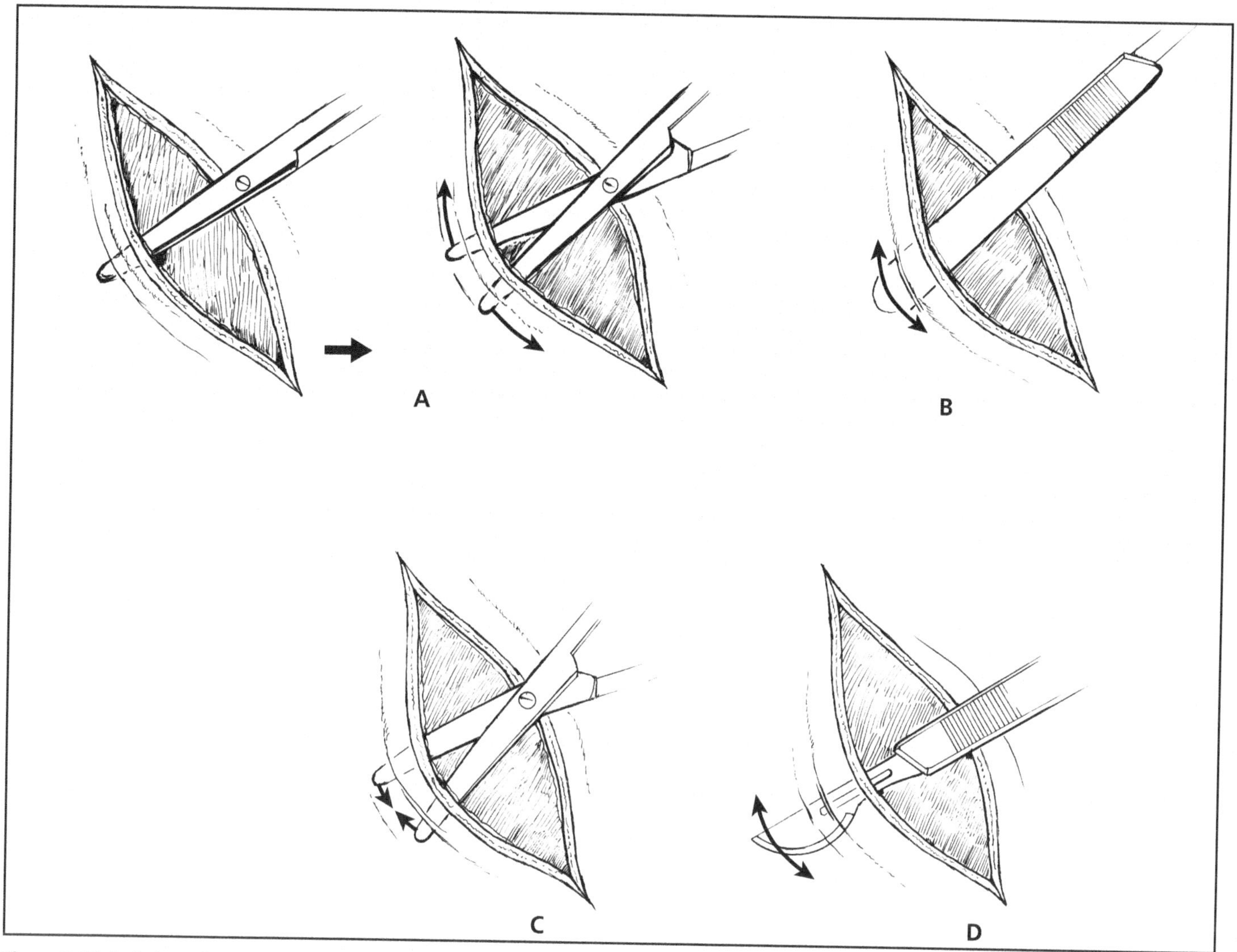


**Figure 3-24.** Techniques for undermining. **A.** Blunt undermining with scissors. **B.** Blunt undermining with a scalpel handle. **C.** Sharp undermining with scissors. **D.** Sharp undermining with a scalpel blade. (After Swaim SF, Henderson RA: Small Animal Wound Management, 2nd ed.: Baltimore: Williams & Wilkins, 2997, 151.)

the skin edge. If skin is undermined too thin through this scar tissue, its vasculature may be damaged.

When undermining is to be done around a wound that is being treated by secondary closure, it is necessary to free the skin edges from their attachment to underlying granulation tissue. This is done by incising and removing any epithelial tissue that is present at the wound edge. The epithelium is incised around the wound at its attachment to the granulation tissue and at its juncture with haired skin. A number 15 scalpel blade can then be used to undercut the epithelium for its removal. The cleavage plain between the dermis and underlying structures is located and undermining continues in this plain. Granulation tissue in the center of the wound is left intact and wound closure is over it.

When undermining skin, atraumatic surgical technique should be used. Crushing instruments such as Allis tissue forceps should be avoided. Brown-Adson thumb forceps, skin hooks, or stay sutures should be used to manipulate skin. A simple skin hook can be made by bending the point of a hypodermic needle with needle holders to form a hook. The hooked needle is held in needle holders to serve as a skin hook (Figure 3-25).

As undermining progresses, periodic attempts should be made to approximate the wound edges to determine if tension relief is adequate. Excessive bleeding may be controlled by electrocoagulation or ligation. However, skin tension and bandaging usually control hemorrhage and prevent seromas. If there is concern whether these will control hemorrhage, or whether dead space will result in a seroma or hematoma, a ¼-inch diameter Penrose drain should be placed under the undermined skin to help prevent seroma or hematoma formation.

## Aftercare

An absorbent bandage should be placed over the wound area to protect the wound. If a drain has been

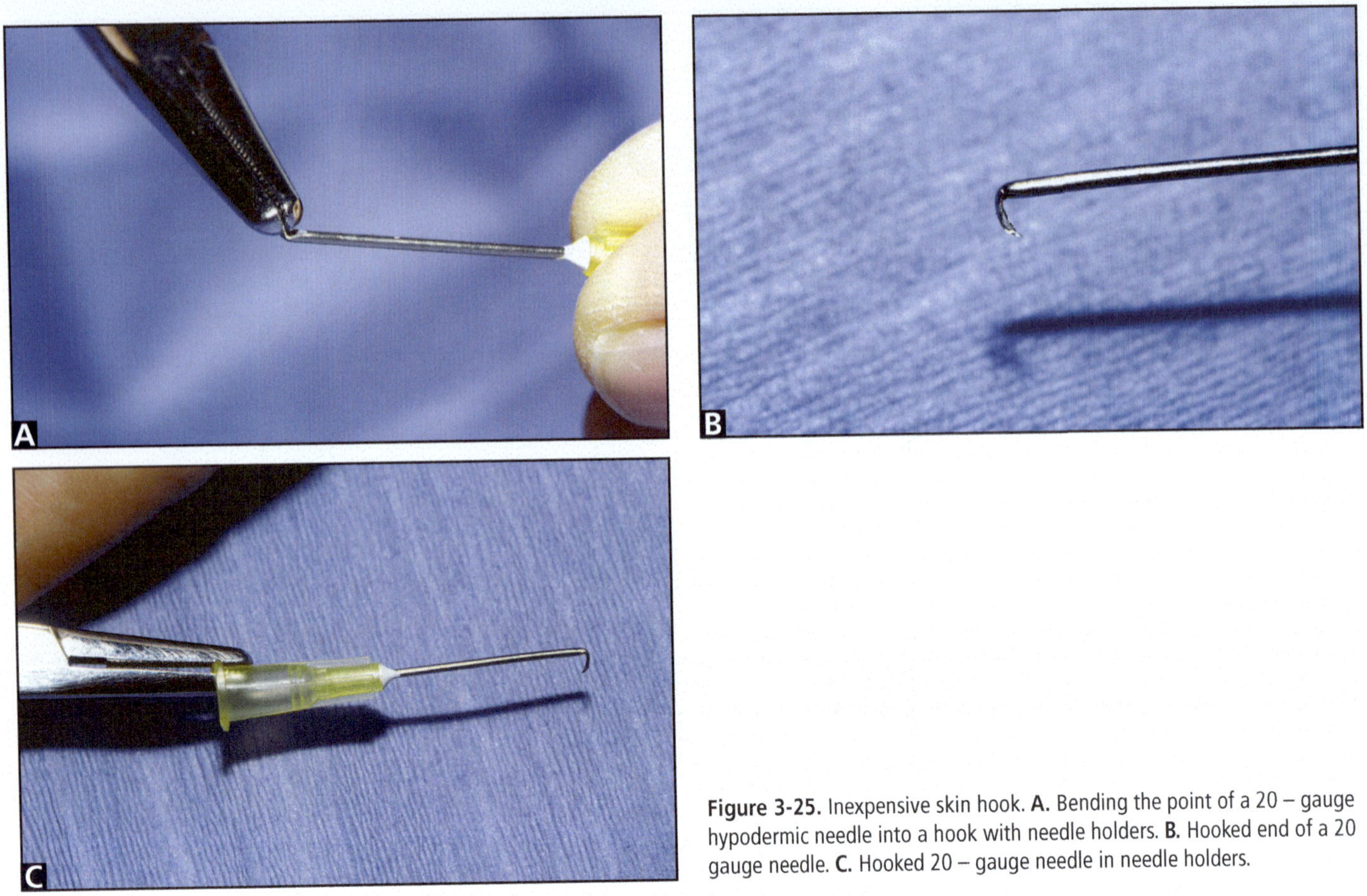

**Figure 3-25.** Inexpensive skin hook. **A.** Bending the point of a 20 – gauge hypodermic needle into a hook with needle holders. **B.** Hooked end of a 20 gauge needle. **C.** Hooked 20 – gauge needle in needle holders.

placed, the bandage will also absorb drainage from the area. The drain is removed 3 to 4 days after placement when drainage has become minimal.

## Advantages and Disadvantages

Undermining is the simplest technique to relieve tension. The skin is released from underlying structures by undermining; thus, the surgeon can take advantage of its elasticity to advance it for closing a wound. In some instances, undermining may provide enough laxity to allow wound closure without additional relaxing skin incisions or grafts. Since scar tissue contracts during healing, the scar tissue that forms in the plane of undermining may provide strength to hold a wound together as healing occurs. However, when dense scar tissue underlies the skin of a chronic wound, some form of relaxing incision may be necessary with undermining to gain tissue laxity for wound closure.

Because of the sparsity of skin on a dog and cat's distal limbs, the amount of gain by undermining is not as great as on other areas of the body where skin is more abundant. Undermining recently traumatized skin could cause additional insult to skin vasculature and result in slough. Undermining could create dead space that could lead to seroma or hematoma formation. If skin tension and bandaging are not sufficient to obliterate the dead space, it may be necessary to place a drain. Vessels and nerves could be severed if care is not used when isolating these structures with sharp-sharp scissors or when doing sharp dissection through dense scar tissue. If sharp undermining in dense scar tissue is too shallow, the undermined skin is too thin with vasculature damage and resulting avascular necrosis.

# Suggested Readings

1. Bohling MW, Swaim SF: Management of the traumatic wound by primary closure. In Birchard SJ, Sherding RG, eds.: Saunders Manual of Small Animal Practice, 3rd ed.: St. Louis: Saunders – Elsevier, 2006, 541.
2. Bennett RG: Fundamentals of Cutaneous Surgery. St. Louis: CV Mosby, 1988, 355.
3. Fahie MA: Primary wound closure. In Tobias KM, Johnston SA, eds.: Veterinary Surgery, Small Animal, Vol. 2: St. Louis: Elsevier – Saunders, 2012, 1197.
4. Fowler D: Tension relieving techniques and local skin flaps. *In* Fowler D, Williams JM, eds.: BSAVA Manual of Canine and Feline Wound Management and Reconstruction. Shurdington, Cheltenham, UK: BSAVA, 1999, 56.
5. Hedlund CS: Surgery of the integumentary system. *In* Fossum TW, ed.: Small Animal Surgery, 2nd ed.: St. Louis: Mosby, 2002, 134.
6. Hedlund CS: Surgery of the integumentary system. In Fossum TW, ed.: Small Animal Surgery, 3rd ed.: St. Louis: Mosby, 2007, 159.
7. Johnston DE: Tension relieving techniques. Vet Clin North Am Small Anim Pract 20:67, 1990.
8. MacPhail CM: Surgery of the integumentary system. In Fossum TW, ed.: Small Animal Surgery, 4th ed.: St. Louis: Mosby, 2013, 190.
9. Mayhew, P: Tension – relieving techniques and local skin flaps.

In Williams J, Moores A, eds.: BSAVA Manual of Canine and Feline Wound Management and Reconstruction, 2nd ed.: Glouster (UK): BSAVA, 2009. 69.
10. McGuire MF: Studies of the excisional wound: I Biomechanical effects of undermining and wound orientation on closing tension and work. Plast Reconstr Surg 66:419, 1980.
11. Pavletic MM: Undermining for repair of large skin defects in small animals. Mod Vet Pract 67:13, 1986.
12. Pavletic MM: Atlas of Small Animal Reconstructive Surgery, 2nd ed.: Philadelphia: WB Saunders, 1999, 131.
13. Pavletic MM: Atlas of Small Animal Wound Management and Reconstructive Surgery, 3rd ed.: Ames, IA: Wiley – Blackwell, 2010, 241.
14. Scardino MS, Swaim SF, Henderson RA, et al: Enhancing wound closure on the limbs. Compend Contin Educ Pract Vet 18:919, 1996.
15. Stanley BJ: Tension – relieving techniques. In Tobias KM, Johnston SA, eds.: Veterinary Surgery, Small Animal, Vol. 2: St. Louis: Elsevier – Saunders, 2012, 1221.
16. Swaim SF: Management of skin tension in dermal surgery. Compend Contin Educ Pract Vet 2:758, 1980.
17. Swaim SF, Henderson RA: Small Animal Wound Management, 2nd ed.: Baltimore: Williams and Wilkins, 1997, 143.
18. Trout NJ: Principles of plastic and reconstructive surgery. *In* Slatter DH, ed.: Textbook of Small Animal Surgery, 3rd ed.: Philadelphia: WB Saudners, 2003, 274.

# Intradermal Closure - Tension Sutures

(See Wounds with Apposable Edges – No Tension, Intradermal Closure in this chapter)

# Simple Interrupted Tension Sutures

## Definition and Indications

A simple interrupted suture is one loop of suture material passed at right angles to the wound edge. The suture ends emerge on opposite sides of the wound. This type of suture is indicated for closing wounds that have minimal or no tension on the wound edges.

## Technique

(See Carpal-Metacarpal/Tarsal-Metatarsal Wounds, Wounds with Apposable Edges - No Tension, Closure-Sutures/Staples, Simple Interrupted Sutures.)

Simple interrupted sutures may be used as tension sutures when there is slight tension on the wound edges. They are placed using alternating wide bites and narrow bites with 3-0 to 2-0 suture material. The narrow bite sutures serve as apposition sutures, while the wide bite sutures serve as apposition and tension sutures (Figure 3-26A). If the skin edges cannot be closely apposed with thumb forceps and mild tension, there may be too much skin tension to use this type of suture pattern. An alternative for placing these sutures is to pass the widely spaced sutures through segments of soft rubber tubing to help prevent them from cutting into the skin. These sutures are used in combination with apposition sutures placed alternately with narrow bites (Figure 3-26B).

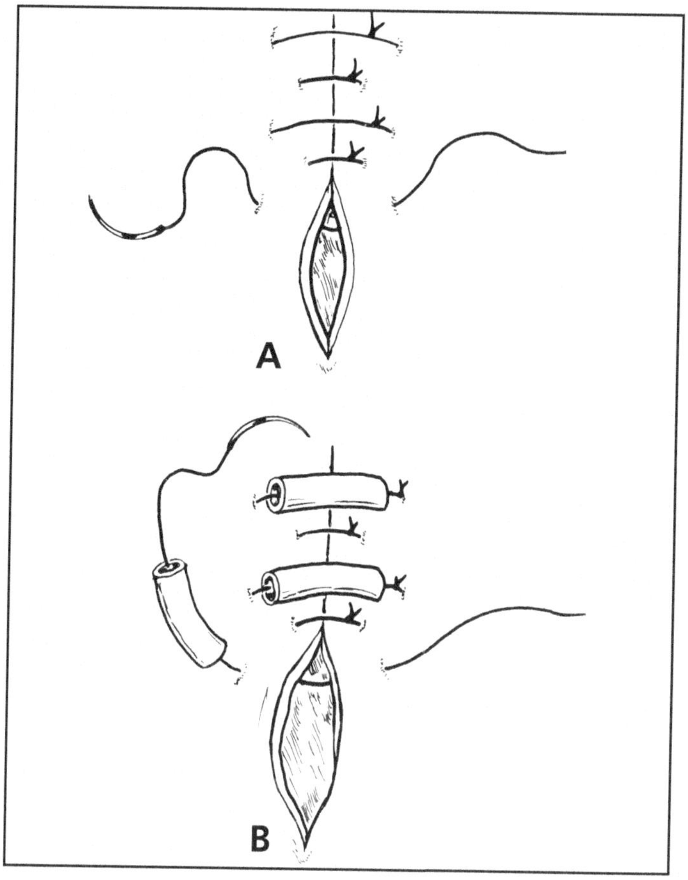

**Figure 3-26.** Alternating wide and narrow bites with simple interrupted sutures. **A.** Placing sutures. **B.** Widely placed sutures passed through tubing segments to prevent sutures from cutting into the skin.

## Aftercare

These sutures are usually removed 7 to 10 days after surgery. If segments of tubing have been used with the wide bite sutures, they are usually removed 3 to 5 days postoperatively.

## Advantages and Disadvantages

When there is minimal tension associated with wound closure, these sutures provide simple and effective closure. The surgeon can adjust the tension of each suture at areas along the wound according to the separating forces that are present. These sutures have the advantage of other interrupted sutures in that failure of one suture does not cause the entire suture line to fail.

Too much tension applied when tying the sutures may invert the skin edges when slight eversion is generally more desirable. In addition, if the closure tension is too great, the suture may tend to cut through the skin. This leaves an uncosmetic "cross-hatched" appearance. If segments of firm rubber tubing are used with the sutures, there may be pressure injury under the segments if the sutures are tied under too much tension.

## Suggested Readings

1. Johnston DE: Tension-relieving techniques. Vet Clin North Am Small Anim Pract 20:67, 1990.
2. Pavletic MM: Atlas of Small Animal Reconstructive Surgery, 2nd ed.: Philadelphia: WB Saunders, 1999, 131.
3. Pavletic MM: Atlas of Small Animal Wound Management and Reconstructive Surgery, 3rd ed.: Ames, IA: Wiley – Blackwell, 2010, 241.
4. Swaim SF: Management of skin tension in dermal surgery. Compend Contin Educ Pract Vet 2:758, 1980.
5. Swaim SF, Henderson RA: Small Animal Wound Management, 2nd ed.: Baltimore: Williams and Wilkins, 1997, 143.
6. Trout NJ: Principles of plastic and reconstructive surgery. *In* Slatter DH, ed.: Textbook of Small Animal Surgery, 3rd ed.: Philadelphia: WB Saudners, 2003, 274.

# Interrupted Vertical Mattress Sutures

### Definition and Indications

The vertical mattress suture is a loop of suture material inserted at a right angle to the wound edge with both suture ends emerging on the same side of the wound. These sutures are indicated for closing wound edges under tension.

### Technique

An interrupted vertical mattress suture of 3-0 or 2-0 nonabsorbable suture material is placed by inserting the needle approximately 8 mm from the skin edge. It is then passed across the wound to exit at a corresponding point on the opposite side of the wound. From this point, the needle is inserted back into the skin on the same side of the wound only 4 mm closer to the wound edge in line with its point of emergence. The needle is taken back across the wound to a point 4 mm from the skin edge on the original side of the wound (Figure 3-27A). The second or near bite may be altered by splitting the thickness of the skin as the needle passes from one side of the wound to the other. Another alteration in suture placement is to place the second bite deeper to catch a small amount of subcutaneous tissue as the needle goes from one side of the wound to the other. Thus, as the suture is tied it helps close dead space under the wound edges. These sutures are placed about 5 mm apart; however, placement will vary depending upon the animal and the thickness of the skin being sutured. Simple interrupted sutures may be used along with interrupted vertical mattress sutures for final skin apposition. Wound closure can also be accomplished by the alternate placement of vertical mattress and simple interrupted sutures. If considerable wound tension is present, rubber tubing may be placed under the vertical mattress sutures to help prevent them from cutting into the tissues (Figure 3-27B & C). Soft latex rubber tubing (Penrose drain tube) is preferred.

### Aftercare

The vertical mattress tension sutures should be removed on the third or fourth day postoperatively. When a bandage is placed over the sutures that have rubber tubing under them, it should be loosely applied because pressure bandages may tend to increase the incidence of pressure necrosis under the tubing.

### Advantages and Disadvantages

Vertical mattress sutures can serve as both appositional to tension sutures. They effectively relieve tension on wound edges, and they slightly evert the wound edges. Vertical mattress sutures are stronger under tension than horizontal mattress sutures. The sutures do not tend to interfere with circulation at the wound edges because all components of the suture lie in a linear plane; whereas, components of a horizontal mattress suture lie in different planes, forming a box which could obstruct circulation at the wound edge. Placement of vertical mattress sutures is relatively time consuming. Vertical mattress tension sutures concentrate tension near the wound edges. This can result in the sutures cutting into the skin if no rubber tubing is used under the sutures. If rubber tubing is used under the sutures there may be areas of pressure injury under the tubing at the time of suture removal. However, these are usually not severe.

## Suggested Readings

1. Bellenger CR: Sutures. Part II: the use of sutures and alternative methods of closure. Compend Contin Educ Pract Vet 4:587, 1982.
2. Bennett RG: Fundamentals of Cutaneous Surgery. St. Louis: CV Mosby, 1988, 445.
3. Bohling MW, Swaim SF: Management of the traumatic wound by primary closure. In Birchard SJ, Sherding RG, eds.: Saunders Manual of Small Animal Practice, 3rd ed.: St. Louis: Saunders – Elsevier, 2006, 541.
4. Boothe H: Intrument and tissue handling techniques. In Tobias KM, Johnston SA, eds.: Veterinary Surgery, Small Animal, Vol. 1: St. Louis: Elsevier – Saunders, 2012, 201.
5. Fahie MA: Primary wound closure. In Tobias KM, Johnston SA, eds.: Veterinary Surgery, Small Animal, Vol. 2: St. Louis: Elsevier – Saunders, 2012, 1197.
6. Fossum TW: Biomaterials, suturing, and hemostasis. In Fossum TW, ed.: Small Animal Surgery, 2nd ed.: St. Louis: Mosby, 2002, 43.
7. Fossum TW: Biomaterials, suturing and hemostasis. In Fossum

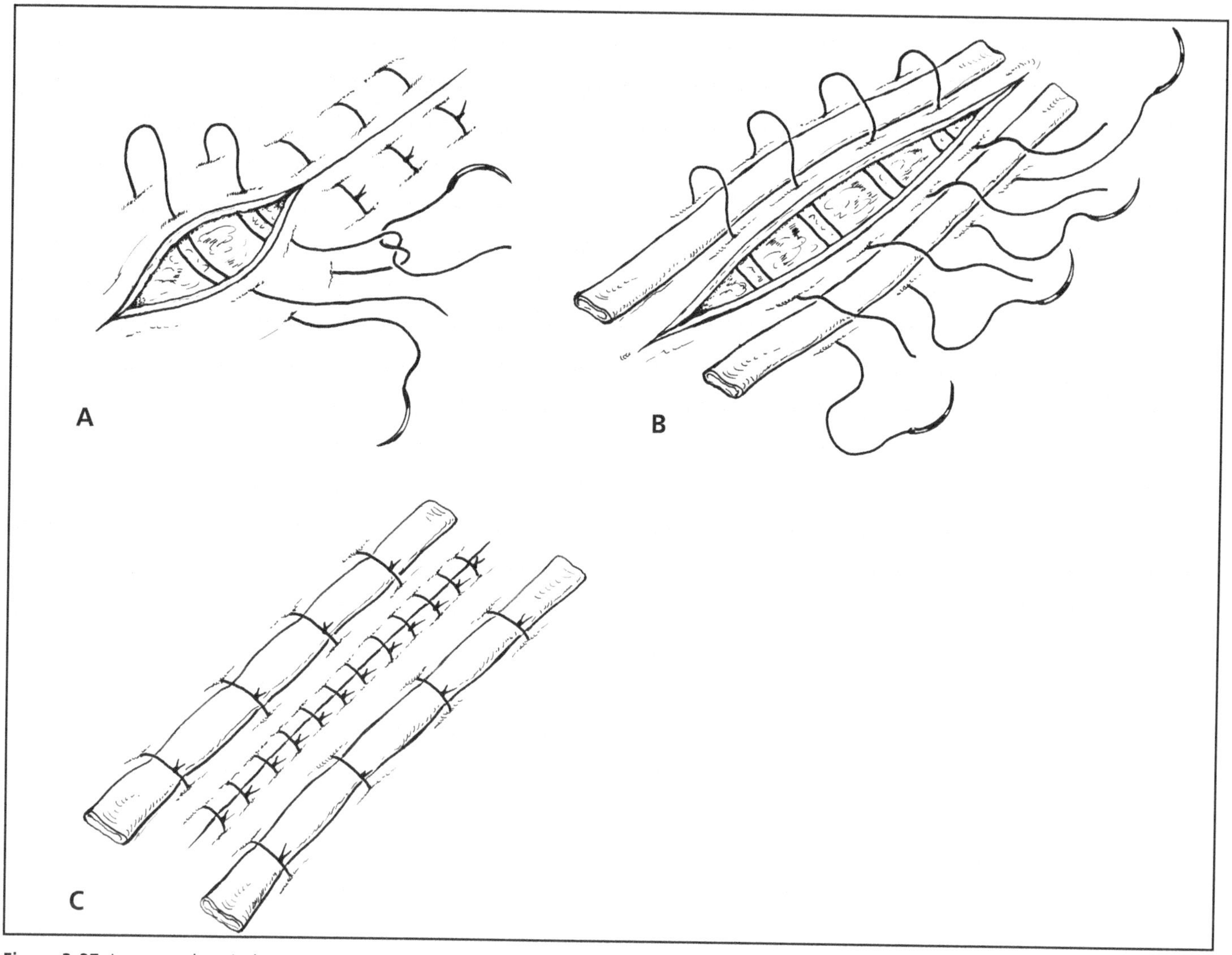


**Figure 3-27.** Interrupted vertical mattress tension sutures. **A.** Suture placement. **B.** Suture placement over segments of soft rubber tubing. **C.** Vertical mattress sutures tied and simple interrupted skin apposition sutures placed for final wound closure.

TW, ed.: Small Animal Surgery, 3rd. ed.: St. Louis: Mosby, 2007, 57.
8. Jankauskas S, Cohen IK, Grabb WC: Basic technique of plastic surgery. In Smith JW, Aston SJ, eds.: Plastic Surgery, 4th ed.: Boston: Little, Brown, 1991, 3.
9. Knecht CD, Allen AR, Williams DJ, et al: Fundamental Techniques in Veterinary Surgery, 3rd ed.: Philadelphia, WB Saunders, 1987, 54.
10. MacPhail CM: Surgery of the integumentary system. In Fossum TW, ed.: Small Animal Surgery, 4th ed.: St. Louis: Mosby, 2013, 190.
11. Pavletic MM: Atlas of Small Animal Reconstructive Surgery, 2nd ed.: Philadelphia: WB Saunders, 1999, 131.
12. Pavletic MM: Atlas of Small Animal Wound Management and Reconstructive Surgery, 3rd ed.: Ames, IA: Wiley = Blackwell, 2010, 241.
13. Scardino MS, Swaim SF, Henderson RA, et al: Enhancing wound closure on the limbs. Compend Contin Edu Pract Vet 18:919, 1996.
14. Swaim SF: Management of skin tension in dermal surgery. Compend Contin Educ Pract Vet 2:758, 1980.
15. Swaim SF: Management of the traumatic wound by primary closure. In Birchard SJ, Sherding RG, eds.: Saunders Manual of Small Animal Practice, 2nd ed.: Philadelphia: WB Saunders, 2000, 392.
16. Swaim SF, Henderson RA: Small Animal Wound Management, 2nd ed.: Baltimore: Williams and Wilkins, 1997, 143.
17. Trout NJ: Principles of plastic and reconstructive surgery. In Slatter DH, ed.: Textbook of Small Animal Surgery, 3rd ed.: Philadelphia: WB Saudners, 2003, 274.
18. Williams J: Decision – making in wound closure. In Williams J, Moores A, eds.: BSAVA Manual of Canine and Feline Wound Management and Reconstruction, 2nd ed.: Glouster (UK): BSAVA. 2009, 25.

# Far-Near-Near-Far and Far-Far-Near-Near Sutures

## Definition and Indicaitons

Far-near-near-far and far-far-near-near sutures are combinations of apposition and tension sutures that are placed in the order that their names imply. They are a variation of the interrupted vertical mattress suture. The far components of these sutures supply the tension while the near components appose the skin edges. These sutures are indicated for closing wounds in which tissue tension must be overcome to appose the wound edges. They are also indicated for closing wounds where tension on the wound edges cyclically increases and decreases during movement, such as over the flexion surface of the carpus or tarsus or in lacerated paw pads.

## Techniques

### Far-Near-Near-Far

Nonabsorbable 3-0 to 2-0 suture material is used, taking the first bite of the suture 5 to 7 mm from the wound edge. The needle is passed through the skin and subcutaneous tissue. It crosses the wound and exits through the skin on the opposite side of the wound about 1 to 3 mm from the edge. The needle is returned back across the wound externally for insertion through the skin 1 to 3 mm from the wound edge. It is then passed through the skin and subcutaneous tissue back across the wound, exiting 5 to 7 mm from the wound edge. All entrance and exit points of the suture in the skin are in a straight line (Figure 3-28A). The distance for placing these sutures varies depending on the location of the wound and tissues being sutured.

### Far-Far-Near-Near

This suture is placed by inserting the needle 5 to 7 mm back from the wound edge, passing it across the wound to a corresponding point on the opposite side of the wound where it penetrates the skin from deep to superficial. After passing through the skin, the needle is returned across the wound externally and is passed through the skin 1 to 3 mm from the wound edge on the original side of the wound. The needle again crosses the wound to penetrate the skin from deep to superficial 1 to 3 mm from the wound edge. All entrance and exit points for the suture in the skin are in a straight line (Figure 3-28B).

## Aftercare

The sutures are removed 7 to 10 days postoperatively unless the surgeon believes that wound tissue movement may be slowing the healing, and then the sutures can be left in place for 14 days or longer if warranted, based on clinical judgment. For example, the sutures may need to be left in the paw pads longer on a heavy dog.

## Advantages and Disadvantages

Both of the sutures provide apposition and tension relief in one suture. They apply necessary tension for wound edge apposition without placing tension on the wound edge itself. Over tightening the sutures may result in inversion of the skin which may impair healing. These sutures place a large amount of suture material in one area with double sutures in an overlapping pattern in the skin.

# Suggested Readings


1. Bohling MW, Swaim SF: Management of the traumatic wound by primary closure. In Birchard SJ, Sherding RG, eds.: Saunders Manual of Small Animal Practice, 3rd ed.: St. Louis: Saunders – Elsevier, 2006, 541.
2. Knecht CD, Allen AR, Williams DJ, et al: Fundamental Techniques in Veterinary Surgery, 3rd ed.: Philadelphia: WB Saunders, 1987, 54.
3. Pavletic MM: Atlas of Small Animal Reconstructive Surgery, 2nd ed.: Philadelphia: WB Saunders, 1999, 131.
4. Pavletic MM: Atlas of Small Animal Wound Management and Reconstructive Surgery, 3rd ed.: Ames, IA: Wiley – Blackwell, 2010, 241.


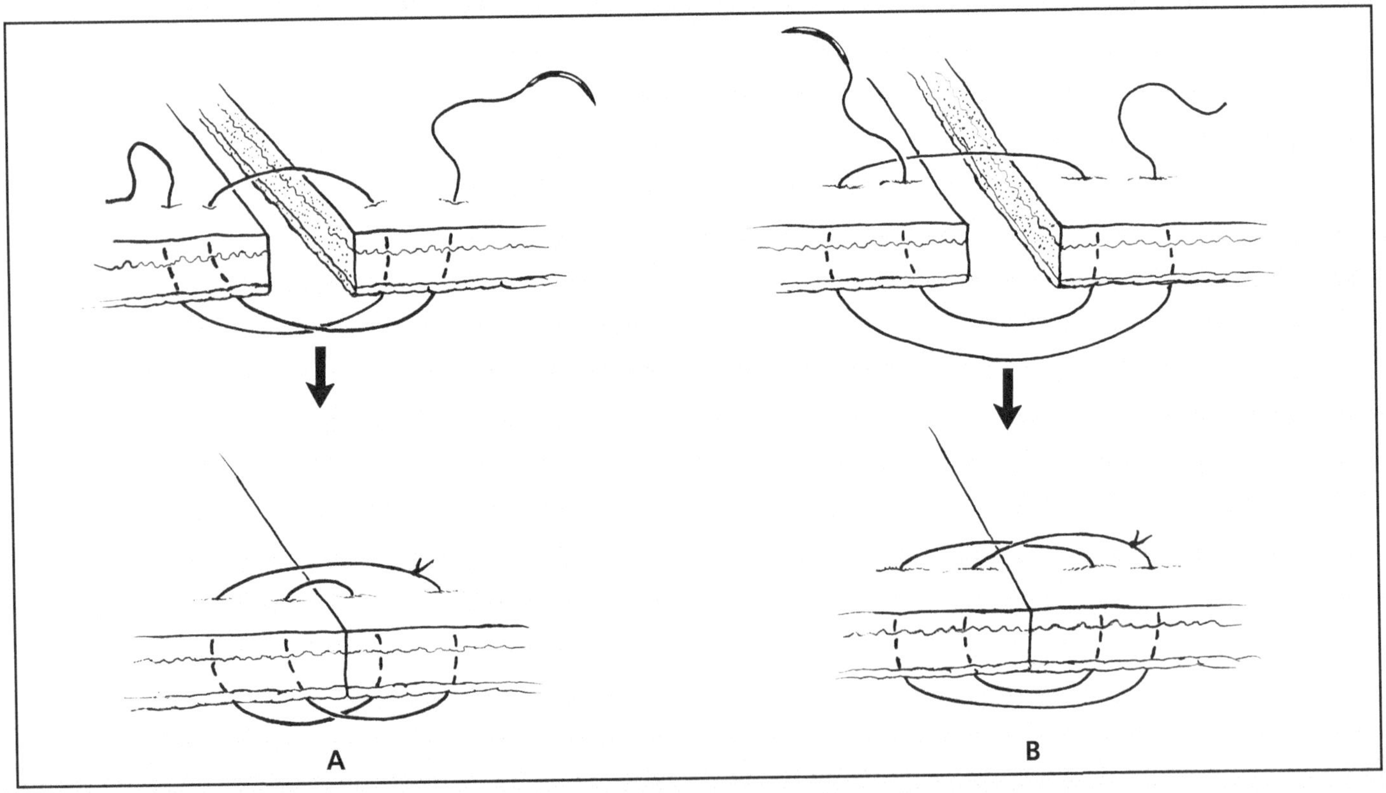


**Figure 3-28.** Combination tension and apposition sutures. **A.** Far-near-near-far suture. **B.** Far-far-near-near suture.

5. Scardino MS, Swaim SF, Henderson RA, et al: Enhancing wound closure on the limbs. Compend Contin Educ Pract Vet 18:919, 1996.
6. Stanley BJ: Tension – relieving techniques. In Tobias KM, Johnston SA, eds.: Veterinary Surgery, Small Animal, Vol. 2: St. Louis: Elsevier – Saunders, 2012, 1221.
7. Swaim SF: Management of skin tension in dermal surgery. Compend Contin Educ Pract Vet 2: 758, 1980.
8. Swaim SF: Management of the traumatic wound by primary closure. In Birchard SJ, Sherding RG, eds.: Saunders Manual of Small Animal Practice, 2nd ed.: Philadelphia: WB Saunders, 2000, 392.
9. Swaim SF, Henderson RA: Small Animal Wound Management, 2nd ed.: Baltimore: Williams and Wilkins, 1997, 143.
10. Trout NJ: Principles of plastic and reconstructive surgery. In Slatter DH, ed.: Textbook of Small Animal Surgery, 3rd ed.: Philadelphia: WB Saudners, 2003, 274.
11. Williams J: Decision – making in wound closure. In Williams J, Moores A, eds.: BSAVA Manual of Canine and Feline Wound Management and Reconstruction, 2nd ed.: Glouster (UK), BSAVA, 2009, 25.

# Presutures

## Definition and Indications

Presutures are Lembert sutures that are placed with bites in healthy skin on either side of a lesion. The sutures are effective in areas where elastic skin is limited, such as on the limbs. They bridge the incision and stretch the skin on each side of the lesion by mechanical creep and stress relaxation so it can be used for wound closure. They are placed several hours (up to 24 hours) prior to excising or debriding a lesion. Presutures are usually indicated for limb wounds where the skin edges cannot be initially apposed or where a lesion (e.g. tumor) will be excised that will result in such a wound. Presutures can also be used when wound edges will appose but there will be tension on the closure (Figure 3-29A-D). If, in the surgeon's judgement, the wound will close without use of a graft or flap, presutures should be considered.

## Technique

Following administration of a tranquilizer or neuroleptanalgesic, the skin around the lesion is prepared for aseptic surgery. A local analgesic is then injected around the lesion. As an alternative, general anesthesia could be used. Either 1-0 or 2-0 nonabsorbable synthetic monofilament suture material is used to take Lembert-type suture bites in the skin, with the number of sutures varying with the length of the surgical site. Sutures are placed 3 to 5 cm from a wound edge or proposed incision site. The bites bridge the lesion (Figure 3-30A). The sutures are tied with tension as they are placed to imbricate the skin (Figure 3-30B and See Figure 3-29B).

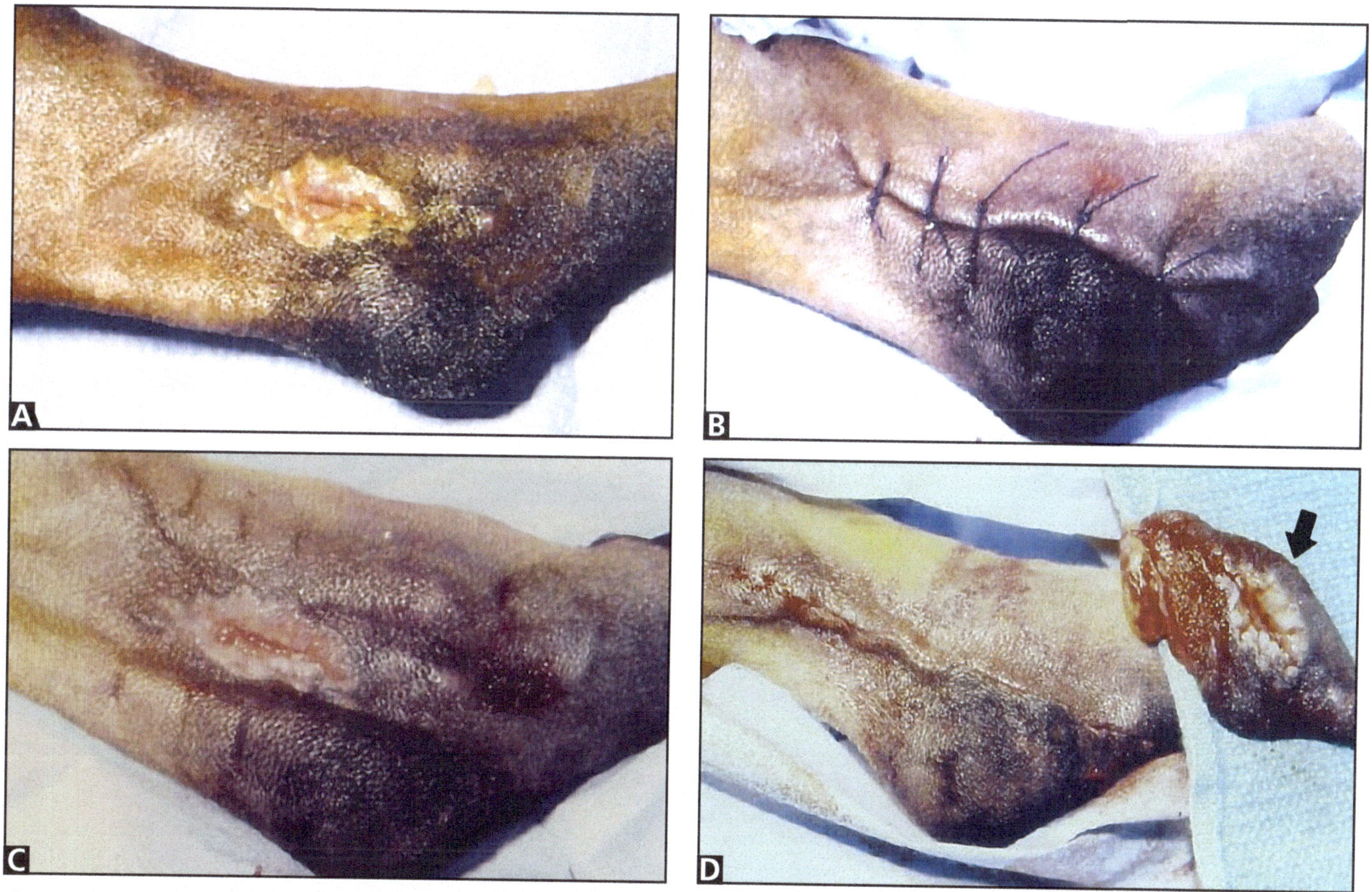

**Figure 3-29.** Presutures. **A.** Lesion on the lateral pelvic limb at the level of the hock. **B.** Presutures placed to stretch the surrounding skin. Lesion is under the skin that has been pulled over it by sutures. **C.** Presutures have been removed. Note suture marks. **D.** The lesion *(arrow)* has been removed and the resulting defect has been closed. ( After Swaim SF, Henderson RA: Small Animal Wound Management, 2nd ed.: Baltimore: Williams & Wilkins, 1997, 174.)

The sutures are placed such that the direction of stretch is in the anticipated direction of tension. This is usually perpendicular to the long axis of the limb. Presutures are usually placed in the late afternoon and placed under a bandage overnight. An Elizabethan collar may be needed to prevent bandage and wound molestation. In addition, an analgesic medication may be necessary.

## Aftercare

The final wound closure after use of presutures to stretch the skin could be considered as the aftercare. The morning after presutures have been placed, the animal is anesthetized and the presutures are removed (See Figure 3-29C). The limb is prepared for aseptic surgery. After the wound is debrided or the lesion is removed, the wound is closed using the prestretched skin (Figure 3-30C and See Figure 3-29D).

## Advantages and Disadvantages

The main advantage of presutures is that they simply and economically prestretch skin so it can be used for wound closure. In addition, they can be used in conjunction with other tension-relieving techniques when the presutures themselves do not provide the relaxation needed for wound closure.

Presutures have the potential disadvantage of not being adjustable and causing a biologic tourniquet. If such constriction does occur, it can be relieved by removing the sutures. If signs of impaired circulation occur, it is a forewarning that primary skin closure after use of presutures only may not be possible or advisable. Additional relaxing techniques such as relaxing incisions or an adjustable horizontal mattress suture may be considered. If it appears these will be insufficient, skin grafts or flaps may be necessary for wound closure.

# Suggested Readings


1. Bohling MW, Swaim SF: Management of the traumatic wound by primary closure. In Birchard SJ, Sherding RG, eds.: Saunders Manual of Small Animal Practice, 3rd ed.: St. Louis: Saunders – Elsevier, 2006, 541.
2. Bohling MW, Swaim SF: Paw and distal limb skin reconstructive and salvage techniques. In Bojrab MJ, ed.: Current Techniques in Small Animal Surgery, 5th ed.: Jackson, WY: Teton NewMedia 2014, 628.
3. Fowler D: Tension relieving techniques and local skin flaps. *In* Fowler D, Williams JM, eds.: BSAVA Manual of Canine and Feline Wound Management and Reconstruction. Shurdington,


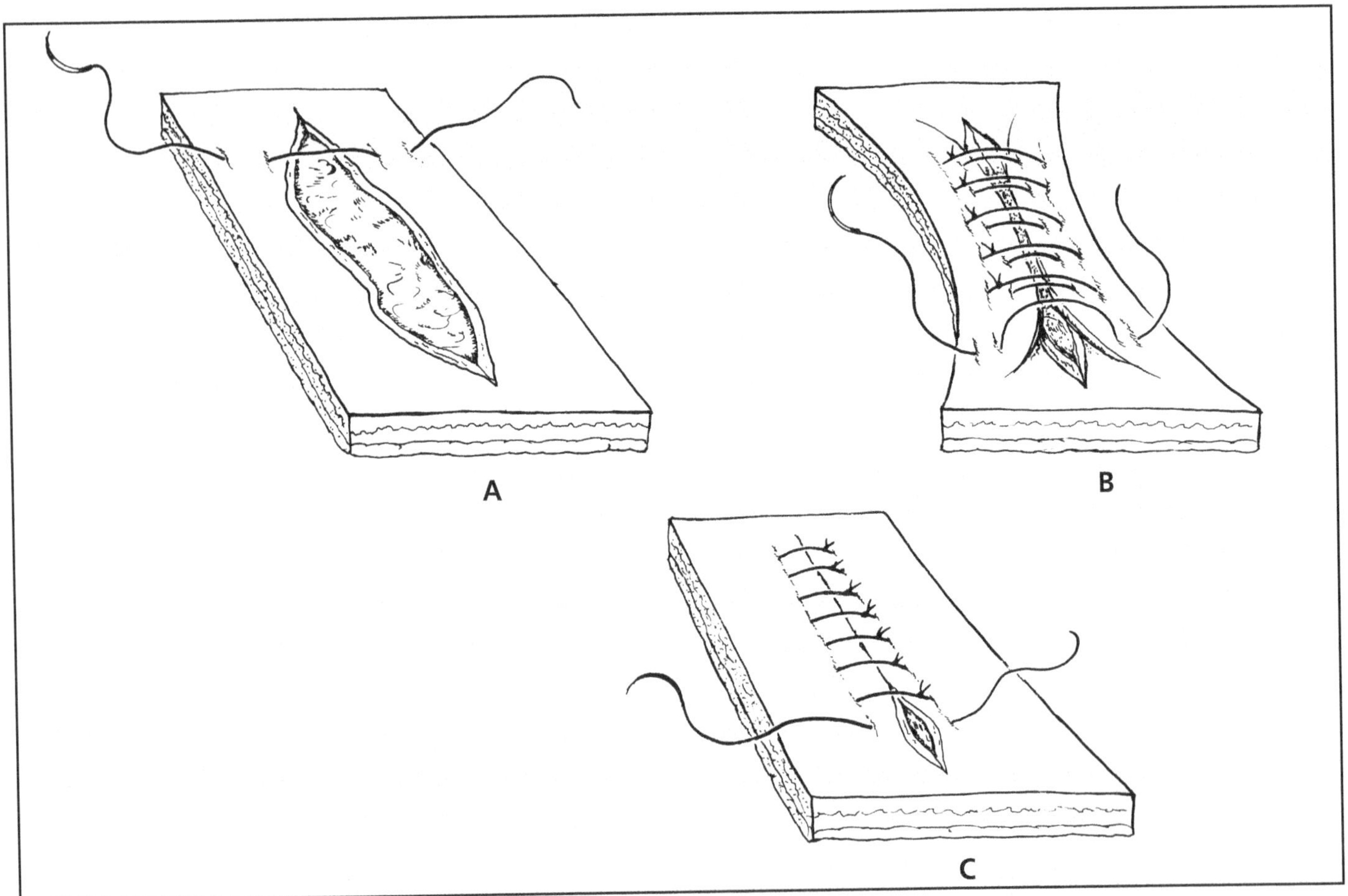


**Figure 3-30.** Presutures. **A & B.** The day before definitive surgery Lembert – type sutures are placed in the skin adjacent to the lesion. The sutures are tied under tension pulling the skin over the lesion. **C.** Before definitive surgery, presutures are removed, and the wound is debrided. The wound is closed using the prestretched skin made available by the presutures.

Cheltenham, UK: BSAVA, 1999, 57.
4. Fowler D: Distal limb and paw injuries. Vet Clin No Am Small Anim Pract 36: 819, 2006.
5. Hedlund CS: Surgery of the integumentary system. *In* Fossum TW, ed.: Small Animal Surgery, 2nd ed.: St. Louis: Mosby, 2002, 134.
6. Hedlund CS: Surgery of the integumentary system. In Fossum TW, ed.: Small Animal Surgery, 3rd ed.: St. Louis: Mosby, 2007, 159.
7. Laing MD, Briggs P, Heckler FR, et al: Presuturing, a new technique for closing large skin defects: clinical and experimental studies. Plast Reconst Surg 81:694, 1988.
8. MacPhail CM: Surgery of the integumentary system. In Fossum TW, ed.: Small Animal Surgery, 4th ed.: St. Louis: Mosby, 2013, 190.
9. Pavletic MM: Atlas of Small Animal Reconstructive Surgery, 2nd ed.: Philadelphia: WB Saunders, 1999, 173.
10. Pavletic MM: Atlas of Small Animal Wound Management and Reconstructive Surgery, 3rd ed.: Ames, IA: Wiley – Blackwell, 2010, 287.
11. Scardino MS, Swaim SF, Henderson RA, et al: Enhancing wound closure on the limbs. Compend Contin Educ Pract Vet 18:919, 1996.
12. Stanley BJ: Tension – relieving techniques. In Tobias KM, Johnston SA, eds.: Veterinary Surgery, Small Animal, Vol. 2: St. Louis: Elsevier – Saunders, 2012, 1221.
13. Swaim SF, Henderson RA: Small Animal Wound Mangement, 2nd ed.: Baltimore: Williams and Wilkins, 1997, 143.
14. Swaim SF, Scardino MS: Paw and distal limb salvage and reconstructive techniques. In Bajrab MJ, ed.: Current Techniques in Small Animal Surgery, 4th ed.: Baltimore: Williams and Wilkins, 1998, 625.
15. Swaim SF: Management of the traumatic wound by primary closure. *In* Birchard SJ, Sherding RG, eds.: Saunders Manual of Small Animal Practice, 2nd ed.: Philadelphia: WB Saunders, 2000, 392.
16. Trout NJ: Principles of plastic and reconstructive surgery. *In* Slatter DH, ed.: Textbook of Small Animal Surgery, 3rd ed.: Philadelphia: WB Saunders, 2003, 274.
17. Williams J: Decision – making in wound closure. In Williams J, Moores A, eds.: BSAVA Manual of Small Animal Wound Management and Reconstruction, 2nd ed.: Glouster (UK), BSAVA, 2009, 25.

# Various Shaped Wounds

There are numerous shaped wounds and these may occur on the distal limb. The following is not an exhaustive coverage of the techniques to close these wounds. However, it covers some of the wound shapes that may be commonly encountered, explaining the source of these wounds. Although there will be specific descriptions of closure techniques, the most important thing is for the surgeon to use his/her hands and imagination in planning closure. In so doing, it may be found that a specific technique may not be applicable for a certain shaped wound, and a modification may be necessary. Other wounds will have no specific shape, again the hands and imagination come into play in designing wound closure. *The important underlying factors in planning wound closure on the distal limb, where skin is at a premium, are to relieve or avoid tension, reduce or avoid removing extra normal skin (e.g. "dog-ears"), and use "dog-ear" skin when possible to help with wound closure.*

## Chevron, Crescent and Triangular-Shaped (Y-Closure)

### Definition and Indications

Chevron-shaped wounds are basically V-shaped, and they have an angular flap of skin associated with them. Some wounds may have a crescent – like shape with a curved rather than angular flap of skin. Such wounds usually occur when a limb is pushed down into or pulled up against a sharp edge (Figure 3-31 and Figure 3-32). The entire flap may be viable in some wounds. In some wounds, part of the flap may have been lost as a result of necrosis or debridement of the flap. This flap loss may have been severe enough that the entire flap is missing. This results in a triangular-shaped defect.

If the entire flap is viable, it can be sutured back in place. However, if a distal portion of the flap is missing, the resulting chevron-shaped defect may be closed in the shape of a Y. Because the flap is free, it does not require any undermining.

The flap of skin associated with a chevron-shaped or crescent - shaped wound should be evaluated for viability. The size, position and length of the flap are important with regard to the blood supply to the flap. In some flaps, the blood supply to the entire flap may be intact. However, a large ventrally based flap that has folded back on itself as the result of gravity may have a greater tendency for impaired circulation due to the kinking of blood vessels at its base than a smaller or dorsally based flap (Figure 3-33). If a ventrally based flap has been present for any length of time, there is more tendency for impaired circulation.

### Technique

The flap should be carefully evaluated before a decision is made on a technique for reconstruction. If the entire flap is viable and it has a sharp angle at its tip, it may be repositioned and sutured in place. The tip is sutured in place with a half-buried horizontal mattress suture to help preserve blood supply at the tip of the flap. The suture is passed through the full-thickness of skin on the outside edge on one side of the wound, through the tip of the flap as an intradermal suture, and then full-thickness out through the skin edge on the other side of the wound. The suture is tied to pull the flap tip into position (Figure 3-34A), followed by suturing the 2 remaining arms of the defect. If it is necessary to trim the edge of the flap slightly and it still has an angular tip, there may be some tension associated with closure. To help alleviate tension, the V-shaped chevon is closed in the shape of a Y. The 2 sides of the point of the defect are sutured until tension develops, forming the

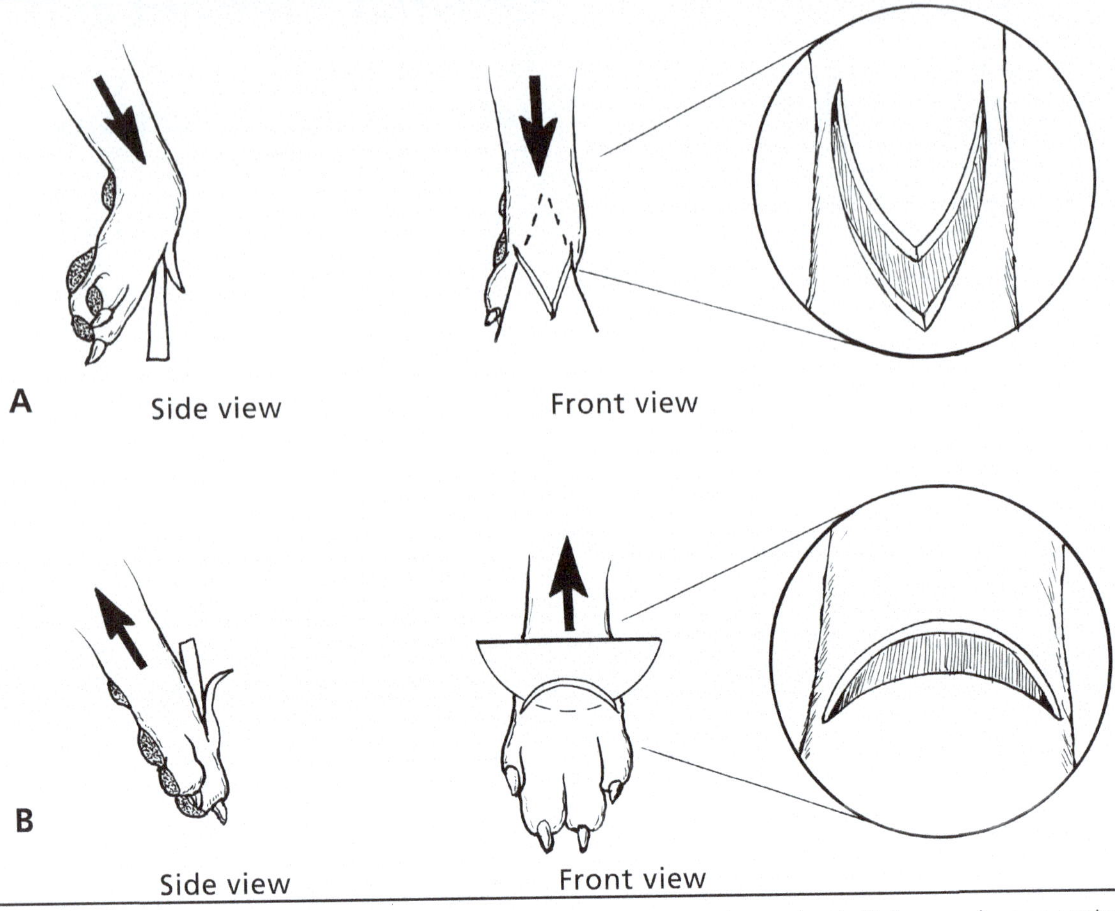


**Figure 3-31.** Dynamics of chevron and crescent – shaped wounds. **A.** Chevron – shaped wound created as the limb comes down on a pointed cutting object with sharp edges. **B.** Crescent – shaped wound created as the limb comes up under a curved cutting edge.

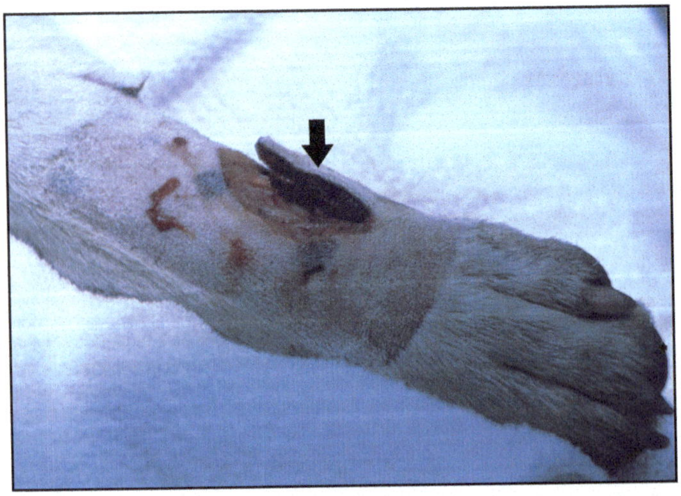

**Figure 3-32.** Flap of skin *(arrow)* elevated from the distal limb by a sharp object.

stem of the Y. Then the 2 arms are sutured, beginning at their ends and suturing toward the stem of the Y. At the juncture of the 3 suture lines, a half-buried horizontal mattress suture is placed (Figure 3-34B). Alternatively, the 2 sides of the defect can be closed first until tension develops followed by closure of the stem of the Y.

A flap with a sharp line of demarcation across it with discolored tissue distal to the line generally has a poor prognosis for viability of the flap. It may be necessary to debride the edge of the flap progressively until fresh hemorrhaging is observed at the wound edge before suturing the remaining tissue back in place (Figure 3-35A & B).

The skin on each side of the remaining defect should be undermined. Suturing is performed as described as in closing a Y shaped defect (Figure 3-35C & D).

When avascular necrosis and/or debridement requires amputation of the flap, a triangular defect is formed (Figure 3-36A). Skin around the defect should be undermined and the defect should be closed either by closing the stem on a Y and then the arms or with

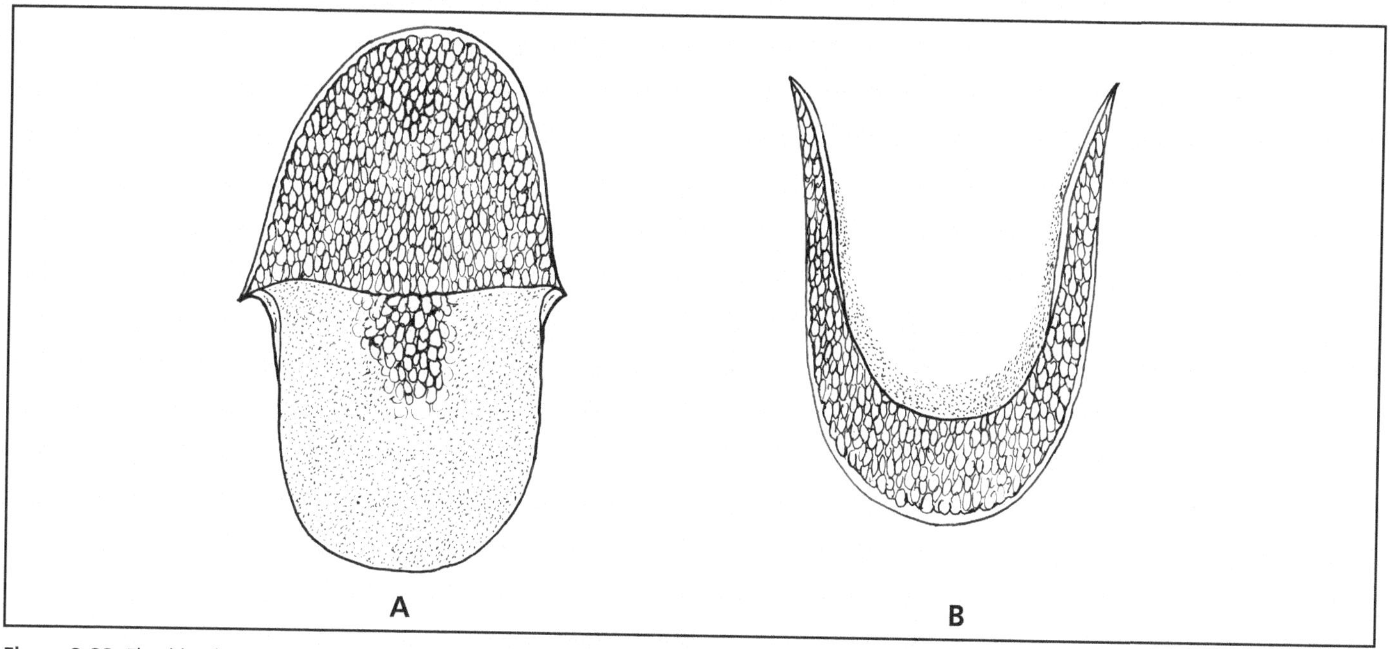


**Figure 3-33.** Flap blood supply and viability. **A.** A ventrally based flap folded back resulting in impaired circulation to a larger area *(stippled area)*. **B.** Dorsally based flap with less impaired circulation *(stippled area)*. (After Swaim SF, Henderson RA: Small Animal Wound Management, 2nd ed.: Baltimore: Williams & Wilkins, 1997, 273.)

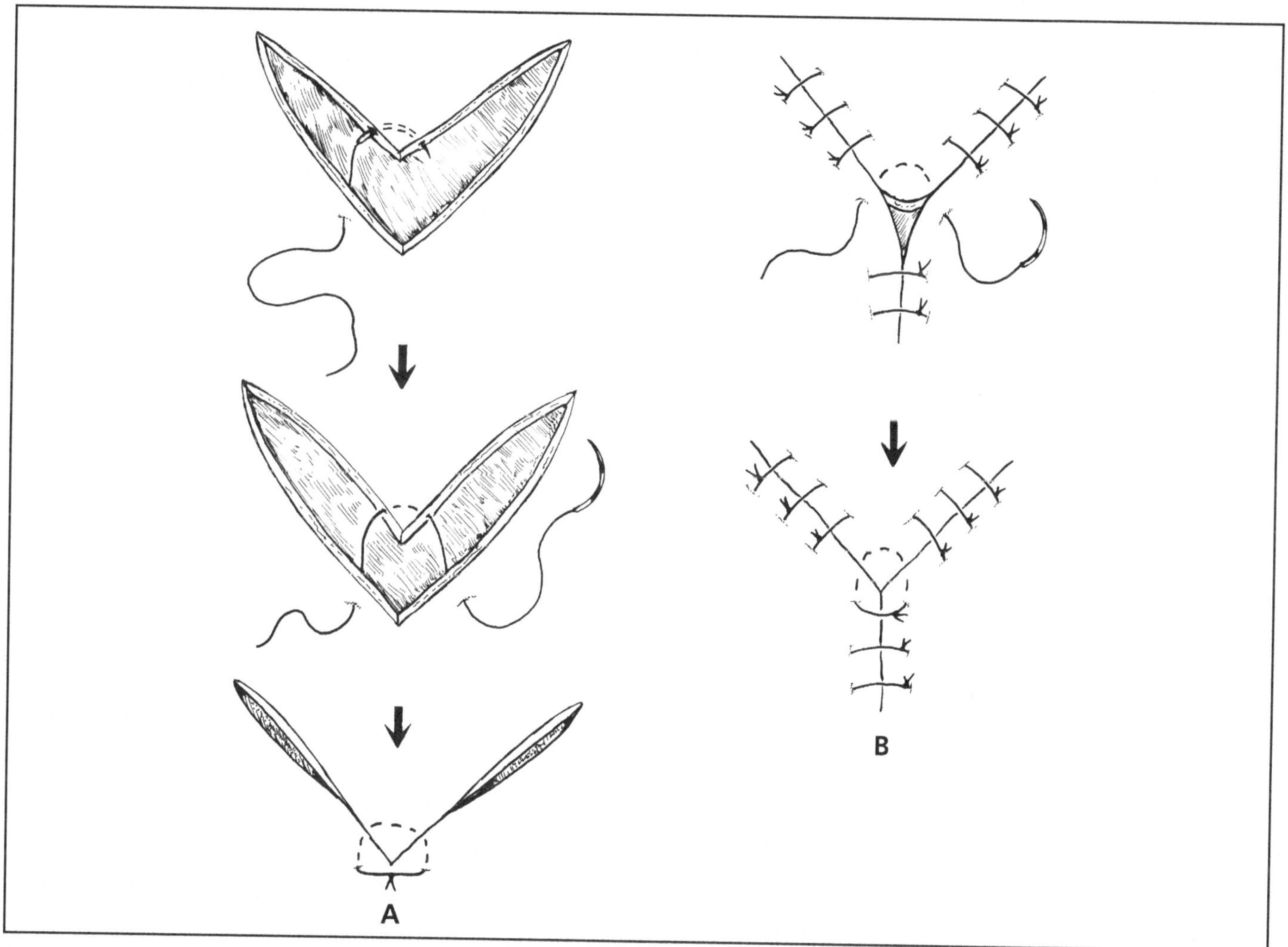


**Figure 3-34.** Viable chevron – shaped wound with sharp angular tip of the flap. **A.** Half – buried horizontal mattress suture is placed at flap tip. Suture passed through full – thickness skin on the outside edge of one side of the wound, intradermally through the flap tip, and then out full – thickness through the skin edge of the other side of the wound. The suture is tied to pull the flap tip into place. **B.** With slight trimming of the flap edge and a remaining angular flap tip, Y – shaped closure may be used with a half – buried horizontal mattress suture at the junction of the suture lines.

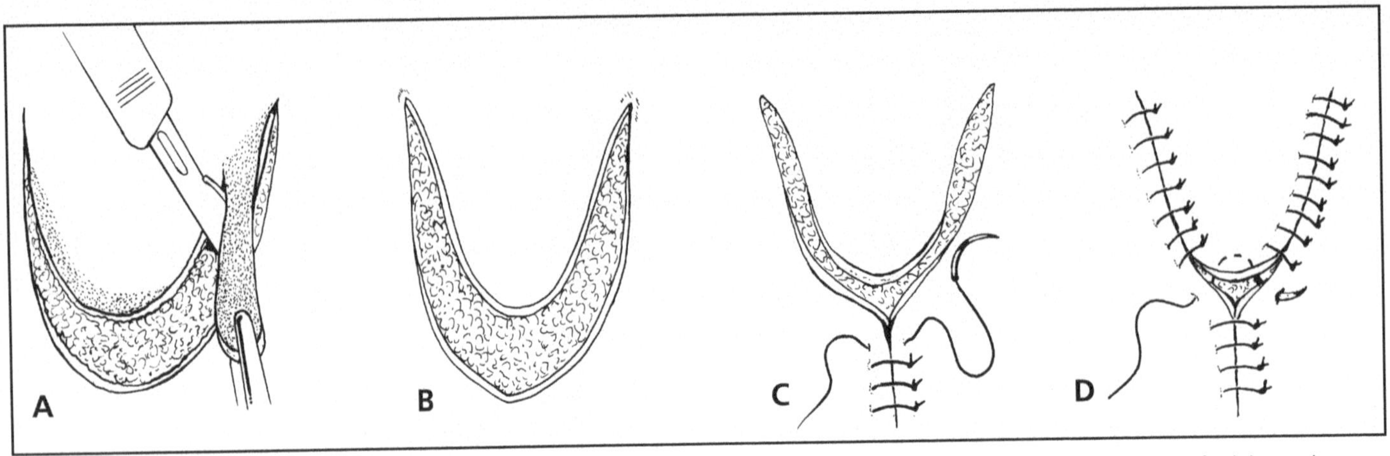


Figure 3-35. Debridement and Y – shaped closure of a chevron – shaped wound. A. Debriding the edge of the flap progressively until fresh hemorrhage is seen at wound edge. B. Viable tissue flap. C. Suturing is started at the point of the chevron until tension develops. D. Arms of the Y are sutured and a half – buried horizontal mattress suture is placed at the juncture of the arms and stem of the Y. (After Swaim SF, Henderson RA: Small Animal Wound Management, 2nd ed.: Baltimore: Williams & Wilkins, 1997, 273.)

centripetal suture placement. Again, at the junction of the 3 suture lines, a half-buried horizontal mattress suture should be placed (Figure 3-36B-D).

## Aftercare

Y-shaped closure of chevron-shaped wounds and centripetal closure of triangular-shaped defects require no special aftercare.

## Advantages and Disadvantages

Y-shaped closure of chevron-shaped wounds and centripetal closure of triangular defects provide simple techniques for closing such wounds. With centripetal closure of triangular-shaped wounds there may be slight elevation of the skin at the wound corners which are not true "dog-ears". These usually flatten with time. If there is suture line breakdown in these wounds, it usually begins at the junction of the 3 suture lines. However, the half-buried horizontal mattress suture helps prevent this.

# Suggested Readings


1. Boothe HW: Instrument and tissue handling techniques. In Tobias KM, Johnston SA, eds.: Veterinary Surgery, Small Animal, Vol. 1: St. Louis: Elsevier – Saunders, 2012, 201.
2. Hedlund CS: Surgery of the integumentary system. *In* Fossum TW, ed.: Small Animal Surgery, 2nd ed.: St. Louis: Mosby, 2002, 134.
3. Hedlund CS: Surgery of the integumentary system. In Fossum TW, ed.: Small Animal Surgery, 3rd ed.: St. Louis: Mosby, 2007, 159.
4. MacPhail CM: Surgery of the integumentary system. In Fossum TW, ed.: Small Animal Surgery, 4th ed.: St. Louis: Mosby, 2013, 190.
5. Pavletic MM: Atlas of Small Animal Reconstructive Surgery, 2nd ed.: Philadelphia: 1999, 131.
6. Pavletic MM: Atlas of Small Animal Wound Management and Reconstructive Surgery, 3rd ed.: Ames, IA: Wiley – Blackwell, 2010, 241.
7. Stanley BJ: Tension – relieving techniques. In Tobias KM, Johnston SA, eds.: Veterinary Surgery, Small Animal, Vol. 2: St. Louis: Elsevier – Saunders, 2012, 1221.
8. Swaim SF, Henderson RA, Sutton HH: Correction of triangular and wedge-shaped skin defects in dogs and cats. J Amer Anim Hosp Assoc 16:225, 1980.
9. Swaim SF, Henderson RA: Small Animal Wound Mangement, 2nd ed.: Baltimore: Williams and Wilkins, 1997, 235.
10. Trout NJ: Principles of plastic and reconstructive surgery. *In*


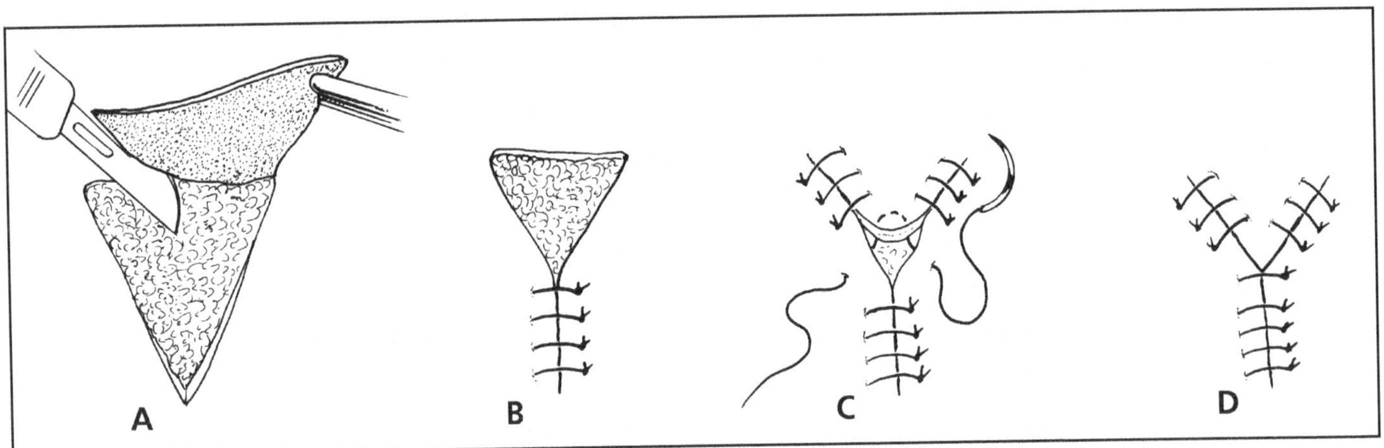


Figure 3-36. Debridement and Y – shaped closure of a triangular wound. A. Debriding nonviable skin. B. Viable tissue remains and suturing is started at the point of the triangle. It continues until tension develops. C and D. Arms of the Y are sutured and a half – buried horizontal mattress suture is placed at the juncture of the arms and stem of the Y.

Slatter DH, ed.: Textbook of Small Animal Surgery, 3rd ed.: Philadelphia: WB Saunders, 2003, 274.
11. Williams J: Decision – making in wound closure. In Williams J, Moores A, eds.: BSAVA Manual of Canine and Feline Wound Management and Reconstruction, 2nd ed.: Glouster (UK): BSAVA, 2009, 25.

# Circular (Linear Closure)

## Definition and Indications

With a circular wound all points of the wound edge are an equal distance from the wound center. Small circular wounds lend themselves best to linear closure. These are wounds that would most commonly result from excision of a lesion. Circular excision is the most tissue conserving configuration for removing a lesion.

Linear closure of a circular wound entails suturing one side of the wound to the other side, with "dog-ear" removal as needed. The size of the "dog ear" will be dependant upon the laxity of the skin and size of the circular defect. Linear closure should be used when edge-to-edge closure can be done with a small amount of tension and it results in little or no "dog-ear" formation i.e. small circular wounds.

## Technique

The skin around a circular defect should be manipulated to ascertain how much is available for closure and the potential for "dog-ear" formation with closure. The direction of tension line pull on the skin is first determined, and the sides of the wound which are parallel to the direction of pull are sutured together at their midpoint (Figure 3-37A & B). A 3-0 to 2-0 interrupted non - absorbable suture is placed using a pattern that is appropriate to the tension on the wound. The two resulting elliptical defects are then sutured. If "dog ears" result, they are removed and the resulting defects are sutured (Figure 3-37C & D).

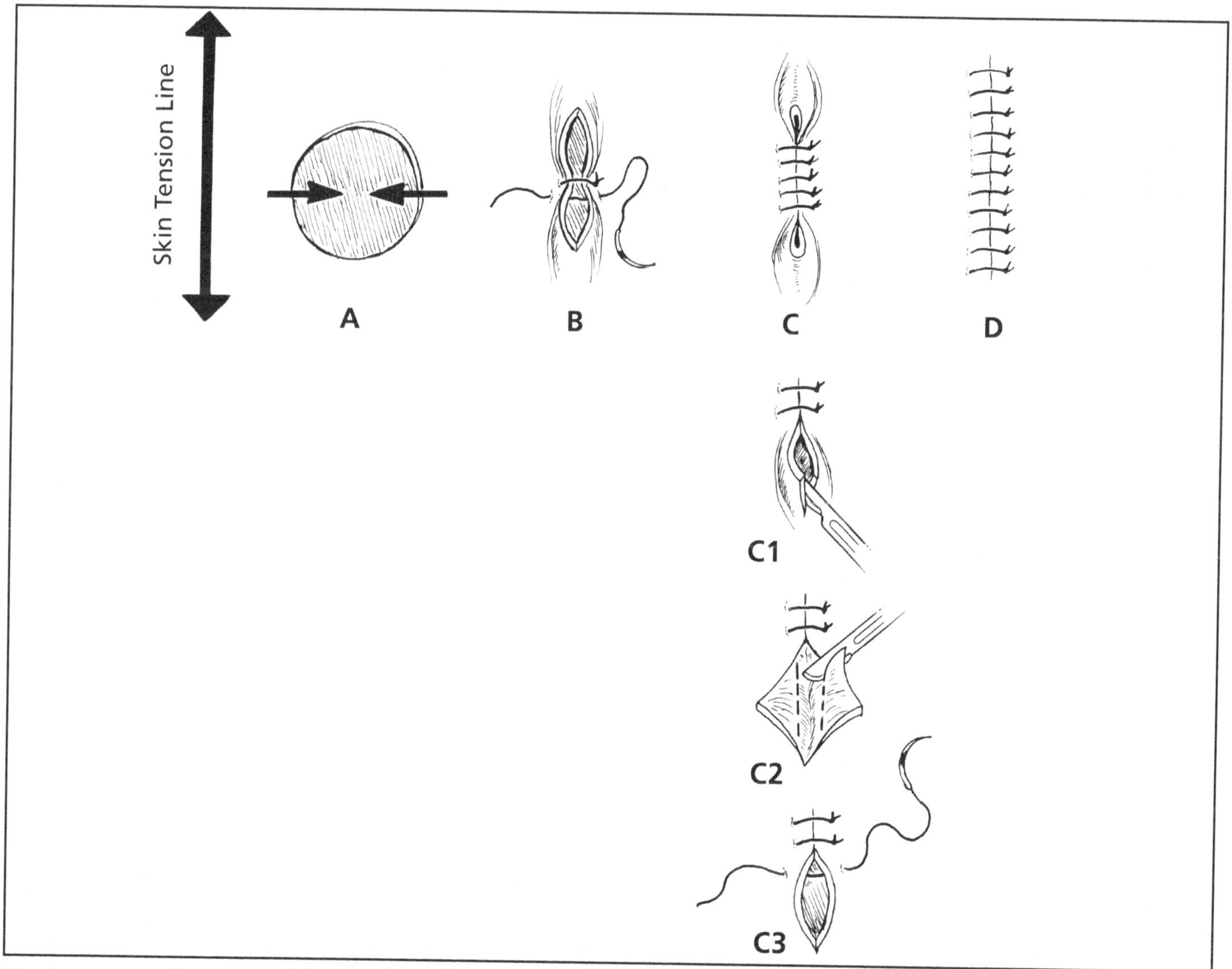


**Figure 3-37.** Linear closure of a circular defect. **A.** Circular defect with sides that are to be apposed *(arrows)*. **B.** One suture in the center of the defect leaving 2 small fusiform defects to be closed. **C.** Wound closed with resulting "dog ears" at the ends. **C1.** Splitting out the "dog ears" with a scalpel blade. **C2.** Removing the resultant triangular flaps. **C3.** Closing the remaining defects. **D.** Completed closure.

## Aftercare

No special aftercare is required with linear wound closure.

## Advantages and Disadvantages

Linear closure of a circular wound is the simplest and least time consuming technique for closure. It may require removing some extra normal skin when "dog-ears" are excised; however, the amount should be small if wound assessment was performed adequately, and in some instances "dog-ear" removal may not be necessary.

# Suggested Readings

1. Hedlund CS: Surgery of the integumentary system. *In* Fossum TW, ed.: Small Animal Surgery, 2nd ed.: St. Louis: Mosby, 2002, 134.
2. Hedlund CS: Surgery of the integumentary system. In Fossum TW, ed.: Small Animal Surgery, 3rd ed.: St. Louis: Mosby, 2007, 159.
3. MacPhail CM: Surgery of the integumentary system. In Fossum TW, ed.: Small Animal Surgery, 4th ed.: St. Louis: Mosby, 2013, 190.
4. Pavletic MM: Atlas of Small Animal Wound Management and Reconstructive Surgery, 3rd, ed.: Ames, IA: Wiley – Blackwell, 2010, 241.
5. Stanley BJ: Tension – relieving techniques. In Tobias KM, Johnston SA, eds.: Veterinary Surgery, Vol. 2: St. Louis: Elsevier – Saunders, 2012, 1221.
6. Swaim SF, Henderson RA: Small Animal Wound Management, 2nd ed.: Baltimore: Williams and Wilkins, 1997, 235.
7. Swaim SF, Lee AH, McGuire JA: Techniques for reconstructing circular skin defects in dogs. Vet Surg 13:18, 1984.
8. Trout NJ: Principles of plastic and reconstructive surgery. *In* Slatter DH, ed.: Textbook of Small Animal Surgery, 3rd ed.: Philadelphia: WB Saunders, 2003, 274.

# Circular (Combined - V Closure)

## Definition and Indications

Combined-V closure of a circular wound entails creating two V-shaped flaps on opposite sides of the circular wound to be used for closure of the defect. The technique is indicated for closure of circular defects such as would occur following removal of a relatively large lesion when there is little extra skin adjacent to the defect to be used for closure, and all of the skin must be used to close the defect. None of the skin will be removed as "dog-ears".

## Technique

Two V-shaped flaps are designed on opposite sides of the circular defect. The flaps are designed as if making equilateral triangles. First, the direction of skin tension line pull on the defect is determined to establish the long axis of the defect. The central axis of each triangle is then designed 45 degrees from the long axis of the defect, with the apex of each triangle pointing toward the center of the circle. The height of each triangle is equal to the radius of the circle. To create the V-shaped flaps, only two sides of each triangle are cut with the vortex of the V pointing back to the long axis of the defect (Figure 3-38A & B). The flaps are incised and undermined. They are then moved and sutured into new positions (Figure 3-38C-E). The angular tips of the flaps may be sutured with half-buried horizontal mattress sutures, thus helping preserve blood supply to the tips of the flaps. The tips of the V-shaped flaps are sutured to the side of the circular defect, and the angular tips at the edge of the circle are sutured at the base of the V-shaped flap. This should be done such that small fusiform defects are formed with sides that are equal in length. This converts the original circular defect into smaller fusiform defects (Figure 3-38D).

The skin of each of the flaps is used to close the larger central fusiform defect. The central suturing techniques may be used to distribute the skin of each flap to close its half of the fusiform. A central suture is placed between the center of each flap and the corresponding concave side of the wound. A suture is then placed in the center of each of the resulting defects. This pattern of suture placement is continued until closure of the defect is complete (See Figure 3-38, inset 1). Alternatively, a "fudging" suture technique can be used to provide a smooth closure. With this, simple interrupted sutures are placed so they are closer together on the convex side of the wound and further apart on the concave side of the wound. This evenly distributes any "dog-ears" that might form all along the suture line (See Figure 3-3, inset 2 ). Simple interrupted 3-0 nonabsorbable sutures are used.

## Aftercare

No special aftercare is needed with combined-V closure of circular defects.

## Advantages and Disadvantages

The combined-V technique provides circular defect closure without the excision of extra normal skin. The skin of the flaps, that would be "dog ear" skin, is used to help close the defect. This technique is advantageous for circular wound closure on the limbs where skin is not as abundant for "dog-ear" removal as on the trunk. It takes a little longer to plan and perform the procedure than it does for the linear closure.

# Suggested Readings

1. Alverado A. Reciprocal incision for closure of circular skin defects. Plast and Reconst Surg 67:482, 1981.

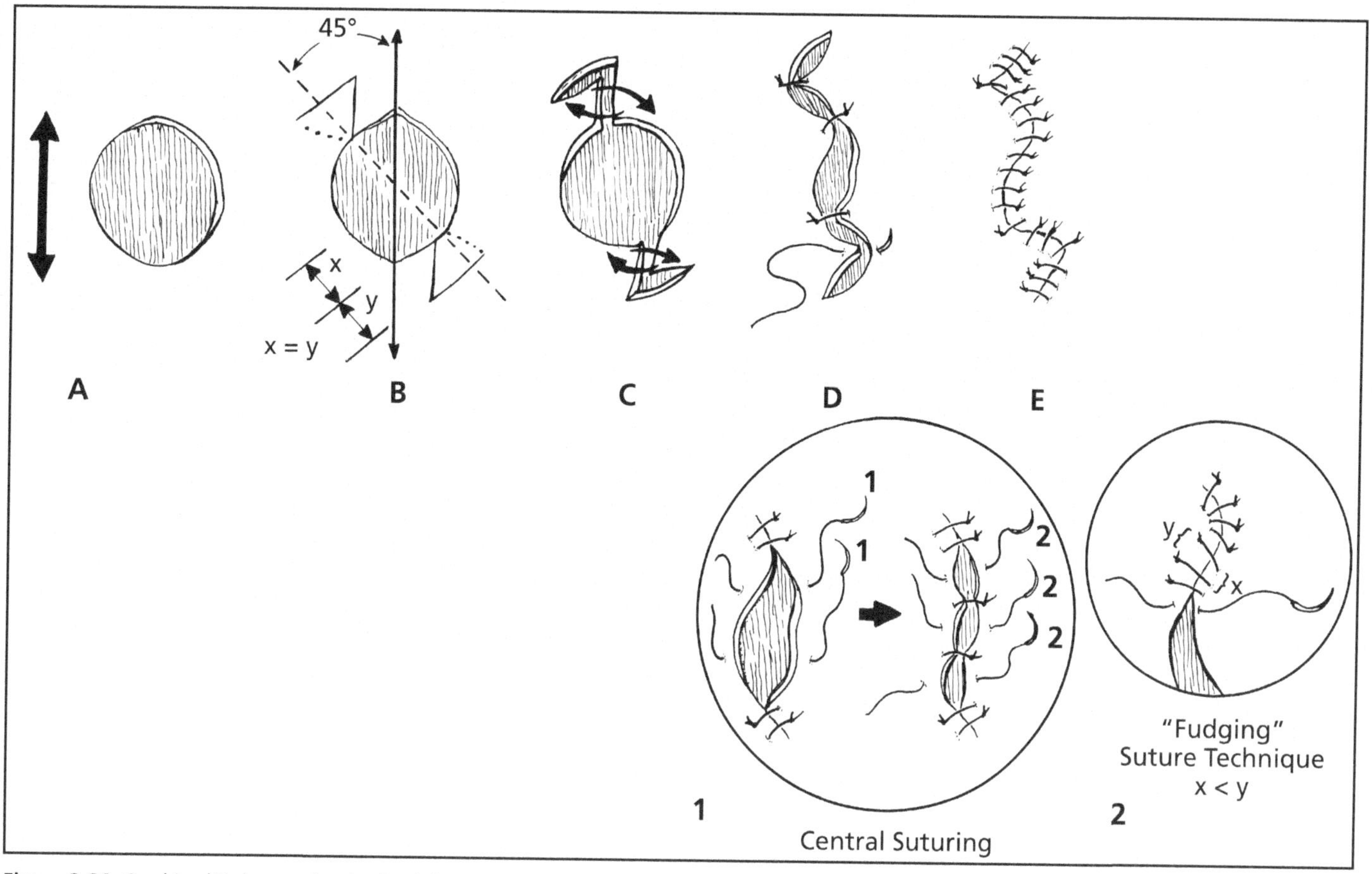


**Figure 3-38.** Combined V closure of a circular defect. **A.** Circular defect. **B.** V – shaped flaps designed 45 degrees off of the tension line pull as two sides of an equilateral triangle. The flap points are directed back toward the line of tension. The height of each flap is equal to the radius of the circular defect *(x=y)*. **C.** The flaps will be transposed into their new positions *(arrows)*. **D.** Transposition and suturing the tips of the flaps converts the circular defect into smaller fusiform defects. **E.** The skin of each flap essentially closes half of the circular defect. *(Inset 1)* Central suturing. Sutures are placed between the center of each flap and its corresponding concave side of the wound, (1,1) then in the center of the 3 remaining defects (2,2,2). This pattern of closure is continued until the wound is closed. *(Inset 2)* "Fudging" suture technique. Sutures are closer together on the convex side of the wound and further apart on the concave side of the wound *(x<y)*. (After Swaim SF, Lee AH, McGuire JA: Techniques for reconstructing circular skin defects in dogs. Vet Surg 13:22, 1984.

2. Fowler D: Tension relieving techniques and local skin flaps. *In* Fowler D, Williams JM, eds.: BSAVA Manual of Canine and Feline Wound Management and Reconstruction. Shurdington, Cheltenham, UK: British Small Animal Veterinary Association, 1999, 57.
3. Hedlund CS. Surgery of the integumentary system. *In* Fossum TW, ed.: Small Animal Surgery, 2nd ed.: St. Louis: Mosby, 2002, 134.
4. Hedlund CS: Surgery of the integumentary system. In Fossum TW: Small Animal Surgery, 3rd ed.: St. Louis: Mosby, 2007, 159.
5. MacPhail CM: Surgery of the integumentary system. In Fossum TW, ed.: Small Animal Surgery, 4th ed.: St. Louis: Mosby, 2013, 190.
6. Mutaf M, Sunay M, Bulut O: The "reading man" procedures: A new technique for closure of circular skin defects. Ann Plast Surg 60: 420, 2008.
7. Stanley BJ: Tension – relieving techniques, in Tobia KM, Johnston SA, eds.: Veterinary Surgery, Small Animal, Vol. 2: St. Louis: Elsevier – Saunders, 2012, 1221.
8. Swaim SF, Henderson RA: Small Animal Wound Management, 2nd ed.: Baltimore: Williams and Wilkins, 1997, 235.
9. Swaim SF, Lee AH, McGuire JA: Techniques for correcting circular skin defects in dogs. Vet Surg 13:18, 1984.
10. Trout NJ: Principles of plastic and reconstructive surgery. *In* Slatter DH, ed.: Textbook of Small Animal Surgery, 3rd ed.: Philadelphia: WB Saunders, 2003, 274.

# Crescent-Shaped ("Fudging" Suture, Central Suture, and Linear Closure)

## Definition and Indications

Crescent-shaped wounds have one side longer than the other side. Such wounds may occur when a limb is pulled up into or pushed down against a sharp edge (See Figure 3-31B). Necrosis or wound edge debridement may result in a discrepancy between the length of the wound edges. With slight discrepancy between the edges of the wound, the "dog-ears" resulting from closure will be small. Larger discrepancies between wound edge length result in larger "dog-ears". With small "dog-ears", they may be distributed in small increments all along the suture line using the "fudging" suture pattern or the central suture pattern. The "fudging" technique should not be used if the discrepancy between wound edges is greater than 10% to 20%. If the discrepancy between the wound edges is large and will result in larger "dog-ear" formation, linear closure with "dog-ear" removal is indicated.

## Techniques

### "Fudging" Suture

The wound edge should be debrided of nonviable tissue as needed. Nonabsorbable 3-0 simple interrupted sutures are placed so they are slightly closer together on the short side of the wound and further apart on the long side of the wound (Figure 3-39 inset 1).

### Central Suture

When the central suture technique is used, a suture is placed in the center of the wound followed by central placement of a suture in the two remaining defects (Figure 3-39 inset 2). This pattern of central suture placement is continued until closure is complete.

A closure with the "fudging" and central suture technique distributes "dog ear" skin all along the suture line in small increments.

## Linear Closure

Simple interrupted 3-0 nonabsorbable sutures may be placed alternately from either end of the defect toward its center. As the "dog-ear" forms in the center of the suture line, it is removed and the defect is closed (Figure 3-40A). Alternatively, suturing may start at one end of the defect and progress to the other end with "dog-ear" removal at that end of the defect (Figure 3-40B). Suturing may also begin in the center of the defect and progress toward the ends, with removal of the "dog ears" at both ends of the suture line (Figure 3-40C).

## Aftercare

No special aftercare is needed with the "fudging," central suturing or linear closure techniques for closure of crescent-shaped defects.

## Advantages and Disadvantages

The "fudging" and central suturing techniques allow closure of crescent-shaped wounds without removing extra normal skin as "dog-ears". However, careful placement of sutures may be necessary to distribute "dog-ear" skin evenly along the suture line with either technique. Linear closure of crescent-shaped wounds with "dog-ear" removal results in removal of extra normal skin.

# Suggested Readings


1. Bennett RG: Fundamentals of Cutaneous Surgery, St. Louis: CV Mosby, 1988, 473.
2. Borges AF. Dog-ear repair. Plast Reconstr Surg 69:707, 1982.
3. Fahie MA: Primary wound closure. In Tobia KM, Johnston SA, eds.: Veterinary Surgery, Small Animal, Vol. 2: St. Louis: Elsevier –


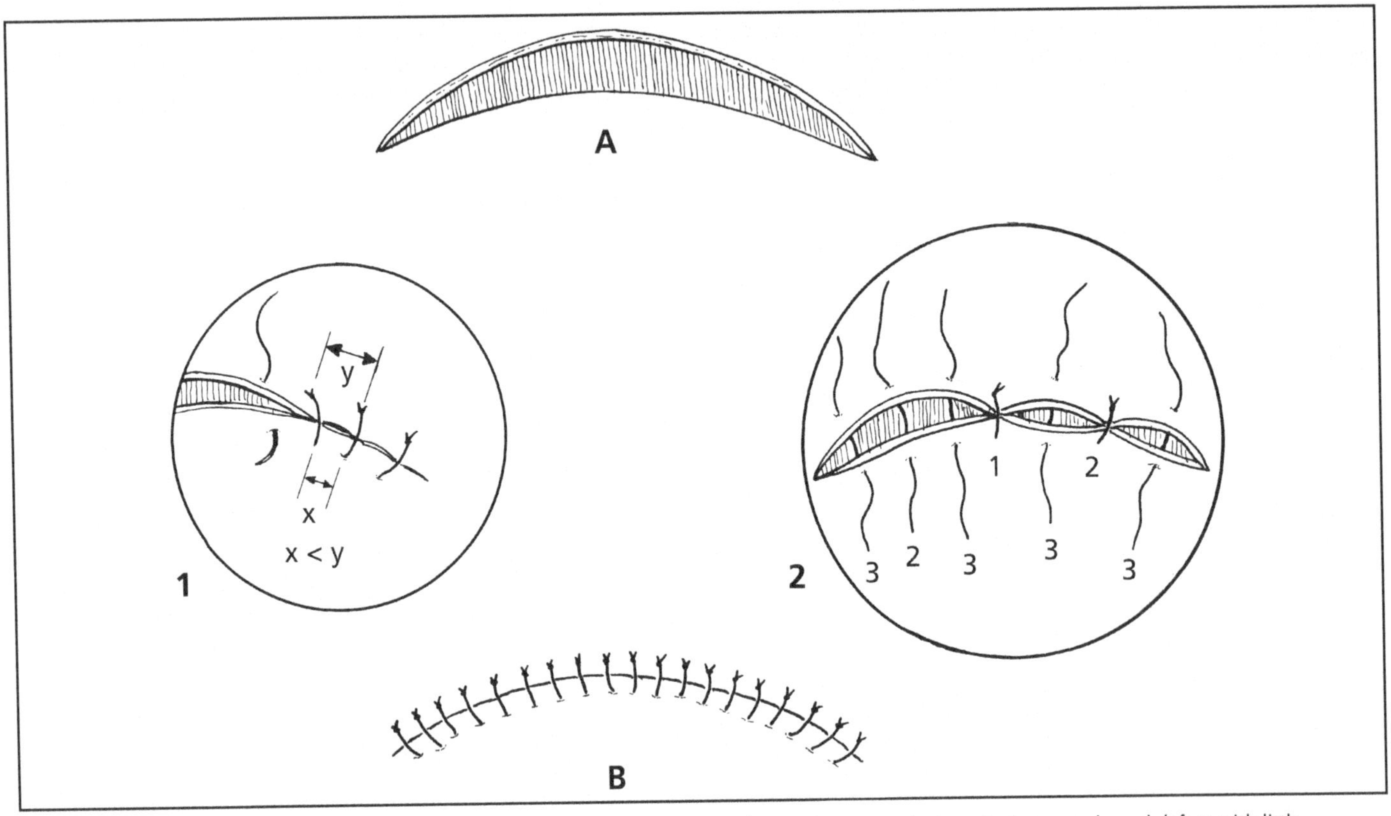


**Figure 3-39.** Closure of a crescent shaped defect – "fudging" suture technique and central suture technique. **A.** Crescent shaped defect with little difference between the lengths of the wound edges. *(Inset 1)* "Fudging" suture technique. Sutures are placed closer together on the short side of the defect and further apart on the long side of the defect *(x<y)*. *(Inset 2)* Central suture technique. A central suture is placed in the wound *(1)*, followed by sutures in the center of the 2 resulting defects *(2,2)*. This pattern of central suture placement is continued *(3,3,3,3)* etc. **B.** Completed wound closure. (After Swaim SF, Henderson RA: Small Animal Wound Management, 2nd ed.: Baltimore: Williams & Wilkins, 1997, 269.

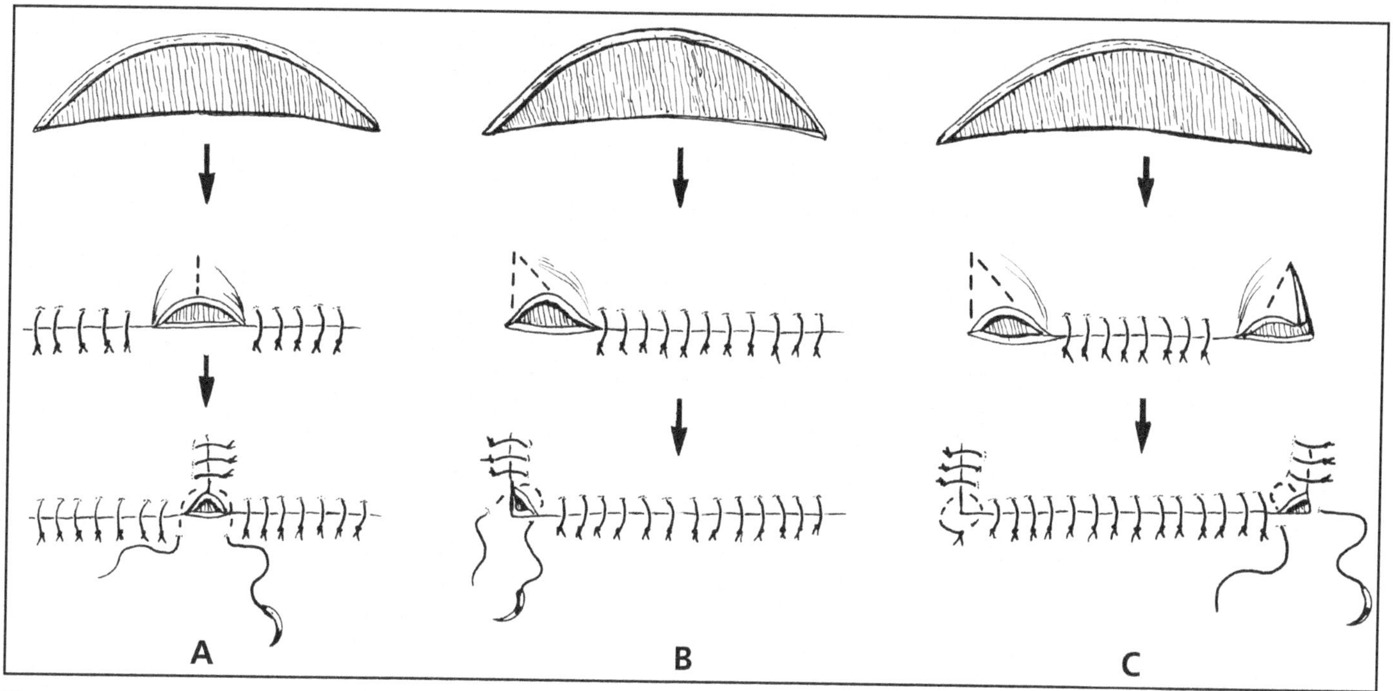


Figure 3-40. Closure of crescent – shaped defect. A. Linear closure with "dog ear" removal in the center. B. Closure from one end with "dog ear" removal at the opposite end. C. Closure from the center toward each end with "dog ear" removal at each end. (After Trout NJ: Principles of plastic and reconstructive surgery. In Slatter DH, ed.: Textbook of Small Animal Surgery, 3rd ed.: Philadelphia: WB Saunders, 2003, 288.)

Saunders, 2012, 1197.
4. Gorney M: Tissue dynamics and surgical geometry. In Kernahan DA, Vistnes LM, eds.: Biological Aspects of Reconstructive Surgery. Boston: Little, Brown, 1977, 265.
5. Hedlund CS: Surgery of the integumentary system. *In* Fossum TW, ed.: Small Animal Surgery, 2nd ed.: St. Louis: Mosby, 2002, 134.
6. Hedlund CS: Surgery of the integumentary system. In Fossum TW, ed.: Small Animal Surgery, 3rd. ed.: St. Louis: Mosby, 2007, 159.
7. MacPhail CM: Surgery of the integumentary system. In Fossum TW, ed.: Small Animal Surgery, 4th ed.: St. Louis: Mosby, 2013, 190.
8. Pavletic MM: Atlas of Small Animal Wound Management and Reconstructive Surgery, 3rd ed.: Ames, IA: Wiley – Blackwell, 2010, 241.
9. Stanley BJ: Tension – relieving techniques. In Tobias KM, Johnston SA, eds.: Veterinary Surgery, Small Animal, Vol. 2: St. Louis: Elsevier – Saunders, 2012,1221.
10. Swaim SF, Henderson RA: Small Animal Wound Management, 2nd ed.: Baltimore: Williams and Wilkins, 1997, 235.
11. Trout NJ: Principles of plastic and reconstructive surgery. *In* Slatter DH, ed.: Textbook of Small Animal Surgery, 3rd ed.: Philadelphia: WB Saunders, 2003, 274.

# Wounds Over The Carpus and Tarsus - Apposable Edges Extension Surfaces

## Definition and Indications

Wounds with apposable edges over the extension surface of the carpus or tarsus may be subject to tension stresses that can impair healing, whether they are closed with or without tension. If the wounds do not have apposable edges, and they require some form of reconstruction other than primary closure, i.e. skin graft, they may also be subject to tension stresses. When the joint is flexed, tension may be placed on the wound (Figure 3-41A Also See Figure 3-42A).

Two techniques may be helpful in preventing tension damage. First, reconstructive wound repair may be indicated to help prevent tension damage. Second, immobilization of the joint is indicated.

## Techniques

### Wounds Over the Carpal Extension Surface

If a wound extends horizontally across the carpus and has apposable edges, it may be beneficial to reconstruct the wound by changing its direction so that it runs vertically and will be less prone to disruption by carpal flexion. This can be done by use of a Z-plasty. The wound is used as the central limb of the Z-plasty. The arms of the Z-plasty are designed off of the ends of the central limb at 60 degree angles, with one arm on each side of the central limb (Figure 3-41B). After incising the arms of the Z, the flaps of the Z-plasty are transposed into their new position and sutured in place (Figure 3-41C & D). This changes the direction of the central limb of the Z so that it is parallel to the long axis of the limb. In this position, it is less prone to disruption if the carpus is flexed (Figure 3-41E).

### Wounds Over the Tarsal Extension Surface

Wounds of this area are over or near the prominence of the calcaneal tuberosity (Figure 3-42A), and flexion of the joint results in separation of the wound edges (Figure 3-42B). It may be possible to appose the wound

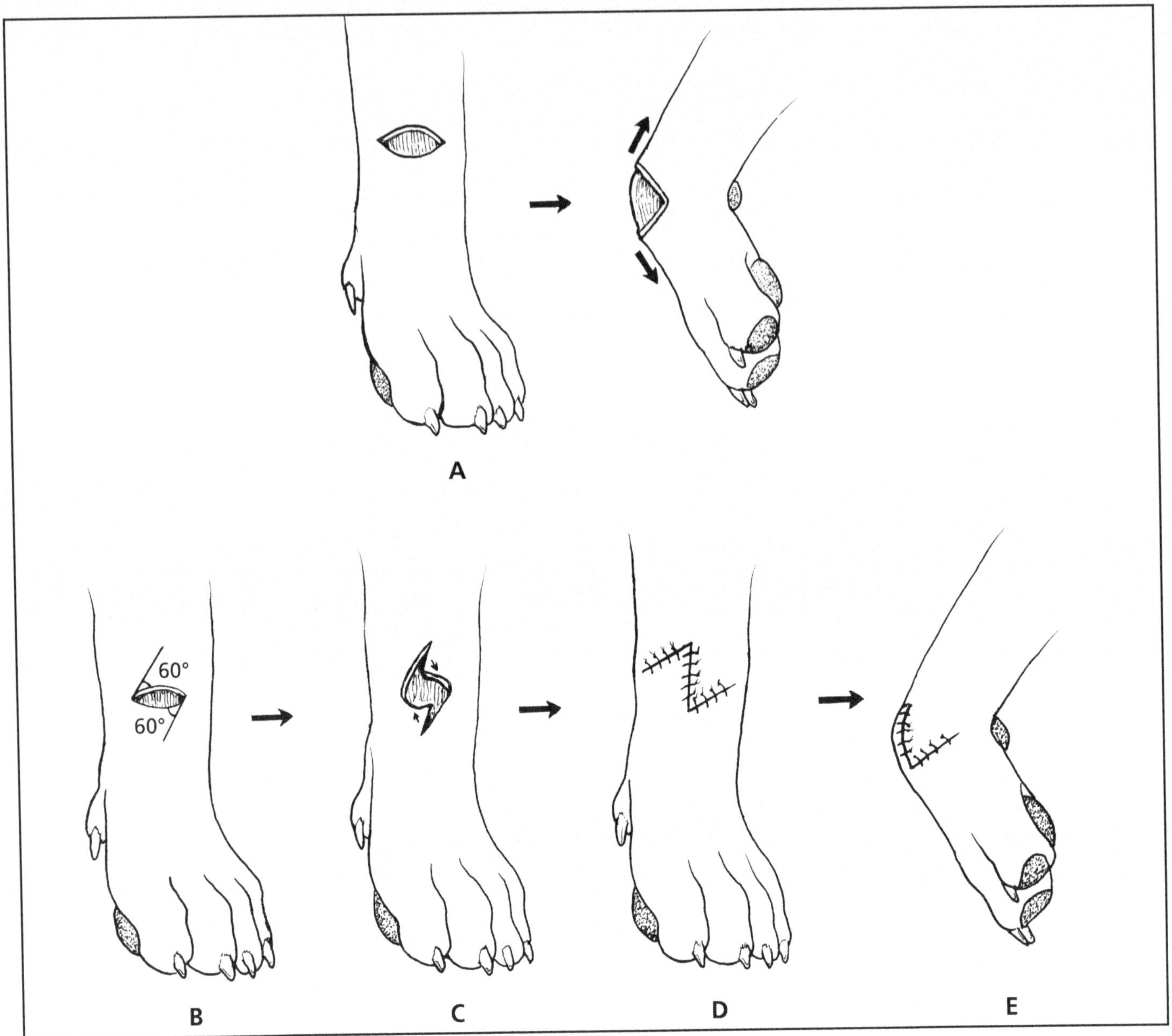


**Figure 3-41.** Horizontal wound across the extension surface of the carpus. **A.** Carpal flexion further separates the wound edges. **B.** A Z – plasty designed with the wound as the central limb of the Z and arms designed at 60 degree angles off of the central limb. **C.** Arms have been incised and will be transposed. **D.** Completed Z – plasty. **E.** Less tendency for wound separation with carpal flexion. (After Swaim SF, Henderson RA: Small Animal Wound Management, 2nd ed.: Baltimore: Williams & Wilkins, 1997, 145.

edges with some wounds if the tarsal joint is placed in extension (Figure 3-42C).

Skin grafts may be necessary to reconstruct the carpal and tarsal extension surface with some wounds (See Carpal – Metacarpal/Tarsal – Metatarsal Wounds, Wounds With Nonapposable Edges – No Potential for Apposition, Mesh Grafts).

## Aftercare

### Wounds Over the Carpal Extension Surface

After closure of a defect over the extension surface of the carpus, the carpal joint should be immobilized to prevent flexion. This can be done by incorporating a splint on the flexion surface of a limb bandage. The author (SFS) prefers a metal splint of the Mason metasplint design (Mason Metasplints, Jorgensen Labs, Inc., Loveland, CO). The bandage and splint should extend the length of the leg to help alleviate the pressures of a short splint (Figure 3-43A). If the splint is too short, immobilization will not be sufficient, and weight bearing tends to lever the top of the splint caudally away from the limb and place bandage pressure on the cranial surface of the limb (Figure 3-43B). The bandage and splint should be maintained for at least 10 days, with periodic changes, to allow for adequate healing of the wound.

### Wounds Over the Tarsal Extension Surface

After closure of a wound over the tarsal extension

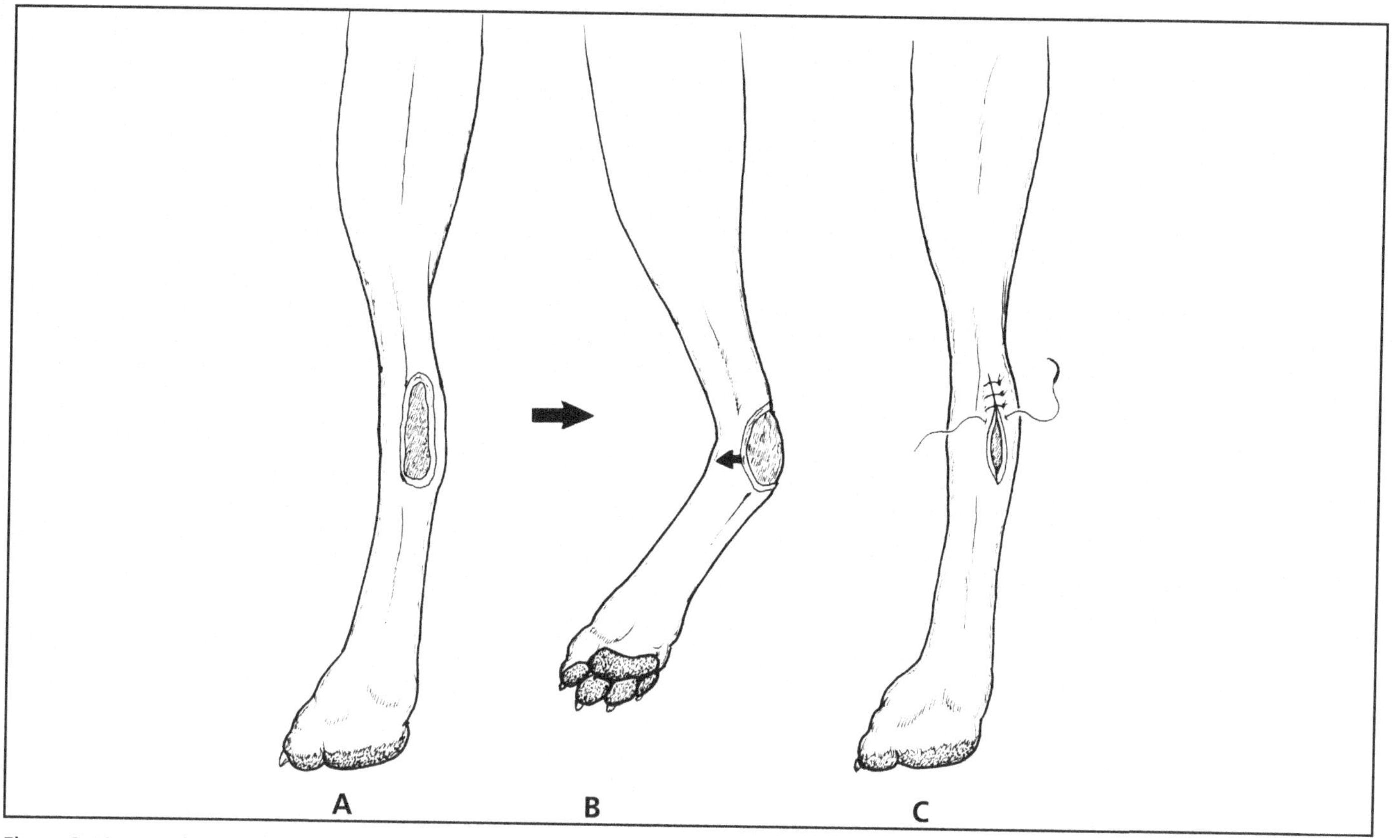


**Figure 3-42.** Wounds over tarsal extension surface. **A.** Wound over the point of the hock. **B.** When joint is flexed wound edges separate. **C.** Joint extended and wound can be sutured.

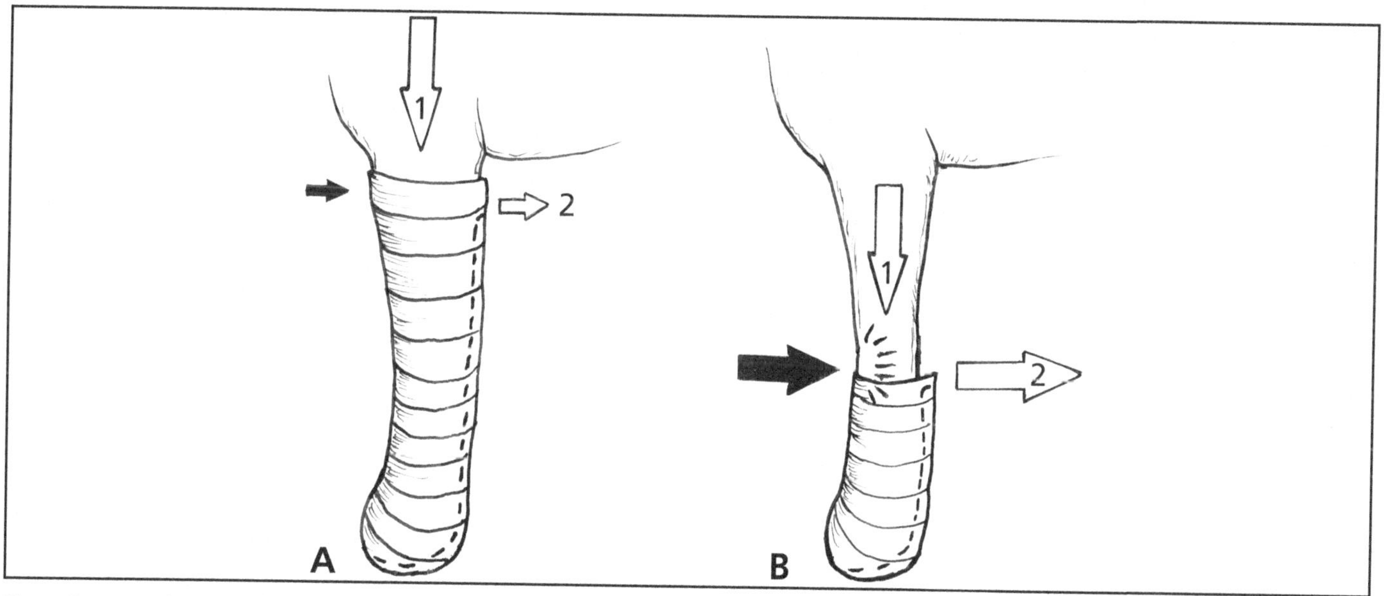


**Figure 3-43.** Bandaging and splinting the forelimb. **A.** Proper technique – bandage/splint applied to the length of the forelimb. **B.** Improper technique – bandage/splint applied to partial length of the limb. As weight is borne on the limb *(open arrow 1)* the top of the splint tends to move caudally *(open arrow 2)*. The result is pulling of the tape on the front of the bandage caudally causing pressure on the front of the limb *(closed arrow)*. The pressure is greater *(larger arrows)* for a partial length bandage/splint.

surface, the joint should be immobilized to prevent flexion. This can be done by incorporating a splint in the flexion (cranial) surface of a limb bandage. Fiber glass casting tape can be used to make the splint This type of immobilizer molds well to the angulation of the pelvic limb. The bandage and splint should extend to near the stifle for proper immobilization of the area (Figure 3-44A). The bandage and splint should be maintained for at least 10 days, with periodic changes to allow for adequate healing of the wound.

## Advantages and Disadvantages

Wound healing over the carpal and tarsal extension surfaces may be enhanced by changing the direction

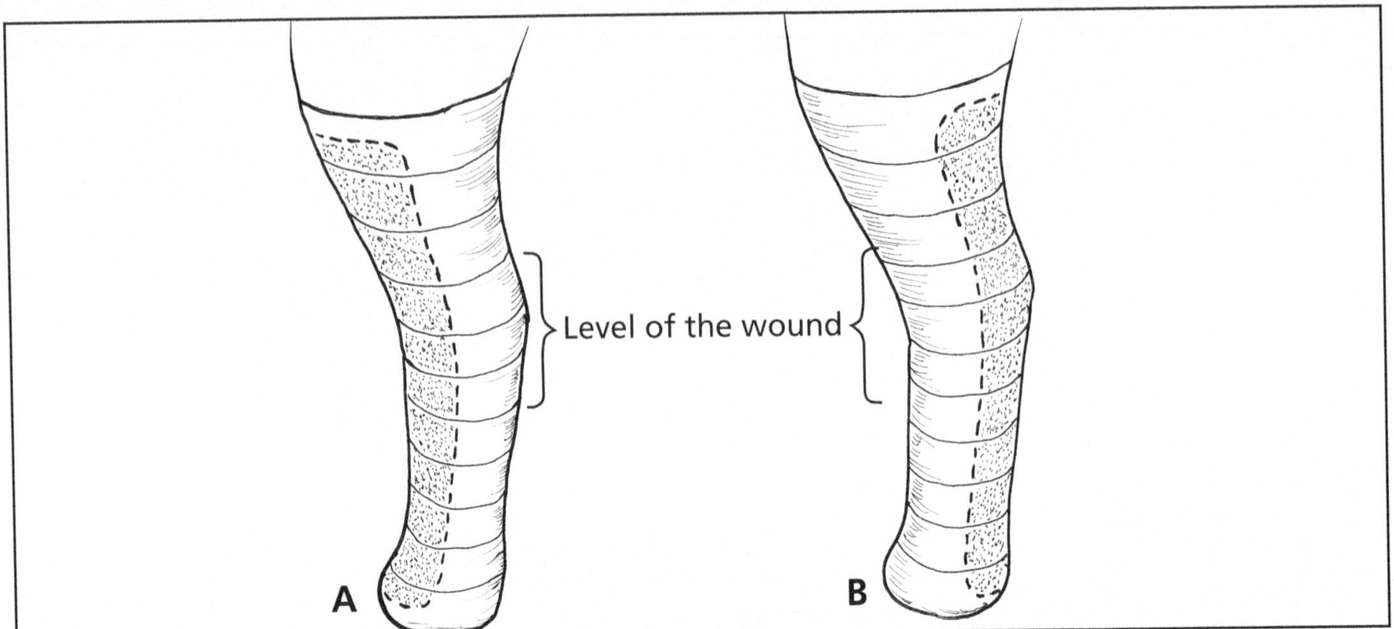


**Figure 3-44.** Bandaging and splinting the pelvic limb. For wounds at the tarsal level. **A.** With a wound on the extension surface a fiberglass immobilizer is incorporated in the flexion surface of the bandage *(stippled area)*. **B.** With a wound on the flexion surface a fiberglass immobilizer is incorporated in the extension surface of the bandage *(stippled area)*.

of a horizontal wound, e.g. Z-plasty over the extension surface of the carpus, or by placing the limb in extension to provide skin laxity for wound closure, e.g. wounds over the tarsal extension surface. These procedures plus immobilizing the joints in extension may require more time in initial wound management. However, they may help prevent continued wound disruption and development of a nonhealing wound.

# Suggested Readings

1. Campbell BG: Dressings, bandages and splints for wound management in dogs and cats. Vet Clin No Am Small Animal Pract 36: 759, 2006.
2. Fowler D: Tension relieving techniques and local skin flaps. In Fowler D, Williams JM, eds.: BSAVA Manual of Canine and Feline Wound Management and Reconstruction. Shurdington Cheltenham, UK: British Small Animal Veterinary Association, 1999, 57.
3. Hedlund CS: Surgery of the integumentary system. *In* Fossum TW, ed.: Small Animal Surgery, 2nd ed.: St. Louis: Mosby, 2002, 134.
4. Hedlund CS: Surgery of the integumentary system. In Fossum TW, ed.: Small Animal Surgery, 3rd ed.: St. Louis: Mosby, 2007, 159.
5. Jankauskas S, Cohen IK, Grabb WC: Basic technique of plastic surgery. *In* Smith JW, Aston SJ, eds.: Plastic Surgery, 4th ed.: Boston: Little, Brown, 1991, 3.
6. Mayhew P: Tension – relieving techniques and local skin flaps. In Williams J, Moores A, eds.: BSAVA Manual of Canine and Feline wound Management and Reconstruction, 2nd ed.: Glouster (UK): BSAVA, 2009, 69.
7. McGregor IA: Fundamental Techniques of Plastic Surgery, 8th ed.: Edinburgh: Churchill Livingstone, 1989, 23.
8. Pavletic MM: Atlas of Small Animal Reconstructive Surgery, 2nd ed.: Philadelphia: WB Saunders, 1991, 131.
9. Pavletic MM: Atlas of Small Animal Wound Management and Reconstructive Surgery, 3rd ed.: Ames, IA: Wiley – Blackwell, 2010, 241.
10. Stanley BJ: Tension – relieving techniques. In Tobias KM, Johnston SA, eds.: Veterinary Surgery, Small Animal, Vol. 2: Elsevier – Saunders, 2012, 1221.
11. Swaim SF: Surgery of Traumatized Skin: Management and Reconstruction in the Dog and Cat, Philadelphia: WB Saunders, 1980, 395.
12. Swaim SF, Henderson RA: Small Animal Wound Management, 2nd ed.: Baltimore: Williams and Wilkins, 1997, 235.
13. Swaim SF, Henderson RA, Sutton HH: Correction of triangular and wedge-shaped skin defects in dogs and cats. J Amer Animal Hosp Assoc 16:225, 1980.
14. Swaim SF, Renberg WC, Shike KM: Small Animal Bandaging, Casting and Splinting Techniques. Ames, IA: Wiley – Blackwell, 2011, 43.
15. Trout NJ: Principles of plastic and reconstructive surgery. *In* Slatter DH, ed.: Textbook of Small Animal Surgery, 3rd ed.: Philadelphia: WB Saunders, 2003, 274.

# Flexion Surfaces

## Definition and Indications

Wounds over the flexion surface of the carpus or tarsus may be subject to movement and tension stresses that could be detrimental to healing whether the wounds were closed under tension or not. When the joints are moved tension may be placed on wounds (Figure 3-45 and Figure 3-46). Immobilization of the joints is necessary to help reduce movement and tension on the repair site.

### Techniques

The surgeon should utilize his/her hands and imagination in assessing the wound and deciding upon the best means of closure, e.g. use of tension sutures, relaxing incisions, grafts or flaps. The reader is referred to the sections of the text that deal with these subjects for information on their use.

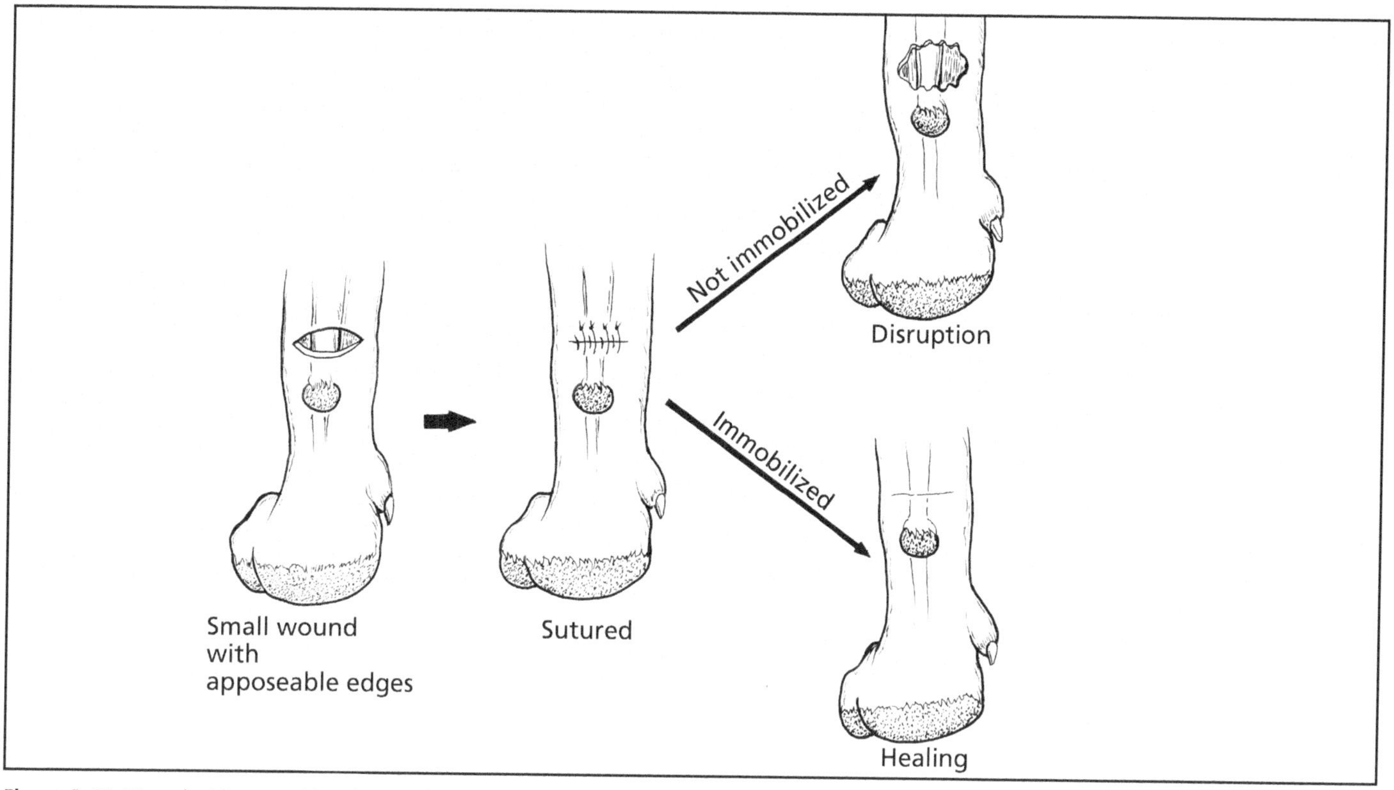


**Figure 3-45.** Wound with apposable edges on the carpal flexion surface may have tension placed on it with movement, resulting in disruption. With immobilization, the wound may heal.

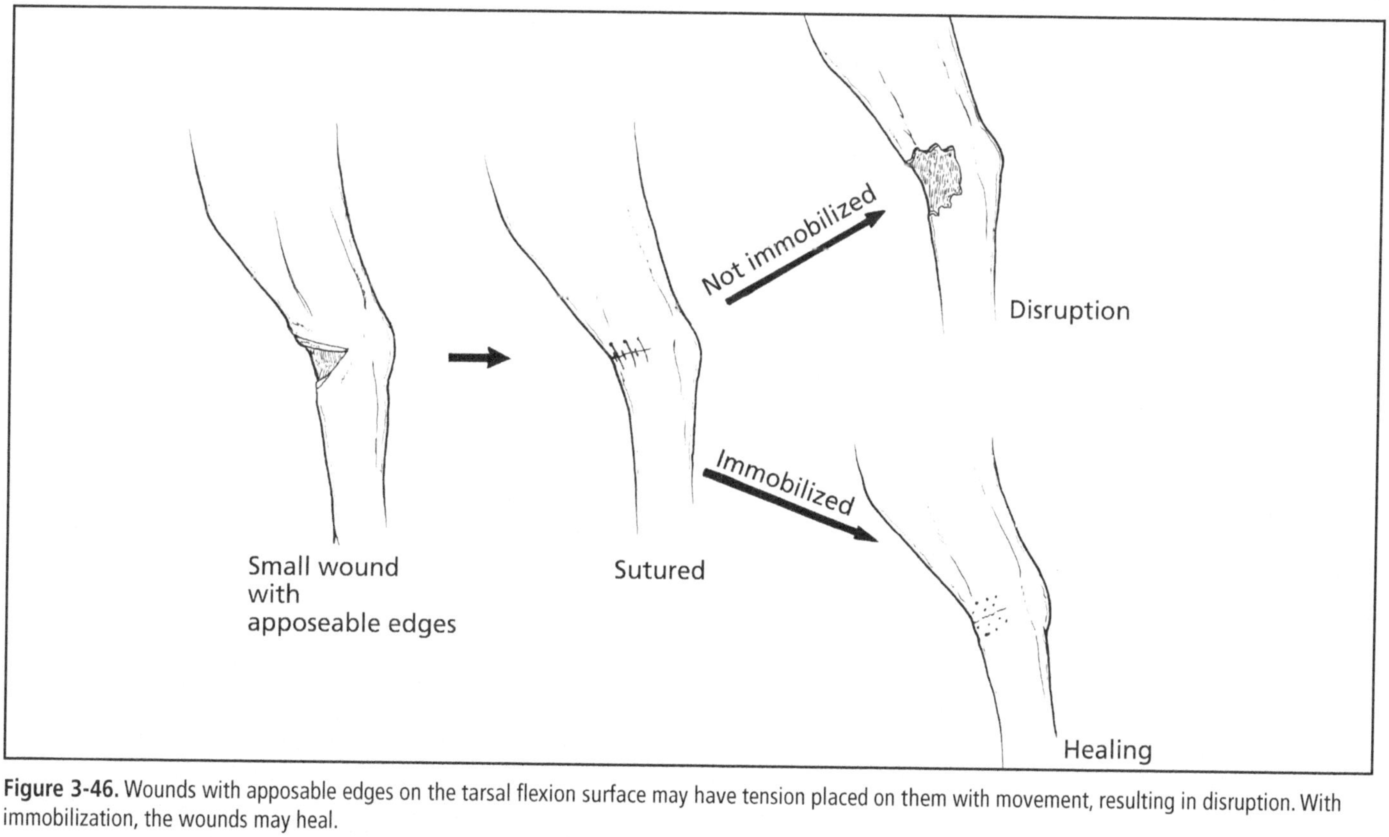


**Figure 3-46.** Wounds with apposable edges on the tarsal flexion surface may have tension placed on them with movement, resulting in disruption. With immobilization, the wounds may heal.

## Aftercare

### Wounds Over the Carpal Flexion Surface

Following closure of a wound over the flexion surface of the carpus, the joint should be immobilized. Because of the relatively straight configuration of this joint in a standing position, the splint incorporated into the bandage may be placed on the flexion surface of the limb. Bandaging and splinting are as described for aftercare of wounds on the carpal extension surface (See Figure 3-43A & B). The bandage and splint should be maintained at least 10 days with periodic changes.

### Wounds Over the Tarsal Flexion Surface

Immobilization of the tarsal area should be accomplished by incorporating a splint in the bandage. However, due to the normal angulation of the joint and the potential dynamics of the area as the animal ambulates, it is best to place the splint on the caudal surface of the limb. This helps prevent passive pressure of the splint against the cranial tarsal area which could interfere with healing (See Figure 3-44B). The bandage and splint should be maintained for at least 10 days, with periodic changes.

## Advantages and Disadvantages

Wound healing over the carpal and tarsal flexion surfaces is enhanced by immobilizing the areas. Bandage and splint maintenance may require more time, but this may help prevent wound disruption and development of a nonhealing wound. Open wounds on the flexion surface of a joint have the potential for developing wound contracture deformities which limit joint extension especially with large wounds (See Figure 1-13). Thus, efforts should be made to prevent their development by splinting them in extension.

# Suggested Readings


1. Campbell BG: Dressings, bandages and splints for wound management in dogs and cats. Vet Clin No Am Small Animal Pract. 36: 759, 2006.
2. Pavletic MM: Atlas of Small Animal Reconstructive Surgery, 2nd ed.: Philadelphia: WB Saunders, 1999, 11.
3. Swaim SF, Hinkle SH, Bradley DM: Wound Contraction: Basic and clinical factors. Compend Contin Educ Vet Pract 23:20, 2001.
4. Swaim SF, Henderson RA: Small Animal Wound Management, 2nd ed.: Baltimore: Williams and Wilkins, 1997, 13.
5. Swaim SF, Lee AH, Henderson RA: Mobility vs immobility in the healing of open wounds. J Amer Anim Hosp Assoc. 25:91, 1989.
6. Swaim SF, Renberg WC, Shike KM: Small Animal Bandaging, Casting and Splinting Techniques. Ames, IA: Wiley – Blackwell, 2011, 43.


# Wounds with Nonapposable Edges - Potential for Apposition and Relief of Tension - Related Scars

## Potentially Apposable Wound Edges and Tension-Related Scars

### General Information

Distal limb wounds with relatively large amounts of skin missing are common. In some of these wounds, initial apposition of the skin edges may not be possible. However, it may be possible to use techniques whereby the skin can be stretched over a period of time to allow closure without the use of grafts or flaps. Various types of relaxing incisions may also be used in the skin adjacent to the wound to allow wound edge apposition. In some instances stretching procedures can be used in conjunction with relaxing incisions to attain skin edge apposition.

Extension restricting and constricting scars can result when some wounds with large skin deficits heal as open wounds, i.e. contractural scars across flexion surfaces, and circumferential scars, respectively. It may be possible to use Z-plasties to relieve the tension related scars.

## Undermining

See Carpal-Metacarpal/Tarsal-Metatarsal Wounds, Wounds with Apposable Edges-Tension, Undermining.

## Closure-Tension Sutures

### Presutures

See Chapter III, Carpal-Metacarpal/Tarsal-Metatarsal Wounds, Wounds with Apposable Edges-Tension, Presutures.

# Adjustable Horizontal Mattress Sutures

## Definition and Indications

The adjustable horizontal mattress suture is a continuous intradermal suture. It is anchored at one or both ends such that it can be tightened periodically, thus gradually advancing the wound edges closer together or into apposition. This suture is indicated in fresh wounds after proper debridement has been accomplished and in wounds in the repair stage of healing with the presence of granulation tissue and contraction. The skin's biomechanical properties of creep and stress relaxation are utilized in that skin held under tension will gradually stretch. The suture is primarily used on limb wounds when the skin edges cannot be apposed initially; however, in the surgeon's clinical opinion, the wound will eventually close without using a graft or flap.

## Technique

A synthetic 1-0 or 2-0 monofilament suture (polypropylene or nylon) on a cutting or reverse cutting needle is used for the adjustable horizontal mattress suture. The suture is started at one end of the wound by passing the needle through the full-thickness of the skin. The suture is pulled through the skin until approximately 2 inches protrude beyond the skin. This end of the suture is passed through a sewing button, and 2 small adjustable fishing weights [split shot], (Removable Split Shot, (Non – Lead Weights) Eco – Friendly, Eagle Claw Fishing Tackle, Denver, Co) are placed on the suture adjacent to the button (Figure 3-47 and Figure 3-48). The suture is then placed as an intradermal horizontal mattress suture along the wound. It is important that adequate bites be taken in the dermis, thus taking advantage of its dense collagenous composition to ensure sufficient holding strength of the suture in the dermis. As the suture is placed, each bite is advanced slightly so the suture passes across the wound at a slight angle rather than passing directly perpendicular to the wound's long axis. Such placement allows the suture to slide through the tissue with greater ease when it is tightened. When this suture is being used on a wound that is in the repair stage of healing, care is taken not to disrupt the skin's attachment to the granulation tissue because, in this case, the adjustable horizontal mattress suture is being used to enhance wound contraction (Figure 3-49). At the opposite end of the wound the last

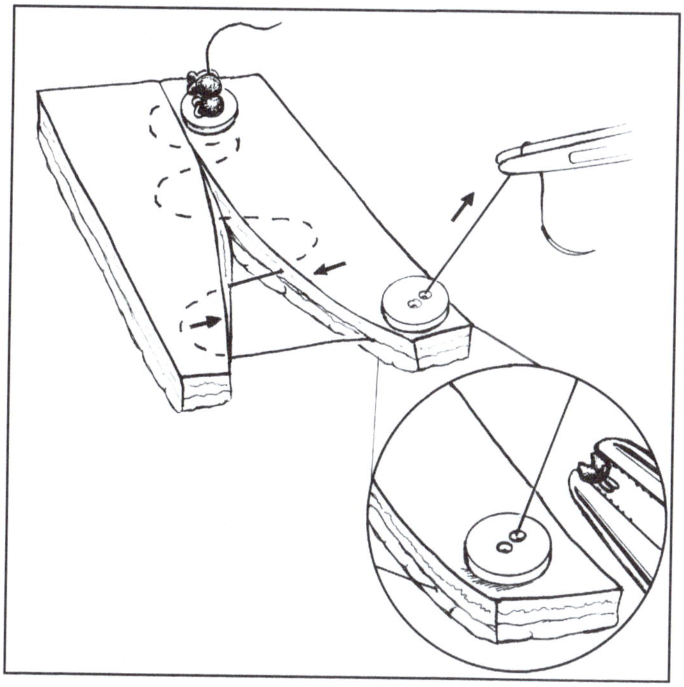

**Figure 3-48.** Adjustable horizontal mattress suture. A sewing button and split shots placed on the beginning of the suture. Suture is placed intradermally. At opposite end of the wound, the suture goes through the skin and another sewing button. Upward traction on the suture *(arrow near suture)* pulls the wound edges toward each other *(arrows on skin)*. *(Inset)* Split shot is applied to the other suture end to maintain tension on wound edges.

passage of the needle is through the entire thickness of the skin and through a hole in a sewing button. With the monofilament nature of the suture material, upward traction on it advances the wound edges toward each other as the suture slides through the dermis (See Figure 3-48). To maintain the advancement of the skin edges, a split shot is placed on the suture adjacent to the button (See Figure 3-48 inset). A second weight is placed against the first one to prevent slippage. Excess suture material is cut off about 2 inches beyond the weights, and a bandage is placed over the wound.

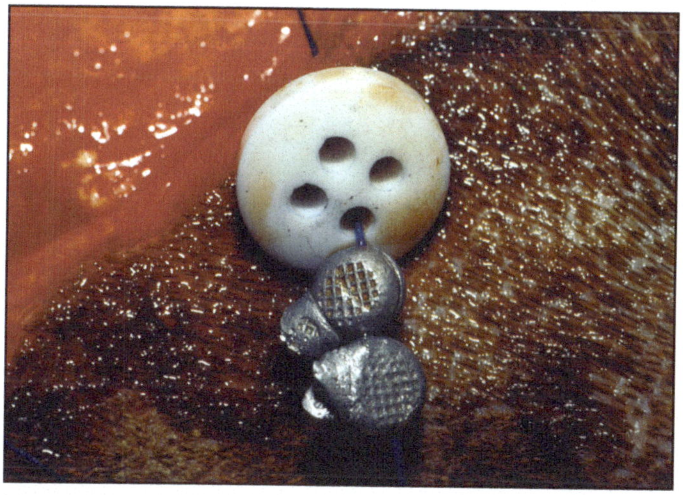

**Figure 3-47.** Adjustable horizontal mattress suture. A sewing button and 2 split shots placed on the beginning of the suture.

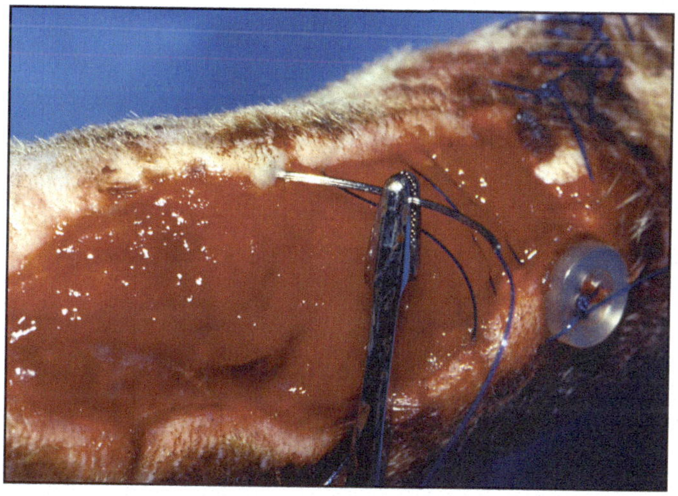

**Figure 3-49.** On wounds that have a granulation tissue bed, the skin attachment to the granulation tissue is not disturbed as the suture is placed with a secure intradermal bite. (From Swaim SF, Henderson RA: Small Animal Wound Management, 2nd ed.: Baltimore, Williams & Wilkins, 1997, 172.)

The split shot should be made of tin ("Environmentally Friendly") rather than lead to avoid the possibility of lead toxicosis in case the animal molests the wound and ingests the split shot. The split shots are designed with a "tongue-in-groove" arrangement to hold the sutures secure (Figure 3-50). They are adjustable in that they can be placed on the suture by squeezing a needle holder or hemostat jaws on the ball of the split shot (Figure 3-51). To remove the split shot from the suture, the needle holder or hemostat jaws squeeze the 2 tabs on the split shot to open it (Figure 3-52).

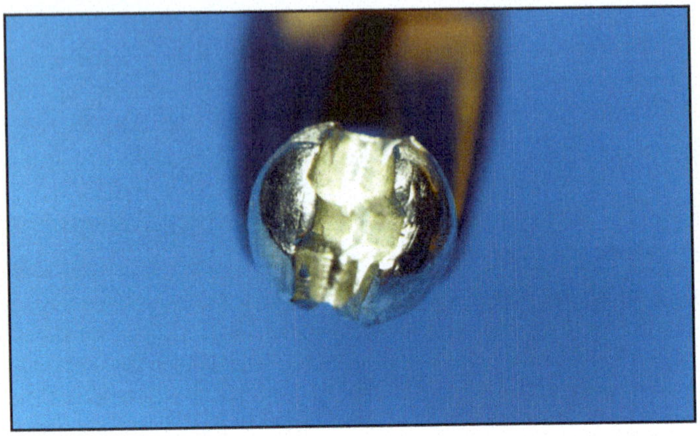

**Figure 3-50.** Holding ability of the split shot on the suture comes from the "tongue – in – groove" design of the split shot.

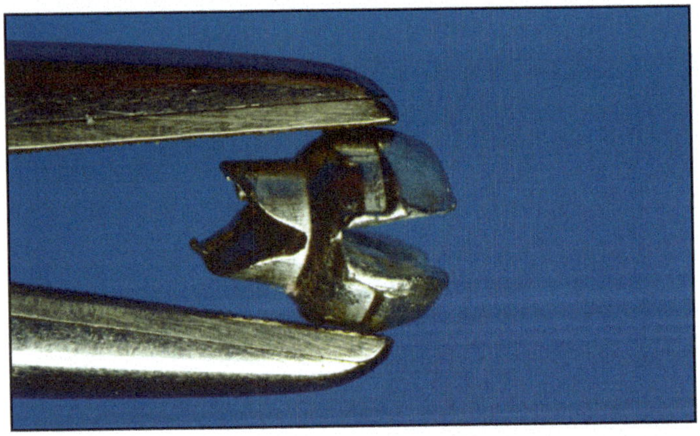

**Figure 3-51.** A split shot is placed on the suture by squeezing the ball of the split shot with needle holders or hemostats.

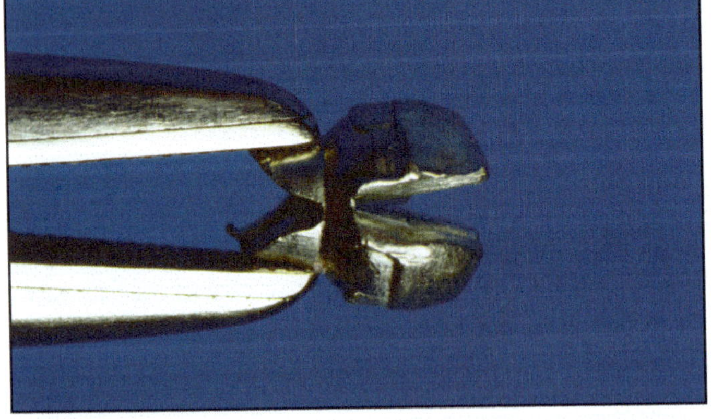

**Figure 3-52.** A split shot is removed from the suture by squeezing the 2 tabs on the split shot to open it.

With longer wounds, or wounds with an angle in them 2 adjustable horizontal mattress sutures can be placed (Figure 3-53). Thus, for long wounds the suture can be tightened from both ends, and for angled wounds the suture in each arm of the angle can be tightened. This can be advantageous because the tightening capability of the suture decreases as you move away from the suture's ends in long wounds and around curves in angled wounds.

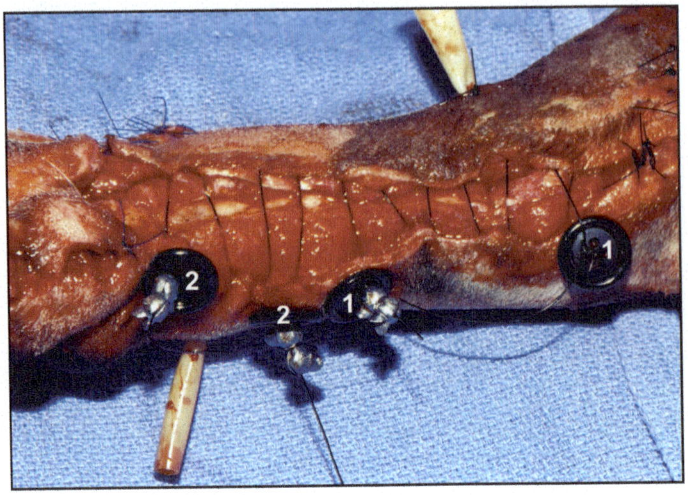


**Figure 3-53.** A long wound on which 2 adjustable horizontal mattress sutures have been used. *"1"* indicates one suture. *"2"* indicates second suture.

## Aftercare

The wound is bandaged after suture tightening using a nonadherent contact layer, an absorbent wrap, and adhesive tape or elastic tape. The bandage is changed daily. At the time of bandage change, the suture beyond the split shot is grasped with hemostats, and the jaws of a needle holder with a new split shot are used to hold the button down. Upward traction is placed on the end of the suture while the limb is steadied. As the original split shots move away from the button and the suture slides through the dermis, the wound edges will be observed to advance toward each other. When sufficient advancement of the wound edges has occurred, the split shot in the needle holders against the button is applied to the suture. The amount of wound edge advancement can be determined by the distance between the original split shot and the button. It may be necessary to administer a neuroleptanalgesic drug to make suture tightening more comfortable for the animal.

If the limb distal to the adjustable horizontal mattress suture becomes edematous, the paw feels hypothermic, and/or the base of the nails appears cyanotic on dogs with light colored nails, it indicates that the closure is too tight and a "biologic tourniquet" has been created. The suture can then be loosened. To aid in evaluating the effects of suture tension, the limb can be bandaged such that the third and fourth digits remain exposed to observe for these signs.

In some instances of early severe distal limb trauma, where the surgeon believes the limb will swell significantly within 1 to 2 days of trauma, the surgeon may elect to place the adjustable horizontal mattress suture immediately after debridement. However, daily suture tightening may not begin until the edema starts to subside.

Skin edge advancement is usually greatest during the first 2 to 3 days after tightening has begun due to the skin's inherent elasticity. When the wound edges are apposed, or they have advanced to their limit (i.e. tension does not result in further advancement), the suture should be left in place a few days to allow the collagen deposition of the repair stage of healing to secure the wound edges in place.

## Advantages and Disadvantages

The technique utilizes the extensibility of the skin to advance it gradually to close the wound (Figure 3-54). Thus, a graft or flap may not be necessary. Even if a graft is needed its size will be smaller after using this technique. If wound contraction has started, this technique will enhance the process and shorten the time for wound closure. The technique has the additional advantage that it can be used in combination with some form of relaxing incision to attain wound closure. However, the adjustable horizontal mattress suture should be used first. The technique has the disadvantage that it can create a "biologic tourniquet" if the suture is tightened too much. This, however, can be easily corrected by loosening the suture. If tightening the suture is uncomfortable for the animal a neuroleptanalgesic may be needed prior to tightening. If these sutures are placed in wound edges that are too widely separated on the limbs, tightening could result in sutures cutting into the tissues as they are tightened across the curvature of the wound.

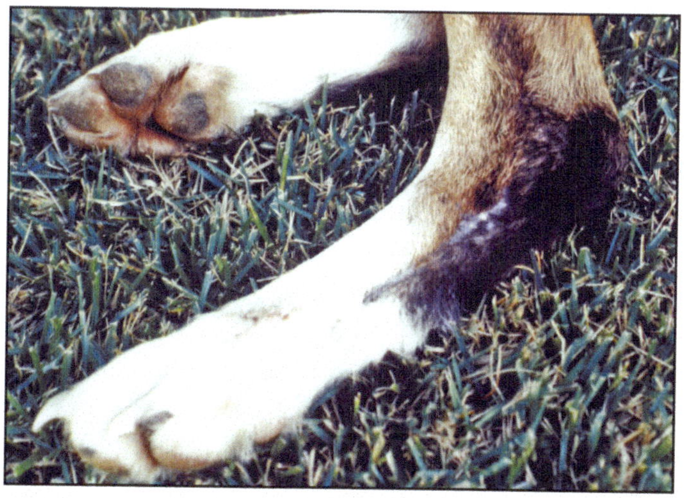

**Figure 3-54.** Limb of dog shown in figure 3-53 with healed wound after advancing skin over the wound with an adjustable horizontal mattress suture.

# Suggested Readings


1. Bohling MW, Swaim SF: Management of the traumatic wound in primary closure. In Birchard SJ, Sherding RG, eds.: Saunders Manual of Small Animal Practice, 3rd ed.: St. Louis: Saunders – Elsevier, 2006, 541.
2. Bohling MW, Swaim SF: Paw and distal limb skin reconstructive and salvage techniques. In Bojrab MJ, ed.: Current Techniques in Small Animal Surgery, 5th ed.: Jackson, WY: Teton NewMedia, 2014, 628.
3. Fowler D: Distal limb and paw injuries: Vet Clin No Amer Small Animal Pract 36: 819, 2006.
4. Hedlund CS: Surgery of the integumentary system. *In* Fossum TW, ed.: Small Animal Surgery, 2nd ed.: St. Louis: Mosby, 2002, 134.
5. Hedlund CS: Surgery of the integumentary system. In Fossum TW, ed.: Small Animal Surgery, 3rd ed.: St. Louis: Mosby, 2007, 159.
6. MacPhail CM: Surgery of the integumentary system. In Fossum TW, ed.: Small Animal Surgery, 4th ed.: St. Louis: Mosby, 2013, 190.
7. Scardino MS, Swaim SF, Henderson RA, et. al.: Enhancing wound closure on the limbs. Compend Contin Educ Pract Vet 18:919, 1996.
8. Stanley BJ: Tension – relieving techniques. In Tobias KM, Johnston SA, eds.: Veterinary Surgery, Small Animal, Vol. 2: St. Louis: Elsevier – Saunders, 2012, 1221,
9. Swaim SF, Henderson RA: Small Animal Wound Management, 2nd ed.: Baltimore: Williams and Wilkins, 1997, 143.
10. Swaim SF, Scardino MS: Paw and distal limb salvage and reconstruction techniques. *In* Bojrab MJ, ed.: Current Techniques in Small Animal Surgery, 4th ed.: Baltimore: Williams and Wilkins, 1998, 625.
11. Trout NJ: Principles of plastic and reconstructive surgery. *In* Slatter DH, ed.: Textbook of Small Animal Surgery, 3rd ed.: Philadelphia: WB Saunders, 2003, 274.


# Closure - Simple Relaxing Incision

## Definition and Indications

A simple relaxing incision is made adjacent, and usually parallel, to a wound to allow the skin between the wound and the relaxing incision to close the wound without tension. After wound closure, the resulting relaxing incision defect, which is over vascularized noncompromised tissue (e.g. muscle), is allowed to heal as an open wound. The procedure is generally more applicable on wounds that are parallel to the long axis of the limb.

On the distal limb, simple relaxing incisions are indicated for closing wounds that are too large to close by using extensive undermining and on which skin stretching techniques such as adjustable horizontal mattress sutures or presutures have not provided enough skin relaxation to close the wound. These are generally wounds that are not of a nature or size to warrant more involved reconstructive procedures. These relaxing incisions are also indicated to close wounds that have exposed bone, surgical implants, or vital structures (tendons, ligaments, nerves, or blood vessels).

Wounds that are susceptible to external trauma and infection, and chronic nonhealing wounds such as occur from recurrent trauma or radiation may heal primarily by using the flap(s) created by a relaxing incision(s). However, the nature of the wound must be assessed and the presence of healthy well vascularized adjacent skin must be assured before using this procedure.

## Technique

When using a simple relaxing incision to close a wound that is not surrounded by loose elastic skin, an attempt is made to appose the center of the wound or the area of greatest tension using a pair of towel forceps. Starting at this point of greatest tension, the relaxing incision is started. It is usually at a distance from the wound edge equal to the width of the wound (Figure 3-55A). The incision is made incrementally, with gentle undermining of the flap being created (Figure 3-55B). After sufficient skin has been freed to allow closure, wound closure is then started using a 3-0 absorbable continuous subcutaneous suture if there is sufficient subcutaneous tissue for suturing. The skin is then closed with simple interrupted 3-0 nonabsorbable skin sutures (Figure 3-55C).

An alternative technique is to begin undermining at the edge of the defect at the point of greatest skin tension and continue until the edges can be apposed with tension Figure 3-56A & B). The skin is then closed using a 3-0 absorbable continuous subcutaneous suture and simple interrupted 3-0 nonabsorbable skin sutures (Figure 3-56C) A relaxing incision is made at the point where undermining stopped or where tension lines are observed. The incision should begin at the area of maximum skin tension and extend as necessary to relieve excess tension(Figure 3-56D & E). If the location and size of the wound indicate it, relaxing incisions can be made bilaterally. Any defects that remain after closing the original wound are left to heal as open wounds. These generally heal within 21 to 30 days.

## Aftercare

The suture line and open donor site wounds from the relaxing incisions should be bandaged using a nonadherent wound contact dressing, absorbent wrap, and adhesive tape. In the early stages of healing, bandage changes should be daily and become less frequent in the later stages of healing of the relaxing incision sites. Bandaging is discontinued after the relaxing incision site has fully healed.

If the animal is inclined to molest, i.e. lick the wound area persistently after bandaging is discontinued, bandaging should be resumed for another 2 to 4 weeks to protect the area and let the healed wound tissue further mature. Periodic attempts should be made during this time to discontinue bandages while observing whether the dog tends to lick at the wound.

The open wound that remains after using a relaxing incision should be observed as it heals for the development of a "biologic tourniquet" as the result of contraction and epithelialization. If it appears that this is developing, removal of the constricting scar tissue and reconstruction of the area with a graft or flap will be necessary.

## Advantages and Disadvantages

The technique allows closure of wounds that would otherwise have tension on them. Vital structures or

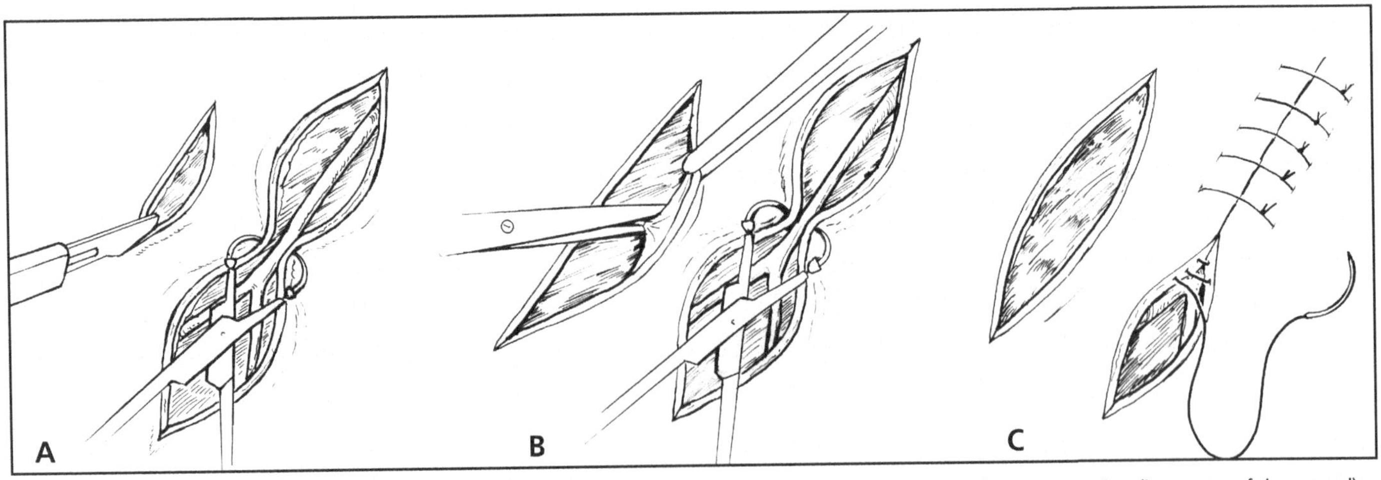


**Figure 3-55.** Simple relaxing incision. **A.** Towel forceps are used to try to appose wound edges at their point of greatest tension (i.e. center of the wound). An incision is made at this point with the distance from the wound edge equal to the width of the wound. **B.** The incision is made incrementally with undermining of the resulting flap. **C.** Wound closure with a continuous absorbable subcutaneous suture and simple interrupted nonabsorbable sutures.

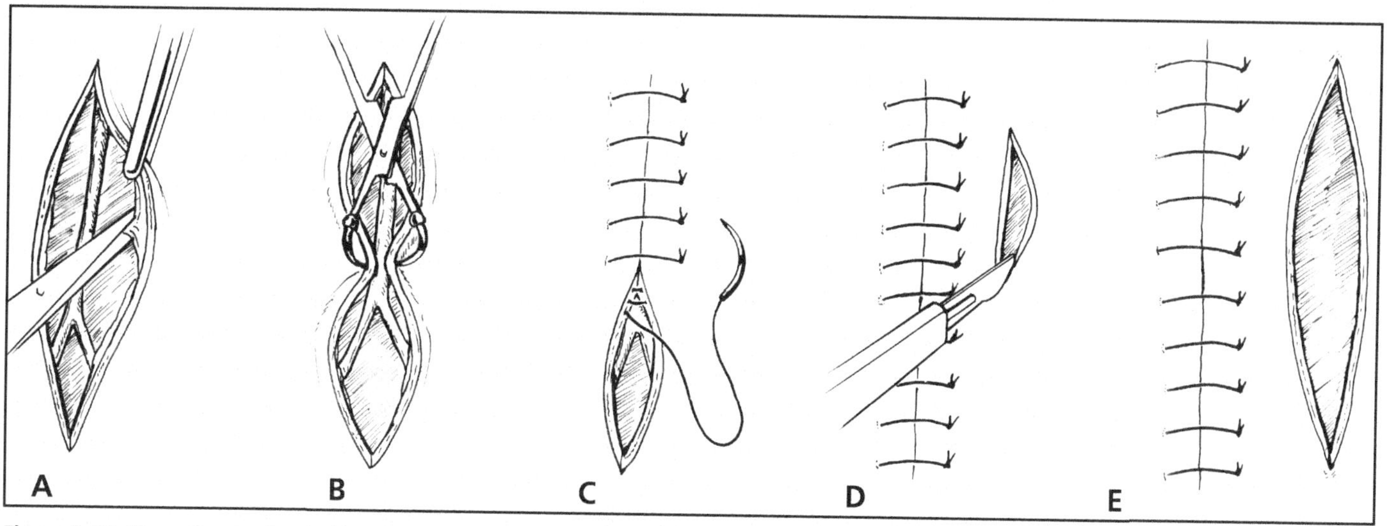


**Figure 3-56.** Alternative simple relaxing incision technique. **A & B.** Undermining along one edge of the wound until the edges can be apposed by towel forceps with tension. **C.** Wound closure with a continuous absorbable subcutaneous suture and simple interrupted nonabsorbable sutures. **D & E.** Relaxing incision is made at the point where undermining stopped and is extended as needed to relieve excess tension.

surgical implants that may have been exposed in the original wound can be covered by the bipedicle flap of skin created by the simple relaxing incision, while the relaxing incision defect is in an unobtrusive location where second intention healing can readily take place. When used to close wounds that are susceptible to external trauma and infection as well as chronic nonhealing wounds, the flap(s) created by the relaxing incision(s) may provide adequate blood supply for healing while the relaxing incision defect is in a region with sufficient circulation for second intention healing.

A potential disadvantage of the simple relaxing incision is that the central portion of the flap created by the incision may necrose if the flap is too long and has insufficient vascularization to its central portion. The procedure entails making wounds to close wounds. Thus, the procedure should be reserved for instances when simple undermining, skin stretching sutures, and tension suture techniques are not effective.

Relaxing incisions may concern the surgeon after closure of the original wound because there is a new wound the same size as the original wound on another surface of the limb. These defects may be in an area less subject to trauma than the original wound and they may have a better blood supply than the original wound area. As a result, such wounds usually heal uneventfully in time. However, if the animal tends to molest the wound early in the post-healing period there is the possibility that a chronic nonhealing wound will develop. Thus, a longer period of protective bandaging may be indicated. There is also the possibility that scar tissue in the area may form a "biologic tourniquet" as the wound heals.

# Suggested Readings

1. Bohling MW, Swaim SF: Management of the traumatic wound by primary closure. In Birchard SJ, Sherding RG, eds.: Saunders Manual of Small Animal Practice, 3rd ed.: St. Louis: Saunders – Elsevier, 2006, 541.
2. Fowler D: Tension relieving techniques and local skin flaps. *In* Fowler D, Williams JM, eds.: BSAVA Manual of Canine and Feline Wound Management and Reconstruction. Shurdington, Cheltenham, UK: BSAVA, 1999, 57.
3. Hedlund CS: Surgery of the integumentary system. *In* Fossum TW, ed.: Small Animal Surgery, 2nd ed.: St. Louis: Mosby, 2002, 134.
4. Hedlund CS: Surgery of the integumentary system. In Fossum TW, ed.: Small Animal Surgery, 3rd ed.: St. Louis: Mosby, 2007, 159.
5. Johnston DE: Tension-relieving techniques. Vet Clin North Am Small Animal Pract 20:67, 1990.
6. MacPhail CM: Surgery of the integumentary system. In Fossum TW, ed.: Small Animal Surgery, 4th ed.: St. Louis: Mosby, 2013, 190.
7. Mayhew P: Tension relieving techniques and local skin flaps. In Williams J, Moores A, eds.: BSAVA Manual of Canine and Feline Wound Management and Reconstruction, 2nd ed.: Glouster (UK): BSAVA, 2009, 69.
8. Pavletic MM: Atlas of Small Animal Reconstructive Surgery, 2nd ed.: Philadelphia: WB Saunders, 1999, 131.
9. Pavletic MM: Skin flaps in reconstructive surgery. Vet Clin North Am Small Animal Pract 20:81, 1990.
10. Pavletic MM: Atlas of Small Animal Wound Management and Reconstructive Surgery, 3rd ed.: Ames, IA: Wiley – Blackwell, 2010, 241.
11. Scardino MS, Swaim SF, Henderson RA, et al: Enhancing wound closure on the limbs. Compend Contin Educ Pract Vet 18:919, 1996.
12. Stanley BJ: Tension – relieving techniques. In Tobias KM, Johnston SA, eds.: Veterinary Surgery, Small Animal, Vol. 2: St. Louis: Elsevier – Saunders, 2012, 1221.
13. Swaim SF: Management of skin tension in dermal surgery. Compend Contin Educ Pract Vet 2:758, 1980.
14. Swaim SF: Management of the traumatic wound by primary closure. *In* Birchard SJ, Sherding RG eds.: Saunders Manual of Small Animal Practice, 2nd ed.: Philadelphia: WB Saunders, 2000, 392.
15. Swaim SF, Henderson RA: Small Animal Wound Management, 2nd ed.: Baltimore: Williams and Wilkins, 1997, 143.
16. Trout NJ: Principles of plastic and reconstructive surgery. *In* Slatter DH, ed.: Textbook of Small Animal Surgery, 3rd ed.: Philadelphia: WB Saunders, 2003, 274.

# Multiple Punctate Relaxing Incisions

## Definition and Indications

Multiple punctate relaxing incisions are multiple small parallel staggered incisions made unilaterally or bilaterally in the skin adjacent to a wound as a tension-relieving technique during wound closure. This technique can be used if necessary after undermining, presutures or an adjustable horizontal mattress suture has been used.

## Technique

Following undermining, multiple punctate relaxing incisions may be considered if it is not possible to appose the skin edges. Beginning at one end of the wound, a continuous intradermal tension suture of 2-0 or 3-0 absorbable suture material is placed and tightened as it is placed. If the wound edges do not appose as the suture is tightened or if they appose with tension, punctate relaxing incisions 0.5 to 1 cm long and 1 to 2 cm appart are made in the skin adjacent to the wound edges on one or both sides of the wound as the suture is placed and tightened. The initial incisions are made parallel to the long axis of the wound and usually no closer than 1 cm from the wound edge. If additional incisions are needed for relaxation they are made in staggered fashion in rows parallel to the first incisions. These incisions are 0.5 to 2 cm from the initial row (Figure 3-57A & B and Figure 3-58A). Generally, more incisions are needed at the widest area of the defect because of the greater tension in this area. Punctate incisions are made as they are needed to provide wound edge apposition. This approach helps prevent making more incisions than are necessary. The greater the number of incisions, the greater are the chances of interfering with the blood supply to the skin adjacent to the wound, thus increasing the potential for tissue necrosis in the area. Final skin sutures are placed with simple interrupted 3-0 nonabsorbable suture (Figure 3-57C and Figure 3-58B).

## Aftercare

The surgical site is covered with a nonadherent contact bandage. An absorbent wrap and adhesive tape complete the bandage. During the early stages of healing bandage changes should be done daily and less often as healing progresses. The punctate incisions are usually healed in 14 to 21 days.

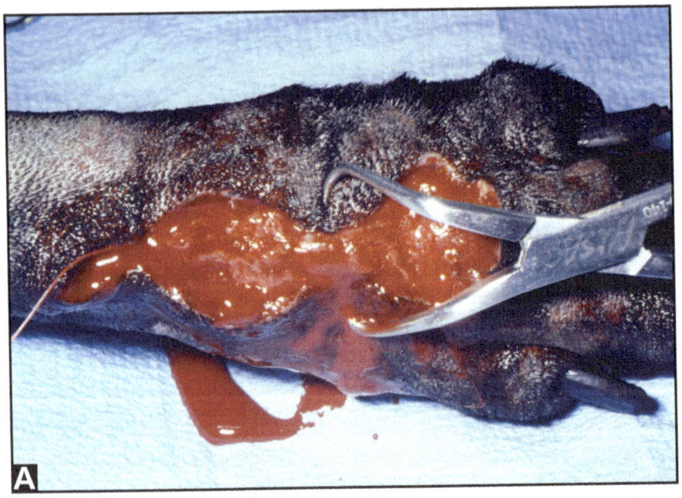
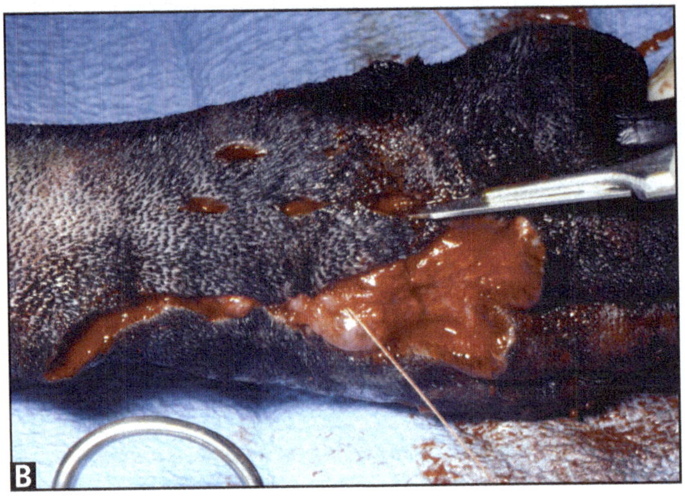
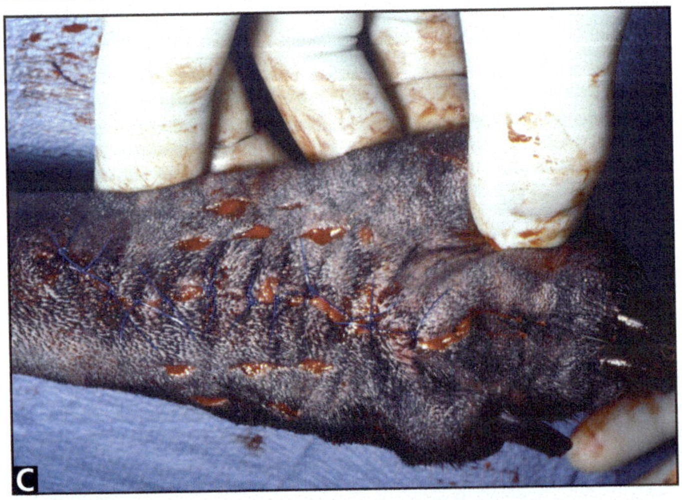

**Figure 3-57.** Multiple punctuate relaxing incisions. **A.** Distal limb wound with a continuous absorbable intradermal suture started, and towel forceps attempting to appose wound edges. **B.** As the intradermal suture is placed and tightened, staggered rows of punctuate incisions are made parallel to the long axis of the wound. **C.** Final skin apposition with nonabsorbable sutures.

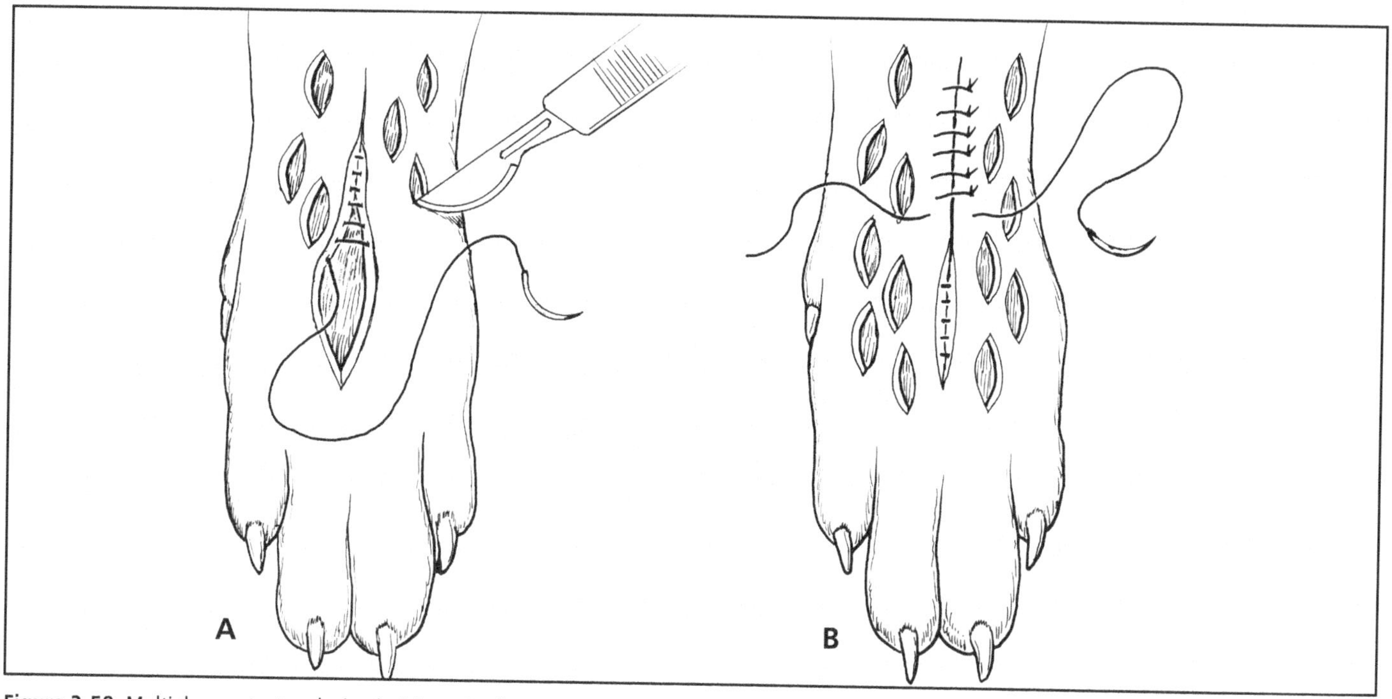


**Figure 3-58.** Multiple punctuate relaxing incisions. **A.** Placing continuous absorbable intradermal suture and making parallel staggered rows of punctuate incisions with suture placement. **B.** Placing final nonabsorbable skin apposition sutures.

If the limb distal to the area of wound closure becomes edematous, the paw feels hypothermic and/or the base of the nails appears cyanotic on dogs that have light colored nails, it indicates the closure is too tight and a "biologic tourniquet" has been created. The surgeon should consider removing the sutures to relieve the tourniquet effect, i.e. the viability of the distal limb should not be jeopardized in order to have a closed wound. An adjustable horizontal mattress suture should be considered to provide gradual wound closure.

If the animal is inclined to molest, i.e. lick the wound area persistently after the bandaging is discontinued, bandaging should be resumed for another 2 to 4 weeks to protect the area and let the healed wound tissue further mature. Periodic attempts should be made to discontinue bandaging while observing whether the dog tends to lick at the wound.

## Advantages and Disadvantages

When compared to simple relaxing incision(s), multiple punctate relaxing incisions are more cosmetic and they heal more quickly than the large wounds created by simple relaxing incisions. Thus, they are more acceptable to the pet owner. Staggering the rows of incisions help ensure vascular supply to the skin edges.

These incisions require making wounds to close a wound, and the amount of relaxation may not be as great as that resulting from simple relaxing incision(s). If punctate incisions are too great in number or size, the danger of vascular insufficiency in the skin adjacent to the wound is increased, which could result in sloughing of the skin. If the sutures are too tight even with the relaxing incisions, a "biologic tourniquet" can result.

# Suggested Readings


1. Bohling MW, Swaim SF: Management of the traumatic wound by primary closure. In Birchard SJ, Sherding RG, eds.: Saunders Manual of Veterinary Practice, 3rd ed.: St. Louis: Saunders – Elsevier, 2006, 541.
2. Bohling MW, Swaim SF: Paw and distal limb reconstructive and salvage techniques. In Bojrab MJ, ed.. Current Techniques in Small Animal Surgery, 5th ed.: Jackson, WY: Teton NewMedia 2014, 268.
3. Bailey JV, Caron JP, Lees MJ: Wound closure by mesh-expansion in 2 equine skin wounds. Mod Vet Pract 67:355, 1986.
4. Bailey JV, Jacobs KA: The mesh expansion method of suturing wounds on the legs of horses. Vet Surg 12:78, 1983.
5. Fowler D: Tension relieving techniques and local skin flaps. *In* Fowler D, Williams JM, eds.: BSAVA Manual of Canine and Feline Wound Management and Reconstruction. Shurdington, Cheltenham, UK: BSAVA, 1999, 57.
6. Fowler D: Distal limb and paw injuries. Vet Clin No Am Small Animal Practice 36: 819, 2006.
7. Hedlund CS: Surgery of the integumentary system. *In* Fossum TW, ed.: Small Animal Surgery, 2nd ed.: St. Louis: Mosby, 2002, 134.
8. Hedlund CS: Surgery of the integumentary system. In Fossum TW: Small Animal Surgery, 3rd ed.: St. Louis: Mosby, 2007, 159.
9. MacPhail CM: Surgery of the integumentary system. In Fossum TW, ed.: Small Animal Surgery, 4th ed.: St. Louis: Mosby, 2013, 190.
10. Mayhew P: Tension – relieving techniques and local skin flaps. In Williams J, Moores A, eds.: BSAVA Manual of Canine and Feline Wound Management and Reconstruction, 2nd ed.: Glouster (UK): BSAVA, 2009, 69.
11. Pavletic MM: Atlas of Small Animal Reconstructive Surgery, 2nd ed: Philadelphia: WB Saunders, 1999, 131.
12. Pavletic MM: Atlas of Small Animal Wound Management and Reconstructive Surgery, 3rd ed.: Ames, IA: Wiley – Blackwell, 2010, 241.

13. Scardino MS, Swaim SF, Henderson RA, et al: Enhancing wound closure on the limbs. Compend Contin Educ Pract Vet 18:919, 1996.
14. Stanley BJ: Tension – relieving techniques. In Tobias KM, Johnston SA, eds.: Veterinary Surgery, Small Animal, Vol. 2: St. Louis: Elsevier – Saunders, 2012, 1221.
15. Swaim SF: Wound Management of the distal limbs and paws: Reconstruction and salvage. Vet Med Rep 2:128, 1990.
16. Swaim SF: Management of the traumatic wound by primary closure. *In* Birchard SJ, Sherding RG, eds.: Saunders Manual of Small Animal Practice, 2nd ed.: Philadelphia: WB Saunders, 2000, 392.
17. Swaim SF, Henderson RA: Small Animal Wound Management, 2nd ed.: Baltimore: Williams and Wilkins, 1997, 143.
18. Swaim SF, Scardino MS: Paw and distal limb salvage and reconstruction techniques. *In* Bojrab MJ, ed.: Current Techniques in Small Animal Surgery, 4th ed.: Baltimore: Williams and Wilkins, 1998, 625.
19. Trout NJ: Principles of plastic and reconstructive surgery. *In* Slatter DH, ed.: Textbook of Small Animal Surgery, 3rd ed.: Philadelphia: WB Saunders, 2003, 274.
20. Vig MM: Management of integumentary wounds of extremities in dogs. An experimental study. J Am Anim Hosp Assoc 21:187, 1985.

# Z-Plasty

## Definition and Indications

Z-plasty is a relaxing incision that changes the direction of tension adjacent to a wound, thus providing laxity of the skin to close the wound. A Z-plasty is composed of a central limb, 2 arms, and 2 angles where the arms join the central limb. The general design of Z-plasty is that the arms and central limb are of equal length. The Z-plasty angles can be any size between 30 and 90 degrees, and the angles can be equal in size or any combination of sizes. The most workable angle in skin is 60 degrees, with both angles of this size since larger angles tend to produce greater tension on surrounding tissue (Figure 3-59). Angles less than 45 degrees produce narrow flaps with insufficient blood supply.

The dynamics of a Z-plasty involve transposing 2 interdigitating triangular skin flaps (Figure 3-60).

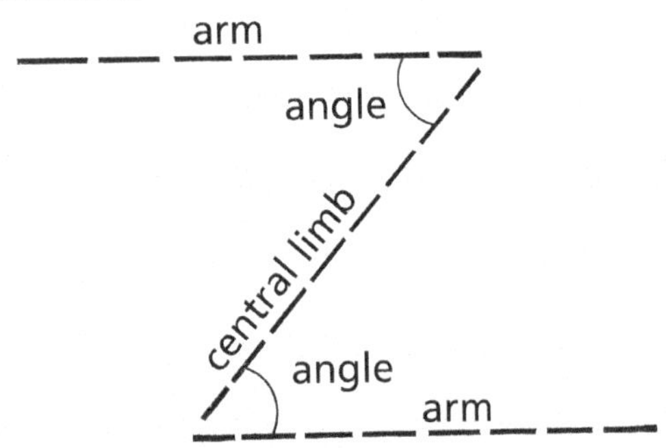


ARM LENGTH = CENTRAL LIMB LENGTH
ANGLES = FROM 30° - 90°. (60° is most common)

**Figure 3-59.** Components and general rules of Z-plasty. (After Swaim SF, Henderson RA: Small Animal Wound Management, 2nd ed.: Baltimore: Williams & Wilkins, 1997, 182.)

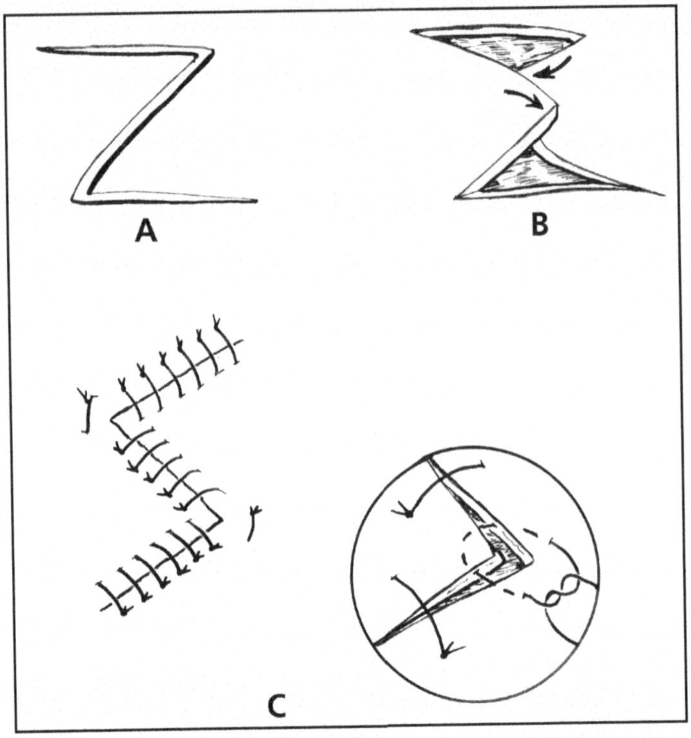


**Figure 3-60.** Dynamics of Z-plasty. **A.** Z incised. **B.** Undermining and transposition of flaps. **C.** Flaps sutured in their new position. Inset: half – buried horizontal mattress suture at flap tips. (After Swaim SF, Henderson RA: Small Animal Wound Management, 2nd ed.: Baltimore: Williams & Wilkins, 1997, 183.)

These dynamics can be utilized for 3 types of tension relief on the distal limb. First, the technique can be effective in providing skin relaxation for wound closure of small to medium sized wounds on the distal limbs. Second, it can be used to relieve tension along a thin bowstring scar that restricts extension of a joint, and third, Z-plasty can relieve the circumferential constricting tension of a scar that is causing a "biologic tourniquet". These scars usually result from circumferential skin loss in a limited area with intact skin proximal and distal to the defect or from circumferentially constricting strings or bands.

In all 3 types of tension relief, the principle involved is gaining length or relaxation in the direction of the original central limb of the Z when the Z-plasty flaps are transposed. The gain in length (relaxation) in one direction is caused by shortening of the skin along the opposite sides of the Z-plasty (Figure 3-61). Thus, there must be some skin laxity perpendicular to the line of tension to allow rotation of the Z-plasty flaps.

In some instances, a single Z-plasty cannot be used on a long scar because of the length of the scar - i.e. the arms cannot be made equal in length to the central limb because structures are in the area that interfere with their design or the small circumference of the limb does not allow the design of arms equal in length

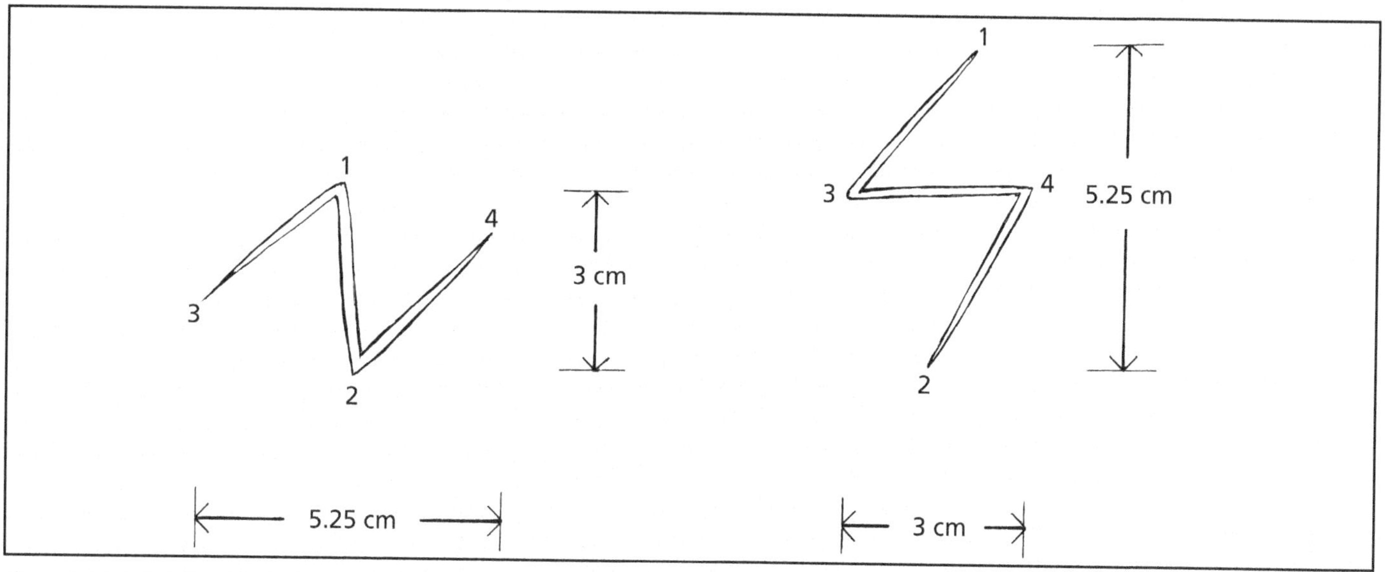


**Figure 3-61.** Principles of Z-plasty as a relaxing incision. There is an increase in length in the direction of the original central limb when flaps are transposed. The gain in length is caused by shortening the skin length along the opposite sides of the Z-plasty, i.e. the distance between 1 and 2 lengthens as the distance between 3 and 4 shortens. (After Swaim SF, Henderson RA: Small Animal Wound Management, 2nd ed.: Baltimore: Williams & Wilkins, 1997, 183.)

to the central limb. In such instances, multiple small Z-plasties may be designed for tension relief because their effect tends to be additive.

Either the size of the angles of the Z-plasty or the length of the central limb may be used to govern the length gained in the direction of the central limb of the Z-plasty. The larger the angle size, the greater will be the length gain; and the longer the central limb length, the greater will be the length gain (Figure 3-62 & Figure 3-63). It is important however, to remember that scar tissue in the area will affect the actual amount of length gained using a Z-plasty.

## Techniques

In all procedures requiring a Z-plasty, drawing of the

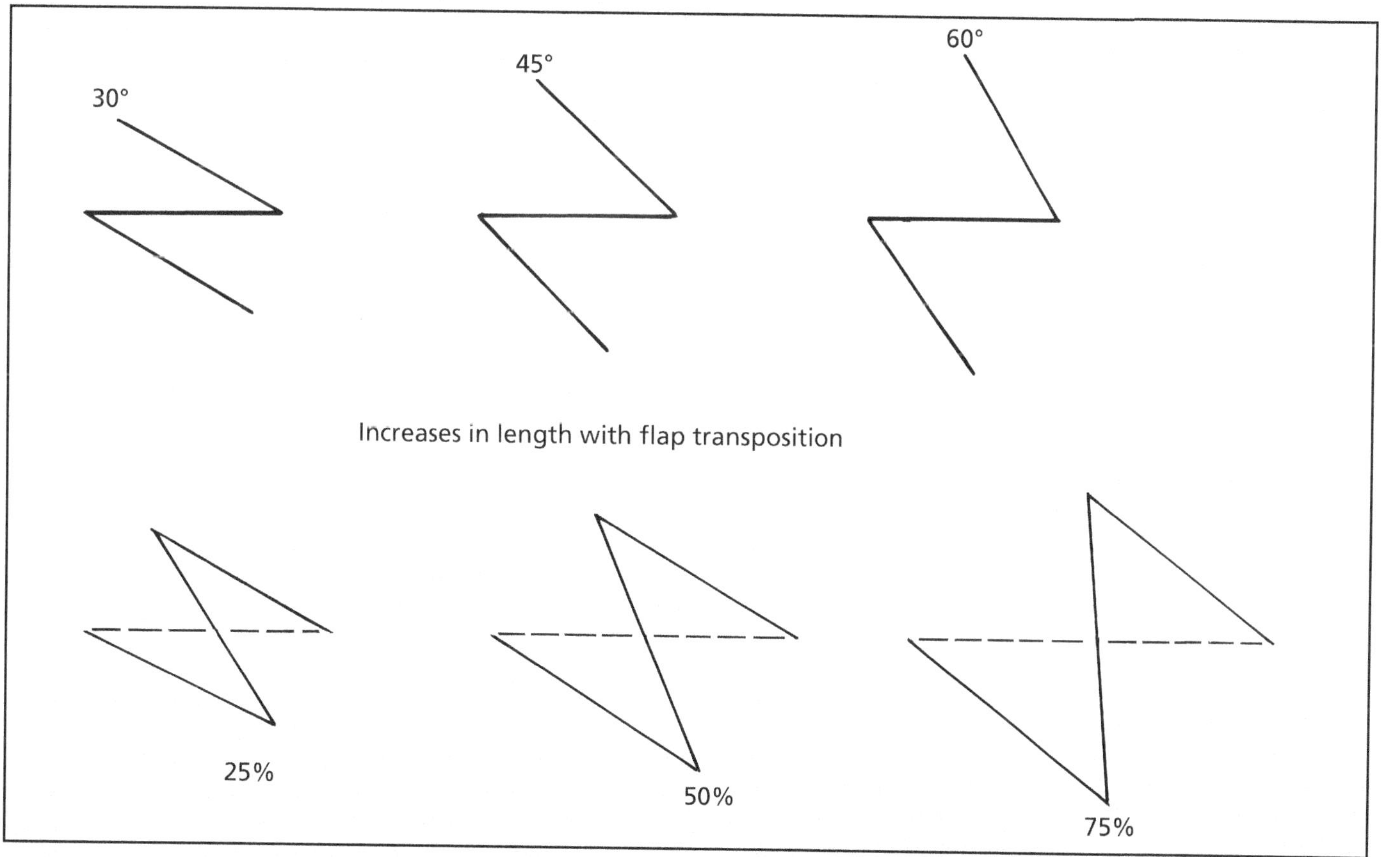


**Figure 3-62.** Percentage increase in length in the direction of the original central limb of the Z based on angle size. (After Jankauskas S, Cohen IK, Grabb WC: Basic techniques of plastic surgery, 4th ed.: Boston: Little Brown, 1991, 73.)

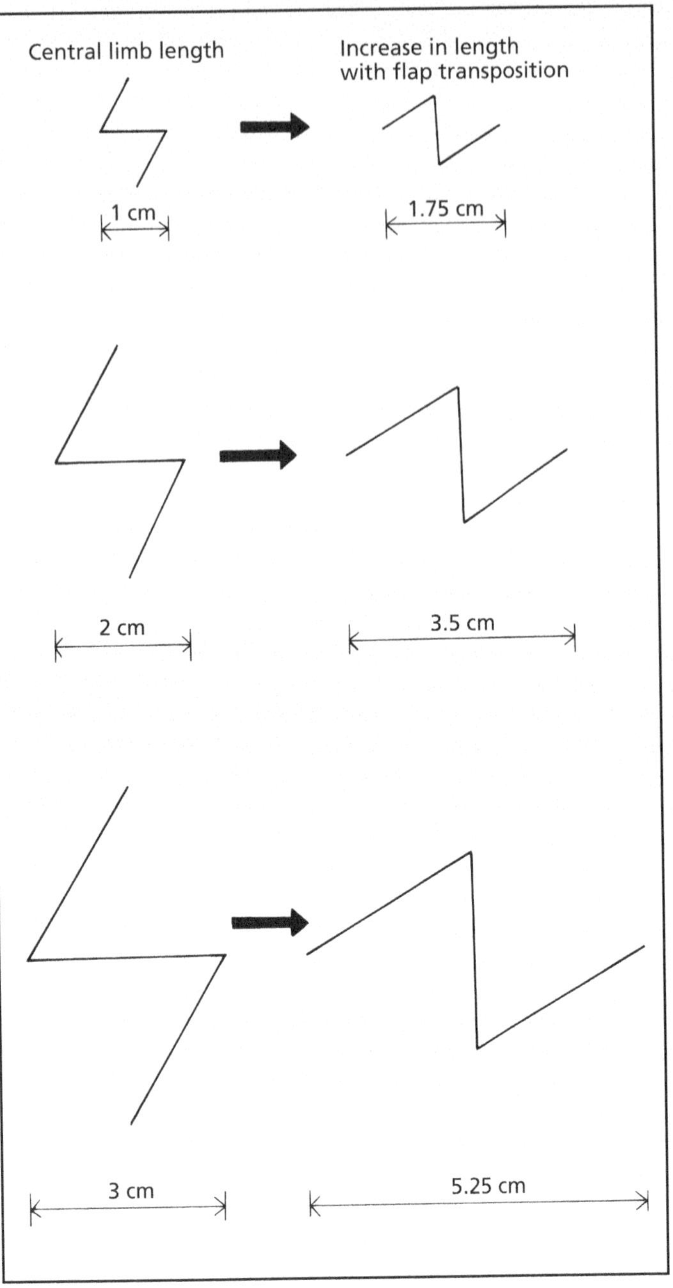


**Figure 3-63.** Increase in length in the direction of the original central limb of the Z based on different lengths of the central limb and 60 degree angles. (After Jankauskas S, Cohen IK, Grabb WC: Basic techniques of plastic surgery, 4th ed.: Boston. Little, Brown, 1991, 74.)

Z-plasty(ies) may be done with a splintered cotton-tipped applicator or tooth pick dipped in sterile methylene blue. A commercial skin marking pen can also be used to draw the Z-plasty(ies).

## Z-plasty Relaxing Incision

Prior to using a Z-plasty as a relaxing incision, the skin around the defect should be manipulated to determine whether there is sufficient skin in one plane to allow the necessary relaxation in the perpendicular plane. If skin is available for the procedure, a Z-plasty with 60 degree angles is designed adjacent to the wound. If the skin is taut, slightly smaller angles, e.g. 45 degrees, and a longer central limb can be used to gain length without resulting in too much tension. The Z is made with the central limb in the direction that relaxation is needed. The arms of the Z-plasty are then designed off the ends of the central limb (Figure 3-64A-D). If there is scar tissue in the area, the flaps should be designed so there is no scar tissue across the base of a flap which could restrict circulation. To design 60 degree angles for a Z-plasty, the angle size can be easily estimated. A 90 degree angle can be readily visualized. By dividing the 90 degree angle into thirds and taking 2/3's of the right angle, measured from the central limb, a 60 degree angle is attained (Figure 3-65). The Z-plasty is then incised (Figure 3-66A). The flaps of the Z and the skin between the Z and the wound are undermined (See Figure 3-64 B). Undermining at the base of the Z-flaps should be done with care to avoid damage to the blood supply of the flaps. The relaxation provided allows the skin to be advanced toward the opposite side of the defect. If necessary, underlying tacking or "walking" sutures of 3-0 absorbable suture material can be used to advance the skin edge toward the opposite side of the wound. The wound is closed with some form of tension suture, e.g. continuous intradermal 3-0 absorbable suture, as needed, and 3-0 nonabsorbable simple interrupted skin sutures. As the wound is closed, the flaps of the Z-plasty tend to transpose into their new positions for final suturing (See Figure 3-64 C). The Z-plasty defect is sutured. The tips of the flaps are sutured first with half-buried horizontal mattress sutures of 3-0 or 4-0 nonabsorbable material. Alternatively, a simple interrupted suture can be placed in the center of the new central limb, followed by suturing the flap tips. When suturing is completed the central limb of the Z should be 90 degrees from its original position (See Figures 3-64D & 3-66B).

## Z-plasty to Release a Bowstring Scar

To relieve the tension of a bowstring scar that is restricting extension of a joint the scar and tissue around the scar should be assessed in deciding on the procedure to be used. If the restricting scar is narrow and relatively short and there is loose skin adjacent to the scar, a single Z-plasty may be considered for use to correct the defect. When the scar is long and narrow and there is loose skin adjacent to the scar, multiple Z-plasties should be considered because constructing arms equal in length to the central limb may be difficult. If the scar is wide and/or there is little loose skin adjacent to it, scar removal and reconstruction with a flap or graft are indicated.

If a single Z-plasty can be used, it is constructed with the central limb of the Z along the scar. The arms

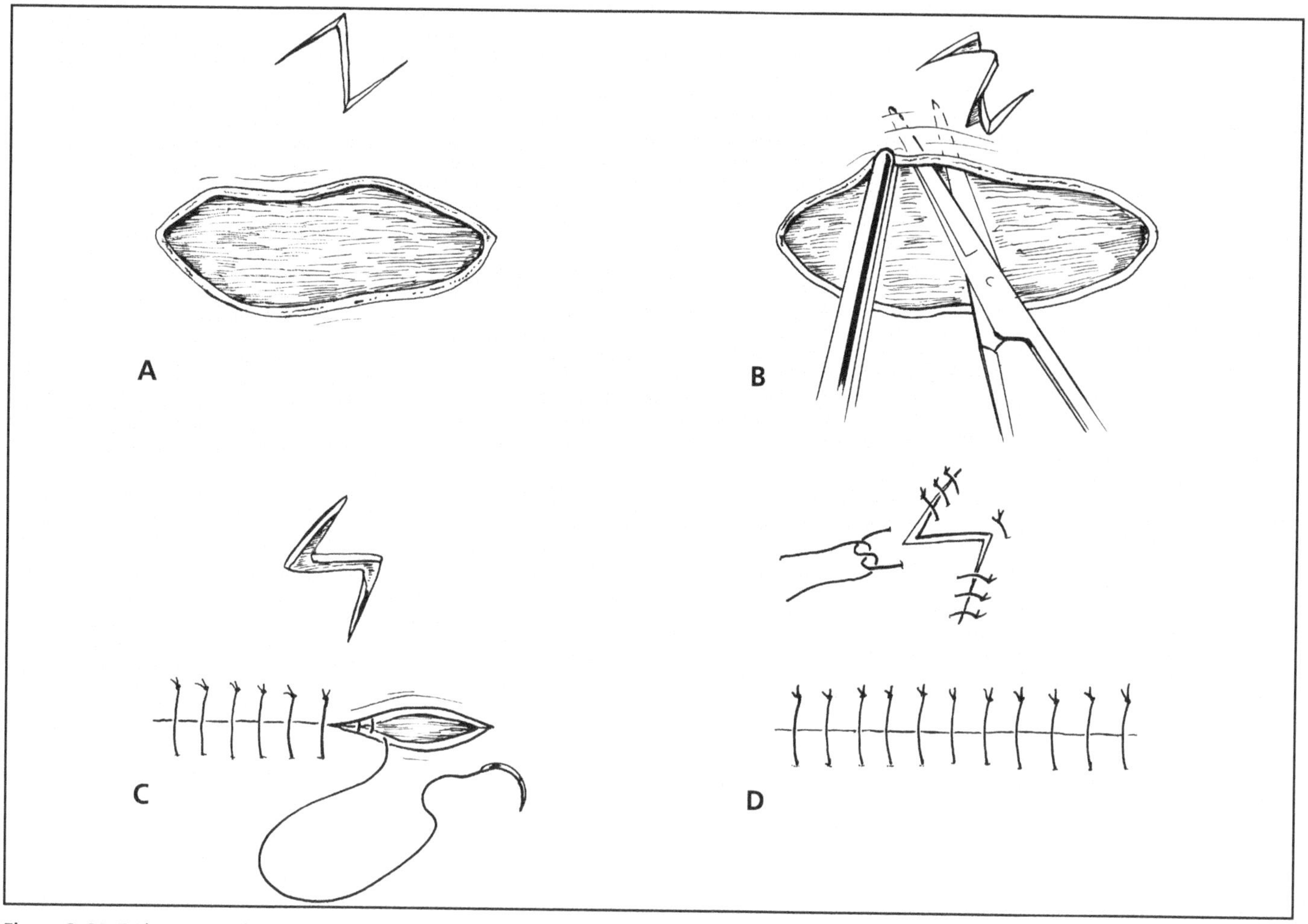


**Figure 3-64.** Z-plasty as a relaxing incision for wound closure. **A.** A 60 degree angle Z – plasty is designed adjacent to the wound with the central limb in the direction relaxation is needed. **B.** After incising the Z-plasty, its flaps and surrounding skin are undermined. **C.** Closure of the defect with continuous absorbable intradermal suture, if needed, and simple interrupted nonabsorbable sutures. The Z-plasty flaps tend to move into their new positions. **D.** Suturing the Z-plasty flaps, including half – buried horizontal mattress sutures at the flap tips.

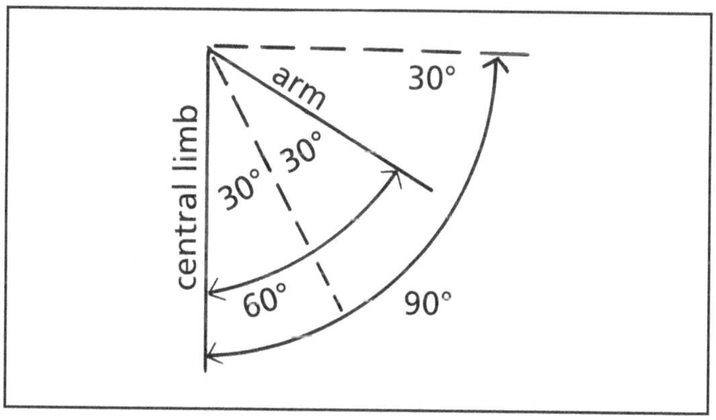


**Figure 3-65.** Designing a 60-degree angle for Z-plasty angles. A 90-degree angle can be readily visualized. This angle is divided into thirds (three 30-degree angles). Taking 2/3's of the 90-degree angle measured from the central limb gives the desired 60-degree angle.

are designed off of either end of the central limb at 60 degrees and are equal in length to the central limb (Figure 3-67A). However, if there is considerable tension within the line of the central limb and less tension laterally where the arms will be incised, the central limb may be made longer than the arms. It may be up to 22% longer. After the flaps of the Z are incised and undermined, excess scar tissue is excised from under the flaps as needed. If there is any dead space under the flaps after removing this tissue, a few 3-0 interrupted absorbable tacking sutures can be considered to help immobilize the flaps in place when they are transposed into their new positions. Simple interrupted nonabsorbable 3-0 skin sutures are used to suture the skin edges with a half-buried horizontal mattress suture of 3-0 or 4-0 nonabsorbable material used to suture the flap tips. Completion of the technique gives relaxation in the direction of the original central limb of the Z with relief of tension by the bowstring scar (Figure 3-67B).

If a linear restricting scar is long (Figure 3-68A), designing the arms of a single Z-plasty would be difficult. If there is loose skin adjacent to the scar then multiple Z-plasties should be considered for reconstruction. The central limb of the Z-plasties is designed along the linear scar (Figure 3-68B). A piece of developed x-ray film is cut in the shape of an equilateral triangle (all sides equal in length and all angles 60

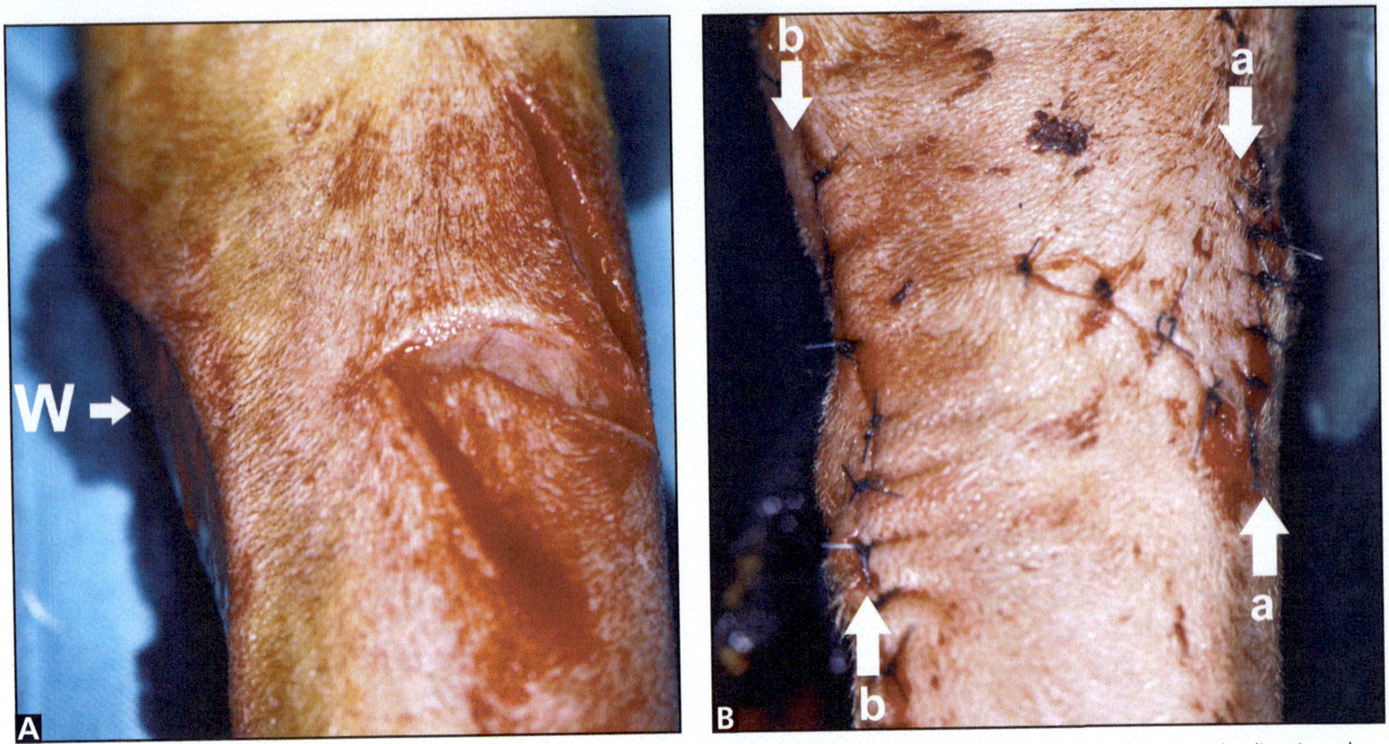


**Figure 3-66.** Z-plasty as a relaxing incision for wound closure. **A.** Z-plasty incised adjacent to a limb wound *(W)* with the central limb in the direction relaxation is needed. **B.** The wound and Z-plasty have been closed. The central limb of the Z is rotated 90 degrees from its original position and is now parallel *(a arrows)* to the closed wound *(b arrows)*.

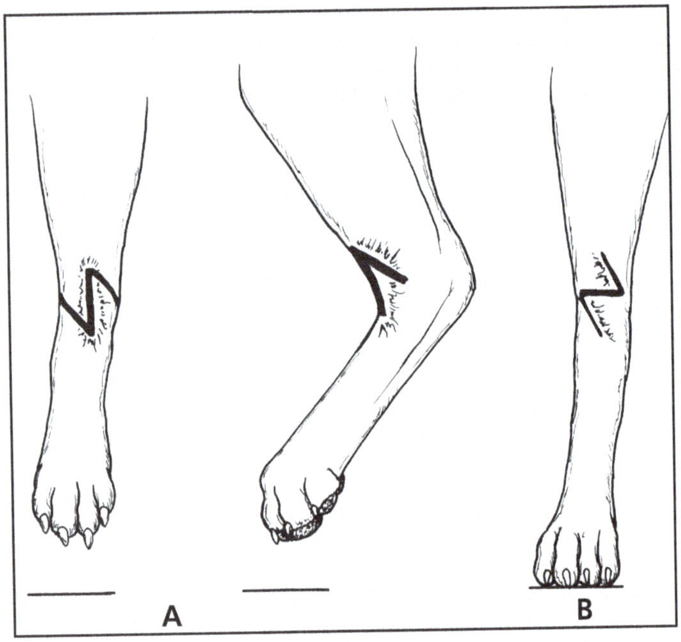


**Figure 3-67.** A – Z plasty to release a short bowstring scar across the flexion surface of the tarsus. **A.** Frontal and lateral view – the central limb of the Z is along the scar. Arms equal in length to the central limb are designed at 60 degrees off of the ends of the central limb. **B.** After incision and transposition of the Z flaps, there is relaxation in the original direction of the central limb of the Z with relief of tension caused by the bowstring scar, i.e. the tarsal joint can be extended (B-sutures not shown).

degrees). It will be used as a template to design the arms of the Z-plasties. The length of the sides of the triangle is dependent upon the amount of skin medial and lateral to the bowstring scar that is available for transposition. One edge of the triangle is laid along the line that has been drawn along the scar, and a limb of a small Z-plasty is drawn along an appropriate edge of the triangle (Figure 3-68C). The triangle is placed back and forth on opposite sides of the central limb line, and several small 60 degree angle Z-plasties are designed along the line (Figure 3-68D & E).

The small Z-plasties are operated one at a time. Each Z-plasty is incised, the 2 skin flaps are undermined and reflected, and any underlying scar tissue is excised. The flaps of the Z-plasty are then transposed and sutured in their new positions. This procedure is performed on each Z-plasty, with the final result being an increase in length along the linear scar, i.e. release of flexion restriction (Figure 3-68F & G). Skin from either side of the scar has been used to release the constriction. It is important that the entire Z-plasty technique be completed on each Z-plasty before doing the next one. To cut more than one Z-plasty at a time makes proper flap transposition very difficult.

## Z-plasty to Release Circumferential Constriction

To relieve circumferential constricting tension (Figure 3-69A) of a scar that may be causing a "biologic

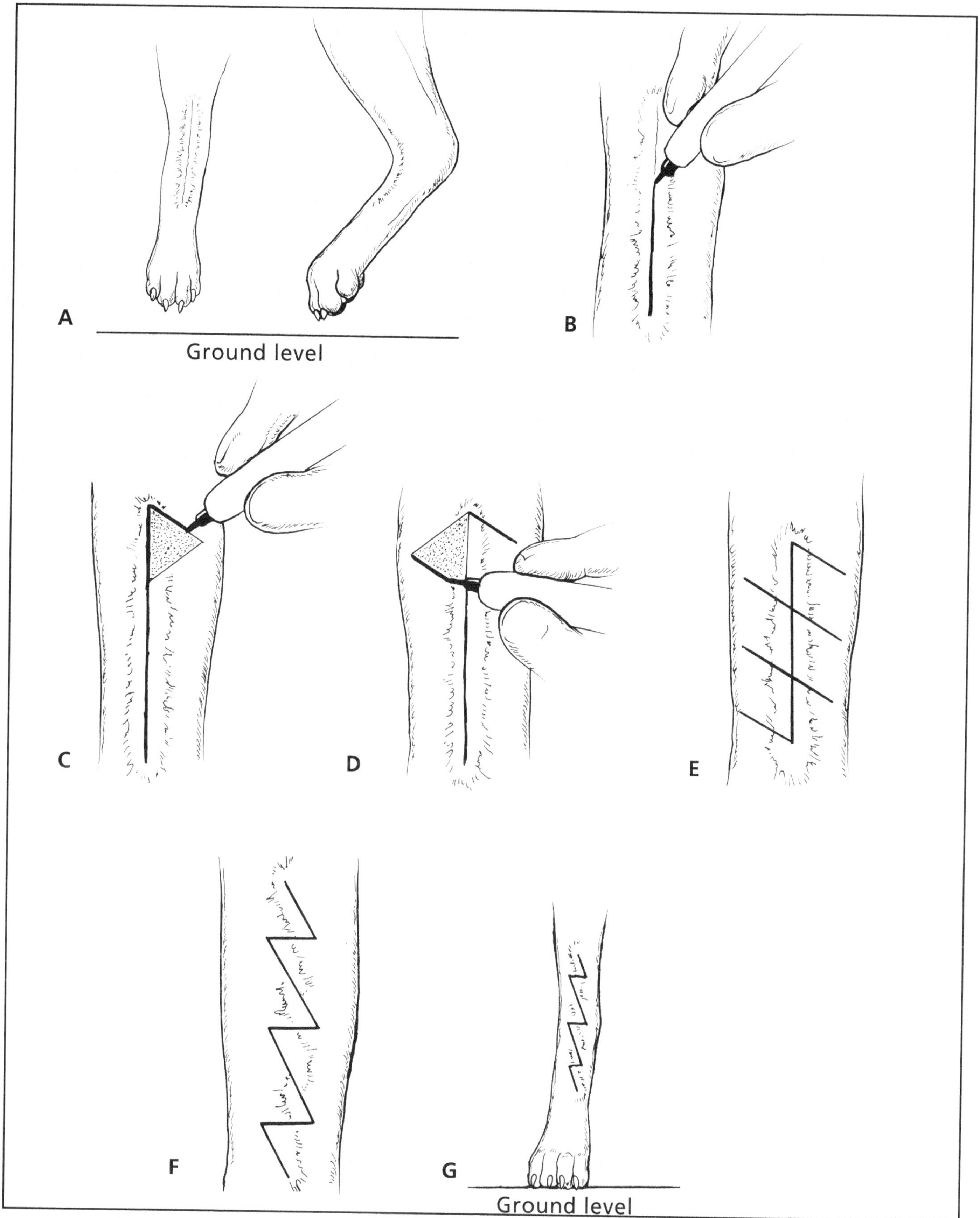


**Figure 3-68.** Multiple Z-plasties to release a long bowstring scar across the flexion surface of the tarsus. **A.** Frontal and lateral view of the bowstring scar. **B.** Drawing the central limb of Z's along the scar. **C.** One limb of a small Z being drawn along an edge of an equilateral triangle template. **D.** Second limb of the small Z being drawn along an edge of the template. **E.** Three small Z-plasties in line along the central limb of the bowstring scar. **F.** Completed transposition of the Z-plasty flaps. **G.** Relaxation in the original direction of the central limb of the Z's with relief of tension caused by the bowstring scar, i.e. the tarsal joint can be extended (F and G-sutures are not shown).

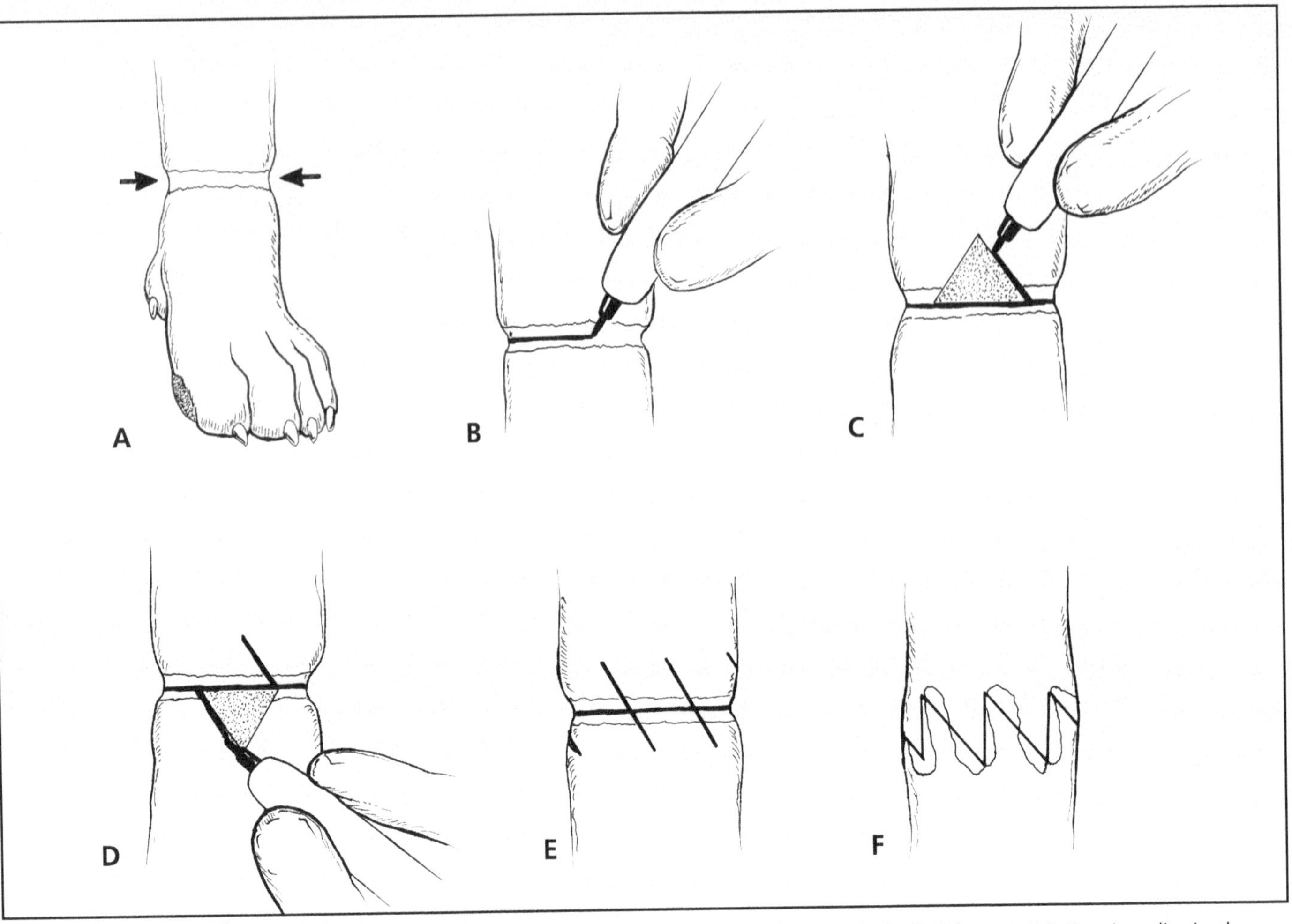


**Figure 3-69.** Z-plasties to release a circumferential constriction. **A.** Circumferential constricting scar at the level of the carpus. **B.** Drawing a line in the scar (central limb of the Z's). **C.** One limb of a small Z being drawn along an edge of an equilateral triangle template. **D.** Second limb of the small Z being drawn along an edge of the template. **E.** Completed small Z's around the limb. **F.** Completed transposition of all Z-plasty flaps with relief of circumferential constriction (F-sutures not shown).

tourniquet", a line is drawn in the circumferential scar (Figure 3-69B). This serves as the central limb for numerous small Z-plasties. A piece of developed x-ray film is cut in the shape of an equilateral triangle (all sides equal in length and all angles 60 degrees) to be used to design the arms of the small Z-plasties. The length of the sides of the triangle depends on the availability of skin proximal and distal to the circumferential scar that can be used for reconstruction. This is determined by manipulation of this skin. One edge of the triangle is laid along the line that has been drawn in the circumferential scar, and a limb of a small Z-plasty is drawn along an appropriate edge of the triangle. The triangle is placed on the opposite side of the circumferential line to draw the second arm of the Z-plasty (Figure 3-69C & D). By placing the triangle back and forth on opposite sides of the circumferential line, many small 60 degree angle Z-plasties are designed around the limb (Figure 3-69E and Figure 3-70A).

Surgery is done on the Z-plasties one at a time (Figure 3-70B). The Z-plasty is incised, the 2 skin flaps are undermined and reflected, and any underlying scar tissue is removed. The flaps of the Z-plasty are then transposed and sutured in place. This procedure is performed on each Z-plasty. The final result is increased diameter of the limb in the area where the constricting circumferential scar had been, using skin above and below the scar for this purpose (Figure 3-69F and Figure 3-70C). It is important that the entire Z-plasty procedure be completed on each Z-plasty before doing the next Z-plasty. If more than one Z-plasty is incised at a time, it becomes very difficult to determine the proper positioning for the flaps.

## Aftercare

When Z-plasty has been used as a relaxing technique for wound closure, the area which was undermined to create the Z-plasty should be observed for any accumulation of serum or blood beneath the skin. If this occurs, a Penrose drain or strip of one side of a Penrose drain should be placed for drainage. However, there is usually sufficient tension on the area to obliterate any dead space and effect subcutaneous hemostasis. In addition, if tacking or "walking" sutures

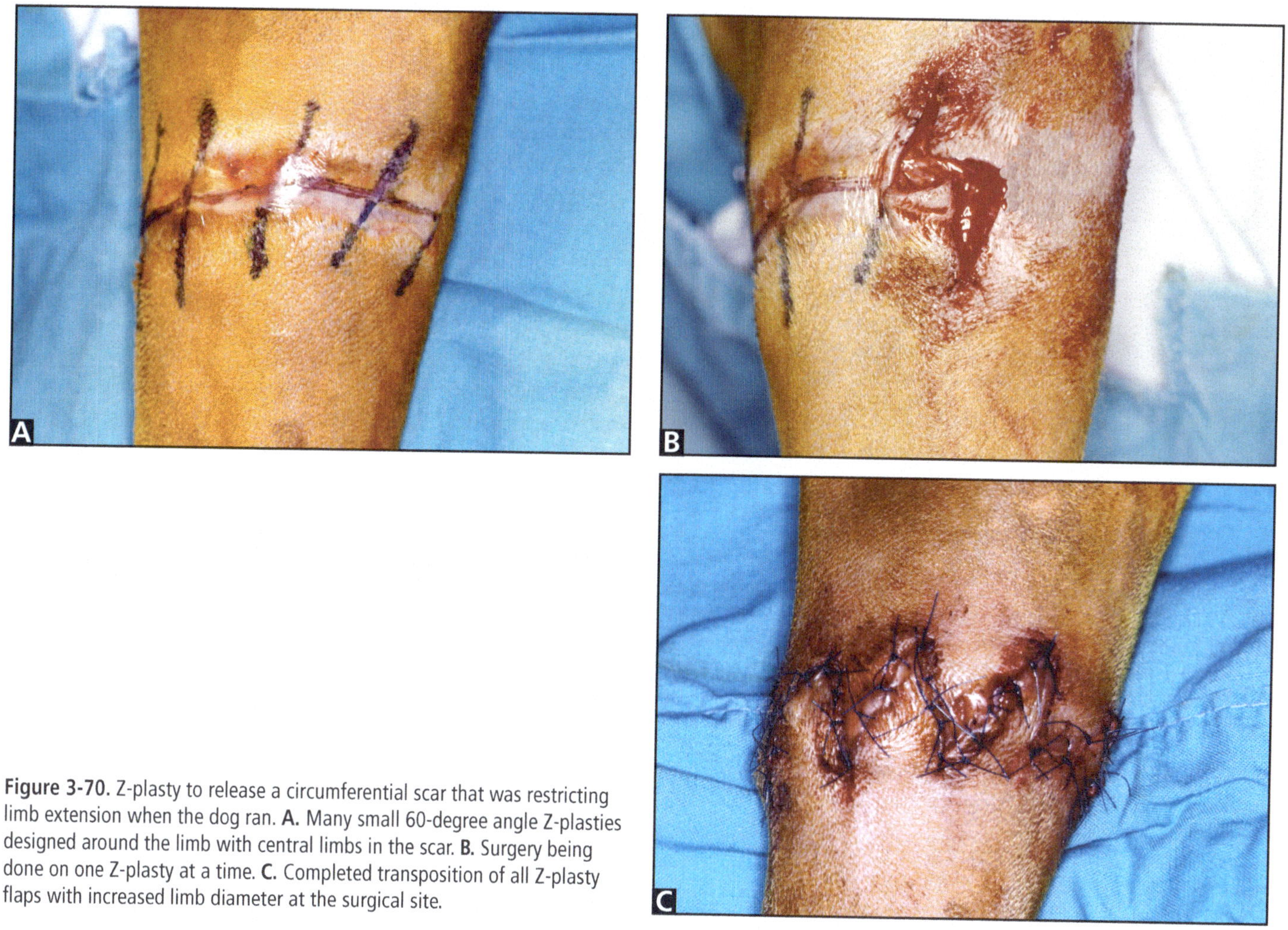

**Figure 3-70.** Z-plasty to release a circumferential scar that was restricting limb extension when the dog ran. **A.** Many small 60-degree angle Z-plasties designed around the limb with central limbs in the scar. **B.** Surgery being done on one Z-plasty at a time. **C.** Completed transposition of all Z-plasty flaps with increased limb diameter at the surgical site.

have been used to move the skin over the wound, they help reduce the chance of seroma or hematoma. When Z-plasty has been used to relieve the tension of a bowstring scar over the flexion surface of a joint or to relieve a circumferential constricting scar, the area should be placed in an immobilization bandage for 7 to 10 days, especially when surgery was done to relieve a bowstring scar. Placing a splint in the bandage helps prevent movement of the area which could interfere with healing of the suture lines. Sutures can be removed from the skin at 7 to 14 days, depending upon the purpose of the Z-plasty. If the Z-plasty was used to relieve the tension of a bowstring scar where there will be movement of the area, the sutures should be left in longer. If clinical judgement indicates it, flap tip sutures can be left in a little longer.

## Advantages and Disadvantages

Z-plasty provides relief of tension to allow wound closure; however, it requires creating a wound to close a wound. Although a Z-plasty with two 60 degree angles theoretically provides a 75 percent increase in length in the direction of the central limb of the Z, actual increase is less. The increase may vary from 41 to 63 percent depending on skin elasticity and wound location. When the technique is used to relieve the tension of a bowstring scar, it has the advantage of allowing correction without the removal of any tissue. If there is a long scar (linear or circumscribing) multiple Z-plasties can be used to relieve tension with the advantage of causing less tissue distortion in the areas of high tension and less total contracture. However, multiple Z-plasties have the disadvantages of being technically more difficult to perform and the gain in length may not be as great as with a single Z-plasty with the same central limb length. With use of Z-plasty over joints there is the possibility of wound disruption if there is no immobilization of the underlying joint for 7 to 10 postoperative days. If there is significant scar tissue in the area, the actual gain in length with a Z-plasty may not be as much as the theoretical gain.

# Suggested Readings


1. Bohling MW, Swaim SF: Management of the traumatic wound by primary closure. In Birchard SJ, Sherding RG, eds.: Saunders Manual of Small Animal Practice, 3rd ed.: St. Louis: Saunders – Elsevier, 2006, 541.
2. Bosworth G, Tobias KM: Skin reconstruction techniques: Z-plasty as an aid in tension-free wound closure. Vet Med 99:892, 2004.
3. Burke M: Z-plasty, How, When and Why. Aust Fam Phys 26:1027, 1997.

4. Crawford ME, Dockery GL: Use of Z-plasty in scar revisions and skin contractures of the lower extremity. J Amer Podia Med Assoc 85:29, 1995.
5. Fowler D: Tension relieving techniques and local skin flaps. *In* Fowler D, Williams JM, eds.: BSAVA Manual of Canine and Feline Wound Management and Reconstruction. Shurdington, Cheltenham, UK: BSAVA, 1999, 57.
6. Fowler D: Distal limb and paw injuries. Vet Clin No Am Small Animal Pract. 36: 819, 2006.
7. Hedlund CS: Surgery of the integumentary system. *In* Fossum TW, ed.: Small Animal Surgery, 2nd ed.: St. Louis: Mosby, 2002, 134.
8. Hedlund CS: Surgery of the integumentary system. In Fossum TW, ed.: Small Animal Surgery, 3rd ed.: St. Louis, Mosby, 2007, 159.
9. Hudson DA: Some thoughts on choosing a Z-plasty: The Z-plasty made simple. Plast Reconst Surg 106:665, 2000.
10. Jankauskas S, Cohen IK, Grabb WC: Basic technique of plastic surgery. *In* Smith JW, Aston SJ, eds.: Plastic Surgery, 4th ed.: Boston: Little, Brown, 1991, 3.
11. MacPhail CM: Surgery of the integumentary system. In Fossum TW, ed.: Small Animal Surgery, 4th ed.: St. Louis: Mosby, 2013, 190.
12. Mayhew P: Tension – relieving techniques and local skin flaps. In Williams J, Moores A, eds.: BSAVA Manual of Canine and Feline Wound Management and Reconstruction, 2nd ed.: Glouster (UK): BSAVA, 2009, 69.
13. McGregor IA: Fundamental Techniques of Plastic Surgery, 8th ed.: Edinburgh: Churchill Livingston, 1989, 23.
14. Pavletic MM: Atlas of Small Animal Reconstructive Surgery, 2nd ed.: Philadelphia: WB Saunders, 1999, 131.
15. Pavletic MM: Atlas of Small Animal Wound Management and Reconstructive Surgery, 3rd ed.: Ames, IA: Wiley – Blackwell, 2010, 241.
16. Rohrich RJ, Zbar RI: A simplified algorithm for the use of Z-plasty. Plast Reconst Surg 103:1513, 1999.
17. Scardino MS, Swaim SF, Henderson RA, et. al.: Enhancing wound closure on the limbs. Compend Contin Educ Pract Vet 18:919, 1996.
18. Stanley BJ: Tension – relieving techniques. In Tobias KM, Johnston SA, eds.: Veterinary Surgery, Small Animal,Vol. 2: St. Louis: Elsevier – Saunders, 2012, 1221.
19. Swaim SF: Management of skin tension in dermal surgery. Compend Contin Educ Pract Vet 2:758, 1980.
20. Swaim SF: Management of the traumatic wound by primary closure. *In* Birchard SJ, Sherding RG, eds.: Saunders Manual of Small Animal Practice, 2nd ed.: Philadelphia: WB Saunders, 2000, 392.
21. Swaim SF, Henderson RA: Small Animal Wound Management, 2nd ed.: Baltimore: Williams and Wilkins, 1997, 143.
22. Swaim SF, Renberg WC, Shike KM: Small Animal Bandaging, Casting and Splinting Techniques, Ames, IA.: Wiley – Blackwell, 2011, 43.
23. Trout NJ: Principles of plastic and reconstructive surgery. *In* Slatter DH, ed.: Textbook of Small Animal Surgery, 3rd ed.: Philadelphia: WB Saunders, 2003, 274.
24. Vig MM: Management of experimental wounds of the extremities in dogs with Z-plasty. J Am Anim Hosp Assoc 28:553, 1992.

# V-to-Y-Plasty

## Definition and Indications

V-to-Y-plasty is a form of relaxing incision that creates a bipedicle advancement flap of skin to cover a defect. The technique is indicated to relieve minor tension in small areas, and for chronic wounds surrounded by inelastic tissue.

## Techniques

A V-shaped incision is made in the skin adjacent to the wound, usually approximately 3 cm from the wound, with the point of the V pointing away from the wound. The skin between the V-incision and the wound is undermined Figure 3-71A) and advanced over the defect. If it is needed, underlying tacking or "walking" sutures of 3-0 absorbable suture material can be used to advance the skin edge toward the opposite side of the wound. The wound is closed with some form of tension suture, e.g. continuous intradermal 3-0 absorbable suture as needed, and 3-0 nonabsorbable simple interrupted apposition sutures (Figure 3-71B). The remaining defect is closed in a Y-shape. For this closure, suturing is started at the ends of the arms of the V, placing sutures alternately on one side then the other to form the arms of the Y. When tension starts to develop with closure, the remaining defect is closed as the stem of the Y (Figure 3-71C & D).

An alternative technique to perform a V-to-Y-plasty is to suture the stem of the Y first beginning at the tip of the V incision. This pushes the inner triangle of the skin flap toward the wound to reduce the tension of wound closure (Figure 3-72A & B). The wound is closed as previously described followed by closure of the arms of the Y (Figure 3-72C & D). A modification of this technique entails closing the wound first followed by closure of the Y stem and then the Y arms (Figure 3-73).

## Aftercare

The skin that was undermined between the wound and the V incision should be observed for the accumulation of blood or serum under the skin. A Penrose drain can be placed under the area if this occurs. However, if tacking or "walking" sutures have been used for advancing the skin to close the wound, the chance of seroma or hematoma is reduced. In addition, tension in the area usually obliterates dead space in which blood or serum could accumulate.

## Advantages and Disadvantages

V-to-Y-plasty provides tension relief for closing wounds that have tension associated with closure. However, it requires creating a wound to close a wound.

# Suggested Reading

1. Bohling MW, Swaim SF: Management of the traumatic wound by primary closure. In Birchard SJ, Sherding RG, eds.: Saunders Manual of Small Animal Practice, 3rd ed.: St. Louis: Saunders – Elsevier, 2006, 541.
2. Fowler D: Tension relieving techniques and local skin flaps. *In* Fowler D, Williams JM, eds.: BSAVA Manual of Canine and Feline Wound Management and Reconstruction. Shurdington,

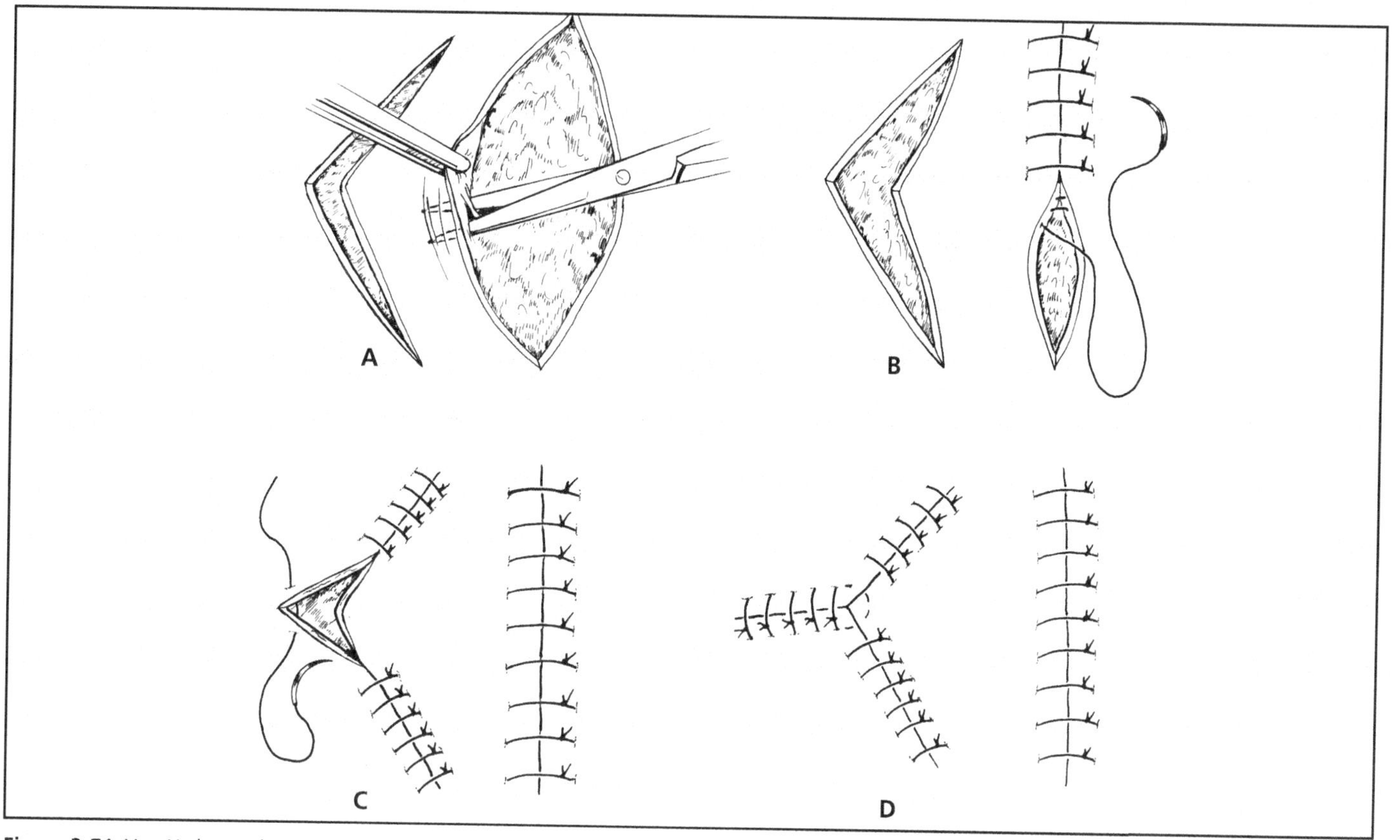


**Figure 3-71.** V-to-Y plasty relaxing incision. **A.** A V-shaped incision is made adjacent to the wound with the point of the V away from the wound. The skin between the V-incsion and the wound is undermined. **B.** The wound is closed with an absorbable continuous intradermal suture and simple interrupted apposition sutures. **C.** Closure of the V-incision beginning at the ends and placing sutures alternately on one side and then the other until tension develops; thus, forming the arms of the Y. The stem of the Y is closed beginning at its end. **D.** Completed closure of the wound and relaxing incision. (After Swaim SF, Henderson RA: Small Animal Wound Management, 2nd ed.: Baltimore: Williams & Wilkins, 1997, 181 & 182.)

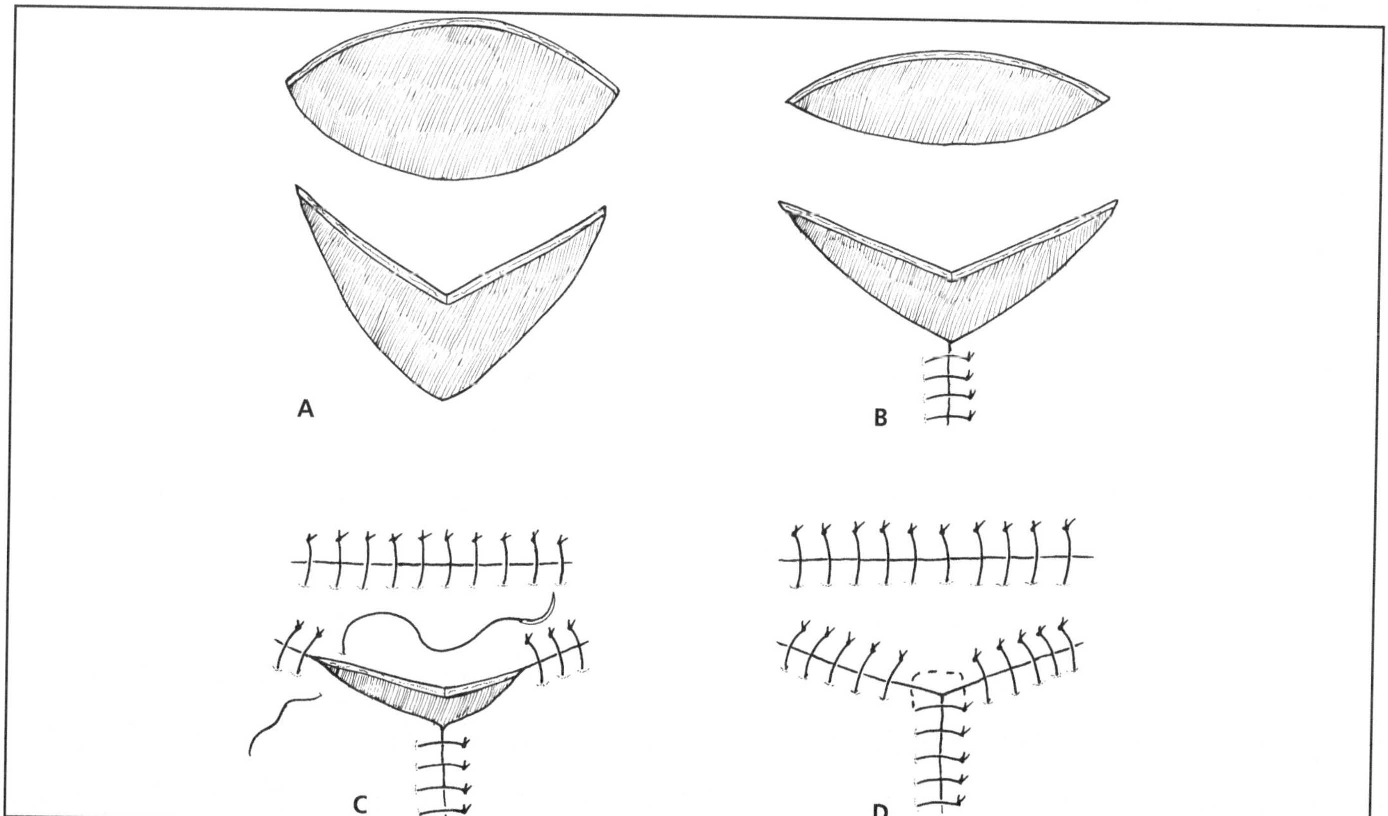


**Figure 3-72.** Alternate technique 1 for V – to – Y plasty relaxing incision. **A.** V – incision made adjacent to the wound. **B.** Stem of the Y is sutured first, followed by **C.** closure of the wound then closure of the arms of the Y. **D.** Completed closure of the wound and relaxing incision.

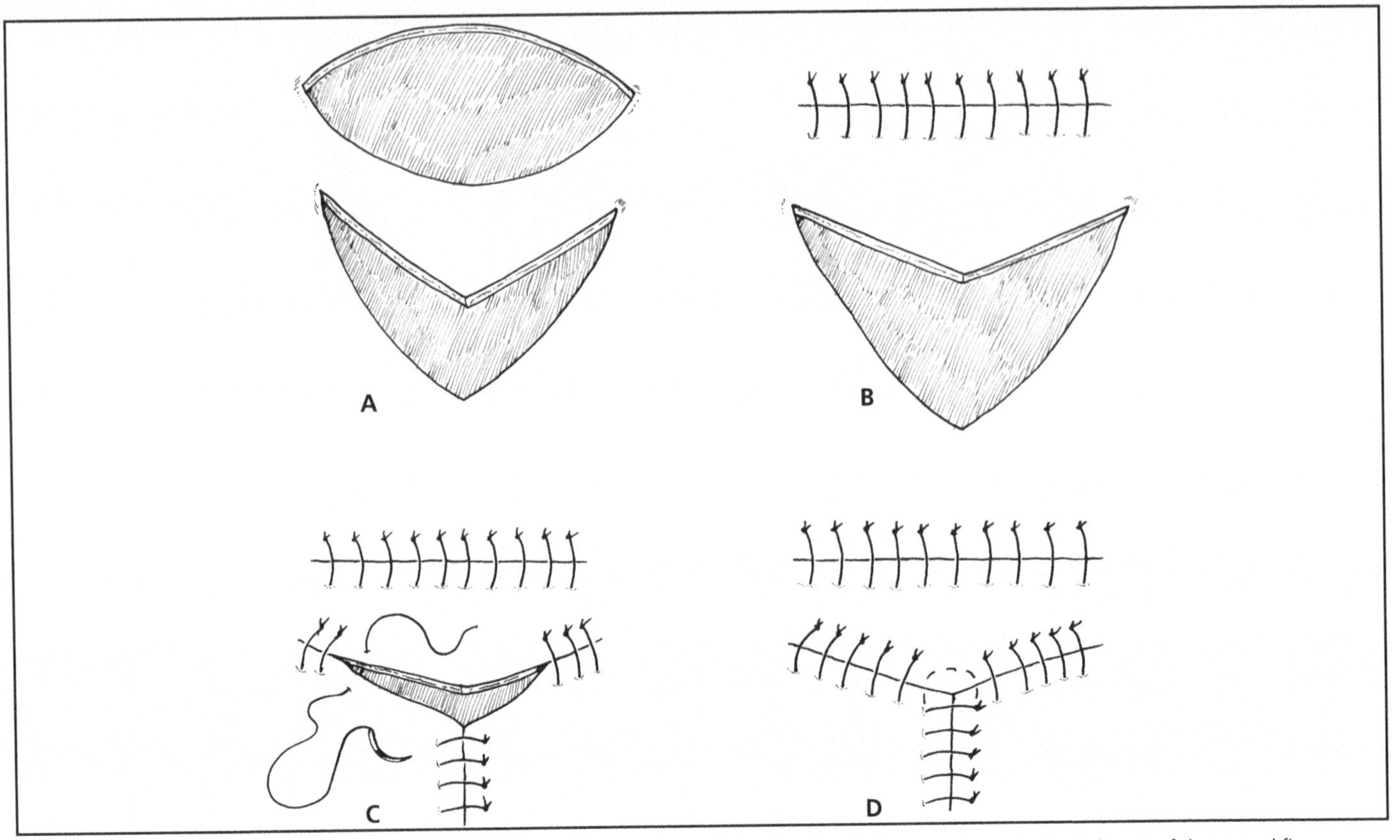


Figure 3-73. Alternate technique 2 for V – to – Y plasty relaxing incision. A. V – incision made adjacent to the wound. B. Closure of the wound first, followed by C. Closure of the stem of the Y then by closure of the arms. D. Completed closure of the wound and relaxing incision.

Cheltenham, UK: BSAVA, 1999, 57.
3. Fowler D: Distal limb and paw injuries. Vet Clin No Am Small Animal Pract. 36: 819, 2006.
4. Hedlund CS: Surgery of the integumentary system. *In* Fossum TW, ed.: Small Animal Surgery, 2nd ed.: St. Louis: Mosby, 2002, 134.
5. Hedlund CS: Surgery of the integumentary system. In Fossum TW, ed.: Small Animal Surgery, 3rd ed.: St. Louis: Mosby, 2007, 159.
6. MacPhail CM: Surgery of the integumentary system. In Fossum TW, ed.: Small Animal Surgery, 4th ed.: St. Louis: Mosby, 2013, 190.
7. Mayhew P: Tension – relieving techniques and local skin flaps. In Williams J, Moores A, eds.: BSAVA Manual of Canine and Feline Wound Management and Reconstruction, 2nd ed.: Glouster (UK): BSAVA, 2009, 69.
8. Pavletic MM: Atlas of Small Animal Reconstructive Surgery, 2nd ed: Philadelphia: WB Saunders, 1999, 131.
9. Pavletic MM: Atlas of Small Animal Wound Management and Reconstructive Surgery, 3rd ed.: Ames, IA: Wiley – Blackwell, 2010, 241.
10. Stanley BJ: Tension – relieving techniques. In Tobias KM, Johnston SA, eds.: Veterinary Surgery, Small Animal, Vol. 2: St. Louis: Elsevier – Saunders, 2012, 1221.
11. Swaim SF: Management of skin tension in dermal surgery. Compend Contin Educ Pract Vet 2:758, 1980.
12. Swaim SF: Management of the traumatic wound by primary closure. *In* Birchard SJ, Sherding RG, eds.: Saunders Manual of Small Animal Practice, 2nd ed.: Philadelphia: WB Saunders, 2000, 392.
13. Swaim SF, Henderson RA: Small Animal Wound Management, 2nd ed.: Baltimore: Williams and Wilkins, 1997, 143.
14. Trout NJ: Principles of plastic and reconstructive surgery. *In* Slatter DH, ed.: Textbook of Small Animal Surgery, 3rd ed.: Philadelphia: WB Saunders, 2003, 274.

# Wounds Over the Carpus and Tarsus - Nonapposable Edges Extension Surfaces

## Definition and Indications

Wounds over the extension surface of the carpus or tarsus may be large enough that the wound edges cannot be apposed, but they have the potential for apposition.

## Techniques

The surgeon should use his/her hands to manipulate the skin and clinical judgement to decide what, if any, of the tension sutures or relaxing incisions could be used to close such wounds. Another option is use of a flap or graft for closure (Figure 3-74 and Figure 3-75).

## Aftercare

The aftercare described for the various tension sutures, relaxing incisions, flaps and grafts would apply for wounds over the extension surface of the carpus and tarsus. However, it is crucial that immobilization of the area in extension be maintained to prevent wound disruption. The techniques for immobilization of these areas in the previous section (Wounds with Apposable Edges-Tension) are applicable for wounds with nonap-

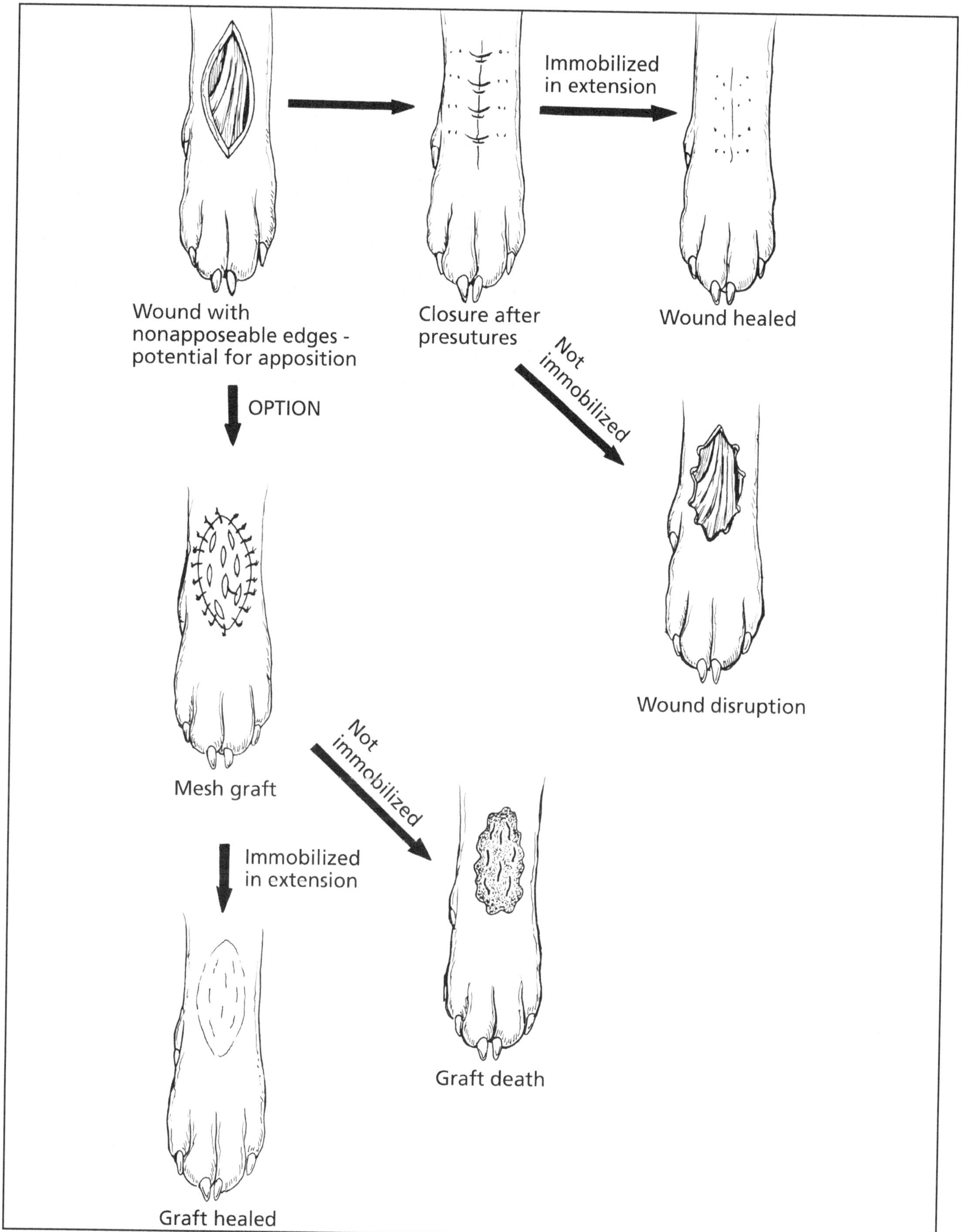


**Figure 3-74.** Wound on the extension surface of the carpus with nonapposable edges that have the potential for apposition. Wound edges are apposed after using presutures. Immobilization of the joint in extension may result in healing. With no immobilization wound disruption may occur. Option – mesh grafting the wound with immobilization may result in healing, but lack of immobilization may lead to graft death.

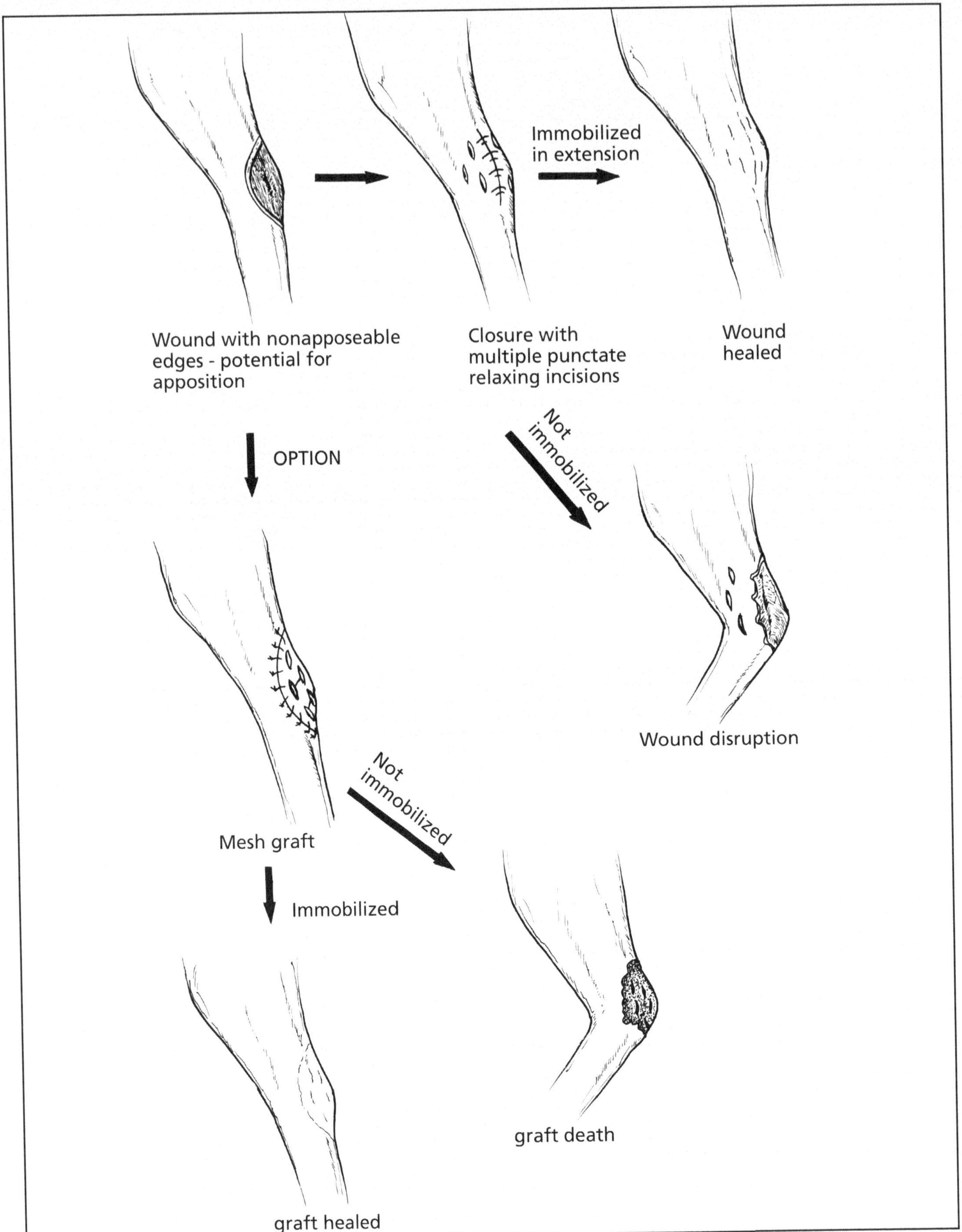


**Figure 3-75.** Wound on the extension surface of the tarsus with nonapposable edges that have the potential for apposition. Wound edges are apposed by using multiple punctuate relaxing incisions. Immobilization of the joint in extesnison may result in healing. With no immobilization wound disruption may occur. Option – mesh grafting the wound with immobilization may result in healing, but lack of immobilization may lead to graft death.

posable edges that have been apposed by tension sutures, relaxing incisions, flaps and grafts. After healing has occurred, gradual increases in exercise/movement should take place to help prevent wound disruption.

### Advantages and Disadvantages

The advantages and disadvantages for the various tension sutures, relaxing incisions, flaps and grafts also apply for wounds over the extension surface of the carpus and tarsus. A major disadvantage for these wounds is the increased tendency for disruption with joint movement/flexion.

## Suggested Readings

(See Suggested Reading for the various Tension Sutures, and Relaxing Incisions, Flaps and Grafts in this chapter.)

## Flexion Surfaces

### Definition and Indications

As with wounds over the extension surface of the carpus or tarsus, wounds over the flexion surface of the carpus or tarsus may also be large enough that the wound edges cannot be apposed, but they have the potential for apposition.

### Techniques

A primary technique that can be considered for closure of carpal or tarsal flexion surface wounds with nonapposable edges that have the potential for closure is flexion of the joint to ascertain if closure can be accomplished with the joint flexed. Using clinical judgement, the surgeon may choose to use one of the tension suture or relaxing incision techniques in combination with joint flexion for wound closure. Another option is to use a graft or flap for closure (Figure 3-76 and Figure 3-77).

### Aftercare

The aftercare described for the various tension sutures, relaxing incisions, flaps and grafts would apply for wounds over the flexion surface of the carpus and tarsus. However, it is crucial that immobilization of the area of flexion be maintained to prevent wound disruption. The techniques for immobilization of these areas stated in the previous section (Wounds with Apposable Edges-Tension) are applicable for wounds with nonapposable edges that have been apposed by tension sutures, relaxing incisions, flaps and grafts.

### Advantages and Disadvantages

The advantages of the various tension sutures, relaxing incisions, flaps and grafts apply for wounds over the flexion surface of the carpus and tarsus. A major disadvantage for these wounds is the increased tendency for disruption with joint movement/extension.

## Suggested Readings

(See Suggested Reading for the various tension sutures, relaxing incisions, flaps and grafts.)

## Wounds with Nonapposable Edges - No Potential for Apposition

### General Information

Some distal limb wounds are of such magnitude that there is not sufficient skin to close the wound, even if stretching or relaxing procedures are used. These wounds will require skin replacement in the form of a graft or flap for wound closure. A flap is a segment of skin which remains attached to a blood supply while it is being placed over a wound. A graft is a segment of skin removed from one area of the body and placed on a different area where it develops a new blood supply.

## Skin Flaps

## Pouch Flaps and Hinge Flaps

### Definition and Indications

Pouch flaps and hinge flaps are double or single pedicle flaps of skin, respectively, that are direct, distant flaps created on the body. They are used to reconstruct defects on the distal limb, to include metacarpal and metatarsal pad replacement on cats, by advancing the limb to the flap (Figure 3-78A & B). The flaps lend themselves best to correcting defects that involve the lateral aspect of the limb. For the thoracic limbs, these flaps work best for small dogs and cats because bandaging the animal's limb along the thoracic area is more comfortable for smaller animals than for larger breeds of dogs. Because of their size, limb flexibility and skin elasticity, cat anatomy particularly lends itself to this type of flap. When considering the pelvic limb, these flaps work best on cats and small female dogs, because using them on large or male dogs is more difficult due to the dog's size or the presence of genitalia that must be bandaged around. It has been suggested that pouch flaps be used for larger or nearly circumferential lesions and hinge flaps be used for smaller or less than circumferential lesions. These flaps require a cooperative animal and owner.

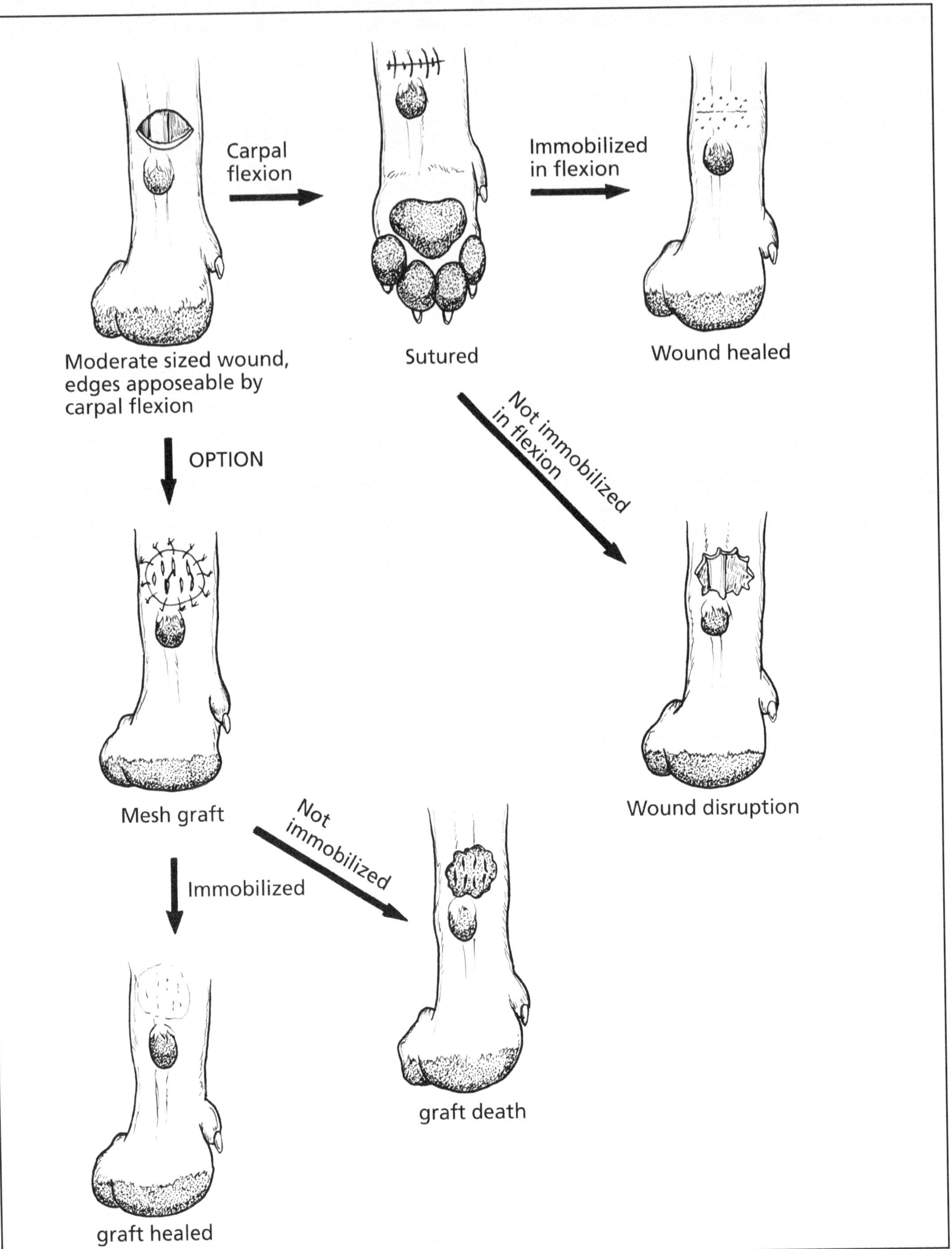


**Figure 3-76.** Wound on the flexion surface of the carpus with noapposable edges that have the potential for apposition. Wound edges are apposed by flexion of the carpus and suturing. Immobilization of the joint in flexion may result in healing. With no immobilization, wound disruption may occur. Option – mesh grafting the wound with immobilization may result in graft healing, but lack of immobilization may lead to graft death.

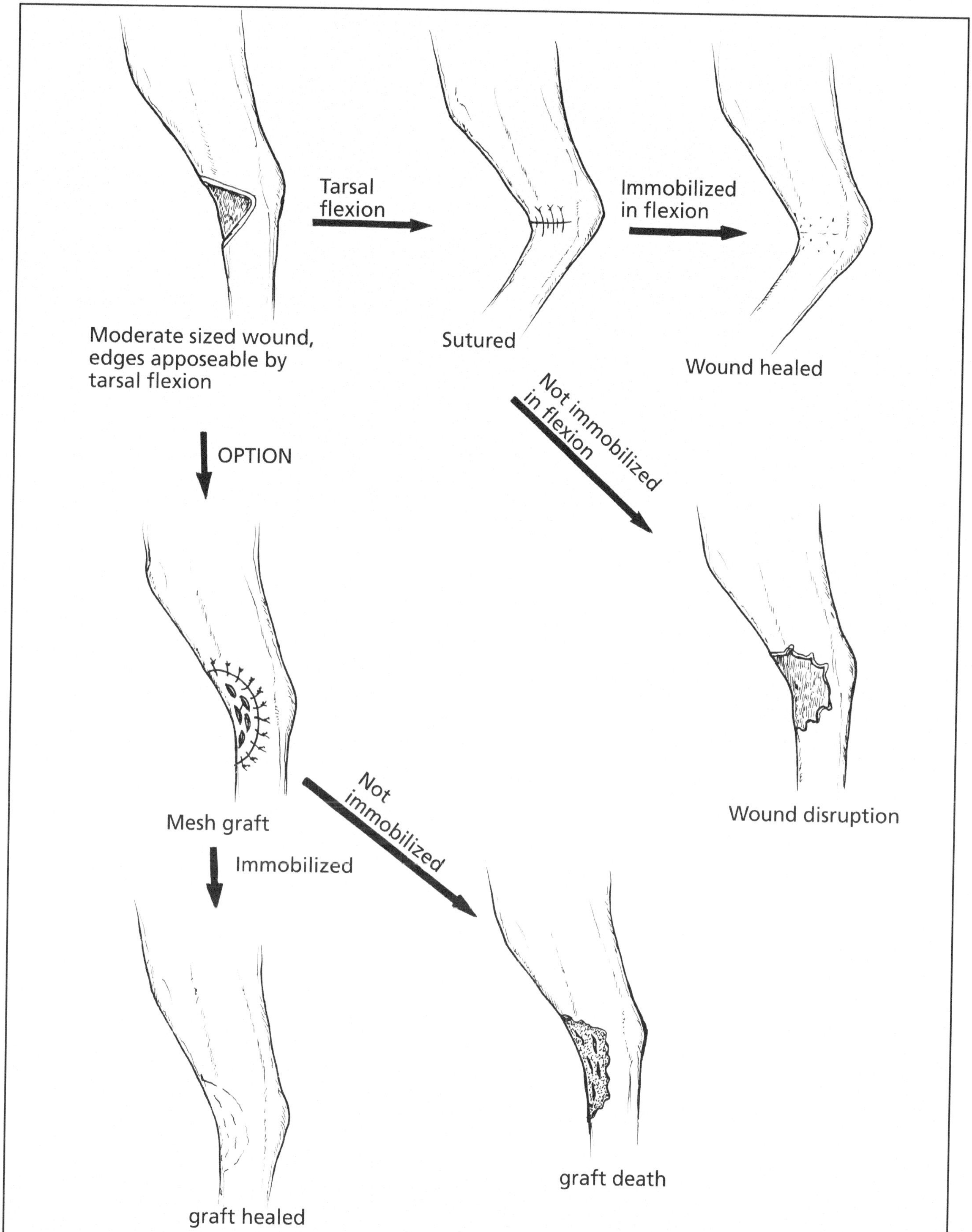


**Figure 3-77.** Wound on the flexion surface of the tarsus with noapposable edges that have the potential for apposition. Wound edges are apposed by flexion of the tarsus and suturing. Immobilization of the joint in flexion may result in healing. With no immobilization wound disruption may occur. Option – mesh grafting the wound with immobilization may result in graft healing, but lack of immobilization may lead to graft death.

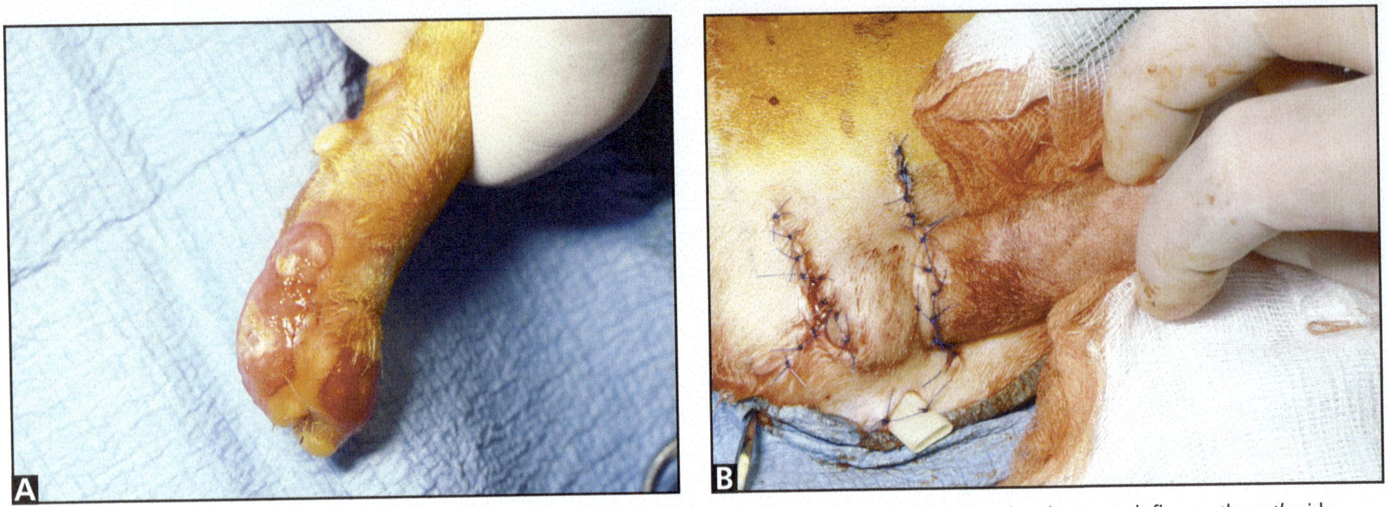

Figure 3-78. Pouch flap for reconstructing a paw defect on a cat. A. Defect on the cat's forepaw. B. Defect placed under a pouch flap on the cat's side.

## Techniques

If it is uncertain whether an animal will tolerate its limb being positioned along its trunk for maintaining a pouch flap or hinge flap, the wounded limb should be bandaged along the animal's side for 2 to 3 days before surgery. If the animal will not tolerate its limb being immobilized along its side, then another type of reconstruction must be considered.

The lateral thoracoabdominal area on the side of the limb wound should be prepared for aseptic surgery, as should the entire wounded limb to include the paw.

The animal is placed in lateral recumbency with the affected limb uppermost. If the wound has a bed of granulation tissue with epithelium advancing from the wound edge, the epithelium is removed. The surface of the granulation tissue is cleared of any coagulum on its surface by wiping it with a surgical sponge soaked in a 1:40 dilution of chlorhexidine diacetate (Nolvasan solution, Ft. Dodge Animal Health, Ft. Dodge, IA) or gluconate (ChlorhexiDerm Disinfectant, Dermatologics in Veterinary Medicine Pharmaceuticals, Inc., Miami, FL) solution. The affected limb is then placed along the animal's side in the most comfortable position which minimizes stress on the joints.

### Pouch flaps

For a double pedicle pouch flap, the level of the proximal edge of the defect is marked along the animal's side perpendicular to the long axis of the limb. An incision is made in the skin along this mark to extend through the cutaneous trunci muscle. A second incision is made parallel to the first incision. It is usually 1 to 2 cm longer than the length of the defect to allow for primary contraction of the flap and the skin stretching that will be necessary to place the limb under the flap (Figure 3-79A).

When a wound completely encircles a limb the flap is undermined beneath the cutaneous trunci muscle, the limb is flexed, and the paw is passed under the flap. The limb is positioned so that the wound is covered by the flap. Simple interrupted 3-0 nonabsorbable monofilament sutures are placed to appose the edges of the flap and edges of the wound (Figure 3-79B). If a wound involves only the lateral aspect of the limb, with intact skin on the medial side of the limb, the flap is undermined and elevated. With the flap held away from the body, skin on either side of the donor site is advanced beneath the flap using "walking" sutures. The edges of skin are then sutured together with simple interrupted 3-0 monofilament nonabsorbable sutures (Figure 3-79 inset). After cleaning and/or scraping the wound surface, the limb is passed under the flap. This places the intact skin on the medial side of the leg in contact with the sutured skin under the flap rather than the subcutaneous tissue of the donor site. The raw undersurface of the flap is thus in contact with the wound on the lateral aspect of the limb.

The edges of the flap are sutured to the wound edges. Several tacking sutures should be placed through the flap into underlying wound tissue to immobilize the flap against the wound to help assure adequate vascular and connective tissue adherence to the wound. A ¼-inch diameter Penrose drain may be placed in the most dependent base of the flap (Figure 3-79C). This provides for drainage of any fluid that may accumulate in the space around the flap and limb. Drain placement is especially important if the wound is circumferential around the limb and the adjacent skin edges have not been sutured together under the flap. Another option to allow for drainage is to leave an area open for drainage at the ventralmost area of the junction of the flap with the most distal aspect of the defect.

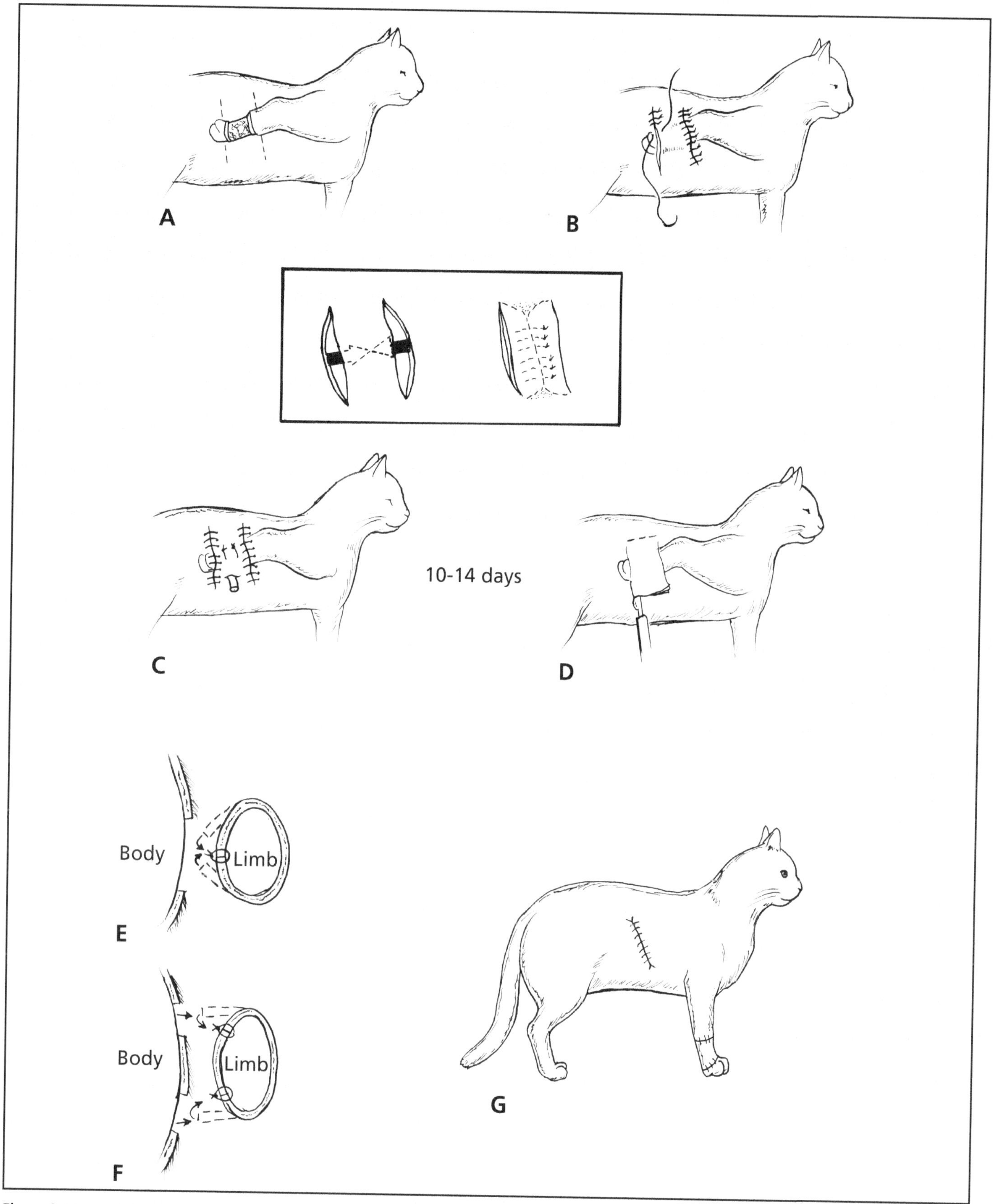


**Figure 3-79.** Pouch flap for distal forelimb wound repair. **A.** Limb in position with proposed flap site *(broken line)*. **B.** Suturing the flap to the wound. **Inset:** Suturing adjacent skin edges together under the flap. **C.** Placement of a drain under the limb/flap area and 2 tacking sutures through flap. **D.** Cutting the pedicles of the flap. **E.** Final transfer of the flap when the wound encircles the limb. **F.** Final transfer of the flap when the wound does not encircle the limb. **G.** Flap transferred to the limb; donor site sutured.

## Hinge flaps

For a hinge flap, the procedures are essentially the same; to include making the flap 1 to 2 cm wider than the length of the wound. The single base of the flap may be either dorsally or ventrally located. The flap is carefully designed, with the flap length being determined from the desired location of the flap base to the most distant edge of the wound. To help in designing the flap, a sterile cloth template may be used. The template is made in the desired size and shape of the flap. It is held firmly in place at its base (Figure 3-80A). The limb is placed in position, and the template is laid over the wound to determine if the proposed flap will be of the correct size (Figure 3-80B). Once the size and shape have been determined, the flap is placed on the donor site and traced. It is then cut on 3 sides and undermined (Figure 3-80C).

After cutting and elevating the flap, the donor site is closed as much as possible with 3-0 absorbable "walking" sutures and 3-0 nonabsorbable simple interrupted sutures (Figure 3-80D). After cleaning and/or scraping the surface of the limb wound, the limb is placed in position, and the flap is sutured to the edges of the defect with 3-0 nonabsorbable simple interrupted sutures (Figure 3-80E).

The limb can be held in position against the body to prevent it from shifting ventrally to put tension on the flap. To accomplish this, large tacking or support sutures may be placed between areas of intact skin on the limb and similar skin on the trunk of the animal for both pouch and hinge flaps.

After the flap has had sufficient time to revascularize and establish a connective tissue bond to the wound, usually about 14 days, the base(s) of the flap(s) is/are incised. When cutting the flap free from the trunk, sufficient skin should be taken at the bases of the flap to provide skin for closure of the remaining wound on the medial side of the limb if it was a circumferential defect (Figure 3-79D and Figure 3-80F). A delaying procedure can be utilized in helping assure that a pouch flap has an adequate blood supply. For this, the bases of the flap are incised in stages. For a pouch flap, the ventral pedicle is incised one half to one third of the way across at 10 to 14 days, followed by severance of the remaining portion of the flap at 2 to 3 day intervals. This is followed by incising the dorsal pedicle in a similar fashion. An alternative procedure for performing the delaying procedure is to sever one pedicle followed by severing the second pedicle 3 to 5 days later. With a hinge flap, the delaying procedure can be started at 10 to 14 days with incision of half of the pedicle followed by incision of the remaining half 2 to 3 days later. Some surgeons do not believe that the delaying procedure is critically beneficial, and it is time consuming.

With a pouch flap and a circumferential limb wound, the medial surface of the limb will be adhered to the body wall, and it will be necessary to dissect it free to proceed. The 2 edges of the flap are then wrapped around the remaining defect on the medial side of the limb. The edges of the flap are trimmed appropriately and sutured together using simple interrupted 3-0 nonabsorbable sutures (Figure 3-79E). If the defect did not completely encircle the limb, the 2 edges of the flap are then sutured to the remaining freshly debrided skin edges of the defect using the above described suture material and pattern (Figure 3-79F).

For a hinge flap, the single pedicle may be lengthened slightly at the time it is severed from the trunk to help assure sufficient skin to cover any remaining defect (Figure 3-80G). However, long pedicle extensions may result in some flap tip necrosis due to insufficient circulation.

If the donor site has excessive granulation tissue, it should be trimmed. The donor site on the trunk of the animal is then closed by undermining and advancing the skin edges together with "walking" sutures and continuous subcuticular sutures of 3-0 absorbable suture material. Final skin apposition is with 3-0 simple interrupted nonabsorbable sutures (Figure 3-79G and Figure 3-80H).

## Aftercare

Two phases are involved in aftercare of pouch and hinge flaps. First, there is care of the limb while it is in the flap on the trunk. Second, there is care of the limb after the flap has been finally transposed to the limb.

The limb is bandaged against the body for about 10 to 14 days after the limb is sutured under the flap. Extra, absorbent primary bandage material (i.e. surgical gauze sponges) is placed over the flap in areas where there will be drainage. Cotton may be placed between the body and limb in areas of intact skin as padding. Care should be taken to avoid bandage pressure on skin over the olecranon and possibly over the extension surface of the carpus depending on the position of the limb. Modified donut-type bandages of soft cast padding material can be used for this purpose (Figure 3-81A). It should be remembered that the cast padding material of this bandage becomes compressed after 2 to 3 days. Thus, it will

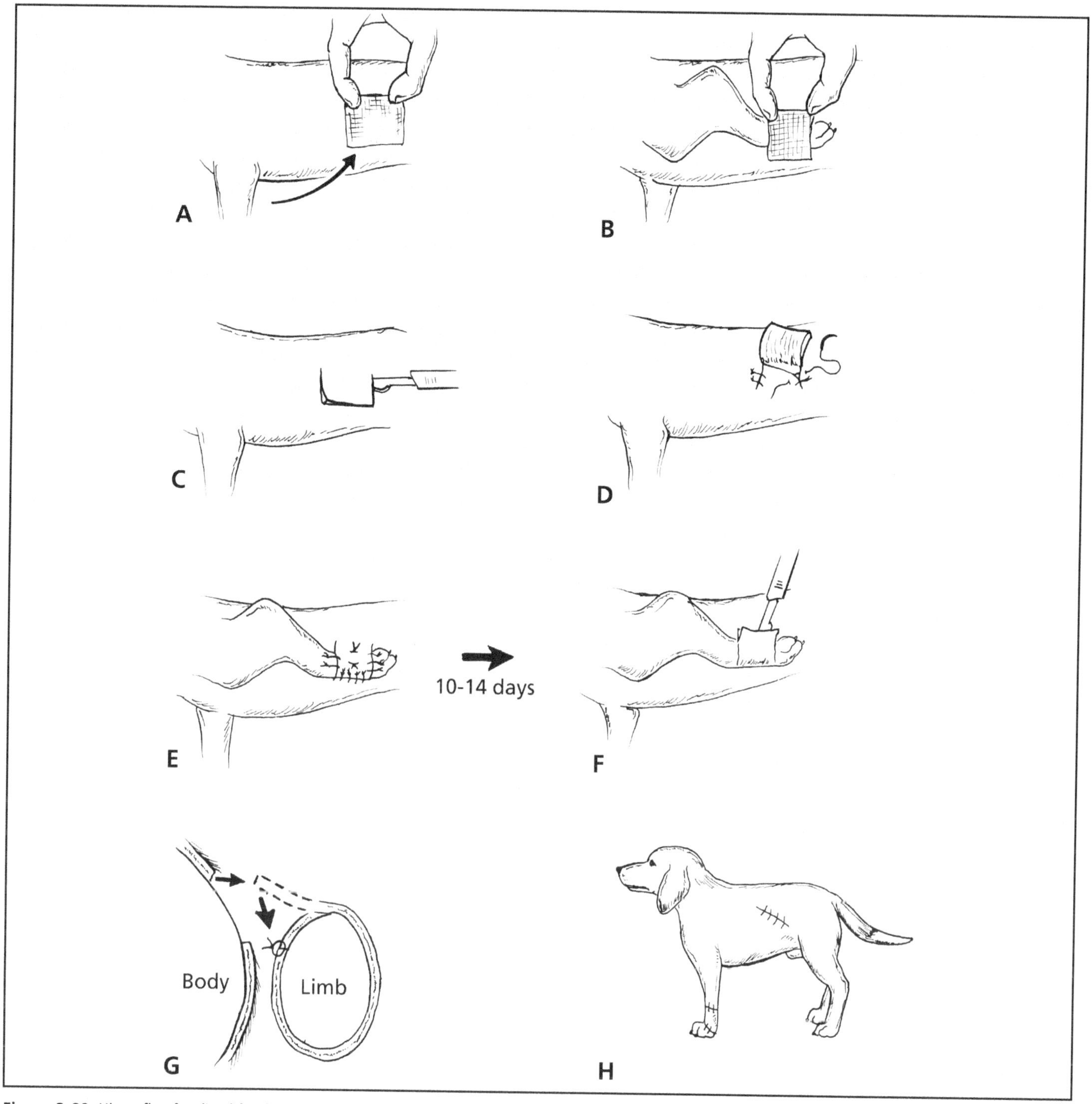


**Figure 3-80.** Hinge flap for distal forelimb wound repair. **A.** Cloth pattern of a hinge flap held along dog's side at proposed flap site. Forelimb will be moved back under the pattern to determine exact location for the flap *(arrow)*. **B.** Distal limb wound placed under the cloth pattern. **C.** Cutting and elevating the flap. **D.** Flap reflected upward and donor site being sutured. **E.** Flap sutured over the wound. **F.** Cutting flap pedicle. **G.** Final transfer of the flap. **H.** Flap transferred to the limb; donor site sutured.

be necessary to replace it periodically. The bandage is completed with circumferential absorbent secondary wrap and tertiary wrap of adhesive tape or elastic adhesive tape. Because limbs bandaged against the body have a tendency to rotate outward, careful bandaging is necessary to help reduce this. To avoid daily bandage changes of the entire bandage, an access window may be cut in the bandage over the flap to allow the flap to be attended as it heals in place (Figure 3-81B). A patch bandage is placed over the access window between treatments. In the early stages of healing when drainage is copious, bandages over the flap should be changed frequently. Following this, bandages can be changed every 2 to 3 days as drainage decreases.

After the flap has been transferred to the limb it should be protected with a bandage for another 7 to 10 days.

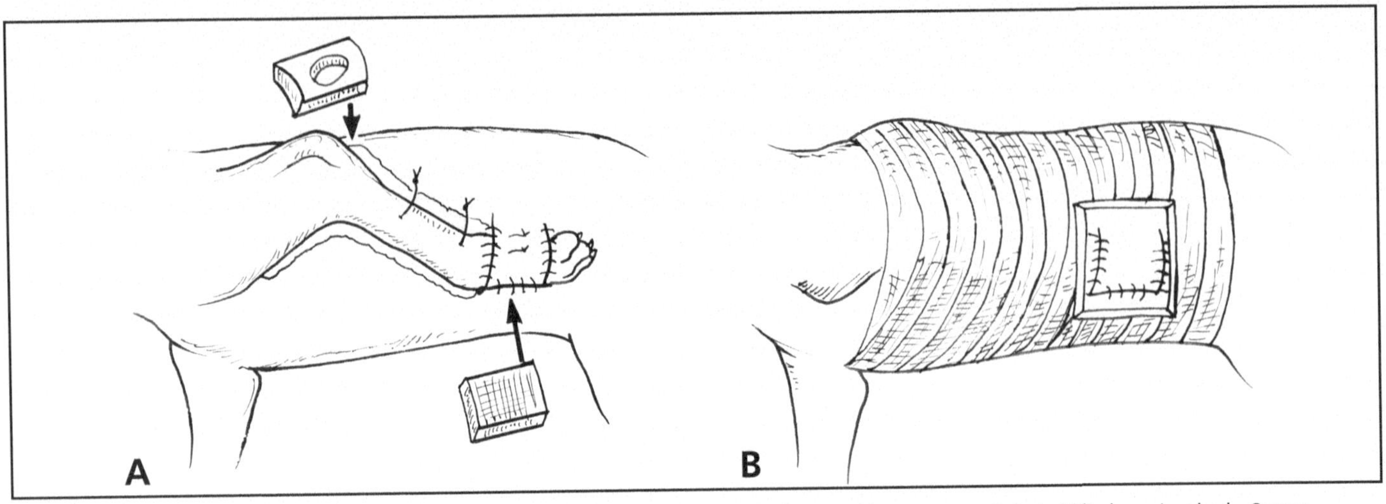


**Figure 3-81.** Bandaging a forelimb against the body for pouch and hinge flaps. **A.** Two large tacking sutures to help hold limb against body. Cotton between the limb and body. Modified "donut" – type bandage to be placed over elbow. Absorbent gauze sponges to be placed over the surgical site. **B.** Access window cut in the immobilizing bandage for observation of the surgical site.

## Advantages and Disadvantages

Pouch and hinge flaps are relatively cosmetic in that they provide a full-thickness, fully-haired segment of skin for wound repair. The direction of hair growth is generally acceptable on the forelimbs. Pouch and hinge flaps are thicker than surrounding skin following transfer. This is due to inclusion of the cutaneous trunci muscle in the flap, inflammation and fibrous connective tissue deposition. However, the flaps will shrink in time and become more cosmetic.

The full-thickness fully-haired skin of a pouch flap or hinge flap is functional because it will withstand the trauma to which it may be subjected on the distal limb. Pouch flaps with 2 pedicles are advantageous because they support the limb against the body better than a hinge flap while vascular and connective tissue connection develops between the flap and the wound. These flaps are best suited for the thoracic limbs of small dogs and cats because bandaging the thoracic limb along the animal's side is more comfortable for smaller animals than for larger breeds of dogs. For distal limb and paw wounds, a pouch flap is the flap of choice. A hinge flap should be considered if the wound extends from the paw to the radial-humeral area and if it will be difficult to flex the forelimb joints sufficiently to insert the paw in the cranial-most pouch incision.

Because of the multiple stages of the procedure, there is an increase in the time and expense of its performance. If a window is not cut in the bandage to allow flap treatment and the entire body bandage is changed each time the flap is tended, there will be a further increase in cost of bandaging.

When used on larger dogs, it may be difficult to immobilize the limb against the body. In addition, use of a pouch flap or hinge flap on the pelvic limb is more difficult on a male dog because of the genitalia and the necessity of bandaging around them.

The cosmetic results of a pouch flap or hinge flap on the pelvic limb may not be as favorable as on the forelimb. The direction of hair growth on the hind limb flap is usually opposite that on the remainder of the leg (Figure 3-82).

The body bandage required for limb and flap immobilization may be a problem on cats, resulting in marked loss of proprioception. Thus, there is an inability to walk for a while after bandaging, and an intolerance of the bandage.

Although the flap carries its blood supply with it, it must establish vascular connections from the wound site so the pedicle(s) of the flap can be severed as the flap is finally transferred to the limb. Sufficient immobilization of the limb in the flap is important so that these connections can take place. Excess movement of the limb in the flap jeopardizes healing. Another factor in attaining adequate vascular connections is the condition of the wound being repaired. If a flap is used to repair a distal limb wound that has exposed bone, it may be at risk if the pedicles are severed too soon, i.e. before granulation tissue has formed over the bone (under the flap) to provide adequate flap vascularization. Therefore, leaving the flap in place a few more days to assure adequate vascular connections before pedicle severance will prolong aftercare slightly.

Related to this is placement of a pouch flap or hinge flap over a distal limb wound after a tumor has been removed and the resulting wound has been irradiated. The vascularity of the wound will be tenuous and the

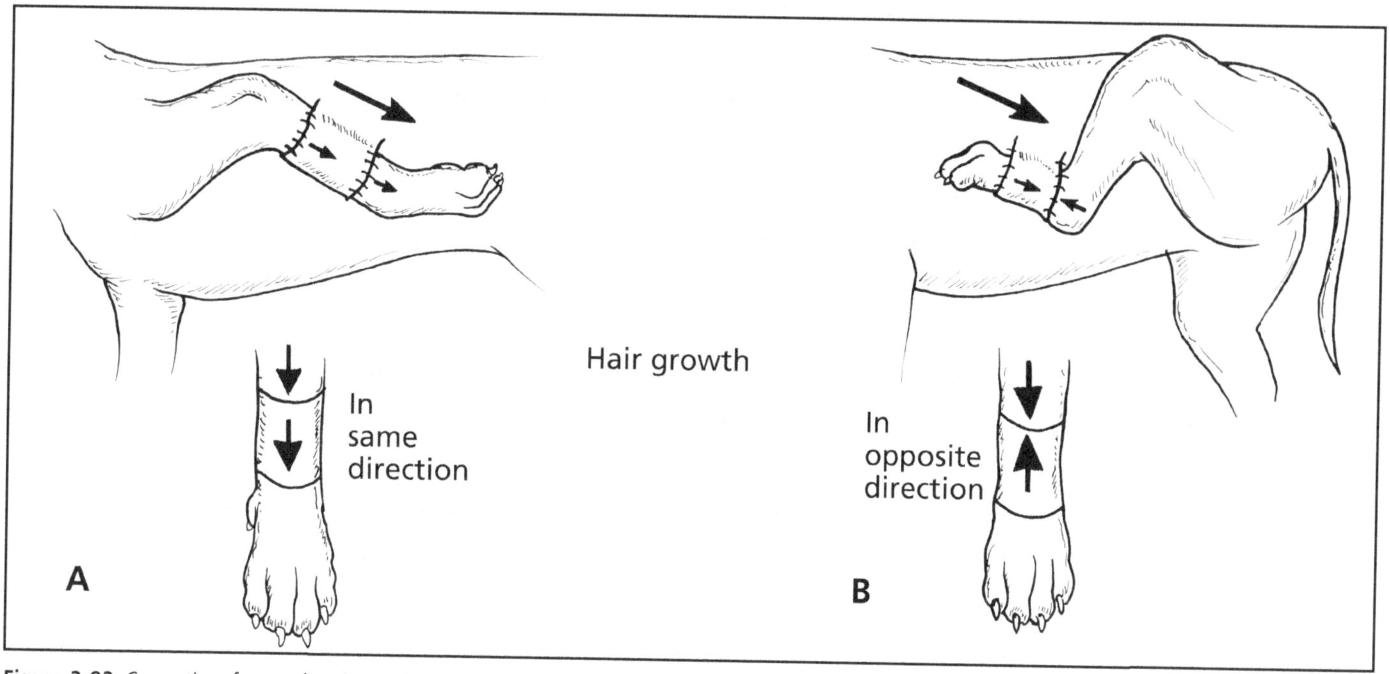


**Figure 3-82.** Cosmetics of a pouch or hinge flap. **A.** Direction of hair growth on the lateral thoraco – abdominal area and the forelimb is usually similar *(arrows)*. **B.** Direction of hair growth on the distal aspect of the pelvic limb is usually different from that on the lateral thoraco – abdominal area. (After Swaim SF, Henderson RA: Small Animal Wound Management, 2nd ed.: Baltimore: Williams & Wilkins, 1997, 328.

successful healing of such a flap will be jeopardized.

After the flap pedicle(s) are severed to transfer the flap to the leg and the limb is released from the body, the animal may be lame for a period of 7 to 10 days. This is accompanied by mild muscle atrophy until normal limb use is regained.

# Suggested Readings

1. Basher A: Foot injuries in dogs and cats. Compend Contin Educ Pract Vet 16:1159, 1994.
2. Birchard SJ, Smeak DD: Selected skin graft and reconstructive techniques. *In* Birchard SJ, Sherding RG, eds.: Saunders Manual of Small Animal Practice, 2nd ed.: Philadelphia: WB Saunders, 2000, 404.
3. Birchard SJ, Smeak DD: Selected skin graft and reconstructive techniques. In Birchard SJ, Sherding RG. eds.: Saunders Manual of Small Animal Practice, 3rd ed.: St. Louis: Saunders – Elsevier, 2006, 557.
4. Fowler D: Distal limb and paw injuries. Vet Clin No Am Small Anim Pract 36: 819, 2006.
5. Hedlund CS: Surgery of the integumentary system. *In* Fossum TW, ed.: Small Animal Surgery, 2nd ed.: St. Louis: Mosby, 2002, 134.
6. Hedlund CS: Surgery of the integumentary system. In Fossum TW, ed.: Small Animal Surgery, 3rd ed.: St. Louis: Mosby, 2007, 159.
7. Hunt GB: Local or subdermal plexus flaps. In Tobias KM, Johnston SA, eds.: Veterinary Surgery, Small Animal, Vol. 2: St. Louis: Elsevier – Saunders, 2012, 1243.
8. Johnston DE: The repair of skin loss on the foot by means of a double-pedicle abdominal flap. J Am Anim Hosp Assoc 12:593, 1976.
9. Lemarié RJ, Hosgood G, Read RA, et al: Distant abdominal and thoracic pedicle skin flaps for treatment of distal limb skin defects. J Small Anim Pract 36:255, 1995.
10. MacPhail CM: Surgery of the integumentary system. In Fossum TW, ed.: Small Animal Surgery, 4th ed.: St. Louis: Mosby, 2013, 190.
11. Mayhew P: Tension – relieving techniques and local skin flaps. In Williams J, Moores A, eds.: BSAVA Manual of Canine and Feline Wound Management and Reconstruction, 2nd ed.: Glouster (UK): BSAVA, 2009, 69.
12. Pavletic MM: Skin flaps in reconstructive surgery. Vet Clin North Am 20:81, 1990.
13. Pavletic MM: Atlas of Small Animal Reconstructive Surgery, 2nd ed: Philadelphia: WB Saunders, 1999, 219.
14. Pavletic MM: Pedicle grafts. Slatter DH, ed.: Textbook of Small Animal Surgery, 3rd ed.: Philadelphia: WB Saunders, 2003, 292.
15. Pavletic MM: Atlas of Small Animal Wound Management and Reconstructive Surgery, 3rd ed.: Ames, IA: Wiley – Blackwell, 2010, 337.
16. Pope ER, Swaim SF: Shifting tissue and using flaps. Vet Med 81:512, 1986.
17. Swaim SF: Foot salvage techniques in dogs and cats: Options: "do's" and "don'ts". J Am Anim Hosp Assoc 21:511, 1985.
18. Swaim SF, Henderson RA: Small Animal Wound Management. 2nd ed.: Baltimore: Williams and Wilkins, 1997, 295.
19. Sykes GP: Pouch graft: Resurfacing the distal extremity of a dog. Canine Pract 7:28, 1980.
20. Yturraspe DJ, Creed JE, Schwach RP: Thoracic pedicle skin flap for repair of lower limb wounds in dogs and cats. J Am Anim Hosp Assoc 12:581, 1976.

# Tubed Pedicle Flaps

## Definition and Indications

Tubed pedicle flaps are multistaged indirect flaps which have the pedicle sutured into a tube before its eventual transfer to the wound on the distal limb using the delaying procedure in the transfer process. The procedure is indicated for transferring skin from the proximal to the distal portion of the limb when there is no immediate need to cover a wound. It is generally indicated when simpler means of skin transfer are unable to close the defect. In addition, it can provide full-thickness fully-haired skin as a weight-bearing tissue on a cat, i.e. replacement of pad tissue (Figure 3-83A-C). It can be used on any sized dog or cat. The flap lends itself to use on the pelvic limb more than on the forelimb due to the greater abundance of skin relatively close above the tarsus which can be moved distally in one stage. Whereas, on the forelimb skin for constructing a flap is relatively sparse above the carpus.

A tubed pedicle flap may be a simple tubed pedicle where a portion of the tube itself is used to cover the wound. A second form of the flap is the tubed pedicle and "pancake", where a segment/"pancake" of skin is created by the delaying procedure on the proximal end of the tubed pedicle. This is done to provide a larger amount of skin to repair a distal limb wound.

## Techniques

### Simple Tubed Pedicle

The entire limb is prepared for aseptic surgery. The animal is placed in lateral recumbency with the affected limb uppermost.

The flap is planned using a ruler and piece of sterile cloth. To help assure the survival of the flap, it should be planned such that only one movement of the flap will be needed to transfer skin from the donor site to the distal limb wound. Using digital manipulation skin is pinched up along the long axis of the limb above the wound to determine how much can be used to construct the flap and yet close the resulting defect without creating a biologic tourniquet on the limb. Since the flap lends itself to hind limb use, the flap design is usually done on the medial or lateral surface of the tibial area. The flap should be designed long enough to permit the proximal end to eventually be swung/"tumbled" distally to cover the wound. To further assure proper design of the flap, a piece of sterile cloth can be cut to the length and width of the proposed flap. It is placed over the donor site, and the two ends of the cloth are pinched together from side to side to simulate the tubing of the ends of the flap (Figure 3-84A). Holding the distal end of the cloth pattern tightly in place, the proximal end is swung distally to assure that it will reach the distal end of the wound (Figure 3-84B). Once the surgeon is certain that the length, width, and location of the flap are correct, the cloth pattern is laid over the donor site and the long edges of the pattern are drawn on the skin, i.e. two parallel lines parallel to the long axis of the limb (Figure 3-84C). It is wise to make the flap slightly

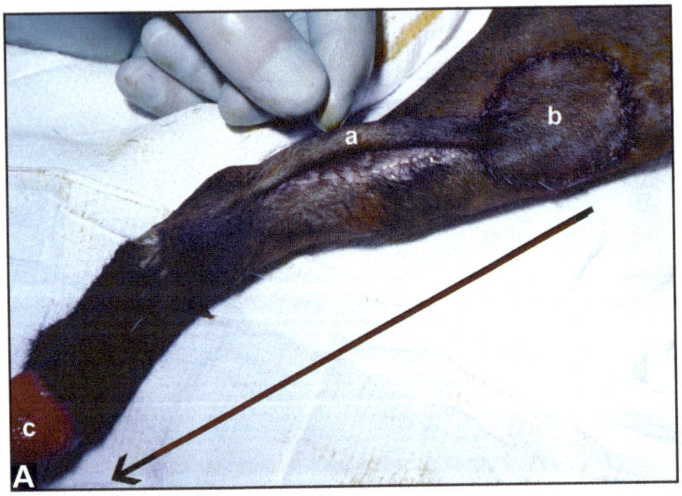


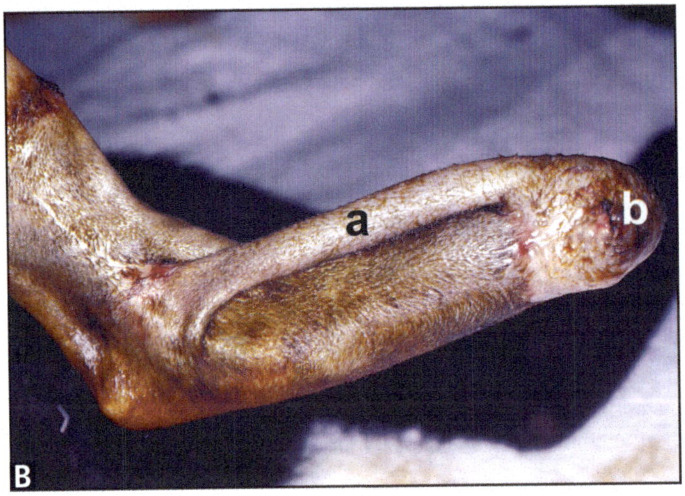


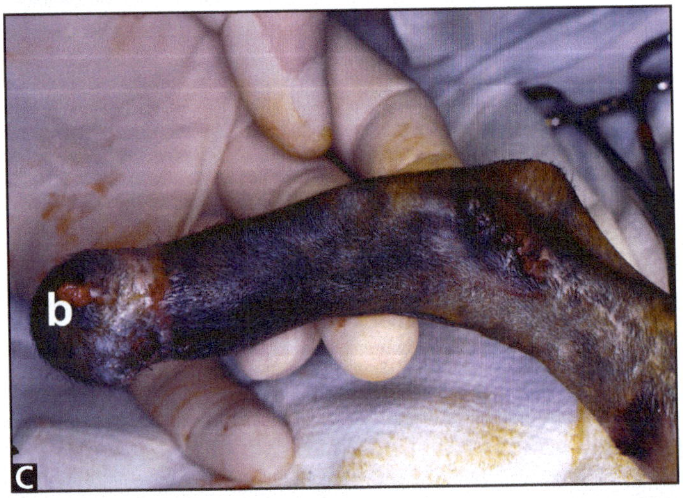


**Figure 3-83.** Tubed pedicle and "pancake" to replace paw tissue on a cat. **A.** Tubed pedicle *(a)*, "pancake" *(b)*, paw defect *(c)*, and proposed "pancake" rotation to cover paw defect *(arrow)*. **B.** Tubed pedicle *(a)* "pancake" over paw defect *(b)*. **C.** "Pancake" in place *(b)* after excision of tubed pedicle.

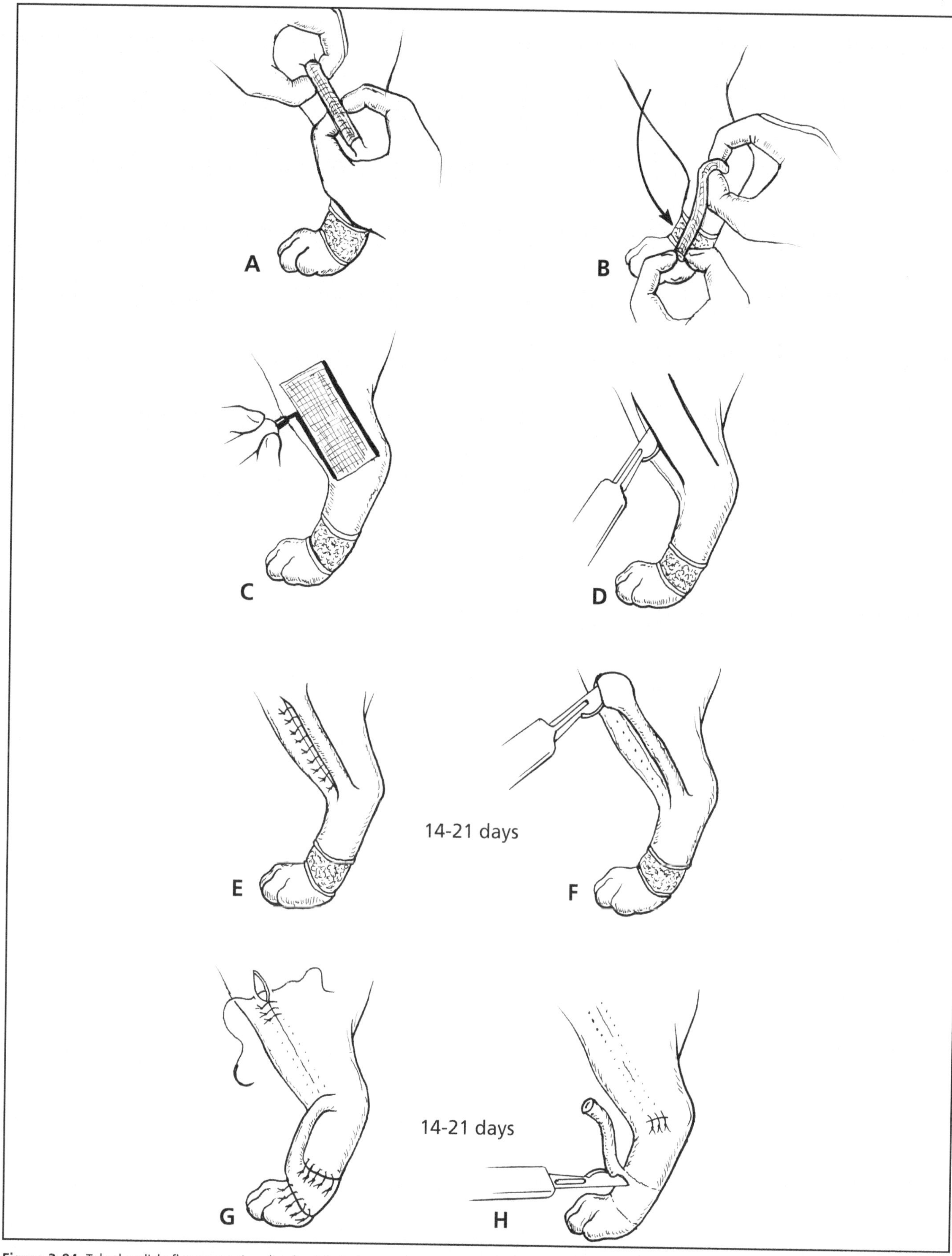


**Figure 3-84.** Tubed pedicle flap to repair a distal pelvic limb wound on a cat. **A.** Planning the tubed pedicle – pinching a piece of cloth pattern and underlying skin together in proposed donor area on the lateral aspect of the limb. **B.** Transposing the cloth pattern assessing its ability to reach the lesion. **C.** Tracing the parallel long edges of the cloth pattern on the skin. **D.** Incising the flap. **E.** Flap sutured into a tube, and donor site closed. **F.** Cutting the proximal end of the tube with a small amount of extra skin. **G.** Tube transposed and skin of its proximal end sutured over wound. **H.** Excising the tubed pedicle.

longer than is necessary to reach the wound to allow for some shrinkage which will occur during the healing period. Some surgeons recommend that the length and width of the flap be increased by 2 to 3 cm. However, discretion and clinical judgment should be used, e.g. such increases cannot be made on a cat's limb.

The two lines are incised and the skin is undermined (Figure 3-84D). The 2 edges of the flap are sutured together with simple interrupted sutures of 3-0 nonabsorbable monofilament suture to form a tubed pedicle which is attached to the skin of the leg at each end. The donor defect under the tube is sutured with the same suture material and pattern with which the tube was sutured (Figure 3-84E).

The wound on the distal limb is bandaged appropriately. The bandage may be extended proximally to cover the tubed pedicle to keep the animal from molesting it. The part of the bandage over the tube should not be tight to prevent compression of the tube and thus a compromise of its circulation. Cotton padding may be placed under the flap to support it and keep it from being kinked during bandaging. A restraint collar can also be used to prevent molestation of the tube.

Fourteen to 21 days following creation of the tubed pedicle, the involved limb is prepared for aseptic surgery. Any epithelium that is advancing from the wound edge over granulation tissue that is on the wound is removed. The surface of the granulation tissue is cleared of any coagulum on its surface by wiping it with a surgical sponge soaked with a 1:40 dilution of chlorhexidine diacetate (Nolvasan solution, Ft. Dodge Animal Health, Ft. Dodge, IA) or gluconate (ChlorhexiDerm Disinfectant, Dermatologics in Veterinary Medicine, Pharmaceuticals, Inc., Miami, FL) solution. The proximal end of the tubed pedicle is severed from the skin of the leg. If needed, a small area of surrounding skin at the end of the tube can be taken with the tubed pedicle (Figure 3-84F). However, it should be remembered that if too large a piece is taken to transfer immediately to the wound, the blood supply via the tube may not be sufficient to sustain it, and a portion of it may necrose. To help assure adequate vascularization of the tubed pedicle from its distal end the proximal end can be incised in stages. Half of the tube is incised and resutured in place, then 2 days later these sutures are removed and the remaining half of the tube is transected. After the proximal end of the tube is separated, the separated end of the tube is incised along the scar line where the skin edges were originally sutured together and the tube is opened flat using judicious incisions in the subcutaneous tissue to avoid severe damage to the blood supply of the skin. Skin hooks can be used to apply traction on the skin edges as the flap is untubed. The opened end of the flap is then transferred distally and laid over the wound. Its edges are trimmed and sutured to the wound edges with 3-0 simple interrupted sutures of monofilament nonabsorbable suture material. The area where the proximal end of the tubed pedicle was severed is trimmed and sutured with like suture material and pattern (Figure 3-84G).

The distal limb is bandaged to include coverage of the tubed pedicle. Care should be taken not to compress the tubed pedicle and thus compromise its blood supply. Cotton may be placed under the tubed pedicle to support it and help prevent a sharp kink at its distal end which could obstruct flap vasculature. The bandage is changed periodically.

Fourteen to 21 days following transfer of the flap to the wound, the tubed pedicle is severed at its former distal attachment and the edges of the remaining wound are trimmed and sutured with the above described suture material and pattern. The tubed pedicle is then severed at its attachment to the skin of the flap that was used for wound repair (Figure 3-84H). The edges of the remaining wound are trimmed and sutured with the above described suture material and pattern (See Figure 3-87H). The remnants of the tubed pedicle are discarded. The sutures from the flap transfer 18 to 21 days earlier are removed, and bandaging is continued as needed until the sutures placed at the time of flap severance are removed at 7 to 10 days.

### Tubed Pedicle and "Pancake"

This procedure is the same as a simple tubed pedicle; however, it has an additional stage where a segment of skin/"pancake" is created by the delaying procedure on the proximal end of the tubed pedicle. After the first 14 to 21 day period following creation of the tubed pedicle, a segment of skin is incised at the proximal end of the tubed pedicle. Following incision, the skin is sutured again (Figure 3-85A & B). This segment has thus been cut off from peripheral blood supply and will become more dependent on vascularization coming from the tubed pedicle. The wound, tubed pedicle and "pancake" of skin are bandaged for another period of 14 to 21 days. At the end of this period, the sutures are removed from the "pancake" segment of skin, it is reincised, undermined, transferred to the wound and sutured in place (Figure 3-85C). At this point the procedure continues as with the simple tubed pedicle procedure (Figure

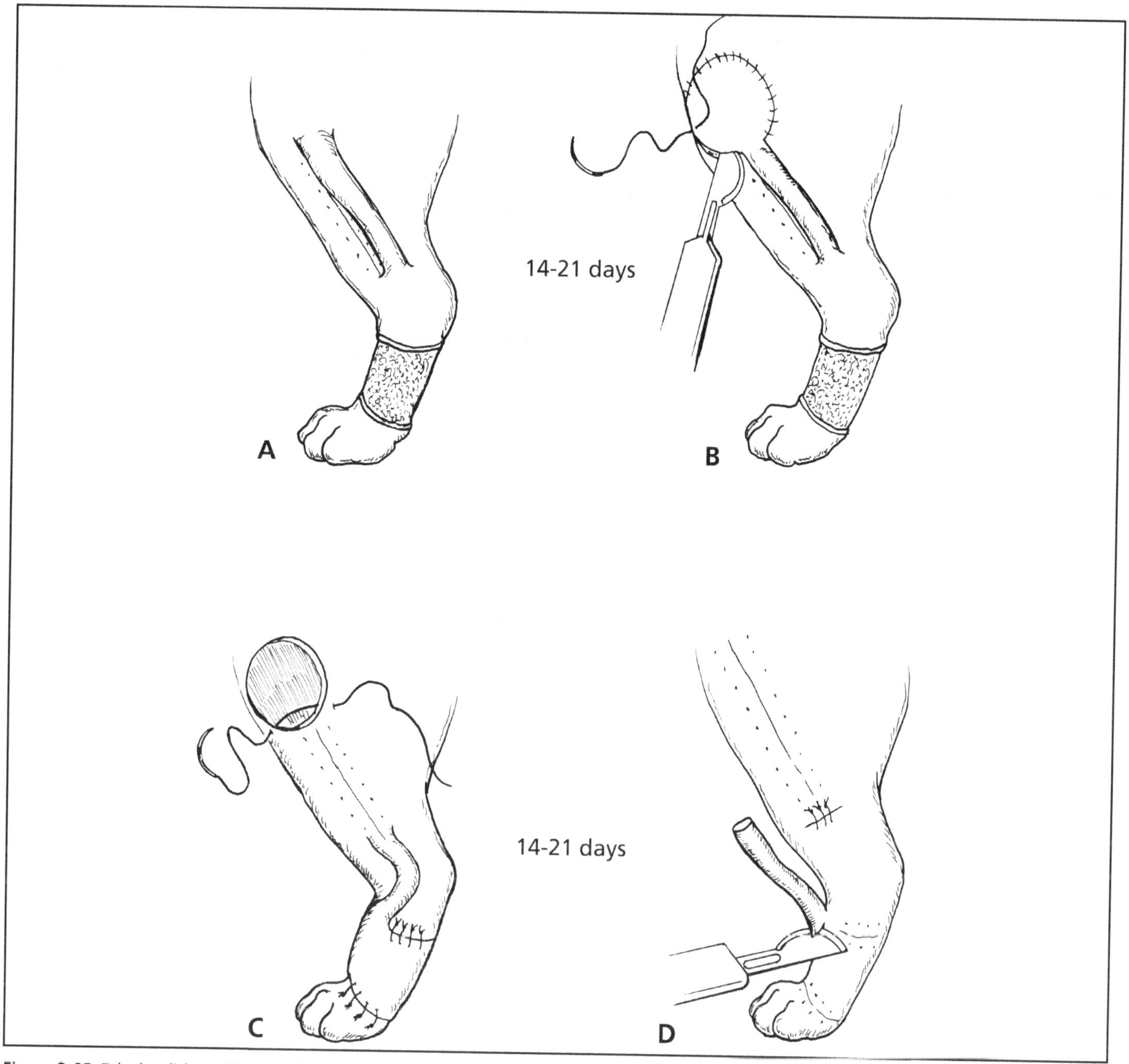


**Figure 3-85.** Tubed pedicle and "pancake" to repair a distal pelvic limb wound on a cat. **A.** Tubed pedicle on the lateral aspect of the limb. **B.** Cutting a "pancake" segment of skin on the proximal end of the tubed pedicle and suturing it back in place. **C.** "Pancake" segment of skin transposed on tubed pedicle to the wound with suturing it in place and closing the donor site. **D.** Excising the tubed pedicle.

3-85D). Thus, the procedure for a tubed pedicle and "pancake" is like that for a simple tubed pedicle with the addition of another 14 to 21 day period for the delay procedure of the segment/"pancake".

## Aftercare

Because the tubed pedicle flap procedures are multi-staged with aftercare associated with each stage, the aftercare was included with the "Technique" section to make progression of the procedures easier to follow.

## Advantages and Disadvantages

Tubed pedicle repair of distal limb wounds provides full-thickness, fully-haired skin for reconstruction; however, the direction of hair growth will be different from the surrounding area due to the transposition of the end of the flap as it is transferred from proximal to distal. The full-thickness, fully-haired properties of the skin provide durability to withstand any stress or trauma to which the area may be subjected. These flaps have an advantage over the pouch flaps and hinge flaps in that it is not necessary to bandage the limb along the animal's side while the procedure is being performed. Thus, there may be more comfort for the animal as it is able to use its limb without the muscle atrophy or lameness associated with pouch flaps and hinge flaps.

The main disadvantage of the tubed pedicles is the long time necessary to complete the procedure because of the 14 to 21 day delay period between each stage of creating and moving the flap. With prolonged time comes the disadvantage of maintaining protection of the flap from molestation by bandaging or using a restraint collar. In addition, during this time the tubed pedicle can become kinked or twisted compromising its blood supply. There is also the chance of infection during this time.

These flaps, as all other flaps, carry their blood supply with them. Because of the delay periods associated with using them, there is usually a good bed of granulation tissue on the wound. Thus, when it is transferred to the wound there is adequate vascular tissue from which it can revascularize. However, if the flap is placed over a wound that has been irradiated after a tumor removal, the vascularity of the wound will be tenuous and the successful healing of the flap will be jeopardized.

# Suggested Readings


1. Basher A: Foot injuries in dogs and cats. Compend Contin Educ Prac Vet 16:1159, 1994.
2. Hedlund CS: Surgery of the integumentary system. *In* Fossum TW, ed.: Small Animal Surgery, 2nd ed.: St. Louis: Mosby, 2002, 134.
3. Hedlund CS: Surgery of the integumentary system. In Fossum TW, ed.: Small Animal Surgery, 3rd. ed.: St. Louis: Mosby, 2007, 159.
4. Hunt GB: Local or subdermal plexus flaps. In Tobias KM, Johnston SA, eds.: Veterinary Surgery, Small Animal, Vol. 2: St. Louis: Elsevier – Saunders, 2012, 1243,
5. MacPhail CM: Surgery of the integumentary system. In Fossum TW, ed.: Small Animal Surgery, 4th ed.: St. Louis: Mosby, 2013, 190.
6. Pavletic MM: Atlas of Small Animal Reconstructive Surgery, 2nd ed: Philadelphia: WB Saunders, 1999, 220.
7. Pavletic MM: Pedicle grafts. In Slatter DH, ed.: Textbook of Small Animal Surgery, 3rd ed.: Philadelphia: WB Saunders, 2003, 292.
8. Pavletic MM: Atlas of Small Animal Wound Management and Reconstructive Surgery, 3rd ed.: Ames, IA: Wiley – Blackwell, 2010, 337.
9. Swaim SF, Garrett PD: Foot salvage techniques in dogs and cats: Options: "do's" and "don'ts". J Am Anim Hosp Assoc 21:511, 1985.


# Reverse Saphenous Conduit Flap

## Definition and Indications

The reverse saphenous conduit flap has branches of the saphenous artery and medial saphenous vein. These supply and drain the overlying skin by means of direct cutaneous vessels. When vascular connections with the femoral artery and vein are cut, blood flow is maintained in reverse by distal anastomotic connections between the cranial branch of the saphenous artery and the perforating metatarsal artery via the medial and lateral plantar arteries and the cranial branch of the medial saphenous vein and cranial branch of the lateral saphenous vein, along with other venous connections with the cranial and caudal branches of the medial saphenous veins distal to the tibiotarsal joint.

This flap has potential for use in repairing major wounds at or below the tarsus. It is particularly suited for wounds overlying the cranial surface of the metatarsus.

## Technique

Measurements are taken, and the flap is designed over the craniotibial area to reach and cover the distal limb defect. It is necessary to taper the flap width distally because of the limited skin available in this area to develop the flap pedicle. The incision for the distal end of the flap is generally made across the central third of the medial femoral area. This is at or slightly above the level of the patella (Figure 3-86A). Using Metzenbaum scissors for blunt dissection, the saphenous artery, medial saphenous vein, and nerve are isolated, ligated, and divided at the level of the femoral artery and vein. Two incisions are then made distally in convergent style from the ends of the transverse incision. They are 0.5 to 1.0 cm cranial and caudal to the branches of the saphenous artery and medial saphenous vein, respectively. The flap is then undermined under the saphenous vasculature to include the vasculature with the flap. The flap is undermined progressively, and a portion of the medial gastrocnemius muscle fascia is included with the flap to prevent injury to the caudal branch of the saphenous artery and medial saphenous vein. Below this point, the tibial nerve merges with the descending caudal branches of the saphenous artery and medial saphenous vein. It can be preserved by careful dissection between these structures. The peroneal artery and vein are ligated and divided to facilitate raising the flap. To complete elevation of the flap, it is undermined proximal to the anastomosis between the cranial branch of the medial saphenous vein and the caudal branch of the lateral saphenous vein (Figure 3-86B).

The donor site is closed using interrupted subcutaneous sutures of 3-0 absorbable suture material. Simple interrupted nonabsorbable skin sutures complete closure of the area (Figure 3-86C).

The flap pedicle (portion between the base of the flap and the portion to be sutured over the wound) may be handled in one of 2 ways. First, it can be tubed by suturing the flap edges together with simple interrupted sutures of 3-0 nonabsorbable material, thus forming a skin tube that traverses the skin between the donor site and the wound (Figure 3-86C & D). The second option is to make a "bridge incision" between the base of the donor site and the proximal end of the wound (Figure 3-86E & F). The edges of the pedicle are sutured to the edges of the "bridge incision".

If the wound has a bed of granulation tissue, the surface of the wound is cleared of any coagulum that is present by wiping it with a surgical sponge soaked with a 1:40 dilution of chlorhexidine diacetate (Nolvasan Solution, Ft. Dodge Animal Health, Ft. Dodge, IA) or gluconate (ChlorhexiDerm Disinfectant, Dermatologics in Veterinary Medicine, Pharmaceuticals, Inc., Miami, FL) solution. If epithelium is advancing over the granulation tissue, from the wound edges, it is removed. The distal end of the flap is trimmed appropriately to fit the wound and is sutured over

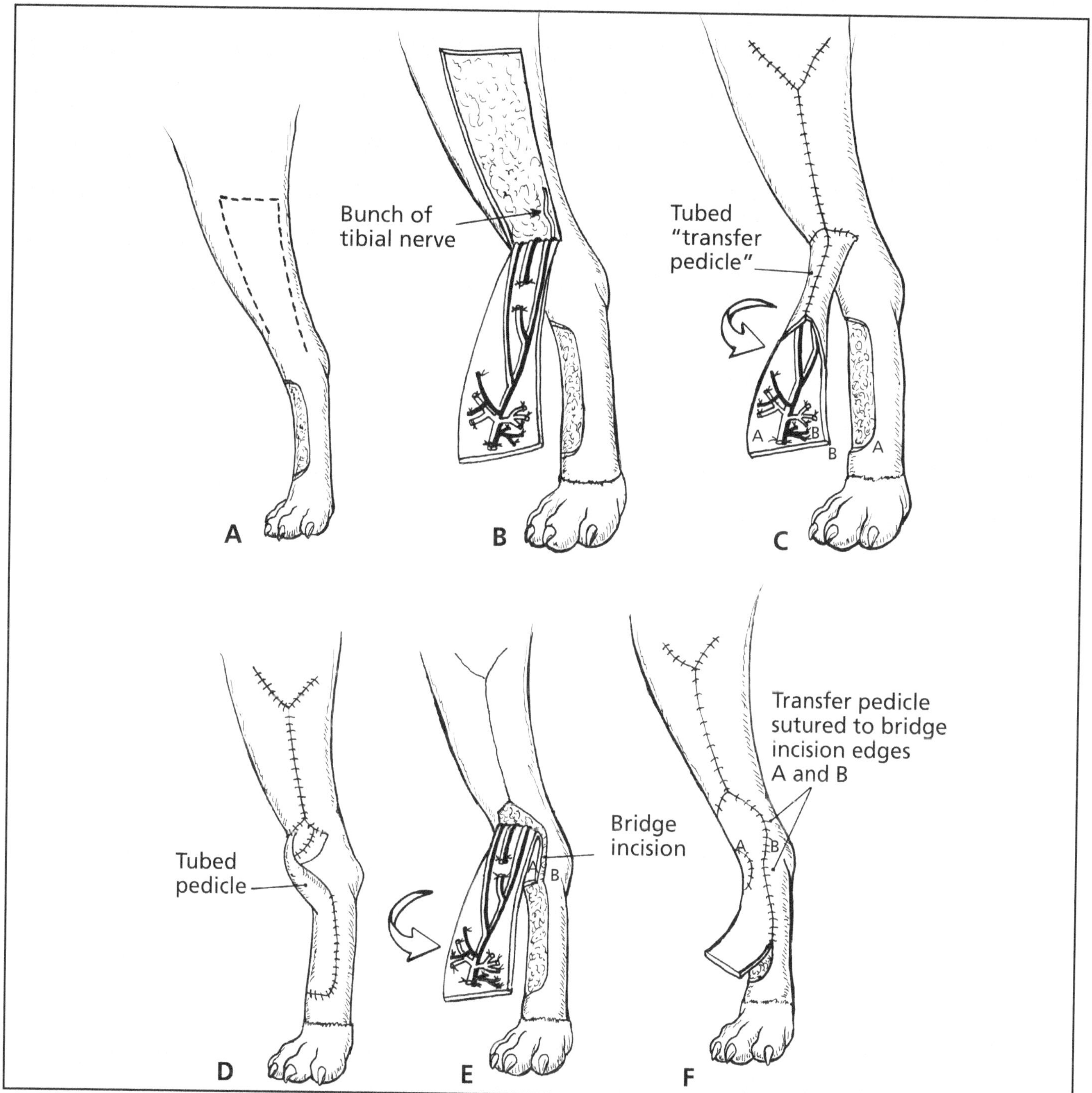


**Figure 3-86.** Reverse saphenous conduit flap. **A.** Outline of the flap over the craniomedial tibial area. **B.** Reflection of the flap beneath the saphenous vasculature with appropriate vessel ligations and divisions (see text). **C.** Option 1 – Pedicle of the flap is tubed and donor site is sutured. Distal end of the flap will be rotated *(arrow)* to cover the wound. **D.** Distal end of the flap sutured over wound with tubed pedicle. **E.** Option 2 – A "bridge incision" is made between flap base and wound. Distal end of flap will be rotated *(arrow)* to cover the wound. **F.** Flap being sutured in place with edges of pedicle sutured to edges of "bridge incision". (From Pavletic MM: Atlas of Small Animal Wound Management and Reconstructive Surgery, 3rd ed.: Ames,IA: Wiley-Blackwell, 2010, 243.)

the wound with 3-0 simple interrupted monofilament nonabsorbable material.

## Aftercare

The distal limb should be bandaged, and the bandage can cover the donor site. If the pedicle of the flap has been tubed, the bandage should be placed so that it does not compress the tube and compromise the flap's circulation. If necessary, cotton can be placed under or around the tube to help prevent kinking of the tube. The bandage is changed periodically. Sutures are removed at 7 to 10 days postoperatively. After 14 to 21 days, when the flap has developed a good vascular connection to the wound, the tube can be excised followed by trimming and suturing of the 2 attachment areas. If the pedicle of the flap was sutured to the edges of the "bridge incision", the sutures are removed from the entire surgical area at 7 to 10 days postoperatively.

## Advantages and Disadvantages

Reverse saphenous conduit flaps provide fully-haired skin for wound repair; however, the direction of hair growth will be different from the area around the wound due to the transposition of the end of the flap as it is transferred from proximal to distal. The full-thickness, fully-haired skin provides durability to withstand any stress or trauma to which the area may be subjected. These flaps have the advantage that they do not require the limb to be bandaged along the animal's side for flap placement as do the pouch flaps and hinge flaps. The animal may thus be more comfortable in using the limb, and the muscle atrophy and lameness associated with pouch flaps and hinge flaps are averted. Because pouch flaps and hinge flaps do not lend themselves well to use on the pelvic limbs, especially on large dogs and male dogs, this technique offers a means of distal pelvic limb reconstruction on these dogs.

Another advantage of the reverse saphenous conduit flap over pouch, hinge and tubed pedicle flaps is that they are transferred to the wound in one stage. Thus, this flap does not have the increased time and expense associated with it as with the other flaps.

A disadvantage of this flap is that it requires exact knowledge of the vascular and nerve structures in the area, and proper management of these is vital to survival of the flap. If the tibial nerve is cut while creating the flap an atrophic ulcer may develop on the anesthetic metatarsal pad and adjacent skin in an active dog. When there has been extensive trauma to the distal pelvic limb, angiography should be considered to determine whether anastomotic connections are intact and that the saphenous artery and medial saphenous vein are not the major circulatory supply to the distal limb.

# Suggested Readings

1. Cornell K, Salisbury K, Jakovljevic, et al: Reverse saphenous conduit flap in cats: An anatomic study. Vet Surg 24: 202, 1995.
2. Degner DA, Bauer MS, Cozens M: Reverse saphenous conduit flap: A case report in a cat. Vet Comp Orthop Traum 6:175, 1993.
3. Fowler D: Distal limb and paw injuries. Vet Clins No Am Small Anim Pract 36: 819, 2006.
4. Hedlund CS: Surgery of the integumentary system. In Fossum TW, ed.: Small Animal Surgery, 2nd ed.: St. Louis: Mosby, 2002, 134.
5. Hedlund CS: Surgery of the integumentary system In Fossum TW, ed.: Small Animal Surgery, 3rd ed.: St. Louis: Mosby, 2007, 159.
6. MacPhail CM: Surgery of the integumentary system. In Fossum TW, ed.: Small Animal Surgery, 4th ed.: St. Louis: Mosby, 2013, 190.
7. Mayhew P: Tension – relieving techniques and local skin flaps. In Williams J, Moores A, eds.: BSAVA Manual of Canine and Feline Wound Management and Reconstruction, 2nd, ed.: Glouster (UK): BSAVA, 2009, 39.
8. Pavletic MM, Watters J, Henry RW, et al: Reverse saphenous conduit flap in the dog. J Am Vet Med Assoc 182:380, 1983.
9. Pavletic MM: Atlas of Small Animal Reconstructive Surgery, 2nd ed: Philadelphia: WB Saunders, 1999, 275.
10. Pavletic MM: Atlas of Small Animal Wound Management and Reconstructive Surgery, 3rd ed.: Ames, IA: Wiley – Blackwell, 2010, 357.
11. Remedios AM, Fowler JD: Axial pattern flaps in the cutaneous reconstruction of lower limb wounds. Compend Contin Educ Pract Vet 17:1356, 1995.
12. Remedios AM: Axial pattern flaps. In Fowler D, Williams JM, eds.: BSAVA Manual of Canine and Feline Wound Management and Reconstruction. Shurdington, Cheltenham, UK: British Small Animal Veterinary Association, 199, 69.
13. Swaim SF: Wound management of the distal limbs and paws: Reconstruction and salvage. Vet Med Rep 2:128, 1990.
14. Wardlaw JL, Lanz OI: Axial pattern and myocutaneous flaps. In Tobias KM, Johnston SA, eds.: Veterinary Surgery, Small Animal, Vol. 2: St. Louis, Elsevier – Saunders, 2012, 1256.

# Skin Grafts

# Mesh Grafts

## Definition and Indications

A mesh graft is a piece of full-thickness skin which has had numerous slits cut in it in parallel staggered rows. These grafts are indicated to repair wounds when there is insufficient skin for wound closure by moving local tissue or using a skin flap. These grafts are frequently used on the distal limbs (Figure 3-87A-C and Figure 3-88A). Mesh grafts are indicated for fresh wounds and excision sites that have tissue that is vascularized sufficiently so that it will produce granulation tissue. They are also indicated for a wound that has a healthy bed of granulation tissue which has started to epithelialize from the wound edges.

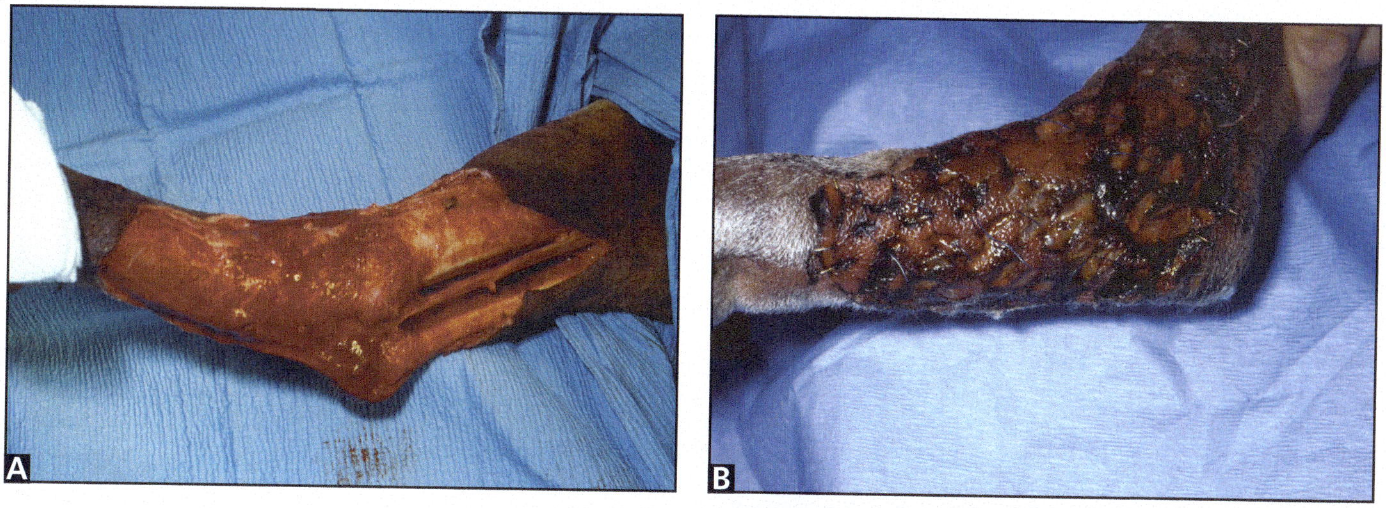

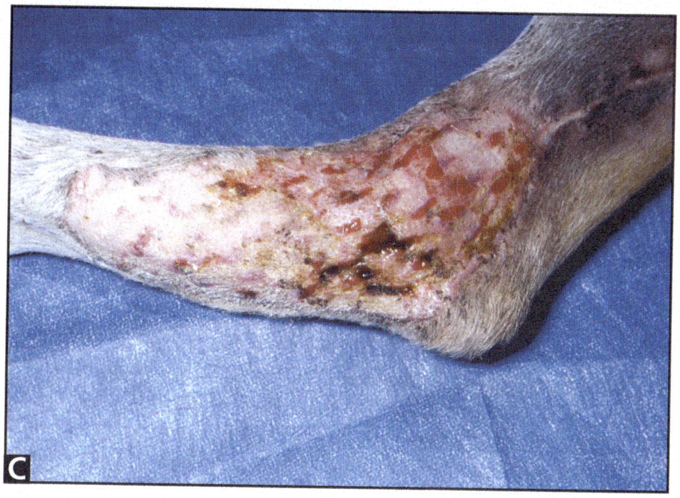

**Figure 3-87.** Full – thickness mesh skin graft to repair a wound over the tarsal area after tumor removal. **A.** Original wound. **B.** Mesh graft – 5 days postoperatively showing the cyanosis and edema of plasmatic imbibition. **C.** Mesh graft healed at – 21 days.

## Technique

Wounds that are trauma-induced, contaminated, and/or infected should receive staged debridement, if needed, and wound lavage. They should be treated with a topical antibiotic or antibacterial medication for a few days prior to grafting. Silver sulfadiazine or 0.2% nitrofurazone ointment have been found effective for the antimicrobial treatment. A wound healing stimulant (CarraVet Acemannan Wound Gel, Inc., Newnan, GA.; Intracell, Macleod Pharmaceuticals, Ft. Collins, CO; or Iamin Hydrating Gel Wound Dressing, Folica, Dayton, NJ) may also be used to stimulate formation of granulation tissue on the wound, especially if there is exposed bone. With the animal under general anesthesia or under the influence of a neuroleptanalgesic, the surface of the granulation tissue should be scraped with a No. 10 scalpel blade the day prior to surgery. This helps remove the surface microbial flora that are in the superficial 1 mm of this tissue and any unhealthy granulation tissue. After attaining hemostasis by pressure on the wound bed, it is bandaged with a nonadherent semiocclusive bandage (Telfa "Ouchless" Adhesive Pads, Covidien, Tyco/Health Care, Kendall, Mansfield, MA) that has a thin coating of gentamicin sulfate antibiotic ointment (Gentamicin sulfate ointment 0.1%, Fougera, Melville, NY). An absorbent secondary bandage wrap and tertiary adhesive tape wrap are applied. A metal splint is incorporated in the bandage. The bandage/splint should extend well above the carpus or tarsus, especially if the wound is over the carpus or tarsus.

At the time of surgery, the animal is placed in lateral recumbency with the wound exposed. The wound is protected with a sterile saline moistened surgical sponge. The distal limb and the lower craniolateral thoracic area are prepared for aseptic surgery.

If epithelium has begun to grow from the wound edges out over the granulation tissue, it is generally considered an indication that the granulation tissue is healthy enough to support a graft. Thumb forceps and a number 15 scalpel blade are used to remove any epithelium that has started to grow over the granulation tissue from the wound edges. The scalpel blade is used to incise vertical to the skin at the juncture of the haired skin with epithelium. After incising around the circumference of the wound, the scalpel blade is inserted horizontally under the leading edge of the epithelium parallel to the wound surface and back to the level of the vertical incision. The scalpel blade is advanced under

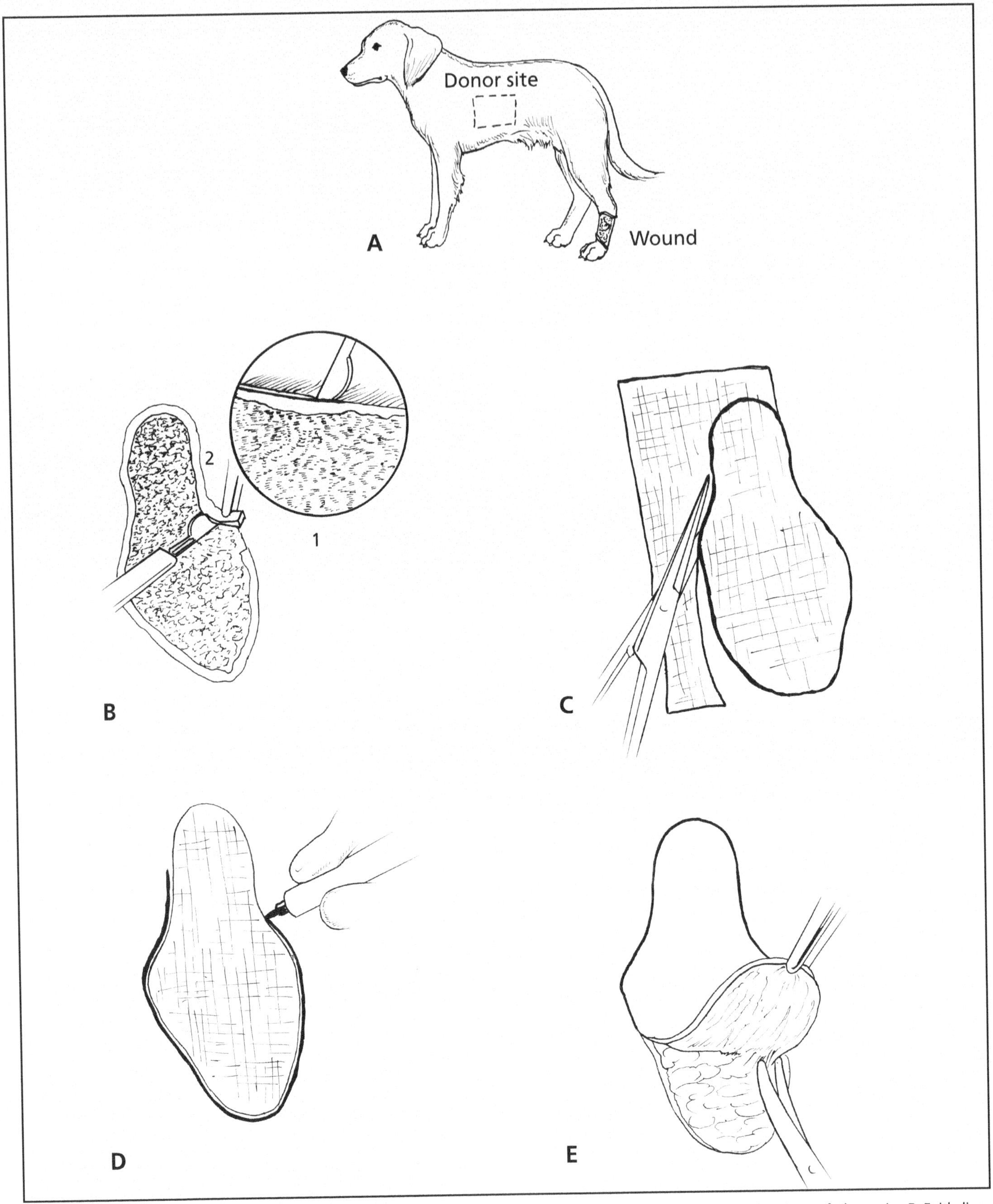


**Figure 3-88.** Full – thickness mesh graft to repair a distal pelvic limb skin defect. **A.** Dog with distal pelvic limb wound showing graft donor site. **B.** Epithelium being removed from wound edge. *Inset: (1)* Verticle incision at juncture of epithelium and haired skin. *(2)* Horizontal incision under the epithelium. **C.** Cutting a wound pattern from cloth. **D.** Tracing cloth pattern on the donor site. **E.** Removing the graft from the donor site.

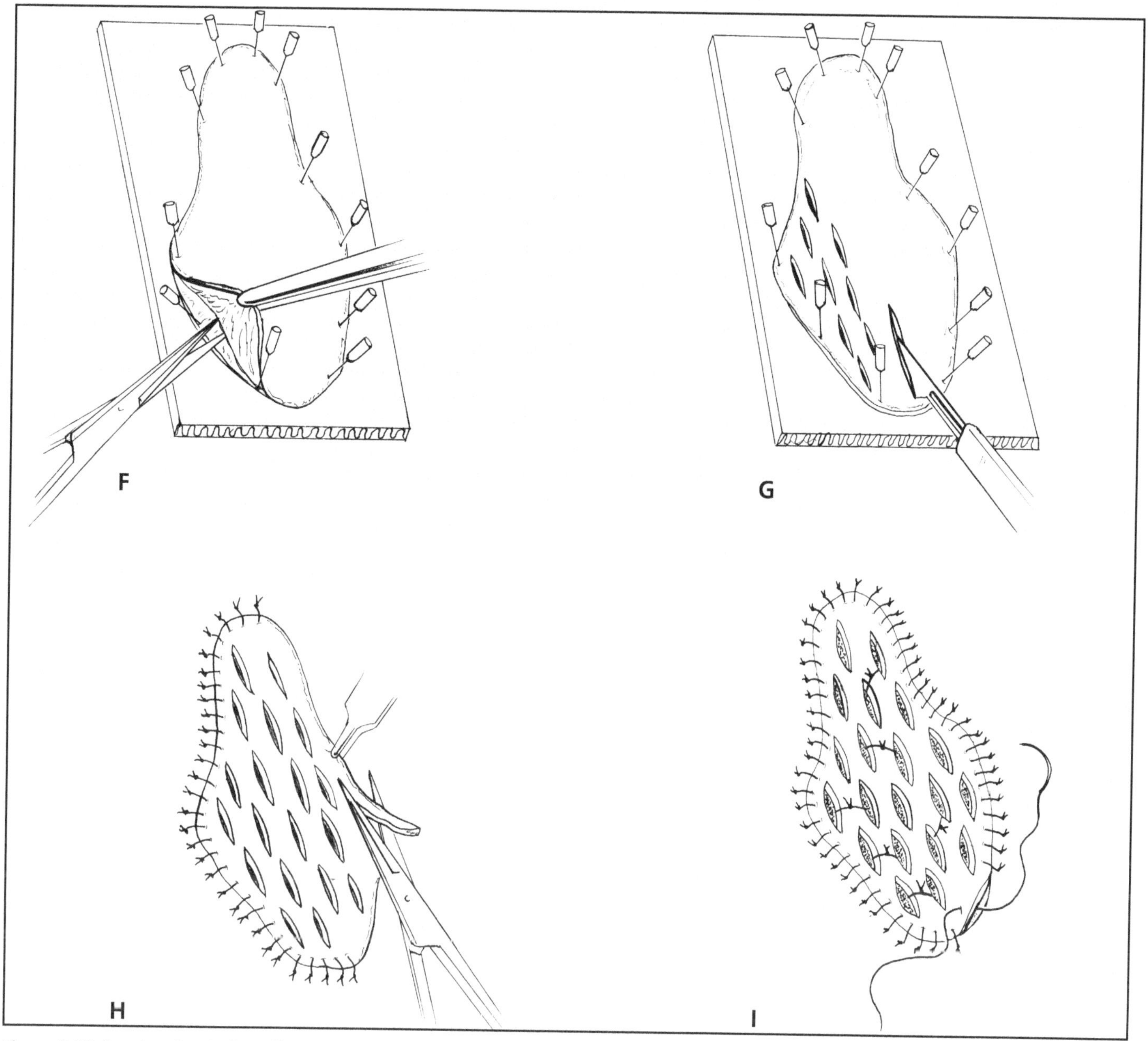


**Figure 3-88.** (continued) **F.** Graft is affixed to corrugated cardboard by hypodermic needles. Removing the subcutaneous tissue from the graft. **G.** Cutting mesh holes in the graft. **H.** Trimming the remaining edge of the graft after one edge is sutured. **I.** Graft being sutured in place with tacking sutures to immobilize it to the wound surface.

the epithelium around the wound while elevating the freed epithelium with thumb forceps (Figure 3-88B and insert). A piece of sterile cloth is then placed over the wound to obtain a blood imprint of the wound. The imprint of the wound edge will be especially prominent since it has just been freshened by removing the epithelium. The cloth is then cut with scissors so that it exactly matches the shape of the wound (Figure 3-88C). The cloth "pattern" is transferred to the lower craniolateral thoracic area, being careful not to turn the pattern over as it is transferred. A saline moistened gauze sponge is placed over the wound to keep it moist while the graft is harvested.

The pattern is positioned so that the direction of hair growth on the graft will be the same as the hair growth direction on the skin surrounding the wound. The edge of the pattern is then traced on the skin with a sterile skin marker, a sterile toothpick or sterile, splintered wooden applicator stick dipped in sterile methylene blue (Figure 3-88D).

After removing the pattern from the donor area, the traced line is incised with a No. 15 or 10 scalpel blade, and the graft is removed using thumb forceps and Metzenbaum scissors (Figure 3-88E). The graft is then placed dermal side up on a piece of sterile corrugated cardboard (i.e. piece of cardboard box). It is stretched and fixed to the cardboard with sterile hypodermic needles. All subcutaneous tissue is removed from the graft starting at one edge and advancing across the graft (Figure 3-88F). If subcutaneous tissue has been removed sufficiently, the dermis will have a cobblestone appearance when the graft is held under a surgery light and tilted back and forth. The bulbs of hair follicles give the dermis this cobblestone appearance.

With the graft still on the cardboard, a No. 11 scalpel blade is then used to cut parallel rows of staggered incisions in the graft. Stretching the graft across the bottom of a stainless steel surgical tray and cutting incisions while holding segments of skin under tension with the thumb and index finger of the opposite hand has been described. The incisions are made by starting at one edge of the graft and proceeding across the graft, making incisions approximately 1 cm long and 0.5 to 1.0 cm apart (Figure 3-88G) (See Figure 3-89). An alternative to hand meshing a graft is to remove it from the cardboard and place it dermal-side down on a mesh graft expansion unit. The unit is composed of parallel rows of notched blades. A teflon roller is rolled over the graft's epidermal surface to force it onto the blades, thus cutting parallel rows of staggered incisions in the graft (Figure 3-90). If incisions can be made parallel to the direction of hair growth, then hair regrowth will be more cosmetic on the graft because incisions will not have been made across hair follicles which damages more follicles. Thus, when the graft is placed on the limb, the direction of hair growth and direction of mesh incisions are generally parallel to the long axis of the limb. During the time that subcutaneous tissue is being removed and mesh incisions are being cut in the graft, it should be kept moist with physiologic saline.

If a graft has been hand meshed, it is removed from the cardboard and properly oriented on the wound,

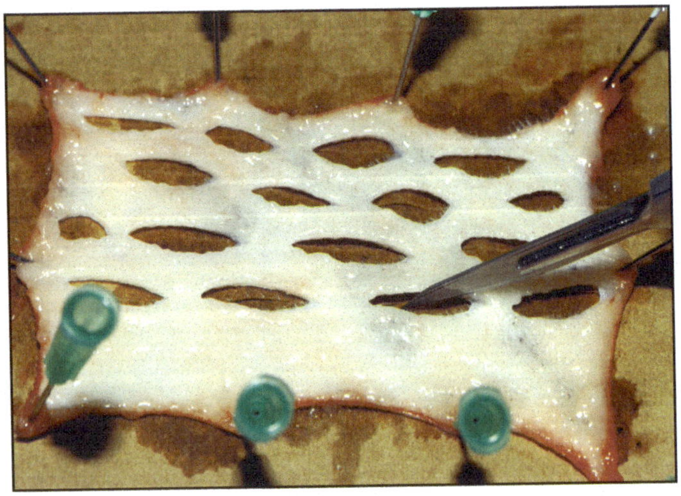

**Figure 3-89.** No. 11 scalpel blade being used to cut parallel staggered rows of slits in a full – thickness skin graft. (From Swaim SF: Skin grafts. In Slatter DH, ed.: Textbook of Small Animal Surgery, 3rd ed.: Philadelphia: WB Saunders, 2003, 328.

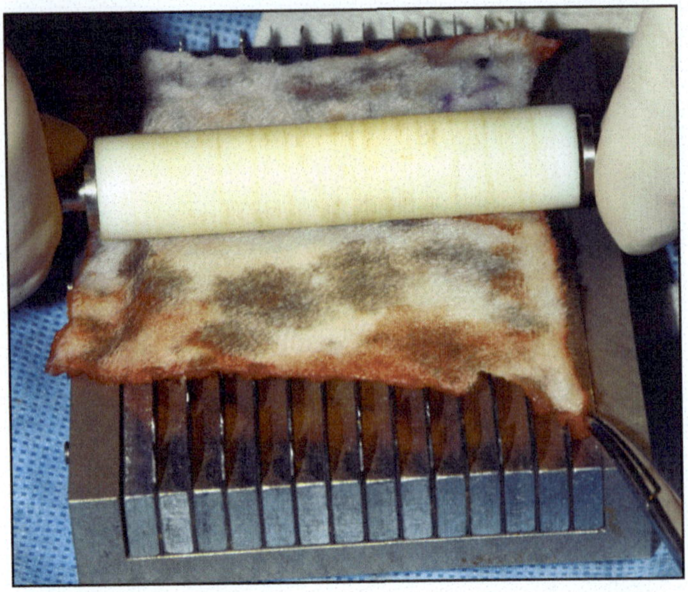

**Figure 3-90.** A skin graft on a mesh graft expansion unit with the Teflon roller to be passed over the graft to cut parallel rows of staggered incision.

3-0 monofilament nonabsorbable suture in a simple interrupted or simple continuous pattern is used to suture one edge of the graft to its corresponding wound edge. As an alternative, skin staples may be used to fix the graft edge in place. The graft is smoothed over the wound and affixed to the other wound edges at various points with a few simple interrupted tacking sutures or staples. It may be necessary to manipulate the graft slightly when placing these sutures to establish the best position for the graft. If the graft mesh incisions are not open after the graft has been tacked at the other edges, the tacking sutures or staples are removed and 2 to 3 mm of skin are trimmed from this edge of the graft before it is sutured or stapled in place (Figure 3-88H). This ensures expansion of the mesh incisions to allow fluid drainage from under the graft, thus allowing contact of the graft with the wound.

Further immobilization of the graft to the wound is accomplished by 3-0 monofilament nonabsorbable simple interrupted tacking sutures between adjacent slits at intermittent places in the graft. These tacking sutures are especially important at areas where a graft lies over a concavity on the wound to pull the graft in contact with the underlying wound bed to allow adequate vascularization of the graft at this area (Figure 3-88I).

The donor site is closed by undermining and advancing the skin edges together with "walking" sutures of 3-0 or 2-0 absorbable suture material, a simple continuous subcutaneous suture of 3-0 or 2-0 absorbable suture, and finally simple interrupted skin sutures of 3-0 or 2-0 monofilament nonabsorbable suture material or staples.

## Aftercare

A sterile absorbent nonadherent primary dressing pad (Telfa "Ouchless" Adhesive Pads, Covidien, Tyco Health Care, Kendall, Mansfield, MA) with a thin coating of gentamicin sulfate antibiotic ointment (Gentamicin sulfate ointment 0.1%, Fougera, Mellvile, NY) is placed over the graft. If the graft is on the forelimb, a modified "donut" bandage made from a soft padding material (Specialist Cast Padding, BSN Medical, Rutherford, NC) is placed over the carpal pad to keep pressure from the outer bandage and splint off of this pad. A similar modified "donut" bandage is placed over the area of the calcaneal tuberosity when the graft is on the pelvic limb to keep pressure off of the point of the hock. A secondary wrap of absorbent material (Kerlix Roll, Covidien, Tyco/ HealthCare Kendall, Mansfield, MA) is wrapped over this. Two-inch wide adhesive tape (Curity Standard Porous Tape, Covidien/Tyco HealthCare Kendall, Mansfield, MA) is used for the tertiary bandage layer. A metal splint with a paw cup is incorporated in the bandage to help immobilize the grafted area, especially if the graft is over the carpal area. The bandage and splint should extend to at least the midradial level. If the grafted area is over the tarsal or metatarsal area of the pelvic limb, a fiberglass casting tape splint (Vetcast Plus, Veterinary casting tape, 3M, St. Paul, MN) should be molded over the bandage to extend from the paw to the proximal tibial area. The splints are generally only needed for the first 10 to 14 days after grafting.

On subsequent bandage changes, if an animal tends to struggle during bandage changes, some form of sedation may be necessary in the early postoperative period to avoid movement of the graft. The bandage is changed daily for the first 7 postoperative days. For the first 2 days after grafting, grafts may appear anemic. Following this, the grafts may become cyanotic and edematous. During the healing process, they become less edematous and less cyanotic with a change in color to a deep red then pink. Occasionally, a graft will progress from the anemic appearance to a red or pink color without having a deep cyanotic color phase. In general, cyanosis is an acceptable color for a graft as long as its color progresses to red and pink. Colors that indicate a poor prognosis for the graft are black and white which indicate avascular necrosis. In addition, a hard crust or a macerated graft with lack of normal skin turgor are poor prognostic signs.

As mesh grafts heal, granulation tissue grows up into each of the mesh holes of the graft. Once granulation tissue is up in the mesh holes, epithelial tissue from the adjacent epidermis grows across the surface of the granulation tissue. As a result, drainage from the mesh holes decreases and bandage changes can be less frequent: every other day, then every third or fourth day, based on clinical judgement. Generally, bandaging is discontinued after 21 days. An alternative bandaging technique is to change bandages every other day for 10 days, followed by changes as needed for 2 more weeks. Sutures and/or staples at the graft edge and tacking sutures are removed at 7 to 10 days postoperatively.

When bandaging is discontinued, the dog will want to lick at the grafted area. Some initial licking at the graft is acceptable; however, continuous licking at the graft can cause damage to it. It is recommended that bandaging be discontinued in the morning of the first of 2 or 3 days (i.e. a weekend) when the owner can spend time with the animal to deter it from molesting the graft, e.g. walking or playing with a dog. If the animal persists in licking at the graft when bandaging is discontinued at 21 days, it may be an indication of abnormal sensations in the graft which could be related to reinnervation of the graft. Keeping the graft under a bandage for another 7 to 10 days may be helpful in situations such as this.

Infection does not occur often. When it is encountered, it is characterized by a tenacious exudate and areas of the graft that are white and do not have normal skin turgor. A culture and sensitivity testing should be performed. As the bandages are removed, any exudate that is present should be very gently removed by blotting with a 1:40 dilution of chlorhexidine diacetate (Nolvasan solution, Ft. Dodge Animal Health, Ft. Dodge, IA) or gluconate (ChlorhexiDerm Disinfectant, Dermatologics in Veterinary Medicine Pharmaceuticals, Inc., Miami, FL) solution. Devitalized graft segments will be very dark or white and nonadherent. These segments should be debrided. An absorbent surgical sponge coated with antibiotic ointment should be placed on the wound followed by the remainder of the bandage as described above. The bandage should be changed twice daily, with staged debridement as needed, until the graft appears normal and the exudate subsides. When culture and sensitivity results become available, the topical antibiotic can be changed as indicated.

Occasionally, a partial-thickness take of a graft occurs. With this, the deeper portion of the dermis revascularizes and heals; however, the superficial portion of the dermis and the epidermis are lost. When this occurs, the superficial slough is debrided as needed at each bandage change. Although it has been recommended to leave nonviable areas until the remainder of the graft has healed, careful removal of such tissue eliminates areas where bacteria could grow. The healed dermis that remains will reepithelialize and provide covering for the wound; however, due to loss of hair follicles in the superficial slough, there will be a sparse hair growth on the graft.

If the full-thickness of a mesh graft is lost, the wound should be treated as an open wound, allowing it to heal by contraction and epithelialization as much as it will. The wound can then be regrafted if healing is not sufficient. An alternative is to treat the wound as an open wound until it begins to reepithelialize from the wound edges, and then regraft the wound.

## Advantages and Disadvantages

The mesh incisions of a mesh graft provide flexibility so that it conforms better to concave and convex surfaces as well as irregular edges. Grafts meshed on a mesh graft expansion unit are more expansible because they expand in more than one direction; whereas, those meshed by hand expand in only one direction. The tacking sutures through the mesh incisions immobilize the graft to the wound surface, making it more stable. The granulation tissue plugs that grow up into the mesh incisions also help immobilize the graft. In addition, vessels can grow laterally from each granulation tissue plug into the edge of adjacent dermis (Figure 3-91). Thus, the area from which a graft can revascularize is increased with a mesh graft. The mesh incisions allow blood, serum and exudate to drain from under the graft, thus allowing the graft to contact the wound surface better for revascularization. In addition, the mesh incisions also allow expansion of the graft so a smaller segment of skin can cover a larger defect. With proper application and management, survival of mesh grafts may be 90 to 100%. In general, mesh grafts heal quickly on cats. Their skin is thin, and grafts revascularize and heal in place quickly. Thus, the length of time for postoperative bandaging on cats is usually shorter than on dogs.

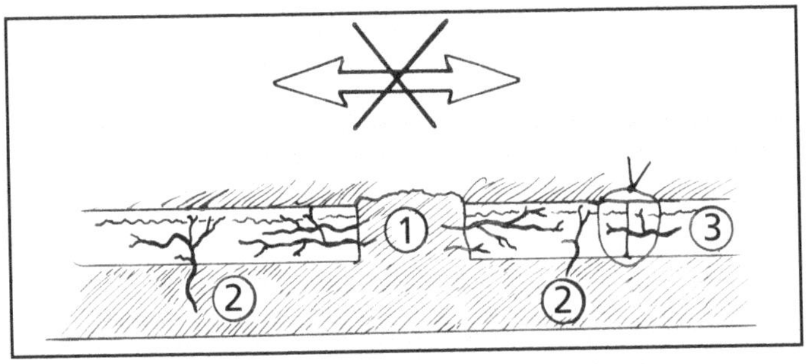


**Figure 3-91.** Cross section of a mesh graft hole. Advantages of mesh grafts. Granulation tissue that grows into mesh holes helps immobilize the graft on the wound *(double headed arrow and "x" indicates no graft movement)*. Grafts have added area for revascularization – *(1)* from edges of granulation tissue in each mesh hole. Grafts also revascularize from *(2)* wound surface and *(3)* dermis at wound edge.

A disadvantage of mesh grafts is their initial uncosmetic appearance early in the wound healing process; however, as the grafts heal, the mesh incisions become less noticeable as they heal by contraction and hair regrows on the graft (Figure 3-92A & B). The more a mesh graft is expanded, the less cosmetic it appears initially, but too little initial expansion may result in poor drainage of blood, serum, and exudate from under the graft which in turn results in poor graft healing. If an animal tends to produce excess granulation tissue, that tissue may grow up through the mesh incisions and partially overgrow the graft surface. This can mechanically impede wound contraction and epithelialization. Topical application of a steroid usually reduces this granulation tissue.

The hair regrowth on a graft is variable and unpredictable. There may be a full regrowth of hair on some grafts. Other grafts will have a sparse regrowth of hair, especially with partial-thickness graft healing.

# Suggested Readings


1. Basher A: Foot Injuries in Dogs and Cats. Compend Contin Educ Pract Vet 16:1159, 1994.
2. Birchard SJ, Smeak DD: Selected skin graft and reconstructive techniques. *In* Birchard SJ, Sherding RG, eds.: Saunders Manual of Small Animal Practice, 2nd ed.: Philadelphia: WB Saunders, 2000, 392.
3. Birchard SJ, Smeak DD: Selected skin graft and reconstructive techniques. In Birchard SJ, Sherding RG, eds.: Saunders Manual of Small Animal Practice, 3rd ed.: St. Louis: Saunders – Elsevier, 2006, 557.
4. Bohling MW, Swaim SF: Skin grafts. In Tobias KM, Johnston SA, eds.: Veterinary Surgery, Small Animal, Vol. 2: St. Louis: Elsevier – Saunders, 2012, 1291.
5. Fowler D: Distal limb and paw injuries: Vet Clin No Am Small Anim Pract. 36: 819, 2006.
6. Gibbs A: Skin reconstruction techniques: Full-thickness mesh grafts. Vet Med 99:882, 2004.
7. Hedlund CS: Surgery of the integumentary system. *In* Fossum TW, ed.: Small Animal Surgery, 2nd ed.: St. Louis: Mosby, 2002, 134.
8. Hedlund CS: Surgery of the integumentary system. In Fossum TW, ed.: Small Animal Surgery, 3rd ed.: St. Louis: Mosby, 2007, 159.
9. MacPhail CM: Surgery of the integumentary system. In Fossum TW, ed.: Small Animal Surgery, 4th ed.: St. Louis: Mosby, 2013, 190.
10. Pavletic MM: Atlas of Small Animal Reconstructive Surgery, 2nd ed: Philadelphia: WB Saunders, 1999, 275.
11. Pavletic MM: Atlas of Small Animal Wound Management and Reconstructive Surgery, 3rd ed.: Ames, IA: Wiley – Blackwell, 2010, 403.
12. Pope ER: Mesh grafting. Vet Clin North Am, Small Anim Pract 20:177, 1990.
13. Pope ER: Mesh skin grafting. *In* Bojrab MJ, ed.: Current Techniques in Small Animal Surgery, 4th ed.: Baltimore: Williams and Wilkins, 1998, 603.
14. Pope ER: Skin grafting in small animal surgery. Part II. Full-thickness skin grafting techniques. Compend Contin Educ Pract Vet 10:1068, 1988.

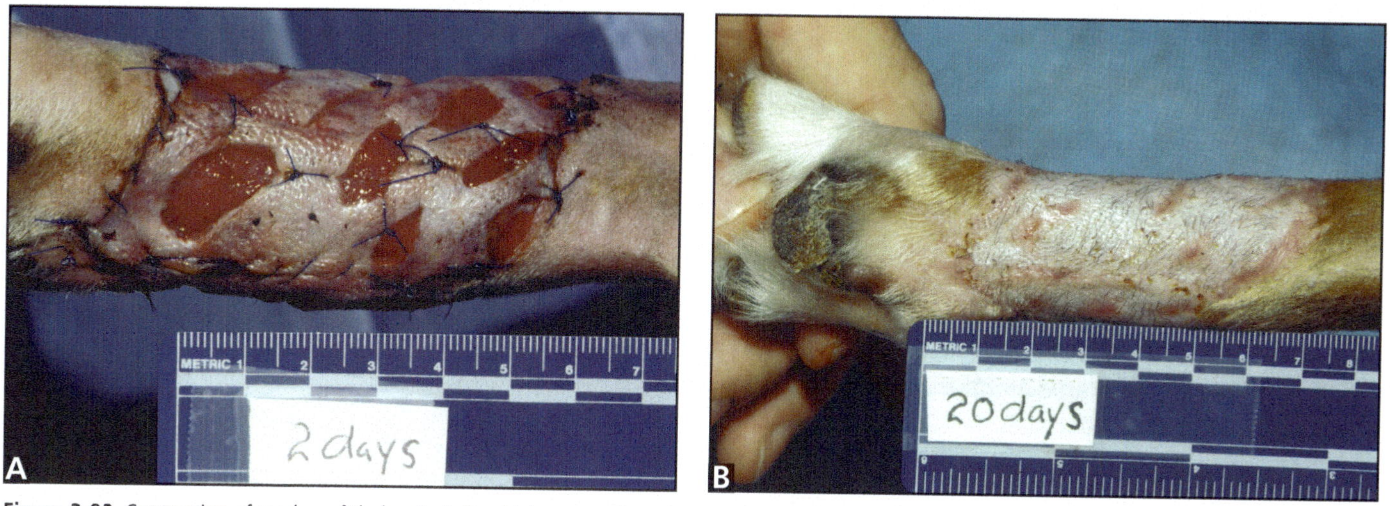


**Figure 3-92.** Contraction of mesh graft holes. **A.** Full – thickness mesh graft on a dog's distal limb with simple interrupted sutures between some mesh holes to anchor the graft to the wound. The graft is expanded with large mesh holes. **B.** Graft after it has healed showing contraction of mesh openings. (From Swaim SF: Skin grafts. In Slatter DH: Textbook of Small Animal Surgery, 3rd ed.: Phiadelphia, 2003, 334.

15. Swaim SF: Principles of mesh grafting. Compend Contin Educ Pract Vet 4:194, 1982.
16. Swaim SF: The full-thickness mesh graft. Vet Med 81:524, 1986.
17. Swaim SF: Wound management of the distal limbs and paws: Reconstruction and salvage. Vet Med Rep 2:128, 1990.
18. Swaim SF: Skin grafts. *In* Slatter DH, ed.: Textbook of Small Animal Surgery, 3rd ed.: Philadelphia: WB Saunders, 2003, 321.
19. Swaim SF: Skin grafts. *In* Harari J, ed.: Small Animal Surgery Secrets. Philadelphia: Hanley and Belfus, 2000, 62.
20. Swaim SF, Henderson RA: Small Animal Wound Management, 2nd ed.: Baltimore: Williams and Wilkins, 1997, 295.
21. Swaim SF, Pope ER, Lee AH, et al: Evaluation of a practical skin grafting technique. J Am Anim Hosp Assoc 20:637, 1984.
22. White RAS: Skin grafting. *In* Fowler D, Williams JM, eds.: BSAVA Manual of Canine and Feline Wound Management and Reconstruction. Shurdington, Cheltenham, UK: BSAVA, 1999, 83.
23. White RAS: Free skin grafting. In Williams J, Moores A, eds.: BSAVA Manual of Canine and Feline Wound Management and Reconstruction, 2nd ed.: Glouster (UK): BSAVA, 2009, 144.

# Strip Grafts

## Definition and Indications

Strip grafts are strips of full-thickness skin that are 5 mm wide. They are placed in linear parallel grooves that have been cut in the granulation tissue of a wound. The grooves are approximately 2 mm deep and 3 to 5 mm apart. These grafts provide skin coverage for defects where local flaps or moving local tissue cannot be used for wound closure, such as distal limb wounds (Figure 3-93A & B and Figure 3-94A). Strip grafts are indicated for wounds with low grade infection or irregular surfaces. Smaller wounds and wounds in areas not subjected to excessive wear or external trauma lend themselves to strip grafts. Wounds that are parallel to the long axis of the limb are particularly suited for strip grafting. A healthy bed of granulation tissue is necessary for strip grafting.

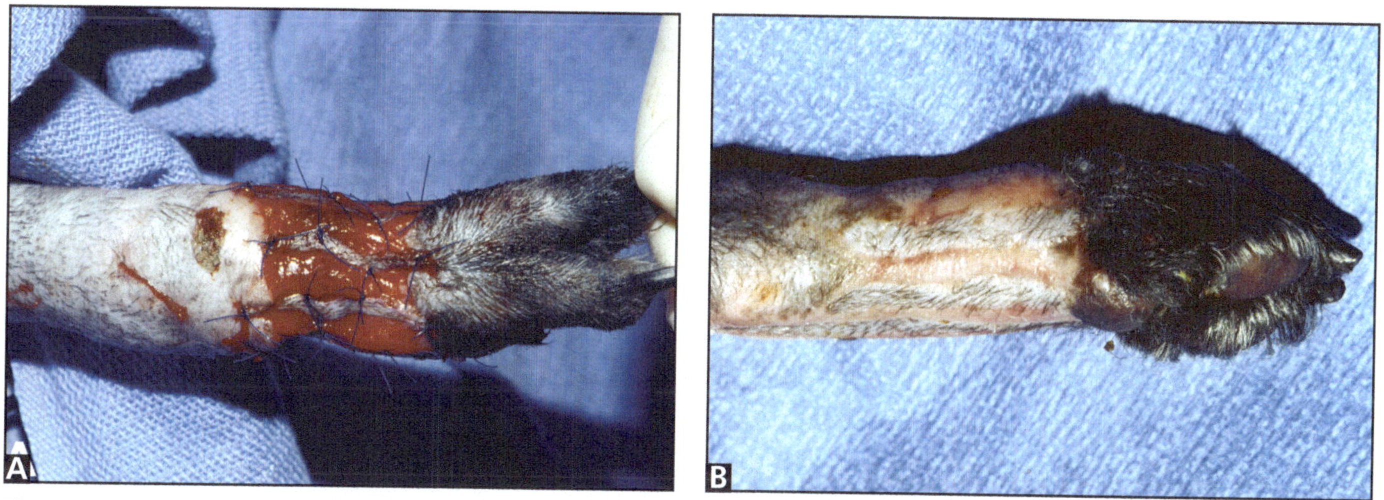


**Figure 3-93.** Strip grafts for distal limb wound repair. **A.** Strip grafts have been placed and sutured in grooves cut in granulation tissue. **B.** Healed strip grafts. Epithelium has covered the area between grafts and grafts are becoming wider. (From Swaim SF: Skin grafts. In Slatter DH, ed.: Textbook of Small Animal Surgery, 3rd ed.: Philadelphia: WB Saunders, 2003, 334).

## Technique

The animal is placed in lateral recumbency with the affected area exposed. The wound surface is wiped with a surgical sponge wet with a 1:40 dilution of chlorhexidine diacetate (Nolvasan solution, Ft. Dodge Animal Health, Ft. Dodge, IA) or gluconate (ChlorhexiDerm Disinfectant, Dermatologics in Veterinary Medicine Pharmaceuticals, Inc., Miami, FL) solution. A surgical sponge moistened with the same solution is used to cover the wound while the area around the wound and the lower craniolateral thoracic area are prepared for aseptic surgery.

The wound is prepared for grafting by incising the granulation tissue with a No. 15 scalpel blade, to create parallel longitudinal incisions about 2 mm deep and approximately 3 to 5 mm apart (Figure 3-94B). As the granulation tissue is incised, it usually retracts, to provide a groove wide enough to accommodate a strip graft. If the granulation tissue does not retract sufficiently, the scalpel blade may be used to widen the groove. Strips of umbilical tape or gauze are compressed into the grooves to control hemorrhage for 5 minutes. The wound should be covered with a sterile saline-soaked sponge while preparing the grafts.

To prepare the grafts, parallel lines 5 mm apart are drawn horizontally on the lower craniolateral thoracic skin. The lines can be drawn with a sterile skin marking pen, a sterile, splintered wooden applicator stick, or a sterile toothpick dipped in sterile methylene blue. For long wounds, they must be the same length as the recipient grooves. The number of strips created will

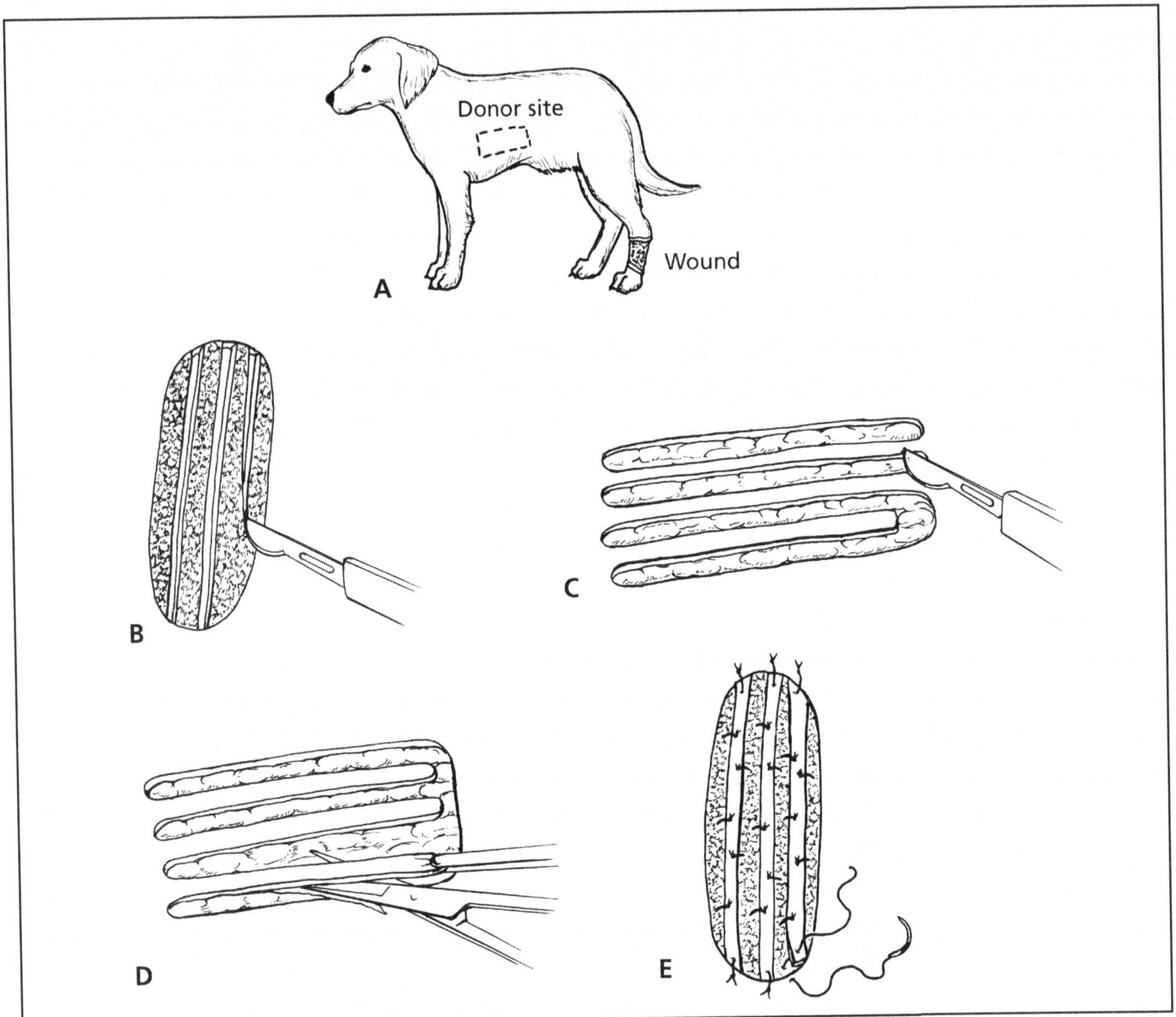


**Figure 3-94.** Strip grafts to repair a pelvic limb wound. **A.** Dog with limb wound and showing donor site of skin strips. **B.** Grooves being cut in granulation tissue. **C.** Strip grafts cut and one end of each strip being cut free. **D.** Subcutaneous tissue being removed from strip grafts with scissors. **E.** Suturing strip grafts into grooves. (After Swaim SF, Henderson RA: Small Animal Wound Management, 2nd ed.: Baltimore: Williams & Wilkins, 1997, 312.

be one less than the number of lines drawn. The strip grafts are created as adjacent parallel lines and one of their connecting ends are incised with a No. 15 scalpel blade (Figure 3-94C). Thumb forceps are used to grasp the cut end of each graft. The graft is elevated by blunt dissection with scissors as traction is placed on the graft with the thumb forceps. Scissors are run down the dermal side of the graft to remove subcutaneous tissue as the graft is held under tension (Figure 3-94D). Although the grafts were measured at 5 mm wide, when cut they will undergo primary contraction to about 2 mm wide. Thus, they will fit into the grooves that have been cut in the granulation tissue of the wound.

An alternative technique for harvesting strip grafts is to excise a rectangular segment of skin from the donor area which is equal in length to the length of the defect. The width of the rectangle is estimated by the number of strips required, the width of the skin strips, and the space between each strip after it is placed in the wound. The rectangle of skin can be affixed to a piece of sterile cardboard in the manner described for preparing mesh grafts. All subcutaneous tissue is removed from the skin and then strips of skin 3 to 5 mm wide are cut from the rectangular segment of skin.

Each strip is placed in a previously cut groove with the direction of the hair growth on the graft being the same as that on the surrounding skin. The graft is anchored in the groove with a simple interrupted 3-0 monofilament nonabosrbable suture placed at each end of the strip. The bandage placed over the wound is usually sufficient to hold the graft in place; however, additional sutures may be placed at intervals along the strips to further anchor each strip into its groove (Figure 3-94E).

The graft donor site on the thorax is closed by undermining and advancing the wound edges together with "walking" suture, of 3-0 or 2-0 absorbable suture material, a simple continuous subcutaneous suture of 3-0 or 2-0 absorbable suture and finally simple interrupted skin sutures of 3-0 or 2-0 monofilament nonabsorbable suture material or staples.

### Aftercare

The aftercare of strip grafts is the same as for mesh grafts (see Mesh Grafts in this chapter).

### Advantages and Disadvantages

No special equipment is needed for strip grafting, and the procedure is easily accomplished. These grafts revascularize quickly because they are in granulation tissue grooves, thus allowing vessel ingrowth from the bottom and sides of the groove. Due to their presence in grooves, strip grafts are less subject to damage from bandage movement on the wound surface. The open nature of the grafts allows fluid to drain from the wound surface for absorption into a bandage. As the grafts heal, they tend to widen, and epithelium grows from the edge of each graft to cover the granulation tissue between the strips. As they mature, they become more cosmetic; however, the final cosmetic appearance of strip grafts may not be as good as that of a mesh graft.

## Suggested Readings

1. Bohling MW, Swaim SF: Skin grafts. In Tobias KM, Johnston SA, eds.: Veterinary Surgery, Small Animal, Vol. 2: St. Louis: Elsevier – Saunders, 2012, 1271
2. Hedlund CS: Surgery of the integumentary system. *In* Fossum TW, ed.: Small Animal Surgery, 2nd ed.: St. Louis: Mosby, 2002, 134.
3. Hedlund CS: Surgery of the integumentary system. In Fossum TW, ed.: Small Animal Surgery, 3rd ed.: St. Louis, Mosby, 2007, 159.
4. MacPhail CM: Surgery of the integumentary system. In Fossum TW, ed.: Small Animal Surgery, 4th ed.: St. Louis: Mosby, 2013, 190.
5. Pavletic MM: Atlas of Small Animal Reconstructive Surgery, 2nd ed: Philadelphia: WB Saunders, 1999, 275.
6. Pavletic MM: Skin grafting techniques. Bojrab MJ, ed.: Current Techniques in Small Animal Surgery, 4th ed.: Baltimore: Williams and Wilkins, 1998, 585.
7. Pavletic MM: Atlas of Small Animal Wound Management and Reconstructive Surgery, 3rd ed.: Ames, IA: Wiley – Blackwell, 2010, 403.
8. Swaim SF: Skin grafts. Vet Clin North Am Small Anim Pract 20:147, 1990.
9. Swaim SF: Wound management of the distal limbs and paws: Reconstruction and salvage. Vet Med Rep 2:128, 1990.
10. Swaim SF: Skin grafts. *In* Slatter DH, ed.: Textbook of Small Animal Surgery, 3rd ed.: Philadelphia: WB Saunders, 2003, p 321.
11. Swaim SF: Skin grafts. *In* Harari J, ed.: Small Animal Surgery Secrets. Philadelphia: Hanley and Belfus, 2000, 62.
12. Swaim SF, Lee AH, Newton JC, McGuire JA: Evaluation of strip skin grafts in dogs. J Am Anim Hosp Assoc 23:115, 1987.
13. Swaim SF, Henderson RA: Small Animal Wound Management, 2nd ed.: Baltimore: Williams and Wilkins, 1997, 295.

## Wounds with Exposed Bones and Joints

### General Information

It is not uncommon to have distal limb wounds that have exposed bones and joints. These wounds often, but not necessarily, have nonapposable edges that have no potential for apposition. Due to the close proximity of the bones and joints to the overlying skin, trauma and surgical procedures may leave these structures exposed. A common source of injury resulting in exposed bones and joints is the anatomical degloving wound; whereby, an automobile tire passes over the limb. Shearing forces are applied to the skin and subcutaneous tissue that separate them from underlying muscle and fascia. Forces are often such that all soft tissue is sheared from the bones (Figure 3-95). In addition, crushing and abrasion are also associated with the injury. Crushing can result in single or multiple fractures and damage to blood vessels and nerves. Abrasion grinds away skin and underlying soft tissue as well as bone. When abrasion involves joints, the loss of ligamentous support and joint capsules results in an unstable, open joint.

Physiologic degloving occurs when the skin and subcutaneous tissue on the distal limb are damaged, usually by an automobile tire. However, the skin is still intact, but it has been damaged to the extent that is will slough after a few days. Fractures and damage to blood vessels and nerves can accompany this type of injury.

Another situation that can result in exposed bones and joints is radical soft tissue tumor excision on the distal limb.

The techniques indicated for treatment of wounds with exposed bones and joints vary with the condition. Techniques to stabilize fractures and unstable joints are covered in the orthopedic section of the text (Part Two: Orthopedic Injuries). Techniques indicated to cover exposed bones and joints include allowing the wound to heal by second intention, moving local skin, or using grafts or flaps. With these techniques, it is necessary to have the bone or joints covered with granulation tissue, especially if second intention healing or a skin graft is to be used.

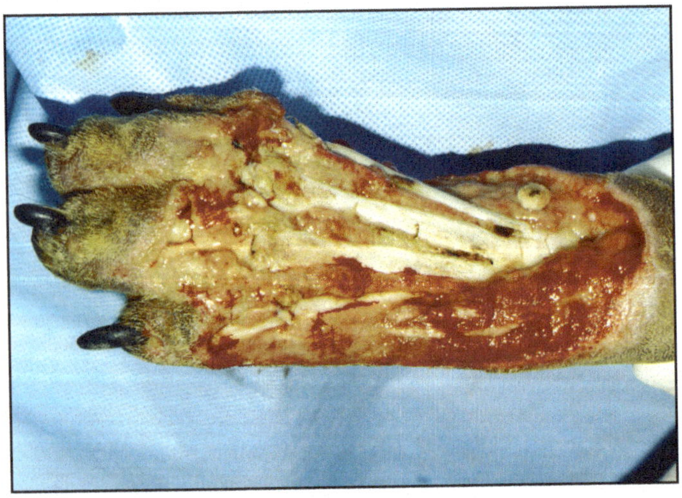

**Figure 3-95.** Distal limb degloving wound with soft tissue sheared off of bone, exposing metatarsal bones.

# Bone Coverage by Granulation Tissue

## Definition and Indications

Bone drilling (ferrage) entails drilling small holes in the bone to the level of the marrow cavity and allowing a clot to form over the bone. The clot is well attached to the bone at the drill holes (Figure 3-96A-C). Fibroblasts and capillaries invade the clot's fibrin network as it serves as a lattice for fibroplasia and neovascularization of the granulation tissue.

## Technique

After lavage and staged debridement of the wound a topical antibiotic or antibacterial medication is placed on the wound with a bandage cover. In addition, the dog is started on systemic antibiotics (e.g. cefadroxil [Cefatabs, Ft. Dodge Animal Health, Ft. Dodge, IA] and enrofloxacin [Baytril, Bayer Corp., Shawnee Mission, KS]). Bandaging, with daily change, is continued until healthy granulation tissue has developed around the exposed bone, forming a depression with bone at the bottom. This usually takes place in 7 to 10 days.

After granulation tissue is present, a 1.5 mm diameter drill bit and twist drill are used to drill a series of holes in the exposed bone (See Figure 3-96A). The holes are approximately 5 mm apart. When drilling a metacarpal or metatarsal bone, the holes should be centered in the bone to allow maximum exposure of the medullary canal and they should be oriented along the length of the bone. Drilling should be done judiciously, taking into consideration the size of the bone and the condition and severity of the wound. When abrasion has weakened the bone due to loss of cortical bone, drilling can predispose to fracture. To enhance the formation of a clot over the bone, blood can be drawn from a peripheral vein, placed in the depression over the holes and allowed to clot (Figure 3-96B).

## Aftercare

After the bone has been drilled, the wound should be bandaged with a topical gentamicin sulfate antibiotic ointment (Gentamicin sulfate ointment 0.1%, Fougera, Melville, NY) on a nonadherent semiocclusive pad (Telfa "Ouchless" Adhesive Pads, Covidien, Tyco/Health Care, Kendall, Mansfield, MA). The bandage should be changed daily, leaving any clot over the bone undisturbed (See Figure 3-96C). Extensions of the clot down through the ferrage holes help secure the clot to the bone surface. The clot may not completely fill the defect or it may contract over 7 days. However, the clot is converting to granulation tissue during the 7 to 10 day

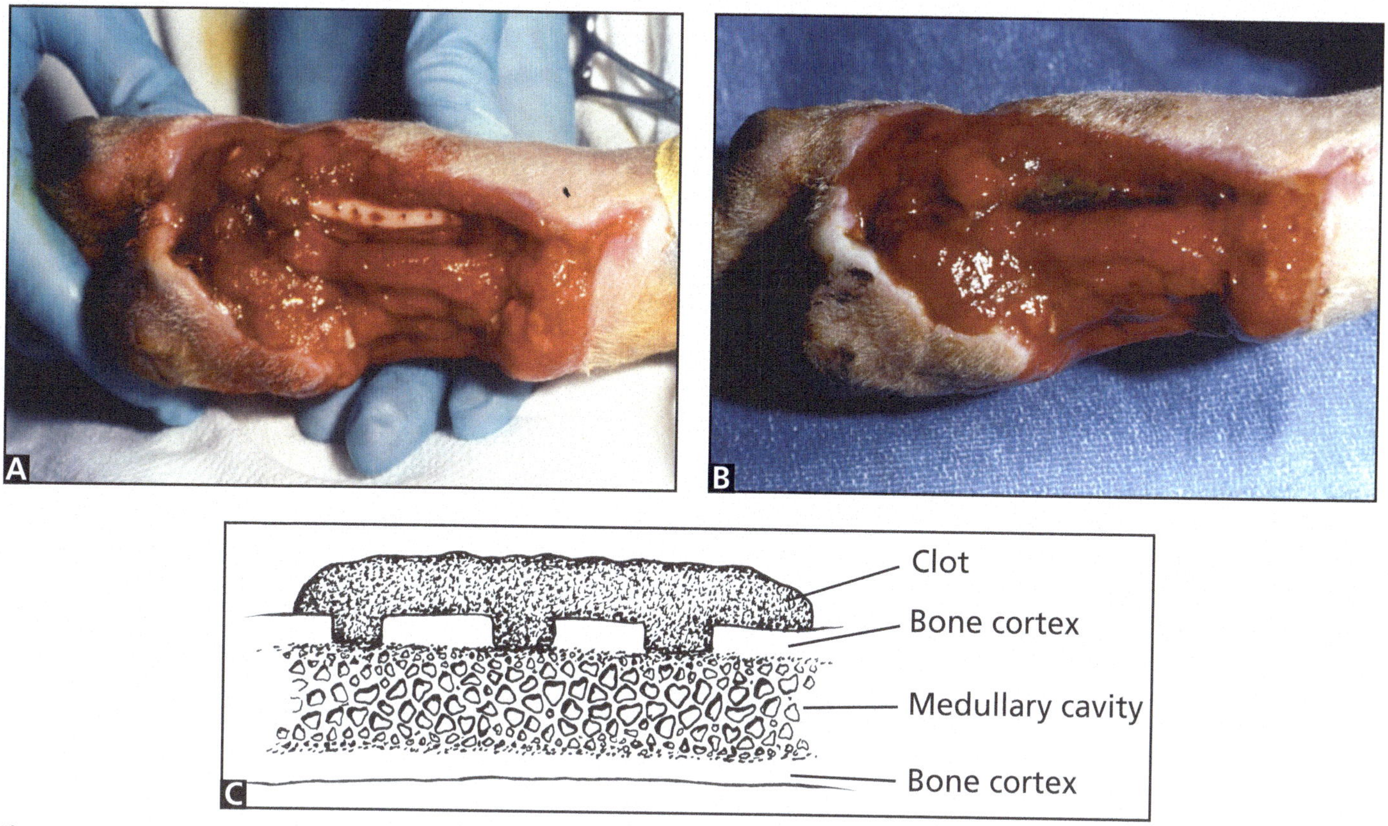


**Figure 3-96.** Coverage of exposed bone. **A.** Holes have been drilled in a metatarsal bone. **B.** A clot has formed over the bone. **C.** The clot is attached over the bone by extensions down through the drill holes. (From Swaim SF, Pope ER: Early management of limb degloving injuries. Sem Vet Med Surg (Small Anim) 3:274, 1988.

period. At this time, the edges of the granulation tissue may be scraped to allow another clot to form. It will also be converted to granulation tissue. In addition, a wound healing stimulant (CarraVet Acemannan Wound Gel, Carravet, Inc., Newnan, GA) can be applied topically to enhance granulation tissue formation. Systemic antibiotics should be continued for 7 to 10 days after drilling.

## Advantages and Disadvantages

Ferrage provides bone coverage and protection, first by a clot then by granulation tissue. If the wound is to heal by second intention, contraction proceeds more rapidly once granulation tissue is continuous within the wound. The time necessary for bandaging is thus shortened. For reconstruction, the granulation tissue provides a vascular base for graft or flap placement.

The technique has the disadvantage that it may predispose to a fracture of the drilled bone, especially if it is weakened by abrasion in the initial trauma, and in cats where the bones are smaller.

If bone protrudes above the level of the wound, it will usually not cover with granulation tissue. Exposed, desiccated bone that is not necessary to the salvage of the limb should be excised below the surface of the granulation bed and treated accordingly until granulation tissue covers the area.

# Suggested Readings

1. Clark GN: Bone perforation to enhance wound healing over exposed bones in dogs with shearing injuries. J Amer Anim Hosp Assoc 37:215, 2001.
2. Lee AH, Swaim SF, Newton JC, et al: Wound healing over denuded bone. J. Am Anim Hosp Assoc 23:75. 1987
3. Pavletic MM. Atlas of Small Animal Reconstructive Surgery, 2nd ed.: Philadelphia: WB Saunders, 1999, 41.
4. Pavletic MM: Atlas of Small Animal Wound Management and Reconstructive Surgery, 3rd ed.. Ames, IA: Wiley – Blackwell, 2010, 31, 127.
5. Swaim SF, Pope ER: Early management of limb degloving injuries. Sem Vet Med Surg (Small Anim) 3:274, 1988.
6. Swaim SF, Gillette RL: An update on wound medications and dressings. Compend Contin Educ Pract Vet 20:1133, 1998.
7. Swaim SF, Henderson RA: Small Animal Wound Management, 2nd ed.: Baltimore: Williams and Wilkins, 1997, 295.

# Chapter 4

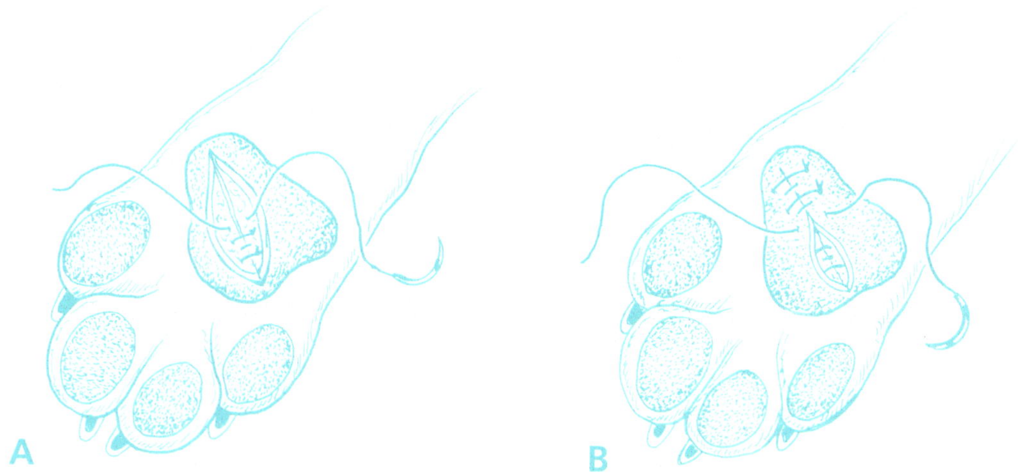


## Paw Wounds

Steven F. Swaim, D.V.M., M.S.

# General Information

## Hemostasis

A bloodless surgical field facilitates any procedures being performed. The following techniques may be used for hemostasis.

1. For procedures that last 30 minutes or less, a tourniquet can be applied on the limb just below the tarsus or proximal to the carpus by drawing a ½-inch-diameter Penrose drain around the limb and clamping it adjacent to the limb with hemostatic forceps (Figure 4-1A & B).

2. For procedures that take longer than 30 minutes, a sterile elastic bandage (Vetrap, 3M Animal Care Products, St. Paul, MN) can be wrapped from the paw up onto the limb to the radial humeral or the femoral-tibial area. An incision is made through the elastic bandage down to the surgical site (Figure 4-1C & D). A pneumatic tourniquet or pediatric blood pressure cuff can also be used for hemostasis.

3. The paw should be elevated above the level of the heart during surgery by placing padding under the limb (Figure 4-2).

# Dorsal Digital Wounds

Occasionally there will be damage to the skin dorsal surface of individual digits. The practitioner should assess the extent of the wound, i.e. the size of the defect and the amount of tissue available for reconstruction. Depending on the size of the wound, the techniques to be used for reconstruction would be those described for wounds of the carpal-metacarpal/tarsal-metatarsal areas or modifications thereof. Often wounds on the dorsum of the digits involve multiple digits. If there is sufficient interdigital skin remaining, its use in reconstructing the dorsal digital surfaces should be considered (Figure 4-3). If there is not sufficient interdigital skin, it will be necessary to consider a mesh graft or some form of flap for reconstructing the area. When interdigital skin is present in a small amount, it should be removed, thus making it like a paw where circumstances have resulted in loss of both dorsal paw and interdigital skin (Figure 4-4). This will allow the axial and abaxial surfaces of the involved adjacent digits to heal together (fuse) while the graft or flap on the dorsal surface of the digits heals in place. To enhance the fusion of the axial and abaxial digital surfaces interrupted absorbable sutures can be used judiciously to suture the digits together. However, care should be taken to try to avoid incorporating the

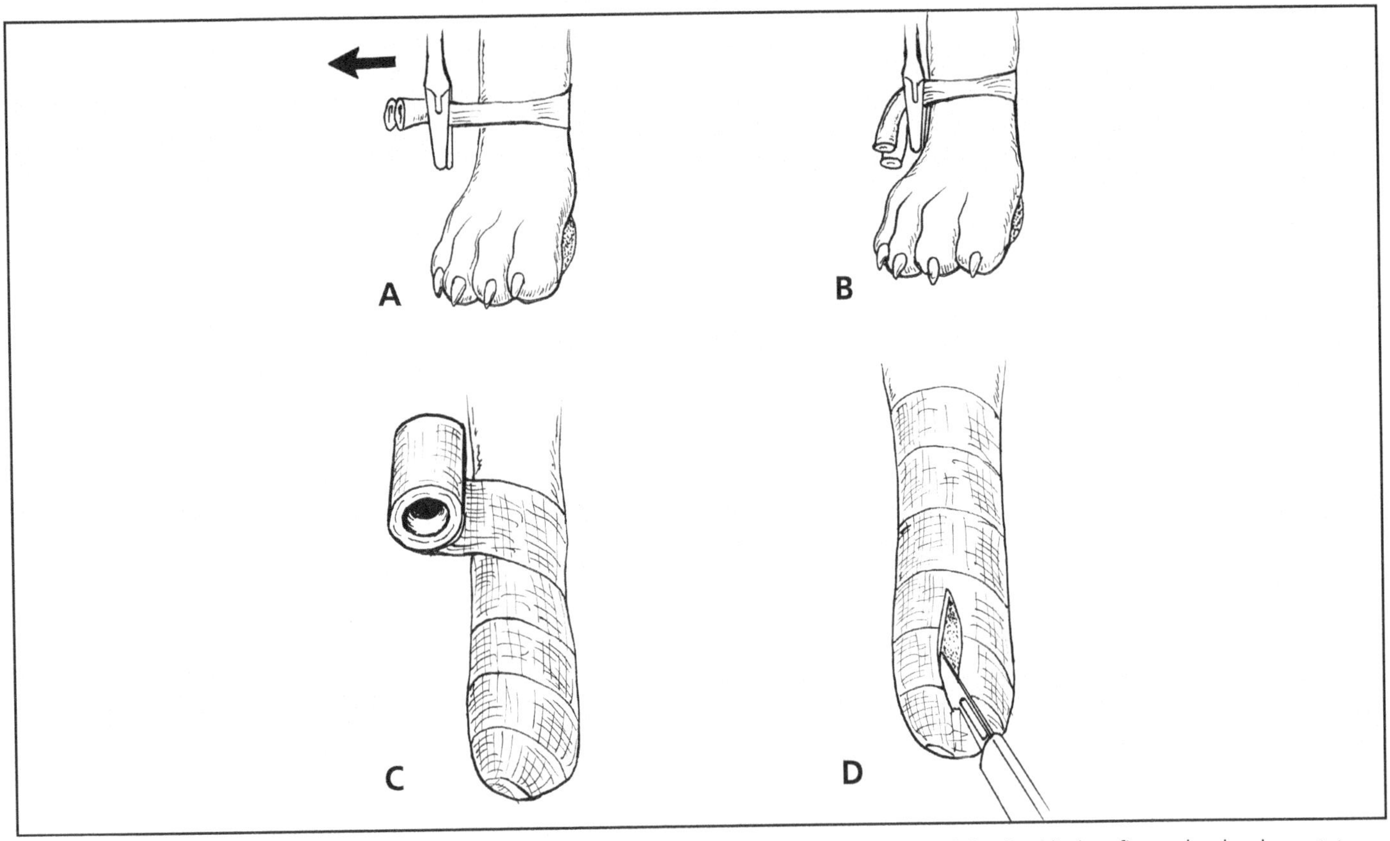


**Figure 4-1.** Application of hemostatic devices for paw surgery. **A.** ½ inch wide Penrose drain pulled around the distal limb to fit snugly when hemostats are applied. **B.** Hemostats clamped across the stretched drain adjacent to the limb. **C.** Sterile elastic bandage wrapped onto the limb tightly from the digits proximally. **D.** An incision is made through the elastic bandage to expose the surgical site. (After Swaim SF, Henderson RA: Small Animal Wound Management, 2nd ed.: Baltimore: Williams & Wilkins, 1997, 335.

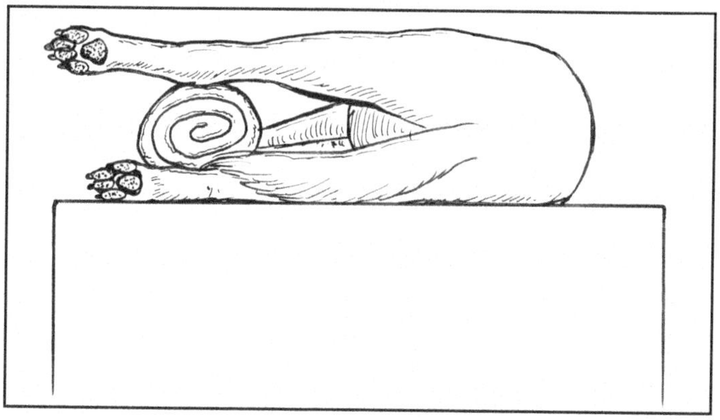

Figure 4-2. Positioning the limb and paw for surgery. With dog in lateral recumbency, the affected limb and paw are elevated. (After Swaim SF, Henderson RA: Small Animal Wound Management, 2nd ed.: Baltimore: Williams & Wilkins, 1997, 335.

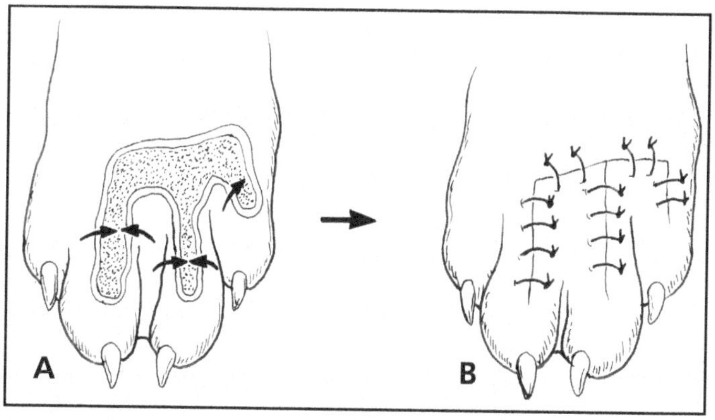


Figure 4-3. Closure of a wound on the dorsal surface of the digits using interdigital skin. A. Skin is moved as shown by arrows. B. Wound closed.

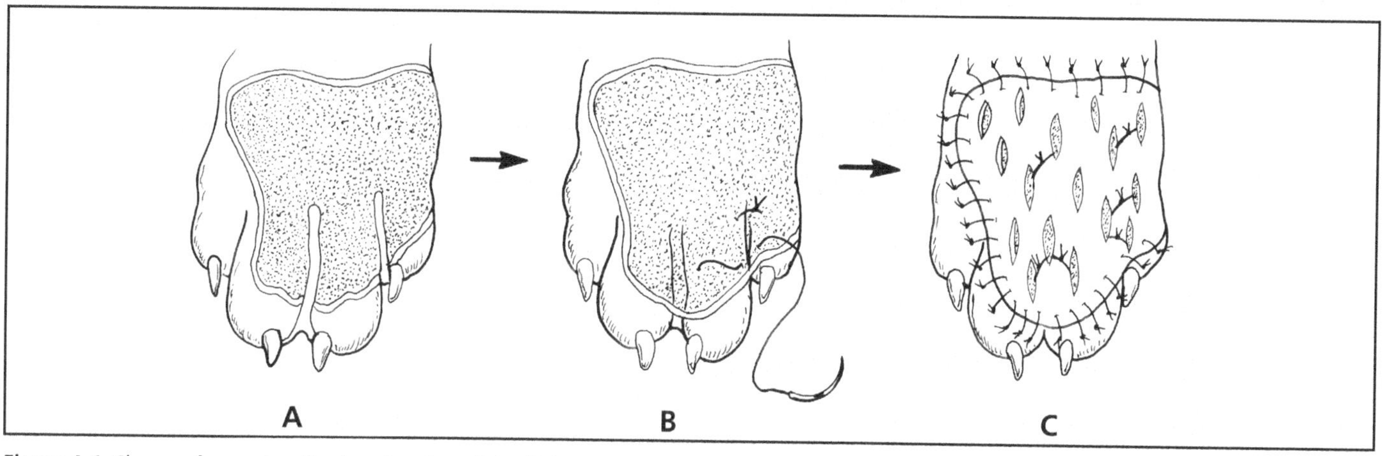


Figure 4-4. Closure of wound on the dorsal surface of the digits. A. Large wound on dorsum of the digits with thin strips of interdigital skin between 3 digits. B. Strips of interdigital skin removed and digits fused together with absorbable sutures. C. A mesh skin graft placed on the wound.

dorsal and palmar/plantar common digital vessels, or the axial and abaxial dorsal proper and palmar/plantar proper digital vessels in the sutures, thus ligating them. It is important not to place a graft over the dorsal surface of the digits, covering intact interdigital skin.

# Palmar/Plantar Pad Wounds - Pad Surface Wounds - Superficial Abraisions and Burns: Bandaging

## Definition and Indications

Superficial abrasion injury of the pads may involve the superficial epidermal layers. A specific superficial injury is loss of all or part of the stratum corneum which exposes the underlying deeper epidermal layers (Figures 4-5 & 4-6).

This type of injury usually results from a dog walking or running for a prolonged period, usually on a rough surface. This injury is seen in dogs that have led a sedentary life for a period and which are taken for a prolonged walk or run before the pads are conditioned to the stress to which they will be exposed. The injury is commonly seen in athletic dogs early in their training programs before their pads have toughened.

Superficial pad burns may result from chemical or thermal sources. One source of superficial pad burns on cats comes from the cat jumping onto the top of a hot wood-burning stove. Such wounds are characterized by pain, erythema, desquamated epidermis and blistering (Figure 4-6).

With superficial pad injuries, bandaging with a topical medication that will stimulate re-epithelialization should be the first line of therapy. An alternative is to use a cyanoacrylate glue to affix a local patch bandage over the area of abrasion.

## Technique

With superficial abrasion and burn injuries the wounds are generally clean. For chemical burns; the area should be lavaged with copious quantities of

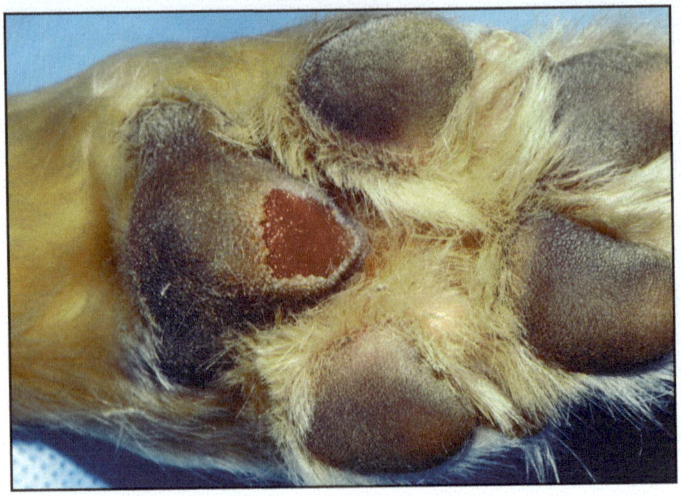

Figure 4-5. Superficial pad abrasion with loss of the stratum corneum from a metacarpal pad which exposes the underlying sensitive deep epidermal layers.

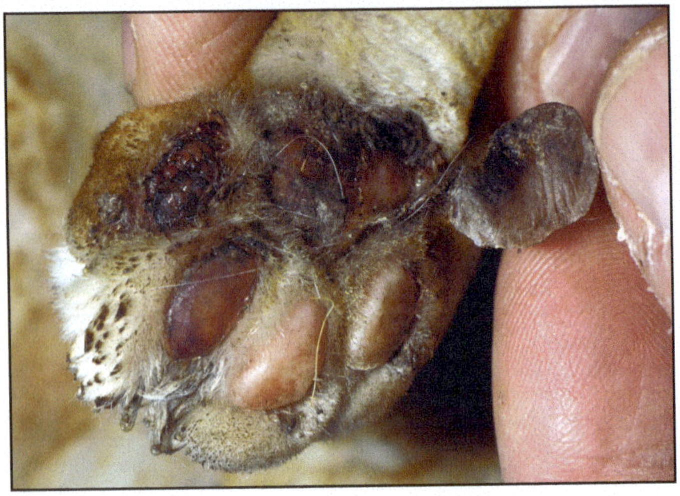

Figure 4-6. Superficial burn of a cat's pads with desquamation of burned superficial epidermis.

water. Any unattached superficial epidermis (Figure 4-7) should be removed back to the point where it is adherent to underlying epidermis using thumb forceps and scissors. Prior to bandaging, a small amount of cotton or cast padding should be placed in the interpad space between the digits and metacarpal/metatarsal pad to help keep the area dry.

Re-epithelialization occurs most rapidly between 2 surfaces (e.g. between the wound surface and a bandage) and in a moist environment (Telfa "Ouchless" Adhesive Pads, Covidien, Tyco/ Health Care/Kendall, Mansfield, MA). Thus, a semiocclusive nonadherent dressing pad should be used for bandaging. It may be coated with an Acemannan-containing hydrogel wound dressing (CarraVet Acemannan Wound Gel, CarraVet, Inc., Newman, GA) which has been found to stimulate healing of pad wounds. A thick, absorbent bandage wrap followed by porous adhesive tape or elastic tape complete the bandage. The paw cup portion of a metal splint may be incorporated in the

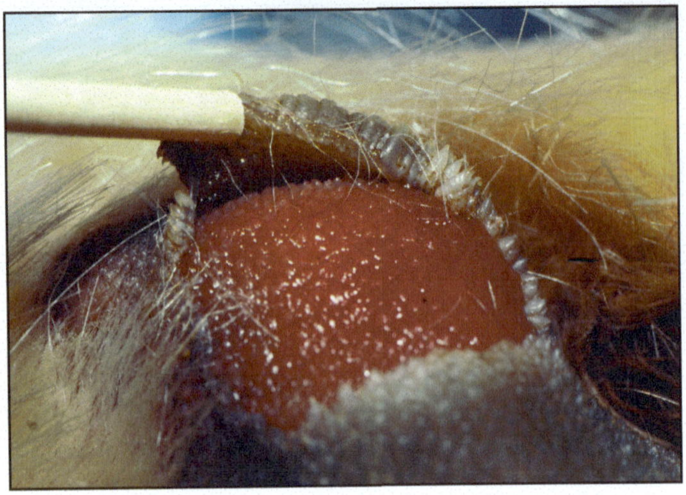

Figure 4-7. Unattached superficial epidermis associated with a superficial pad abrasion on a dog.

bandage, to help support the healing tissue. However, splints are probably not needed on small dogs or cats.

An alternative technique for providing coverage of a superficial abrasion that is used on athletic dogs is to place cyanoacrylate glue on unaffected pad tissue around the abrasion. This is followed by placing a piece of mole skin over the abrasion which will adhere to the glue. However, the author has not used this form of therapy.

## Aftercare

The bandage should be changed daily until the superficial epidermal layers have regenerated and some keratinization has occurred on the wound (Figure 4-8). This may occur as early as 7 to 10 days. Exercise should be restricted while the paw is bandaged, and early after the bandage has been removed. If the cyanoacrylate-mole skin patch local bandage is used, it is observed daily with replacement as needed as it wears.

The pads are monitored as exercise is gradually increased. After bandaging is discontinued the animal should be kept on a relatively clean, nonabrasive surface. The length of time for monitoring should be determined by examination of the paw and clinical judgment. Periodic application of a bootie may be helpful during the transition between bandaging and no bandaging when indicated.

The author has used a topical pad-toughening medication (Paw Pad Toughener, Island Pharmacy, Woodruff, WI) for about a week to help toughen the pads on dogs after they have healed/re-epithelialized. This should be applied daily with some sort of cover (bandage or bootie) to help keep it in contact with the pads. Otherwise it will be "walked" off or licked off soon after application and not be effective.

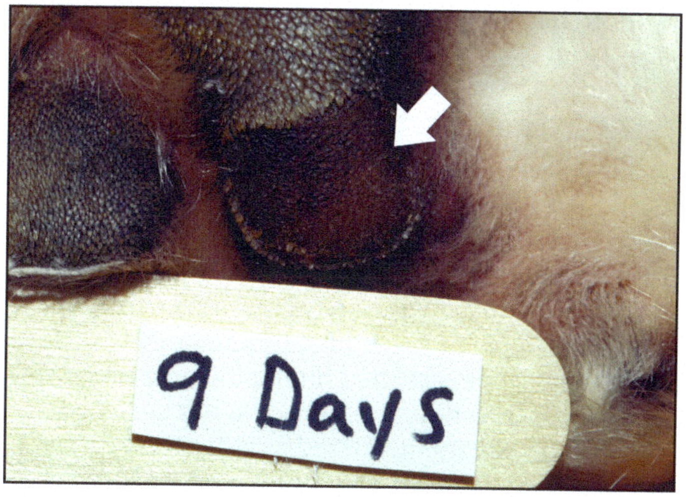


**Figure 4-8.** Superficial pad abrasion 9 days past injury. The pad is healing with regeneration of superficial epidermal layers *(arrow)*.

### Advantages and Disadvantages

The main advantage of nonadherent bandage therapy with the Acemannan-containing hydrogel wound dressing is that this treatment provides a moist environment and a wound healing stimulant medication to enhance re-epithelialization of the wound. The mole-skin patch provides a simple covering for the area. However, the animal may chew or lick it off.

## Suggested Readings


1. Basher A: Foot injuries in dogs and cats. Compend Contin Educ Pract Vet 16:1159, 1994.
2. Bohling MW: Burns. In Tobias KM, Johnston SA, eds.: Veterinary Surgery, Small Animal, Vol. 2.: St. Louis: Elsevier – Saunders, 2012, 1291.
3. Davis PE: Toe and muscle injuries of the racing greyhound. New Zealand Vet J 21:133, 1973.
4. Farrell M, Dunn A, Marchevsky A: Case report. Surgical reconstruction of canine footpads burned by sodium hypochlorite drain cleaner. Compendium 33:, 2012.
5. Fowler D: Distal limb and paw injuries. Vet Clin No Am Small Anim Pract 36: 819, 2006.
6. Hedlund CS: Surgery of the integumentary system. *In* Fossum TW, ed.: Small Animal Surgery, 2nd ed.: St. Louis: Mosby, 2002, 134.
7. Hedlund CS: Surgery of the integumentary system. In Fossum TW, ed.: Small Animal Surgery, 3rd ed.: St. Louis, Mosby, 2007, 159.
8. Hosgood G: Open wounds. In Tobias KM, Johnston SA, eds.: Veterinary Surgery, Small Animal, Vol. 2.: St. Louis: Elsevier – Saunders, 2012, 1220.
9. MacPhail CM: Surgery of the integumentary system. In Fossum TW, ed.: Small Animal Surgery, 4th ed.: St. Louis: Mosby, 2013, 190.
10. Posch AJ, McDonald G: Thermal burns in cats. Mod Vet Pract 58:937, 1977.
11. Swaim SF: Management and bandaging of soft tissue injuries of dog and cat feet. J Am Anim Hosp Assoc 21:329, 1985.
12. Swaim SF, Riddell KP, McGuire JA: Effects of topical medication on the healing of open pad wounds in dogs. J Am Anim Hosp Assoc 28:499, 1992.
13. Swaim SF: Paw injuries: Special wounds needing special attention. Int Sled Dog Vet Med Assoc Rep 1:1, 1995.
14. Swaim SF, Henderson RA: Small Animal Wound Management. 2nd ed.: Baltimore: Williams and Wilkins, 1997, 295.
15. Swaim SF, Renberg WC, Shike KM: Small Animal Bandaging, Casting and Splinting Techniques. Ames, IA: Wiley – Blackwell, 2011, 43.
16. White R. A. S.: Surgical treatment of specific skin disorders. *In* Slatter DH, ed.: Textbook of Small Animal Surgery, 3rd ed.: Philadelphia: WB Saunders, 2003, 339.


## Deep Abrasions, Partial Avulsions and Deep Burns: Bandaging/Splinting

### Definition and Indications

Deep abrasions may remove the entire thickness of pad skin, exposing the underlying fibroadipose padding tissue of the pad. Partial avulsion of a pad may result in loss of a large full-thickness portion of pad skin and possibly a portion of the underlying fibroadipose padding tissue. Deep burns may result in loss of full-thickness skin.

Deep pad abrasions can occur when a dog is accidentally dragged behind a vehicle or encounters some other form of severe abrading force on the pad. Partial avulsion of a pad may result from a severe laceration where a large portion of pad skin and possibly fibroadipose tissue are missing or have such a tenuous attachment that they will necrose, thus warranting complete surgical removal of the avulsed tissue. Deep burns may be the result of chemical or thermal exposure.

With deeper pad injuries, bandaging and splinting should be done to reduce pressure on the healing tissue. Topical medication that will stimulate wound contraction and re-epithelialization should be used along with the bandage/splint.

An important factor associated with deep abrasions, partial avulsions and deep burns is the presence of some normal pad tissue at the periphery of the wound. From this pad tissue, epithelium can advance over the granulation tissue that will form on the fibroadipose tissue to provide a functional pad. Open wound management is indicated for this type of wound before deciding whether more involved surgical procedures are necessary.

### Technique

The wound should be lavaged and debrided of nonviable tissue and debris. After drying the paw, a small amount of cotton should be placed between the digits and in the interpad space between the digits and the metacarpal/metatarsal pad to help keep these areas dry. A semiocclusive nonadherent dressing pad (Telfa "Ouchless" Adhesive Pads, Covidien, Tyco/HealtCare/Kendall, Mansfield, MA) should be used for bandaging. The pad may be coated with an Acemannan-containing hydrogel wound dressing (CarraVet Acemannan Wound Gel, CarraVet, Inc., Newnan, GA). This medication has been found to enhance the healing of pad wounds. The bandage is completed by a thick absorbent bandage wrap followed by a porous adhesive tape or elastic tape outer layer.

Because wound contraction and re-epithelialization both play a role in healing deeper pad wounds, it is important to relieve pressure on the wound because it will counteract contraction. For a medium-sized dog, a donut-type foam sponge pad (Confor™ foam, Lincoln, NE) can be incorporated in the bandage to distribute pressure around the wound. For a large dog, a "clam shell" splint can be used as a localized crutch to keep pressure off of the wounded pad. If all weight-bearing is to be avoided a Velpeau sling, carpal flexion splint or carpal sling can be used on the forelimb or a 90/90 sling can be used on a pelvic limb. Because small dogs and cats are lighter and do not place as much weight on their pads as larger dogs, a well padded bandage without a "donut"-type foam sponge pad should be sufficient (See Chapter 2 for informationon the various pads, splints, and slings).

## Aftercare

The bandage should be changed daily until the wound is healed. This may take 21 days or longer depending upon the severity of the wound (Figure 4-9A-D). Exercise should be restricted during the time of bandaging and early after bandaging has been discontinued. The pads are monitored as exercise is gradually increased. The animal should be kept on a relatively clean nonabrasive surface after bandaging is discontinued. The length of the monitoring period should be determined by examination of the pads and clinical judgement. Application of a commercial dog bootie periodically may be beneficial during the transition between bandaging and no bandage.

After the pads have healed, the author has used

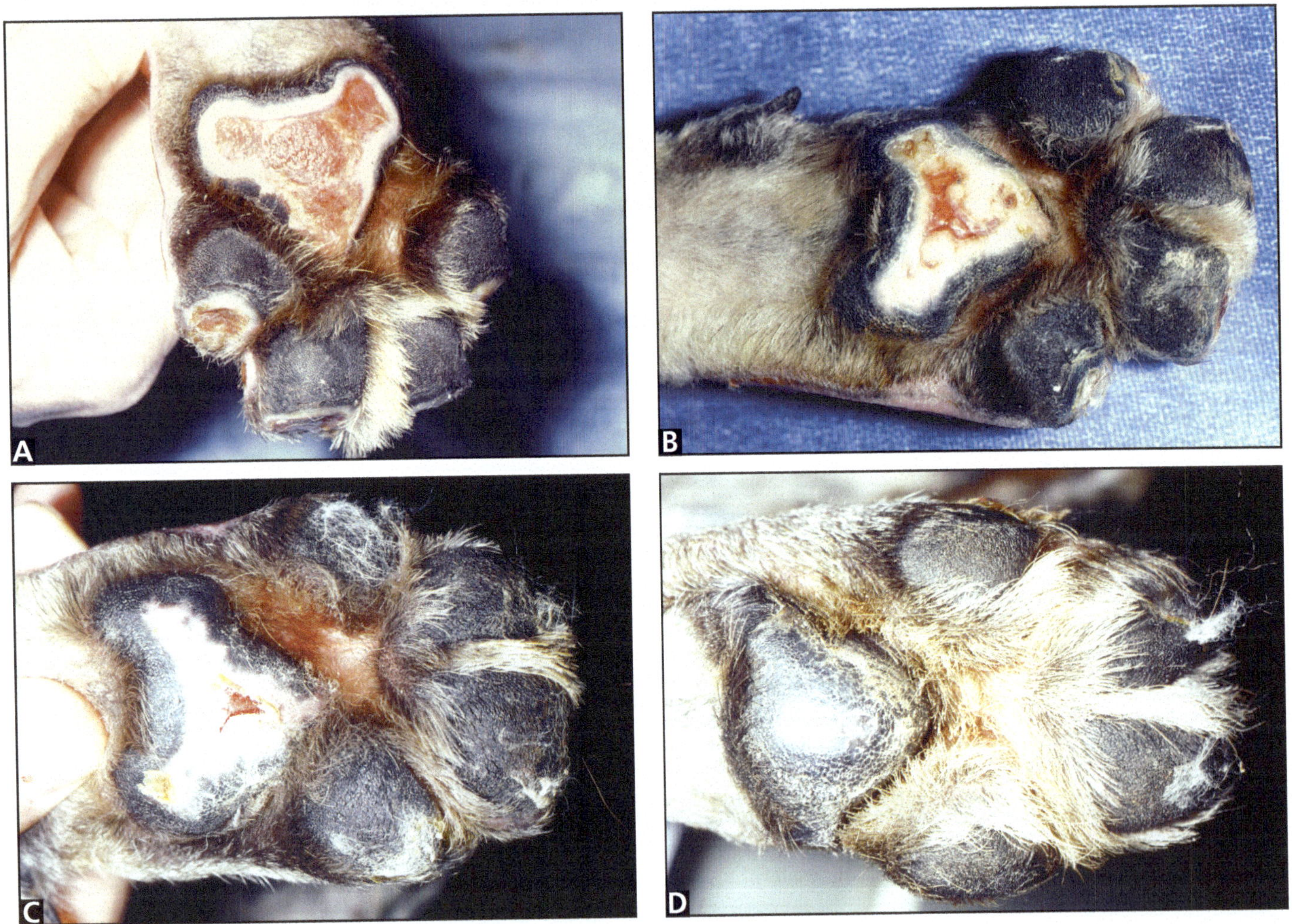


**Figure 4-9.** Deep pad abrasion and its healing. **A.** Digital and metacarpal pad deep abrasion wounds with some normal pad tissue remaining at the pad edges. **B.-D.** Progression of healing of the metacarpal pad by re-epitheliazation and keratinization. ( After Swaim SF, Henderson RA: Small Animal Wound Management, 2nd ed.: Baltimore: Williams and Wilkins, 1997, 341.)

a topical pad-toughening medication (Paw Pad Toughener, Island Pharmacy, Woodruff, WI) to help toughen the pads. The medication is applied daily with some type of cover (bandage or bootie) to help keep it in contact with the pads for about a week.

### Advantages and Disadvantages

The advantage of a pressure relief bandage/splint is that it relieves pressure on the wound which would counteract wound contraction. In addition, the nonadherent bandage with the Acemannan-containing hydrogel wound dressing provides a moist environment and a wound healing stimulant medication to enhance both contraction and re-epithelialization of the wound. Unlike the epithelium that surfaces wounds on other parts of the body, the epithelium that originates from pad skin is a tough keratinized epithelium that will withstand the stress placed on pad skin. Although the contraction portion of healing may result in a smaller pad, with time the tissue spreads to serve its intended function.

## Suggested Readings


1. Basher A: Foot injuries in dogs and cats. Compend Contin Educ Pract Vet 16:1159, 1994.
2. Bohling MW: Burns. In Tobias KM, Johnston SA, eds.: Veterinary Surgery, Small Animal, Vol. 2.: St. Louis: Elsevier – Saunders, 2012, 1291.
3. Farrell M, Dunn A, Marchevsky A: A case report: Surgical reconstruction of canine footpads burned by sodium hypochlorite drain cleaner. Compendium 33:, 2011.
4. Fowler D: Distal limb and paw injuries. Vet Clin No Am Small Animal Pract 36: 819, 2006.
5. Hedlund CS: Surgery of the integumentary system. *In* Fossum TW, ed.: Small Animal Surgery, 2nd ed.: St. Louis: Mosby, 2002, 134.
6. Hedlund CS: Surgery of the integumentary system. In Fossum TW. Ed.: Small Animal Surgery, 3rd ed.: St. Louis: Mosby, 2007, 159.
7. Hosgood GE: Open wounds. In Tobias KM, Johnston SA, eds.: Veterinary Surgery, Small Animal, Vol. 2: St. Louis: Elsevier – Saunders, 2012, 1210.
8. Swaim SF: Management and bandaging of soft tissue injuries of dog and cat feet. J Am Anim Hosp Assoc 21:329, 1985.
9. Swaim SF, Riddell KP, McGuire JA: Effects of topical medication on the healing of open pad wounds in dogs. J Am Anim Hosp Assoc 28:499, 1992.
10. Swaim SF: Paw injuries: Special wounds needing special attention. Int Sled Dog Vet Med Assoc Rep 1:1, 1995.
11. Swaim SF, Vaughn DM, Kincaid SA, et al: Effects of locally injected medications on healing of pad wounds in dogs. Am J Vet Res 57:394, 1996.
12. Swaim SF, Henderson RA: Small Animal Wound Management. 2nd ed.: Baltimore: Williams and Wilkins, 1997, 295.
13. Swaim SF, Hinkle SH, Bradley DM: Wound contraction: Basic and clinical factors. Compend Contin Educ Pract Vet 23:20, 2001.
14. Swaim SF, Marghitu DB, Rumph PF, et al: Effects of bandage configuration on paw pad pressure in dogs: A preliminary study. J Am Anim Hosp Assoc 39:209, 2003.
15. Swaim SF, Renberg WC, Shike KM; Small Animal Bandaging, Casting and Splinting Techniques. Ames, IA: Wiley – Blackwell, 2011, 43.
16. Waldron DR, Zimmerman-Pope N: Superficial skin wounds. *In* Slatter DH, ed.: Textbook of Small Animal Surgery, 3rd ed.: Philadelphia: WB Saunders, 2003, 259.


## Pad Punctures: Open Wound Management

### Definition and Indications

Pad punctures result from a sharp pointed object (e.g. stick) penetrating the pad either partial or full-thickness. Glass fragments are more common in urban animals; whereas, sharp organic material (sticks) are more common in rural areas and in working dogs. Superficial damage is usually minimal. Damage to deeper structures may be considerable, especially if there is movement of the penetrating object in the tissues. This in conjunction with bacterial contamination may result in infection. The object may only penetrate and be removed, or it may penetrate and remain in the wound as a foreign body (Figure 4-10A & B). A sinus tract with or without a surrounding nonhealing wound that has been present for a while may indicate a retained foreign body that entered via a puncture wound.

With uncomplicated puncture wounds, palpation, radiography or ultrasound exploration, lavage, systemic antibiotic and bandaging are indicated in the treatment as an open wound. With an infected puncture wound the same procedures are indicated, but more involved surgical exploration and debridement may be needed.

### Technique

If a puncture wound is not present, but a foreign body is suspected, i.e. a foreign body is present, but the puncture wound tract has healed, eliciting pain on palpation may identify the involved pad. Two-dimensional radiography may help locate radiopaque objects and sometimes glass. However, ultrasonography or magnetic resonance imaging may be necessary to locate radiolucent objects (e.g. thorns).

A single small pad wound may indicate a puncture wound. Initially, the wound should be explored with a pair of hemostatic forceps to determine if a foreign body is retained within the pad.

Following simple tract exploration with forceps, with or without foreign body removal, the wound should be thoroughly lavaged with a 0.05% chlorhexidine diacetate (Nolvasan Solution, Ft. Dodge Animal Health, Ft. Dodge, IA) or gluconate (ChlorhexiDerm Disinfectant, Dermatologics in Veterinary Medicine Pharmaceuticals, Inc., Miami, FL) solution.

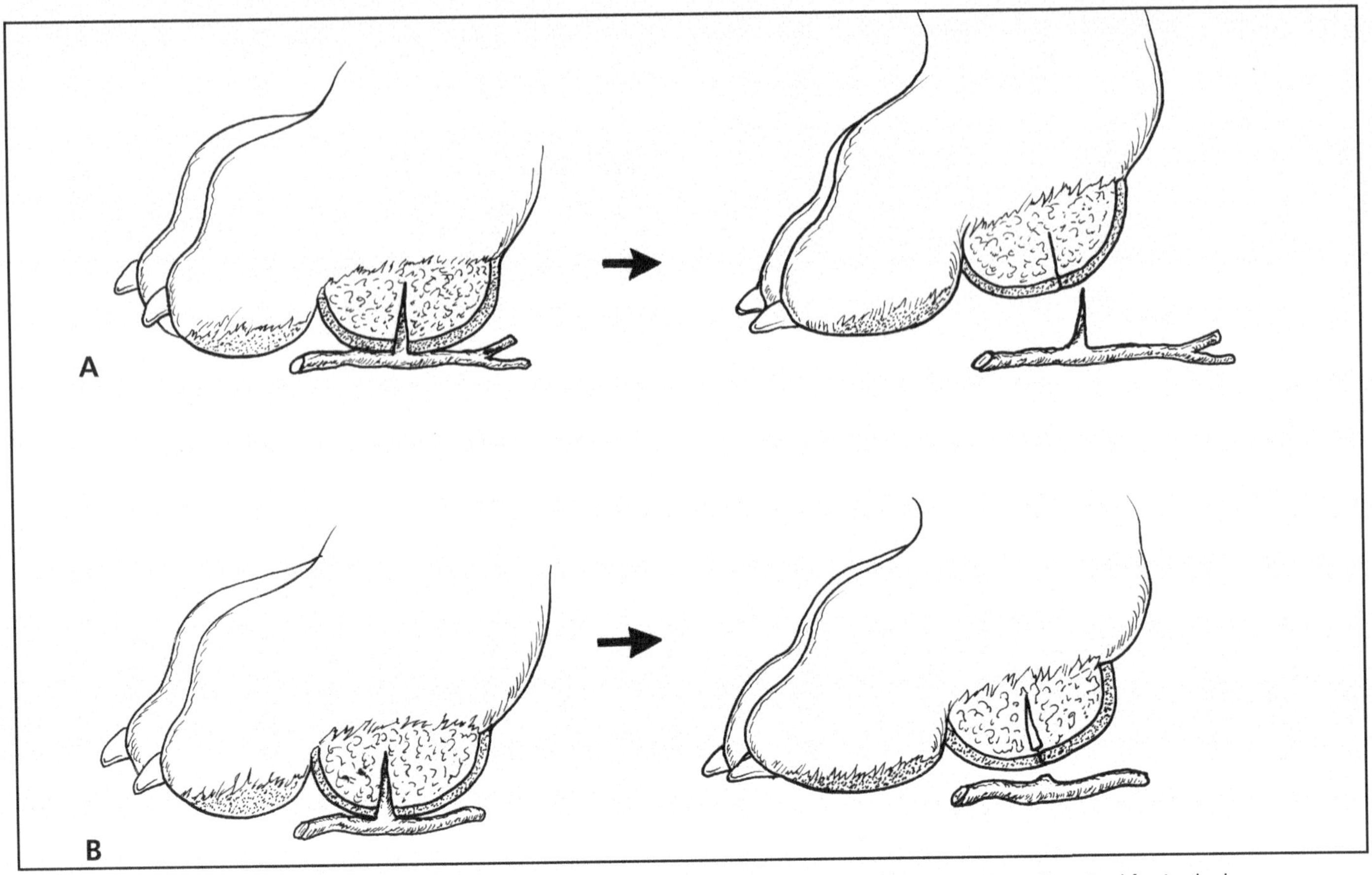


Figure 4-10. Pad puncture wounds. A. Deep puncture wound with no retained foreign body. B. Deep puncture wound with retained foreign body.

Although not as critical in the healing of simple puncture wounds as in the healing of large open or sutured wounds, pressure relief on puncture wounds can be beneficial in their healing. A "donut"-type foam rubber pad can be incorporated in the bandage to distribute pressure around the wound.

If it is necessary to surgically explore the pad to remove the foreign body, the approach should be through the pad surface. If the tissues are healthy, closure as described for pad lacerations may be done. However, if the area is infected, open wound management may be indicated utilizing the "donut"-type foam rubber pad in the bandage or a "clam shell" bandage.

## Aftercare

For simple puncture wounds without a retained foreign body or from which a foreign body has been removed, the animal should be placed on a systemic antibiotic, because of the deeper penetrating nature of the wound. If the wound is fresh the antibiotic selected should be effective against the organisms that are expected to be in the wound, namely *Staphylococcus* and *Streptococcus* spp. The cephalosporins [e.g. cephalexin (Keflex, Dista Products Co., Division of Eli Lilly & Co., Indianapolis, IN) or cephadroxil (Cefa-Drops or Cefa-Tabs, Ft. Dodge Animal Health, Ft. Dodge, IA)] could be considered. Other possible antibiotics could be an amoxicillin (Amoxi-Drops, Amoxi-Inject, Amoxi-Tabs, Pfizer Animal Health Group, Exton, PA) or an amoxicillin-trihydrate and clavulanate potassium combination (Clavamox tablets or drops, Pfizer Animal Health Group, Exton, PA) (See Microbial Evaluation and Therapy, Chapter 1).

'Bandaging should consist of a semiocclusive nonadherent pad (Telfa "Ouchless" Adhesive Pads, Tyco Health Care, Kendall, Mansfield, MA), absorbent secondary wrap and porous adhesive tape or elastic tape. Frequency of bandage change will vary with the severity of the wound. It will be less with simple foreign body retrieval, but will be more frequent following excision of a foreign body with the wound being left open. Because the wound is left open, drainage is good and should decrease daily, as will be noted in the bandages as they are changed. Exercise should be limited during the time of bandaging and early after bandaging has been discontinued.

At the time of bandage changes, the pad and surrounding tissue should be observed for evidence of infection (heat, swelling, hyperemia, and pain). Occasionally, "pseudohealing" can take place whereby the skin heals but, due to underlying contamination and tissue damage, an abscess forms beneath the

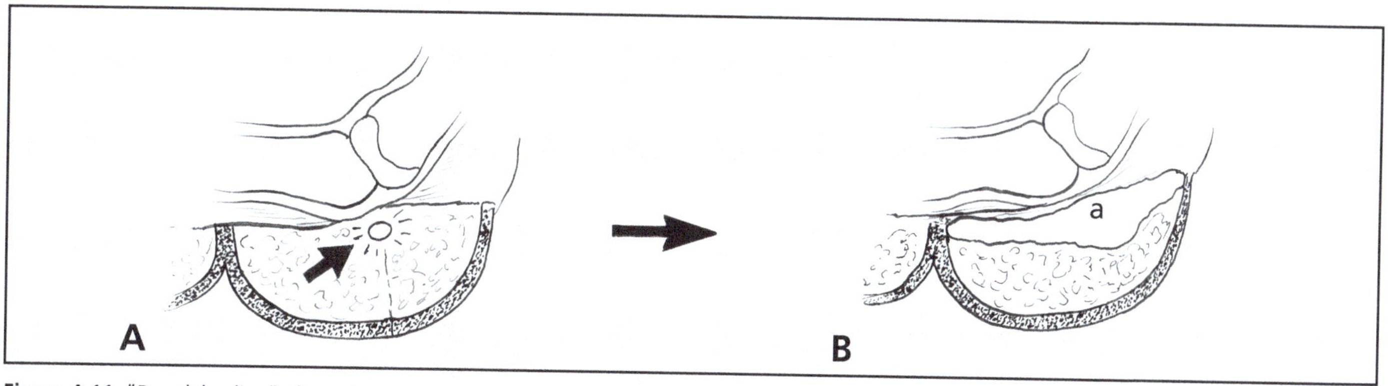


Figure 4-11. "Pseudohealing" of a pad puncture wound. **A.** Healed puncture wound with a small area of contamination at the end of the puncture tract *(arrow)*. **B.** Small area of contamination develops into a large abscess under the pad *(a)*.

healed skin. Left unchecked, the result can be loss of a large amount of tissue (Figure 4-11 and Figure 4-12). "Pseudohealing" is more common following simple foreign body retrieval via the puncture wound. If there is evidence of infection, the area should be explored by needle aspiration to check for exudate or by incision to check for exudate and possibly an earlier undetected retained foreign body. Culture and sensitivity of any exudate or necrotic tissue should be done. An incised wound should be left open to heal as an open wound or for delayed primary closure after infection is under control, to include antibiotic change.

Bandaging following an infection should be aimed at relieving pressure on the wound, using a pressure relief bandage such as incorporating a "donut"-type foam rubber pad in the bandage or using a "clam shell" splint as a local crutch. If all weight-bearing is to be avoided, i.e. with a larger open wound on sutured wound, a Velpeau sling, carpal flexion splint or carpal sling can be used on the forelimb or a 90/90 sling on the hind limb.

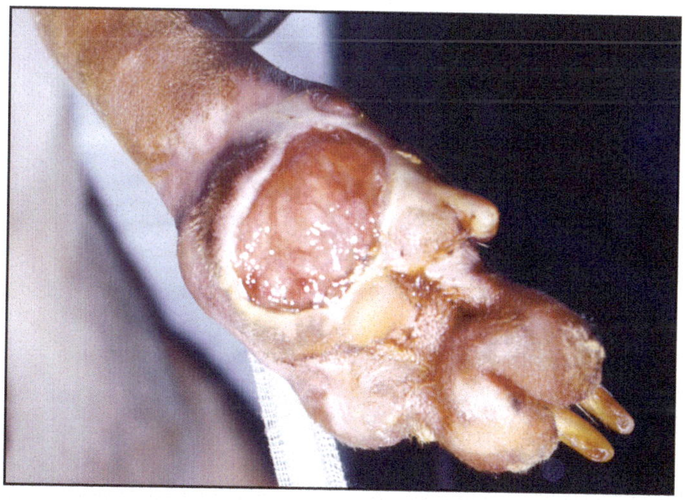

**Figure 4-12.** Loss of a metatarsal pad as the result of "psuedohealing" and abscess formation under the pad.

### Advantages and Disadvantages

Barring complications, puncture wounds heal quickly because of the minimal tissue damage with a simple puncture wound. If excision of the foreign body is necessary and the wound is left open to heal by second intention, healing time will be prolonged. If "pseudohealing" occurs and goes unobserved, the resulting tissue slough can be serious especially with loss of part or all of a metacarpal or metatarsal pad.

## Suggested Readings


1. Hosgood G: Open wounds. In Tobias KM, Johnston SA, eds.: Veterinary Surgery, Small Animal, Vol. 2: St. Louis, Elsevier – Saunders, 2012, 1210.
2. Swaim SF, Henderson RA: Small Animal Wound Management. 2nd ed.: Baltimore: Williams and Wilkins, 1997, 13.
3. Swaim SF, Marghitu DB, Rumph PF, et al: Effects of bandage configuration on paw pad pressure in dogs: A preliminary study. J Am Anim Hosp Assoc 39:209, 2003.
4. Swaim SF, Renberg WC, Shike KM: Small Animal Bandaging, Casting and Splinting Techniques. Ames, IA: Wiley – Blackwell, 2011, 43.
5. White RAS: Surgical treatment of specific skin disorders. *In* Slatter DH, ed.: Textbook of Small Animal Surgery, 3rd ed.: Philadelphia: WB Saunders, 2003, 239.


## Pad Lacerations: Suturing

### Definition and Indications

Material in this section applies primarily to lacerations of the metacarpal and metatarsal pads. However, the general principles also apply to digital pad lacerations.

A laceration is a wound caused by tearing of tissue with a variable amount of damage to superficial and underlying tissue. Pad lacerations of dogs and cats have variable causes. The resulting wound may be superficial or deep. It is important to determine the depth of lacerations in deciding on the proper therapy. Pad wounds are subject to considerable contamination because of the location of the wounds and an animal's tendency to place weight on the paw after injury, especially a canine athlete or working dog (Figure 4-13). Thus, thorough debridement and lavage of pad wounds is necessary. Because pads serve as shock absorbers, pressure on them results in spreading of the pad. For this reason, proper suturing, bandaging and splinting of the pads are important to prevent the wound edges from separating, which causes sutures to cut through tissues and result in delayed or lack of healing.

## Technique

With the animal under general anesthesia, the surface of the wound should be observed for dirt and debris. This will give some indication as to the degree of contamination of the wound. The blades of small hemostatic forceps are placed into the wound and spread to assess the depth of the laceration. The deeper portion of the fibroadipose tissue of the lacerated pad may appear to be apposed. However, this maneuver will reveal the true depth of the laceration. If the laceration has extended through the full thickness of the pad, digital flexor tendons may be observed in the depths of the wound as the forceps are opened (Figure 4-14A-D and Figure 4-15). Digital flexor tendons may have been lacerated. This is reflected by abnormal weight bearing and an extended position of the affected digit(s). In such cases, some form of tendon repair or compensatory surgical procedure will eventually be needed. Abnormal weight bearing and possible pad ulceration may result if surgical correction is not done. Repair of digital flexor tendons can be difficult and is often unsuccessful. However, if it is to be performed, it should be done as early as possible. In the presence of a contaminated wound with lacerated tendons, it would be best to do a temporary tendon repair, leaving long suture tags. Thus, the wound can be treated by staged debridement and lavage for delayed primary closure. The temporary tenorrhaphy prevents further retraction of tendon ends and the long suture tags make it easier to relocate the tendon

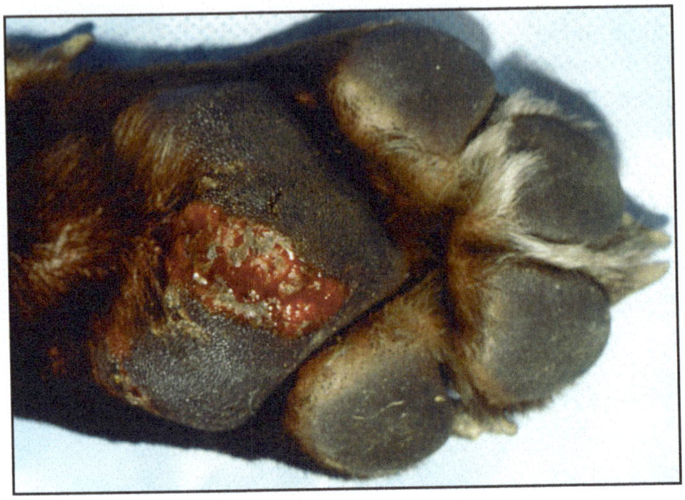

**Figure 4-13.** Deep metatarsal pad laceration with gross contamination of the exposed fibroadipose tissue of the pad.

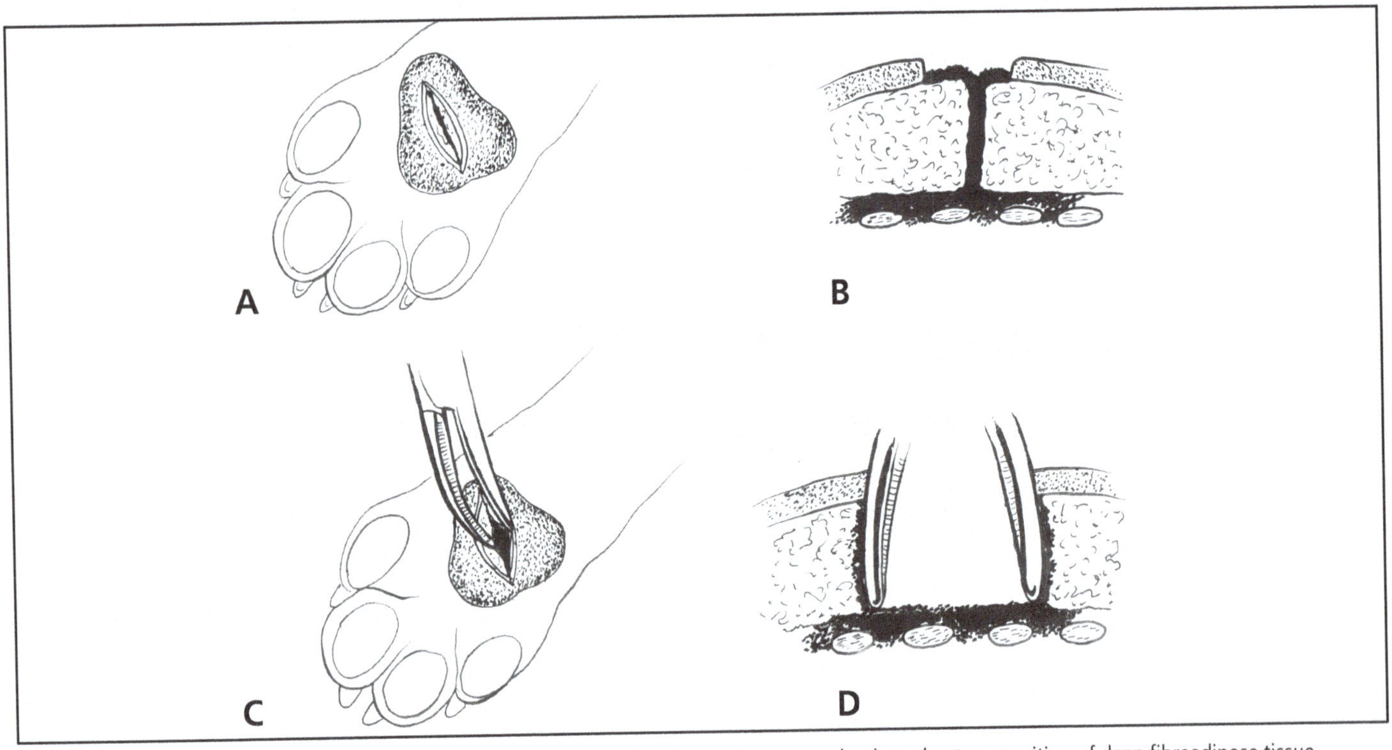


**Figure 4-14.** Evaluating the depth of a pad laceration. **A.** & **B.** Laceration does not appear to be deep due to apposition of deep fibroadipose tissue. However, **B.** laceration extends through the full-thickness of the pad, with contamination of the fibroadipose tissue and the underlying area including digital flexor tendons. **C.** & **D.** Depth of the wound assessed by placing hemostatic forceps in the wound and spreading them. (After Swaim SF, Henderson RA: Small Animal Wound Management, 2nd ed.: Baltimore: Williams & Wilkins, 1997, 336.)

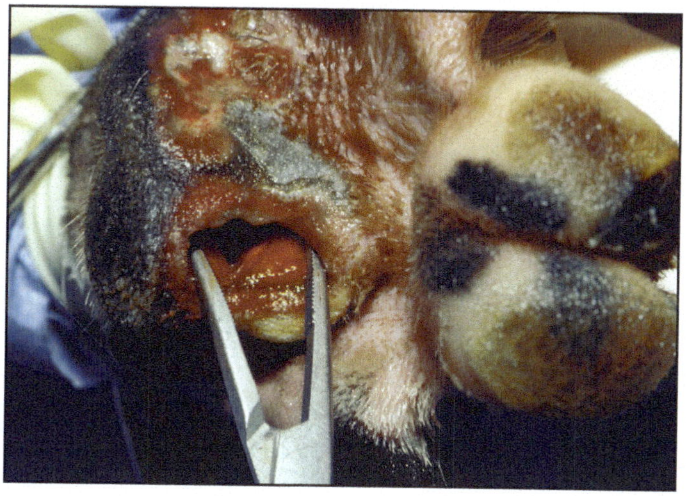

Figure 4-15. Hemostatic forceps in a deep pad wound to assess wound depth and status of underlying tissue.

for definitive repair. If tendon repair fails, fusion podoplasty may be considered as a salvage procedure.

Wounds should be thoroughly debrided and lavaged with a 1:40 dilution of chlorhexidine diacetate (Nolvasan Solution, Ft. Dodge Animal Health, Ft. Dodge, IA) or gluconate (ChlorhexiDerm Disinfectant, Dermatologics in Veterinary Medicine Pharmaceuticals, Inc., Miami, FL) solution to free them of embedded dirt and debris. When the wound has extended through the entire thickness of the pad, a segment of Penrose drain should be placed under, not through, the pad (Figure 4-16A & B & Figure 4-17).

If a pad laceration has been present for a period of time and the tissues are infected, staged debridement and lavage should be performed with delayed primary closer once the wound is free of infection.

To suture a pad laceration, simple interrupted sutures of 3-0 or 4-0 absorbable monofilament suture material are placed in the fibroadipose tissue of the lacerated pad (Figure 4-18A). Final apposition of the wound edges is accomplished with simple interrupted sutures, placed widely from the skin edges, or far-near-near-far sutures using monofilament 3-0 nonabsorbable suture material (Figure 4-18B). Alternatively, on medium to large dogs, vertical mattress sutures with large bites of pad tissue with 2-0 suture material have been described. Another technique for final apposition of the cut edges requires digital apposition of the edges. Cyanoacrylate glue is placed on intact skin on each side of the wound, but not between the wound edges. Segments of 3-0 nonabsorbable suture material are then laid across the wound and into the glue. More glue can be placed over the suture ends for security. The author prefers suturing in layers with far-near-near-far sutures for final skin apposition.

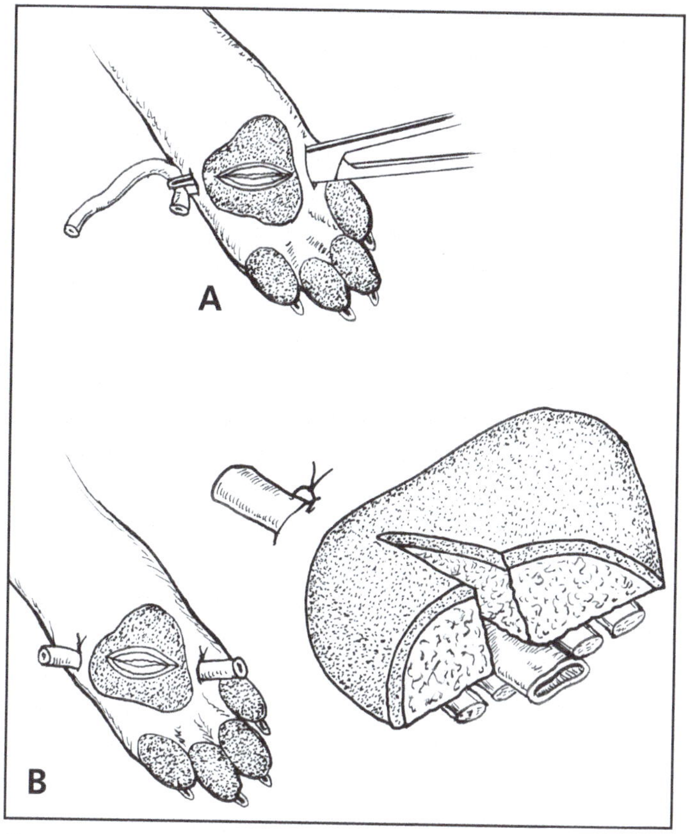


Figure 4-16. Penrose drain placed under a lacerated pad. A. Hemostatic forceps placed under a metacarpal/metatarsal pad via incisions at the edges. Forceps grasp a ¼ inch diameter Penrose drain to pull it under the pad. B. Penrose drain placed under the pad with suture anchors at each end. (After Swaim SF, Henderson RA: Small Animal Wound Management 2nd ed.: Baltimore: Williams & Wilkins, 1997, 337.)

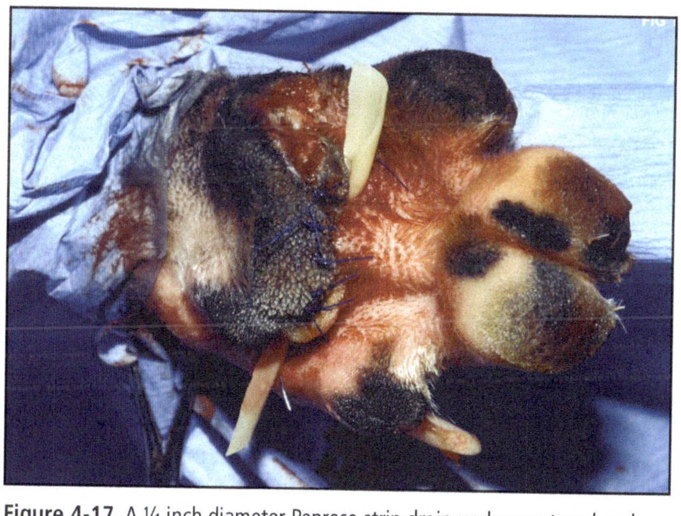

Figure 4-17. A ¼ inch diameter Penrose strip drain under a sutured pad laceration.

## Aftercare

To keep the interdigital and interpad areas dry small amounts of cotton should be placed between the digits and in the space between the digits and metacarpal/ metatarsal pad. A semiocclusive nonadherent dressing pad (Telfa "Ouchless" Adhesive Pads, Covidien, Tyco Health Care, Kendall, Mansfield, MA) should be placed over the wound. A thick absorbent bandage wrap is

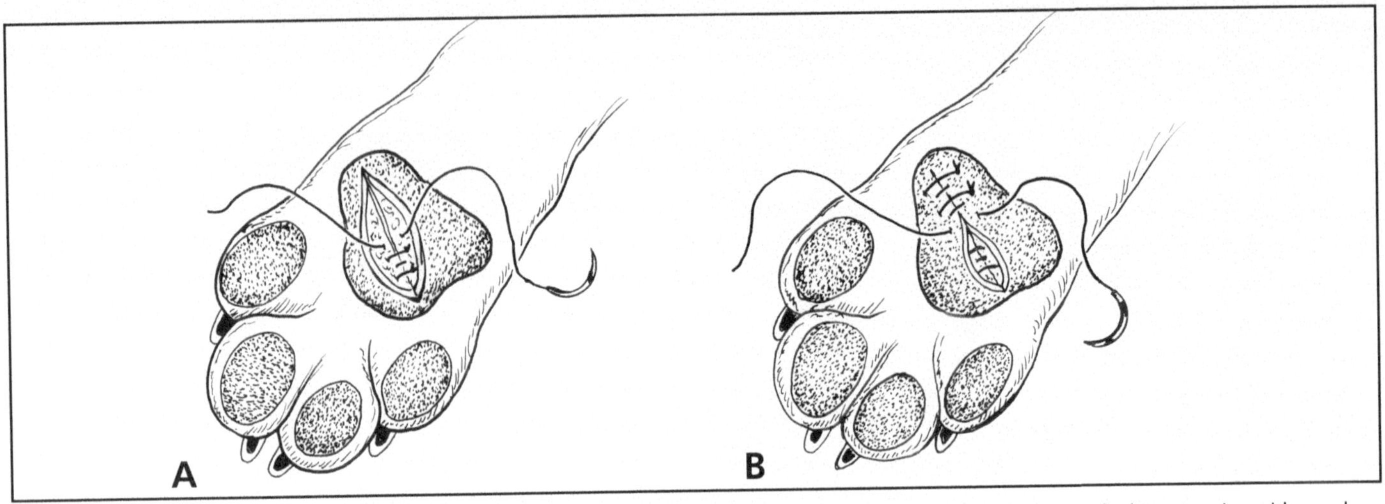


**Figure 4-18.** Suturing a pad laceration. **A.** Simple interrupted absorbable sutures in deep fibroadipose tissue. **B.** Final wound edge appostion with nonabsorbable far-near-near-far sutures. (After Swaim SF, Henderson RA: Small Animal Wound Management, 2nd ed.: Baltimore: Williams & Wilkins, 1997, 338.)

placed on the paw followed by a porous adhesive tape or elastic tape outer layer. Because pressure on the pad will result in the pad spreading and the sutures cutting through the tissues, it is important to relieve pressure on the pad. For a medium-sized dog, a "donut"-type foam rubber pad and metal splint cup can be incorporated in the bandage to distribute pressure around the wound. For a large dog, a "clam shell" splint can be used as a localized crutch to help keep pressure off of the sutured pad. In very large dogs total prevention of weight bearing can be provided by a Velpeau sling, carpal flexion splint or carpal sling for the forelimb or a 90/90 sling for the hindlimb. Because cats and small dogs are lighter and do not place as much weight on the pads as on larger dogs, a well padded bandage without a "donut"-type foam rubber pad should be sufficient.

Due to the contaminated or infected nature of pad lacerations, the animal should be placed on a systemic antibiotic. The antibiotic selected should be effective against the organisms that are expected to be in the wound. These would commonly be *Staphylococcus* and *Streptococcus* spp. The cephalosporins [e.g. cephalexin (Keflex, Dista Products Co., Division of Eli Lilly & Co., Indianapolis, IN) or cephadroxil (Cefa-Drops or Cefa-Tabs, Ft. Dodge Animal Health, Ft. Dodge, IA)] could be considered. Other possible antibiotics could be an amoxicillin (Amoxi-Drops, Amoxi-Tabs, Amoxi-Inject, Pfizer Animal Health Group, Exton, PA) or an amoxicillin-trihydrate and clavulanate potassium combination (Clavamox tablets or drops, Pfizer Animal Health Group, Exton, PA) (See Microbial Evaluation and Therapy, Chapter 1).

Depending upon the amount of drainage, the bandage should be changed every 1 to 3 days for 10 to 14 days following surgery. If drains have been placed, they should be removed when the amount of drainage is minimal. It is desirable to leave sutures in place for about 14 to 21 days to allow for adequate healing. If sutures are removed at 14 days, it is advisable to continue bandaging, possibly with a "donut"-type foam rubber pad, until the surgeon believes healing is adequate to allow paw use without a bandage. A commercial dog bootie may also be used in the transition time from full bandaging to no bandage. The length of time sutures remain in place, the frequency of bandage changes, the time of drain removal, and the length of time bandages or a bootie are needed will vary according to the severity of the wound, the animal's size, and level of activity. Clinical judgment is used in these matters.

## Advantages and Disadvantages

Pad lacerations that are properly sutured tend to heal faster (i.e. there is an earlier gain in wound strength) than lacerations that are only bandaged. In addition, they have a better cosmetic appearance than unsutured pad lacerations allowed to heal as open wounds. When pads are not sutured, bandaged or splinted properly, the wound edges may separate and sutures tear through the tissues when weight is placed on the pad. The result is delayed or lack of healing. If deep or full-thickness pad lacerations are not adequately examined, debrided, lavaged, and drained (if necessary), the superficial tissues may heal, but a deep abscess may form ("pseudohealing") and pad slough may occur (See Figure 4-12).

# Suggested Readings

1. Basher A: Foot injuries in dogs and cats. Compend Contin Educ Pract Vet 16:1159, 1994.
2. Bohling MW, Swaim SF: Paw and distal limb skin reconstructive and salvage techniques. In Bojrab MJ, ed.: Current Techniques in

Small Animal Surgery, 5th ed.: Jackson, WY: Teton NewMedia 2014, 628.
3. Davis PE: Toe and muscle injuries of the racing greyhound. New Zealand Vet J 21:133, 1973.
4. Fowler D: Distal limb and paw injuries. Vet Clin No Am Small Animal Pract 36: 819, 2006.
5. Hedlund CS: Surgery of the integumentary system. *In* Fossum TW, ed.: Small Animal Surgery, 2nd ed.: St. Louis: Mosby, 2002, 134.
6. Hedlund CS: Surgery of the integumentary system. In Fossum TW, ed.: Small Animal Surgery, 3rd ed.: St. Louis: Mosby, 2007, 159.
7. Hosgood G: Open wounds. In Tobias KM, Johnston SA, eds.: Veterinary Surgery, Small Animal, Vol. 2: St. Louis: Elsevier – Saunders, 2012, 1210.
8. Newman ME, Lee AH, Swaim SF, Redding RW: Wound healing of sutured and nonsutured canine metatarsal footpad incisions. J Am Anim Hosp Assoc 22:757, 1986.
9. MacPhail CM: Surgery of the integumentary system. In Fossum TW, ed.: Small Animal Surgery, 4th ed.: St. Louis: Mosby, 2013, 190.
10. Pavletic MM: Atlas of Small Animal Reconstructive Surgery, 2nd ed: Philadelphia: WB Saunders, 1999, 365.
11. Pavletic MM: Atlas of Small Animal Wound Management and Reconstructive Surgery, 3rd ed.: Ames, IA: Wiley – Blackwell, 2010, 535.
12. Swaim SF: Management and bandaging of soft tissue injuries of dog and cat feet. J Am Anim Hosp Assoc 21:329, 1985.
13. Swaim SF: Paw pad injuries: Special wounds needing special attention. Int Sled Dog Vet Med Assoc Rep 1:1, 1995.
14. Swaim SF, Scardino MS: Paw and distal limb salvage and reconstructive techniques. *In* Bojrab MJ, ed.: Current Techniques in Small Animal Surgery, 4th ed.: Baltimore: Williams and Wilkins, 1998, 625.
15. Swaim SF, Hinkle SH, Bradley DM: Wound contraction: Basic and clinical factors. Compend Contin Educ Pract Vet 23:20, 2001.
16. Swaim SF, Marghitu DB, Rumph PF, et al: Effects of bandage configuration on paw pad pressure in dogs: A preliminary study. J Am Anim Hosp Assoc 39:209, 2003.
17. Swaim SF, Renberg WC, Shike KM: Small Animal Bandaging, Casting and Splinting Techniques. Ames, IA: Wiley – Blackwell, 2011, 43.
18. Waldron DR, Zimmerman-Pope N: Superficial skin wounds. *In* Slatter DH, ed.: Textbook of Small Animal Surgery, 3rd ed.: Philadelphia: WB Saunders, 2003, 259.
19. White RAS: Surgical treatment of specific skin disorders. *In* Slatter DH, ed.: Textbook of Small Animal Surgery, 3rd ed.: Philadelphia: WB Saunders, 2003, 239.

# Metacarpal/Metatarsal Pad Loss

# Deep Pad Ulceration: Bandaging

## Definition and Indications

Pad ulcerations usually occur on the metacarpal or metatarsal pads; however, digital pad ulcerations can also be present. The ulcers are usually the result of tendon malfunction, bone malalignment, or peripheral nerve damage. There is an inordinate amount of pressure placed on pad skin as the skin is compressed between the surface the dog walks on and underlying bone.

On the forelimb, one such ulceration occurs at the proximolateral aspect of the metacarpal pad as the result of ulnar nerve paralysis with the production of a ulcer in the pad (Figure 4-19). It is theorized that the ulceration develops when skin circulation is interrupted by compression between a bony prominence and an external surface. The denervation results in interruption of sensory pathways and there are no reflex or volitional movements that relieve prolonged soft tissue compression as in normal animals. The time between first compression and degeneration of subcutaneous tissue is considerably shorter in these denervation type ulcers. In addition, with ulnar paralysis, the flexor muscles (flexor carpi ulnaris and the deep digital flexor) innervated by the nerve are not functioning properly, thus the posture of the metacarpo-phalangeal area is altered with the animal having a "dropped" appearance in the caudolateral metacarpo-phalangeal area (Figure 4-20). With this abnormal posture, the metacarpo-phalangeal articulation of the fifth digit places considerable pressure on the proximolateral aspect of the metacarpal pad. Thus, as a result of the above-described abnormalities, an ulcer forms. Other defining characteristics of ulnar paralysis are denervation atrophy of the flexor muscles innervated by the nerve when palpated in comparison to the opposite limb, and lack of sensory innervation over the area when gently pinched with hemostatic forceps.

Another type of ulcer, observed by the author, may be found on the metacarpal pad subsequent to radial-carpal arthrodesis to provide the animal with a weight-bearing limb as a salvage procedure. In some cases, as the animal ambulates there is twisting of the paw when there is full weight on it due to lack of carpal flexion. The resulting friction between the metacarpal pad and the surface the animal is ambulating on plus pressure on the pad causes an ulcer.

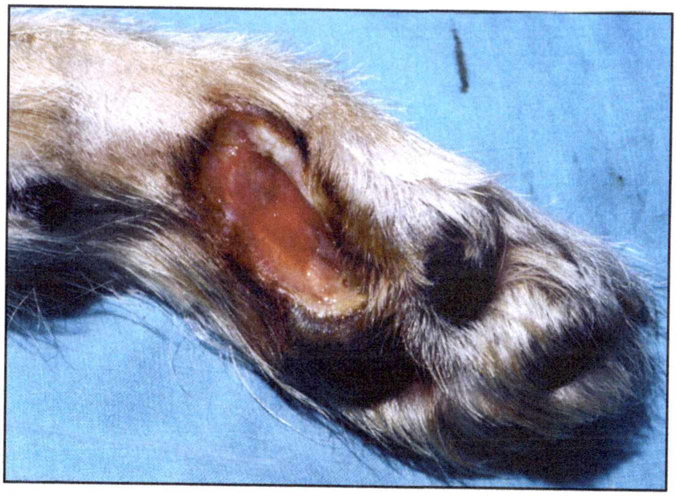

**Figure 4-19.** Trophic ulcer at the proximolateral aspect of the metacarpal pad resulting from ulnar nerve paralysis.

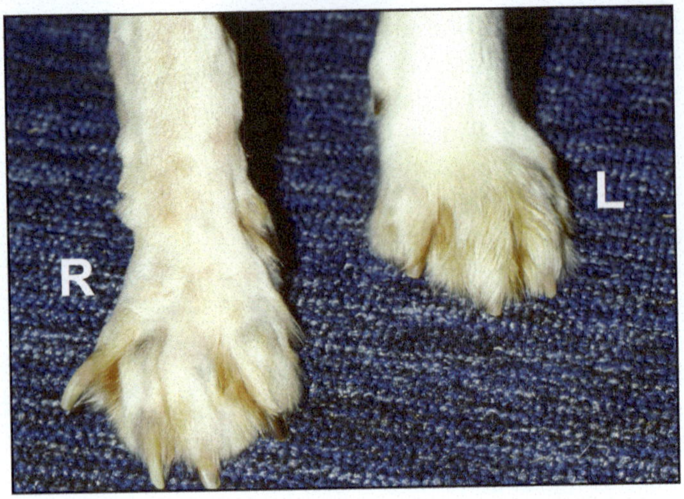


Figure 4-20. Right forelimb with ulnar paralysis. Paw has a dropped appearance caudally and laterally.

The strategy for treating the above described ulcers is to try the simple approach first and go to more involved procedures as necessary.

## Technique

Deep pad ulcers heal as open wounds in the same way deep pad abrasions, partial avulsions, and deep burns heal by contraction and epithelialization. The treatment is the same as for those wounds. (See Palmar/Plantar Pad Wounds, Pad Surface Wounds, Deep Abrasions, Partial Avulsions and Deep Burns: Bandaging/Splinting in this chapter.)

Deep pad ulcers have usually been present for a period of time. Thus, the ideal would be to biopsy the lesion to check for infection with an unusual organism or the presence of a neoplastic condition. However, in the interest of economics for the pet owner, treatment is usually undertaken for about 1 week. If the ulcer has started to heal in this time, healing usually continues. If healing has not started, biopsies should be taken for culture and histopathologic evaluation.

## Aftercare

(See Palmar/Plantar Pad Wounds, Pad Surface Wounds, Deep Abrasions, Partial Avulsions and Deep Burns: Bandaging/Splinting in this chapter.)

If the ulcer begins to form again after it has healed, pad toughener may be used. Exercise may be increased gradually to toughen the pad, or a surgical procedure should be considered for pad replacement.

## Advantages and Disadvantages

(See Palmar/Plantar Pad Wounds, Pad Surface Wounds, Deep Abrasions, Partial Avulsions and Deep Burns: Bandaging/Splinting in this chapter.)

Another advantage of this approach for treatment is that the bandage therapy, pad toughener, and gradual increase in exercise may result in functional healing of the wound without more involved surgical procedures. It should be borne in mind that this approach is most effective on smaller dogs that do not place as much weight/stress on the pad as do larger dogs Figure 4-21A & B).

# Suggested Readings

1. Read RA: Probable trophic pad ulceration following traumatic denervation: Report of two cases in dogs. Vet Surg 15:40, 1986.

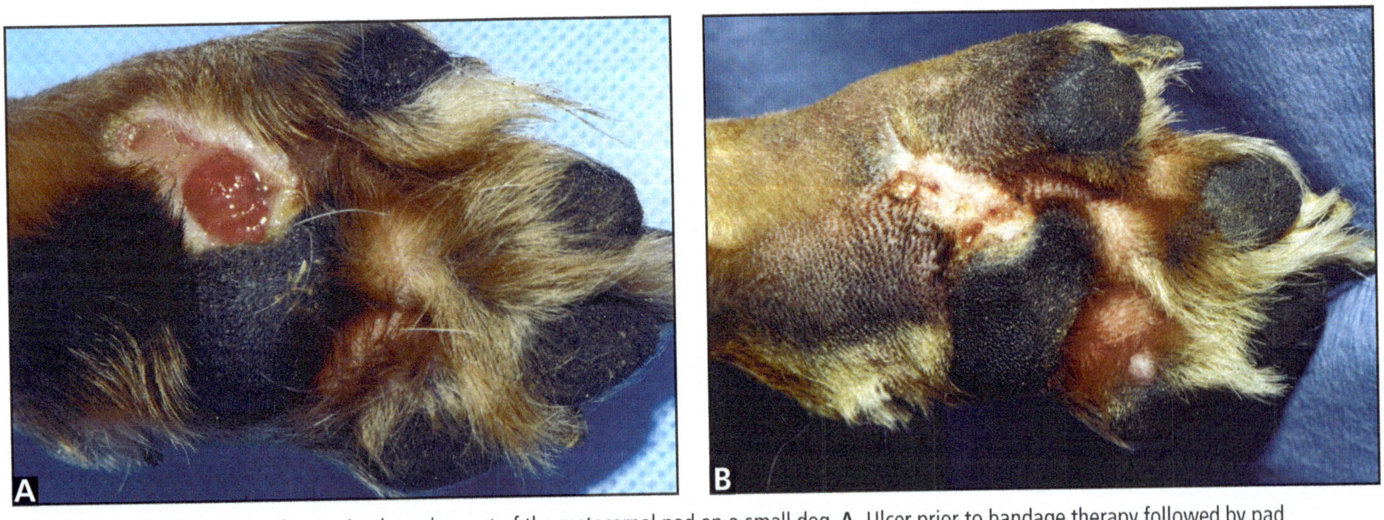


Figure 4-21. Trophic ulcer at the proximolateral aspect of the metacarpal pad on a small dog. A. Ulcer prior to bandage therapy followed by pad toughener. B. Ulcer after one month of treatment. (From Swaim SF: Pressure – Related Wounds: Prevention and Treatment. Clinician's BriefDec: 8, 2003.)

# Pad Replacement: Phalangeal Fillet

## Definition and Indications

Phalangeal fillet is the removal of the proximal, middle, and distal phalanges from a digit, usually the second or fifth digit, to free its pad to be used to replace part of the metacarpal or metatarsal pad using the digital skin as a flap (Figure 4-22). The technique is indicated when large amounts of the metacarpal/ metatarsal pad are missing to include deep pad ulceration, when management of the wound by bandaging and medication, use of pad toughener, and gradual increase in exercise have not resulted in effective healing of the pad by re-epithelialization from the pad that remains. The technique is also indicated to replace the metacarpal or metatarsal pad when it has been completely lost (Figure 4-23). However, it should be borne in mind that the third and fourth digits bear considerable weight. There may be instances where the metacarpal or metatarsal pad are missing and these two digits can bear enough weight that replacement of the missing metacarpal or metatarsal pad may not be needed. This would most likely be on a smaller dog and/or when a metatarsal pad is missing since less weight is borne on the pelvic limbs.

## Techniques

Animals with a chronic nonhealing wound of the metacarpal or metatarsal pad that does not have a known cause (e.g. known trauma, or tumor removal) should receive a thorough examination prior to surgery. A cytologic examination, fungal and bacterial culture and sensitivity as well as histopathologic examination should be performed on the wound tissue. If a fungal infection or a neoplasm is found, appropriate medical and surgical therapy should be performed. This may range from limb amputation to amputation and replacement of only the pad (phalangeal fillet technique). If histopathologic examination reveals the chronic granulomatous tissue of a nonhealing wound, the wound should be thoroughly debrided in case the chronic granulation tissue has foreign material (i.e. dirt and/or sand) embedded in it caused by the animal walking on the wound without a bandage.

### Palmar/Plantar Fillet

The digit nearest the metacarpal or metatarsal pad defect is selected for filleting. This is usually the second or fifth digit, because the third and fourth digits are more important for weight-bearing. When it is necessary to replace an entire metacarpal or metatarsal pad, it is advisable to let all wounds on the paw heal with a bandage or protective commercial bootie covering. This protective covering is left off of the paw for increasingly longer periods of times to allow the animal use of the paw. During this time, the palmar/plantar surface of the paw is observed for early signs of wear or ulceration. In this way, the primary weight-bearing area of the injured paw can be detected, and the second or fifth digit, whichever is nearest the lesion, can be selected for filleting.

A rectangular segment of skin is removed from the palmar/plantar interpad skin which lies between the selected digital pad and the edge of the metacarpal or metatarsal pad defect (Figure 4-24A). The proximal, middle and distal phalanges of the digit are removed by first incising the joint capsules and ligamentous attachments to the phalanges. Using blunt dissection, all 3 bones and the nail are then removed from the digit (Figure 4-24B). The blood and nerve supply to the soft tissues of the digit are thus preserved. If the

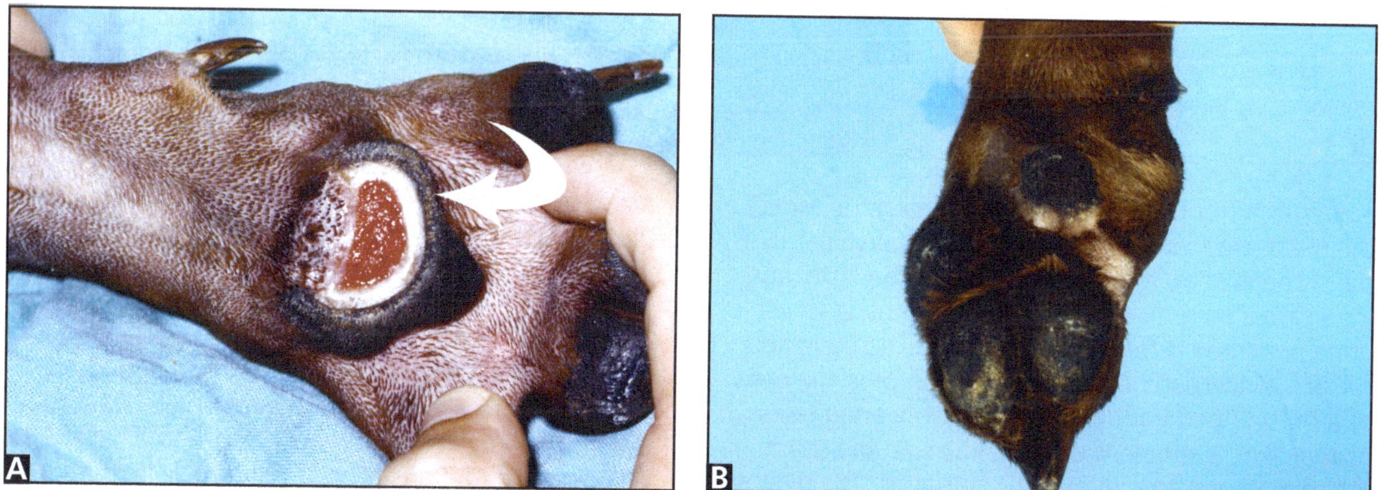


**Figure 4-22.** Phalangeal fillet technique to correct a metacarpal pad defect. **A.** Large nonhealing metacarpal pad wound. After the phalanges and nail are removed from the second digit, the digital pad will be folded back into the defect *(arrow)*. **B.** Completed pad transposition. (From Swaim SF, Garrett PD: Foot salvage techniques for dogs and cats: Options, "do's" and "don'ts". J Am An Hosp Assoc 21: 511, 1985.)

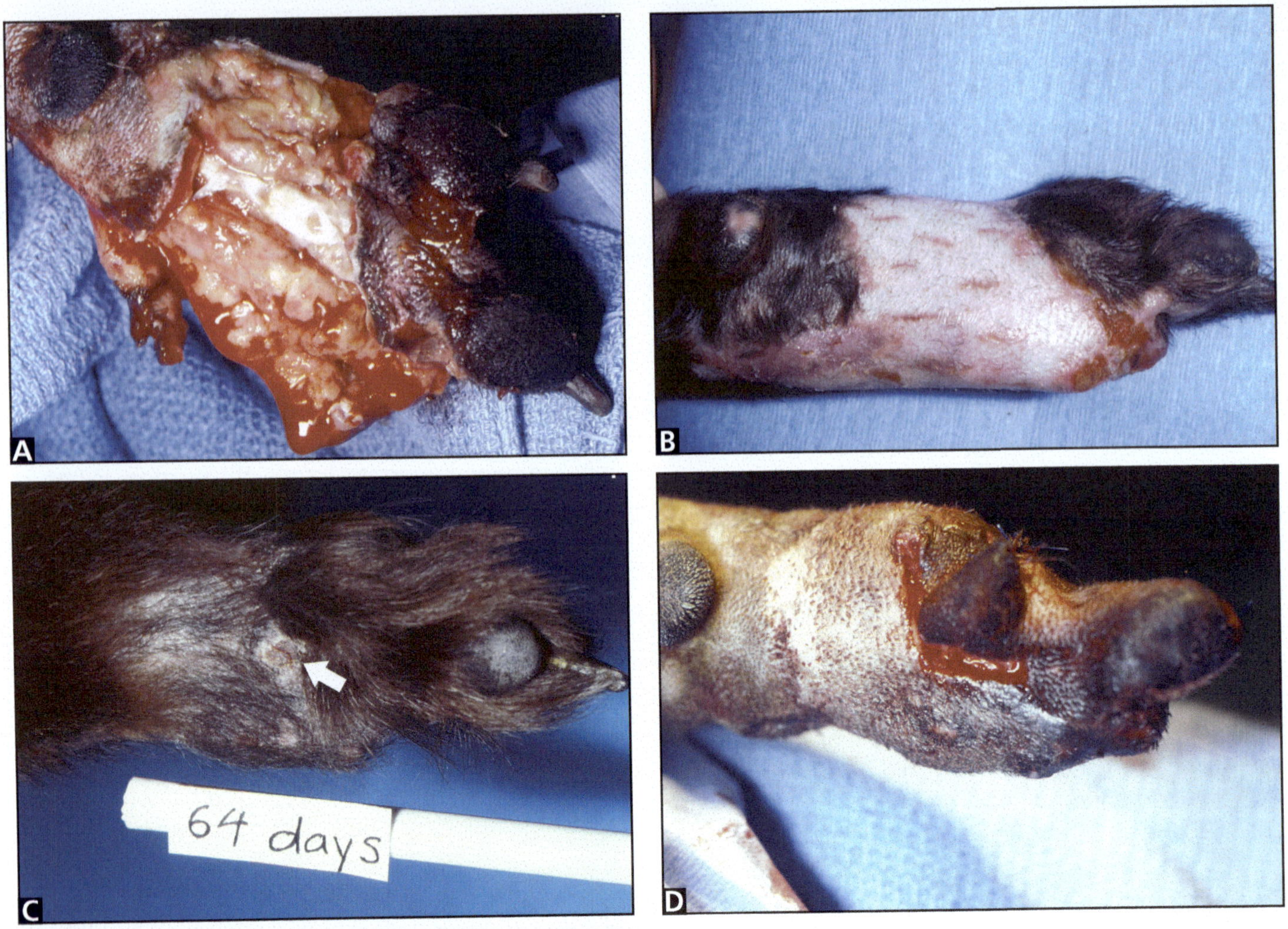


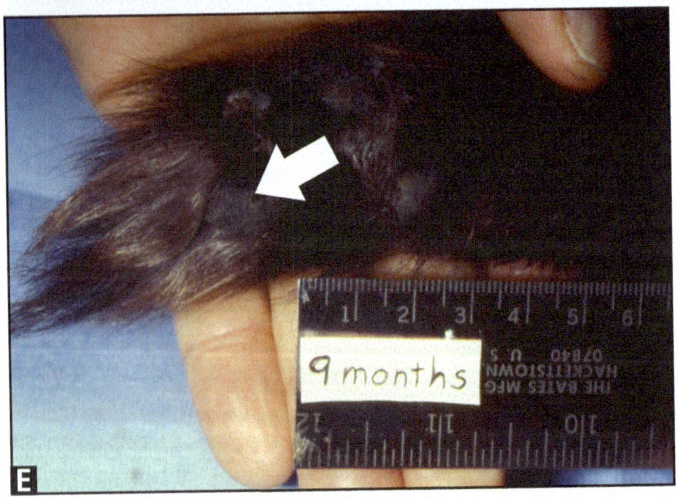


**Figure 4-23.** Mesh skin graft and palmar phalangeal fillet to replace a metacarpal pad. **A.** Forepaw degloving wound with metacarpal pad absent. **B.** Mesh graft reconstruction of the wound. **C.** Small palmer ulcer *(arrow)* beginning 64 days after skin graft. **D.** Fifth digit has been filleted and its pad will be sutured over the ulcerated area. **E.** Nine months after phalangeal fillet, the fifth digital pad is bearing weight functionally with no palmar ulcer *(arrow)*. (A & E from Bradley DM, Shealy PM, Swaim SF: Meshed skin graft and phalangeal fillet for paw salvage: A case report. J Am An Hosp Assoc 29:427, 1993. B and D from Swaim SF, Henderson RA: Small Animal Wound Management, 2nd ed.: Baltimore: Williams & Wilkins, 1997, 344.)

wound is a trophic ulcer at the proximolateral aspect of the metacarpal pad as a result of ulnar nerve paralysis, the surgeon should consider removing the distal end of metacarpal bone five using rongeurs. Thus, a source of bone pressure on the area is removed. The edge and surface of the pad defect are debrided, or in the case of a missing pad with an early weight-bearing lesion in palmar skin, a segment of tissue the size and shape of the second or fifth digital pad is removed. The digital pad of the filleted digit is then transposed back on its neurovascular pedicle of skin to fill the defect in the metacarpal or metatarsal pad or to cover the area of the early weight-bearing lesion (Figure 4-24C). Using 3-0 monofilament nonabsorbable suture material, the edges of the digital pad are sutured to the edges of the defect with a simple interrupted or far-near-near-far pattern (Figure 4-24D). The pedicle of digital skin may form "dog ears" as the pad is folded into position. If there is a question regarding removal of these "dog ears" for fear of jeopardizing the blood supply to the pad or distal end of the pedicle, their edges should be sutured together. After the pad has had an opportunity to establish a blood supply in its new location (about 14 days) and if the "dog ears"

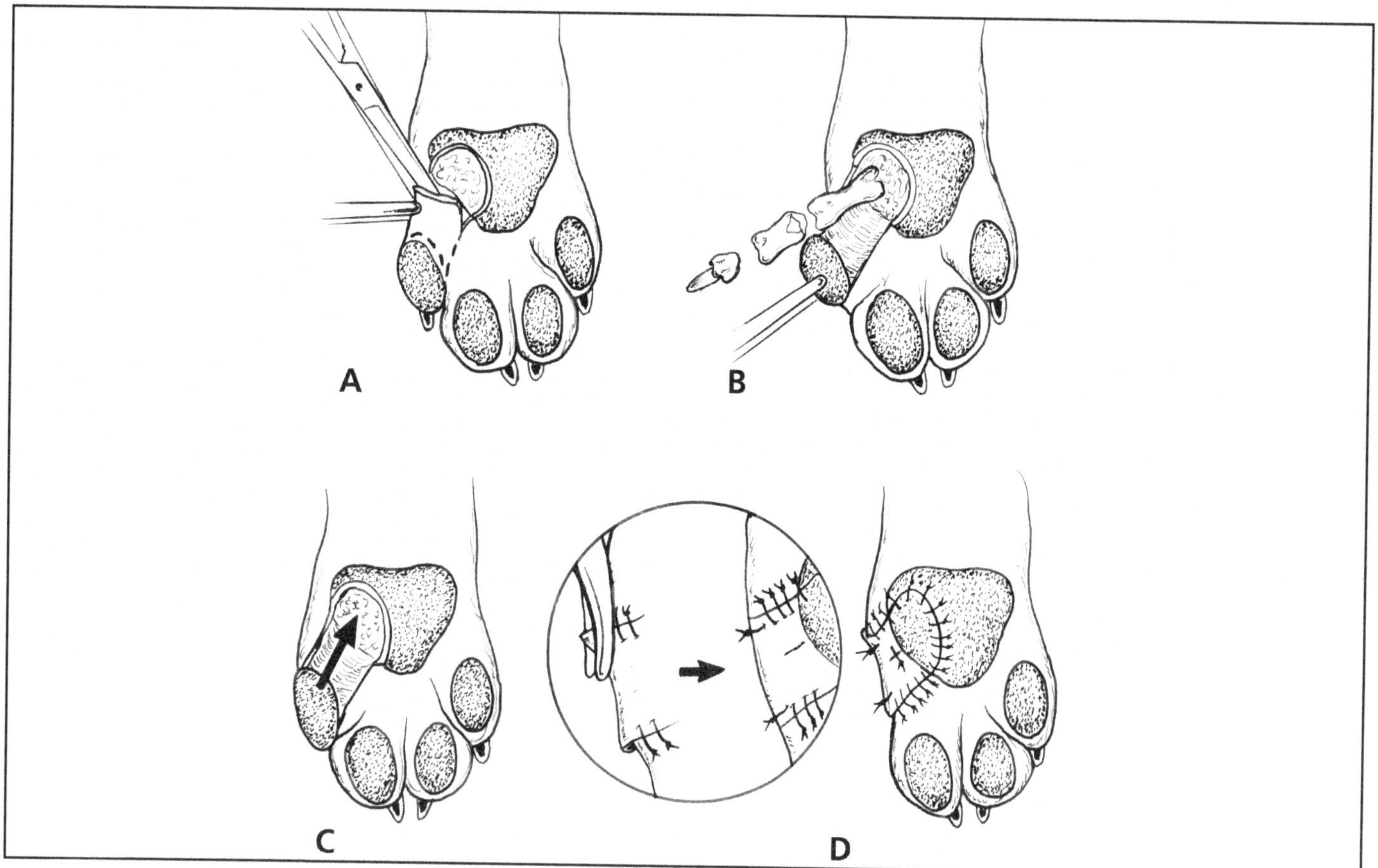


**Figure 4-24.** Palmar/plantar phalangeal fillet technique to fill a metatarsal pad defect. **A.** A rectangle of skin being removed from between the metatarsal pad defect and the fifth digital pad. **B.** Removing the proximal, middle, and distal phalanges and nail. **C.** The fifth digital pad will be folded back into the metatarsal pad defect *(arrow)*. **D.** The fifth digital pad sutured in place with small "dog ears" at the level of the flap fold. *(Inset)* "dog ear" removal for smooth closure. (After Swaim SF, Henderson RA: Small Animal Wound Management 2nd ed.: Baltimore: Williams & Wilins, 1997, 345.)

have not regressed sufficiently, they can be surgically excised (Figure 4-24D inset).

### Dorsal Fillet

Another technique for performing phalangeal fillet is to remove the phalanges from the second or fifth digit via a single longitudinal incision on the dorsum of the digit (Figure 4-25A & B). Following removal of the bones, the skin is sutured with simple interrupted sutures of 3-0 monofilament nonabsorbable suture material. To provide drainage, the incision is left open where the nail was removed (Figure 4-25C and Figure 4-26).

The paw is bandaged with periodic bandage changes for 14 days while the dorsal incision heals. At this time, the rectangle of palmar/plantar interdigital skin is removed from between the metacarpal/metatarsal pad defect and the digital pad. The digital pad is transposed back into the metacarpal/metatarsal pad defect and sutured into place as described previously (Figure 4-25D-F and Figure 4-27).

## Aftercare

The paw is bandaged. Small amounts of cotton or cast padding can be placed in the remaining interdigital areas and in the palmar/plantar interpad area to keep the areas dry. Absorbent gauze sponges are placed over the surgical site. A thick absorbent bandage wrap is placed on the paw, followed by a porous adhesive tape or elastic tape outer layer. To help keep pressure off of the transposed digital flap, which could result in sutures tearing through the skin, a "donut"-type foam rubber pad and metal splint cup can be incorporated in the bandage to distribute pressure around the flap area. A "clam shell" splint can be used as a localized crutch to help keep pressure off of the sutured pad in large dogs. If all weight bearing is to be avoided a Velpeau sling, carpal flexion splint, or carpal flexion sling can be used on the forelimb or a 90/90 sling on the hind limb. Cats and small dogs are lighter and do not place as much weight on their pads as larger dogs. For them, a well padded bandage without a "donut"-type foam rubber pad or metal splint cup should be sufficient. (See Palmar/Plantar Pad Wounds, Deep Pad Wounds, Pad Lacerations: Suturing in this chapter.)

## Advantages and Disadvantages

Filleting a digit from the palmar/plantar surface has the advantage of taking less time because it is a one-step procedure. The digit is filleted and the pad is moved into

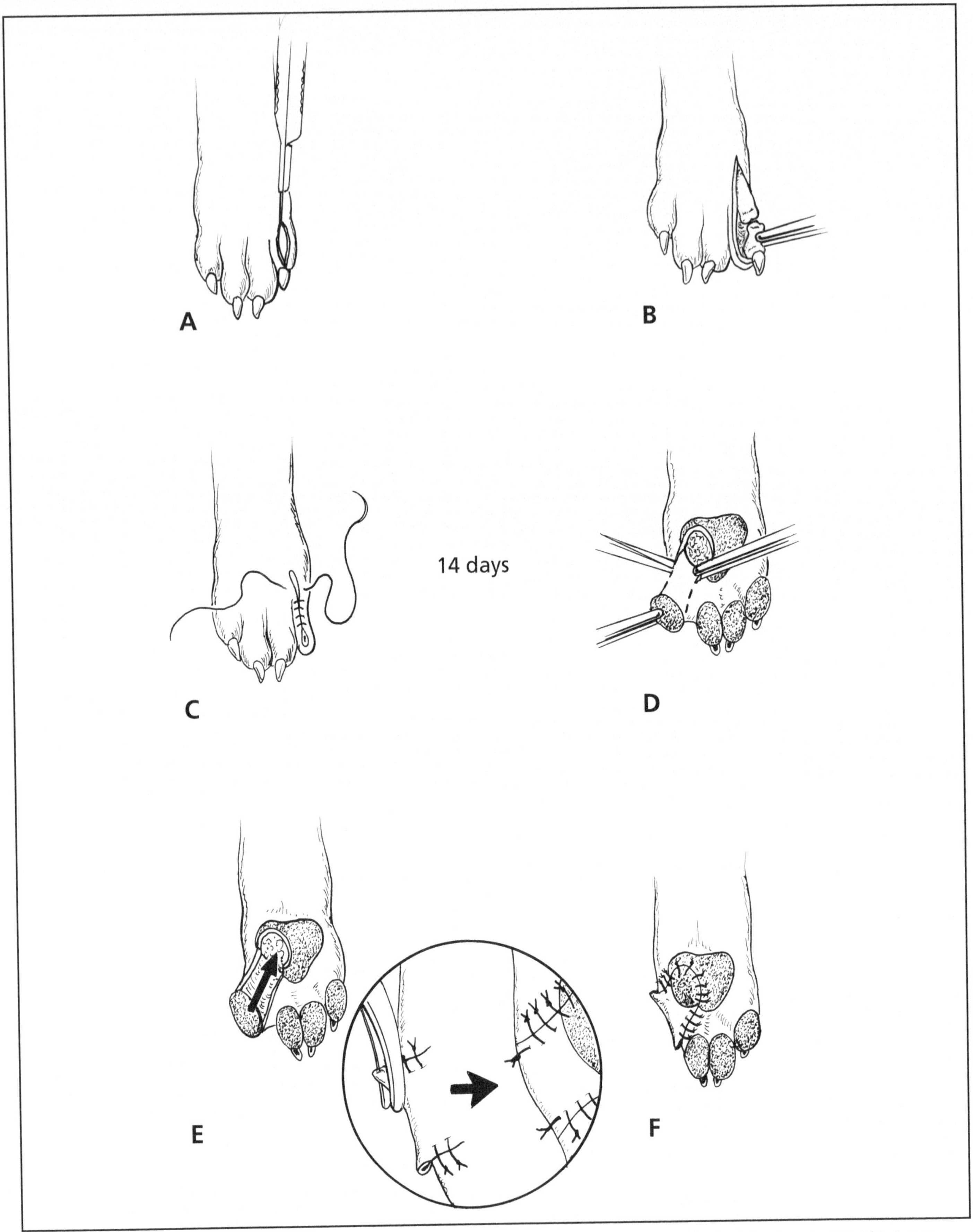


**Figure 4-25.** Dorsal phalangeal fillet technique to fill a metatarsal pad defect. **A.** A longitudinal incision is made along the dorsum of the fifth digit. **B.** Proximal, middle and distal phalanges and nail are removed. **C.** Longitudinal incision is sutured. **D.** Removing a rectangle of skin between the metatarsal pad defect and the fifth digital pad. **E.** The fifth digital pad will be folded back into the metatarsal pad defect *(arrow)*. **F.** The fifth digital pad folded in place with small "dog ears" at the level of the flap fold. *(Inset)* "dog ear" removal for smooth closure. (After Swaim SF, Henderson RA: Small Animal Wound Management 2nd ed.: Baltimore: Williams & Wilkins, 1997, 346.)

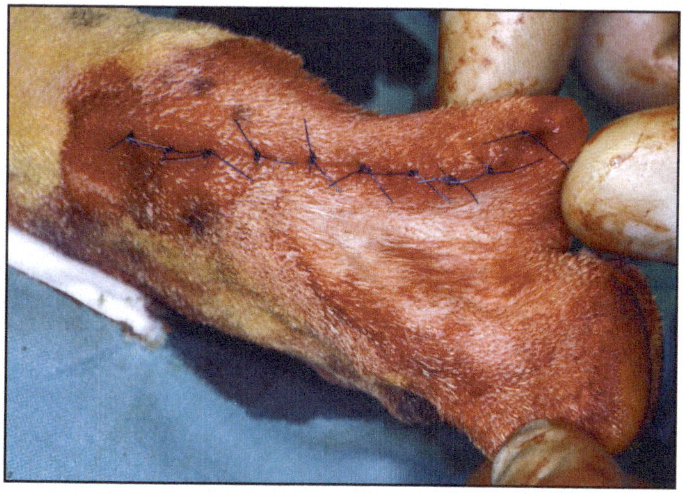

**Figure 4-26.** Dorsally filleted digit with skin edges sutured leaving the distal end of the suture line open for drainage.

position in the same operation. The procedure, however, has the disadvantage of being a little more difficult to perform than the dorsal fillet approach, and there is more potential for damaging the blood supply to the pad. Filleting a digit from the dorsal approach is easier, but the technique takes longer because it is a two-step procedure - filleting the digit, and moving the digital pad into position 14 days later. The digital pad is small when it is used to replace the metacarpal or metatarsal pad; however, when weight is borne on the healed pad, it tends to spread out to serve its intended function.

There may be cases in which the digital pad transposition may be unsuccessful if the pad is transposed into a wound caused by abnormal paw position resulting from tendon malfunction, bone malalignment, or peripheral nerve damage. Unless the cause is corrected, the new pad may wear through as did the original pad. If a transposed pad begins to show signs of breaking down, pad toughener (Paw Pad Toughener, Island Pharmacy, Woodruff, WI) may be used to try to avert loss of the pad.

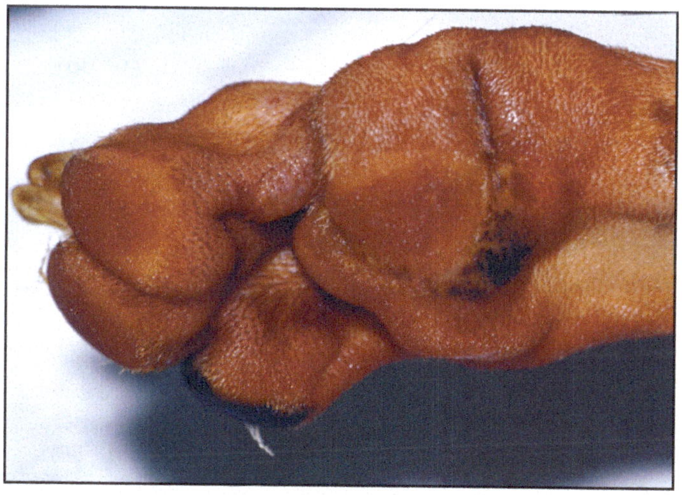

**Figure 4-27.** Digital pad healed in place to replace part of a metacarpal pad.

# Suggested Readings


1. Basher A: Foot injuries in dogs and cats. Compend Contin Educ Pract Vet 16:1159, 1994.
2. Bohling MW, Swaim SF: Paw and distal limb skin reconstructive and salvage procedures. In Bojrab MJ, ed.: Current Techniques in Small Animal Surgery, 5th ed.: Jackson, WY: Teton NewMedia 2014, 628.
3. Bradley DM, Shealy PM, Swaim SF: Meshed skin graft and phylangeal fillet for paw salvage: A case report. J Am Anim Hosp Assoc 29:427, 1993.
4. Farrell M, Dunn A, Marchevsky A: A case report: Surgical reconstruction of canine foot pads burned by sodium hypochlorite drain cleaner. Compendium 33:, 2011.
5. Fearnside SM, Straw RC: Transposition of first digital pad for reconstruction of a palmar antebrachium soft tissue defect in a cat. Aust Vet 81: 50, 2003.
6. Fowler D, Williams JM: Case examples. *In* Fowler D, Williams JM, eds.: BSAVA Manual of Canine and Feline Wound Management and Reconstruction. Shurdington, Cheltenham, UK: BSAVA, 1999, 145.
7. Fowler D: Distal limb and paw injuries. Vet Clin No Am Small Animal Pract 36: 819, 2006.
8. Hedlund CS: Surgery of the integumentary system. In Fossume TW, ed.: Small Animal Surgery, 2nd ed.: St. Louis: Mosby, 2002, 134.
9. Hedlund CS: Surgery of the integumentary system. In Fossum TW, ed.: Small Animal Surgery, 3rd ed.: St. Louis, Mosby, 2007, 159.
10. Hunt GB: Local or subdermal plexus flaps. In Tobias KM, Johnston SA, eds.: Veterinary Surgery, Small Animal, Vol. 2: St. Louis: Elsevier – Saunders, 2012, 1243.
11. MacPhail CM: Surgery of the integumentary system. In Fossum TW, ed.: Small Animal Surgery, 4th ed.: St. Louis: Mosby, 2013, 190.
12. Neat BC, Smeak DD: Reconstructive weight – bearing surfaces: digital pad transposition. Compend Contin Edu Pract Vet 29: 39, 2007.
13. Niles JD: Special considerations in wound management. In Williams J, Moores A, eds.: BSAVA Manual of Canine and Feline Wound Management and Reconstruction, 2nd ed.: Glouster (UK) BSAVA, 2009, 223.
14. Olsen D, Straw RC, Withrow SJ, et al: Digital pad transposition for replacement of the metacarpal or metatarsal pad in dogs. J Am Anim Hosp Assoc 33:337, 1997.
15. Pavletic MM: Atlas of Small Animal Reconstructive Surgery, 2nd ed: Philadelphia: WB Saunders, 1999, 365.
16. Pavletic MM: Atlas of Small Animal Wound Management and Reconstructive Surgery, 3rd ed.: Ames, IA: Wiley – Blackwell, 2010, 535.
17. Prassinos NN, Sideri A, Papazoglou LG: Conservative management of complete loss of a metatarsal pad in a dog. Vet Comp Ortho Trauma 4: 325, 2009.
18. Rahal SC, Mortari AC, Filho MMM: Mesh skin graft and digital pad transfer to reconstruct the weight – bearing surface in a dog. Can Vet J 48: 1258, 2007.
19. Swaim SF, Garrett PD: Foot salvage techniques for dogs and cats: Options, "do's" and "don'ts". J Am Anim Hosp Assoc 21:511, 1985.
20. Swaim SF: Wound management of distal limbs and paws: Reconstruction and salvage. Vet Med Rep 2:128, 1990.
21. Swaim SF, Marghitu DB, Rumph PF, et al: Effects of bandage configuration on paw pad pressure in dogs: A preliminary study. J Am Anim Hosp Assoc 39:209, 2003.
22. Swaim SF, Scardino MS: Paw and distal limb salvage and reconstructive techniques. *In* Bojrab MJ, ed.: Current Techniques in Small Animal Surgery, 4th ed.: Baltimore: Williams and Wilkins, 1998, 625.
23. Swaim SF, Renberg WC, Shike KM: Small Animal Bandaging, Casting and Splinting Techniques. Ames, IA: Wiley – Blackwell, 2011, 43.

24. White RAS: Surgical treatment of specific skin disorders. *In* Slatter DH, ed.: Textbook of Small Animal Surgery, 3rd ed.: Philadelphia: WB Saunders, 2003, 239

# Pad Replacement: Pouch Flap (For use on cats only)

## Definition and Indications

(See Chapter 3.)

Pouch and hinge flaps may be used to cover skin defects on the dorsum and lateral aspects of the distal limb and paws on dogs and cats for wounds that have nonapposable edges and no potential for apposition. They may also be used to replace the metacarpal and metatarsal pads on cats (Figure 4-28 and See Figure 3-78A & B and Figure 3-79).

A common cause of loss of skin, including pad tissue, on the paw of a cat is tight bandaging to control hemorrhage after onchyectomy. The end result is avascular necrosis. The defect left by this necrosis is an open wound that encircles the distal limb/ paw. There may or may not be some retained digital pad tissue. Although a hinge flap could be used for reconstruction, a pouch flap lends itself well to reconstruction of this wound. Thus, the pouch flap will be described for reconstructing this wound.

For house cats that will walk primarily on carpets, the skin from the body placed on the paw as a pouch or hinge flap will undergo sufficient hyperplasia to function as a pad replacement. In general, skin from the body should not be used for pad replacement on dogs because it does not withstand the stress a dog places on the skin. It is prone to ulceration.

## Technique

(See Chapter 3.)

Any viable pad tissue, i.e. digital pads, that remains on the limb should be left undisturbed. The cat is placed in lateral recumbency with the affected limb uppermost. If the wound is composed of a bed of granulation tissue with advancing epithelium coming from the wound edge, the epithelium is removed. The surface of the wound is cleaned of any coagulum on its surface by wiping the surface with a surgical sponge moistened with a 0.05% chlorhexidine diacetate (Nolvasan Solution, Ft. Dodge Animal Health, Ft. Dodge, IA) or gluconate (ChlorhexiDerm Disinfectant, Dermatologics in Veterinary Medicine Pharmaceuticals, Inc., Miami, FL) solution. The affected limb is then placed along the cat's side in the most comfortable position that minimizes stress on the limb. Two parallel dorsoventral incisions are made in the lateral thoracoabdominal skin at the location of the paw wound along the cat's side. The distance between the incisions is slightly longer than the length of the defect to allow for primary skin contraction and the skin stretching that will be necessary to place the paw under the flap.

The flap is undermined beneath the cutaneous trunci muscle, the limb is flexed and the paw is placed under the flap. Simple interrupted sutures of 3-0 monofilament nonabsorbable suture material are used to suture the edges of the flap to edges of the defect. To help assure adequate vascular and connective tissue adherence to the wound, several tacking sutures should be placed through the flap into underlying tissue (Figure 4-28B & C).

When there is no digital pad tissue at the end of the stump, only one incision is made in the thoracoabdominal skin. The adjacent skin and cutaneous trunci muscle are undermined to accommodate the paw stump. They are undermined cranially for a hind paw defect and caudally for a forepaw defect. The wound edge is sutured to the edge of the incision as described above (Figure 4-28F & G).

To help assure adequate vascular and connective tissue adherence to the wound several tacking sutures should be placed through the flap into underlying wound tissue. A ¼-inch diameter Penrose drain may be placed in the most dependent base of the flap to provide drainage of any fluid that may accumulate in the space around the flap and limb (Figure 4-28C & G). Another option is to leave an area open for drainage at the ventralmost area of junction of the flap with the distal-most aspect of the defect.

To help hold the limb in position against the body, large tacking or support sutures can be placed between areas with intact skin on the limb and similar skin on the cat's trunk. When the flap has had sufficient time to revascularize and establish a connective tissue bond to the wound, usually about 14 days, the flap bases are incised. Sufficient skin should be taken with the bases of the flap to allow for coverage of the remaining wound on the medial side of the paw (Figure 4-28D & H). If it is necessary to assure an adequate blood supply to the flap, the flap may be incised in stages with 2 to 3 day intervals between incisions. Some surgeons do not believe this delaying procedure is critically beneficial.

The medial surface of the paw may be adhered to the cat's body wall. It will be necessary to dissect it free

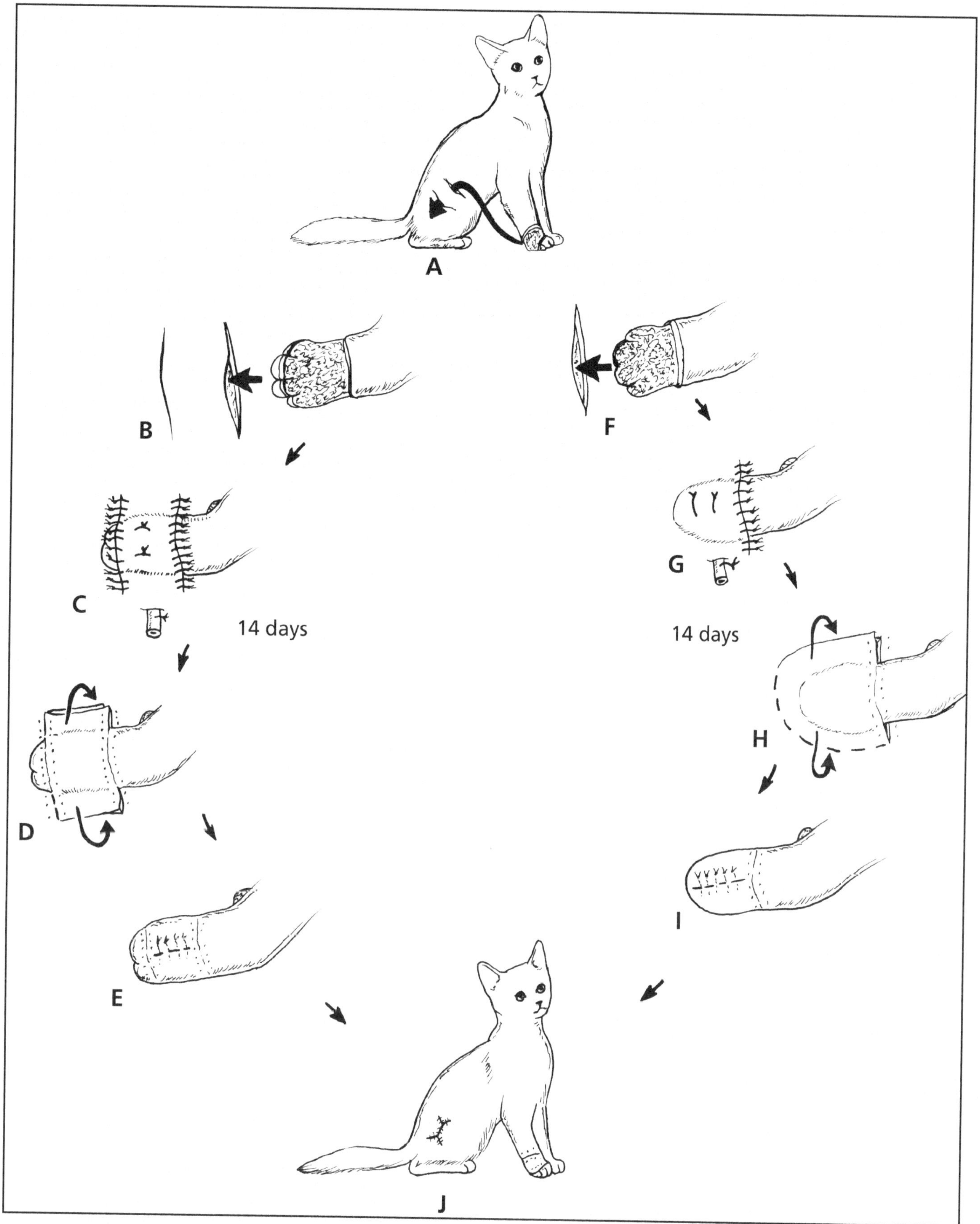


**Figure 4-28.** Pouch flaps to replace pads on cats. **A.** Paw defect, with missing pads, to be placed under a pouch flap on cat's side *(arrow)*. **B.** When some digital pad tissue remains, two dorsal-ventral parallel incisions are made in the lateral throacoabdominal skin, and the skin is undermined. **F.** when no digital pad tissue remains, one dorsal-ventral incision is made in the lateral thoracoabdominal skin, and the skin is undermined – caudally for a forelimb lesion and cranially for a pelvic limb lesion. **C.** & **G.** Paw defect is placed under the flap and sutured in place. A drain is placed. **D.** & **H.** Excision of the flap from the body. **E.** & **I.** Flap wrapped around the paw and sutured in place. **J.** Flap transferred to paw and donor site closed. (After Swaim SF, Henderson RA: Small Animal Wound Management, 2nd ed.: Baltimore: Williams & Wilkins, 1997, 350.)

to continue with the procedure. The 2 ends of the flap are wrapped around the remaining defect on the medial side of the paw. They are trimmed appropriately and sutured together with simple interrupted 3-0 nonabsorbable sutures (Figure 4-28E & I).

The donor site on the cat's side is closed by undermining and advancing the skin edges together with "walking" sutures and continuous subcuticular sutures of 3-0 absorbable suture material. Skin apposition is with 3-0 simple interrupted nonabsorbable sutures (Figure 4-28J).

### Aftercare

(See Chapter 3.)

The limb is bandaged against the body for about 14 days following suturing of the paw under the flap. If necessary, extra, absorbent surgical sponges can be placed over the flap in areas where there will be drainage. Cotton may be placed between the limb and body in areas of intact skin for padding. On the forelimb, care should be taken to avoid bandage pressure on skin over the olecrannon and possibly the extension surface of the carpus depending on the limb's position. A small modified "donut"-type bandage of soft cast padding material can be used for this purpose. However, this may not be critical on cats. Due to their light weight a small amount of pressure is placed on the area. A circumferential absorbent secondary wrap and a tertiary wrap of adhesive tape or elastic bandage complete the bandage. Bandaging should be done carefully to help reduce outward limb rotation. An access window may be cut in the bandage over the flap to allow the flap to be attended to during healing (See Figure 3-81B). Although drainage is usually not copious from cats, the bandage should be changed frequently to monitor drainage and to change dressings overlying the flap as needed.

After the flap has been transferred to the limb it should be protected with a bandage for another 7 to 10 days.

### Advantages and Disadvantages

(See Chapter 3.)

## Suggested Readings

(See Chapter 3)

## Pad Replacement: Tubed Pedicle Flap (For use on cats only)

(See Chapter 3)

## Pad Replacement: Carpal Pad-Single and Bipedicle Advancement Flaps

### Definition and Indications

The carpal pad can be used to construct a weight-bearing tissue under the carpometacarpal area following distal limb amputation using 2 techniques. First, a dorsally-based single pedicle advancement flap can be designed on the palmar surface of the distal limb to include the carpal pad on the distal end of the flap. The flap/carpal pad is rotated under the caudodistal aspect of the carpal bones after amputation at the carpal-metacarpal joint. Second, a horizontally-oriented bipedicle flap can be designed on the palmar surface of the distal limb to include the carpal pad in the center of the flap. The flap/carpal pad is rotated under the carpometacarpal area after amputation in this area.

The 2 carpal pad transposition techniques are indicated as limb salvage procedures when there is significant trauma or destruction of the pads, digits, and distal metacarpal area warranting distal limb amputation at the carpal-metacarpal level. The 2 techniques have been described as case reports* and the practitioner should consider them in selected cases following assessment of the animal's wounds, availability of tissue, the animal's size, it's level of activity and the owner's expectations. The technique has potential for use on large dogs; however, correct positioning of the advanced pad may be more critical considering the greater weight to be borne.

### Techniques

#### Single Pedicle Advancement Flap

A dorsally-based single pedicle flap of skin is created on the palmar surface of the affected limb to include the carpal pad in the distal aspect of the flap. There should be sufficient skin on the flap distal to the carpal pad to allow suturing of the flap to the dorsal limb skin after the flap is advanced into position. After designing the flap it is incised and dissected from underlying structures. The prominence of the accessory carpal bone is removed after transecting the flexor carpiulnaris insertion on it (Figure 4-29A). The distal limb is amputated at the carpal-metacarpal joint. It is advisable to remove the distal articular surfaces of the exposed carpal bones using rongeurs or preferably a pneumatic drill and burr. The flap is then advanced distally until the carpal pad is situated at the caudodistal end of the amputated area, or further if possible to place the carpal pad under the carpal bones as much as possible.

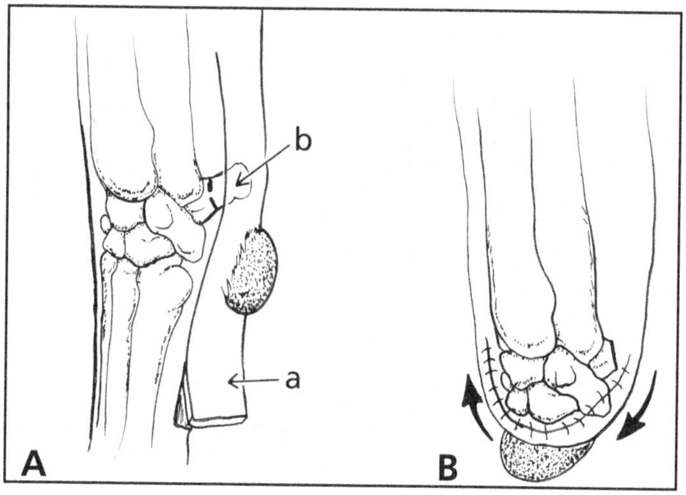


**Figure 4-29.** Single pedicle advancement flap to construct a weight-bearing tissue on the the forelimb. **A.** A dorsally-based single pedicle advancement flap designed on the palmar surface of affected limb with a carpal pad near the distal end of the flap *(a)*. Prominence of the accessory carpal bone will be removed *(broken line (b)*. **B.** Prominence of the accessory carpal bone removed. Distal limb amputated at the carpal-metacarpal articulation. Single pedicle advancement flap advanced and sutured in place with the carpal pad under the carpal bones. (After Barclay CG, Fowler JD, Basher AW: Use of the carpal pad to salvage the forelimb in a dog and cat: An alternative to total limb amputation. J Am Anim Hosp Assoc 23: 527, 1987.)

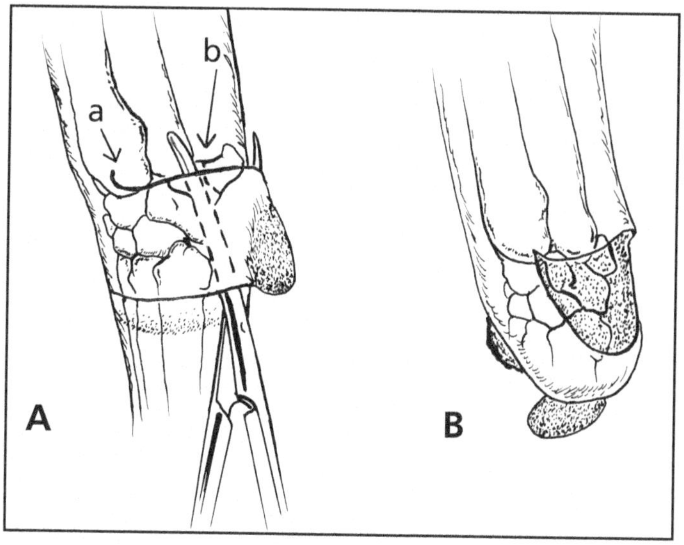


**Figure 4-30.** Bipedicle advancement flap to construct a weight-bearing tissue on the forelimb. **A.** A horizontally-oriented bipedicle skin flap designed on the palmar surface of the affected limb, including the carpal pad in the center of the flap. Incisions are proximal and distal to the carpal pad. Ends of proximal incision are curved proximally 2-3 mm *(a)*. Flap is undermined (scissors). Prominence of accessory carpal bone will be removed *(broken line (b)*. **B.** Prominence of accessory carpal bone removed. Distal limb amputated at the carpal-metacarpal area. Bipedicle advancement flap advanced under the end of the stump. (After Barclay CG, Fowler JD, Basher AW: Use of carpal pad to salvage the forelimb in a dog and cat: An alternative to total limb amputation. J Am Anim Hosp Assoc 23:257, 1987.)

The flap is sutured in place using subcutaneous simple interrupted sutures of 3-0 absorbable suture material to anchor the pad in place. The skin is sutured with simple interrupted sutures of 2-0 to 3-0 nonabsorbable suture material (Figure 4-29B).

### Bipedicle Advancement Flap

A horizontally-oriented bipedicle skin flap is created on the palmar surface of the affected limb to include the carpal pad in the center of the flap. Two parallel horizontal incisions, one proximal and one distal to the carpal pad, are made, with the ends of the proximal incision curved proximally 2 to 3 mm to facilitate flap movement. The flap is undermined (Figure 4-30A). The attachment of the flexor carpiulnaris to the accessory carpal bone is severed, and the prominence of the bone is removed. Amputation at the carpal-metacarpal articulation is performed at this time, if it has not already been performed. If the distal articular surfaces of the carpal bones are exposed with a carpal-metacarpal amputation, they should be removed with rongeurs or preferably with a pneumatic drill and burr. The flap is then advanced into position so the carpal pad is under the amputation stump (Figure 4-30B). The cranial edge of the flap may be sutured to the skin edge on the dorsum of the limb, and the palmar donor area can be allowed to heal as an open wound. Another option is to place a small mesh graft on the palmar donor area.

For both techniques, a semiocclusive nonadherent bandage pad (Telfa "Ouchless" Adhesive Pads, Covidien, Tyco Health Care/Kendall, Mansfield, MA) can be placed over the surgical area followed by an absorbent bandage wrap and a tertiary layer of porous adhesive tape or elastic tape. A "clam shell" splint can be applied to serve as a localized crutch to keep pressure off of the flap as it heals.

## Aftercare

The bandage/splint should be changed every 2 to 3 days, depending on the amount of drainage from the surgical area. Healing may be complete by 14 to 21 days. During this time and early after bandaging has been discontinued, exercise should be limited. The carpal pad should be monitored as exercise is gradually increased after bandaging is discontinued. The length of the monitoring period should be determined by pad examination and clinical judgment.

## Advantages and Disadvantages

The single and double pedicle carpal pad flaps have the primary advantage of offering the practitioner a salvage technique that can be offered to pet owners to salvage a forelimb and avert amputation when there has been severe distal limb trauma. Although the carpal pad is small when it is placed in a weight-bearing position, it will spread out to serve its intended function as weight is placed on the pad. When the procedure is performed on only one forelimb, that limb will be significantly shorter than the other forelimb. Thus, the animal may tend to carry the limb or use it only intermittently. To use the forelimb, the animal would necessarily have to straighten the scapulo-humeral and radio-humeral joints resulting in a straight or "post-legged" posture. Over time, this could conceivably result in orthopedic/arthritic pathology, especially in large dogs.

# Suggested Readings

*1. Barclay CG, Fowler JD, Basher AW: Use of the carpal pad to salvage the forelimb in a dog and cat: An alternative to total limb amputation. J Am Anim Hosp Assoc 23:527, 1987.
2. Basher A: Foot injuries in dogs and cats. Compend Contin Educ Pract Vet 16:1159, 1994.
3. Bohling MW, Swaim SF: Paw and distal limb skin reconstructive and salvage techniques. In Bojrab MJ, ed.: Current Techniques in Small Animal Surgery, 5th ed.: Jackson, WY: Teton NewMedia, 2014, 628.
4. Fowler D: Distal limb and paw injuries. Vet Clin No Am Small Animal Pract 36: 819, 2006.
5. Pavletic MM: Atlas of Small Animal Wound Management and Reconstructive Surgery, 3rd ed.: Ames, IA: Wiley – Blackwell, 2010, 535.
6. Swaim SF: Wound management of distal limbs and paws: Reconstruction and salvage. Vet Med Rep 2:128, 1990.
7. Swaim SF, Scardino MS: Paw and distal limb salvage and reconstructive techniques. *In* Bojrab MJ, ed.: Current Techniques in Small Animal Surgery, 4th ed.: Baltimore: Williams and Wilkins, 1998, 265.
8. Swaim SF, Marghitu DB, Rumph PF, et al: Effects of bandage configuration on paw pad pressure in dogs: A preliminary study. J Am Anim Hosp Assoc 39:209, 2003.
9. Swaim SF, Renberg WC, Shike KM: Small Animal Bandaging, Casting and Splinting Techniques. Ames, IA: Wiley – Blackwell, 2011, 43.
*Primary reference

# Pad Replacement: Pad Grafts

## Definition and Indications

Pad grafts are small rectangular segments of full-thickness pad skin taken from other pads on the same animal. The grafts are placed in rectangular recipient sites the same size as the grafts that have been prepared around the edge of a granulation tissue bed that has developed where the metacarpal/metatarsal pads are missing. The pad grafts heal by wound contraction, epithelialization, and hyperplasia.

Pad grafts are indicated when loss of digits on the paw precludes the use of phalangeal fillet to replace the pad or when it may not be desired or indicated to use a phalangeal fillet to replace a metacarpal or metatarsal pad. If all the digits and the metacarpal or metatarsal pad are missing, the animal's size and level of activity should be considered prior to using pad grafts as a salvage procedure to furnish weight-bearing tissue. The grafts are less likely to be successful on active large dogs. This is especially true when the entire paw is missing, and the pad grafts are placed on the ends of the metacarpal or metatarsal stump. However, with proper conditioning of healed pad grafts, they have worked well in large active dogs.

## Technique

The paw wound is treated as an open wound until a healthy bed of granulation has formed in the area to be grafted. The graft donor and recipient areas are prepared for aseptic surgery. Using a sterile splintered applicator stick dipped in sterile methylene blue and rectangular template of x-ray film with a 6 mm x 8 mm aperture in its center, rectangular tissue segments are traced at intervals around the wound periphery (Figure 4-31A). Graft sizes of 10 to 15 mm x 5 to 10 mm have also been described. A No. 11 scalpel blade is used to incise the rectangles in the granulation tissue. Thumb forceps and iris scissors are then used to remove the tissue. This leaves several rectangular depressions about 2 mm deep around the periphery of wound (Figure 4-31B inset & C).

The splintered applicator stick, methylene blue and template are used to trace the same number and size of rectangular pad grafts in the center of other digital pads or accessory pads on the same animal and possibly the same paw (Figure 4-31C). The grafts are incised with a No. 11 scalpel blade. Then thumb forceps and iris scissors are used to remove the grafts (Figure 4-31D). All subcutaneous tissue is removed from the grafts.

A graft is sutured into each rectangular depression using a 5-0 monofilament nonabsorbable suture in each corner of the graft (Figure 4-31E and Figure 4-32A).

## Aftercare

Small pieces of cotton or cast padding are placed in the interdigital and interpad areas. A nonadherent bandage pad (Telfa "Ouchless" Adhesive Pads, Covidien, Tyco HealthCare/ Kendall, Mansfield, MA) with a thin layer of gentamicin sulfate antibiotic ointment (Gentamicin sulfate ointment, 0.1%, Fougera, Melville, NY) is placed over the grafts. An abundant amount of absorbent secondary wrap is placed followed by a porous adhesive tape or elastic outer layer. To help keep pressure off of the grafts as they become established, a "clam shell" splint should be used as a localized crutch, even on medium and small dogs. A carpal flexion splint or carpal sling can be used on the forelimb for the same purpose. The

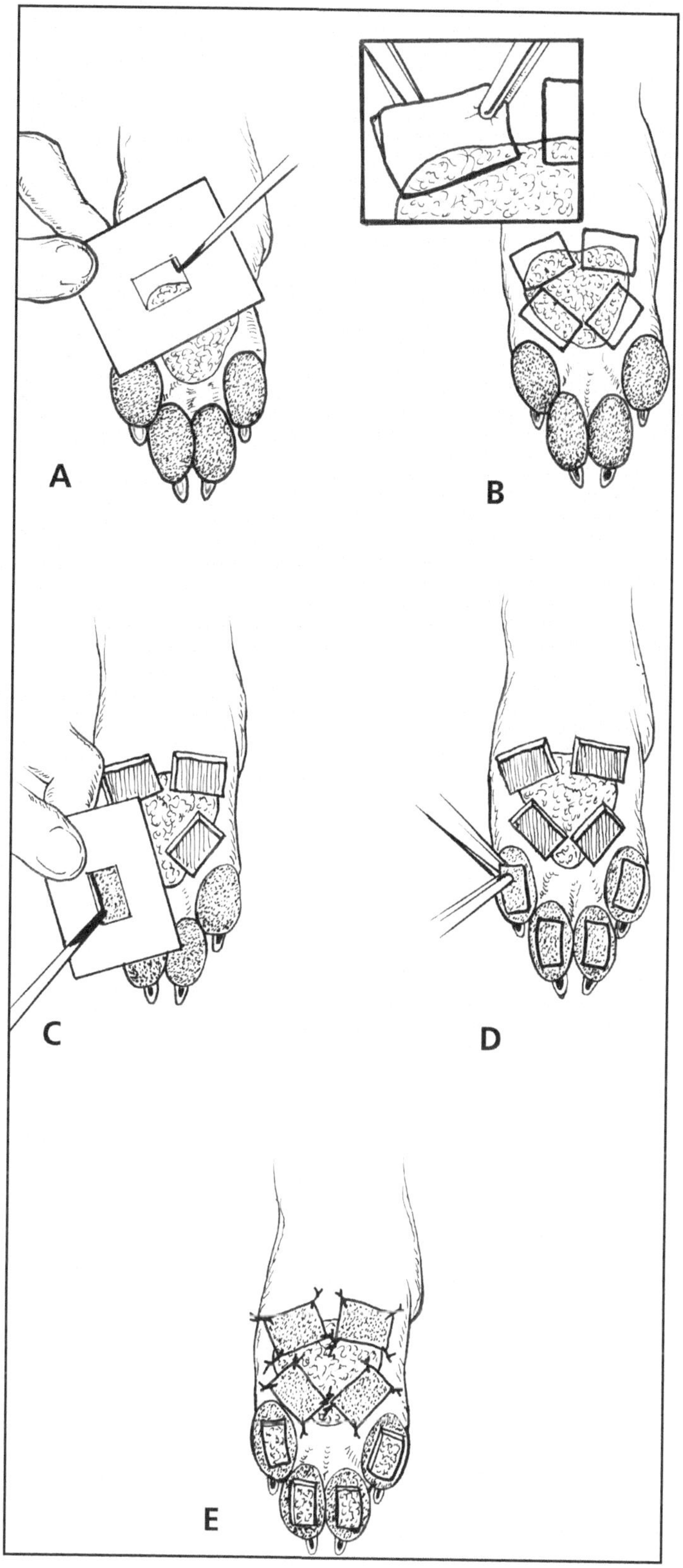


Figure 4-31. A. A piece of x-ray film with a 6x8 mm hole in its center is used with a splintered applicator stick dipped in sterile methylene blue to trace graft recipient sites around the wound. B. *(Inset)* Traced rectangles of tissue are removed from recipient sites with iris scissors and thumb forceps. C. Segmental pad grafts are traced using x-ray film pattern, splintered applicator stick and methylene blue. D. Grafts are excised with iris scissors and thumb forceps. E. Grafts are sutured in recipient sites with simple interrupted sutures of 5-0 polypropylene at each corner of the graft. (After Swaim SF, Bradley DM, Steiss JE, Buxton DF: Free segmental paw pad grafts in dogs. Am J Vet Res 54:2161, 1993.)

graft donor sites should be bandaged the same as a deep pad abrasion. However, if it is necessary to take the pad grafts from another paw it is best to use a foam rubber pad under the metacarpal/metatarsal pad in the bandage to relieve pressure on the digital wounds, because it would be difficult for the animal to ambulate with 2 "clam shell" splints or carpal flexion splints or carpal slings. If the remaining pad tissue around the donor sites is pliable enough the donor sites may be sutured with far-near-near-far sutures of 3-0 monofilament nonabsorbable suture. Bandaging is the same as if the wounds were allowed to heal as open wounds.

The initial bandage after grafting is changed 3 days postoperatively and then every other day until 21 days after surgery. A commercial bootie may be used in the transitional period between bandage and no bandage if it is deemed necessary. The bootie should be of a soft material.

Graft sutures are removed between 10 and 14 days postoperatively. At the time of suture removal, the hard dark stratum corneum will lift off of the grafts, and a viable underlying graft will be present which will form a new stratum corneum.

## Advantages and Disadvantages

Pad grafting offers an alternative to phalangeal fillet for replacing weight-bearing pads. Initially, in the healing process, a tough keratinized epithelium grows from the graft edges to cover the remaining wound. Later wound contraction provides the advantage of coalescing the grafts together thus forming a durable weight-bearing tissue (Figures 4-32B). The pad spreading phenomenon is an advantage; whereby, the grafted area may be small initially, but weight-bearing results in enlargement of the area to compensate and provide a durable weight-bearing tissue (Figure 4-33A-C).

When an entire paw has been lost and pad grafts are placed over the distal ends of metacarpal/metatarsal bones, there is no fibroadipose tissue under the grafts. They heal, epithelialize and coalesce as previously described (Figure 4-34A & B). In addition, with the use of pad toughener and gradual increase in stress on the pads, they become extremely hard to compensate for the lack of fibroadipose tissue and provide a durable weight-bearing tissue (Figure 4-35A & B).

Pad grafting requires making wounds to harvest the grafts in order to salvage or reconstruct a paw area. This requires additional paw bandaging. A slightly longer postoperative time may be required for pad grafts on large active dogs where the grafts are over bone. Use of pad toughener and a gradual increase of pad stress can produce the extremely hard durable pad tissue required.

## Suggested Readings

1. Basher A: Foot injuries in dogs and cats. Compend Contin Educ Pract Vet 16:1159, 1994.
2. Bohling MW, Swaim SF: Skin grafts. In Tobias KM, Johnston SA, eds.: Veterinary Surgery, Small Animal, Vol. 2: St. Louis: Elsevier – Saunders, 2012, 1271.
3. Bohling MW, Swaim SF: Paw and distal limb skin reconstruction and salvage techniques. In Bojrab MJ, ed.: Current Techniques in Small Animal Surgery, 5th ed.: Jackson, Wy: Teton NewMedia, 2014, 628.
4. Bradley DM, Swaim SF, Alexander CN, Jull BA: Autogenous pad grafts for reconstruction of a weight-bearing surface: A case report. J Am Anim Hosp Assoc 30:533, 1994.
5. Bradley DM, Scardino MS, Swaim SF: Construction of a weight-

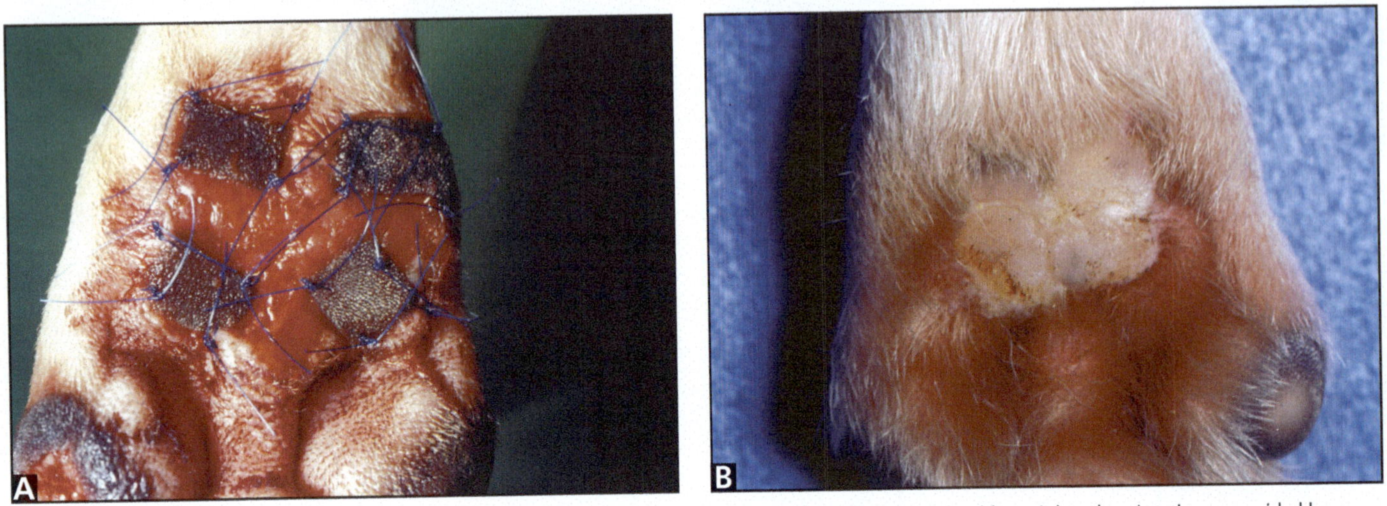


**Figure 4-32.** Pad grafts. **A.** Four pad grafts sutured around the periphery of a metatarsal pad defect. **B.** A durable weight – bearing tissue provided by coalescing of the four pad grafts. (From Swaim SF, Bradley DM, Steis JE, Powers RD, Buxton DF: Free segmental paw pad grafts in dogs. Am J Vet Res 54:2161, 1993.)

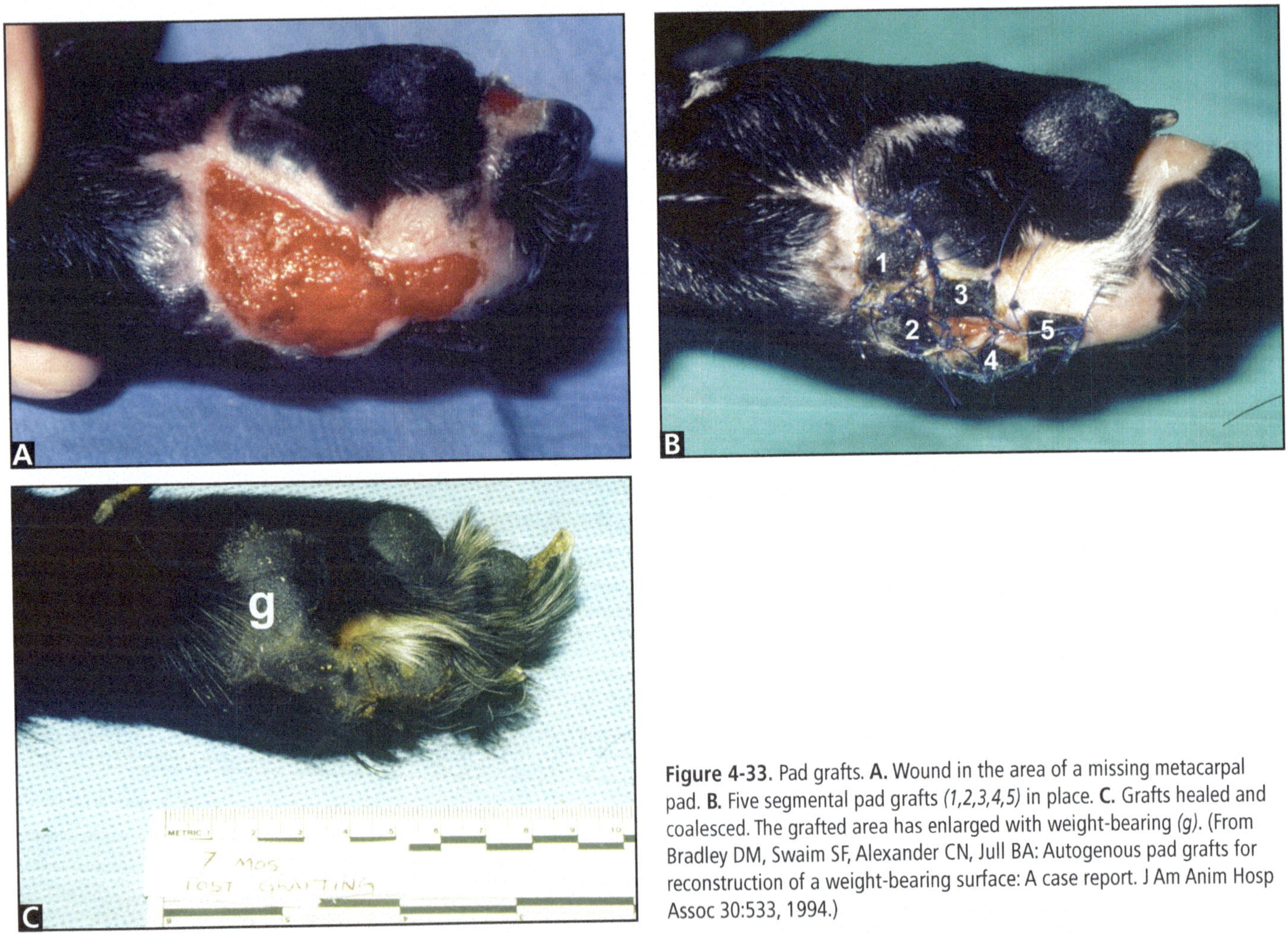


**Figure 4-33.** Pad grafts. **A.** Wound in the area of a missing metacarpal pad. **B.** Five segmental pad grafts *(1,2,3,4,5)* in place. **C.** Grafts healed and coalesced. The grafted area has enlarged with weight-bearing *(g)*. (From Bradley DM, Swaim SF, Alexander CN, Jull BA: Autogenous pad grafts for reconstruction of a weight-bearing surface: A case report. J Am Anim Hosp Assoc 30:533, 1994.)

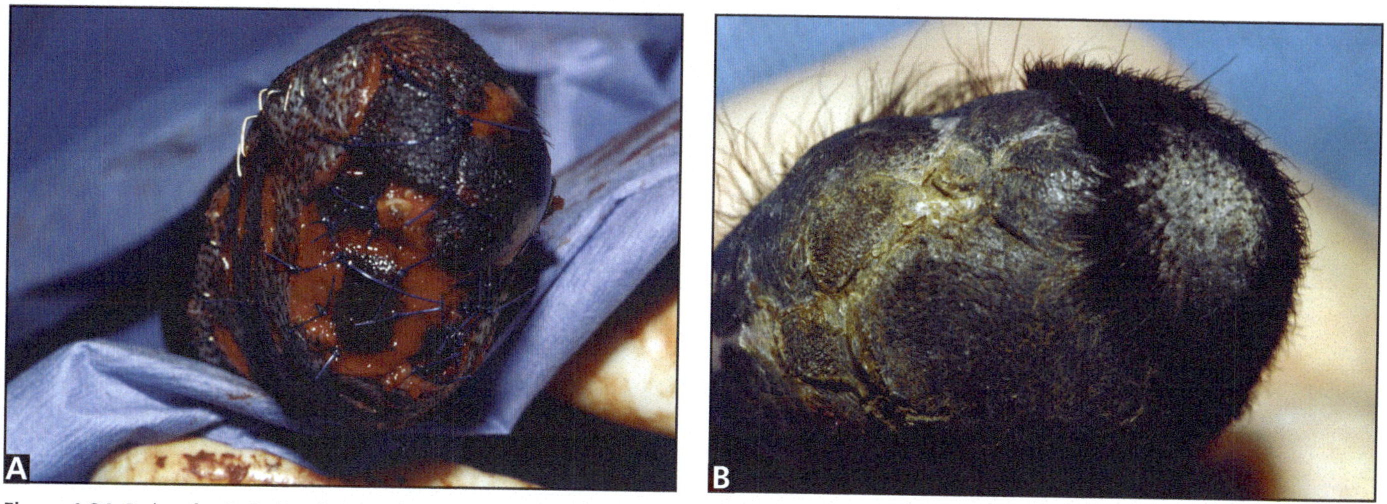


**Figure 4-34.** Pad grafts. **A.** Pad grafts immediately after being placed in granulation tissue over a metacarpal stump following loss of the paw. **B.** Two months after graft placement, showing coalescence and a durable weight-bearing tissue.

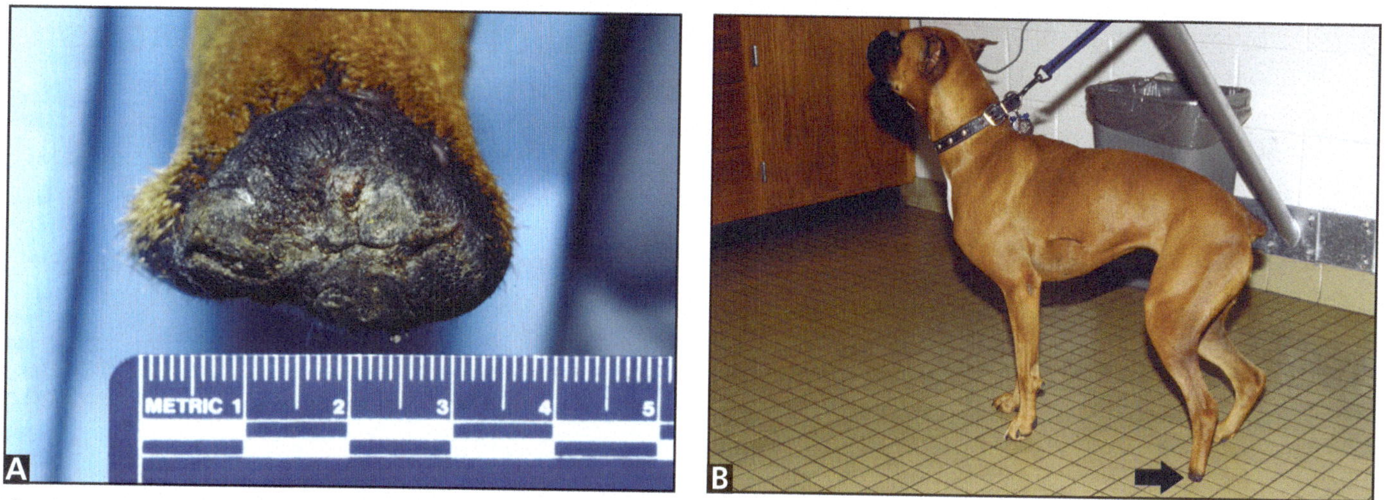


**Figure 4-35.** Pad grafts. **A.** Extremely hard coalesced pad grafts over a metatarsal stump resulting from use of pad toughener and gradual increase in stress of the area. **B.** Dog actively used the limb/stump *(arrow)* after graft healing. (From Bradley DM, Scardino MS, Swaim SF: Construction of a weight-bearing surface on a dog's distal pelvic limb. J Am Anim Hosp Assoc 34:387, 1998.)

bearing surface on a dog's distal pelvic limb. J Am Anim Hosp Assoc 34:387, 1998.
6. Fowler D: Distal limb and paw injuries. Vet Clin No Am Small Animal Pract 36: 819, 2006.
7. Hedlund CS: Surgery of the integumentary system. *In* Fossum TW, ed.: Small Animal Surgery, 2nd ed.: St. Louis: Mosby, 2002, 134.
8. Hedlund CS: Surgery of the integumentary system. In Fossum TW, ed.: Small Animal Surgery, 3rd ed.: St. Louis: Mosby, 2007, 159.
9. MacPhail CM: Surgery of the integumentary system. In Fossum TW, ed.: Small Animal Surgery, 4th ed.: St. Louis: Mosby, 2013, 190.
10. Niles JD: Special considerations in wound management. In Williams J, Moores A, eds.: BSAVA Manual of Canine and Feline Wound Management and Reconstruction, 2nd ed.: Glouster (UK): BSAVA, 2009, 223.
11. Pavletic MM: Foot salvage by delayed reimplantation of severed metatarsal and digital pads by using a bipedicle direct flap technique. J Am Anim Hosp Assoc 30:539, 1994.
12. Pavletic MM: Atlas of Small Animal Reconstructive Surgery, 2nd ed: Philadelphia: WB Saunders, 1999, 365.
13. Pavletic MM: Atlas of Small Animal Wound Management and Reconstructive Surgery, 3rd ed.: Ames, IA: Wiley – Blackwell, 2010, 535.
14. Swaim SF, Riddell KP, Powers RD: Healing of segmental grafts of digital pad skin in dogs. Am J Vet Res 53:406, 1992.
15. Swaim SF, Bradley DM, Steiss JE, et al: Free segmental paw pad grafts in dogs. Am J Vet Res 54:2161, 1993.
16. Swaim SF, Scardino MS: Paw and distal limb salvage and reconstructive techniques. *In* Bojrab MJ, ed.: Current Techniques in Small Animal Surgery, 4th ed.: Baltimore: Williams and Wilkins, 1998, 265.
17. Swaim SF: Skin grafts. In Slatter DH, ed.: Textbook of Small Animal Surgery, 3rd ed.: Philadelphia: WB Saunders, 2003, 321.
18. Swaim SF, Renberg WC, Shike KM: Small Animal Bandaging, Casting and Splinting Techniques. Ames, IA: Wiley – Blackwell, 2011, 43.

# Pad Replacement: Mesh Grafts (For use on cats only)

## Definition and Indications

Mesh grafts may be used to repair large skin defects on the dorsum of the paws of dogs and cats. However, in cats these grafts may also be used to replace pad tissue (Figure 4-36A & B). If a cat is a house cat that will primarily be walking on carpets, the skin of a mesh

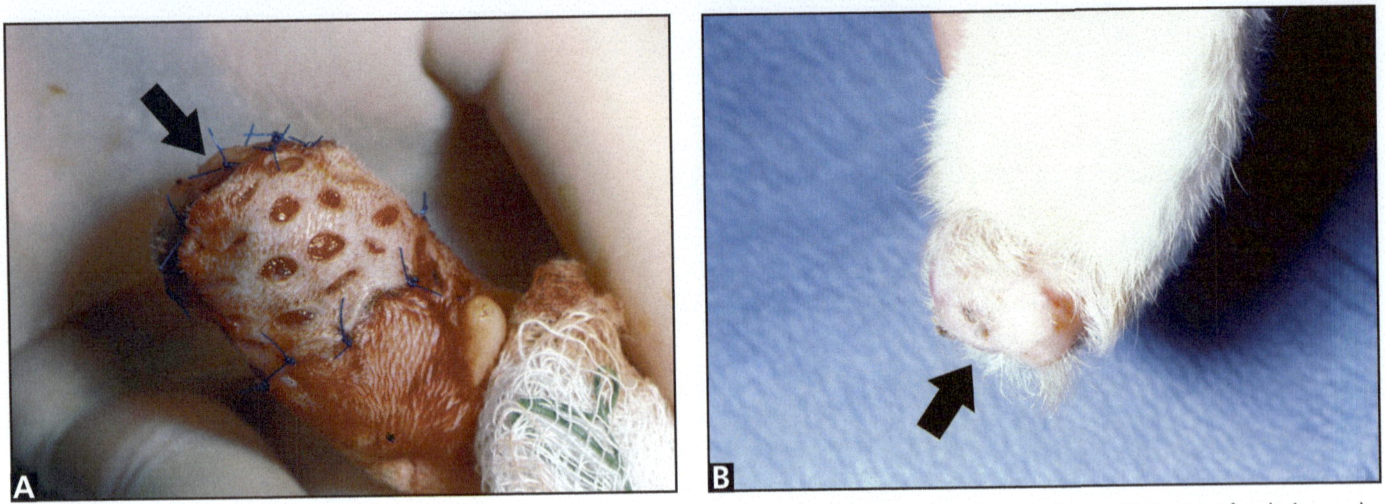


**Figure 4-36.** Mesh graft pad placement on cats. **A.** Full-thickness mesh graft immediately after placement to replace pad tissue. Remnants of pads *(arrow)*. **B.** Graft healed in place. Remnants of pads *(arrow)*. (From Swaim SF: Principles of mesh skin grafting. Compend Contin Educ Pract Vet 4:198, 1982.)

graft will usually undergo sufficient hyperplasia to function as a pad replacement. In general, mesh grafts should not be used to replace the pad skin of dogs because they will not withstand the stress that a dog places on the skin. It is prone to ulceration.

### Technique
(See Chapter 3)

### Aftercare
(See Chapter 3)
Bandaging should be continued after 21 days; however, the bandage should be left off of the paw for increasingly longer periods each day, thus allowing the skin to undergo gradual hyperplasia until it is able to function as pad replacement skin. Clinical judgement is used in deciding when bandaging can be discontinued.

### Advantages and Disadvantages
(See Chapter 3)

## Suggested Readings
(See Chapter 3)

## Interdigital Wounds
Interdigital pododermatitis (interdigital pyoderma) is known by other terms to include interdigital granuloma, interdigital acne, furunculosis, bacterial interdigital granuloma, and pedal folliculitis. It is a multifaceted complex condition that is frustrating to diagnose and treat. Superficial and deep interdigital lacerations are also examples of interdigital wounds.

## Interdigital Pododermatitis
### Definition and Indications
Male dogs of the short – coated breeds are more commonly affected with the condition. These include English Bulldogs, Great Danes, bassets, mastiffs, bull terriers, boxers, dachshunds, dalmations, German Shepherds and Weimaraners. The lesions are granulomatous and not cystic in nature. The condition may manifest itself with widespread involvement of all interdigital skin on all paws or it may be one isolated lesion (Figure 4-37A & B). The lesions may appear erythematous, hyperpigmented, edematous, nodular, ulcerated, and fistulated with a serosanguineous or seropurulent exudate. The paws may be swollen, alopecic, and moist with brown staining from continual licking with widespread involvement. Varying degrees of paronychia, pruritis and pain may be present. The nails may be overly long because it is painful for the dog to walk and wear them down. When interdigital nodules are present, in some cases they may be sensitive and unresponsive to therapy and there may be scars from previous lesions. The dogs are also lame.

Etiologic factors for interdigital lesions are numerous. If only one paw is involved, the penetration of foreign bodies such as "foxtails", thorns, seeds and wood splinters into the interdigital space should be suspected. Neoplasia or local trauma should also be considered if only one interdigital space is involved. When trauma is involved in the etiology, the front paws may be more affected. Field and hunting dogs are subject to interdigital trauma from briars, sand, stones, stubble and breaking through crusts of ice and snow. Animals that work in sticky substances may accumulate masses of sand, stone, and tar in the hair in the interdigital areas. Ice balls can accumulate in this area on sled dogs. Clipper burns, housing on

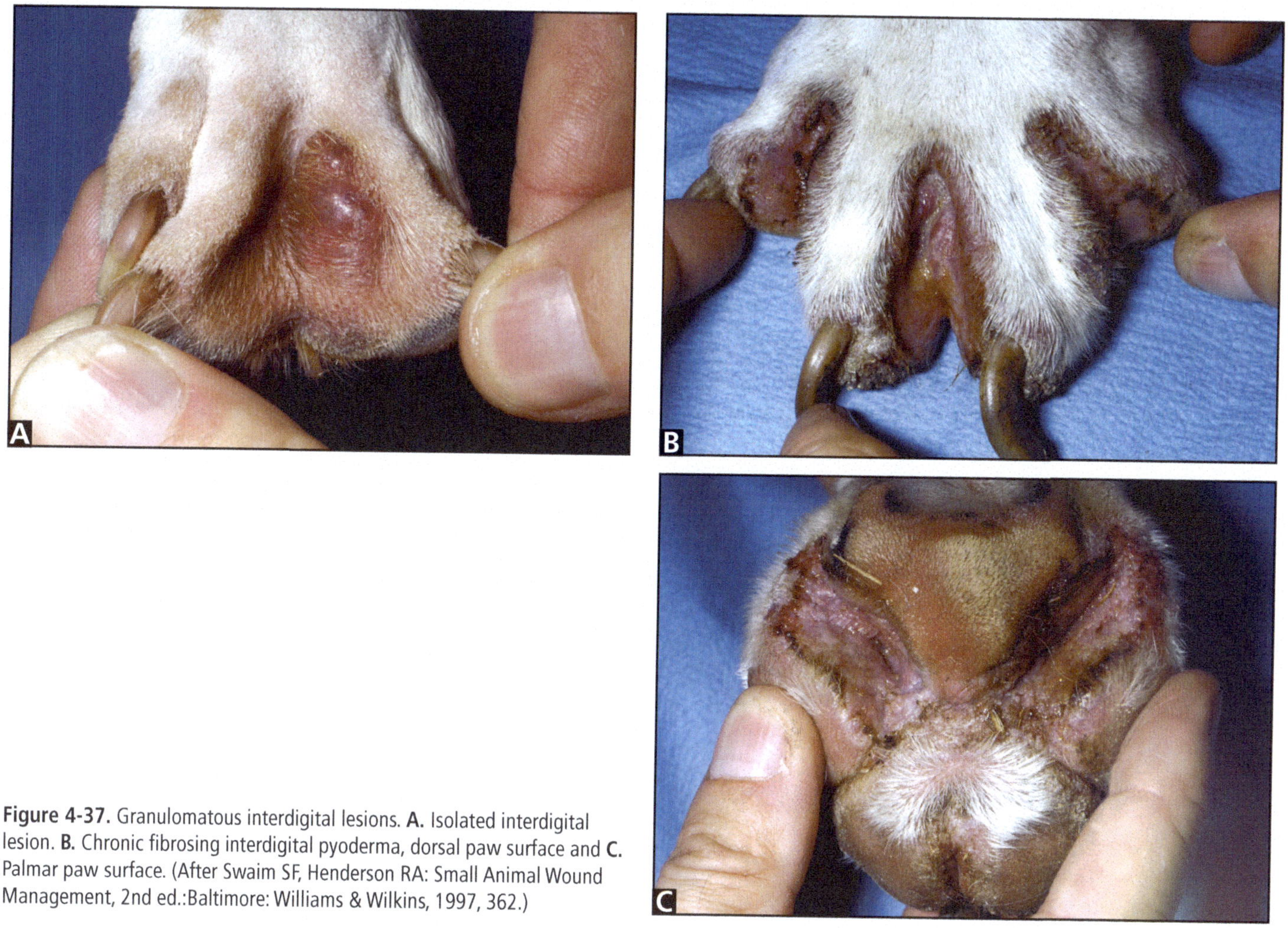

**Figure 4-37.** Granulomatous interdigital lesions. **A.** Isolated interdigital lesion. **B.** Chronic fibrosing interdigital pyoderma, dorsal paw surface and **C.** Palmar paw surface. (After Swaim SF, Henderson RA: Small Animal Wound Management, 2nd ed.:Baltimore: Williams & Wilkins, 1997, 362.)

wire and rough stones are examples of other physical factors that can cause interdigital irritation. Interdigital granulomas have been associated with hair penetrating the skin and breaking off. This could be related to the intertrigenous nature of the area. Contact with irritating chemicals, fertilizers and weed killers may result in irritation of the interdigital area. Contact, inhalant, or food hypersensitivities can initiate interdigital dermatitis as can Staphylococcal allergies and autoimmune conditions (pemphigus, pemphigoid and lupus erythematosus). Numerous bacterial and fungal organisms can cause interdigital lesions. Fungal infection should be suspected when lesions are resistant to antibiotic therapy. The most common parasitic cause of pododermatitis is demodicosis. Other parasitic agents include Pelodera strongyloides, Ancylostoma spp, and Uncinaria stenocephala. Ticks and chiggers favor interdigital areas and can initiate an inflammatory reaction. Other factors reported to cause interdigital dermatitis include psychogenic dermatitis with excessive paw licking, local neoplasia, underlying osteomyelitis, hypothyroidism, and immunodeficient states. Some interdigital lesions may be sterile pyogranulomas. Adverse cutaneous drug reactions, zinc-responsive dermatitis, necrolytic migratory erythema, and canine distemper have also been associated with pododermatitis lesions. In spite of all the possible etiologic possibilities and contributing factors, a substantial number of cases are idiopathic, recurrent bacterial infections and are exceedingly frustrating to manage.

## Techniques

In light of the numerous etiologic factors that can cause interdigital lesions (interdigital pododermatitis), it is essential that a thorough diagnostic evaluation be made on the animal. This would be followed by appropriate therapy. The reader is referred to small animal dermatology text books.

### Diagnostic Techniques

Because of the complex pathogenesis of interdigital pododermatitis, several diagnostic techniques may be necessary in an effort to establish a diagnosis. A thorough history and physical examination (including probing of tracts if foreign bodies are suspected) should be performed. A hematologic examination, serum biochemistry profile, and urinalysis should be performed. Other diagnostic tests should include multiple skin scrapings and exudative cytology. Direct smears of the lesion's surface may provide clues of the cause. However, deep (from the lesion biopsy samples) bacterial and fungal biopsies should be done for accurate wound assessment. Chronic wounds often have surface contaminants that do not interfere with healing. It is necessary to differentiate these from microorganisms causing infection. The wound surface should be thoroughly cleansed using a presurgical scrub technique before taking the biopsy. Cultures should be for aerobes, anaerobes, and fungi. Antibiotic sensitivity tests should be done on these deep biopsy samples. Histopathologic examination should also be done on these deep biopsies. These can help document foreign bodies (including free hair shafts and keratin in the tissues), bacteria, parasites, fungi, and neoplastic tissue. Radiographs can be used to check for bony changes and radiopaque foreign bodies. Ultrasonography can be used to check for radiolucent foreign bodies. Sometimes evaluation of the immune status is indicated and should include hemogram, serum immunoglobulin quantitation, and evaluation of the thyroid and adrenal glands.

## Conservative Medical Therapy

If specific underlying etiologic factors are identified by diagnostic procedures, medical or surgical therapy should be directed accordingly. For draining lesions, paw soaks for 10 to 15 minutes twice daily are indicated until drainage ceases. Magnesium sulfate (Epsom salts) soaks are effective. A 1:40 chlorhexidine diacetate (Nolvasan Solution, Ft. Dodge Animal Health, Ft. Dodge, IA) or gluconate (ChlorhexiDerm Disinfectant, Dermatologics in Veterinary Medicine, Pharmaceuticals, Inc., Miami, FL) solution may also be used for soaking. The author has used a combination of the chlorhexidine and magnesium sulfate by making a 1:40 chlorhexidine dilution and adding magnesium sulfate granules to the solution. Prolonged antibiotic therapy for 8 to 12 weeks is not unusual. Palpation of the interdigital areas is important in monitoring the progress of therapy because the surface lesions may heal weeks before the deep lesions are resolved. Palpable nodules or thickened cords deep to a healed skin surface is indicative of residual deep infection. The lesions may be tender to deep palpation. As long as these lesions are present and are becoming smaller, treatment should continue. An important part of therapy is restriction of exercise and protection of the paw by a bootie or bandage.

Pododermatitis can be self-perpetuating and thus frustrating to deal with. As lesions heal with scarring, the paw becomes more susceptible to future infections. Such scarring can lead to mechanical problems that in turn cause irritations and/or infections (See Figure 4-41A). When treatment of the infection is delayed, increased scarring potential occurs, thus, diagnostic and therapeutic effort should be maximal in such cases. Some cases are resistant to medical therapy alone, especially those with a secondary gram-negative infection. Surgical debridement of all involved tissue may make medical therapy more effective.

## Conservative Incisional or Excisional Therapy.

This form of therapy should be performed when diagnostic techniques reveal a condition that can be treated by simple incision or excision of the affected area. It has been termed a separation podoplasty. These lesions are usually isolated, few in number, and often only involve one paw (e.g. foreign bodies, or neoplasias).

Removal of a solitary foreign body entails insertion of small hemostatic forceps or alligator forceps through the opening in the indurated interdigital skin to explore the wound cavity. If a foreign body is retrieved, the opening may be enlarged to allow drainage (Figure 4-38A & B).

If a palpable cord-like sinus tract extends from the skin opening, the tract may be removed by excisional dissection. An incision is made around the opening. The incised skin is grasped with tissue forceps to apply traction to it. The tract is dissected out using electrosurgery, $CO_2$ laser, scalpel, or fine pointed scissors. Blunt and sharp techniques are used alternatively until the sinus tract and foreign body are isolated (Figure 4-39A). It is necessary to extend the skin incision or excise tissue associated with the tract to obtain adequate exposure. The subcutaneous tissue is closed with a 4-0 absorbable simple continuous suture followed by skin closure using 3-0 monofilament

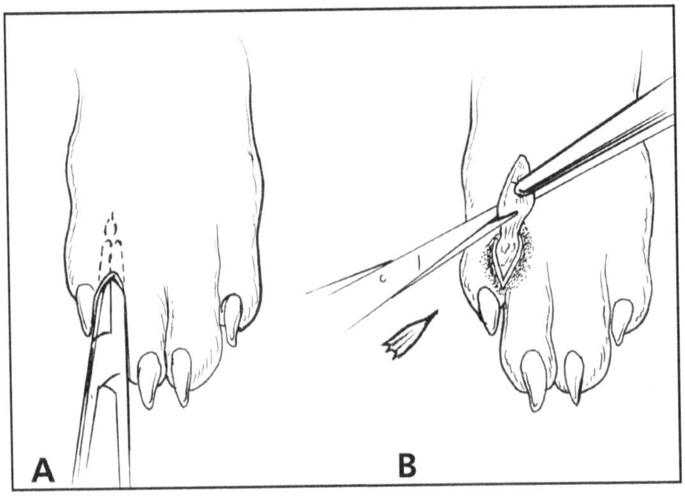


**Figure 4-38.** Interdigital plant seed removal. **A.** Hemostatic forceps used to explore and remove the interdigital foreign body. **B.** The wound opening is enlarged to allow drainage. (After Swaim SF, Henderson RA: Small Animal Wound Management 2nd ed.:Baltimore: Williams & Wilkins, 1997, 364.)

nonabsorbable simple interrupted sutures. The distal end of the excision wound is left open for drainage as the wound heals (Figure 4-39B).

## Moderate Excisional Therapy (Web Excision)

If all or the majority of an interdigital web has a chronic isolated lesion, moderate excisional therapy is indicated. Some neoplasias that involve the interdigital area require moderate excisional therapy and possibly digit amputation according to the guidelines for adequate removal of the tumor.

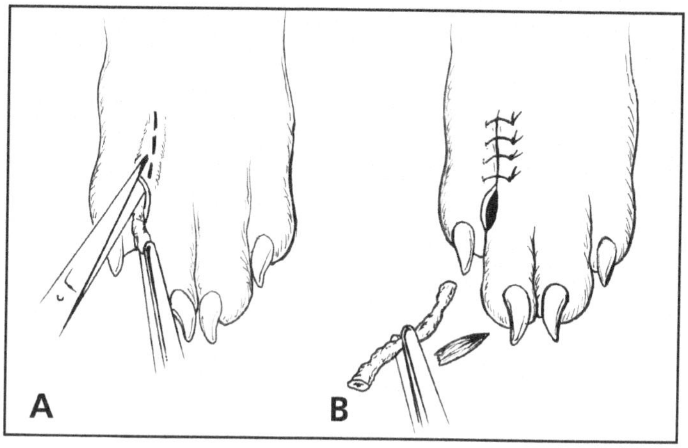


**Figure 4-39.** Interdigital fistulous tract and plant seed removal. **A.** Fistulous tract being dissected. **B.** Wound closure following tract and plant seed removal. Small opening left distally for drainage. (After Swaim SF, Henderson RA: Small Animal Wound Management 2nd ed.:Baltimore: Williams & Wilkins, 1997, 365.)

When just the web skin between 2 digits is involved, dorsal and palmar/plantar skin incisions are made at the junction of the interdigital skin with the adjacent 2 digits (Figure 4-40A & B). All interdigital skin between the two digits (i.e. the entire web) is excised. Hemorrhage is controlled by electrocoagulation, $CO_2$ laser, or ligation with 3-0 absorbable suture material. If sufficient skin is available, the dorsal wound edge is sutured to the palmar/plantar wound edge with 3-0 monofilament nonabsorbable simple interrupted sutures (Figure 4-40C & D). When sufficient skin is not available to suture the dorsal and palmar/plantar wound edges together on each digit, the palmar/plantar skin edges of the 2 adjacent digits are sutured together followed by suturing the dorsal skin edges of the 2 digits together. This fuses the two digits together with no interdigital space (Figure 4-40E & F).

In some cases the skin on the palmar/plantar surface of digits 2 or 5 may be affected along with the interdigital skin between digits 2 and 3 or 4 and 5 (Figure 4-41A). In such instances, the affected skin is excised to include the skin on the cranial surface of the adjacent area of the metacarpal/metatarsal pad (Figure 4-41B). Suturing

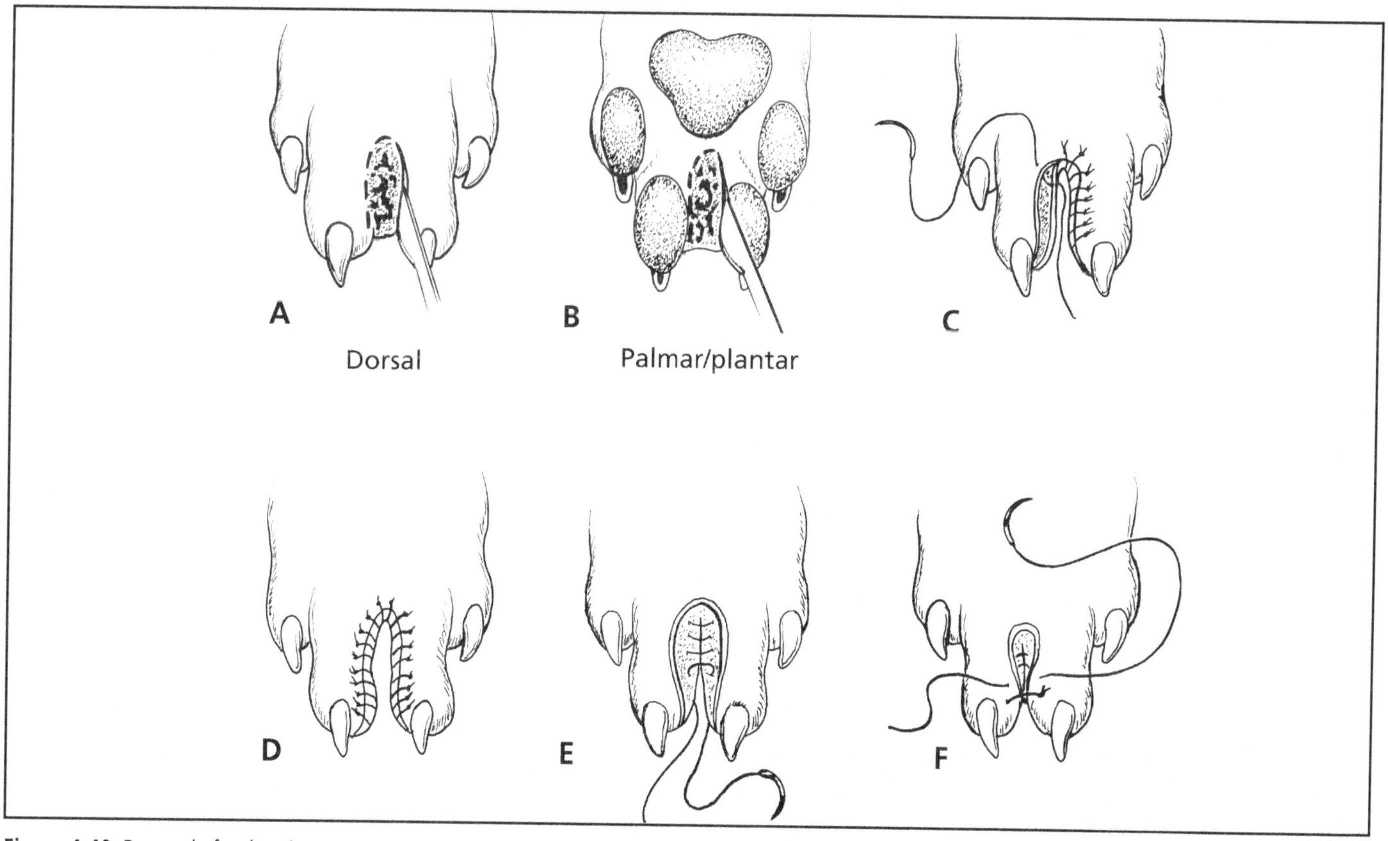


**Figure 4-40.** Removal of a chronic unresponsive interdigital lesion. **A.** Incising the dorsum of the interdigital skin. **B.** Incising the palmar/plantar surface of the interdigital skin. **C.** After removing the entire web, suturing the palmar/plantar interdigital skin to the dorsal interdigital skin on each digit. **D.** Skin defect closed. **E.** Suturing the palmar/plantar interdigital skin of adjacent digits. **F.** Suturing the dorsal interdigital skin of adjacent digits. (After Swaim SF, Henderson RA: Small Animal Wound Management, 2nd ed.:Baltimore: Williams & Wilkins, 1997, 366.)

is done with 2-0 or 3-0 monofilament suture material using simple interrupted sutures to unite digits 2 and 3 or digits 4 and 5. The digits are then sutured back against the denuded cranial surface of the metacarpal/metatarsal pad to create a partial fusion podoplasty (Figure 4-41C).

## Radical Excisional Therapy (Fusion Podoplasty)

When other forms of therapy have not been successful, fusion podoplasty can be performed as a salvage procedure. It is indicated when there is extensive chronic involvement of an individual paw or multiple paws with chronic fibrosing interdigital pyoderma. When all four paws are involved, surgery is performed on 2 paws at a time. Usually the forepaws are the most involved, and surgery is performed on them first. Surgery is then done on the hind paws approximately 1 month later. The technique has also been described for use in treating abnormalities associated with severed digital flexor tendons to fuse the digits against the metacarpal or metatarsal pad to provide a functional paw.

Prior to surgery, culture and sensitivity tests should be performed on the paws, and appropriate systemic antibiotic therapy should be started. After performing surgical preparation on the paws, the interdigital skin to be removed is outlined with a sterile marking pen on the dorsum of the paw, lines are drawn on the digits at the junction of normal and affected skin. Near the nails, the lines are drawn such that 2 to 3 mm of skin are left adjacent to the nail on the axial surfaces of the digits. The third and fourth digits extend beyond the second and fifth digits, respectively. Thus, not all the skin on the abaxial surfaces of digits three and four is interdigital, and it is not necessary to remove all the skin on this surface of those digits. Only the portion of skin that is interdigital will be removed. Lines on the abaxial surfaces of the third and fourth digits are drawn so they intersect the edge of the digital pads approximately midway between their cranial and caudal ends. As a result, the skin excisions on the abaxial surfaces of digits three and four match the axial surface excisions on digits two and five, respectively (Figure 4-42A & insets). When excisions are complete, all intertrigenous skin will have been removed from between the digits on the dorsum of the paw.

On the palmar/plantar surface of the paw, the lines are drawn to enclose all skin that is not pad skin;

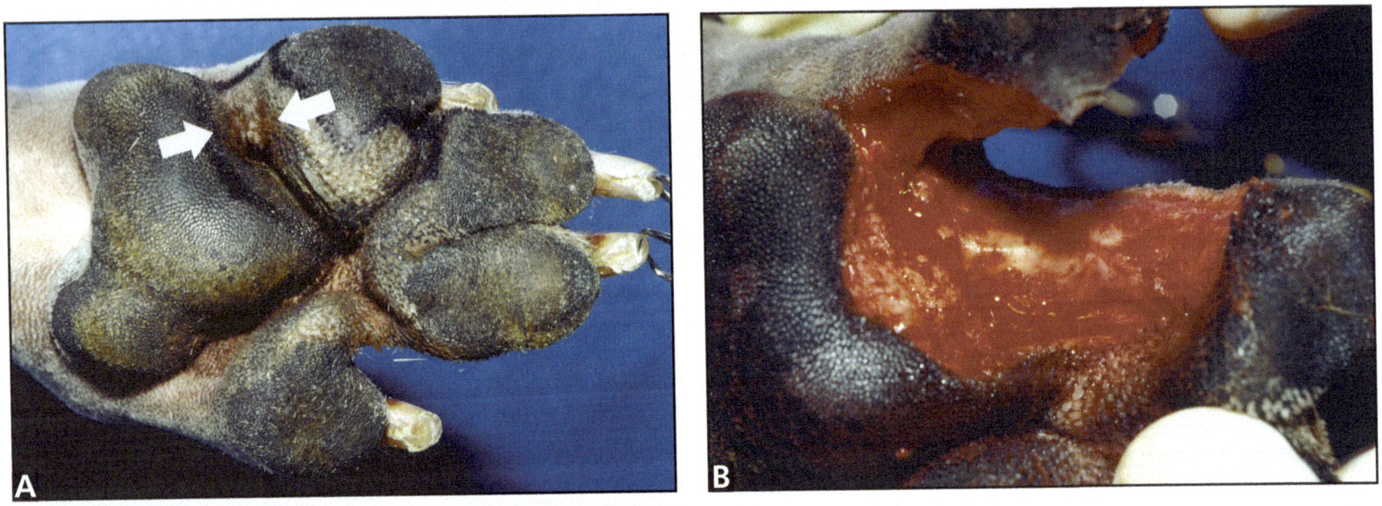


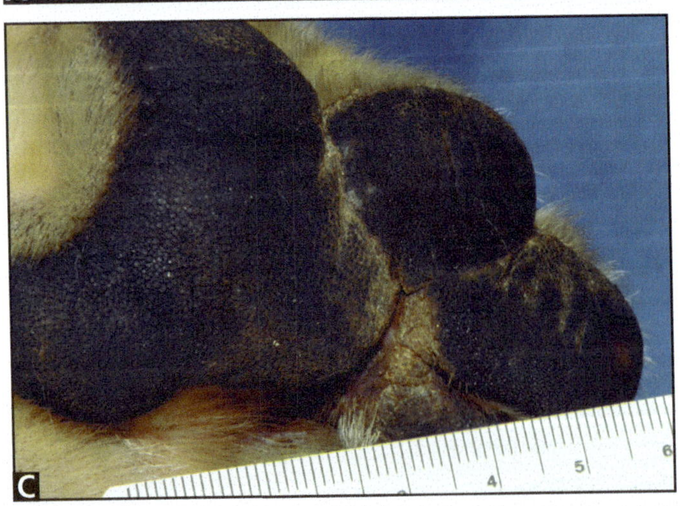


**Figure 4-41.** Partial fusion podoplasty. **A.** Scarring from previous surgery for localized pododermatitis has pulled the palmar surface of the fifth digit into close apposition with the metacarpal pad. Friction between the tissue surfaces resulted in localized irritation and infection (between arrows). **B.** Infected tissue, skin on abaxial surface of fourth digit and skin on axial surface of fifth digit has been removed along with adjacent skin from the cranial surface of the metacarpal pad. **C.** The fourth and fifth digits have been fused together and fused to the adjacent surface of the metacarpal pad – a partial fusion podoplasty.

however, the line does enclose the pad skin on the cranial portion of the metacarpal/ metatarsal pad. The lines are drawn around the caudal edges of the digital pads at the junction of pad skin and haired skin. The lines are not drawn around the cranial edges of the digital pads or around the abaxial surfaces of pads two and five. From the caudoabaxial aspect of the second and fifth digital pads, lines are drawn along the skin folds that extend from this point to the base of the metacarpal/metatarsal pad. The line is then extended across the cranial surface of the metacarpal/ metatarsal pad. Across the front of this pad, the line is approximately 3 to 5 mm cranial to the level at which the caudal edges of the digital pads contact the metacarpal/metatarsal pad when the digits are flexed back against this pad (Figure 4-42B).

A ½-inch diameter Penrose drain tourniquet is applied just distal to the carpus or tarsus to obtain adequate hemostasis. The tourniquet is released twice, for 1 minute each time, during the excisional procedure. It is released after dissection of all interdigital skin from the dorsum of the paw and after dissection of the skin on the palmar/plantar surface.

All of the previously drawn lines are incised with a scalpel, electrosurgical unit, or $CO_2$ laser. Beginning at one interdigital cleft on the dorsum of the paw, the interdigital skin is dissected from the cleft toward the cranial fold of this web of skin. To avoid damage to the axial and abaxial dorsal and palmar/plantar common digital vessels and the axial and abaxial dorsal and palmar/plantar proper digital vessels, dissection is done as close to the dermis as possible. When dense spherical areas of connective tissue (areas of infection surrounded by dense fibrous scar tissue) are encountered, they should be dissected out. As dissection approaches the web fold, it will become difficult and should be discontinued. The skin is then dissected from an adjacent interdigital space in the same manner (Figure 4-42C). After all interdigital spaces have been dissected to the web fold, the paw is turned over. Sharp and blunt dissection is used around the caudal aspects of the digital pads and down the palmar/ plantar aspects of the digits. Dissection is again done as close to the dermis as possible, removing any areas of dense connective tissue surrounding infection. The epidermis and dermis are dissected from the cranial aspect of the metacarpal/metatarsal pad from lateral to medial, leaving the underlying fibroadipose tissue (Figure 4-42D). After tourniquet removal, fine point electrocoagulation or $CO_2$ laser can be used to attain hemostasis. The paw is soaked in a 1:40 dilution of chlorhexidine diacetate (Nolvasan Solution, Ft. Dodge Animal Health, Ft. Dodge, IA) or gluconate (ChlorhexiDerm Disinfectant, Dermatologics in Veterinary Medicine, Pharmaceuticals, Inc., Miami, FL) solution for 1 to 2 minutes. After all infected skin has been removed from the paw the only skin remaining on the paw is the pad skin on the palmar/plantar paw surface (See Figure 4-43) and a thin strip of skin on the dorsum of each digit. The paw is wrapped in a snug pressure bandage, and the same procedures are performed on the opposite paw.

The pressure wrap is removed from the first paw, and simple interrupted sutures of 2-0 or 3-0 monofilament nonabsorbable suture material are used to unite adjacent digital pads (Figure 4-42E). The four united digital pads are then flexed back against the denuded cranial surface of the metacarpal/metatarsal pad. A simple interrupted 2-0 or 3-0 monofilament nonabsorbable suture is placed centrally to begin the fixation of the digital pads back against the front of the metacarpal/metatarsal pad. Similar sutures are placed alternately on either side of the central suture to complete fixation of the united digital pads to the metacarpal/metatarsal pad (Figure 4-42F).

As the sutures hold all the pads together, the fusing/ healing process begins in the deeper tissues. Because of the initial dead space in the deeper tissues, a drain is placed in the area. Prior to placing the final two sutures on either side of the paw, the blades of a curved Carmalt forcep are passed deep to the digital-metacarpal/metatarsal pad sutures across the cranial surface of the metacarpal/metatarsal pad. A ¼-inch diameter Penrose drain is grasped and pulled through the wound. It is cut with approximately ½ inch protruding from each side of the wound. The final skin suture on each side of the paw is then placed, passing each suture through the drain to anchor it (Figure 4-42G & H). The suture should be passed such that it anchors the drain in place but leaves sufficient space around the drain to allow for drainage.

After turning the paw over, the remaining strips of skin on the dorsum of each digit are sutured together with three or four simple interrupted sutures of 3-0 monofilament nonabsorbable suture (Figure 4-42I). Areas at the ends of the digits are not sutured, thus allowing for drainage. After suturing is complete on the first paw, the pressure wrap is removed from the second paw, and it is sutured in the same way.

An alternative to passive drainage of the area with a Penrose drain and open drainage at the ends of the interdigital areas is active closed suction drainage. All

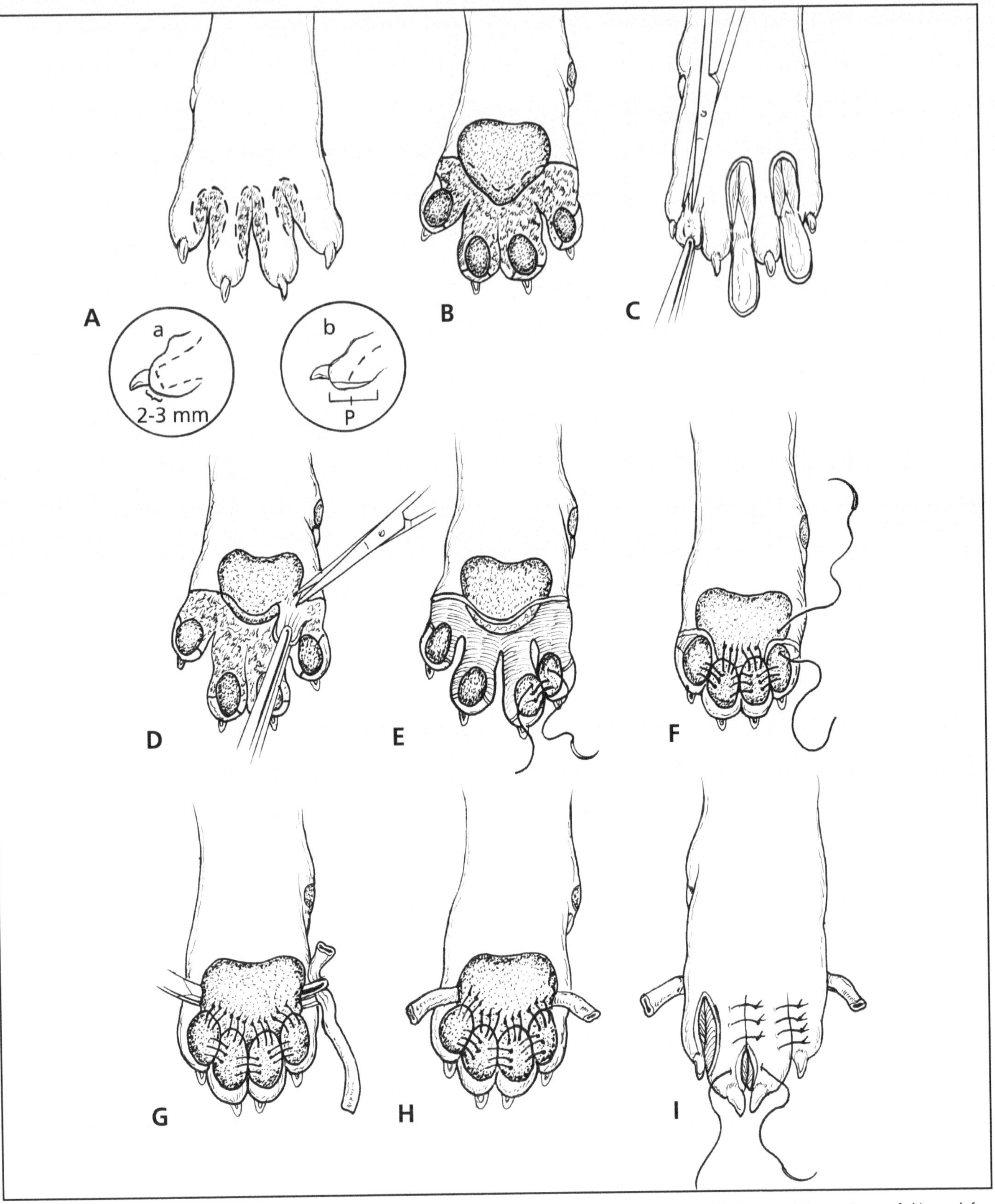


**Figure 4-42.** Fusion podoplasty. **A.** Interdigital tissue to be removed from the dorsal paw surface *(broken lines)*. *(insert a)* Two to 3 mm of skin are left near the nails on the axial digital surfaces. *(insert b)* On the abaxial surfaces of digits 3 and 4 excision lines bisect the length of the pad *(P)*. **B.** Interdigital tissue to be removed from the palmar/plantar paw surface *(broken lines)*. **C.** Dissecting interdigital skin from the dorsal aspect of the paw, dissecting from the cleft to the web fold. **D.** Dissecting interdigital skin from the palmar/plantar paw surface. **E.** Uniting the digital pads with 3 simple interrupted sutures of 2-0 or 3-0 monofilament nonabsorbable suture material. **F.** United digital pads positioned against the metacarpal pad. Suturing progresses alternately to each side from a central suture with simple interrupted sutures of 2-0 or 3-0 monofilament nonabsorbable sutures. **G.** Curved Carmalt forceps passing at the base of the metacarpal pad deep to the sutures to grasp a ¼ inch diameter Penrose drain to be pulled through the area. **H.** Drain in place. **I.** Suturing strips of skin on the dorsal surface of each digit with simple interrupted sutures of 2-0 or 3-0 monofilament nonabsorbable sutures. (After Swaim SF, Lee AH, MacDonald JM, et al: Fusion podoplasty for the treatment of chronic fibrosing interdigital pyoderma in the dog. J Am Anim Hosp Assoc 27:264, 1991.)

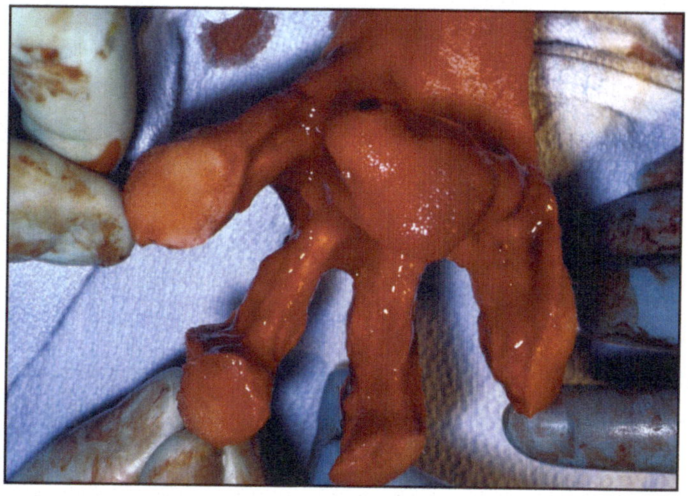

**Figure 4-43.** Appearance of the palmar surface of a paw following removal of all infected skin. (From Swaim SF, Lee AH, MacDonald JM, et al: Fusion podoplasty for the treatment of chronic fibrosing intedigital pyoderma in the dog. J Am Anim Hosp Assoc 27:264, 1991.)

suture lines are sutured completely and a closed suction drain is placed into the interdigital area via a small stab incision in the dorsal paw area. A 19- gauge butterfly catheter can be used for the drain. The syringe adaption part of the catheter is cut off and the tubing is placed through the skin stab incision. A purse string suture is placed around the catheter for a tight seal where it enters the skin. The needled end of the catheter is inserted into a vacuumed blood collection vial to create the suction. The catheter tubing and vial are incorporated in the bandage such that the vial is accessible for replacement periodically as it becomes full.

## Aftercare

### Conservative Medical Therapy

Appropriate antibiotic theraphy should be administered as indicated by diagnostic procedures-culture and sensitivity.

Between times when the paws are soaked, bandages are applied to the paws. When there are draining lesions in the interdigital areas an absorbent surgical sponge should be placed in areas of drainage.

An absorbent secondary wrap is wrapped on the paw followed by an outer wrap of porous adhesive tape or elastic tape. Bandage changes should be done daily, and it should be done until healing is considered adequate.

### Conservative Incisional or Excisional Therapy and Moderate Excisional Therapy

A small amount of cotton or cast padding should be placed between all interdigital areas except those between which surgery has been performed. A piece of semiocclusive nonadherent primary bandage material (Telfa "Ouchless" Adhesive Pads, Covidien, Tyco HealthCare/Kendall, Mansfield, MA) should be placed in (See Figure 2-5) areas of excision or over the suture line where an interdigital web has been removed. The bandage is completed with an absorbent secondary wrap. An outer layer of porous adhesive tape or elastic tape is placed. The need for a large amount of secondary wrap or a "donut"-type foam rubber pad and metal splint cup may not be as great for bandaging these wounds as for bandaging pad lacerations, or phalangeal fillet to replace a metacarpal/metatarsal pad. However, with web excision on a large dog, a "clam shell" bandage may be indicated to keep suture lines from spreading with weight bearing, especially when 2 digits have been sutured together.

Periodic bandage changes should be performed with the frequency dependant upon the amount of drainage that is present. Bandaging is usually continued for approximately 7 to 10 days or until healing is considered adequate.

### Radical Excisional Therapy (Fusion Podoplasty)

Bandaging and splinting play a major role is preventing postoperative problems following fusion podoplasty. A small amount of gentamicin sulfate antibiotic ointment (Gentamicin sulfate ointment 0.1%, Fugera, Melville, NY) is placed over the suture lines. Two absorbent surgical sponges are placed on both the dorsal paw surface and the palmar/plantar surface. A large amount of absorbent secondary wrap is wrapped around the paw. This is followed by an outer layer of porous adhesive tape or elastic tape. On the forelimb this bandage extends to the elbow, and on the pelvic limb it extends to above the hock. It is important to prevent weight-bearing on the operated paws. Thus, the localized crutch effect of a "clam shell" splint is important in bandaging the paws. This puts the paws in a vertical position so that weight-bearing actually pushes the digits back against the metacarpal/metatarsal pad and prevents suture line disruption (Figure 4-44). Such disruption could occur if the digits were allowed to move forward as would occur with other bandage configurations. Bandages are changed daily during the time of significant drainage. This is usually for 10 to 14 days postoperatively. A 0.5% solution of chlorhexidine diacetate (Nolvasan Solution, Ft. Dodge Animal Health, Ft. Dodge, IA) or gluconate (ChlorhexiDerm Disinfectant, Dermatologics in Veterinary Medicine, Pharmaceuticals, Inc., Miami, FL) solution is used to soak the paw at the time of bandage change if there is a characteristic *Pseudomonas* odor at any bandage change. Subsequent bandage changes after the period of heavy drainage progress from every

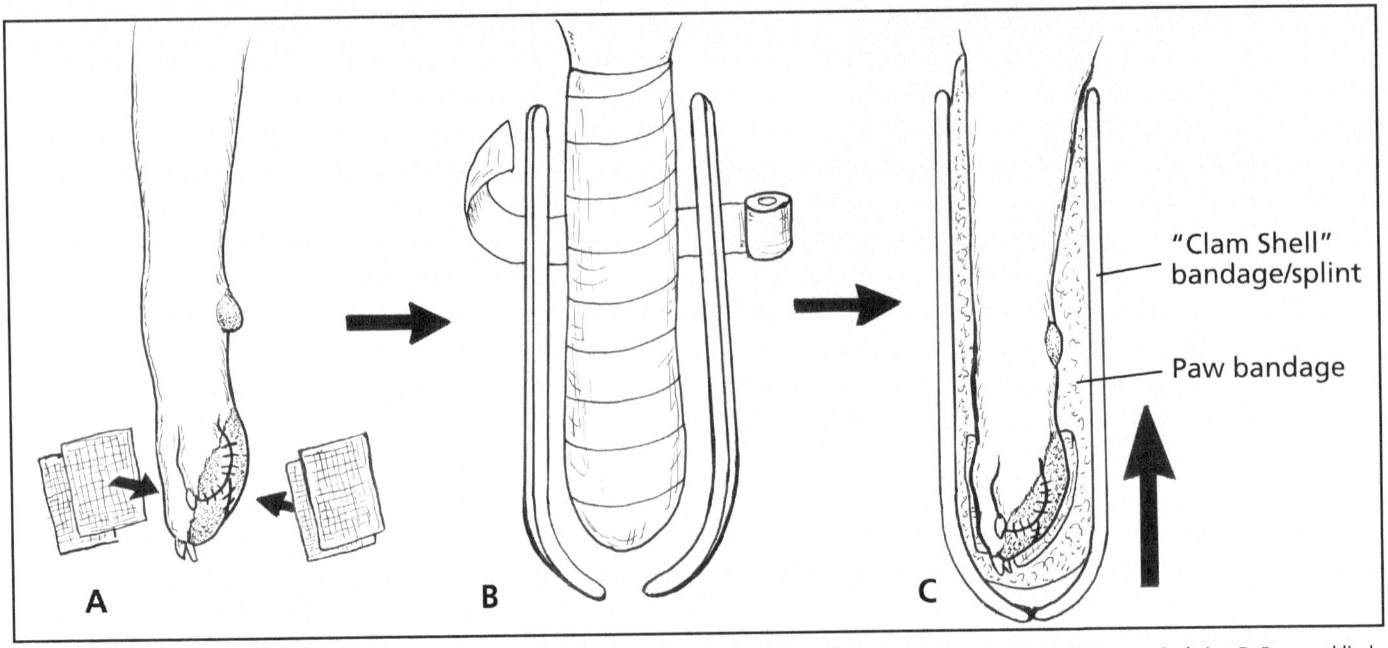


**Figure 4-44.** Splinting a paw after fusion podoplasty. **A.** Completed fusion podoplasty with gauze sponges to be applied over surgical site. **B.** Paw and limb bandaged with "clam shell" splint to be applied to the bandage. **C.** The splint keeps the paw in a vertical position so weight bearing forces the digits back against the metacarpal/metatarsal pad *(arrow)* to prevent wound disruption in the area.

other day changes for about a week to 2 changes during the following week.

At 10 days postoperatively the drain tubes are removed. At 10 to 14 days sutures are removed from the dorsal paw skin and from between the digital pads. The sutures between digital pads and the metacarpal/metatarsal pad are usually removed between 14 and 21 days, usually closer to 21 days. In most instances, all sutures have been removed by 21 days, and the "clam shell" splints have been discontinued. A protective bootie or a light bandage may be indicated for a transitional period between full bandaging and no protective paw cover.

Occasionally some suture separation may occur between the digital pads and the metacarpal/metatarsal pad. This usually exposes an underlying area of healthy granulation tissue. If the sutures in the area are not functioning to hold the tissues in apposition, they are removed. The area of exposed granulation tissue is treated as an open wound with a semiocclusive nonadherent bandage pad (Telfa "Ouchless" Pads, Covidien, Tyco HealthCare/Kendall, Mansfield, MA) and topical Acemannan-containing hydrogel wound dressing (CarraVet Acemannan Wound Gel, CarraVet, Inc., Newnan, GA) until reepithelialization of the area has occurred, usually by 21 days.

Appropriate systemic antibiotic therapy should be continued for 7 to 10 days postoperatively.

## Advantages and Disadvantages

### Conservative Medical Therapy

Conservative medical therapy has the advantage that surgical intervention is not involved in the treatment. The disadvantage of this therapy is that soaks, bandaging and antibiotic therapy may be prolonged, and there is the possibility that the condition may recur following discontinuance of therapy.

### Conservative Incisional or Excisional Therapy

With incisional or excisional therapy to remove a foreign body, the wounds usually heal uneventfully. However, if any foreign material remains in the tissue, the wounds either do not heal, or they heal and break open later to drain. This is an example of "tissue intelligence"; whereby, tissues do not heal as long as a reactive foreign body is present. These wounds require reoperation.

If excisional therapy is performed for removal of an interdigital neoplasm, the advantages and disadvantages would be those associated with the type of neoplasm. Excision of some neoplastic lesions may be considered as moderate excisional therapy or digit amputation dependant upon the guidelines for adequate removal of the neoplasm.

### Moderate Excisional Therapy

Removal of an interdigital web with suturing of the dorsal digital skin to palmar/plantar skin on the same digit may result in a "biologic tourniquet" if the closure is too tight. The resultant hypothermia and/

or swelling of the digit indicates suture removal and second intention healing.

In addition, this procedure will result in a webless space between the digits. This could be considered a minor cosmetic disadvantage. Such a space on the paw of a working field dog could snag on vegetation. Fusing the digits as described in the Techniques section would eliminate the problem.

### Radical Excisional Therapy (Fusion Podoplasty)

The primary advantage of fusion podoplasty is related to the philosophy of the technique "if it is not there to become infected, it cannot become infected." The procedure provides a disease-free, cosmetic, functional paw (Figure 4-45) following long-term unsuccessful therapy of other forms. However, time is involved in attaining the results. If one or 2 paws (usually both fore or both hind paws) are involved, healing is usually complete by one month. If all 4 paws are involved healing usually takes 2 months since surgery is performed on 2 paws at a time. The most affected paws (usually the forepaws) are operated first followed by the remaining 2 paws about a month later after the first 2 paws have healed. The procedure has the disadvantage of being a radical surgical technique. It is quite hemorrhagic in that the chronic fibrosing interdigital pyoderma may have been present for several months to a year or longer prior to surgery and the tissues are very vascular. Postoperatively, there is a tendency for the digits to extend forward as the dog bears weight on the paw if the paw is not adequately splinted. The result may be wound disruption of the suture line between the digital pads and the metacarpal/metatarsal pad. However, the "clam shell" splints usually prevent this. Although the digits may be hyperflexed at the completion of surgery and early in the healing process, it does not appear to affect the dog's gait.

## Suggested Readings


1. Anderson RK: Canine Pododermatitis. Compend Contin Educ Pract Vet 2:361, 1980.
2. Bellah JR: Surgical management of specific skin disorders. *In* Slatter DH, ed.: Textbook of Small Animal Surgery, 2nd ed.: Philadelphia, WB Saunders, 1993, 341.
3. Bohling MW, Swaim SF: Paw and distal limb skin reconstruction and salvage techniques. In Bojrab MJ, ed.: Current Techniques in Small Animal Surgery, 5th ed.: Jackson, WY: Teton NewMedia, 2014, 628.
4. Breathnach RM, Fanning S, Mulcahy G, et al: Canine pododermatitis and idiopathic disease. Vet Jour 176: 146, 2008.
5. Duclos DD, Hargis AM, Hanley PW: Pathogenesis of canine interdigital palmar and plantar comedones and follicular cysts, and their response to laser surgery. Vet Derm 19: 134, 2008.
6. Fowler D: Distal limb and paw injuries. Vet Clin No Am Small Animal Pract 36: 819, 2006.
7. Hedlund CS: Surgery of the integumentary system. *In* Fossum TW, ed.: Small Animal Surgery, 2nd ed.: St. Louis: Mosby, 2002, 134.
8. Hedlund CS: Surgery of the integumentary system. In Fossum TW, ed.: Small Animal Surgery, 3rd ed.: St. Louis: Mosby, 2007, 159.
9. Harvath – Ungerboeck C, van den Broek A: Pedal dermatitis. Part 3: Feline pododermatitis. Compan Anim 16: 44, 2011.
10. Kohler H: Hair as the cause of chronic, purulent dermatitis with abscess formation in dogs. Deutsche Tierarztliche Wochenschrift 90:307, 1983.
11. Krahwinkel DJ, Bone JL: Surgical management of specific skin disorders. In Slatter DH, ed.: Textbook of Small Animal Surgery: Philadelphia: WB Saunders, 1985, 501.
12. MacPhail CM: Surgery of the integumentary system. In Fossum TW, ed.: Small Animal Surgery, 4th ed.: St. Louis: Mosby, 2013, 190.
13. Manning TO, Walton DK, Ford RB: Canine pododermatitis. Dermatol Rep 2:1, 1983.
14. Niles JD: Special considerations in wound management. In Williams J, Moores A, eds.: BSAVA Manual of Canine and Feline Wound Management and Reconstruction, 2nd ed.: Glouster (UK): BSAVA, 2009, 223.
15. Papazoglou LG, Ellison GW, Farese JP, et. al.: Fusion podoplasty for the management of chronic pedal conditions in seven dogs and one cat. J Amer Anim Hosp Assoc 47: 199, 2011.
16. Pavletic MM: Atlas of Small Animal Wound Management and reconstructive Surgery, 3rd, ed.: Ames, IA: Wiley – Blackwell, 2010, 535.
17. Scott DW, Miller WH, Griffin CE: Muller and Kirk's Small Animal Dermatology, 6th ed.: Philadelphia: WB Saunders, 2001, 274.


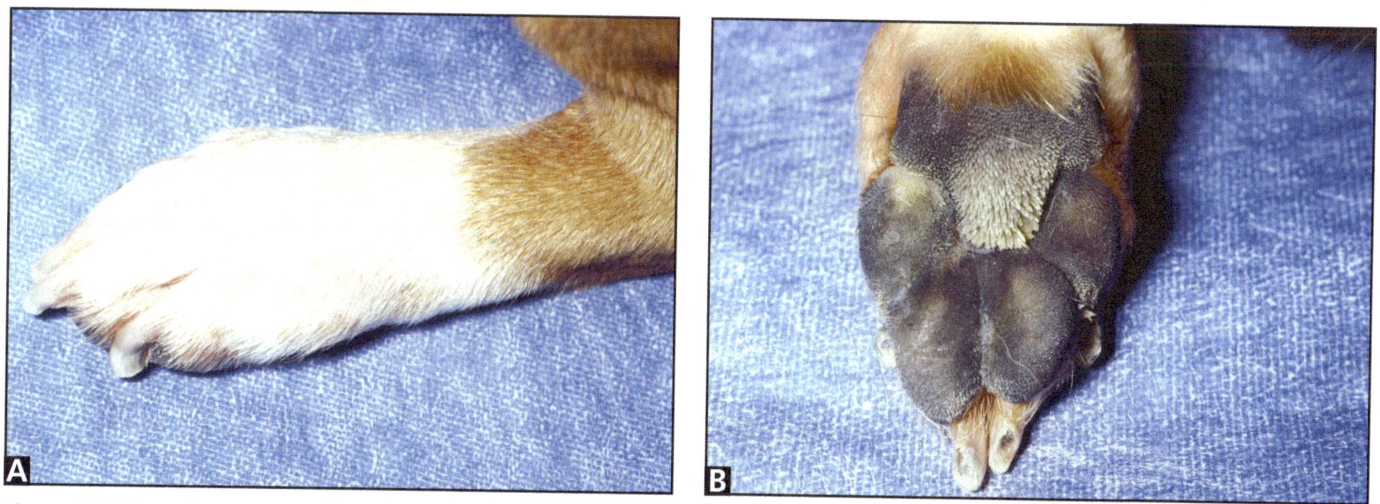


**Figure 4-45.** Cosmetic appearance of a paw following fusion podoplasty. **A.** Dorsal surface. **B.** Plantar surface. (From Swaim SF, Lee AH, MacDonald JM, et al: Fusion podoplasty for the treatment of chronic fibrosing interdigital pyoderma in the dog. J Am Anim Hosp Assoc 21:329, 1985.)

18. Swaim SF, Lee AH, MacDonald JM, et al: Fusion podoplasty for the treatment of chronic fibrosing interdigital pyoderma in the dog. J Am Anim Hosp Assoc 27:264, 1991.
19. Swaim SF, Milton JL: Fusion podoplasty to treat abnormalities associated with severed digital flexor tendons. J Am Anim Hosp Assoc 30:137, 1994.
20. Swaim SF, Henderson RA: Small Animal Wound Management, 2nd ed.: Baltimore: Williams and Wilkins, 1997, 295.
21. Swaim SF, Scardino MS: Paw and distal limb salvage and reconstructive techniques. *In* Bojrab MJ, ed.: Current Techniques in Small Animal Surgery, 4th ed.: Baltimore: Williams and Wilkins, 1998, 625.
22. Swaim SF, Renberg WC, Shike KM: Small Animal Bandaging, Casting and Splinting Techniques. Ames, IA: Wiley – Blackwell, 2011, 43.
23. White RAS: Surgical treatment of specific skin disorders. *In* Slatter DH, ed.: Textbook of Small Animal Surgery, 3rd ed.: Philadelphia: WB Saunders, 2003, 339.
24. White SD: Pododermatitis. Vet Dermatol 1:1, 1989.
25. Whitney JC: Some aspects of interdigital cysts in the dog. J Small Anim Pract 11:83, 1970.
26. van den Broek A, Horvath – Ungerboeck C: Pedal dermatitis in dogs and cats: Part 1 Compan Anim 16: 39, 2011.
27. van den Broek A, Horvath – Ungerboeck C: Pedal dermatitis Part 2: Canine pododermatitis company Anim 16: 41, 2011.
28. Van Nimwegen S, Kirpenstein J: Specific disorders. In Tobias KM, Johnston SA, eds.: Veterinary Surgery, Small Animal, Vol. 2: St. Louis: Elsevier – Saunders, 2012, 1303.

# Superficial Interdigital (Web) Lacerations

## Definition and Indications

Superficial interdigital lacerations can involve the skin on the dorsum of the paw or skin on the palmar/plantar surface of the paw or both paw surfaces (Figure 4-46). The wounds result from coming in contact with sharp objects. Interdigital skin wounds are subject to considerable contamination due to the location of the wounds, especially if they are on the palmar/plantar paw surface. The animal's tendency to place weight on the paw following injury increases contamination. This is especially so with the canine athlete or working dog.

Thorough wound debridement and lavage are indicated. Because the pads and the interdigital skin tend to spread when weight is placed on them, proper suturing, bandaging, and splinting are also indicated to keep wound edges from separating. Such separation results in sutures cutting through tissues and delayed or lack of healing.

## Technique

With the animal under general anesthesia, the area should be prepared for aseptic surgery, and the wound should be explored to ascertain if it is superficial or deep. If it is superficial, it should be thoroughly debrided and lavaged with a 1:40 dilution of chlorhexidine

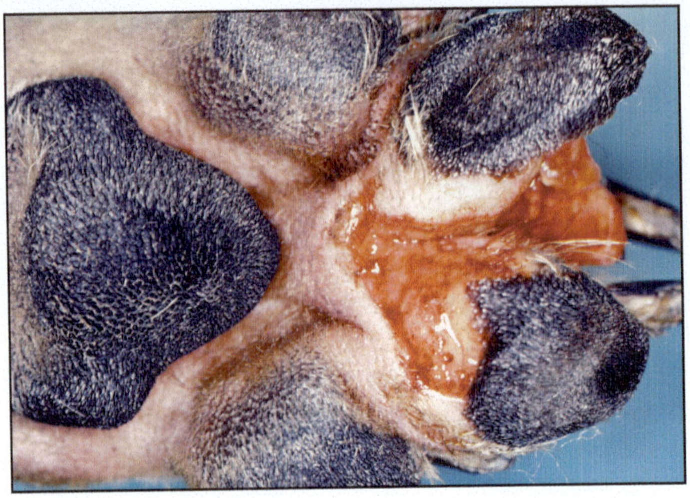

**Figure 4-46.** Laceration of an interdigital space. (From Swaim SF: Management and bandaging of soft tissue injuries of dog and cat feet. J Am Anim Hosp Assoc 21:329, 1985.)

diacetate (Nolvasan Solution, Ft. Dodge Animal Health, Ft. Dodge, IA) or gluconate (ChlorhexiDerm Disinfectant, Dermatologics in Veterinary Medicine, Pharmaceuticals, Inc., Miami, FL) solution. If the laceration has been present for a period of time and the tissues are infected, staged debridement and lavage should be performed. The wound should then be closed by delayed primary closure once infection is cleared.

The wound edges are sutured with simple interrupted sutures placed widely from the wound edges or far-near-near-far sutures of 3-0 monofilament nonabsorbable suture material. If the laceration involves both surfaces of the interdigital skin, the dorsal skin edges are sutured together as are the palmar/plantar edges.

## Aftercare

To help keep interdigital areas dry, small amounts of cotton or cast padding should be placed between digits not involved in the injury and in the space between the digits and the metacarpal/metatarsal pad. A piece of semiocclusive nonadherent dressing pad should be placed over the wound area(s). A thick absorbent bandage wrap is wrapped around the paw followed by a porous adhesive tape or elastic tape outer layer. This bandage wrap will help keep the interdigital area from spreading if the dog bears weight on the paw. For a large dog, a "clam shell" splint can be used as a localized crutch to keep the interdigital areas from spreading with weight bearing.

Because of the contaminated or infected nature of interdigital lacerations, the animal should be placed on a systemic antibiotic. The antibiotic should be effective against the organisms that are expected to be in the wound. These are commonly *Staphylococcus* and *Streptococcus* spp. The cephalosporins [e.g. cephalexin (Keflex, Dista Products Co., Division of Eli Lilly & Co., Indianapolis, IN) or cephadroxil (Cefa-Drops or Cefa-Tabs, Ft. Dodge Animal Health, Ft. Dodge, IA)] can be considered. Other possible antibiotics are an amoxicillin (Amoxi-Drops, Amoxi-Tabs, Amoxi-Inject, Pfizer Animal Health Group, Exton, PA) or an amoxicillin-trihydrate and clavulanate potassium combination (Clavamox tablets or drops, Pfizer Animal Health Group, Exton, PA) (See Microbial Evaluation and Therapy, Chapter 1).

Depending upon the amount of drainage, the bandage can be changed every 1 to 3 days for 10 to 14 days following surgery. It may be desirable to leave the sutures in place for 14 days to allow for adequate healing. If sutures are removed at this time, it is advisable to continue bandaging until the surgeon believes healing is adequate to allow the animal to use the paw without a bandage. A commercial dog bootie may also be used in the transition time between full bandaging and no bandaging, especially if the wound was in interdigital palmar or plantar skin. The length of time sutures remain in place, the frequency of bandage changes, and the length of time bandages and booties are needed will vary according to the severity of the wound, the animal's size, and its activity level. Clinical judgement is used in these matters.

### Advantages and Disadvantages

Interdigital lacerations that are properly sutured, bandaged and/or splinted will heal without complication. When these factors are insufficient, weight-bearing may spread the interdigital spaces which can result in sutures tearing through tissues with delayed or lack of healing.

## Suggested Readings


1. Basher A: Foot injuries in dogs and cats. Compend Contin Educ Pract Vet 16:1159, 1994.
2. Bohling MW, Swaim SF: Management of the traumatic wound by primary closure. In Birchard SJ, Sherding RG, eds.: Saunders Manual of Small Animal Practice, 3rd ed.: St. Louis: Saunders – Elsevier, 2006, 541.
3. Fowler D: Distal limb and paw injuries. Vet Clin No Am Small Anim Pract 36: 819, 2006.
4. Swaim SF: Management and bandaging of soft tissue injuries of dog and cat feet. J Am Anim Hosp Assoc 21:329, 1985.
5. Swaim SF, Henderson RA: Small Animal Wound Management, 2nd ed.: Baltimore: Williams and Wilkins, 1997, 295.
6. Swaim SF, Renberg WC, Shike KM: Small Animal Bandaging, Casting and Splinting Techniques. Ames, IA: Wiley – Blackwell, 2011, 43.
7. Waldron DR, Zimmerman-Pope N: Superficial skin wounds. *In* Slatter DH, ed.: Textbook of Small Animal Surgery, 3rd ed.: Philadelphia: WB Saunders, 2003, 259.


## Deep Interdigital Lacerations (Including Severed Digital Flexor Tendons)

### Definition and Indications

(See Interdigital Wounds, Superficial Interdigital Web Laceration in this chapter.) Wound characteristics for deep interdigital wounds are the same as for superficial wounds; however, deeper structures such as vessels and tendons may also be damaged. Of particular interest are the digital flexor tendons and their management if they have been severed. One cause of lacerated digital flexor tendons is broken glass on the bottom of lakes and ponds near the water edge. Retrievers step on such glass and lacerate palmar/plantar interdigital skin and all or part of the flexor tendons. Another common source of tendon severance is dogs stepping on the unprotected sharp edge of lawn edging material.

### Technique

(See Interdigital Wounds, Superficial Interdigital Web Laceration in this chapter.) Wound management techniques for deep interdigital wounds are the same as those for superficial interdigital wounds. In addition, if digital flexor tendons have been severed, these must receive attention. If the superficial and deep digital flexor tendons have been severed, it is reflected by abnormal weight bearing, flattening of one or more digits and elevation of nails and digital pads. When tendons have been severed, some form of tendon repair or compensatory surgical procedure will eventually be necessary to avoid abnormal weight bearing and possible pad ulceration. Digital flexor tendon repair can be difficult and it is often unsuccessful due to the small size of the tendons, the location of the tendons, and the difficulty in locating their retracted severed ends. Stress applied to repaired tendons also contributes to failure of repair. However, if it is to be performed, it should be done as early as possible. If a contaminated or infected wound has lacerated tendons, it is best to do a temporary tenorrhaphy leaving long suture tags. The wound is treated by staged debridement and lavage until healthy tissue is present for a delayed primary closure. The temporary tendon repair prevents further retraction of the severed tendon ends. The long suture tags make it easier to relocate the tendon for definitive repair (for information on tenorrhaphy see Part 2: Orthopedic Injuries, Sprain Injuries). When tendon repair fails or is not possible, fusion podoplasty may be considered as a salvage procedure to reposition digits in a relatively normal position. See Interdigital Wounds, Interdigital Pododermatitis, Radical Excision Therapy (Fusion Podoplasty).

## Aftercare

[See Interdigital Wounds, Superficial Interdigital Web Lacerations and Interdigital Wounds, Interdigital Pododermatitis, Radical Excision Therapy (Fusion Podoplasty) in this chapter.]

## Advantages and Disadvantages

[See Interdigital Wounds, Superficial Interdigital Web Lacerations and Interdigital Wounds, Interdigital Pododermatitis, Radical Excision Therapy (Fusion Podoplasty) in this chapter.]

The advantage of fusion podoplasty in the treatment of severed digital flexor tendons is that it provides a means of repositioning digits in a relatively normal position and returning the paw and limb to an acceptable degree of function. In addition, the problems of tenorrhaphy and its chance of failure are avoided. The disadvantages of the procedure are the same as those described for its use in treating chronic fibrosing interdigital pyoderma, i.e. it is radical surgery, there is need for careful postoperative bandaging and splinting, and the possibility of wound disruption between the digital and metacarpal/metatarsal pads during healing if such bandaging and splinting is not done.

# Suggested Readings


1. Basher A: Foot injuries in dogs and cats. Compend Contin Educ Pract Vet 16:1159, 1994.
2. Bohling MW, Swaim SF: Management of the traumatic wound by primary closure. In Birchard SJ, Sherding RG, eds.: Saunders Manual of Small Animal Practice, 3rd ed.: St. Louis: Saunders – Elsevier, 2006, 541.
3. Fowler D: Distal limb and paw injuries. Vet Clin No Am Small Anim Pract 36: 819, 2006.
4. Hedlund CS: Surgery of the integumentary system. *In* Fossum TW, ed.: Small Animal Surgery, 2nd ed.: St. Louis: Mosby, 2002, 134.
5. Hedlund CS: Surgery of the integumentary system. In Fossum TW, ed.: Small Animal Surgery, 3rd ed.: St. Louis: Mosby, 2007, 159.
6. Niles JD: Special considerations in wound management. In Williams J, Moores A, eds.: BSAVA Manual of Canine and Feline Wound Management and Reconstruction, 2nd ed: Glouster (UK): BSAVA, 2009, 223.
7. Swaim SF: Management and bandaging of soft tissue injuries of dog and cat feet. J Am Anim Hosp Assoc 21:329, 1985.
8. Swaim SF, Lee AH, MacDonald JM, et al: Fusion podoplasty for the treatment of chronic fibrosing interdigital pyoderma in the dog. J Am Anim Hosp Assoc 27:264, 1991.
9. Swaim SF, Henderson RA: Small Animal Wound Management, 2nd ed.: Baltimore: Williams and Wilkins, 1997, 295.
10. Swaim SF, Milton JL: Fusion podoplasty to treat abnormalities associated with severed digital flexor tendons. J Am Anim Hosp Assoc 30:137, 1994.
11. Swaim SF, Scardino MS: Paw and distal limb salvage and reconstruction techniques. *In* Bojrab MJ, ed.: Current Techniques in Small Animal Surgery, 4th ed.: Baltimore: Williams and Wilkins, 1998, 625.
12. Swaim SF, Renberg WC, Shike KM: Small Animal Bandaging, Casting and Splinting Techniques. Ames, IA.: Wiley – Blackwell, 2011, 43.
13. Waldron DR, Zimmerman-Pope N: Management of superficial skin wounds. *In* Slatter DH, ed.: Textbook of Small Animal Surgery, 3rd ed.: Philadelphia: WB Saunders, 2003, 259.
14. White RAS: Surgical treatment of specific skin disorders. *In* Slatter DH, ed.: Textbook of Small Animal Surgery, 3rd ed.: Philadelphia: WB Saunders, 2003, 339.


# Digit Orthopedic Wounds with Soft Tissue Salvage

## Definition and Indications

Resurfacing digits and the dorsal paw can be done using the phalangeal fillet technique; whereby, damaged phalanges and tendons are removed from a digit(s). The skin of that digit(s) and any available interdigital web skin are used to cover adjacent digits and/or the dorsum of the paw when these areas have sizable skin defects and intact bones (Figure 4-47). The procedure is indicated when paw trauma has resulted in severe damage to the phalanges of a digit(s), yet the skin of that digit(s) is still viable. However, skin from adjacent digit(s) and/or the dorsum of the paw has been badly damaged or is missing but the bone structure is still intact.

## Technique

The wound is carefully debrided and lavaged, and remaining fragments of the proximal, middle, and distal phalanges are removed along with tendon fragments (Figure 4-48A and Figure 4-49A). The skin of the filleted digit(s) along with any viable interdigital webbing skin is incised so it can be used as a flap(s) to resurface adjacent digits with large deficits or the dorsum of the paw (Figure 4-48B & C and Figure 4-49B & C). Sufficient skin and subcutaneous tissue should be maintained at the base of the flaps to provide a blood supply to the flaps. The flaps are sutured to the remaining skin on the adjacent digits or dorsum of the paw using simple interrupted sutures of 3-0 monofilament nonabsorbable suture material (Figure 4-48D and Figure 4-49D).

## Aftercare

A small amount of cotton or cast padding is placed between the remaining intact digits and in the interpad space between the digits and the metacarpal/metatarsal pad to keep the areas dry. Absorbent gauze sponges are placed over the surgical site. A thick absorbent secondary bandage wrap is placed on the paw, followed by a porous adhesive tape or elastic tape outer layer. To help keep pressure and tension off of the transposed digital flaps, which could result in sutures tearing through the skin, a "donut"-type foam rubber pad and metal splint cup can be incorporated in the bandage to distribute pressure around the flap areas. In large dogs, a "clam shell" splint can be used as a localized crutch to help keep pressure and tension

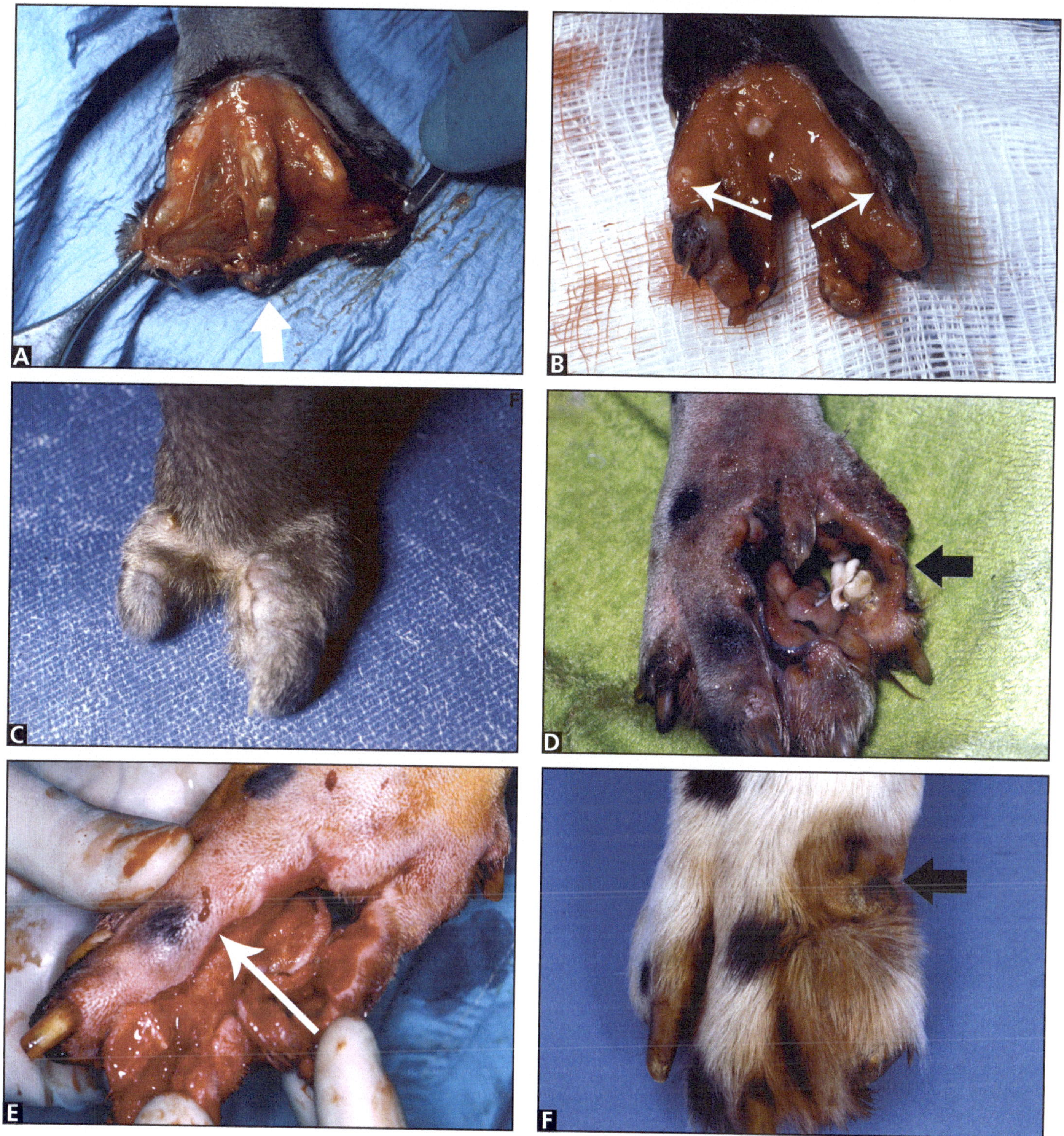


**Figure 4-47.** Phalangeal fillet to resurface digits and dorsum of the paw. **A.** & **D.** Digits with damaged phalanges to be removed *(arrows)*. **B.** & **E.** All phalanges and nails are removed from the injured digits. Skin of digits will cover the adjacent digits **B.** and dorsum of the paw **E.** *(arrows)*. **C.** & **F.** Digital skin flaps healed. Note pad skin on the dorsum of the paw **F.** *(arrow)*. (A., B. & C. courtesy of I. Sanchez; D & E from Swaim SF: Management and bandaging of soft tissue injuries of dog and cat feet. J Am Anim Hosp Assoc 21:329, 340, 1985; F from Swaim SF, Henderson RA: Small Animal Wound Management, 2nd ed.: Baltimore: Williams & Wilkins, 1997, 353.

off of the sutured areas. If all weight bearing is to be avoided, a Velpeau sling, carpal flexion splint or carpal sling can be used on the forelimb or a 90/90 sling on the hind limb. Cats and small dogs which are lighter do not place as much weight on the paws. Thus, a well-padded bandage without a "donut"-type foam rubber pad may be sufficient for them. Bandages are changed periodically for 7 to 10 days. The length of time sutures should remain in place, the frequency of bandage changes, and the length of time bandages are needed are variable factors dependent on wound tension, wound healing rate and amount of drainage.

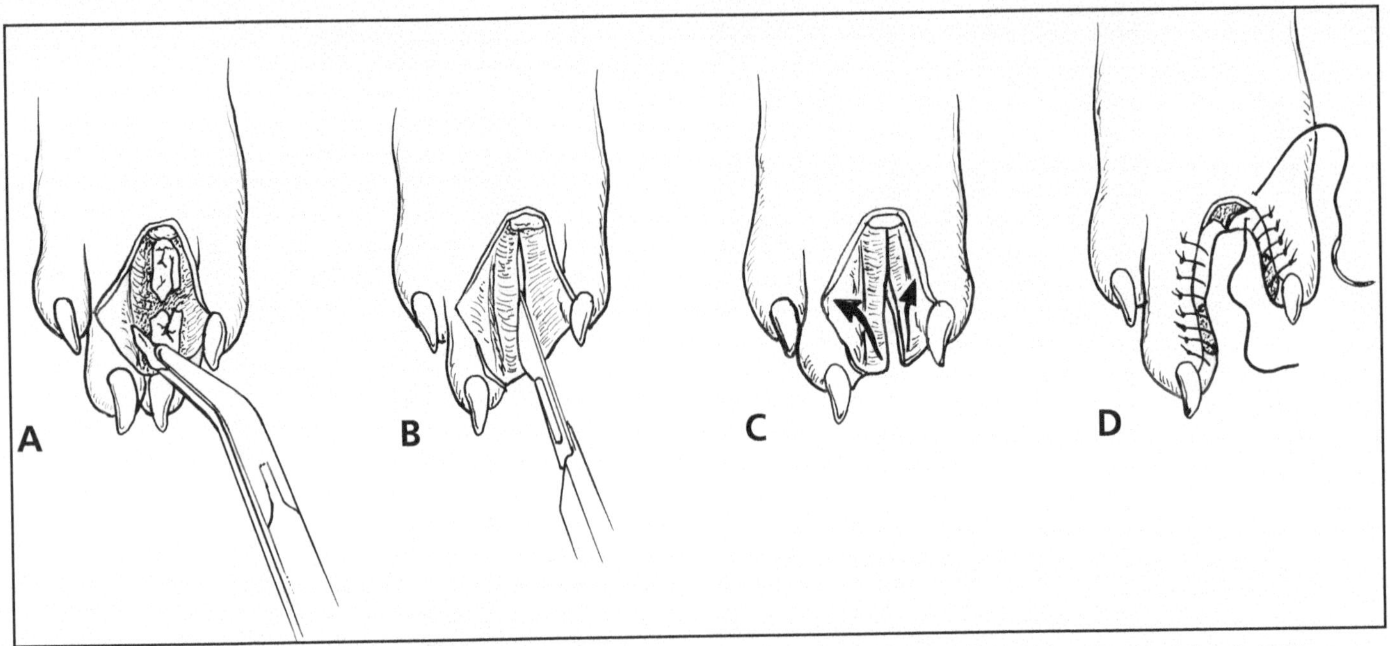


**Figure 4-48.** Phalangeal fillet to resurface adjacent digits. **A.** Removing phalangeal and tendon fragments from a severely damaged digit. **B.** Midline incision made in the skin of the severely damaged digit, creating 2 flaps. **C.** Rotating flaps to resurface adjacent digits *(arrows)*. **D.** Suturing flaps in place. (After Swaim SF, Henderson RA: Small Animal Wound Management, 2nd ed.: Baltimore: Williams & Wilkins, 1997, 354.)

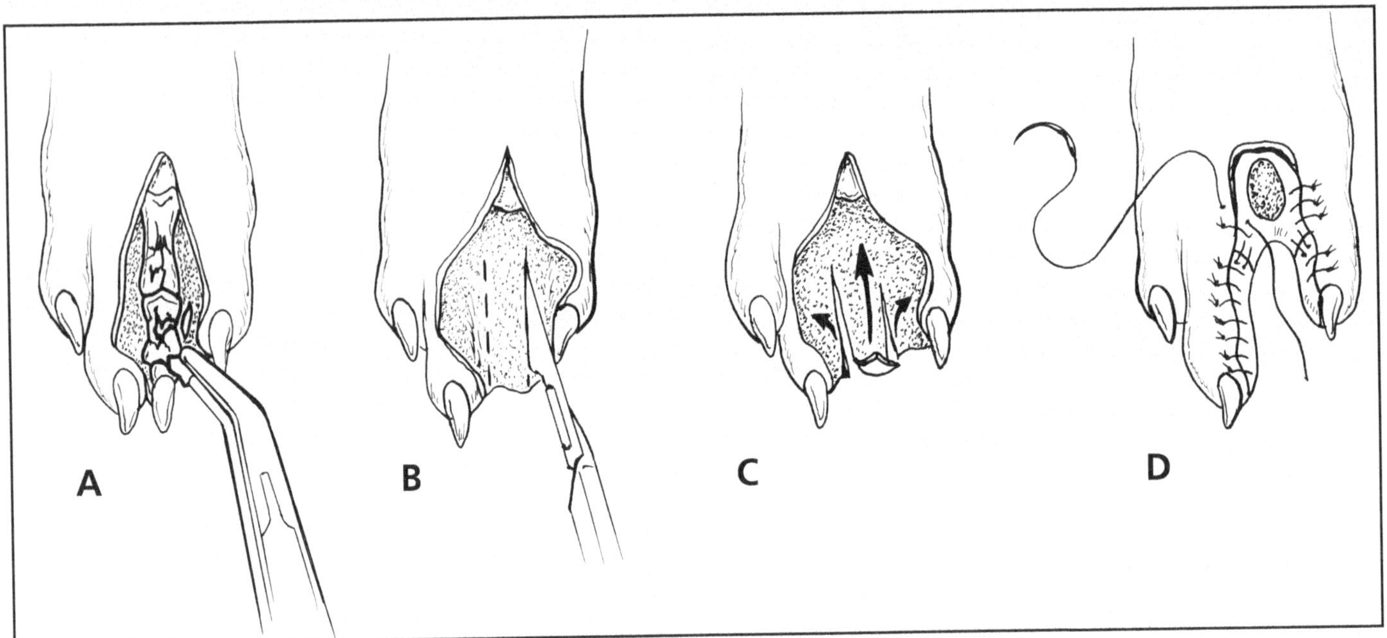


**Figure 4-49.** Phalangeal fillet to resurface adjacent digits and dorsum of paw. **A.** Removing phalangeal and tendon fragments from a severely damaged digit. B. Two skin incisions are made in the skin of the severely damaged digit, creating 3 flaps. **C.** Rotation of the flaps to resurface the adjacent digits and dorsum of the paw *(arrows)*. **D.** Suturing the flaps in place. (After Swaim SF, Henderson RA: Small Animal Wound Management, 2nd ed.: Baltimore: Williams & Wilkins, 1997, 354.)

## Advantages and Disadvantages

The advantage of this phalangeal fillet technique is that locally available skin of digits and their webbing can be used to resurface skin defects on adjacent digits and the dorsum of the paw. The disadvantage of the technique is associated with using digits 3 or 4 (or both) for the procedure. Filleting these digits leaves a cosmetic defect in the center of the paw. In addition, such a defect could cause lameness. If digits 3 and 4 are filleted to resurface digits 2 and 5 or the dorsum of the paw, digits 2 and 5 protrude and may be subject to snagging on vegetation or carpets. If the pads of filleted digits are necessary for the resurfacing procedure they should be left in the skin flap. However, as the flap is in its new position, pad tissue may be on the dorsum of the digits or paw for a less than cosmetic appearance.

# Suggested Readings

(See Paw Wounds, Palmar/Plantar Wounds, Metacarpal/Metatarsal Pad Loss, Pad Replacement: Phalangeal Fillet in this chapter.)

# Digit Space Filling: Phalangeal Fillet

## Definition and Indications

Phalangeal fillet technique for digital space filling requires removing all or some of the phalanges of digits 3 or 4 or both. All soft tissues of these digits are retained as a space filler in the center of the digital area. The technique is indicated when there has been some soft tissue damage and severe osseous damage to the phalanges of digits 3 and 4 (Figure 4-50A), and there is need for cosmetic and/or functional filling of the digital area.

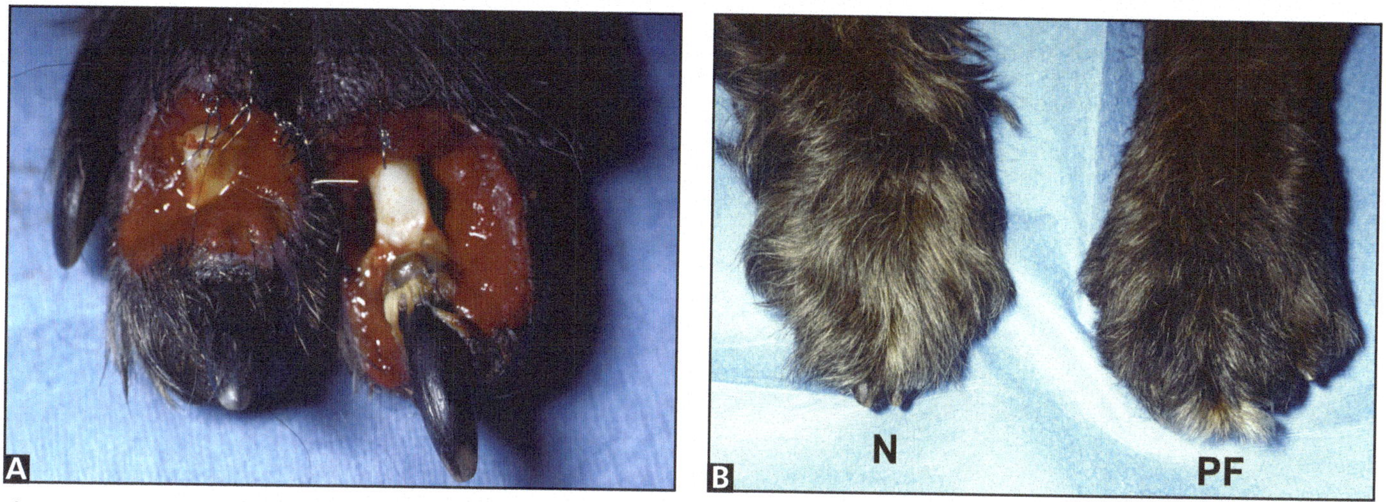


**Figure 4-50.** Phalangeal fillet for space filling. **A.** Traumatized third and fourth digits with nonviable phalanges and viable soft tissues. **B.** After phalangeal fillet, the soft tissues of the third and fourth digits provide space filling in the center of the paw for functional and cosmetic purposes. Right paw – normal *(N)*; Left paw – phalangeal fillet *(PF)*. (From Swaim SF, Henderson RA: Small Animal Wound Management, 2nd ed.: Baltimore: Williams & Wilkins, 1997, 355.)

## Technique

The status of the soft tissues and phalanges of digits 3 and 4 are evaluated to determine if soft tissue and orthopedic repair are indicated. If repair of the phalanges is not possible or feasible but digital soft tissues are viable and useable, partial or total fillet should be considered. The damaged phalanges are removed using forceps, scissors, scalpel and rongeurs (Figure 4-51A,). The soft tissues are debrided and lavaged. The skin edges of the digits are sutured using 2-0 or 3-0 monofilament nonabsorbable simple interrupted sutures (Figure 4-51B). The area of nail removal is left open for drainage.

## Aftercare

(See Wounds, Digit Orthopedic Wounds With Soft Tissue Salvage, Resurfacing: Phalangeal Fillet in this chapter.

## Advantages and Disadvantages

Phalangeal fillet provides a technique to fill a defect in the center of the digital area when it is needed for cosmetic purposes and when it is necessary to prevent a space that could snag on vegetation and carpets (Figure 4-51B). A disadvantage of the technique is the possibility that contraction during healing will pull the digital pads dorsally. This possibility is greatest if all 3 phalanges are removed and less if only the middle and distal phalanges are removed. Some lameness may result following filleting of digits 3 and 4 due to their initial weight bearing function.

# Suggested Readings

(See Paw Wounds, Palmar/Plantar Wounds, Metacarpal/Metatarsal Pad Loss, Pad Replacement: Phalangeal Fillet in this chapter.)

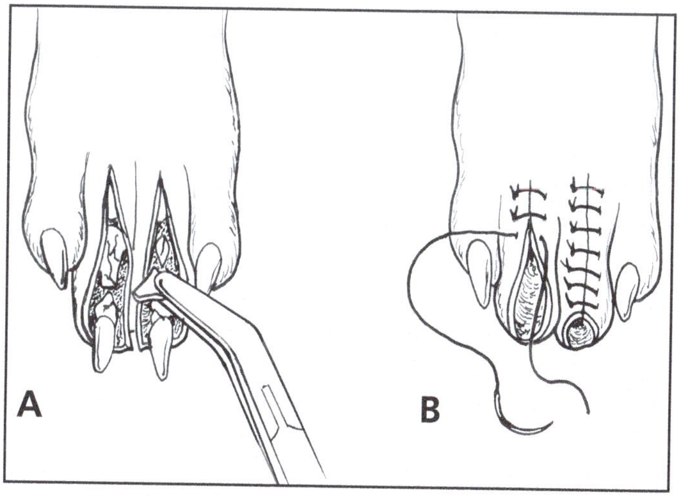


**Figure 4-51.** Phalangeal fillet for space filling. **A.** Removing phalangeal and tendon fragments from traumatized digits, leaving viable soft tissues. **B.** Digital wound edges are sutured, leaving the area of nail open for drainage. (After Swaim SF, Henderson RA: Small Animal Wound Management, 2nd ed.: Baltimore: Williams & Wilkins, 1997, 355.)

# Chapter 5

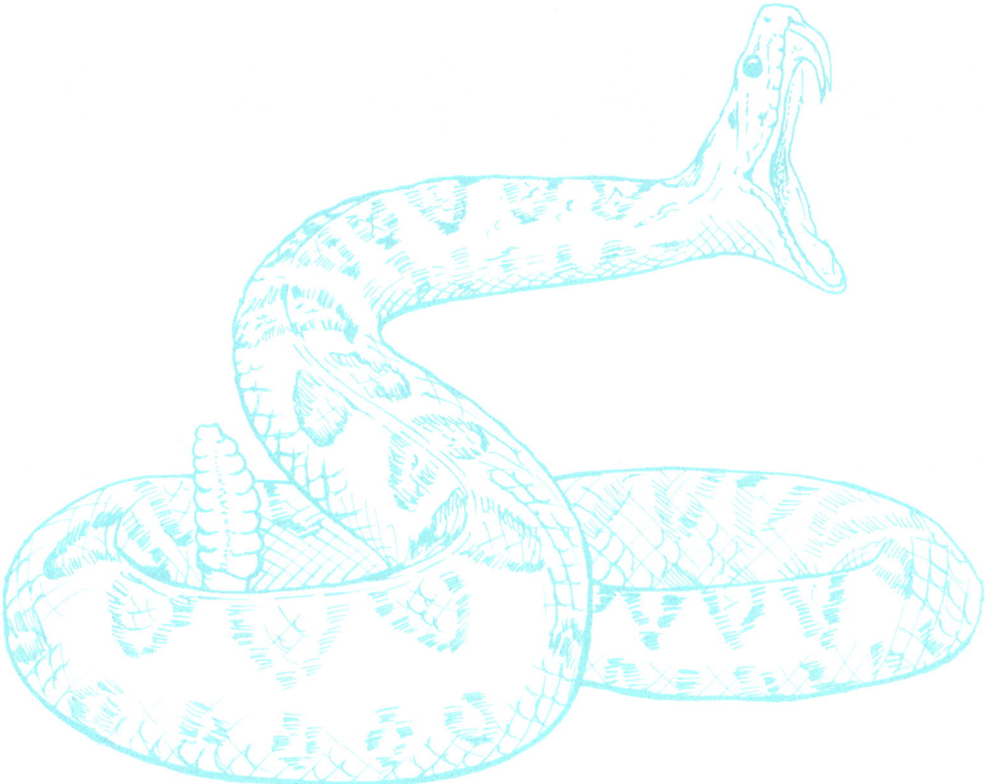

## Specific Wounds - Snake Bite and Acral Lick Dermatitis

Steven F. Swaim, D.V.M., M.S.
Jennifer S. Pendergraft, D.V.M., D.A.C.V.D.
Julia D. Albright, D.V.M., D.A.C.V.B
Janet Welch, D.V.M., D.A.C.V.S.

# Snakebite and Acral Lick Dermatitis

Two specific wounds which affect the soft tissues of the distal limb are venomous snakebite wounds and the wounds associated with acral lick dermatitis. Treatment of both types of wounds may involve more than topical therapy and reconstruction of the wounds.

# Snakebite Wounds

Steven F. Swaim, D.V.M., M.S.

## Definition and Indications

Venomous snakebites which result in wounds are generally caused by bites from snakes of the subfamily Crotalidae (pit vipers). This includes the copperhead, cotton mouth water moccasin and rattlesnake. The eastern diamond back rattlesnake and cotton mouth water moccasin are the most dangerous, with the water moccasin tending to be pugnacious and having more tendency to deliver venom with its bite. Rattlesnakes account for the majority of deaths in animal victims. Bites usually occur on the face and legs.

Snakes control the amount of venom they deliver. Defensive bites tend to have the least amount of venom. Offensive bites deliver more venom, and agonal bites deliver the entire load of venom. A severed head can reflexively bite for up to one hour after decapitation.

Not only can the venom of these snakes cause local tissue wounds, but it can result in systemic abnormalities that can be life threatening. Thus, treatment of envenomizations that have caused soft tissue wounds may require early systemic supportive treatment to save the animal's life prior to wound care. Systemic indications that envenomization has occurred are associated with hemotoxic, vasculotoxic and necrrogenic properties of the venom. These include alterations in the resistance and integrity of blood vessels, blood cell changes (echinocytosis of red cells), coagulation abnormalities, proteinuria, elevated fibrin split products, alterations in cardiac dynamics, changes in nervous system function, and myonecrosis. Clinical signs may be cyanosis, hypotension, bleeding, shock, lethargy, salivation, thirst, lymphangitis, weakness, muscle fasiculations, vomiting, diarrhea, obtundity, seizures, and respiratory depression. Other signs may be coma, tachypnea, urinary and fecal incontinence, and paralysis. Cardiac dysrhythmias, (especially ventricular premature contractions), and depression may be caused by diamond back rattlesnake bites due to a myocardial depressant factor in the venom.

The presence of fang marks indicate that a bite has taken place. It does not indicate envenomization has occurred. Local signs indicating that envenomization has occurred are the presence of one or two fang puncture wounds, which may be hemorrhaging. Bite wounds may also appear as small lacerations, and there can be multiple bites. There is immediate and progressive swelling with tissue discoloration, including ecchymosis, and petechiae formation (Figure 5-1). Tissue damage may extend 1 cm below the skin. There is also immediate and severe pain. However, with time, there is decreased sensitivity. The end result can be local tissue necrosis at the envenomization site. Generally, if there is no pain or swelling at the bite site within 1½ hours of the bite, no envenomization has occurred. It has been stated that absence of pain, swelling, echymoses, systemic symptoms, fasciculations and abnormal laboratory values within 30 to 60 minutes of a pit viper bite precludes the use of an antivenin.

It should be remembered that many factors govern the severity of a snakebite wound and the severity of envenomation cannot be judged by local signs alone. The composition of venom varies between species and individual snakes. The habitat of the snake and season of the year have an effect on the snake's venom as do age, size and motivation of the snake. Other factors are the amount of venom injected in relation to the weight of the victim, the venom injection site, post-bite excitability, the type of tissue injected with venom, the

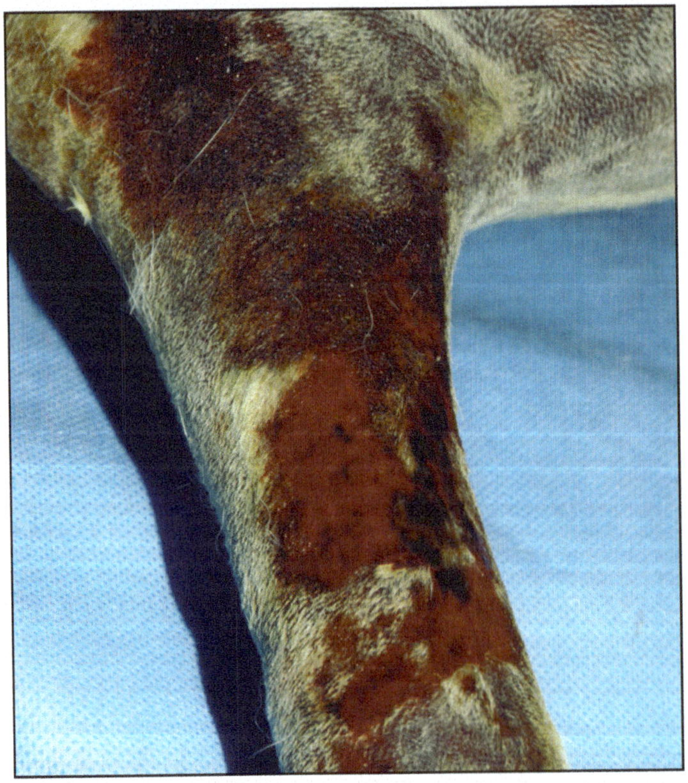

**Figure 5-1.** Pit viper snakebite on a dog's limb with swelling and discoloration as a result of echymosis.

depth of venom injection, and the type of haircoat. The size and health of the victim, preexisting medications, and the time lapse between envenomation and initiation of medical therapy are all governing factors that affect the victim's response to venom. Dogs seem to be more sensitive to the toxic effects of snake venom than cats.

The goals in treating venomous snakebites are neutralization of the venom, treatment of the systemic effects of the venom, and treatment of wound infection with repair of resulting defects in the case of local tissue necrosis.

# Techniques

## Initial (Field) Management

The use of ice, tourniquets, incision and suction, and electrcoshock are of little value in management of snakebites. Although they have been described for treatment, they can cause additional tissue damage, and the stress to the dog or cat can outweigh any potential benefits. Practical early management of snakebite is avoidance of exertion and excitement as well as keeping the bite site below the heart if possible. Rapid transport to veterinary facilities is necessary.

## Animal Monitoring

When a pit viper bite is suspected on the distal limb, the hair should be clipped from the limb. The area of the suspected bite should be examined for fang puncture wounds. However, local edema may obscure puncture wounds. Absence of fang puncture wounds indicates no envenomation by a pit viper. This is an important part of the diagnostic procedure if it is questionable as to the source of the distal limb tissue abnormalities, because antivenin should be administered only if a snakebite is known to have occurred.

Because local tissue reaction may not be adequate for evaluating the severity of envenomization, and because, in some instances, clinical signs of severe envenomation may take several hours to become evident, snakebitten animals should be hospitalized for observation for 6 to 24 hours. To help monitor the progression of clinical envenomation a snakebite severity score (SSS) tool can be used (Table 5-1). Use of this allows more accurate quantification of the patients' condition over time.

The degree and progression of envenomation can be monitored by laboratory tests, which include CBC and differential, coagulation profile (prothrombin time and partial thromboplastin time), platelet count, creatinine phosphokinase, fibrinogen, fibrin degradation products BUN, urinalysis with urine hemoglobin and myoglobin values. These analyses should be performed initially, and at 6 hours after hospital admission, at a minimum. Platelet counts and clotting times can be a sensitive means of monitoring the severity and progression of envenomation, since platelet counts decrease and clotting times are prolonged with pit viper envenomations. A progressive platelet count decrease and prolong clotting time indicates progressive venom activity. Myoglobinuria indicates severe rhabdomyolysis and hemoglobinuria indicates marked hemolysis. An electrocardiogram should be monitored in severe envenomations.

With distal limb bites, circumferential measurements at, above, and below the bite area should be done at half hour intervals to quantify edema progression. When the animal has become clinically stable following antivenin administration, the interval between measurements can be increased.

## Therapy

It is controversial, but use of antihistamines has been advocated in treatment of pit viper envenomization. If it is used, the antihistamine diphenhydramine (Benadryl, Warner-Lambert Division, A Pfizer Co., Morris Plains, NJ) should be administered prior to antivenin therapy – 10 mg for small dogs and cats, 25-50 mg for large dogs. This provides some calming effect on excitable animals. One-half of the antihistamine dose is administered subcutaneously, intravenous catheterization is performed, and the other half of the dose is given intravenously. Lactated Ringer's solution or physiologic saline should be administered intravenously. Aggressive fluid therapy should be used, as most deaths from pit viper bites are due to cardiovascular collapse from marked vascular leakage and pooling of blood.

Antivenin [North American polyvalent antivenin (Crotalidae), Boehringer Ingelheim, Vet Medica, St. Joseph, MO]; or [Crotiladae polyvalent immune, Fab Ovine, Protherics, Inc. Brentwood, TN]. should be administered as soon as possible after the bite to prevent systemic reactions and tissue necrosis. A single vial of antivenin given early is equivalent to several vials given later, and multiple doses given later are costly. The median lethal dose of snake venom is based on the milligrams of venom injected and the victim's weight in kilograms. Thus, smaller animals may require larger doses of antivenin. The average antivenin dose is one to two vials. However, more may be needed. It should be given until serial examinations and coagulation profiles indicate the animal's condition is stable. One vile of antiven is reconstituted by adding

| Table 5-1. Snakebite Severity Score | |
|---|---|
| **Pulmonary System** | |
| Signs within normal limit | 0 |
| Minimal – slight dyspnea | 1 |
| Moderate – respiratory compromise, tachypnea, use of accessory muscles | 2 |
| Severe – cyanosis, air hunger, extreme tachypnea, respiratory insufficiency, or respiratory arrest from any cause | 3 |
| **Cardiovascular System** | |
| Signs within normal limits | 0 |
| Minimal – tachycardia, general weakness, benign dysrhythmia, hypertension | 1 |
| Moderate – Tachycardia, hypotension ( but tarsal pulse still palpable) | 2 |
| Severe – extreme tachycardia, hypotension (non palpable tarsal pulse or Systolic blood pressure < 80mmhg), malignant dysrhythmia or cardiac arrest | 3 |
| **Local Wound** | |
| Signs within normal limits | 0 |
| Minimal – pain, sewlling, ecchymosis, erythema limited to bite site | 1 |
| Moderate – pain, swelling, ecchymosis, erythema involves less than half of extremity and may be spreading slowly | 2 |
| Severe – pain, swelling, ecchymosis, erythema involves most or all of one extremity and is spreading rapidly | 3 |
| Very severe – pains, swelling, ecchymosis, erythema extends beyond effected extremity, or significant tissue slough | 4 |
| **Gastrointestinal System** | |
| Signs within normal limits | 0 |
| Minimal – abdominal pain, tenesmus | 1 |
| Moderate – vomiting, diarrhea | 2 |
| Severe – repetitive vomiting, diarrhea, or hematemesis | 3 |
| **Hematological System** | |
| Signs within normal limits | 0 |
| Minimal – coagulation parameters slightly abnormal, PT<20 sec, PTT <50 sec, platelets 100,000 – 150,000/mm$^3$ | 1 |
| Moderate – coagulation parameters abnormal, PT 20 – 50 sec, PTT 50 – 75 sec, platelets 50,000 – 150,000/mm$^3$ | 2 |
| Severe – coagulation parameters abnormal PT 50 – 100 sec, PTT 75 – 100 sec, platelets 20,000 – 50,000/mm$^3$ | 3 |
| Very severe – coagulation parameters markedly abnormal with bleeding present or the threat of spontaneous bleeding, including PT unmeasurable, PTT unmeasurable, Platelets<20,000/mm$^3$ | 4 |
| **Central Nervous System** | |
| Signs within normal limits | 0 |
| Minimal – apprehension | 1 |
| Moderate – chills, weakness, faintness, ataxia | 2 |
| Severe – lethargy, seizures, coma | 3 |
| **Total Score Possible** | **0 to 20** |

From Peterson ME: Snakebite: Pit Vipers: Part 1, Sci Proc. Central Veterinary Conference: Baltimore: 2008.

the diluent and warming it to body temperature over 10-15 minutes. Physiolgic saline can be added to fill the vial. Mixing should be by a swirling action, not shaking, to prevent foaming. A minimum of one vile of antivenin should be given with subsequent dosage(s) being dependent on clinical signs, laboratory results, and progression or stabilization of the swelling of the limb. In general, smaller animals need a larger dose of antivenin. This will make them more susceptible to delayed serum sickness seven to 14 days after administration. Another factor governing the total dose of antivenin is the pet owner's willingness to have additional vials administered based on cost.

The antivenin is administered slowly with the intravenous fluids. Antivenin should be diluted at a ratio of one vial to 100-250 ml. of crystalloid fluids. The first 10 to 15 ml of antivenin should be given over 5 to 10 minutes with the entire dose being given within a half hour. In a small animal in which an entire container of fluid would result in fluid overload, the fluid infusion volume should be adjusted to prevent such overload. Antivenin should be given slowly through the IV set during fluid administration. As it is administered observation should be made for an allergic reaction. The concave surface of the pinna should be observed for hyperemia. The patient should also be observed for signs of nausea and pruritis as indications of possible allergic reaction. If an allergic reaction (usually anaphylactoid) occurs, antivenin infusion should be stopped and diphenhydramine administration should begin 10 mg for small dogs and cats, 25-50 mg for large dogs. Slow infusion of antivenin should resume after 5 minutes. If the reaction recurs, infusion is stoped and consultaion with a poison control center should be sought. If true anaphylaxis develops, antivenin infusion should stop, and epinephrine and corticosteroids should be given with crystalloid fluids. Epinephrine and resuscitaiton equipment should be available if needed. Although clinical bleeding usually does not develop, low platelet counts may recur 3 to 4 days after antivenin administration. If this occurs, additional antivenin should be considered if platelet levels are lower than 50,000 or if petechiae or ecchymoses develop.

Delayed serum sickness is rare in dogs and cats. If it does occur, it is 7-14 days after antivenin administration. It can be treated with antihistamines and corticosteroids.

Because snakebite wounds are contaminated with oral flora of the snake, to include *Pseudomonas sp* and *Clostridium tetani*, broad-spectrum antibiotics and tetanus toxoids should be administered. Use of corticosteroids is controversial. It has been stated that they can help in treating shock and reducing edema. However, they have also been reported to alter important laboratory values necessary for monitoring the patient's status and increase the severity of toxicity.

If antivenin is not sufficient for pain control, Fentanyl can be administered as a continuous rate infusion (loading dose of 2 mg/kg then 0.5 mg/kg/hour).

## Aftercare

Pit viper envenomation often results in tissue necrosis with loss of tissue. As tissue becomes nonviable, the wound should be managed as an infected wound, to include staged debridement. Primary bandages that support moist wound healing and yet are absorbent should be used (e.g. polyurethane foam). A topical hydrophilic agent (e.g. Intracell – McCloud Pharmaceuticals, Ft. Collins, CO) could be considered. Theoretically, this combination could help remove residual venom from the area of the bite wound. When healthy granulation tissue is present, a decision must be made as to the type of wound closure to be utilized based on the amount of skin remaining on the area.

## Advantages and Disadvantages

It is advantageous to use antivenin as part of pit viper envenomation therapy, because it is difficult to predict the animals' systemic and local response to envenomation. There is the possibility of a hypersensitivity reaction to the antivenin (serum – sickness) as a disadvantage. The cost of antivenin therapy could be considered as a disadvantage; however, if it helps prevent a large tissue slough, and averts a more expensive reconstructive surgical reconstruction, it should be considered as advantageous.

If there is considerable swelling of the limb, it may obscure fang puncture wounds, putting the veterinarian at a disadvantage. The swelling and pain associated with a pit viper bite can also be signs of envenomation by other species, such as stinging insects. The presence of fang puncture wounds is important in deciding whether to use antivenin in the treatment. If there is aquestion as to whether a snakebite bite has occurred, a platelet count can be helpful in deciding. A low platelet count increases the suspicion of pit viper envenomation.

# Suggested Readings

1. Berdoulay P, Schaer M,Starr J: Serum sickness in a dog associated with antivenin therapy for snakebite caused by Croatalus adamanteus. J Vet Emerg Crit Care 15: 206, 2005.
2. Brown D, Wingfield W, et al: Echinocytosis associated with rattlesnake envenomation in dogs. Vet Path 31: 654, 1994.
3. Hackett TB, Wingfield WE, Mazzaferro EM, et. al.: Clinical

findings associate with prairie rattlesnake bites in dogs: 100 cases (1989 – 1998). Am J Vet Res 220: 1675, 2002.
4. Hedlund CS: Surgery of the integumentary system. *In* Fossum TW, ed.: Small Animal Surgery, 2nd ed.: St. Louis: Mosby, 2002, 134.
5. Hedlund CS: Surgery of the integumentary system. In Fossum TW, ed.: Small Animal Surgery, 3rd ed.: St. Louis: Mosby, 2007, 159.
6. Holstege CP, Miller MB, Wermuth M, et al: Crotalid snake envenomation. Crit Care Clin 13:889, 1997.
7. Howe N, Meisenheimer J: Electric shock does not save snake-bitten rats. Ann Emerg Med 17: 254, 1987.
8. Hudelson S, Hudelson P: Pathophysiology of snake envenomization and evaluation of treatments - Part I. Compend Contin Educ Pract Vet 17:889,1995.
9. Hudelson S, Hudelson P: Pathophysiology of snake envenomization and evaluation of treatments - Part II. Compend Contin Educ Pract Vet 17:1035,1995.
10. Hudelson S, Hudelson P: Pathophysiology of snake envenomization and evaluation of treatments - Part III. Compend Contin Educ Pract Vet 17:1385,1995.
11. Johnson E, Kardong K, MacKessey S: Electric shocks are ineffective in treatment of lethal effects of rattlesnake envenomation in mice. Toxicon 25: 1347,1987.
12. MacPhail CM: Surgery of the integumentary system. In Fossum TW, ed.: Small Animal Surgery, 4th ed.: St. Louis: Mosby 2013, 190.
13. Mansfield PD: The management of snake venom poisoning in dogs. Compend Contin Educ Pract Vet 6:988,1984.
14. McCowan JL, Cook KL, Hanel RM, et al: Effect of antivenin dose on outcome from crotalid envenomation: 218 dogs (1988 – 2006). J Vet Emerg Crit Care 19: 603,2009.
15. Pavletic MM: Atlas of Small Animal Wound Management and Reconstructive Surgery, 3rd ed.: Ames, IA: Wiley – Blackwell, 2010, 159.
*16. Peterson ME: Snake bites. *In* Bistner SI, Ford RB, Raffee MR, eds.: Handbook of Veterinary Procedures and Emergency Treatment, 7th ed.: Philadelphia: WB Saunders, 2000, 230.
*17. Peterson ME: Treating Pit Viper Bites. Vet Med: 885, 1998.
*18. Peterson ME: Snake Bite: Pit Vipers. Clinical Techniques In Small Animal Practice 21: 174, 2006.
*19. Peterson ME: Snake Bite: Pit Vipers 1. Sci. Proc. Central Vet Conf: Baltimore: 2008.
*20. Peterson ME: Snake Bite: Pit Vipers 2: Sci. Proc. Central Vet Conf: Baltimore: 2008.
*21. Peterson ME, Matz M, Seibold K, et al: A randomized multicenter trial of Croatalidae polyvalent immune Fab antivenom for the treatment of rattlesnake envenomization in dogs. J Vet Emerg Crit Care 21: 335,2011.
22. Ralidis PM: Medical treatment of reptile envenomation: A review of the current literature. Top Emerg Med 2:16,2000.
23. Schaer M: Eastern diamondback envenomation of 20 dogs. Compend Contin Educ 6: 997, 1984.
24. Scott DW, Miller WH, Griffin CE: Muller and Kirk's Small Animal Dermatology, 6th ed.: Philadelphia: WB Saunders, 2001, 1073.
25. Swaim SF, Henderson RA: Small Animal Wound Management, 2nd ed.: Baltimore: Williams and Wilkins, 1997, 87.
26. Waldron DR, Zimmerman-Pope N: Superficial skin wounds. *In* Slatter DH, ed.: Textbook of Small Animal Surgery, 3rd ed.: Philadelphia: WB Saunders, 2003, 259.
27. Willey JR, Schaer M: Eastern diamondback rattlesnake (Crotalus adamanteus) envenomation of dogs: 31 cases (1982 – 2002). J Am Anim Hosp Assoc 41: 22, 2005.
28. Wingfield WE, Raffe MR: The Veterinary ICU Book. Jackson Hole, WY: Teton NewMedia, 2002, 1034.
*Primary references

# Acral Lick Dermatitis

(Acral Lick Granuloma, Acral Pruritic Nodule, Acropruritic Granuloma)

Jennifer Schissler Pendergraft, DVM, MS
Julia D. Albright, MA, DVM
Janet Welch, DVM, MS

## Definition and Indications

Acral lick dermatitis (ALD), is one of the most challenging and frustrating diseases encountered in canine practice. The genesis and perpetuation of ALD is often multifactorial. Optimal control is achieved by identifying and controlling these factors with a thorough and persistent approach.

ALD is a common disease, characterized by repetitive licking of the skin. Lesions, commonly known as lick granulomas, are well-circumscribed, alopecic,erosive to ulcerative, variably pigmented, and may take the form of nodules or plaques (Figure 5-2). Lesions may fissure and produce purulent, serosanguinous, or hemorrhagic exudates. Rarely, full thickness ulcerations involving subcutaneous tissue, muscle or bone may occur. Lesions are commonly located on the forelimbs, distal to the elbow, but may also involve the distal hind limbs. Patients may have singular or multiple limb involvement. Large breed dogs such as Golden Retrievers, Boxers, Doberman Pinschers and Great Danes appear to be over-represented.

The medical conditions responsible for promoting the licking behavior initially are designated as primary factors. Perpetuating factors are responsible for the progression of the lesions and continuation of the self-trauma, even if the primary factors are controlled. A thorough history, physical examination and

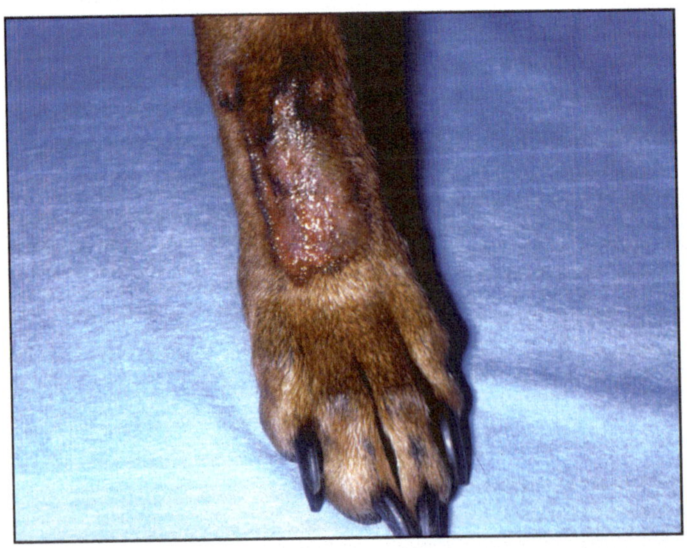

**Figure 5-2.** Acral lick dermatitis lesion on the distal limb of a dog (Courtesy of Dr. D W Angarano).

diagnostic battery are essential to identify the relevant primary and perpetuating factors.

The primary factor most commonly noted in ALD patients is allergic dermatitis: atopic dermatitis, cutaneous adverse food reaction, and flea bite hypersensitivity. Other primary factors of ALD are uncommon and involve both dermatologic and non-dermatologic causes. Dermatologic causes include demodecosis, dermatophytosis (and other deep fungal infections), foreign body, and hypothyroidism (with secondary pruritic bacterial infection). Rarely, neoplasms, including cutaneous lymphoma and mast cell tumors, can mimic ALD. Non-cutaneous primary factors include orthopedic injury, osteoarthritis, orthopedic pin migration, peripheral nerve sheath tumors and peripheral neuropathies. Acral mutilation syndromes of the English Pointer, English Springer Spaniel, and French Spaniels are an extreme example of sensory neuropathy, resulting in self-mutilation starting at a young age that can result in auto-amputation of the digits and distal limbs.

Stereotypic displacement, or attention-seeking behaviors may be a primary or concurrent factor in ALD. Identifying the household circumstances surrounding the behavior at its onset, as well as determining when the licking occurs and whether the licking occurs in the presence or absence of the owner can be helpful. Separation anxiety, lack of mental stimulation, lack of exercise, and interactional conflict between animals should be considered. Changes in the household environment including new human or animal additions, relationship losses, or significant changes in daily household schedule may precipitate ALD.

Perpetuating factors must be addressed, regardless of the primary factor, to halt progression of the ALD and reduce lesion size. Deep infection is the most important and prevalent perpetuating factor in ALD. In a 2008 study of 31 dogs with ALD, the most common bacterial species isolated from lesions were *Staphylococcus* (60%), *Pseudomonas* (8%), and *Enterobacter* (8%). In addition, 50% of cases were multi-drug resistant and 25% were methicillin-resistant. Importantly, cultures from the surfaces of the lesions do not correlate well with those taken by tissue biopsy. Thusly, tissue biopsy for culture is recommended as the best means to culture and subsequently select antibiotic therapy. One may also culture lesions by applying firm pressure, milking exudates from deep within the lesion. The sampling technique is more likely to obtain a representative sample than swabbing the surface of the lesion alone, but is unlikely to be as representative as a sample obtained via multiple tissue biopsies.

Furunculosis (ruptured hair follicles) resulting from self-trauma and bacterial folliculitis fuel the inflammatory fire. The free keratin within the dermis prompts a robust pyogranulomatous inflammatory response, perpetuating further self-trauma and lesion progression. Fibrosis often ensues, further trapping hairs deep within the lesion. These hairs may once again migrate out of the scar, perpetuating the inflammatory response. Apocrine glands also participate in the bonfire, as they dilate and rupture.

Compulsive licking may initiate central, peripheral, and cutaneous neurochemical events that perpetuate the behavior. Compulsive licking may stem from ALD itself without a primary behavioral issue. Licking can prompt release of mood-enhancing endorphins, reinforcing the behavior. Also, patients struggling from anxiety, boredom, or conflict may lick to physiologically self-soothe. Locally, traumatic action of licking perpetuates the sensation of pruritus via release of prostaglandins, leukotrienes and histamine from cutaneous inflammatory cells. Damage to keratinocytes can perpetuate presence and activity of inflammatory cells via release of chemokines and cytokines. It is theorized that chronic pruritic conditions may promote central sensitization of pruritogenic pathways, and may reshape other sensory inputs (heat, cold, pain) to be perceived as itch. Thus, the trauma establishes the spiraling "itch-lick" cycle, perpetuating the lesions, and enhancing their progression.

## Techniques

### Diagnostic Procedures

A thorough history and physical examination are essential in the treatment of ALD to identify the relevant primary and perpetuating factors (Table 5-2).

## Therapy

ALD us a multifactorial disease. Optimal control of the lesions is achieved with multimodal therapy. For patients with extensive lesions, it is very important to educate clients that lifelong therapy is likely required. Recognition and control of both primary and perpetuating factors is essential for lesion control.

The general principles of management of ALD include the following:

1. Obtain a complete history on the animal.
2. Perform a thorough examination of the animal.
3. Conduct diagnostic tests as dictated by history and physical examination as per Table 5-2.

| Table 5-2. Diagnostic Procedures and Rationale | |
|---|---|
| **Diagnostic Procedure** | **Rationale** |
| Thorough history | Determine seasonality: locations, and seasonality of pruritus/otitis that may indicate allergic disease.<br>Determine or eliminate any physical reason for licking.<br>Ascertain presence of any psychogenic factors. (See Psychogenic - Behavior Modification Therapy) |
| Routine clinical pathology (complete blood count, serum chemistries, urinalysis, endocrine function tests) | Establish baseline |
| Dermatologic examination | Observe for signs and locations of other dermatologic lesions that may indicate allergic disease or other primary allergic cause. |
| Deep skin scraping | Assess for *Demodex* (may not be found by scraping in fibrotic lesions). |
| Superficial skin scraping | Assess for *Sarcoptes*, especially if severe pruritus includes the distal limbs, ventrum, and ear margins. (Mites found approximately 30% of cases). |
| Skin/exudates cytology | Assess for presence of bacteria, fungi, and *Demodex* in exudates: and surface *Malassezia* overgrowth. |
| Fungal culture | Assess for dermatophytosis (hair pluck). |
| Tissue bacterial culture and sensitivity | Determine presence of bacterial infection and appropriate systemic antimicrobial therapy. |
| Histopathology | Assess for neoplasia, occult demodicosis, and deep fungal infection. Establish degree of severity, presence of furunculosis, and/or fibrosis. |
| Fine needle aspiration biopsy | Screening for cutaneous neoplasia. Does not replace biopsy. |
| Radiography | Observe for underlying osseous pathology (e.g. arthritis*, osteomyelitis, osteosarcoma, periosteal proliferation**) or radiopaque foreign bodies. Prognostic aid (extensive bony involvement = least likely for satisfactory resolution). |
| Ultrasonography | Check for radiolucent foreign bodies, and cystic structures for aspiration. |
| Electrodiagnostics (nerve conduction velocity, electromyogram) if available | Rule out peripheral neuropathy or nerve root lesion - usually resulting from automobile or other trauma. |
| Elimination diet trial, novel protein/carbohydrate or hydrolysed (8-12 weeks). | Assess for presence of cutaneous adverse food reaction in patients with non-seasonal signs of allergic dermatitis and otitis. |
| Intradermal and *in vitro* allergy tests | Appropriate for patients diagnosed with atopic dermatitis: seasonally pruritic patients, or patients that do not respond to a food trial. Performed in anticipation of allergen specific immunotherapy as allergen avoidance is largely impractical. |
| Adulticidal flea control trial (Topical or long-acting oral***) | Assess for flea bite hypersensitivity in patients with hindlimb pruritus. All cats/dogs in the home should receive adulticidal flea control. |
| Acaridical treatment | Assess for presence of *Sarcoptes scabiei* patients with severe pruritus including the distal limbs, ventrum, and ear margins with a negative superficial skin scrape. |
| T4 +/-TSH, Ft4 by ED | Assess for hypothyroidism |

*Joint disease is not caused by licking. If present it may be the cause of excessive licking.

**Periosteal proliferation is usually caused by licking.

***Spinosad is the only long-acting oral adulticidal flea control product available at the time of writing.

4. Administer appropriate therapy based on identification of a primary cause (e.g. atopic dermatitis).
5. Use other forms of treatment or combinations of treatment as judged appropriate for the animal.
6. Administer long-term systemic antibiotics for deep pyoderma in conjunction with restraint from licking (e.g. Elizabethan collar) to manage perpetuating factors.
7. Periodic tracings of the lesion on transparent acetate with a felt-tipped pen to monitor progress of the treatment process. Digital photography is also helpful for archiving and monitoring.
8. A guarded prognosis should be given because most cases of ALD are chronic with a tendency to recur unless an underlying disease has a good management prognosis. In addition, regardless of the mechanisms involved in causing ALD, a reinforced behavior of chronic licking may be an obstacle that will impede complete resolution of the condition.

Optimal treatment involves a combination of therapies tailored to the individual, almost always involving treatment of secondary infection and controlling the suspected or confirmed primary cause of ALD. Described treatments include: systemic and topical antimicrobials, systemic and topical glucocorticoids, allergy management, osteoarthritis and neuropathic pain management, behavioral modification, deterrents/restraints, $CO_2$ laser debridement, low-level laser therapy (class 111B, IV lasers), acupuncture, cryosurgery, and radiation.

### Systemic Antibiotics

*Staphylococcus pseudintermedius* is the most common agent isolated from ALD. Culture and sensitivity is recommended to guide treatment given the increasing prevalence of antimicrobial resistance, and long duration of treatment required for deep pyoderma (minimum of 8 weeks). Tissue biopsy for culture is recommended as the best means to culture and subsequently select antimicrobial therapy. Surface cultures are not reflective of the organisms present deep within the lesion. Antibiotic therapy for deep infections often requires at least 8 to 12 weeks of treatment. Rechecking the lesion every 2 to 4 weeks is recommended. One should look for re-epithelialization, hair regrowth, and dramatic reduction in dermal thickening. If fibrosis is present, thickening may not completely resolve. The antibiotic therapy should be continued until the lesion resolves or response plateaus. Continue treatment 3 to 4 weeks beyond resolution. If the lesion worsens in the face of antimicrobial therapy, then repeat culture is recommended. Treatment of the underlying cause is recommended to optimize the response, as long-term, intermittent use of antimicrobials may select for growth of antibiotic-resistant bacteria.

### Systemic Glucocorticoids

Glucocorticoids may be prescribed in an attempt to initially control the pathologic changes associated with ALD such as the severe inflammation and foreign body reaction associated with furunculosis, and the fibrosis associated with longstanding trauma and inflammation. Glucocorticoids may also be used to manage atopic dermatitis. Prednisolone/prednisone is often effective starting at 1.0mg/kg to 0.5mg/kg per day for 7 to 14 days, and then tapering to a low, every other day dose.

Intralesional glucorticoid treatment is employed by some practitioners for management of ALD. Triamcinalone acetonide (Vetalog, Fort Dodge Animal Health, Fort Dodge, IA) or methylprednisolone (Depo-Medrol, Pharmacia & Upjohn Co., Kalamazoo, MI) are used. However, such steroid injections should be used with caution in the presence of deep bacterial infection. Systemic side effects may also occur with intralesional administration. This treatment is not recommended for long-term management. Glucocorticoids are best utilized in the initial phases of therapy, particularly in patients with allergic disease, but they are not desirable as a long-term management strategy.

### Allergy management

Flea bite hypersensitivity, cutaneous adverse food reaction, and atopic dermatitis are primary factors in ALD. For patients with hindlimb lesions and pruritus, long-acting adulticidal flea control is recommended, even if fleas or flea feces are not seen. All household dogs or cats should be treated as well. Topical products including impidoclorprid, fipronil/methoprene, selamectin, and dinotefuran are reasonable choices as well as oral spinosad (Comfortis, Trifexis, by Elanco).

Cutaneous adverse food reaction should be suspected for any patient demonstrating non-seasonal cutaneous pruritus and/or otitis externa. An elimination diet involving novel protein/carbohydrate, hydrolysed proteins, or oligopeptides (Anallergenic, Royal Canin) should be performed for a minimum of 8 weeks to assess for cutaneous adverse food reaction. This diet is essential in differentiating cutaneous adverse food reaction from non-seasonal atopic dermatitis. Serological and intradermal tests are not recommended for diagnosis of cutaneous adverse food reaction. Client education is key, as strict adherence to the diet and elimination of flavored medications is required to confidently assess response. If the pruritus is significantly reduced, the patient may be rechallenged with the previous diet to prove that dietary hypersensitivity is present. For responders, the restricted diet should be continued. Non-responders are diagnosed with atopic dermatitis. Atopic dermatitis is diagnosed after flea bite hypersensitivity and cutaneous adverse food reaction have been ruled out, or in patients with historically strict seasonal pruritus and/or otitis. Treatments for atopic dermatitis are numerous and generally involve anti-inflammatory therapy (cyclosporine, glucocorticoids, and antihistamines) and immunotherapy (hyposensitization) as well as topical treatments. For clients wishing to pursue immunotherapy, intradermal and/or serum allergy tests can be performed for allergen selection. It should be noted that immunotherapy may take up to a year to be effective: concurrent treatments are often required in the first year for patient comfort.

## Acaricidal Therapy

Acaricidal therapy is recommended to rule out *Sarcoptes scabiei* for patients with severe pruritus involving the ventrum, distal limbs and/or ear margins. Multiple superficial skin scrapes are recommended for diagnosis. It should be recognized, however, that this method is an insensitive indicator of infestation as patients may suffer from extreme pruritus and very few mites. It is estimated that 30% of superficial skin scrapes are positive for dogs with sarcoptic mange. Thus, acaricidal therapy is recommended for any patient with these signs and negative deep skin scrapes. Treatments include selamectin (Revolution, Pfizer) topically every 2 weeks, or moxidectin and imidocloprid (Advantage multi, Bayer) every 14 days: a total of 3 to 4 applications are typically needed for resolution with these products. Alternatively, ivermectin at 0.03 to 0.04mg/kg per os once weekly for 4 to 6 treatments is a reasonable option for non-herding breeds. Lime sulfur solution at 2 to 3% is very safe and is used once weekly as a dip, a total of 4 to 6 treatments are typically required.

## Topical Therapy

Topical steroids, topical antimicrobials, topical analgesics, and topical deterrents may be used in the management of ALD. Topical medications are often an adjunct to therapy, but may be helpful sole therapy for minor lesions. Commercial or compounded preparations may be used.

Topical solutions may be applied initially once to twice daily. Mechanical restraint or direct supervision is recommended after treatment to prevent the patient from licking off the medication.

• Thiabendazole, dexamethasone, neomycin sulfate solution (Tresaderm, Merial, Iselin, NJ)

• Gentamicin sulfate, betamethasone valerate, clortrimazole ointment (Otomax, Schering-Plough Animal Health Corp., Union, NJ)

• Flucinolone acetonide and dimethyl sulfoxide (DMSO) (Synotic Otic Solution, Fort Dodge Animal Health, Fort Dodge, IA)

• Mupirocin ointment (Bactoderm, Pfizer Animal Health, Exton, PA) may be used as an adjunct in *Staphylococcus* infections.

Compounded solutions have been described:

• Mix equal parts of 90% DMSO solution and a solution of 1% hydrocortisone acetate and 2% Burrow's solution in propylene glycol (Hydro-B-1020, Hydro-Plus).

• Mix an 8ml vial of Synotic Otic Solution with 3ml of flunixin meglumine (Banamine injectable solution, Schering-Plaugh Animal Health Corporation, Union, NJ)

• Mix an 8ml vial of Synotic Otis Solution with 2ml of 22.7 mg/ml injectable enrofloxacin (Baytril, Bayer Animal Health)

Various medications containing the analgesic capsaicin, a substance P inhibitor, have been described for treatment as a deterrent to licking. These treatments are best employed as an adjunct therapy.

• Capsaicin (Zostrix, GenDerm, Corp./Medicis Pharmaceutical Corp., Scottsdale, AZ), an antiarthralgic-myalgic may be applied around the lesion to decrease reinforcing sensations. For greatest efficacy, it must be applied 3 to 4 times daily. It is available as a nonprescription item as either a 0.025% or 0.075% ointment.

• Capsaicin, 0.25% (Dolorac, GenDerm, Corp./Medicis Pharmaceutical Corp., Scottsdale, AZ) in combination with mupirocin ointment (Bactoderm, Pfizer Animal Health, Exton, PA) in a 1:1 ratio may be applied 3 times daily for patients with *Staphylococcus* infections.

• Capsaicin, methylsalicylate, camphor (HEET, MedTech Products, Jackson, WY) in one part combined with bitter apple extract (Grannick's Bitter Apple, Grannick's Bitter Apple Co., Norwalk, CT) in 2 parts can be applied 2 to 3 times daily to early lesions with tapered use as needed. Placing some solution on the nose first allows the dog to lick and smell it simultaneously as the first part of a deterrent procedure. The solution is then placed on the lesion or bandage and the dog will associate the lingering scent with the bitter taste.

### Laser Therapy

$CO_2$ laser ablation therapy may be effective in some cases. This modality vaporizes bacteria, entrapped hairs, and fibrotic tissue. Second intention healing is required post-operatively, therefore mechanical restraint after the procedure is required to allow for wound healing. This therapy is best employed after reduction in lesion size is achieved via management of primary factors and treatment of infection.

"Cold" laser therapy involving Class IIIB and class IV lasers may be of benefit with wound healing as well, however studies investigating function and efficacy of this modality are lacking.

### Neuropathic Pain Management and Acupuncture

For complicated cases of osteoarthritis, a Diplomate of the American College of Veterinary Surgeons could be consulted. Likewise, a Diplomate of the American College of Veterinary Internal Medicine (neurology) could be consulted regarding management of nerve root pain.

Acupuncture has been described as an adjunct to medical management, and physical therapy may also be employed in the treatment of ALD associated with osteoarthritis and neuropathic pain. The authors suggest that a veterinarian trained and certified in acupuncture and/or physical therapy be consulted to perform these respective techniques. Additionally, consultation with a veterinarian who is a Diplomate of the American College of Veterinary Sports Medicine and Rehabilitation is beneficial for complicated cases to optimize therapy and physical performance.

### Cryosurgery

This form of therapy has been advocated as a last resort for very large lesions. Freezing reportedly destroys nerve endings in the area of the lesion and thus blocks the itch-lick cycle. The frozen mass of tissue sloughs over a period of several weeks with new reparative tissue forming in the resulting wound. As with laser therapy, second intention healing is required post-operatively, therefore mechanical restraint after the procedure is required to allow for wound healing. In comparison to $CO_2$ laser, tissue damage is less controlled. It may be necessary to repeat the procedure 2 or 3 times. The procedure should be performed by personnel familiar with cryosurgical techniques.

### Surgical Therapy

Surgical therapy may be considered from two standpoints. First, there may be a surgically approachable underlying cause for the ALD lesion. For instance, if a foreign body is causing subdermal irritation resulting in constant licking, surgical removal of the foreign body should be performed. An arthropathy with a painful unstable joint resulting in continual licking of the overlying skin may benefit from surgical arthrodesis to stabilize the joint.

The second surgical approach involves surgical removal of the ALD lesion. Three forms of reconstruction may be considered following lesion removal: 1) primary suturing, 2) skin grafting, or 3) a skin flap. The amount of skin remaining in the area after removing the lesion will govern the technique used. The reader is referred to other sections of this text for information on closure techniques. Removal of the ALD lesion should be performed judiciously, for if the primary cause of the ALD is not addressed, the patient may create another lesion, or traumatize the site of surgery post-healing.

### Radiation Therapy

Radiation therapy is rarely used and has been reported to have variable efficacy in treating ALD. Effectiveness correlates with the duration and size of the lesion. The best response is seen in early lesions with minimal fibrosis and inflammation: whereas, larger chronic lesions with underlying bone involvement do not respond as well.

### Psychogenic-Behavior Modification Therapy

#### Environmental modifications

When ALD appears to be of psychogenic origin, counseling with the client is the first step in management to determine whether or not there was a psychogenic effect first. Environmental factors can play a major role in the psychogenic aspect of ALD.

Environmental modifications are indicated when the history reveals environmental factors as a cause of anxiety or tension in the dog resulting in excessive licking. A psychogenic component to the condition can be suspected if a new ALD lesion develops after the original lesion has been covered with a bandage. Some common environmental causes of ALD include:

1. The dog is left alone all day.
2. The dog is confined in a crate, cage, kennel or run for long periods without sufficient interaction or enrichment.
3. There is a new baby in the home.

4. There is a new pet in the home.
5. A nearby female dog in estrus is not accessible to the male dog.
6. A new dog has come into the neighborhood.
7. A long-time companion of the dog has died or moved away.

The first step in treatment is recognizing the cause and eliminating management practices, routines, and interaction patterns that have the potential to evoke self-mutilation behavior. Increased human companionship in the form of routine exercise and going to the dog for regular periods of individual attention can help. When possible, taking the dog to the owner's place of employment may be helpful. Gregarious, high-energy patients may respond well to "doggy day care" while the client is away for the day. Consider interactive toys with a food reward component that can occupy their mouths and provide mental stimulation. Encourage the clients to periodically rotate the toys. Avoidance of cages, kennels, and runs can be helpful when ALD appears to be associated with confinement. Introduction of another pet into the household may be helpful if the condition is related to loss of a companion animal, prolonged separation from the owner, or boredom due to the owner having insufficient time to spend with the animal. The owner should be aware that the success of this approach is not guaranteed. It depends on the extent to which a friendship develops between the two dogs. However this should be approached with caution as interactional conflict may worsen the condition.

Once an ALD lesion has developed, alterations of environmental factors alone may not be effective, and other forms of therapy may be needed in addition.

Consultation with a board certified behaviourist (some provide telephone consultations with veterinarians and clients) may be of tremendous help if there is a strong behavioral component. Adjunct medical therapy may also be helpful particularly in conjunction with environmental and behavioral modification.

## Pharmacologic behavior alteration

This form of therapy may be needed for only a short while until behavior modifications or factors causing stress or boredom are eliminated, or may need to be continued long-term. Consultation with a board certified behaviorist is recommended for optimal results. The following drugs have been described:

• *Antidepressants* are suitable for long-term treatment if required for relief. These include doxepin (Sinequan®, Pfizer Animal Health, Exton, PA) at 0.5 to 2.0 mg/kg twice daily. This medication is not only an anti-depressant but is also an antihistamine. In difficult cases, the fluoxetine or clomipramine may be the most effective treatment. Fluoxetine (Prozac, Dista Products Co. [Eli Lilly and Co.], Indianapolis, IN) is a selective serotonin reuptake inhibitor and is dosed orally at 1 to 2 mg/kg once daily. Fluoxetine was proven effective in reducing lesion size and licking in a placebo-controlled trial.

• Clomipramine (Clomicalm Novartis Animal Health U.S., Greensboro, NC) is a tricyclic antidepressant dosed orally at 1 mg/kg daily. The dose can be increased by 1mg/kg daily every two weeks to a maximum dose of at 3 mg/kg daily. Some dogs may experience vomiting or diarrhea initially with clomipramine. In one study using clomipramine for treatment of ALD, the drug was effective, but when stress factors were not removed from the environment there was a relapse of the ALD lesion. Another antidepressant used to treat ALD is imipramine (Tofranil, Geneva Pharmaceuticals, Broomfield, CO) at 2 to 4 mg/kg daily orally.

• Amitriptyline is a tricyclic antidepressant, antipruritic, and neuropathic pain modifier. It is dosed orally at 2.2mg/kg twice daily.

• A lag time of at least 4 to 5 weeks should be expected before any change in excessive grooming behavior is noted with antidepressant drugs.

• *Anxiolytic* drugs such as phenobarbital at 2.2 to 6.6 mg/kg twice daily orally, or diazepam (Valium, Roche Laboratories, Nutley, NJ) at 0.2 mg/kg twice daily orally can be used. They are helpful, but less effective than the antidepressants.

• *Endorphin blockers and endorphin substitutes* have been used to treat ALD. Naltrexone (Trexane, Bristol-Myers-Squibb, New York, NY) at 2.2 mg/kg daily orally has been used for treatment. If the lesion does not heal or licking does not decrease within 10 days, the treatment should be increased to every 12 hours. If licking decreases and the lesion begins to heal, the effective dose should be maintained for one month. Long-term control may be accomplished using reduced doses or longer intervals between doses. The administration of an exogenous source of opiate may reduce the dog's desire to stimulate the release of its own endogenous endorphins. Hydrocodone (Hycodan, du Pont Pharmaceutical Co., Jericho, NY) at 5 mg/20 kg every 12 hours may be used for treatment on a limited basis for up to 16 weeks. A dose of 0.25 mg/kg per os every 12 hours may give a more consistent effect. Ten mg/20 kg three times daily has also been described.

## Nonpharmacologic Behavior Alteration (Physical Restraints)

Physical restraining devices should be considered to keep a dog from self-molestation, especially if the dog is unsupervised. Use of such devices may be employed at the beginning of treatment, but should be gradually reduced. Elizabethan collars or modifications thereof (Figure 5-3A-E) are effective. This is affixed to the dog's collar for added security. The patients should be supervised when Elizabethan collars are used initially as some dogs will use the edge of the Elizabethan collar to more aggressively self-traumatize lesions. Soft, inflatable (Boobooloon), and foam (Soft Elizabethan Collar, Jorgenson Laboratories, Loveland, CO) Elizabethan collars may be better tolerated by the patient and client and cannot be used to self-traumatize.

A rigid, plastic, wrap-around collar with fasteners (Bite Not Collar, Bite Not Products, San Francisco, CA)

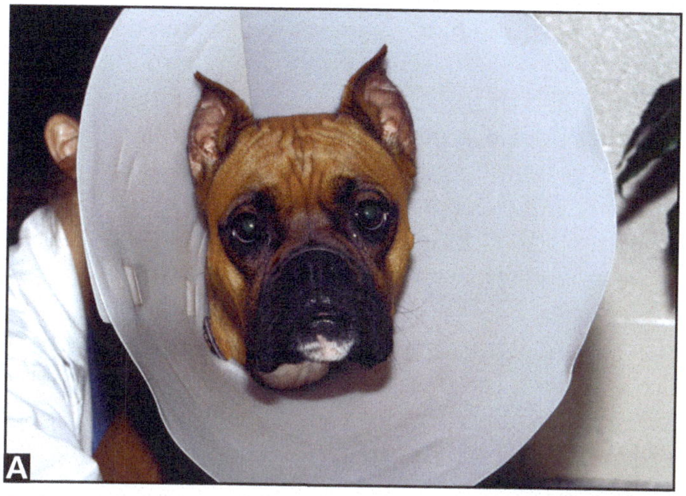

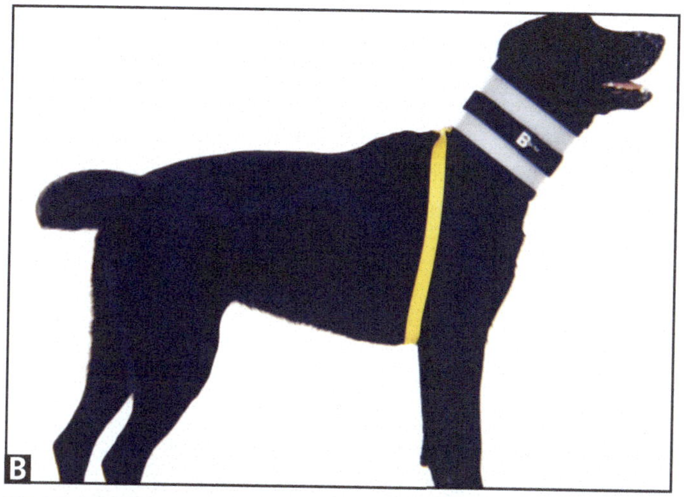

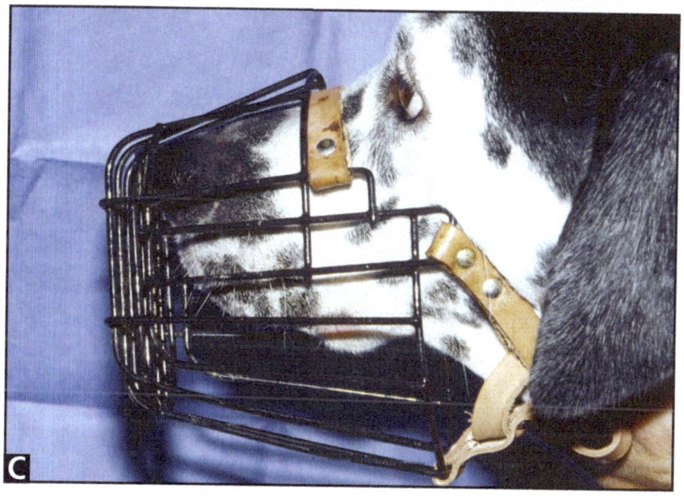

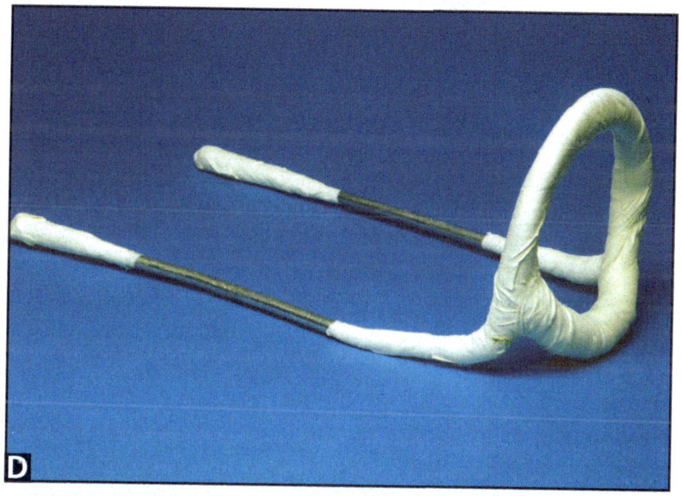

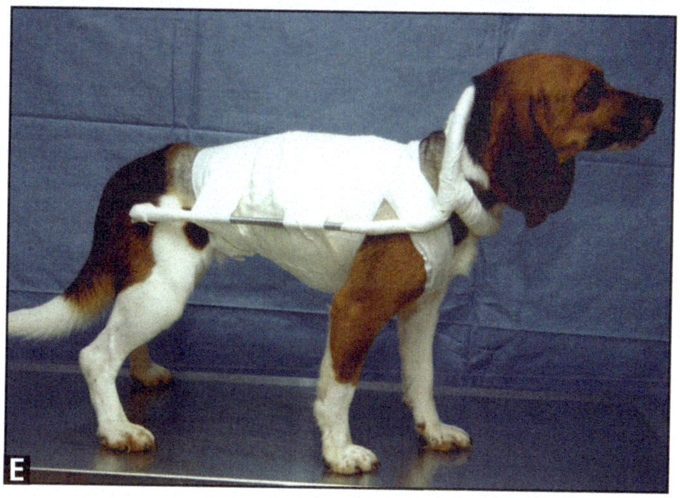

**Figure 5-3.** Physical restraint devices to prevent self – molestation. **A.** Elizabethan collar. **B.** Rigid plastic wrap – around collar. **C.** Wire basket – type muzzle. **D.** Aluminum splint rod side braces. **E.** Aluminum splint rod side braces placed on a dog over a body bandage. (B Courtesy Bite Not Collar Co.) E from Swaim SF, Henderson RA: Small Animal Wound Management, 2nd ed.: Baltimore: Williams & Wilkins, 1997, 121.

can be placed around a dog's neck. Various sizes are available which extend from just behind the ears to the shoulders. To prevent the collar from coming off over the dog's head, a fabric strap attached to the collar goes around the thorax just caudal to the forelimbs. These collars are most effective in preventing an animal from molesting areas caudal to the shoulders. For protection of the distal limbs, they may not be as effective as an Elizabethan collar.

Socks or wraps can be applied and are typically effective for dogs with mild lesions that require a mild deterrent. Socks should be regularly laundered, breathable, and can be secured proximately with Vetwrap (3M Animal Care) and the client instructed about their proper placement to avoid bandage sores and ischemic injury. These coverings should be removed once daily and the limb should be allowed to breathe for approximately an hour a day. During this time, the patient will need to be supervised to prevent further trauma.

Wire basket-type muzzles of various sizes are commercially available. These are effective in preventing molestation of the distal limbs as well as other parts of the body. These should be used in lieu of the canvas and leather muzzles which are designed to prevent animals from biting. The canvas and leather muzzles do not allow the dog to breathe through its mouth, and they become unsanitary when wet with saliva. If a dog tries to pull a wire basket type muzzle off over its nose with its forepaws, the muzzle can be modified by placing a strip of tape or leather from the portion of the muzzle that goes over the nasal area to the strap that goes behind the ears.

Aluminum splint rod side braces can be made to deter a dog from molesting the hind limbs. A ring large enough to fit at the base of the dog's neck is bent in the center of the rod. The lengths of rod that remain are bent at right angles to the ring to form the side braces (Figure 5-4A). If needed, the ring is bent slightly across its center, either caudally or cranially, to better fit the dog's conformation at the base of the neck. The ring and ends of the side braces are padded with cotton held in place by tape. A body bandage that extends from the axillary region to the flank area is usually applied with two pieces of tape crisscrossed over the pectoral area of the dog and attached to the body bandage to keep it from slipping caudally. The dog's head is placed through the ring of the brace, and the two side braces extend along the dogs sides to the area of the hind quarters. Two segments of 2-inch wide porous adhesive tape are placed around the body and over the side braces to keep them along the dog's sides (Figure 5-4B). The body bandage keeps the two pieces of tape from sticking to the dog's hair and thus provides comfort. Side braces may not be as effective as an Elizabethan collar or wire basket muzzle in preventing molestation of the distal limbs.

### Electronic stimulation (Electroshock)

On 5 dogs the use of remote punishment using precisely controlled momentary shock from an electronic training collar revealed promising results. However, a larger scale evaluation of this approach is needed. This technique is best used under the supervision of a board-certified animal behaviorist, as improper use can lead to further behavioral and psychological problems. A bandage can be applied that delivers a mild electrostatic shock when applied (StopLik, Rockway Inc.).

## Aftercare

### Systemic Antibiotics and/or Glucocorticoids

Because of the chronicity of some ALD lesions, antibiotic therapy may need to be prolonged. After

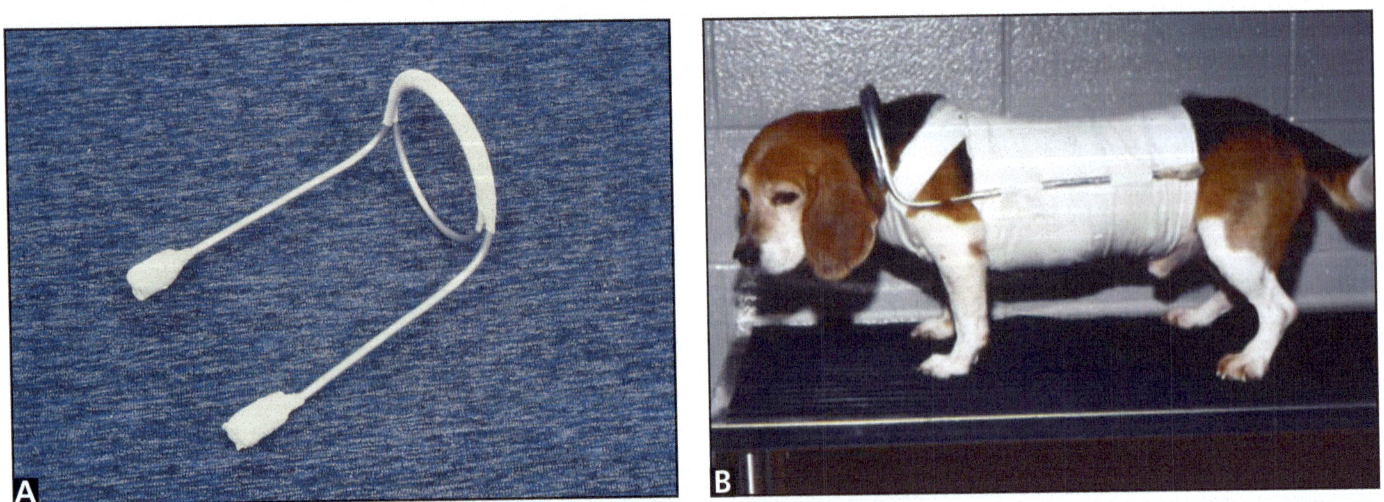

**Figure 5-4. A.** Aluminum splint rod side braces. The circular ring fits at the base of the dog's neck, and the straight rods go along the dog's sides. **B.** Dog with a body bandage and aluminum splint rod side braces in place.

a course of antibiotic therapy it is important to observe the patient for early signs of recurrence of the infection and institute further and possibly different antibiotic therapy.

### Topical Therapy, Laser Therapy, Radiation Therapy and Cryosurgery

Prevention of the animal from licking the ALD wound is an important part of these therapies. A topical medication must remain in contact with the lesion to be effective. Thus, a bandage and/or one of the physical restraint mechanisms are/is indicated when using this form of therapy. When tissues have been disturbed as part of the therapy, i.e. $CO_2$ laser ablation, radiation therapy or cryosurgery, bandaging is indicated to absorb any fluid and tissue debris as well as to protect the wound.

### Allergy Treatment

For flea allergic patients, flea control should be maintained for the patient and housemate dogs and cats. If ALD is related to cutaneous adverse food reaction, the strict diet must be maintained. Patients with atopic dermatitis related to ALD require long-term maintenance therapy which may include anti-inflammatory medications, immunotherapy, and adjunctive topical treatments.

### Surgical Therapy

Aftercare following the surgical approach to ALD is of 2 types. First, if surgery was performed to correct some underlying condition that was causing ALD (e.g. arthrodesis), the aftercare for that surgery is in order. Second, when surgery involves removal of the ALD lesion with repair of the resulting defect, aftercare is specific to the surgical procedure that was used for the repair. It is important to protect the surgical site beyond the time that the wound appears healed (at least a month) to prevent self-molestation and allow for adequate maturation of the healing process.

### Psychogenic-Behavior Modification Therapy

When environmental modifications are part of the therapy, gradual re-exposure to the environmental stimuli that evoked the anxiety-induced ALD should be performed. Acceptable performance by the dog should be rewarded. For example, when time alone is the anxiety-inducing factor, the dog should be left alone for increasingly longer periods. A reward is given for acceptable behavior. Gradual reduction of the dose of pharmacologic agents to a minimum effective dose and frequency can be considered. Gradually reducing the use of physical restraint devices should be considered when they have been used for ALD therapy.

With electroshock therapy, observation of the dog and the owner's compliance in applying the therapy is an important element in treatment/aftercare.

## Advantages and Disadvantages

### Systemic Antibiotics and/or Glucocorticoids

Antibiotics can make an effective contribution in controlling ALD initially. Although often needed in the initial stages of treatment protracted antibiotic therapy may select for antibacterial resistant organisms. Antibiotic therapy alone is not recommended for treatment of ALD.

### Topical Therapy, Laser Therapy, Radiation Therapy and Cryosurgery

Topical chemical deterrents of licking may be effective initially; however, the dog may develop a tolerance to the taste of the chemical and continue to lick the area. When bandaging is a part of the aftercare in these forms of therapy, the cost of bandage materials may be considered a disadvantage to the therapy. For radiation therapy, it is impractical for the majority of cases due to the cost factors and lack of treatment centers. The time involved with sloughing of pathologic tissue and formation of new tissue may be considered a disadvantage of cryosurgery; however, the reported destruction of nerve endings to block the itch-lick cycle may be considered an advantage. The decreased postoperative pain and sterilization of the lesion can be considered advantages of laser therapy.

### Allergy Treatment

Treatment of allergic disease is lifelong and therefore may require significant expense for ongoing management. Client compliance is absolutely necessary for optimal control.

### Surgical Therapy

When an underlying condition has been successfully corrected it may have the advantage of healing spontaneously when the animal stops licking the area because of the comfort provided by surgical correction.

When surgery is performed to remove an ALD lesion, good uneventful healing of the reconstructed area is an advantage of this form of therapy. However, owners should be informed that at some time after removal of bandages and restraint devices the dog may severely damage or destroy the reconstructed area. Gradual removal of restraint devices and discontinuance of bandaging after it has been present a sufficient amount of time, at least a month, may be helpful in allowing maturation of the healed tissues.

## Psychogenic-Behavior Modification Therapy

Time and effort by the pet owner are required when undertaking environmental modifications followed by re-exposure to environmental stimuli. The same is true when teaching the dog substitute behavior. When another pet is added to the environment to help prevent boredom-related licking, initial results may be beneficial. However, this may not be effective after the novelty wears off. Incompatibility between the 2 dogs and competition for attention from the owner may be problems. Occasionally, both dogs will lick at the affected dog's ALD lesion.

When pharmacologic agents are used for a short period while behavior modifications or stress and boredom factors are eliminated, it could be considered an advantage in their use. However, the expense of some medications is a disadvantage, especially if it is necessary to use them for a prolonged period. Fluoxetine and clomipramine may cause lethargy, anorexia, hyperactivity, personality changes and diarrhea. Progestagens may be effective; however, animal owners should be adequately warned when they are used. These drugs are not approved for behavioral therapy in dogs. In addition, they are expensive and should not be used on intact females. It is also possible that their use may correct one behavioral abnormality and induce another one.

Physical restraint devices may be beneficial in treating ALD. However, they require periodic adjustment and removal. Attention must be paid to their fitting and padding to avoid skin irritation. There is the possibility that restraint devices may further frustrate a psychotic dog. Elizabethan collars placed around a dog's neck are effective in preventing wound molestation; however, they are cumbersome and obstruct the dog's peripheral vision. The wrap-around collar does not have these disadvantages; however, it may not be as effective in preventing access to the distal limbs. Physical restraint devices are not appropriate for long term use.

# Suggested Readings


1. Amalsadvala I, Swaim SF: Management of hard – to – heal wounds. Vet Clin No Am Small Animal Pract 36: 693, 2006.
2. Brignac MM: Hydrocodone treatment of acral lick dermatitis. Proceedings - 2nd World Congress on Veterinary Dermatology, Montreal, Canada, 2:50, 1992.
3. Demetriou JL, Shales CJ, Hamilton MH, Sissener IR: Reconstruction of a nonhealing lick granuloma in a dog using phalangeal filler. J Am Anim Hosp Assoc 43: 288, 2007.
4. Denerolle P, White SD, Taylor TS, Vandenabeele SIJ: Organic diseases mimicking acral lick dermatitis in six dogs. J Am Anim Hosp Assoc 43: 215, 2007.
5. Eckstein RA, Hart BL: Treatment of canine acral lick dermatitis by behavior modification using electronic stimulation. J Am Anim Hosp Assoc 32:225, 1996.
6. Gnirs K and Prelaud P: Cutaneous manifestatitons of neurologic diseases: a review of neuropathophysiology and diseases causing pruritus. Vet Dermatol 2005: 16: 137 – 146.
7. Goldberger E, Rapoport JL: Canine acral lick dermatitis: Response to the antiobsessional drug clomiprimine. J Am Anim Hosp Assoc 27:179, 1991.
8. Hedlund CS: Surgery of the integumentary system. *In* Fossum TW, ed.: Small Animal Surgery, 2nd ed.: St. Louis: Mosby, 2002, 134.
9. Hedlund CS: Surgery of the integumentary system. In Fossum TW, ed.: Small Animal Surgery, 3rd ed.: St. Louis: Mosby, 2007, 159.
10. Hewson CJ, Luescher A, Parent JM, et al: Efficiency of clomiprimine in the treatment of canine compulsive disorder. J Am Vet Med Assoc 213:1760, 1998.
11. MacDonald JM, Bradley DM: Acral lick dermatitis. *In* Kirk RW, ed.: Kirk's Current Veterinary Therapy XIII: Small Animal Practice, 13th ed.: Philadelphia: WB Saunders, 2000, 551.
12. MacPhail CM: Surgery of the integumentary system. In Fossum TW, ed.: Small Animal Surgery, 4th ed.: St. Louis: Mosby, 2013, 190.
13. Overall KL: Recognition, diagnosis, and management of obsessive-compulsive disorders: Part I. Canine Pract 17:40, 1992.
14. Overall KL: Recognition, diagnosis, and management of obsessive-compulsive disorders: Part II - a rational approach. Canine Pract 17:25, 1992.
15. Overall KL: Recognition, diagnosis, and management of obsessive-compulsive disorders: Part III - a rational approach. Canine Pract 17:39, 1992.
16. Owen LN: Canine lick granuloma treated with radiation therapy. J Small Anim Pract 30:454, 1989.
17. Paradis M, et.al: Acral mutilation and analgesia in 13 French Spaniels. Vet Dermatol 2005: 16: 87-93.
18. Patel A: Acral lick dermatitis. Compan Anim 15: 43, 2010.
19. Patterson S: Canine acral lick granuloma. Sci Proc Brit Vet Derm Study Group, 17, Spring 2007.
20. Patterson S, Midgley D, Barclay I: Canine acral lick dermatitis. In Pract 29: 328, 2007.
21. Pereira JT, Larsson CE, Ramos D: Environmental, individual and triggering aspects of dogs presenting with psychogenic acral lick dermatitis. J Vet Behav, Clin Appl Rsch 5: 165, 2010.
22. River SB, Walter PA, McKeever PJ: Treatment of canine acral lick dermatitis with radiation therapy: 17 cases (1979-1991). J Am Anim Hosp Assoc 29:541, 1993.
23. Scott DW, Walton DK: Clinical evaluation of a topical treatment for canine acral lick dermatitis. J Am Anim Hosp Assoc 20:565, 1984.
24. Scott DW: Psychogenic skin disease: In Scott DW, Miller WH, Griffin CE, eds.: Muller and Kirk's Small Animal Dermatology. 6th ed.: Philadelphia: WB Saunders, 2001, 1055.
25. Shoulberg N: The efficacy of fluoxetine (Prozac) in the treatment of acral lick and allergic-inhalant dermatitis in canines. Proc. Annual Membership Meeting, Am Acad Vet Dermatol and Am Coll Vet Dermatol 6:31, 1990.
26. Shumaker AK, Angus JC, Coyner KS, et al: Microbiological and histopathological features of canine acral lick dermatitis. Vet Derm 19: 288, 2008.
27. Swaim SF, Henderson RA: Small Animal Wound Management, 2nd ed.: Baltimore: Williams and Wilkins, 1997, 87.
28. Swaim SF, Renberg WC, Shike KM: Small Animal Bandaging, Casting and Splinting Techniques. Ames, IA: Wiley – Blackwell, 2010, 111.
29. J. Van den Broek A, Horvath-Ungerboeck C: Pedal dermatitis in dogs and cats: Part 1 Compan Anim, 16: 39, 2011.
30. Van Nes JJ: Electrophysiological evidence of sensory nerve dysfunction in 10 dogs with acral lick dermatitis. J Am Anim Hosp Assoc 22:157, 1986.
31. Walton DK: Psychodermatoses. *In*: Kirk RW, ed.: Current Veterinary Therapy IX. Philadelphia: WB Saunders, 1986, 557.
32. White RAS: Management of specific skin wounds. Vet Clin No Amer Small Animal Pract 36: 895, 2006.
33. White SD: Naltrexone for treatment of acral lick dermatitis in dog. J AM Vet Med Assoc 196: 1073, 1990.

# Chapter 6

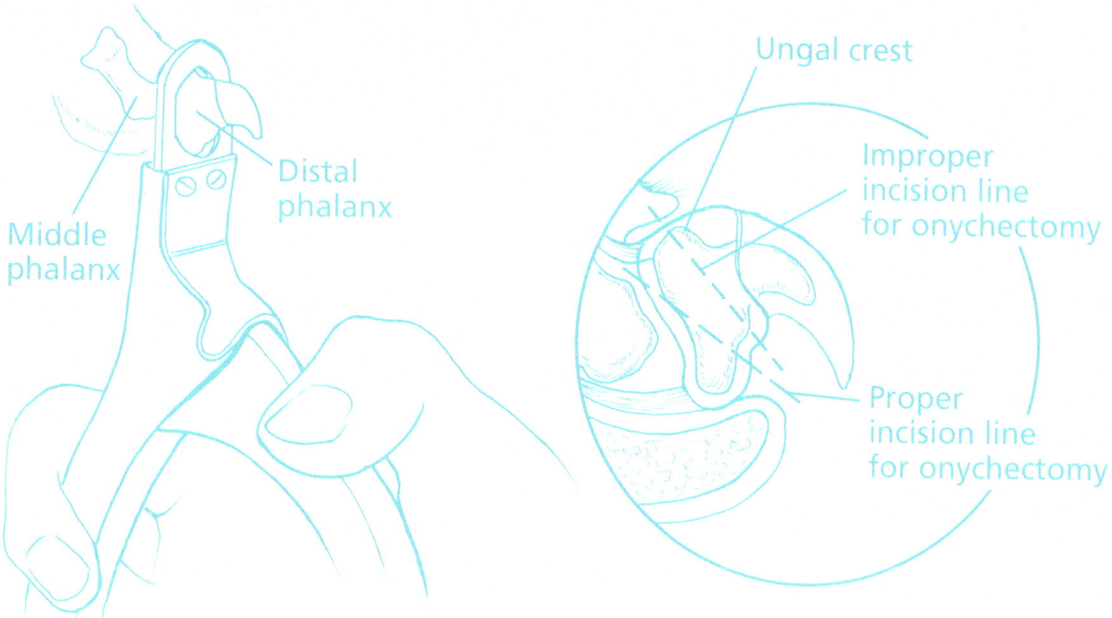


# Onychectomy, Deep Digital Flexor Tenectomy, and Digit Amputation

Steven F. Swaim, D.V.M., M.S.

# Onychectomy

## Definition and Indications

Onychectomy (declawing) is removal of the distal phalanx and nail of the digits. The procedure is usually performed on cats but is occasionally done on dogs. It is generally performed between 3 and 12 months of age to prevent cats from scratching people, other animals and household materials. It is a controversial procedure. The procedure is usually performed on the forelimbs only; however, hind limb claws can be removed also. Onychectomy or more extensive digit amputation is indicated for removal of neoplasms that involve the nail bed such as melanomas, squamous cell carcinomas, soft tissue sarcomas, osteosarcomas, and mast cell tumors. The procedure is also performed for traumatic injuries and bacterial and fungal infections of the nail beds.

## Techniques

The procedure is performed under general anesthesia, using multimodal analgesia (Table 6-1). However, preemptive analgesia can be provided by regional blocks of the radial, median and ulnar nerves at the time of anesthesia and preparation of the paw for onychectomy (See Initial Wound Management of Contaminated and Infected Wounds, Anesthesia and Analgesia). On cats, the hair on the paw is usually not clipped unless the cat has long hair. However, the paw, digits and nails are scrubbed aseptically. On dogs the hair is clipped and the paws are prepared for aseptic surgery. A tourniquet is applied to the limb below the radial-humeral joint to minimize blood loss and improve visualization of the surgical area. Rubber bands should not be used as tourniquets. On cats an alternative for hemostasis can be accomplished by having an assistant compress the brachial artery against the humeral shaft with the thumb or index finger, compressing the vessel just cranial to the triceps muscle on the medial aspect of the brachium.

### Dissection Onychectomy (Cats and Dogs)

The nail is extended by grasping its tip with Allis tissue forceps or by pushing up on the digital pad. A number 15 scalpel blade is used to sharply incise the hairless, cuticle – like skin circumferentially and dissect between the middle and distal phalanx. The common digital extensor tendon and dorsal ligaments are incised. The contour of the proximal end of the distal phalanx is followed while cutting the deep digital flexor tendon and dorsal ligaments and dissecting the phalanx away from the digital pad and other soft tissues in the area (i.e. joint capsule, collateral ligaments and other tendons). Care is taken not to cut the digital pad in the process. On dogs, the articular cartilage on the distal end of the middle phalanx is removed with small rongeurs. The same procedure is repeated on all claws that are to be removed (Figure 6-1). Tourniquets are released. Uniform pressure on the paws for a few minutes may be necessary to attain hemostasis. On dogs electrocoagulation or vessel ligation may be needed to get hemostasis.

On cats the skin edges are apposed as a bandage is applied. Alternatively, a simple interrupted or cruciate suture of 3-0 monofilament synthetic absorbable suture material can be used to appose skin edges using care not to place sutures through the digital pads. If a cyanoacrylate tissue adhesive is used to appose the skin edges, it should be placed sparingly over the apposed skin edges and not between the edges. On dogs, one or 2 sutures, depending on the size of the dog, are used to appose wound edges.

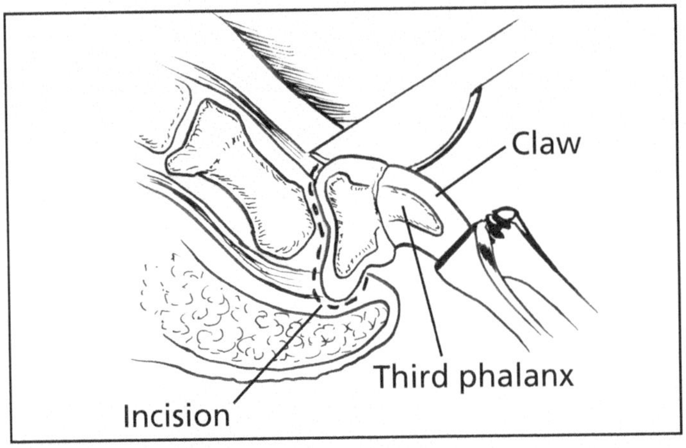


**Figure 6-1.** Dissection onychectomy. Disarticulation of the distal phalanx with a scalpel blade, cutting tendons, ligaments, joint capsule by following the contour of the proximal end of the distal phalnx. Allis tissue forceps extend the nail.

### Nail Clipper Onychectomy (Cats)

The paws are prepared for aseptic surgery as previously described and the nails are clipped to facilitate positioning of the nail clipper. The nail is extended by grasping its tip with Allis tissue forceps or by pushing up on the pad that is being worked on. The front edge of the ring on the sterile nail clipper is positioned in the groove between the distal end of the middle phalanx and the ungual crest of the distal phalanx. The blade of the clipper is positioned just cranial to the digital pad, and it is pushed through the soft tissues over the flexor process (Figure 6-2). If the blade is placed too far cranial on the base of the nail, part of the ungual crest will be left and nail regrowth will occur (See Figure 6-2 inset). With the ring of the nail clipper in position caudal to the ungual crest, the blade is released slightly so that traction applied to the claw causes the flexor process to slip out and above the blade. At this time, the digital flexor tendon is incised and joint disarticulation is completed.

## Table 6-1. Anesthetic Considerations for Onychectomy in Cats**

| | |
|---|---|
| **Preoperative Considerations** | |
| Associated conditions | • Minimal; usually healthy |
| Blood work | • HCT<br>• TP<br>• In patients older than 5-7 yr, consider electrolytes, liver enzymes, BUN, and Cr |
| Physical exam | • Normal |
| Premedications | • Hydromorphone* (0.05-0.1 mg/kg IV, IML **or**<br>• Morphine (0.1-0.2 mg/kg IV or 0.2-0.4 mg/kg IM). **or**<br>• Buprenorphine† (0.005-0.02 mg/kg IV, IM), **or**<br>• Fentanyl patch placed 6-12 hr prior to surgery |
| **Intraoperative Considerations** | |
| Induction | • If premedicated, give:<br>  • Ketamine (5.5 mg/kg IV) with diazepam (0.28 mg/kgIV) **or**<br>  • Propofol (4-8 mg/kg IV), **or**<br>  • Thiopental (8-10 mg/kg IV)<br>• If no premeds given, then:<br>  • Dexmedetomidine‡ (33 µg/kg IM), **plus**<br>  • Butorphanol (0.66 mg/kg IM), **plus**<br>  • Ketamine (6.6 mg/kg IM); use ½, of all doses if given IV |
| Maintenance | • Isoflurane or sevoflurane<br>• Atipamezole (333 µg/kg IM) at end of procedure if reversal of dexmedetomidine is needed. |
| Monitoring | • HR<br>• Respiratory rate<br>• $SpO_2$<br>• Temperature<br>• +/- Blood pressure |
| Blocks | • Digital block (see Chapter 1, page 7) |
| **Postoperative Considerations** | |
| Analgesia | • Morphine (0.1-0.2 mg/kg IV or 0.1-0.5 mg/kg IM q1-4hr), **or**<br>• Hydromorphone* (0.05-0.1 mg/kg IV, IM q3-4hr), **or**<br>• Buprenorphine† (0.005-0.02 mg/kg IV, IM q4-8hr or 0.01-0.02 OTM q6-12hr)<br>• +/- Ketamine CRI (2 µg/kg/min IV. If no previous loading dose, then give 0.5 mg/kg IV prior to CRI) **plus**<br>• Meloxicam§ (0.05-0.1 mg/kg PO, SC once) |
| Monitoring | • $SpO_2$<br>• Blood Pressure<br>• HR<br>• Respiratory rate<br>• Temperature |
| Estimated pain score | • Severe |

HCT, Hematocrit; TP, total protein; Cr, creatinine; HR, heart rate; EBL, estimated blood loss; $SpO_2$, oxygen saturation via a pulse oximeter; CRI, constant rate infusion; OTM, oral transmucosal.

*Monitor for hyperthermia in cats.

†Buprenorphine is a better analgesic than morphine in cats.

‡Use only in young animals.

§Black box warning added by the FDA in October 2010 identified cases of renal failure and death in cats with repeated uses of meloxicam. Meloxicam is approved for single use only in cats in the United States.

** From MacPhail CM: Surgery of the integumentary system. In Fossum TW, ed.: Small Animal Surgery, 4th ed.: St. Louis: Mosby, 2013, 190.

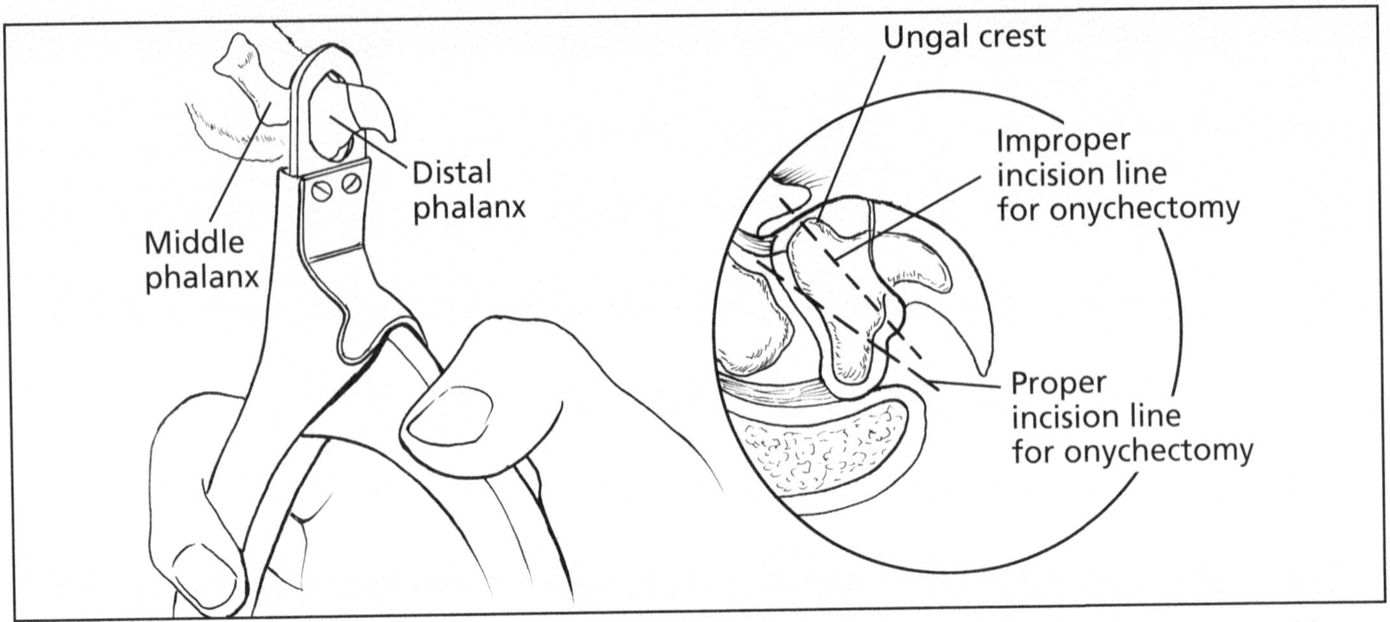


**Figure 6-2.** Nail clipper onychectomy. Front edge of the nail clipper ring positioned in the groove between the distal end of the middle phalanx and the ungal crest of the distal phalanx. *(Inset)* Proper line for onychectomy takes all of ungal crest leaving a remnant of the flexor process. Improper line for onychectomy leaves part of ungal crest. (After MacPhail CM: Surgery of the intergumentary system. In Fossum TW, ed.: Small Animal Surgery, 4th ed.: St. Louis Mosby, 2013, 280).

As an alternative technique, the nail clipper is positioned with the blade dorsally in the groove between the distal end of the middle phalanx and ungual crest of the distal phalanx. The blade is used to transect the digital extensor tendons. The blade is rotated ventrally, keeping it in continuous contact with the skin. Lifting the nail dorsally closes the joint space and deviates the flexor process ventrally. After insuring that the digital pad is proximal to the transection line and that the blade is in the joint space, the nail clipper is closed to amputate the distal phalanx and claw.

After the claw is removed, a small portion of the palmar aspect of the distal phalanx, which is a remnant of the flexor process, remains. It can be removed by grasping it with thumb forceps and carefully dissecting it from the digital pad with sharp-sharp scissors or a scalpel blade. On large cats, this portion of bone can be left to retain deep digital flexor function.

The same procedure is repeated on all claws that are to be removed. Tourniquets are released. Uniform pressure on the paws for a few minutes may be necessary to attain hemostasis.

A bandage can be used to appose skin edges or they may be apposed with either a simple interrupted or cruciate suture of 3-0 monofilament synthetic absorbable suture material. A cyanoacrylate tissue adhesive can also be placed over the apposed skin edges for closure. Care is used not to place sutures in the pads. If skin edges are apposed using cyanoacrylate tissue adhesive care should be used to place it over apposed wound edges and not between them.

### $CO_2$ Laser Onychectomy (Cats)

A $CO_2$ laser can be used for onychectomy. The laser is set at 6W in a continuous-wave mode using a 0.8 mm bore tip. A circumferential incision is made through the redundant tissue at the ungal crest, preserving as much skin as possible. The distal phalanx is then disarticulated with the laser by incising/cutting through the extensor tendon, synovial membrane, colateral ligaments, and flexor tendon. A simple interrupted suture can be placed in the remaining skin. If cyonoacrylate adhesive is used to close the area, it should be used sparingly on the skin surface and not within the wound.

## Aftercare

For postoperative analgesia, pre and postoperative opiods and a single postoperative dose of an NSAID can be used. One recommended regimen is buprenorphine (0.01 to 0.02 mg/kg IM or per os Q 6 hours) or a fentanyl patch (25 µg/hr). One dose of ketoprofen (2 mg/kg IM or SQ) can be given during postoperative recovery. Another postoperative analgesic is meloxicam (0.1 mg/kg PO per day for 3 to 4 days). Other regimens of post operative analgesics have been described. The reader is referred to the opening comment under "Suggested Readings".

A bandage is applied from the paw to the distal antebrachium. A piece of absorbent surgical gauze is placed over the end of the paw as the primary layer. This is followed by a secondary layer of several wraps of a slightly elastic absorbent wrap (Kling, Johnson & Johnson, Inc., Arlington, TX). A tertiary layer of one-inch wide porous adhesive tape completes the bandage. Because the cats have a tendency to shake the paws following recovery from anesthesia in an attempt to get bandages off, it is important to have the bandage tape well affixed to the hair of the limb at the proximal end. This does not mean tightly wrapped, but adhered to the hair. Bandages are left in place 12 to 24 hours. If bleeding persists, rebandaging should be continued for 2 to 3 days. Extreme caution should be used when applying bandages, especially when using elastic wrap materials, to avoid tight bandages that cause ischemia of the paws and result in avascular necrosis. Elastic tubular compression fabric is available for application using a metal cylindrical application device. The bandage material is applied to the distal limb in layers by pulling it off of the applicator onto the limb that has been placed in the applicator.

After bandage removal, no attempt should be made to clean dried blood off of the paw. The cat will do this very effectively. If sutures (especially absorbable sutures) have been used, they are usually removed by the cat within a week.

Shredded paper should replace clay-type litter in litter boxes for 2 weeks while the nail beds heal. Physical activity should be kept to a minimum for 7 to 10 days, during which time the cat is kept on clean dry surfaces.

Aftercare following canine onychectomy is similar to that for cats; however, the bandages have a thicker secondary layer for padding, especially on larger dogs. Bandaging is continued for 7 to 10 days with periodic changes depending upon the amount of hemorrhage in the bandage at bandage changes.

## Advantages and Disadvantages

An advantage of buprenorphine for postoperative pain management is that it is relatively inexpensive and can be given orally by the owner. If a Fentanyl patch is used, it is in place and the owner does not have to administer anything. The patch must be applied at least 6 hours prior to surgery. It can cause dysphoria in some cats.

With feline onychectomy young growing cats have the advantages of less hemorrhage and a shorter convalescent time compared to older or obese cats. Feline onychectomy has the advantages of preventing damage to household materials, and skin scratches to people and other animals. Canine onychectomy can also prevent skin scratches, (e.g. skin damage to elderly people/owners who have very thin skin).

Onychectomy has potential postoperative complications which can be considered disadvantages. These disadvantages include pain, hemorrhage, pad damage, lameness, swelling, infection, claw regrowth, middle phalanx protrusion, and palmigrade stance. Improper tourniquet application can result in neuropraxia, tissue necrosis and lameness. With neuropraxia, the radial nerve is most often affected. Signs usually resolve in 6 to 8 weeks. Postoperative pain may be present and may be more prevalent early following surgery done by dissection compared to nail clipper onychectomy. With $CO_2$ laser onychectomy there is excellent hemostasis with reduced postoperative swelling and pain. Pad laceration during the procedure prolongs pain and lameness. Hemorrhage is most common in older cats and dogs. It is also common in cats when wounds are not sutured. Use of tissue adhesives may cause postoperative lameness (frequently nonweight bearing) and infections with extrusion of the adhesive as a foreign body if it was placed between the wound edges. In general, cats that have had onychectomy do not return to normal activity as quickly as cats that have had deep digital flexor tenectomy.

If bandages are too tight, occluded vasculature and reperfusion injury may occur when they are removed. If elastic tubular compression fabric is used for bandaging, it should be remembered that the compression of the layers is additive. Thus, although each layer does not apply a large amount of pressure, several layers can apply too much pressure and occlude vasculature. The same is true of layers of an elastic wrap. Vasculature is destroyed in the process of reperfusion injury and ischemic necrosis results (Figure 6-3). The paws usually appear normal at bandage removal but become quite swollen within 12 hours followed by progressive loss of tissue.

If the germinal cells of the dorsal aspect of the ungual crest are not completely removed, regrowth of a claw, which is usually malformed, will occur. This may be more common with nail clipper onychectomy. A draining tract in the area is indicative of such a claw. Exposure necrosis of the middle phalanx and abscess associated with retention of portions of the distal phalanx may also occur. Both of these require removal of affected/infected tissue, wound closure and antibiotic therapy as needed.

Lameness occurs after most onychectomies but it usually resolves within a week. Dissection onychectomy causes the longest period of lameness, followed by the nail clipper technique, with $CO_2$ laser causing the least lameness.

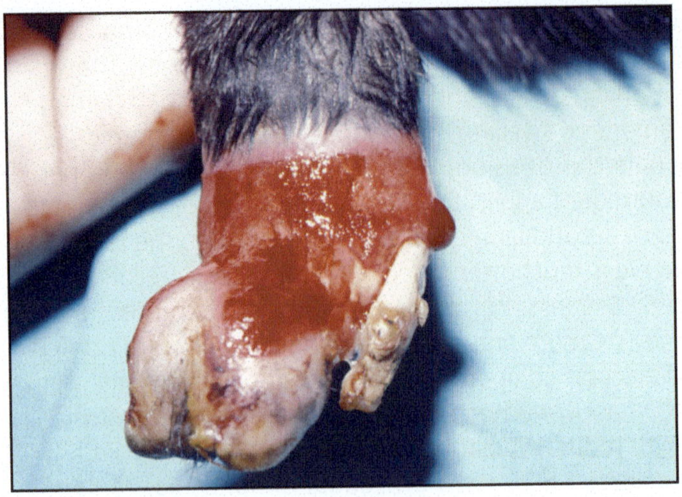

**Figure 6-3.** Slough of paw tissue as a result of a postonychectomy bandage being placed too tight.

Onychectomy on the forepaws may impair a cat's ability to climb if it is outside. However, if the back claws are intact a cat can supinate the forelimbs sufficiently to climb a tree. Cats with onychectomy of all 4 paws should be house cats.

# Suggested Readings

There have been numerous publications on feline onychectomy, with many of these devoted to pain management. The reader should conduct a literature search for more information on the subjects.


1. Bellah JR: Surgical management of specific skin disorders. *In* Slatter DH, ed.: Textbook of Small Animal Surgery, 2nd ed.: Philadelphia, WB Saunders, 1993, 341.
2. Boored MJ, Griffen CE, Rosenkrantz WS: Onychectomy as a therapy for symmetric claw and claw fold disease in the dog. J Am Anim Hosp Assoc 33: 107, 1997.
3. Burns SM, Howerth EW, Rawlings CA, et. al.: Comparison of the carbon dioxide laser and radiofrequency unit for feline onychectomy. J Am Anim Hosp Assoc 46: 375, 2010.
4. Carroll GL, Howe LB, Slatter MR, et. al.: Evaluation of analgesia provided by postoperative administration of butorphenol to cats undergoing onychectomy. J Am Vet Med Assoc 213: 246, 1998.
5. Carroll GL, Howe LB, Peterson KD: Analgesic efficacy of preoperative administration of meloxicam or butorphenol in onychectomized cats. J Am Vet Med Assoc 226, 913, 2005.
6. Curcio K, Bidwell LA, Bohart GV, et. al.: Evaluation of signs of postoperative pain and complications after forelimb onychectomy in cats receiving buprenorphine alone or with bupivacaine administered as a four – point regional nerve block. J Am Vet Med Assoc 228: 65, 2006.
7. Dobbins S, Brown NO, Shaver FS: Comparison of the effects of buprenorphine, oxymorphone hydrochloride, and ketoprophen for postoperative analgesia after onychectomy or onychectomy and sterilization in cats. J Am Anim Hosp Assoc 38: 507, 2002.
8. Ellison GW: Feline onychectomy complications: Prevention and management. North Amer Clin Brief Apr 03, 29.
9. Franks NJ, Boothe HW, Taylor L, et. al.: Evaluation of transdermal fentanyl patches for analgesia in cats undergoing onychectomy. J Am Vet Med Assoc 217: 1013, 2000.
10. Gaynor JS: Chronic pain syndrome of feline onychectomy. Clinicians Brief, Apr.: 11, 2005.
11. Gellasch KL, Kruse – Ellioh T, Osmond CS, et. al.: Comparison of transdermal administration of fentanyl versus intramuscular administration of butorphanol for analgesia after onychectomy in cats. J Am Vet Med Assoc 220, 1020, 2002.
12. Gordon WJ, Conzemius MG: Analgesia after onychectomy in cats: Vet Med 100: 46, 2005.
13. Hardin MS: A better way to bandage paws after routine onychectomy. Vet Med__:413, 1988.
14. Hedlund CS: Surgery of the integumentary system. *In* Fossum TW, ed.: Small Animal Surgery, 2nd ed.: St. Louis: Mosby, 2002, 134.
15. Hedlund CS: Surgery of the integumentary system. In Fossum TW, ed.: Small Animal Surgery, 3rd ed.: St. Louis: Mosby, 2007, 159.
16. Hinkle – Schwartz S: Onychectomy and tendonectomy. Clinicians Breif Mar, 2011.
17. Holmberg DL, Brisson BA: A prospective comparison of postoperative morbidity associated with the use of scalpel blades and lasers for onychectomy in cats. Can Vet J 47: 162, 2006.
18. Jankowski AJ, Brown DC, Duval J, et. al.: Comparison of effects of elective tenectomy or onychectomy in cats. J Am Vet Med Assoc 213: 370, 1998.
19. Landsberg G, Hortwitz D: Feline scratching and declawing. In Behnan A, ed.: Behavior in Dogs and Cats, Question and Answer: Guelph, Ontario, Canada: Lifelearn, Inc., 1998, 107.
20. Landsberg GM: Feline scratching and destruction and effects of declawing. Vet Clin North Am Small Animal Pract 21:265, 1991.
21. Landsberg GM: Declawing revisited - controversy over consequences. Vet Forum 11:94, 1994.
22. MacPhail CM: Surgery of the integumentary system. In Fossum TW, ed.: Small Animal Surgery, 4th ed.: St. Louis: Mosby, 2013, 190.
23. Manley PA: Amputation of the digit. *In* Birchard SJ, Sherding RG, eds.: Saunders Manual of Small Animal Practice, 2nd ed.: Philadelphia: W.B. Saunders, 2000, 1182.
24. Martinez SA, Hauptman J, Walshaw R: Comparing two techniques for onychectomy in cats and two adhesives for wound closure. Vet Med 88:516, 1993.
25. Mison MB, Bohert GH, Walshaw R, et. al.: Use of carbon dioxide laser for onychectomy in cats. J Am Vet Med Assoc 221: 651, 2002.
26. Patronek GJ: Assessment of claims of short and long – term complications associated with onychectomy in cats. J Am Vet Med Assoc 219: 932, 2001.
27. Robinson DA, Romans CW, Gordon – Evans WJ, et. al.: Evaluation of short – term limb function following unilateral carbon dioxide laser or scalpel onychectomy in cats. J Am Vet Med Assoc 230: 353. 2007.
28. Rochat MC: Amputation of the digit. In Birchard SJ, Sherding RG, eds.: Saunders Manual of Small Animal Practice, 3rd ed.: St. Louis: Saunders – Elsevier, 2006, 1167.
29. Romans CW, Gordon WJ, Robinson DA, et. al.: Effect of postoperative analgesic protocol on limb function following onychectomy in cats. J Am Vet Assoc 227: 89, 2005.
30. Schenck CT: The use of surgical glue for declawing cats. Vet Forum 11:62, 1994.
31. Scherk – Nixon M: A study of the use of transdermal fentanyl patch in cats. J Am Anim Hosp Assoc 32: 19, 1996.
32. Swaim SF: The effects of dressings and bandages on wound healing. Seminars in Vet Med and Surg 4:274, 1989.
33. Swiderski J: Onychectomy and its alternatives in the feline patient. Clin Tech Sm Anim Pract 17: 158, 2002.
34. Taylor PM, Kirby JJ, Robinson C, et. al.: A prospective multi – centre clinical trial to compare buprenorphine and butorphenol for postoperative analgesia in cats. J Fel Med Surg 12: 247, 2010.
35. Tobias KS: Feline onychectomy at a teaching institution: A retrospective study of 163 cases. Vet Surg 23:274, 1994.
36. Winkler KP, Greenfield CL, Bensen GJ, et. al.: The effect of wound irrigation with bupivacaine on postoperative analgesia in the feline onychectomy patient. J Am Anim Hosp Assoc 23: 346, 1997.

37. Yeon SC, Flanders JA, Scarlett JM, et al: Attitudes of owners regarding tendonectomy and onychectomy in cats. Am J Vet Rsch 218:43, 2001.
38. Young WP: Feline onychectomy and elective procedures. Vet Clin No Am Small Anim Pract 32: 601, 2002.

# Deep Digital Flexor Tenectomy (Cats)

## Definition and Indications

With tenectomy of the deep digital flexor tendon the claws remain contracted. The technique is an alternative to onychectomy.

## Technique

Following anesthesia the paws are clipped and prepared for aseptic surgery. A tourniquet other than a rubber band is applied to the forelimb below the radial-humeral joint to minimize hemorrhage. A 3 to 5 mm skin incision is made parallel to the long axis of the digit over the palmar surface of the middle phalanx near the proximal interphalangeal joint (Figure 6-4A). The incision will expose the deep digital flexor tendon lying under the skin. Mosquito forceps or iris scissors are used to dissect under the tendon and elevate it (Figure 6-4B). A 5 mm segment of the tendon is excised with a scalpel blade Figure 6-4C). The edges of the skin incision are sutured with a simple interrupted suture of 3-0 monofilament synthetic absorbable suture,(Figure 6-4D) or a cynoacrylate tissue adhesive is placed over, not between, the apposed wound edges. The same procedure is repeated on all claws that are to be operated, and the tips of the claws are trimmed. The tourniquet is released.

## Aftercare

No bandages are used on the paws. Shredded paper should be used in the litter box rather than clay-type litter for 2 weeks. Activity should be limited including jumping for 1 week. It will be necessary for the owners to trim the claws periodically since there will be no natural wear from the cat sharpening the claws.

## Advantages and Disadvantages

The advantages of the technique include shorter hospitalization, no need for bandages, less pain, and return to normal activity within 3 days. A disadvantage of the technique is that if the superficial digital flexor tendon (which inserts on the proximal aspect of the middle phalanx) is excised rather than the deep digital flexor tendon the result is an abnormal flat-footed stance. The nails become thick and blunt and must be trimmed regularly when a deep digital flexor tenectomy has been performed. Other disadvantages include persistent lameness, retained ability to scratch, interphalangeal joint immobility, fibrosis, pain, and

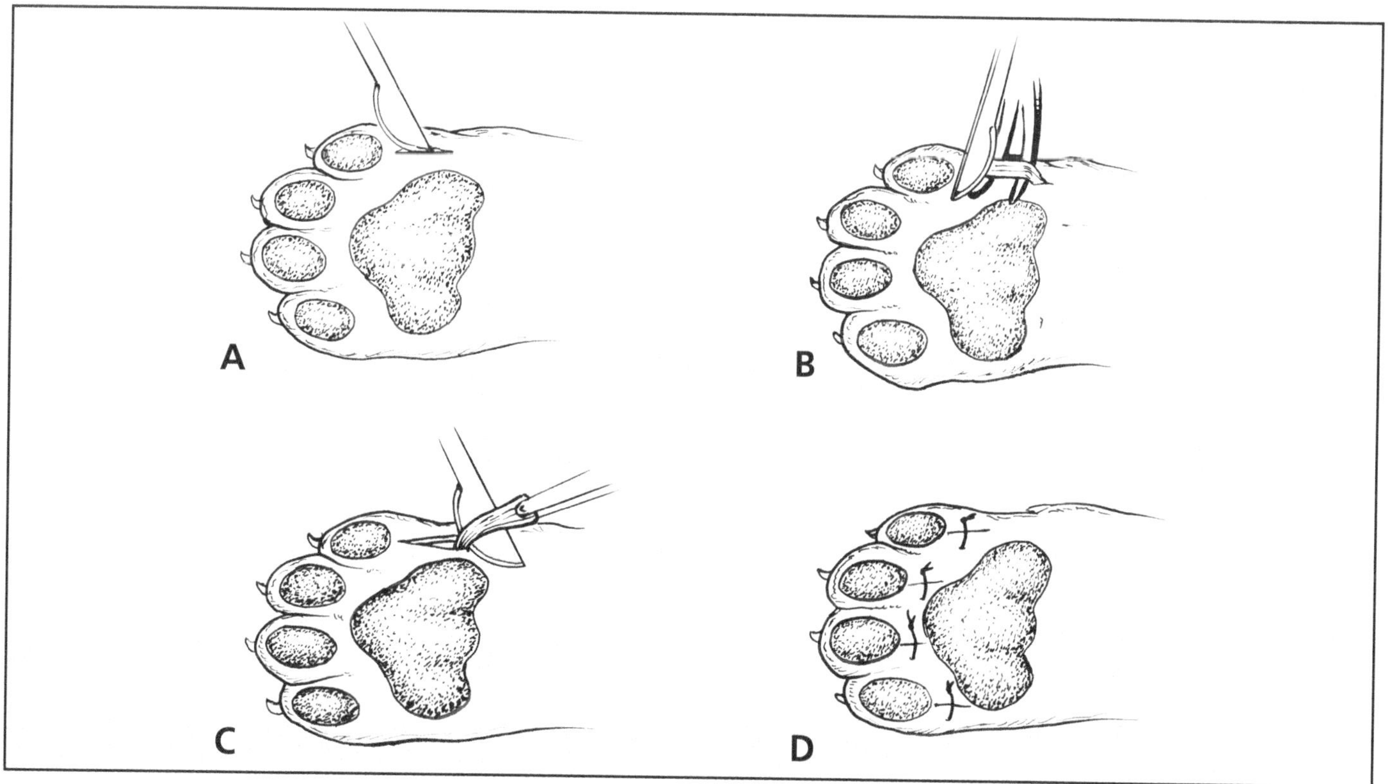


**Figure 6-4.** Deep digital flexor tenectomy. **A.** Three – 5 mm skin incisions parallel to the digit long axis on palmar surface of the middle phalanx near the proximal interphalangeal joint. **B.** Mosquito forceps used to dissect under the tendon and the tendon is cut. **C.** Excision of a 5 mm. section of the deep digital flexor tendon. **D.** Simple interrupted skin sutures close the skin incisions on each digit.

ingrowth of claws into the digital pads. Owners may be dissatisfied with the unaesthetic appearance of the thickened claws and the necessity to clip the nails. Onychectomy may be needed to relieve clinical signs. No significant differences in behavioral problems have been detected between cats having deep digital flexor tenectomy and those having onychectomy.

# Suggested Readings


1. Bellah JR: Surgical management of specific skin disorders. *In* Slatter DH, ed.: Textbook of Small Animal Surgery, 2nd ed.: Philadelphia, WB Saunders, 1993, 341.
2. Hedlund CS: Surgery of the integumentary system. *In* Fossum TW, ed.: Small Animal Surgery, 2nd ed.: St. Louis: Mosby, 2002, 134.
3. Hedlund CS: Surgery of the integumentary system. In Fossum TW, ed.: Small Animal Surgery, 3rd ed.: St. Louis: Mosby, 2007, 159.
4. Hinkle – Schwartz S: Onychectomy and tendonectomy. Clinicians Brief Mar, 2011.
5. Jankowski AJ, Brown DC, Duval J, et al: Comparison of effects of elective tenectomy or onychectomy in cats. J Am Vet Med Assoc 213:370, 1998.
6. MacPhail CM: Surgery of the integumentary system. In Fossum TW, ed.: Small Animal Surgery, 4th ed.: St. Louis: Mosby, 2013, 190.
7. Rife JN: Deep digital flexor tendonectomy - an alternative to amputation onychectomy for declawing cats. J Am Anim Hosp Assoc 24:73, 1988.
8. Yeon SC, Flanders JA, Scarlett JM, et al: Attitudes of owners regarding tendonectomy and onychectomy in cats. Am J Vet Rsch 218:43, 2001.


# Dewclaw Amputation

## Definition and Indication

The dewclaw is the first digit of the canine rear paws; however, the term has also been used for the first digit on the forelimb. The first (proximal) and second (middle) phalanges of the dewclaw are inconsistent. In some dogs dewclaws are absent and in others they may be double such as the Great Pyrenees and briards which must have double rear dewclaws to satisfy breed standards.

Amputation of loosely attached dewclaws is commonly done on toy breeds to prevent injury during grooming. In hunting dogs, they are removed to prevent traumatic injury. In puppies, dewclaws should be removed at 3 to 5 days of age at the same time as caudectomy if it is to be performed.

## Techniques

### Neonates

After aseptic preparation of the medial aspect of the paw, an assistant holds the puppy with that aspect of the paw exposed and immobilized. A local analgesic agent is injected at the base of the dewclaw. For analgesia 0.5 to 0.75 mg/kg of lidocaine (without epinephrine) and 0.25 to 0.5 mg/kg of bupivacaine can be mixed together in a tuberculin syringe. The mixture is injected through a 25 gauge needle. Lidocaine (2 mg/kg) can be divided between the 2 dewclaws. The dewclaw is abducted and the web of skin between the metacarpus/ metatarsus and the dewclaw is cut with scissors (Figure 6-5A). The metatarsal/metacarpal-phalangeal joint is disarticulated or the bone of the phalanx is transected adjacent to the metacarpal/ metatarsal bone with a scalpel blade, electrosurgery, laser, or scissors (Figure 6-5B). Hemostasis is attained by digital pressure, silver nitrate cautery or electrocautery. Sutures are generally not applied; however, if digital pressure or electrocautery have been used, a simple interrupted suture may be placed to appose the skin edges or cyanoacrylate tissue adhesive can be applied over the digitally apposed skin edges.

### Older Dogs

If dewclaw removal was not performed within the first week of life, it should be delayed until 3 months of age to minimize risk of exposure to hospital disease. Under general anesthesia with the dog in lateral recumbency, the areas of the saphenous, peroneal

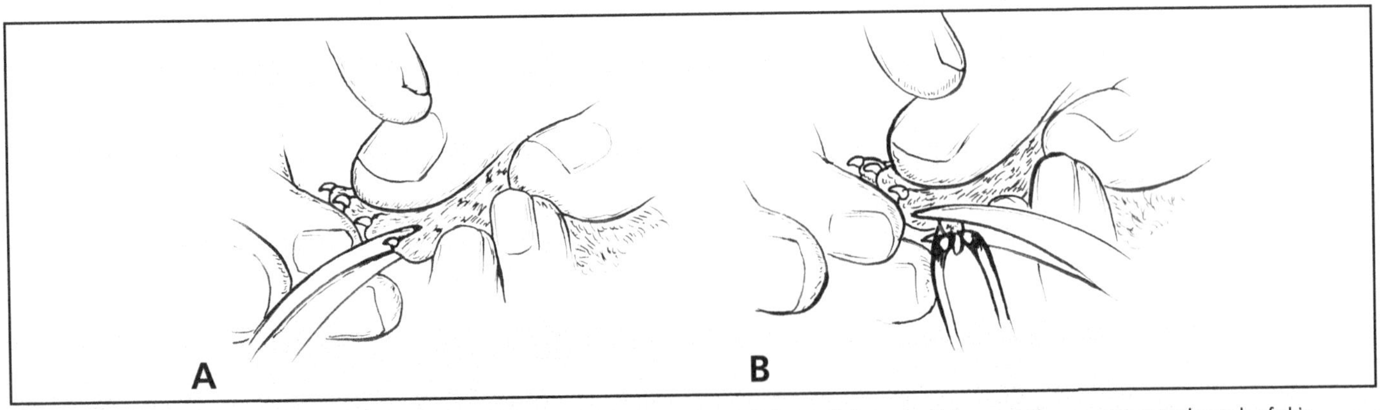


**Figure 6-5.** Dewclaw amputation on neonate. **A.** Assistant holds neonate and exposes the medial aspect of the paw. The surgeon cuts the web of skin between the metacarpus/metatarsus and the dewclaw with scissors. **B.** The metatarsal/metacarpal-phalangeal joint is disarticulated or bone of the phalanx is cut with scissors. (After Bellah JR: Surgical management of specific skin disorders. In Slatter DH, ed.: Textbook of Small Animal Surgery, 2nd ed.: Philadelphia, WB Saunders, 1993, 353.)

and tibial nerves are injected with 0.2 to 0.4 ml of 0.5% bupivacaine. The dewclaw areas are clipped and prepared for aseptic surgery. With a number 15 scalpel blade, an elliptical incision is made around the base of the dewclaw where it articulates with the metacarpal/metatarsal bone (Figure 6-6A). After incising the skin the dewclaw is abducted and the skin and subcutaneous tissue are dissected to the metacarpal/metatarsal-phalangeal joint (Figure 6-6B). If the proximal and middle phalanges are firmly attached, free them with a number 11 scalpel blade. Using 3-0 absorbable suture material, the dorsal common and axial palmar digital vessels are ligated. A scalpel blade is used to disarticulate the metacarpal/metatarsal-phalangeal joint (Figure 6-6C), or bone cutters can be used to transect the proximal phalanx of the dewclaw near the metacarpal/metatarsal-phalangeal joint; however, the results are less cosmetic with the bone transection. The subcutaneous tissues are closed with simple continuous or simple interrupted sutures of 3-0 or 4-0 absorbable suture material. The skin is sutured with simple interrupted sutures of 3-0 or 4-0 monofilament nonabsorbable suture (Figure 6-6D). To discourage licking at the site, simple interrupted 4-0 or 5-0 stainless steel sutures with short tags may be considered.

## Aftercare

Bandages are not usually applied to neonates after dewclaw removal. On older dogs, a soft padded bandage is applied circumferentially around the limb at the level of the surgical site to protect it for 3 to 5 days. Skin sutures are removed in 7 to 10 days. Care must be used not to place bandages too tightly, especially if an elastic wrap is used.

## Advantages and Disadvantages

When dewclaws are removed at 3 to 5 days of age, hemorrhage is minimal and the procedure is easier. Dewclaw removal at a later age requires general anesthesia, hemorrhage control is more involved and the procedure is more complex. Older dogs are prone to molest the surgical site which can result in wound disruption, hemorrhage, infection, and scarring. If the bandage around the surgical site is placed too tightly, swelling or ischemic necrosis can occur.

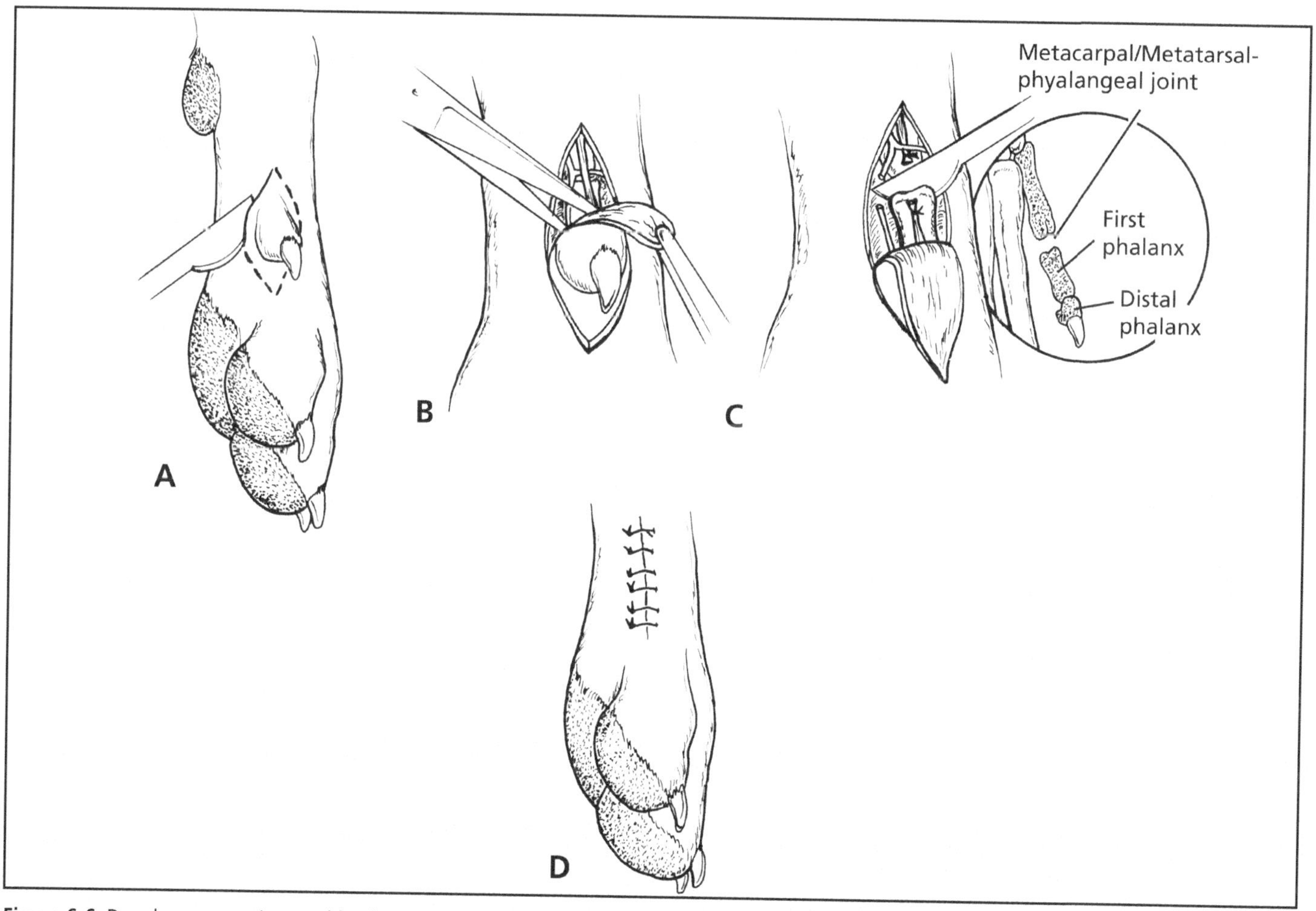


**Figure 6-6.** Dewclaw amputation on older dogs. **A.** Elliptical skin incision made around the base of the dewclaw. **B.** Skin and subcutaneous tissue are dissected to the metacarpal/metatarsal-phalangeal joint. **C.** After ligating and dividing the dorsal common and axial palmar vessels, the metacarpal/metatarsal-phalangeal joint is disarticulated and the dewclaw is removed. **D.** Subcutaneous tissue and skin are sutured. (After MacPhail CM: Surgery of the intergumentary system. In Fossum TW, ed.: Small Animal Surgery, 4th ed.: St. Louis: Mosby, 2013, 284).

# Suggested Readings


1. Bellah JR: Surgical management of specific skin disorders. *In* Slatter DH, ed.: Textbook of Small Animal Surgery, 2nd ed.: Philadelphia, WB Saunders, 1993, 341.
2. Hedlund CS: Surgery of the integumentary system. *In* Fossum TW, ed.: Small Animal Surgery, 2nd ed.: St. Louis: Mosby, 2002, 134.
3. Hedlund CS: Surgery of the integumentary system. In Fossum TW, ed.: Small Animal Surgery, 3rd ed.: St. Louis: Mosby, 2007, 159.
4. MacPhail CM: Surgery of the integumentary system. In Fossum TW, ed.: Small Animal Surgery, 4th ed.: St. Louis: Mosby, 2013, 190.
5. Manley PA: Amputation of the digit. *In* Birchard SJ, Sherding RG, eds.: Saunders Manual of Small Animal Practice, 2nd ed.: Philadelphia: W.B. Saunders, 2000, 1182.
6. Rochat MC: Amputation of the digit. In Birchard SJ, Sherding RG, eds.: Saunders Manual of Small Animal Pract, 3rd ed.: St. Louis: Saunders – Elsevier, 2006, 1167.


# Digit Amputation

## Definition and Indications

Digit amputation is the removal of all or part of one or more digits from an animal's paw. The level of amputation may be at the metacarpal/metatarsal-phalangeal joint, the proximal or distal interphalangeal joint, or by osteotomy of the affected digital bones. The level of amputation is determined by the site of the lesion and disease process. The most common indications for digit amputation are traumatic injuries where the digit is nonfunctional or nonviable due to vascular or cutaneous loss (e.g. trap injury). Comminuted or intra-articular fractures, chronic sprains, tendon injuries and irreparable luxations are also indications for amputation. Other indications for digit amputation are chronic bacterial or fungal infections, osteomyelitis, degenerative joint disease, phlebitis, thromboembolic disease, pressure necrosis from bandages and casts, and severe arthritis. Digits are occasionally amputated to facilitate salvage of a weight – bearing pad.

Neoplasias of the digits are also an indication for amputation. They are most common in large to medium-sized male dogs (10 to 30 kg). Neoplasias occur in older animals (mean age 10 years for dogs and 12.7 years for cats). The common tumors involved include squamous cell carcinomas, malignant melanomas, soft tissue sarcomas, osteosarcomas, and mast cell tumors. Black dogs are predisposed to subungual squamous cell carcinomas.

Digital tumors in cats are frequently metastatic from pulmonary tumors, and commonly involve the weight – bearing digits. They can involve more than one digit.

## Techniques

### Distal Interphalangeal Amputation (Dog)

A circumferential skin incision is made at the base of the nail with a number 15 scalpel blade (Figure 6-7A). The distal interphalangeal joint between the distal and middle phalanges is isolated. Following the contour of the proximal end of the distal phalanx with the blade, the common digital extensor tendon, dorsal ligaments, deep digital flexor tendon, collateral ligaments, and joint capsule are cut and the distal phalanx is dissected away from the digital pad and removed with the nail (Figure 6-7B). Hemorrhage is controlled by ligation of vessels with 3-0 absorbable suture material. The distal one third of the middle phalanx is removed with bone cutters to provide more soft tissue between the pad and bone end (Figure 6-7C). For closure, the extensor tendon can be sutured to the dorsal surface of the pad. One or two 3-0 simple interrupted absorbable sutures can be placed in the subcutaneous tissue to close the dead space over the end of the middle phalanx. The skin is sutured with a simple interrupted or a cruciate suture of 3-0 monofilament nonabsorbable suture material (Figure 6-7D). "Dog-ears" are removed if necessary.

### Proximal Interphalangeal and Metacarpal/ Metatarsal-Phalangeal Amputation

Following administration of general anesthesia, peripheral nerves are blocked with 0.2 to 0.4 ml of 0.5% bupivacaine at each site. For the forelimb, the median, ulnar and radial nerves are blocked. For the pelvic limb, the tibial, peroneal and saphenous nerves are blocked.

For removal of the third or fourth digits, a circumferential incision is made at the level of the proximal interphalangeal joint or metacarpal/metatarsal-phalangeal joint with a short longitudinal incision on the dorsum of the paw adjoining the circumferential incision (inverse "Y" incision) (Figure 6-8A). When amputating the second or fifth digit similar incisions are made; however, the longitudinal incision is made on the side of the paw. The flexor and extensor tendons, ligaments and joint capsule are transected. Digital arteries and veins are ligated with 3-0 or 4-0 absorbable suture. The sesamoid bones are included in the excision at the metacarpal/metatarsal-phalangeal level. The head of the proximal phalanx is removed if amputation is at the proximal interphalangeal joint. The head of the metacarpal/metatarsal bone is removed if amputation is at the metacarpal/metatarsal-phalangeal joint (Figure 6-8B & C). The extensor tendon can be sutured to the dorsal surface of the pad if it is preserved. However, the pad is usually removed

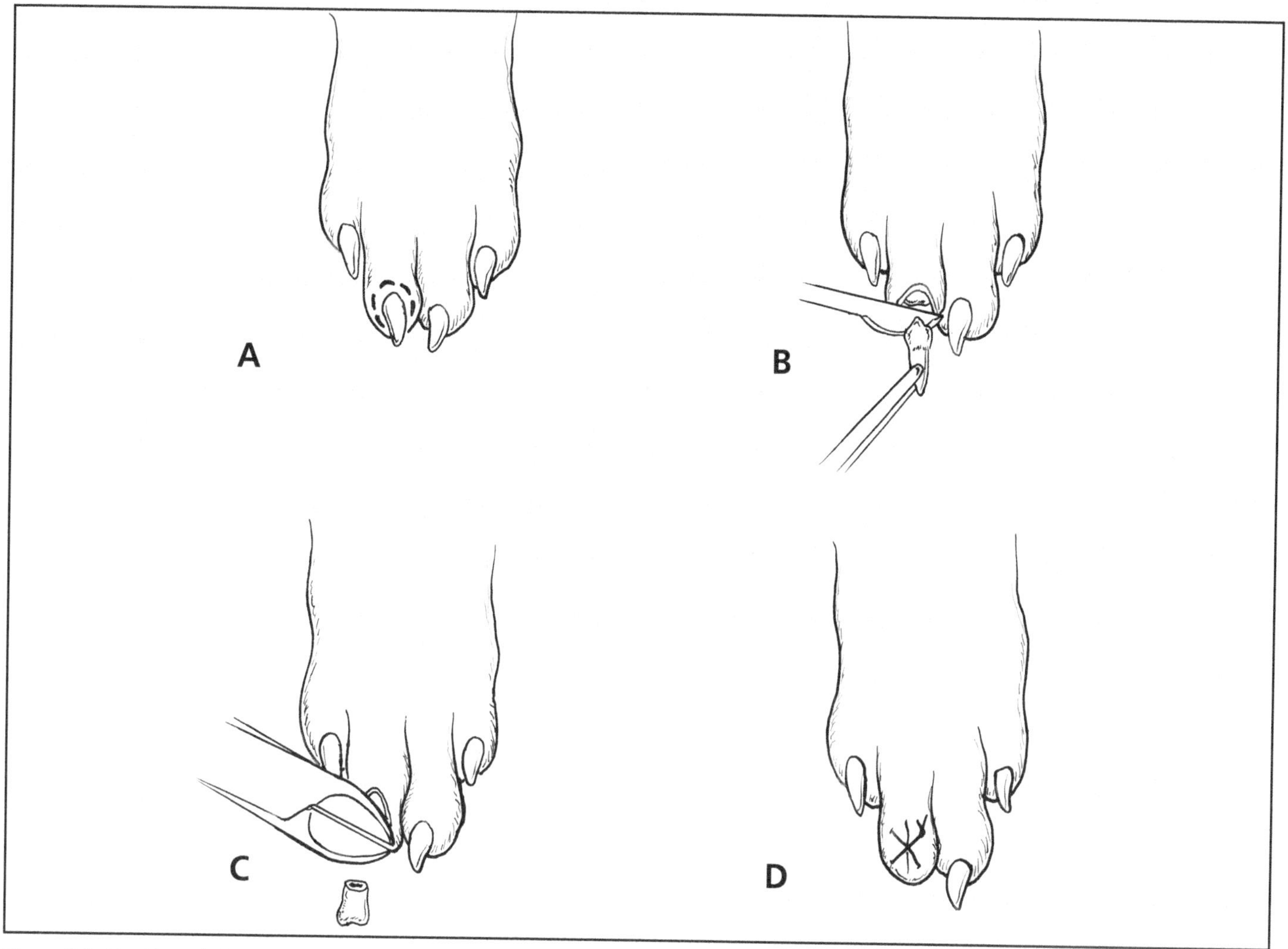


**Figure 6-7.** Distal interphalangeal amputation. **A.** Circumferential skin incision is made at base of the nail. **B.** Distal phalanx and nail are removed by cutting tendons, ligaments, joint capsule and attachment to the digital pad. **C.** Distal 1/3 of the middle phalanx is removed. **D.** After suturing the extensor tendon to dorsal pad surface, subcutaneous tissue and skin are sutured. (After Swaim SF, Henderson RA: Small Animal Wound Management, 2nd ed.: Baltimore: Williams & Wilkins, 1997, 357.)

with these amputations. Subcutaneous tissue is closed over the end of the bone with 3-0 or 4-0 simple interrupted absorbable sutures. The skin is sutured with 3-0 nonabsorbable monofilament simple interrupted or a cruciate suture( Figure 6-8D).

## Pandigital Metacarpal/Metatarsal-Phalangeal Amputation

When all digits have lost or are losing their viability, they should be evaluated to ascertain if amputation is necessary. Signs of impending digital loss include easy epilation of hair from the digit, abnormal turgor (has become extremely soft and moist or hard) of digital skin, nails that are easily pulled off their nail beds, and when no pain is elicited by inserting an 18 gauge needle into the digital pad. When trimming a nail into the quick or inserting an 18 gauge needle into a pad results in no sign of sensation and there is no hemorrhage, slow hemorrhage or very dark blood the prognosis for saving the digit is poor. A sharp line of demarcation between viable and nonviable tissue is a definite indication digits will be lost (Figure 6-9). When evaluating the digital pads, the metacarpal/metatarsal pad should also be evaluated by needle insertion. Occasionally, hemorrhage from these larger pads may be slow, and signs of sensation may be questionable. In these cases, surgery should be performed, utilizing this pad. The philosophy is that if the pad does progress to necrosis, amputation can be performed at that time. Often these metacarpal/ metatarsal pads remain viable and serve nicely in this salvage procedure.

Following administration of general anesthesia, peripheral nerves are blocked with 0.2 to 0.4 ml of 0.5% bupivacaine at each site. For the forelimb, the median, ulnar and radial nerves are blocked. For the pelvic limb, the tibial, peroneal, and saphenous nerves are blocked.

A transverse skin incision is made on the dorsal paw surface at the level of the metacarpal/metatarsal-phalangeal articulation. If a sharp line of demarcation

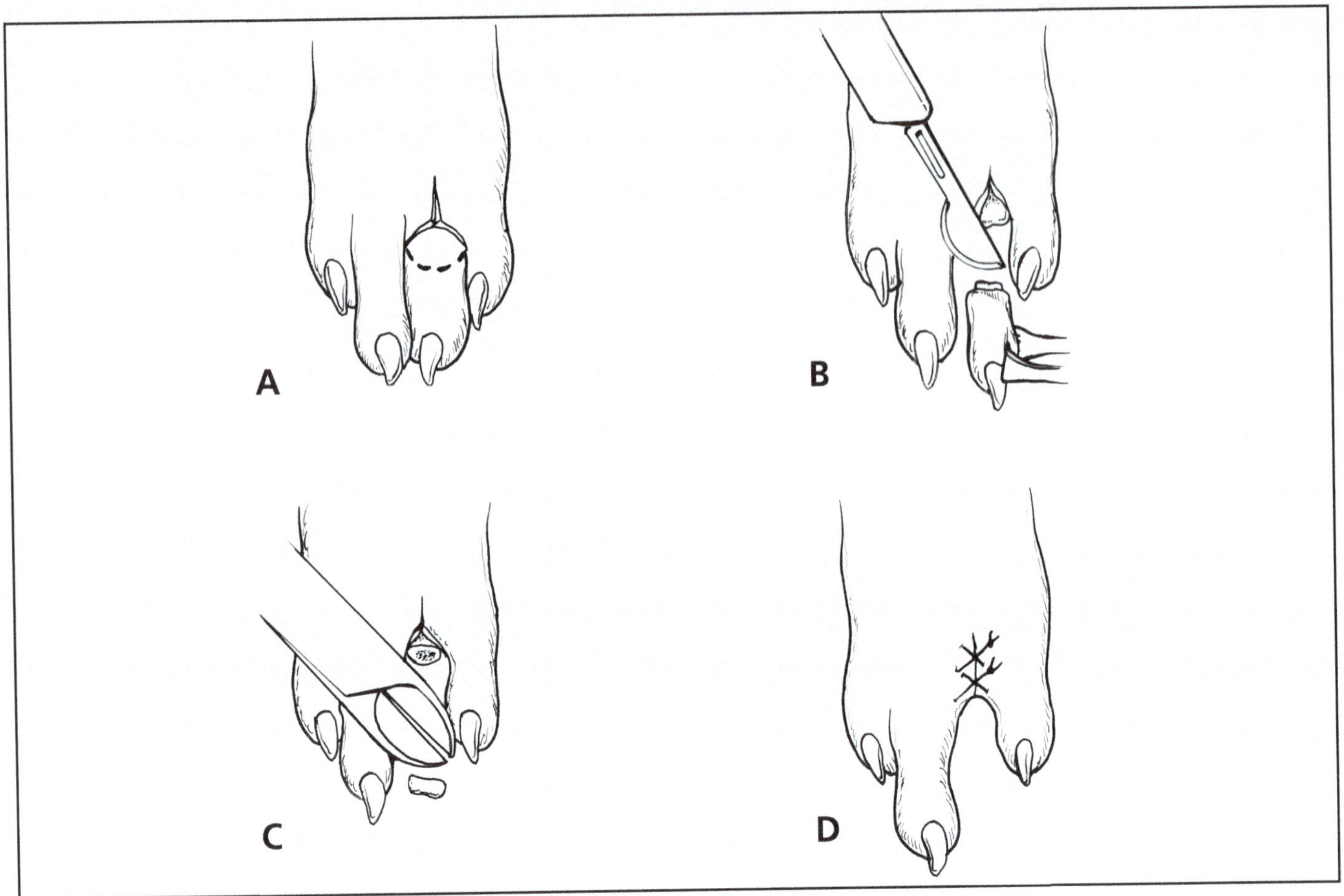


**Figure 6-8.** Proximal interphalangeal or metacarpal/metatarsal-phalangeal amputation. **A.** Circumferential skin incision is made at base of fourth digit with a short longitudinal incision on the dorsum of the paw. **B.** Removal of the fourth digit by cutting tendons, ligaments, vessels and joint capsule. **C.** Removing the head of the proximal phalanx or metacarpal/metatarsal bone. **D.** Subcutaneous tissue and skin are sutured. (After Swaim SF, Henderson RA: Small Animal Wound Management, 2nd ed.: Baltimore: Williams & Wilkins, 1997, 358.)

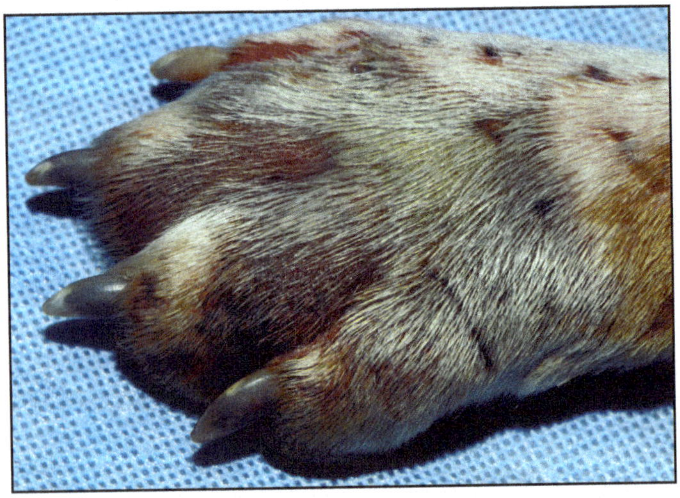

**Figure 6-9.** A sharp line of demarcation between viable and noviable tissue as a strong indication digits will be lost. Three nails are also quite cyanotic.

is present between viable and nonviable tissue, the incision is made approximately 3 mm proximal to the demarcation line (Figure 6-10A and Figure 6-11A). The incision is continued onto the palmar/plantar paw surface, incising at the juncture of the metacarpal/metatarsal pad with the skin between this pad and the digital pads (Figure 6-11B). As with the dorsum of the paw, if there is a line of demarcation cranial to the metatarsal/metacarpal pad, the incision should be made in viable skin approximately 3 mm proximal to the line.

Beginning on the dorsum of the paw, the skin is reflected followed by ligation of the dorsal axial and abaxial common or proper digital vessels with 3-0 absorbable suture material. Vessels are severed distal to the ligatures followed by division of the nerves, extensor tendons, collateral ligaments and metacarpal/metatarsal-phalangeal joint capsules. The paw is then turned over to approach the palmar/plantar surface. The sesamoid ligaments and sesamoid bones are removed. Palmar/plantar common or proper digital vessels are ligated and the vessels are severed distal to the ligations along with severance of the flexor tendons. The digits are removed leaving the metacarpal/metatarsal pad (Figure 6-10B, and Figure 6-11C).

In the absence of infection, the metacarpal/metatarsal heads are removed with rongeurs. Because metacarpals/metatarsals 3 and 4 extend beyond 2 and 5, they do not allow the metacarpal/metatarsal pad to rotate fully under their ends. Thus, rongeurs are

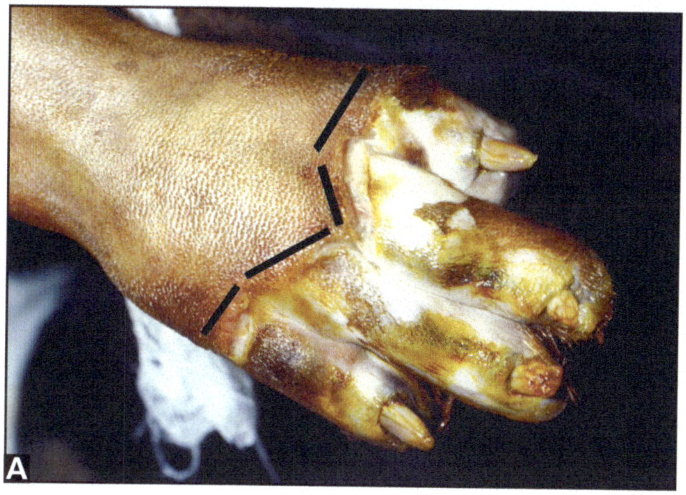


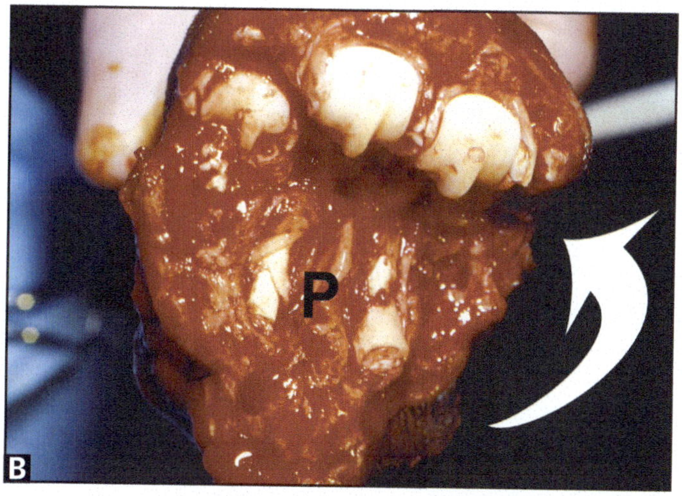


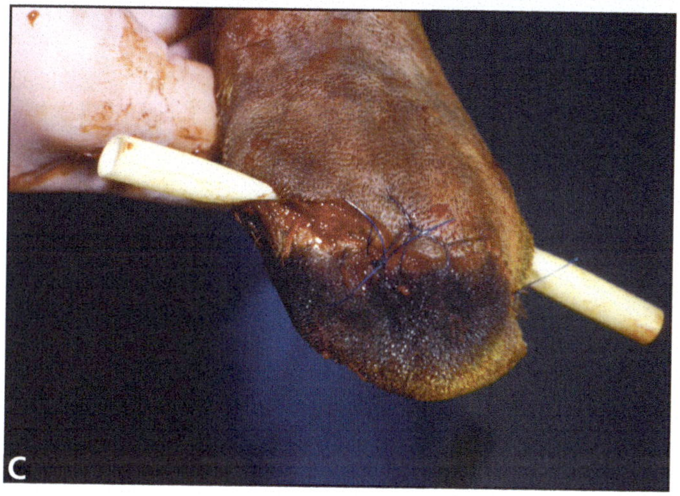


**Figure 6-10.** Proximal metacarpal-phalangeal amputation. **A.** Necrotic digits. Proposed line of excision *(broken line)*. **B.** Following digit removal, the metacarpal pad *(P)* will be rotated *(arrow)* to cover the ends of the metacarpal bones. **C.** Metacarpal pad sutured in place with a Penrose drain in place to allow for drainage. ( After Swaim SF, Henderson RA: Small Animal Wound Management, 2nd ed.: Baltimore: Williams & Wilkins, 1997, 359.)

used to incrementally trim their ends in conjunction with trimming skin on the dorsum of the metacarpal/ metatarsal area (Figure 6-11D) until the metacarpal/ metatarsal pad can be rotated under the ends of these bones with the thickest portion of the pad directly under the bone ends. The heads of the metacarpal/ metatarsal bones should not be removed if there is infection in the area to avoid the possibility of ascending infection into the marrow cavities of the bones. Following control of infection, the area may be reoperated to remove the metacarpal/metatarsal heads and trim the bones as needed.

A ¼-inch diameter Penrose drain is placed at the base of the metacarpal/metatarsal pad and the pad is rotated cranially under the ends of the metacarpal/ metatarsal bones. Interrupted horizontal mattress sutures of 3-0 absorbable suture material are used to join the metacarpal/ metatarsal pad to the subcutaneous tissue on the cranial aspect of the metacarpal/ metatarsal area (Figure 6-11E). Skin closure is completed with 3-0 monofilament nonabsorbable suture material in a far-near-near-far suture pattern. A simple interrupted nonabsorbable tacking suture is placed at each end of the drain to anchor it in place (Figure 6-10C and Figure 6-11F).

## Aftercare

With amputation of individual digits, a small amount of cotton or cast padding is placed between the remaining digits and in the space between the digits and the metacarpal/metatarsal pad. A piece of semiocclusive nonadherent bandage material (Telfa "Ouchless" pads, Covidien, Tyco HealthCare/Kendall, Mansfield, MA) is placed over the suture line. An absorbent secondary wrap and adhesive tape or elastic tape tertiary layer complete the bandage. The amount of secondary wrap and need for special padding and a metal splint are not as great as when bandaging a pad laceration or phalangeal fillet to replace a pad. When a pandigital amputation has been performed, a "clam shell" bandage is indicated to keep pressure off of the area, especially with large dogs.

The length of time sutures remain in place, the frequency of bandage changes, time of drain removal and the duration of bandaging vary depending on the procedure that has been performed, the suture tension, wound healing rate, and drainage. Clinical judgement should be used to assess these factors.

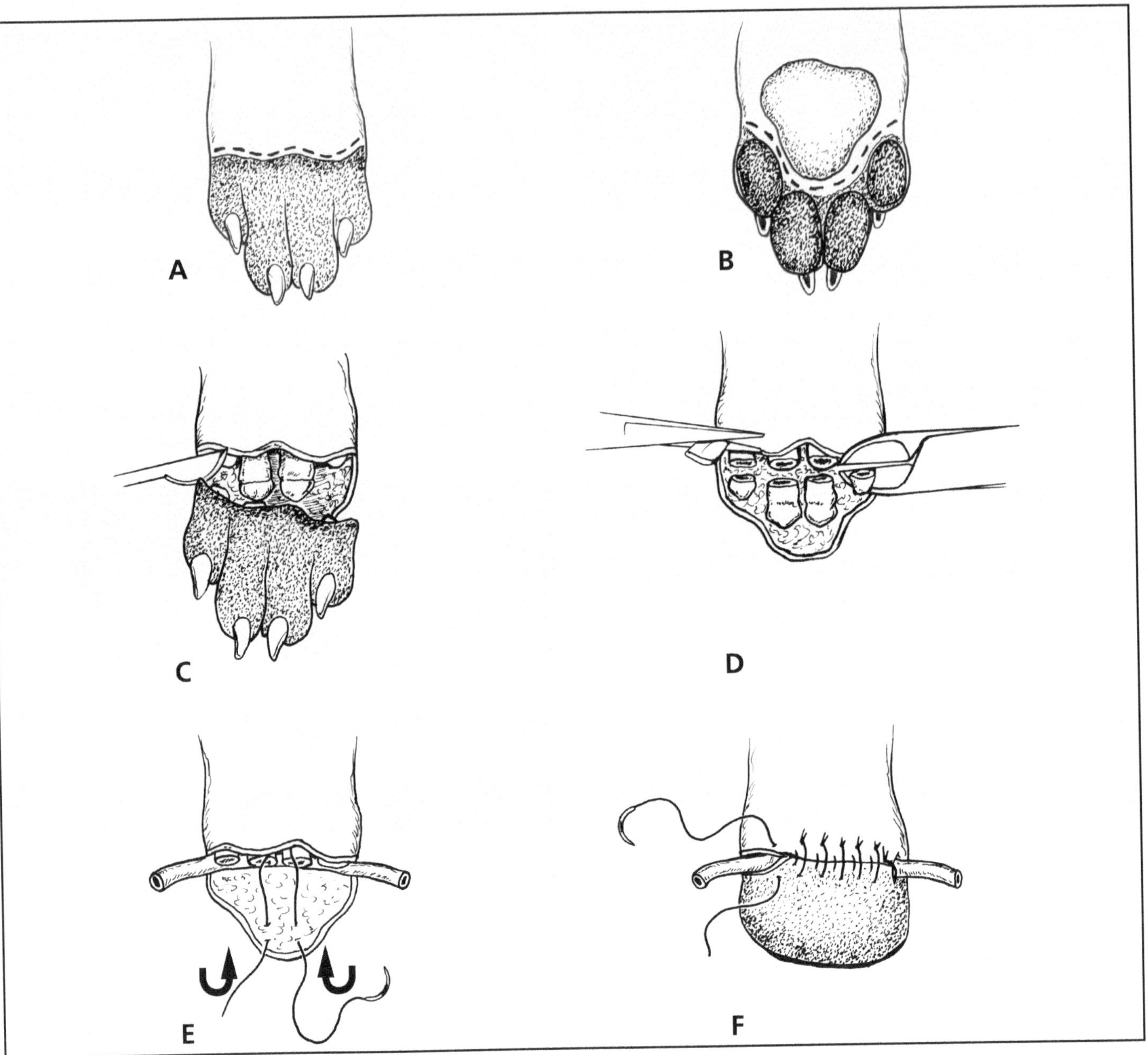


**Figure 6-11.** Proximal pandigital metacarpal/metatarsal-phalangeal amputation. **A.** Transverse incision on the dorsum of the paw just proximal to the demarcation line *(broken line)*. **B.** Incision on the palmar/plantar paw surface at the junction of the metacarpal/metatarsal pad with skin between this pad and the digital pads. **C.** All digits removed. **D.** Metacarpal/metatarsal heads removed. **E.** Penrose drain placed with one of the interrupted horizontal mattress sutures placed to rotate *(arrows)* the pad under the metacarpal/metatarsal bones. **F.** Placing far-near-near-far skin sutures. (After Swaim SF, Henderson RA: Small Animal Wound Management, 2nd ed.: Baltimore: Williams & Wilkins, 1997, 360.)

## Advantages and Disadvantages

Complications following digit amputation include hemorrhage, infection, and dehiscence. When a neoplastic condition has been removed the tumor may recur.

Amputation of one digit usually causes no problem. However, lameness may result if more than 2 digits are removed, or digits 3 or 4 are removed. Low-grade persistent lameness after amputation of digit 3 or 4 may occur with resection through the middle to distal region of the proximal or middle phalanx. This may require a second surgery to remove remnants of the bone. If digits 2 and 5 are removed, leaving digits 3 and 4, animals usually have no problem. However, if digits 3 and 4 are both amputated, leaving digits 2 and 5, the animal may be lame. In addition, removal of the 2 middle digits leaves a space in the center of the paw, and the remaining digits (2 and 5) may be subject to snagging on objects. This can be a problem with working and sporting dogs working in the field. If a dog's paw is relatively small or narrow, it may be possible to fuse digits 2 and 5 after removing 3 and 4, thus eliminating the space in the center of the paw. If all but one digit is amputated, it is best to amputate the one remaining digit to prevent problems with lameness and snagging.

When pandigital amputation and repositioning of the metacarpal/metatarsal pad has been performed without shortening metacarpals/metatarsals 3 and 4, there is increased chance of deep penetration of these bones into the pad, increasing the likelihood of ulceration and discomfort ("bottoming out"). When the procedure has been performed on an animal that has neurological deficits in the operated limb, the animal's gait and limb usage may result in weight not being borne in the center of the transposed pad. Weight may be borne on skin adjacent to the pad as the pad tends to shift out of its intended position with a resultant ulcer in the area. Another reason the transposed pad moves out of position from under the ends of the metacarpal/metatarsal bones is the lack of strong connective tissue attachment to underlying structures which is present in the normal paw.

An attempt can be made to reposition and fix the pad back in the desired position. Sufficient skin may be removed from the area around the pad and ulcer such that when the pad is sutured back to the skin there is enough tension to help hold the pad in place. For additional support, interrupted 2-0 or 3-0 nonabsorbable monofilament sutures may be placed, taking deep bites under the pad in an attempt to anchor it in place to deeper tissues. Repositioning the pad may not be successful in that continual weight-bearing by the animal, especially a large dog, may result in the pad dislocating again.

Another procedure to consider is debridement of the ulcerated area, harvesting pad grafts from other pads on the same dog and placing them in the ulcerated area (Figure 6-12). As the grafts mature and toughen, they tend to withstand the stress the animal places on the area.

# Suggested Readings

1. Bellah JR: Surgical management of specific skin disorders. *In* Slatter DH, ed.: Textbook of Small Animal Surgery, 2nd ed.: Philadelphia, WB Saunders, 1993, 341.
2. Bohling MW, Swaim SF: Paw and distal limb skin reconstruction and salvage techniques. In Bojrab MJ, ed.: Current Techniques in Small Animal Surgery, 5th ed.: Jackson, WY: Teton New Media. 2014, 628.
3. Hedlund CS: Surgery of the integumentary system. *In* Fossum TW, ed.: Small Animal Surgery, 2nd ed.: St. Louis: Mosby, 2002, 134.
4. Hedlund CS: Surgery of the integumentary system. In Fossum TW, ed.: Small Animal Surgery, 3rd ed.: St. Louis: Mosby, 2007, 159.
5. Kapatkin AS, Garcia – Nolan I, Hayashi K: Carpus, metacarpus and digits. In Tobias KM, Johnston SA, eds.: Veterinary Surgery, Small Animal, Vol. 1: St. Louis: Elsevier – Saunders, 2012, 785.

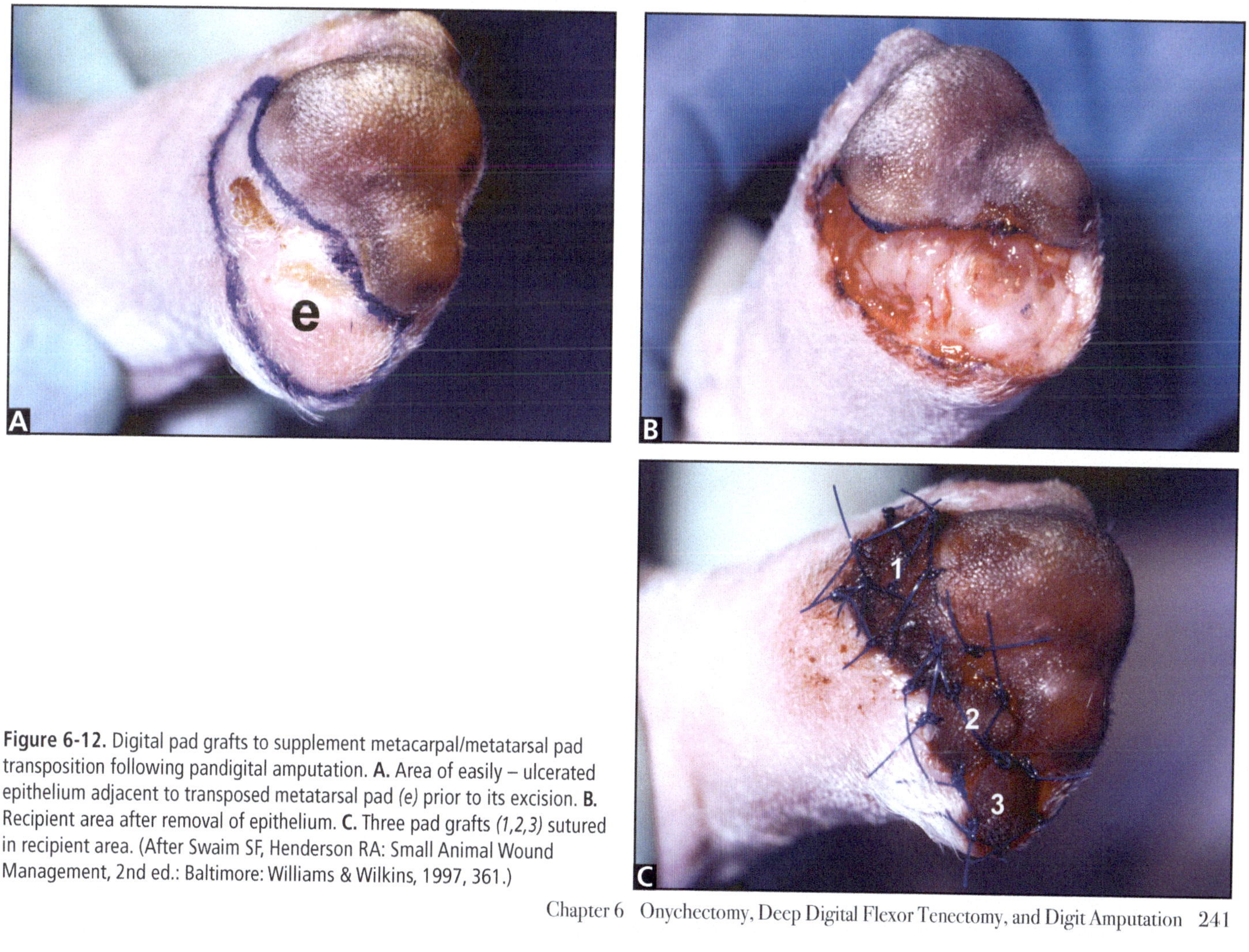


**Figure 6-12.** Digital pad grafts to supplement metacarpal/metatarsal pad transposition following pandigital amputation. **A.** Area of easily – ulcerated epithelium adjacent to transposed metatarsal pad *(e)* prior to its excision. **B.** Recipient area after removal of epithelium. **C.** Three pad grafts *(1,2,3)* sutured in recipient area. (After Swaim SF, Henderson RA: Small Animal Wound Management, 2nd ed.: Baltimore: Williams & Wilkins, 1997, 361.)

6. Kaufman KL, Mann FA: Short- and long-term outcomes after digit amputation in dogs: 33 cases (1999-2011) Jour Am Vet Med Assoc 242: 1249, 2013.
7. MacPhail CM: Surgery of the integumentary system. In Fossum TW, ed.: Small Animal Surgery, 4th ed.: St. Louis: Mosby, 2013, 190.
8. Manley PA: Amputation of the digit. *In* Birchard SJ, Sherding RG, eds.: Saunders Manual of Small Animal Practice, 2nd ed.: Philadelphia: W.B. Saunders, 2000, 1182.
9. Muir P, Pead MJ: Chronic lameness after digit amputation in three dogs. Vet Rec 143:449, 1998.
10. Pavletic MM: Atlas of Small Animal Reconstructive Surgery, 2nd ed.: Philadelphia: W.B. Saunders, 1999, 365.
11. Probst CW, Millis DL: Carpus and digits. *In* Slatter DH, ed.: Textbook of Small Animal Surgery, 3rd ed.: Philadelphia, WB Saunders, 2003, 1974.
12. Rochat MC: Amputation of the digit. In Birchard SJ, Sherding RG, eds.: Saunders Manual of Small Animal Practice, 3rd ed.: St. Louis: Saunders – Elsevier, 2006, 1167.
13. Swaim SF, Garrett PD: Foot salvage techniques in dogs and cats: Options, "do's" and "don'ts". J Am Anim Hosp Assoc 21:511, 1985.
14. Swaim SF, Henderson RA: Small Animal Wound Management, 2nd ed.: Baltimore: Williams and Wilkins, 1997, 295.
15. Swaim SF, Scardino MS: Paw and distal limb salvage and reconstructive techniques. *In* Bojrab MJ, ed.: Current Techniques in Small Animal Surgery, 4th ed.: Williams and Wilkins, 1998, 625.
16. Swaim SF, Renberg WC, Shike KM: Small Animal Bandaging, Casting and Splinting Techniques. Ames, IA Wiley – Blackwell, 2011, 43.
17. White RAS: Surgical treatment of specific skin disorders. *In* Slatter DH, ed.: Textbook of Small Animal Surgery, 3rd ed.: Philadelphia: WB Saunders, 2003, 339.

# Part Two: Orthopedic Injuries

# Chapter 7

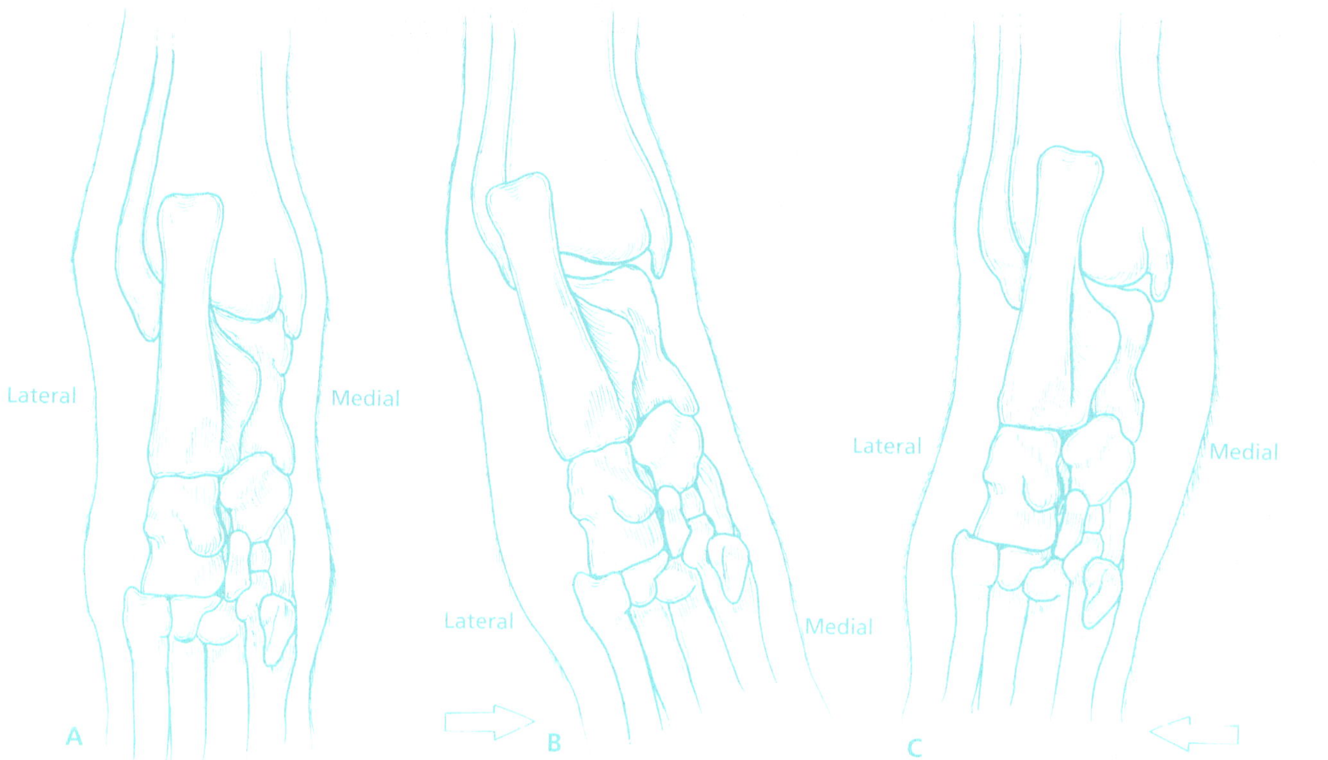


## Orthopedic Injuries of the Tarsal Area

Janet Welch, D.V.M., D.A.C.V.S.

# Introduction

Orthopedic injuries of the distal limbs can involve muscles and tendons, ligaments and bone. Ligamentous injuries often result in significant instability of the tarsal joint or digits. Distal limb fractures that involve an articular surface require prompt and precise repair or, in severest form, arthrodesis to salvage the limb. A review of the pertinent anatomy of orthopedic structures in the distal hind limb follows. The discussion of injuries will be organized according to osseous tissues, ligament, muscle and tendon.

# Anatomy of the Distal Hind Limb

## Osseous Structures

The distal tibia has two grooves that articulate with the ridges of the talus. The medial part of the distal extremity of the tibia is the medial malleolus. The distal fibula forms the lateral malleolus.

The tarsus is composed of seven bones arranged in three irregular rows. The proximal row is composed of a long, laterally located calcaneus and a shorter, medially located talus. The calcaneus is the largest tarsal bone and its proximal half, the tuber calcanei, is the insertion site of the common calcanean tendon. On the medial side of the calcaneus is a projection, the sustentaculum tali. The tendon of the deep digital flexor glides over the plantar surface of this process. The calcaneus articulates with the talus medially and with the fourth tarsal bone distally (Figure 7-1).

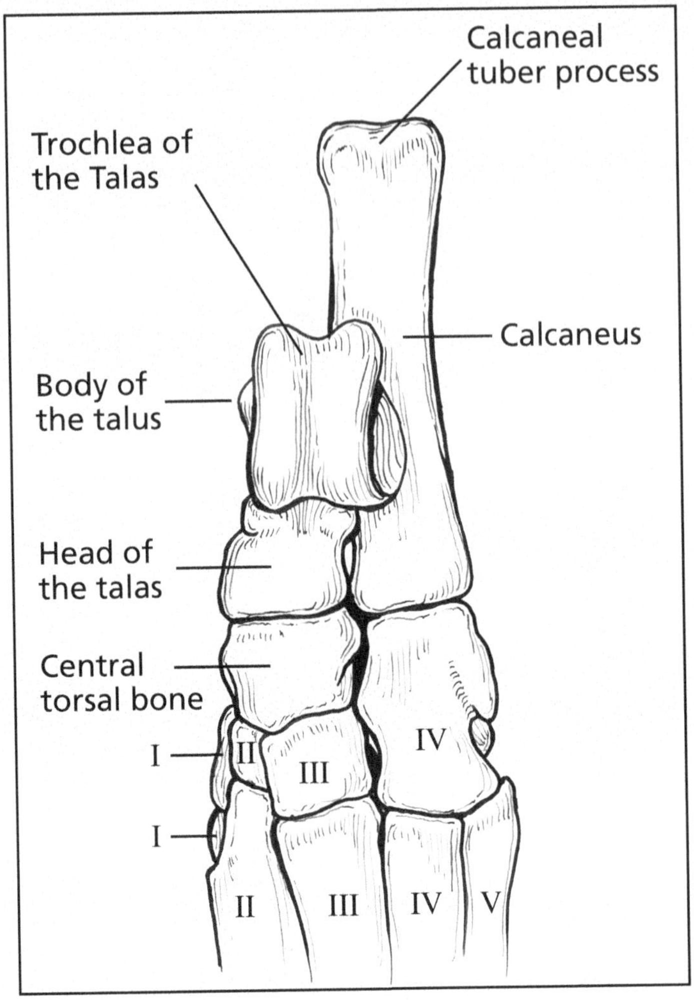

**Figure 7-1.** Osseous structures of the left tarsus, dorsal aspect. Bones are arranged in 3 rows. The talus and calcaneus are proximal, the central and 4th tarsal bones are in the middle, and the first (I) to fourth (IV) tarsal bones are distal. (After Evans HE, Miller's Anatomy of the dog, 3rd ed.: Philadelphia: W B Saunders, 1993).

The talus is the only bone that articulates with the tibia and fibula. It articulates with the tibia and fibula proximally, and with the central tarsal bone distally. The central tarsal bone articulates with all tarsal bones and acts as a buttress or stabilizer for the tarsus. The central tarsal bone lies in the medial part of the tarsus between the proximal and distal rows. The first to third tarsal bones articulate with the central tarsal bone proximally and the metatarsal bones distally. The fourth tarsal bone spans the length of the distal two rows of tarsal bones on the lateral side (See Figure 7-1).

There are 5 metatarsal bones and each is numbered from the medial to the lateral side. Metatarsal bones have 3 anatomic regions. The proximal portion is the base, the midportion is the shaft or body, and the distal portion is the head. The plantar surfaces of metatarsal bones II through IV are covered by the four interosseous muscles. A perforating metatarsal artery passes from the dorsal to plantar side of the paw between metatarsal bones II and III. The primary weight-bearing bones are the third and fourth metatarsal bones and associated digits.

The first metatarsal bone is small and not always present. If present it is typically a small flattened piece of bone attached to a phalanx on the medial aspect of the tarsus and is referred to as the "dew claw." Metatarsal bones II through IV articulate distally with their respective digits. A pair of sesamoid bones is present on the plantar aspect of each metatarsophalangeal joint and are seated in the tendons of insertion of the interosseous muscles. Single smaller dorsal sesamoids are also found at each metatarsophalangeal articulation.

Each of the four main digits (II through V) contains 3 phalanges, referred to as proximal, middle and distal. Each individual phalanx consists of a base proximally and a head distally. Each distal phalanx has a projection of bone from the plantar border of the base which serves as the insertion of the deep digital flexor tendon. The rounded dorsal part of the base is the extensor process on which the common digital extensor tendon inserts. A thin shelf of bone, the ungual crest, overlaps the claw.

## Nomenclature of the Tarsal Joints

The tarsocrural joint is the articulation between the tibia and talus. Distal to this, the tarsus has three levels of joint articulation. The proximal intertarsal joint is more correctly referred to as the calcaneoquartal and talocalcaneocentral joint. The distal intertarsal joint is referred to as the centrodistal joint. The remaining articulation is the tarsometatarsal joint (Figure 7-2).

## Ligaments

The medial and lateral collateral ligaments and the plantar ligaments provide the major ligamentous support for the tarsus. The medial collateral ligament is divided into a long and a short part. The long part originates from the medial malleolus and inserts on the first tarsal bone and the first and second metatarsals. The short part divides and inserts on the talus and first tarsal and metatarsal bones. The lateral collateral ligament also consists of a long and a short part. The long part runs from the lateral malleolus to the base of the fifth metatarsal bone, attaching along its course to the calcaneus and fourth tarsal bones. The short part divides. One band extends to the tuber calcanei and the other goes to the talus (Figure 7-3).

The plantar ligaments are better developed than the ligaments on the dorsal side, allowing them to withstand the tensile stresses exerted on the joint. There are three distinct ligaments: the middle, medial, and lateral plantar ligaments (Figure 7-4).

The ligament between the talus and calcaneus is the talocalcaneal ligament. Numerous short ligaments unite the talus, central tarsal bone, and numbered tarsal bones.

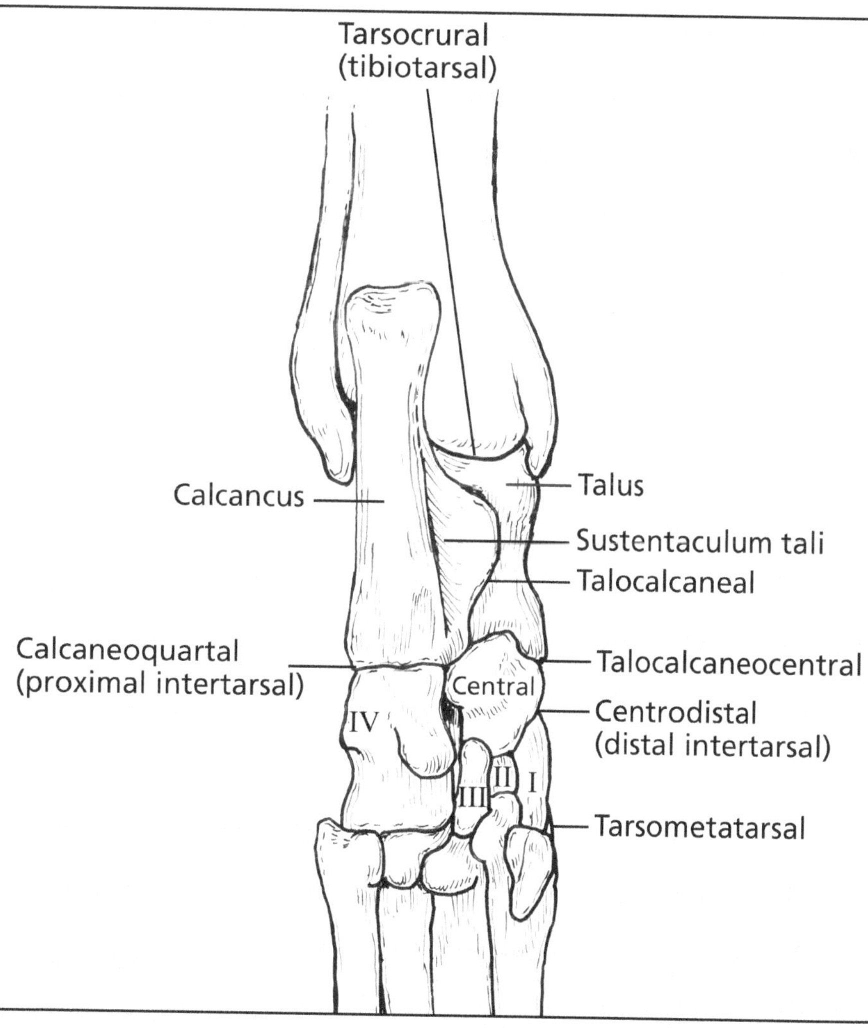


**Figure 7-2.** Left tarsus, plantar aspect. The joint spaces are the tarsocrural, proximal intertarsal (talocalcaneocentral and calcaneoquartal), distal intertarsal (centrodistal) and tarsometatarsal. (After Slatter DH: Textbook of Small Animal Surgery, 2nd ed: W. B. Saunders, 1993).

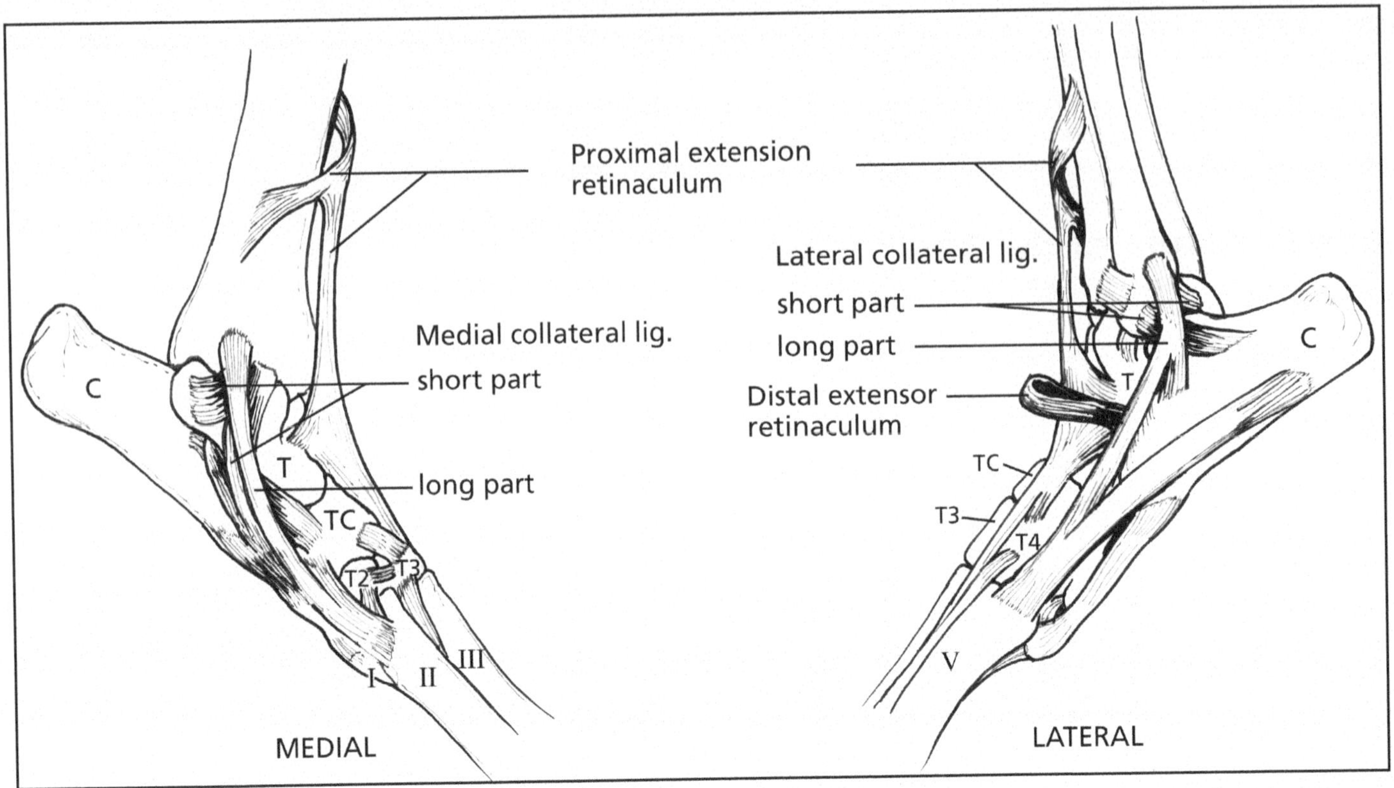


**Figure 7-3.** Left tarsus, medial and lateral aspects. Tarsal ligaments. *T* = talus, *T2, T3, T4* = second, third, fourth tarsal bones. *TC* = central tarsal, *I to V* = metatarsals. (After Evans HE: Miller's Anatomy of the Dog, 3rd ed: Philadelphia: W.B. Saunders, 1993).

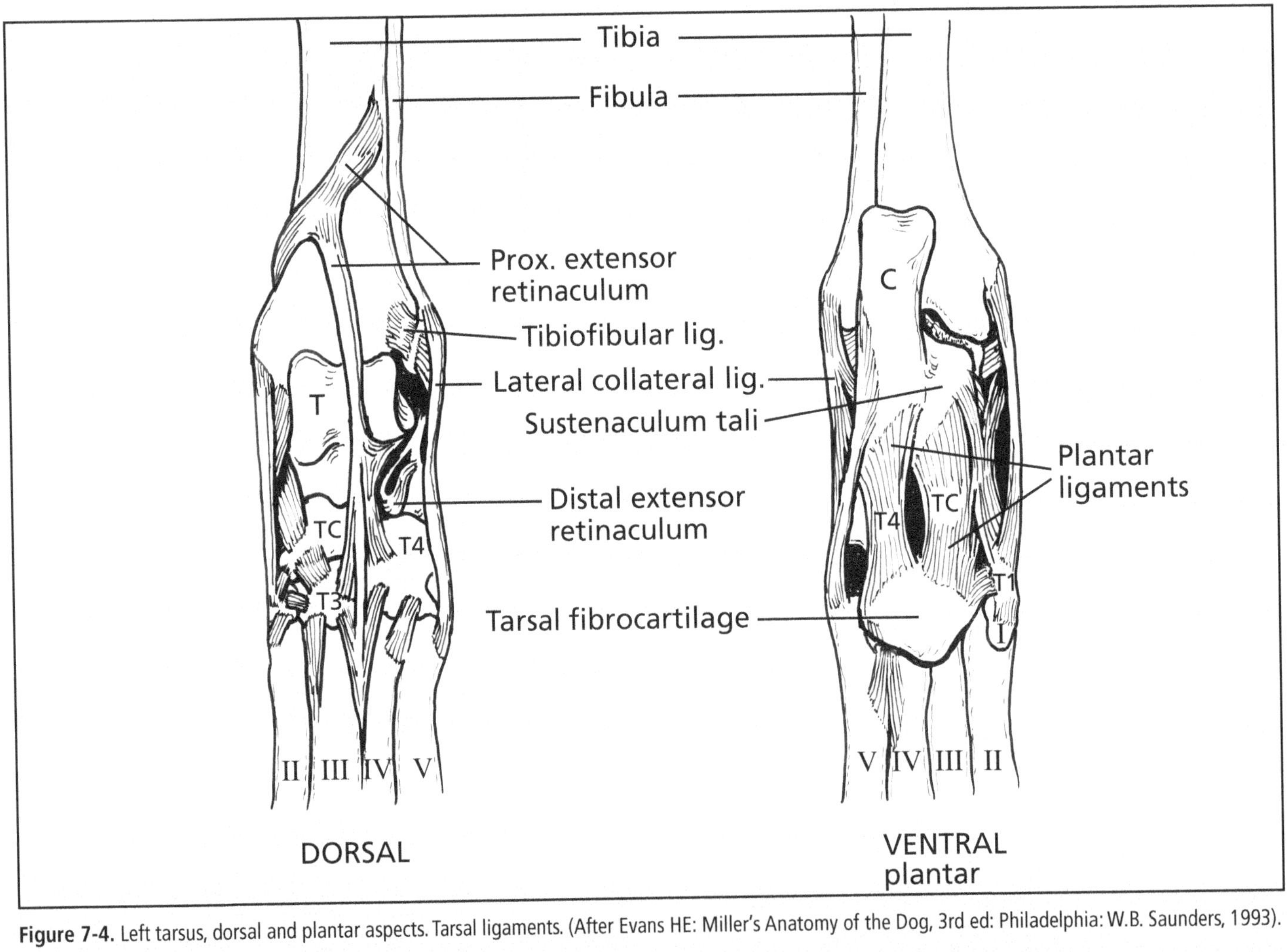


**Figure 7-4.** Left tarsus, dorsal and plantar aspects. Tarsal ligaments. (After Evans HE: Miller's Anatomy of the Dog, 3rd ed: Philadelphia: W.B. Saunders, 1993).

## Tendons

The tendons lying on the dorsal surface of the tarsus are flexors of the tarsus and extensors of the digits. The tendons lying on the plantar surface are extensors of the tarsus and flexors of the digits.

The major tendons located on the plantar surface of the tarsus are the common calcanean tendon and the deep digital flexor tendon. The common calcanean tendon is the most important extensor tendon of the tarsus. The common calcanean tendon is composed of 3 tendons: 1. the gastrocnemius tendon, 2. the combined biceps, gracilis and semitendinosis tendon, and 3. the superficial digital flexor tendon. The gastrocnemius tendon attaches laterally on the calcaneus. The combined tendon of the biceps, gracilis and semitendinosus muscles attaches medially on the calcaneus. The superficial digital flexor tendon caps the tuber calcanei, attaching on each side, and continues distally to insert on the plantar aspect of the second phalanges (Figure 7-5).

The deep digital flexor tendon extends the tarsus and flexes the digits. The deep digital flexor tendon is composed of two parts: the lateral flexor hallucis longus and the medial flexor digitorum longus. At the distal row of tarsal bones, the flexor digitorum longus tendon unites with the flexor hallucis longus. The deep digital flexor tendon inserts on the base of each of the distal phalanges (See Figure 7-5).

The muscles located on the cranial and lateral aspect of the tarsus are, in general, the tarsal joint flexors and digital extensors. These muscles are the cranial tibial, long digital extensor, extensor hallicus longus, peroneus longus, lateral digital extensor and peroneus brevis. The tendon of the cranial tibial muscle inserts on the proximal surface of metatarsals I and II. The long digital extensor tendon originates on the distal femur and inserts on the distal phalanges of digits II, III, IV, and V. The long digital extensor tendon is the most important extensor of the digits. The extensor hallucis longus is a delicate muscle arising from the proximal lateral tibia. Near the distal tibia it becomes a fine tendon that runs between the cranial tibial and long digital extensor tendons and inserts on the second digit. The remaining muscles are referred to as the fibular group: the peroneus longus, lateral digital extensor and peroneus brevis. The peroneus longus tendon inserts on the proximal plantar surface of metatarsals I, II, and V, and acts to rotate the paw laterally. The tendon of the lateral digital extensor runs just in front of the tendon of the peroneus brevis.The peroneus brevis arises from the distal fibula and tibia and its tendon, along with that of the lateral digital extensor, runs in the caudal groove of the lateral malleoulus. The peroneus brevis inserts on the proximal end of metatarsal V. The lateral digital extensor unites with the long digital extensor at the level of the fifth digit (Figure 7-6).

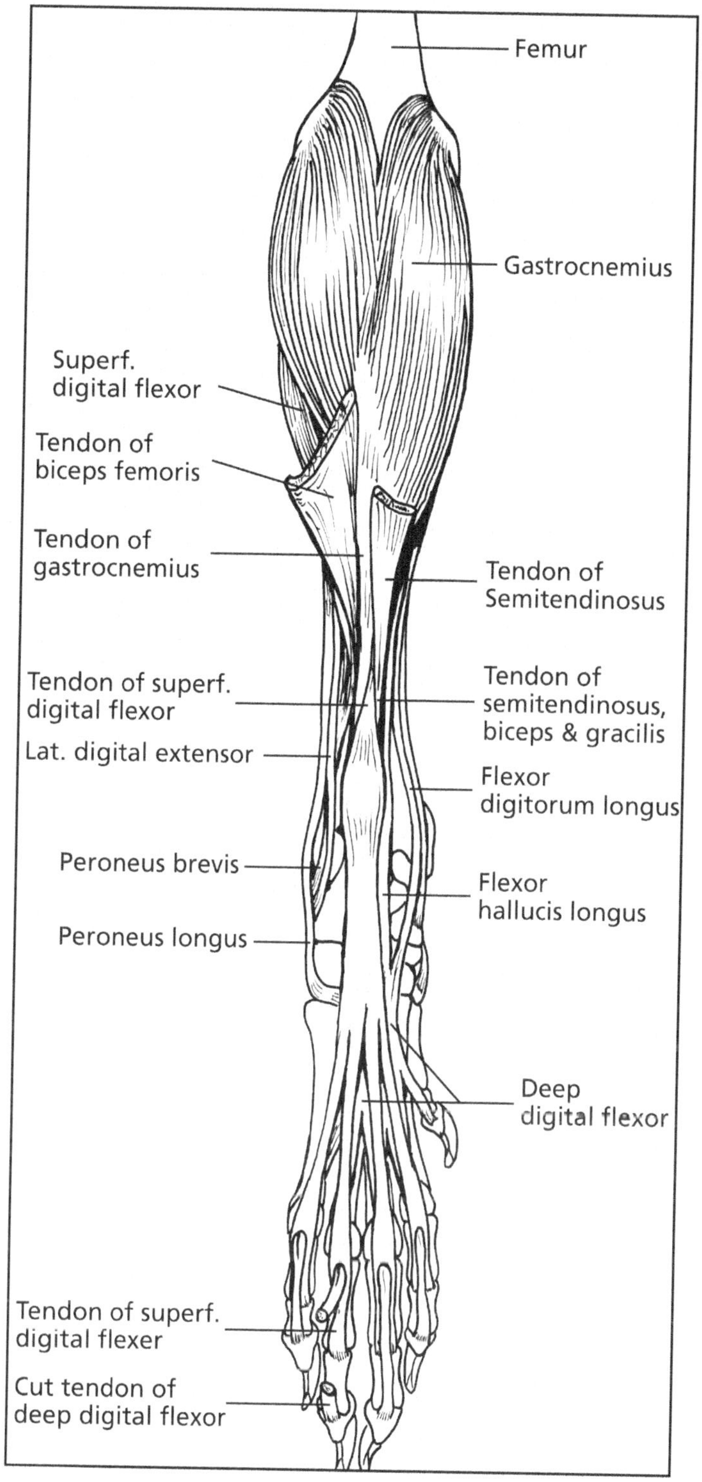


**Figure 7-5.** Tarsus, plantar aspect. Tendons. (After Evans HE: Miller's Anatomy of the Dog, 3rd ed. Philadelphia: W.B. Saunders, 1993).

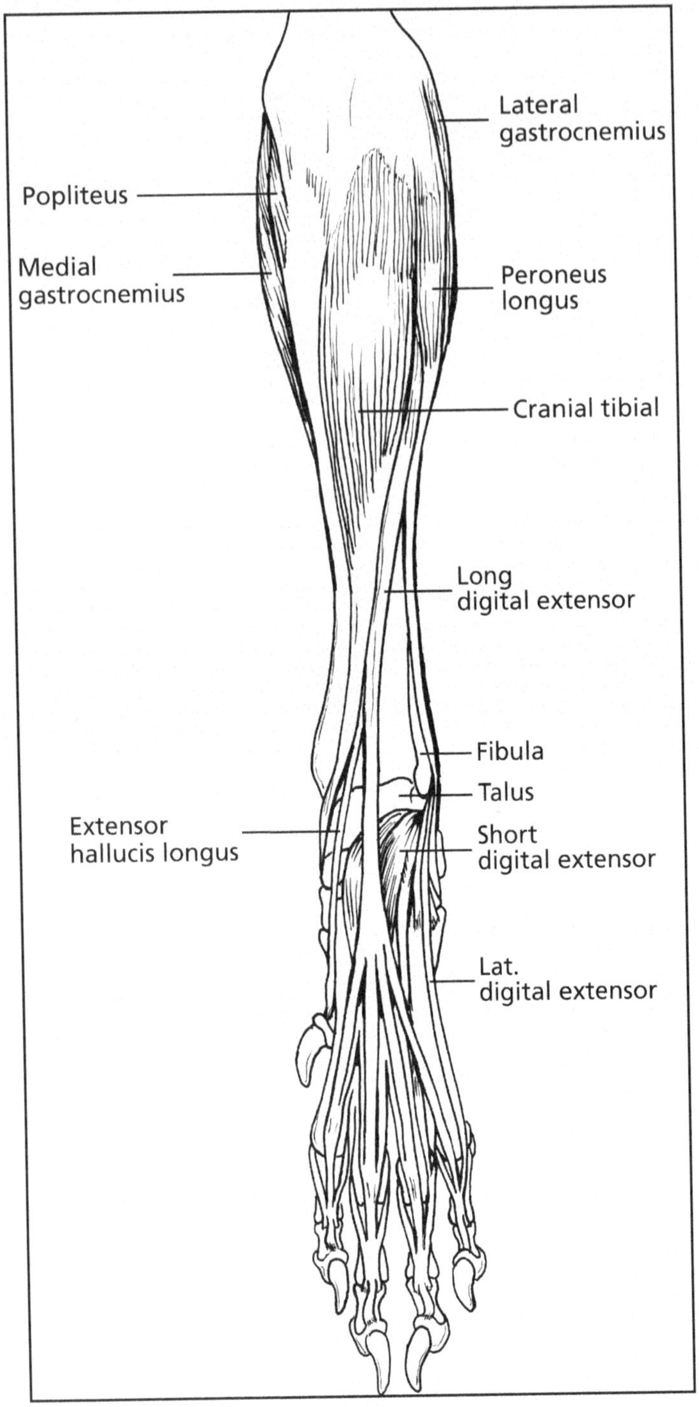


**Figure 7-6.** Tarsus, dorsal aspect. Tendons (After Evans HE: Miller's Anatomy of the Dog, 3rd ed. Philadelphia: W.B. Saunders, 1993).

## Blood Supply

The major blood supply to the hind paw is provided by the cranial tibial artery. This artery is the distal continuation of the popliteal artery and courses between the cranial tibial and long digital extensor muscles. At the level of the tarsocrural joint the cranial tibial artery becomes the dorsal pedal artery which gives rise to dorsal metatarsal arteries and a perforating branch. Just distal to the tarsometatarsal joint, the perforating branch passes in a dorsal to plantar direction between metatarsals II and III. The perforating branch anastomoses with the caudal branch of the saphenous artery to perfuse the plantar surface of the paw.

## Suggested Readings

1. Evans HE, DeLahunta A, Miller ME. Guide to the Dissection of the Dog 5th ed. Philadelphia: W B Saunders, 2000.
2. Evans HE. Miller's Anatomy of the Dog 3rd ed. Philadelphia: Saunders, 1993.

# Ligament and Tendon Injuries

## General Information

Ligaments and tendons are composed of dense groupings of connective tissue consisting primarily of type I collagen. Ligaments connect two or more bones and tendons connect a muscle to a bone. The collagen fibers in ligaments and tendons are crimped so that they can respond to a normal tensile load by stretching. Individual collagen bundles in tendons are surrounded by a loose connective tissue termed endotenon and the entire group of bundles is covered by epitenon. The outermost layer of the tendon unit is the paratenon. Tendons within synovial sheaths lack the typical paratenon.

Tendons surrounded by a paratenon rather than a synovial sheath are able to receive vascular ingrowth more readily when they are damaged. Thus, they can have a better capacity for rapid healing and are referred to as "vascular tendons." Examples of "vascular tendons" are the tendons of insertion of the triceps brachii and gastrocnemius muscles. Examples of sheathed tendons include digital flexor tendons. Sheathed tendons depend on intrinsic blood supply for healing.

When injured, both ligaments and tendons undergo inflammatory, reparative, and maturation phases of healing. However, the dense, organized collagenous structure of tendons and ligaments requires a sustained maturation phase. During the maturation phase, type III collagen is replaced by mechanically superior type I collagen. Water content decreases and collagen fibers become more densely packed and appropriately aligned. As fibers become closer in proximity, there is increased surface area available for cross linking, which improves tensile strength. Tendons and ligaments heal poorly if a gap is present in the tissue. A large gap results in excessive scar tissue formation and obstructs histologically normal collagen bundles from bridging the repair site. The alignment of collagen bundles becomes more organized as the tissue is subjected to stretching forces, but this cannot be instituted too soon after surgery or a gap will be created.

# Sprain Injury

## General Information

Ligamentous injury is referred to as a sprain. A sprain is classified as grade 1 (mild), grade 2 (moderate) and grade 3 (severe). Most grade 2 and all grade 3 injuries require surgical intervention.

## Definition and Indications

### Grade 1 Sprain

A grade 1 injury involves overstretching of the ligament without disruption. Microscopically there is hemorrhage, stretching and tearing of collagen fibers. Clinically there is minimal lameness with mild to moderate soft tissue swelling in the region of the joint. The region is tender on palpation. Treatment options indicated for a first degree sprain include cold therapy, a period of restricted activity, and nonsteroidal anti-inflammatory drugs (NSAIDs) (see techniques).

### Grade 2 Sprain

A grade 2 sprain is a partial ligament rupture. Although there is still continuity of the ligament, the strength is substantially reduced. With this injury, there is more extensive swelling and obvious lameness. There is distinct pain on palpation and resistance to manipulation. Radiographs show soft tissue swelling but bony lesions are rarely seen and instability is not apparent without taking stress radiographs. Treatment options/indications for grade 2 sprains include cold therapy, restricted activity, NSAIDs, chondroprotective agents and splint immobilization. Surgical stabilization is usually indicated for normal function if instability is present on stress radiographs (see techniques). To some degree, the size and activity of a patient influences the need for surgery. A small sedentary animal with a grade 2 sprain may have a satisfactory outcome if treated non-surgically.

### Grade 3 Sprain

A grade 3 sprain is complete disruption of all collagen fibers. The lameness is severe and often non-weight-bearing. There is gross swelling which may involve the entire paw. There is extreme pain on manipulation that is frequently accompanied by crepitus or abnormal mobility. On radiographs bony lesions are frequently present and small avulsion fractures are common. Subluxation may be detected on survey radiographs, but if not, it is evident with stress radiographs (Figure 7-7A, B & C). Treatment options/indications for grade 3 sprains include immediate bandaging for immobilization and comfort, analgesics, chondroprotective agents, and surgical stabilization. Cold therapy can also be applied before and after surgery (see techniques).

## Techniques

## Diagnosis and Nonsurgical Treatment for Sprain Injury

### Stress Radiographs

Stress radiography is done by applying a controlled force on a joint to demonstrate joint instability. The examiner is protected with appropriate lead attire and the animal is given appropriate sedation and analgesia

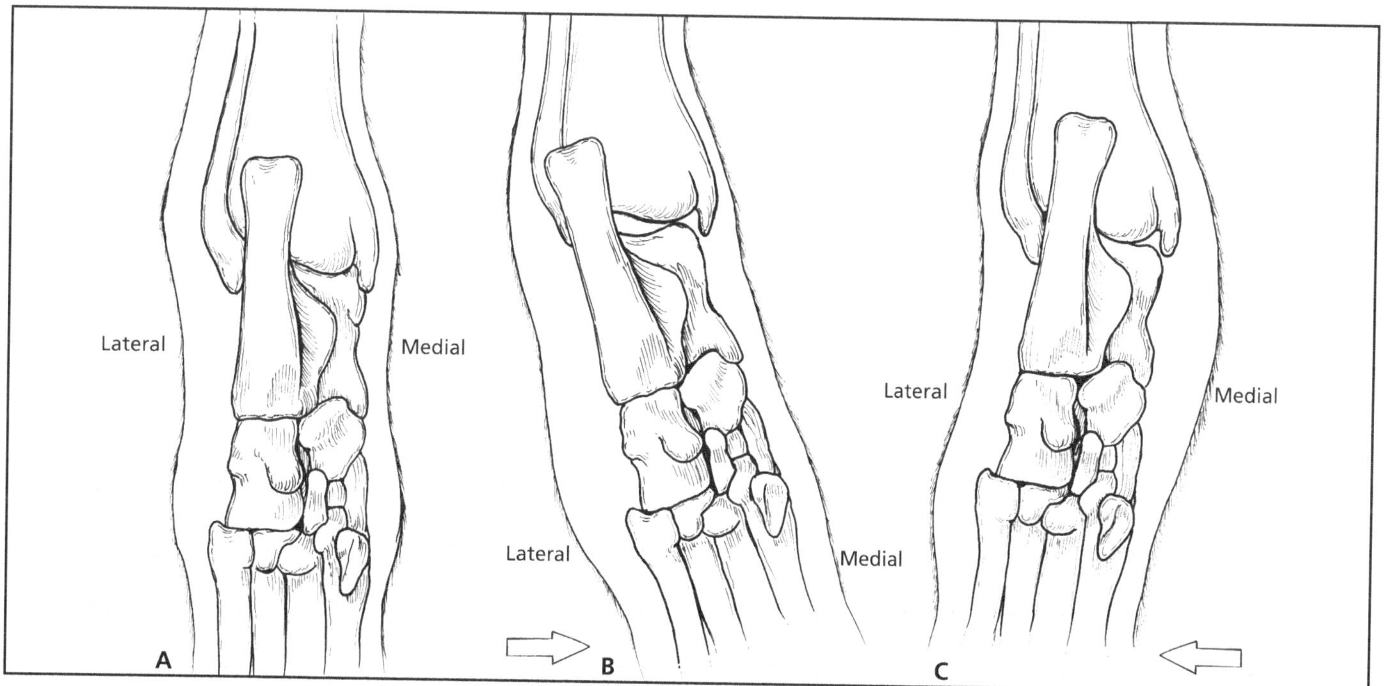


**Figure 7-7.** Stress radiography to check for sprain injury. **A.** Normal position of the tarsus. **B.** Varus stress: metatarsals are pulled medially to check for lateral instability. **C.** Valgus stress: metatarsals are pulled laterally to check for medial instability.

to obtain the radiographs. To test for medial instability of the tarsal joint, the limb is positioned for a cranial-caudal view. The proximal tibia is stabilized with the upper hand, and the distal metatarsals are grasped with the lower hand. A valgus force is placed on the joint by directing the metatarsals laterally. The radiograph is taken and evaluated for excessive opening of the joint surfaces. To test for lateral instability, the tarsus is positioned and held in the same way. The examiner applies a varus stress by pulling the metatarsals medially (See Figure 7-7).

### Cold Therapy

Cold therapy is used during the acute phase of sprain or strain injury; typically for the first 1-2 days following a sprain. The physiologic effects of cold therapy include reduction of edema through vasoconstriction, reduced blood flow and reduced cellular metabolism. Cold therapy also promotes analgesia through decreased nerve conduction velocity and increased duration of the refractory period, the time when a nerve cannot be stimulated by a second impulse.

A common method of applying cold therapy is with ice packs. These can be homemade or manufactured. To make a homemade ice pack, a freezer bag is filled with crushed ice, wrapped in a thin damp cloth (such as a pillowcase), and directly applied over the affected area. Cold packs can also be prepared by mixing 3 parts water to 1 part rubbing alcohol, double bagging with sealed bags, and placing in the freezer prior to application. A slush forms and can be molded around irregular body parts. To prevent skin damage, a towel or cloth is placed between the skin and the ice pack. Commercial cold packs come in different forms. Packs that freeze solid cool the skin more than frozen gel packs, which contain gelatin or antifreeze to make them more moldable. Commercial ice packs are also manufactured in sheets that may be trimmed to fit the extremity and secured with elastic wrap or used with commercial custom-designed wraps (Canineicer, www.canineicer.com).

Cold packs are applied for approximately 20 minutes at a time. Cold therapy treatments are given 3 to 6 times daily during the first 1-2 days after injury. Skin is observed for response to cold therapy. Near the end of a 20 minute session it is normal for skin to appear erythmatous but pale or white skin indicates excessive cold-induced change. Caution is advised with the water-alcohol mix during longer application because there is an increased potential for cold-induced injury.

### Heat Therapy

When the period of acute inflammation has subsided heat therapy is substituted for cold therapy. The purpose of heat application is to vasodilate cutaneous blood vessels. Heat therapy also induces muscle relaxation by decreasing the firing rate of type II muscle spindles and increasing the firing rate of type II fibers of the golgi tendon organs.

Heat can be applied using homemade hotpacks consisting of moistened heated hand towels. Commercial packs can deliver heat for a longer period of time and can function either as cold or hot compresses (www.canineicer.com; FlexiPAC Chattanooga Group Inc, Hixson TN). Heat is applied for 20 minutes 3 to 6 times daily.

Heat therapy is contraindicated during acute inflammation, over an area of subcutaneous or cutaneous hemorrhage, thrombophlebitis, acute edema, or over open wounds.

### Bandaging

Bandaging the limb can reduce edema by compressing lymphatics and blood vessels to limit fluid efflux into the interstitium. A grade 2 or 3 sprain is initially immobilized with a soft padded bandage. If cold therapy is going to be provided, frequency is reduced to correspond with daily bandage changes. A bandage for tarsocrural stability would extend from the digits to the proximal tibia. The bandage must leave only the distal end of middle 2 digits visible since bandages that begin proximal to the digits can have a tourniquet effect. The digits are monitored for increase in swelling. Swelling can indicate that the bandage is too tight and should be changed or removed. A "donut – type" pad of cast padding can be placed over the point of the hock within the bandage to prevent a pressure wound over the point of the hock.

When acute swelling has subsided, a supportive splint may be applied. The splint bandage consists of cast padding (Specialist cast padding, Johnson and Johnson, New Brunswick, NJ), elastic roll gauze (Kling, Sof-Kling conforming bandage, Ethicon, Somerville, NJ) a fiberglass splint, (Delta-Lite and Delta-Lite C splint; BSN Medical, Charlotte, NC) and a tertiary layer of elastic bandage wrap (Vetwrap, 3M, St. Paul, MN) or porous white tape (Zonas tape, Johnson and Johnson, New Brunswick, NJ; Curity Tape, Covidien, Mansfield, MA). The duration of splinting depends on the level of injury.

To apply the splint, the animal is sedated and placed in lateral recumbency. Tape stirrups of 1 inch-wide adhesive tape are applied to the medial and lateral or dorsal and plantar aspects of the limb. Three to 4 layers of cast padding are applied, beginning at the digits and continuing up to the proximal tibia, with about 50% overlap of the preceding wrap. Next, 2 layers of elastic roll gauze are applied. The tape stirrups are twisted and reflected to be placed adhesive side on the bandage. Next, the splint is made from synthetic casting tape and placed on the lateral aspect of the distal limb. The width of casting tape is selected according to the animal's size – 2 inches for cats and small dogs and 3 inches for medium to large dogs. The casting tape is removed from the package and immersed briefly in cold water. Excess water is squeezed from the casting tape and it is unrolled to form a multi-layered splint of the desired length. The splint is placed on the medial or lateral side; according to the location of the sprain. After it has hardened, an additional layer of elastic gauze is placed on top of the splint to stabilize it. A final protective layer of elastic bandage wrap or 2 inch wide adhesive tape is placed (Figure 7-8A through F).

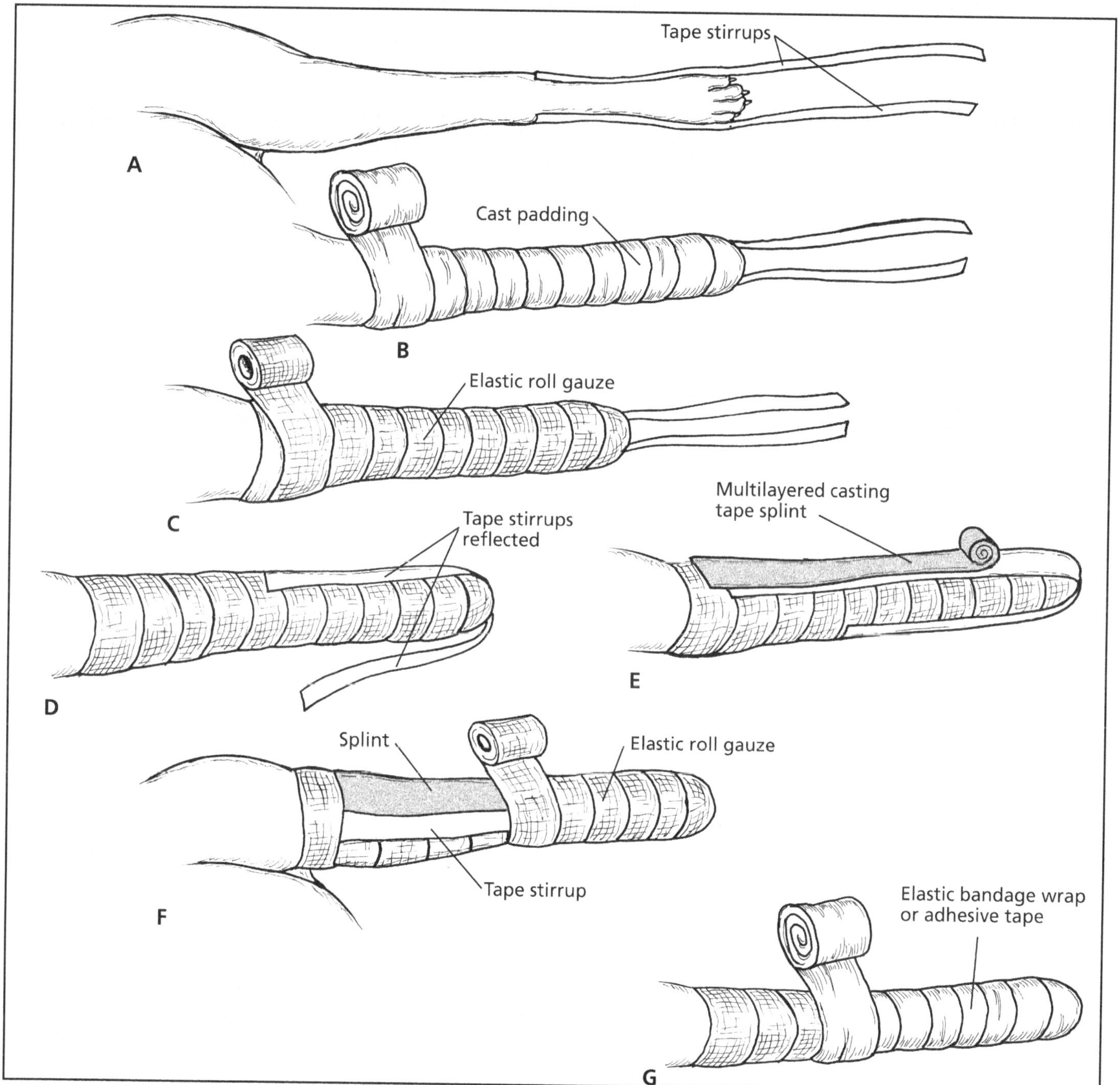


**Figure 7-8.** Application of a distal limb splint. **A.** Tape stirrups of 1 inch-wide adhesive tape are applied to the medial and lateral aspects of the paw. **B.** Three to 4 layers of cast padding are applied, from the digits to the proximal tibia, with about 50% overlap of the preceding wrap. **C.** Two layers of elastic roll gauze are applied. **D.** The tape stirrups are twisted and reflected to be placed adhesive side down on the bandage. **E.** A multilayered synthetic casting tape splint is placed on the lateral aspect of the distal limb. **F.** An additional layer of elastic gauze is placed on top of the splint to stabilize it. A final protective layer of bandage material (Vet-wrap or 2-inch white tape) is placed.

### Nonsteroidal Anti-Inflammatory Drugs

There are several available choices for nonsteroidal anti-inflammatory drugs (NSAIDs). Generally, cyclooxygenase 2 (COX 2) targeted NSAIDs are chosen. One method for administering NSAIDS for a sprain injury is to give a full dose for 1 to 2 weeks, a half dose for 1 to 2 weeks, and then taper as needed.

### Chondroprotective Agents

Chondroprotective agents are available in oral and injectable forms. Injectable polysuflated glycosaminoglycan (Adequan, Novartis Animal Health US) has been shown to reach the synovial fluid within 2 hours after intramuscular injection and remain in the joint for 3 days. The author uses a dose of 4.4 mg/kg intramuscularly (IM) or subcutaneously (SQ) twice weekly for 4 weeks, then once every 2 to 4 weeks. Polysufated glycosaminoglycan has been shown to inhibit destructive inflammatory enzymes within joints and to stimulate cartilage matrix production and hyaluronan production. This medication can be initiated shortly after significant sprain injury and continued throughout the healing process.

Oral chondroprotective agents containing both glucosamine and chondroitin (Cosequin, Nutramax Laboratories, Edgewood, Md) have been shown to decrease inflammation and improve cartilage matrix within joints. Oral chondroprotective agents are administered at a loading dose for the first 4 to 6 weeks and then decreased to a maintenance dose.

## General Information

Complete rupture or avulsion of the collateral ligaments is a grade 3 sprain. This type of injury significantly destabilizes the tarsocrural joint. Medial injuries allow valgus (lateral) deviation of the foot, and lateral injuries allow varus (medial) angulation.

Ruptured ligaments may be primarily repaired using suture patterns such as the locking loop. This alone is an unreliable method of repair because the ligament tends to be extensively frayed with a "crabmeat" appearance. In this circumstance, a prosthetic imbrication technique is useful. This technique anchors non-absorbable suture at the origin and insertion of the ligament using either screws and washers or suture anchors. The suture material provides initial stability and serves as a template for fibroplasia to provide long term stability. A prosthetic imbrication technique can be used as the primary method of repair or can be placed in addition to a locking loop or other suture pattern to provide additional stability.

## Surgical Treatment of Sprain Injuries

Ligament repairs are stabilized postoperatively. A soft padded bandage and splint that extends from the digits to the proximal tibia is placed for 4 to 6 weeks and changed weekly. When the splint is removed a soft padded bandage is placed for 2 weeks.

If areas of pressure irritation are identified during splint changes the position of the splint can be moved. A lateral splint can be moved to the medial side or an area of irritation over a bony prominence such as the tuber calcanei can be covered with a "donut" of bandage material to relieve pressure.

A transarticular external fixator can be placed in lieu of a splint for postoperative stabilization. External fixation provides such rigid immobilization that it should not be kept on for too long and should be managed in a way that gradually confers more movement to the joint. An external fixator can be static or hinged (see Transarticular External Fixation of the Tarsus pgs. 299-305). A hinged external fixator can be locked down initially then loosened to provide controlled motion and a static external fixator can be replaced with a splint and soft padded bandage after 3 to 4 weeks.

Exercise is limited to controlled leash walks for the first 12 weeks after grade 3 sprain repair then gradually increased to normal levels over the next month. Nonsteroidal anti-inflammatory drugs may be administered on a tapering dosage schedule for 2 to 4 weeks after surgery. Glucosamine-chondroitin supplements may be prescribed for 12 to 16 weeks or longer.

Surgical repair of isolated rupture of the short medial or short lateral collateral ligaments is protected with a soft padded bandage and splint for 4 weeks followed by a soft padded bandage alone for 2 weeks.

## Advantages and Disadvantages

The locking loop suture is a simple and straightforward technique for approximating the ends of a torn ligament. Tissues are usually so damaged that this cannot be relied upon as the only method of repair and it is supplemented with prosthetic imbrication. This added step greatly increases the security of the repair.

Suture anchors have advantages over screws and washers for this surgery. Suture anchors eliminate the risk of the suture slipping off, which can occur when using screws and washers. Suture anchors have a lower profile than screws and washers and thus may induce less irritation of surrounding soft tissues. The advantage of using nylon fishing or leader line is that it is historically effective and inexpensive. There are newer versions of synthetic suture material composed of polyethylene or polyethylene and polyester that have increased strength and stiffness in laboratory testing compared with nylon (FiberWire, Arthrex Vet Systems, Bonita Springs, FL, OrthoFiber, Securos Inc., Fiskdale, MA). These materials also create a smaller knot. However differences in testing between sutures may not equate to different outcomes in this application.

Placing an external fixator is more invasive than placing a splint and can induce greater cartilage damage by rigidly immobilizing the joint and thereby decreasing nutrient diffusion into the cartilage. Immobilization by an external fixator for 4 weeks reduces cartilage proteoglycan. The proteoglycan content does increase after remobilization but cartilage damage occurs with rapid, sudden remobilization of joints. Progressive remobilization helps to preserve cartilage integrity and can be accomplished by converting from an external fixator, to a splint, to a soft padded bandage and then no bandage with controlled exercise.

## Diagnosis and Surgical Treatment of Rupture of Both Short and Long Medial and Lateral Collateral Ligaments

### Stress Radiographs

Diagnosis is based on physical examination and stress radiographs. Subluxations may not be seen on standard lateral and craniocaudal radiographs and stress radiography is indicated for full evaluation of joint stability. The examiner applies a valgus stress to show medial collateral ligament rupture and a varus stress to show lateral collateral ligament rupture (See Figure 7-7). A widened joint space indicates collateral ligament instability.

### Locking Loop Suture Pattern

The locking loop pattern creates 4 loops of suture that grasp bundles of tissue when the suture is tightened. There are transverse and longitudinal components to this pattern. To allow the loops to tighten on the ligament bundles, the transverse component must be superficial to the longitudinal one. The first pass of the suture is transverse. This pass is begun on one of the stumps of ligament approximately 1 cm from the torn edge. The suture is passed in a medial to lateral direction. The second pass of the suture is longitudinal. The needle re-enters the ligament directly behind the first entry site of the suture. The needle is directed distally deep to the transverse portion and then parallel to the fibers of the ligament. It exits at the end and then enters the opposite side of the ligament and the pattern is repeated to form the 4 locking loops (Figure 7-9A, B & C). The 2 ends of the suture are tightly tied. The suture material is size 2-0 to 0 in a medium-to large dog. A smooth surface suture material such as nylon or polypropylene is chosen to allow free gliding through the ligament as the knot is tightened. If desired interrupted or horizontal mattress sutures of absorbable 2-0 to 3-0 suture may be placed at the tendon edges. It is possible in larger ligaments to place 2 locking loop patterns side by side. This provides a stronger repair than placing a single suture (Figure 7-10).

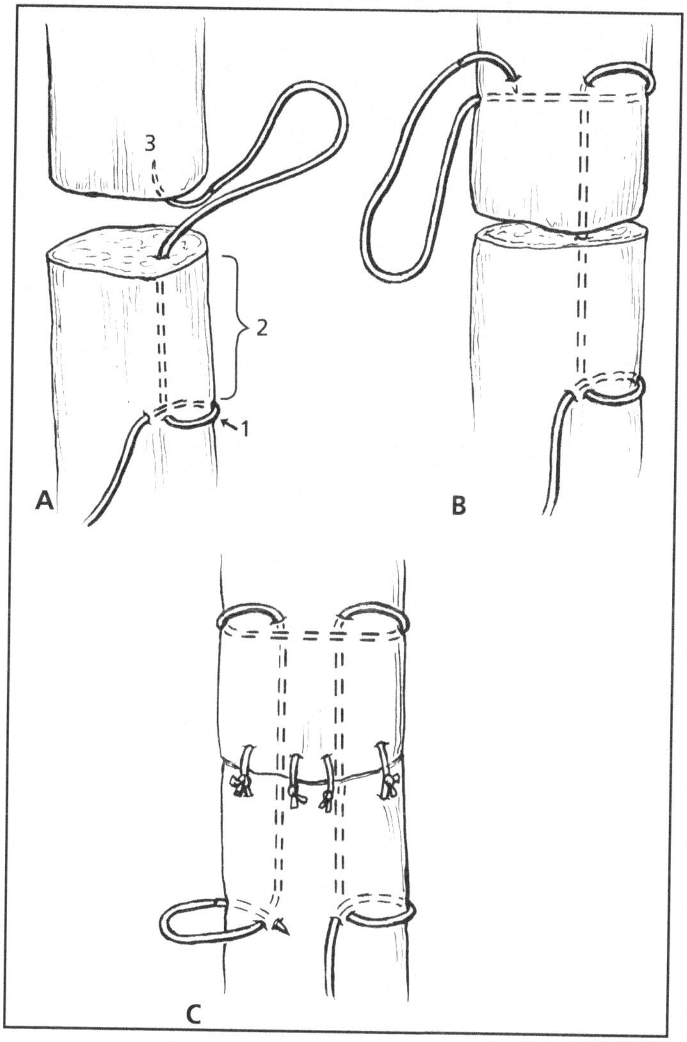


**Figure 7-9.** Locking loop suture. The locking loop pattern has transverse and longitudinal components. To allow the loops to tighten on the ligament bundles, the transverse component must be superficial to the longitudinal one. **A.** The first pass of the suture is transverse. This pass is begun approximately 1 cm from the torn edge of the ligament *(1)*. The second pass of the suture is longitudinal. The needle re-enters the ligament directly behind the first pass of the suture. The needle is directed deep to the transverse portion and then parallel to the fibers of the ligament. The needle enters the opposite side of the ligament. **B.** A longitudinal suture is placed in the opposite side of the ligament followed by a transverse suture. **C.** The pattern is repeated to form the 4 locking loops. Interrupted sutures may be placed between tendon ends to improve apposition. (After Aron D N. A "new" tendon stitch. J Am Anim Hosp Assoc 17:587, 1981).

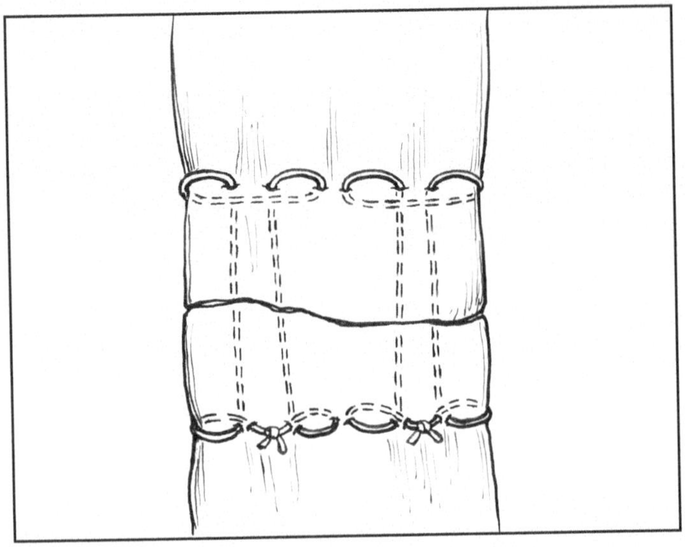

Figure 7-10. Double locking loop suture. Two locking loop suture patterns may be placed side by side in larger ligaments.

### Prosthetic Imbrication

The prosthetic imbrication technique anchors heavy gauge monofilament suture at the origin and insertion of the ligament using either screws and washers or suture anchors. The suture material provides initial stability and serves as a template for fibroplasia to provide long term stability. There are several types of suture anchors designed for use in veterinary patients. (Imex Veterinary, Inc., Longview, TX; Securos Veterinary Orthopedics, Charlton, MA; Arthrex Vet Systems, Bonita Springs, FL). Suture anchors look similar to traditional bone screws in that they have a threaded shaft, but are equipped with a hole at the top for passage of suture material. Most products have specialized screw drivers that fit the suture anchors and are used to implant the device into bone. Traditional screws and washers can also be used as anchor points for suture instead of specialized suture anchors. The suture is a heavy gauge non-absorbable such as 50 to 80 pound test fishing line. Polyethylene blends of suture are also available (FiberWire, Arthrex, Inc., Naples, FL; OrthoFiber, Securos, Inc., Fiskdale, MA).

### Prosthetic Imbrication for Both Short and Long Medial Collateral Ligament Rupture of the Tarsus

The patient is positioned in lateral recumbency with the affected limb down to expose the medial surface. The skin incision is centered over the medial surface of the tarsocrural joint. It extends from the distal fourth of the tibia to the level of the tarsometatarsal joint. The subcutaneous tissue and crural fascia are incised on the same line as the skin and are retracted with the skin. The short and long collateral ligaments are inspected to ascertain the extent of injury. The proximal and distal portions of the ruptured collateral ligaments are usually too damaged to suture together. The medial portion of the talus is exposed by incising the joint capsule (Figure 7-11).

A double prosthetic imbrication technique is used. This technique anchors suture from the origin of the collateral ligament to the distal insertions of both the long and the short portions of the collateral ligament. To place suture anchors, the origin of the medial collateral ligament is located just proximal to the medial malleolus. The surgeon must be aware that the malleolus extends 1 to 2 cm distal to the tarsocrural joint space. The origin anchor is placed as distally in the tibia as possible, without invading the joint space, and just cranial to the midline. For the medial short ligament insertion site, the anchor is placed in the proximal plantar aspect of the medial talus. This anchor should appear to be slightly distal and plantar to the origin anchor. The anchor for the long ligament insertion is placed at the plantar base of the talus. Suture size is chosen according to the size of the animal (Figure 7-12). The suture is a heavy gauge non-absorbable such as 50 to 80 pound test fishing line. Suture from the origin anchor is tied to suture from the short ligament insertion site anchor with the joint in 90 degrees of flexion. Next suture from the origin anchor is tied to suture from the long ligament insertion anchor with the joint held at a normal standing angle. The incision is closed in layers with absorbable suture.

This technique can be performed using screws and metal washers instead of suture anchors. The origin screw is angled 20 degrees proximally to avoid invading the joint (Figure 7-13). The landmarks for placing the screws are as described for suture anchors. The suture is anchored beneath each metal washer. The strand of suture corresponding to the short collateral ligament is tightened with the tarsocrural joint held in 90 degrees of flexion and that for the long ligament is tightened with the joint held at a normal standing angle. Complete tightening of each screw is performed after the suture is tied.

### Prosthetic Imbrication for Both Short and Long Lateral Collateral Ligament Rupture of the Tarsus

Prosthetic imbrication repair for rupture of the lateral collateral ligaments is based on the same premise as medial collateral ligament repair. The suture is anchored at the origin and insertion sites for the long and short collateral ligaments. The patient is positioned in lateral recumbency with the affected limb up. The skin incision is centered over the lateral surface of the tarsocrural

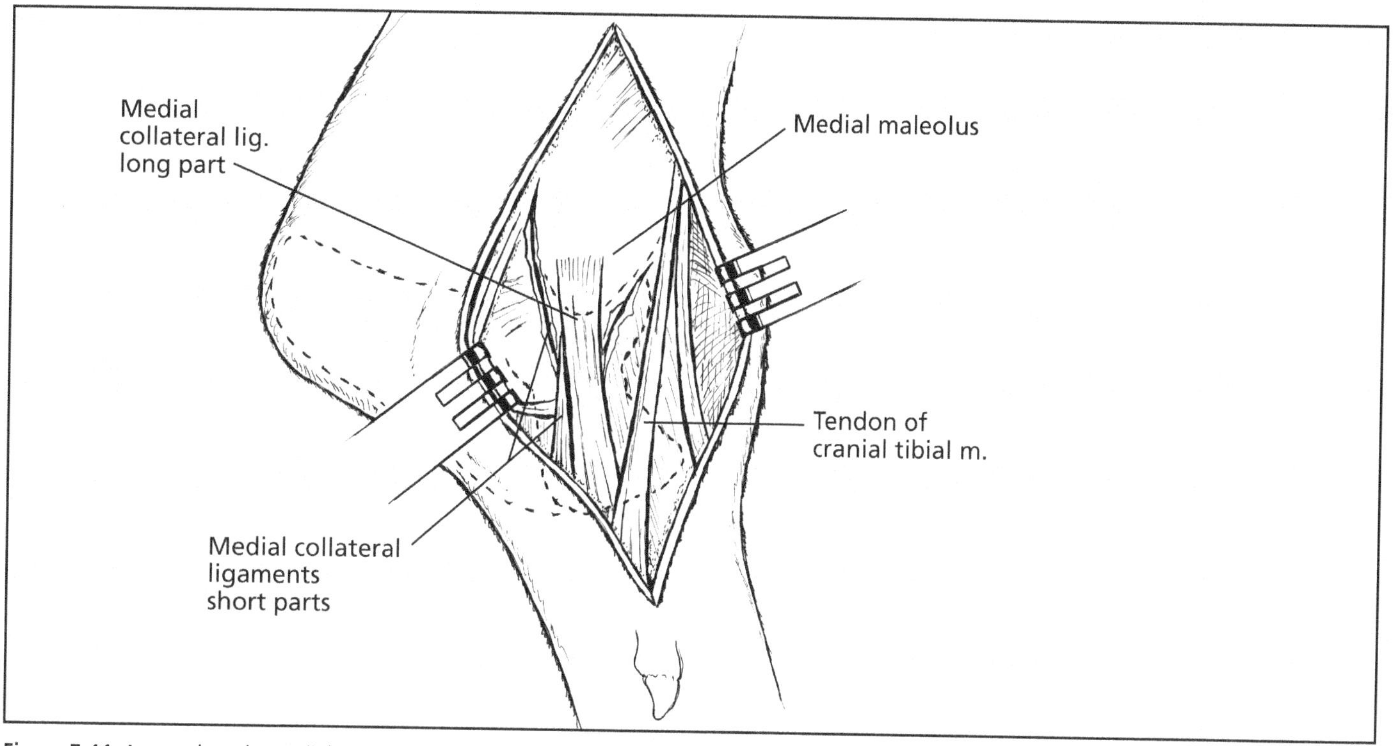


**Figure 7-11.** Approach to the medial tarsal bones. The skin incision is centered over the medial surface of the tarsocrural joint. It extends from the distal fourth of the tibia to the level of the tarsometatarsal joint. The subcutaneous tissue and crural fascia are incised on the same line as the skin and are retracted with the skin. The medial collateral ligaments are visualized. (After Piermattei DL, Johnson KA. An Atlas of Surgical Approaches to the Bones and Joints of the Dog and Cat 4th ed. Philadelphia: Saunders, 2004, 389).

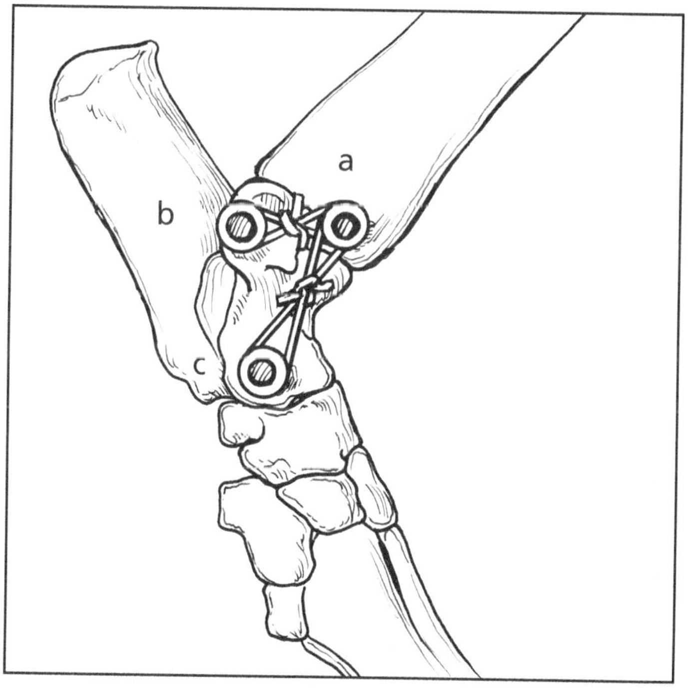


**Figure 7-12.** Prosthetic imbrication of the medial aspect of the tarsus. This procedure may be done using screws and washers or suture anchors. The origin anchor is placed as distally in the tibia as possible, without invading the joint space and just cranial to midline *(a)*. The anchor for the short ligament insertion site is placed in the proximal plantar aspect of the medial talus. This anchor should appear to be slightly distal and plantar to the origin anchor *(b)*. The anchor for the long ligament insertion is placed at the plantar base of the talus *(c)*. The origin anchor is sutured to both insertion anchors using heavy gauge suture. (After Aron DN, Purinton PT. Replacement of the collateral ligaments of the canine tarsocrural joint: a proposed technique. Vet Surg 14:178, 1985).

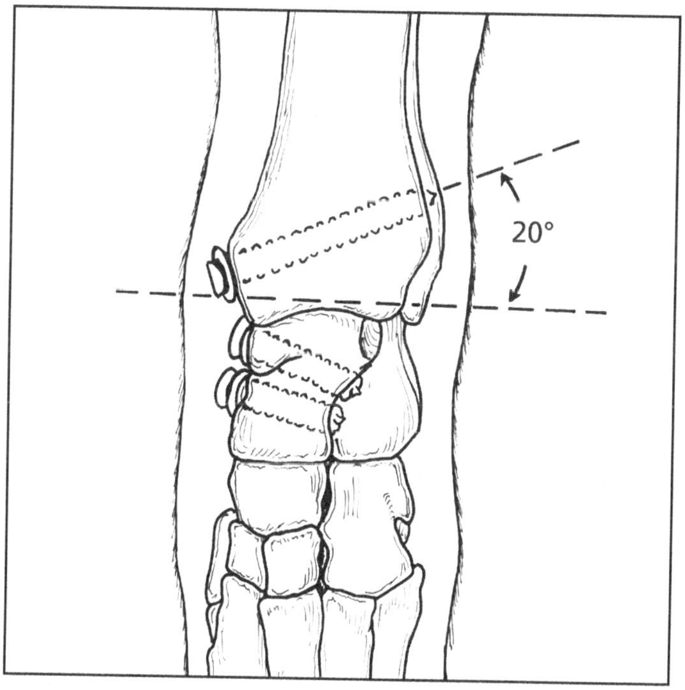


**Figure 7-13.** Prosthetic imbrication of the medial aspect of the tarsus using screws, craniocaudal view. The origin screw is angled 20 degrees proximally to avoid invading the joint.

joint. It extends from the level of the lateral saphenous vein down to the level of the tarsometatarsal joint. The subcutaneous tissue and crural fascia are incised on the same line and are retracted with the skin (Figure 7-14). The tendon of the peroneus longus muscle is seen on the cranial aspect of the lateral malleolus and the lateral digital extensor and peroneus brevis tendons are caudal to the malleolus. The extensor retinaculum overlying the lateral malleolus is incised parallel to the peroneus longus tendon so the tendon can be retracted cranially. The short and long collateral ligaments are inspected to ascertain the extent of injury.

Suture is anchored from the origin of the lateral collateral ligament to the distal insertions of both the long and the short portions of the ligament. The origin suture is anchored just proximal to the lateral malleolus. The surgeon must be aware that the malleolus extends 1 to 2 cm distal to the tarsocrural joint space. The origin anchor is placed through the distal fibula and into the tibia. The location is more caudal than that of the corresponding screw for medial collateral ligament imbrication. The insertion anchor for the short portion of the ligament is placed in a position just proximal and plantar to the articular surface of the calcaneus. The insertion anchor for the long portion of the ligament is placed through a tubercle located at the dorsal extent of the base of the calcaneus (Figure 7-15). Suture size is chosen according to the size of the animal. The suture is a heavy gauge non-absorbable such as 50 to 80 pound test fishing line. Suture from the origin anchor is tied to suture from the short collateral ligament insertion anchor with the joint held in 90 degrees of flexion. Next suture from the origin anchor is tied to suture from the long ligament insertion anchor with the joint held at a normal standing angle. The incision is closed in layers with absorbable suture.

This technique can be performed using screws and metal washers instead of suture anchors as described for medial collateral ligament rupture.

## General Information

The short collateral ligaments limit rotational movement of the tarsocrural joint with the joint in flexion. The ligament can undergo sprain injury or avulsion of its attachment to bone.

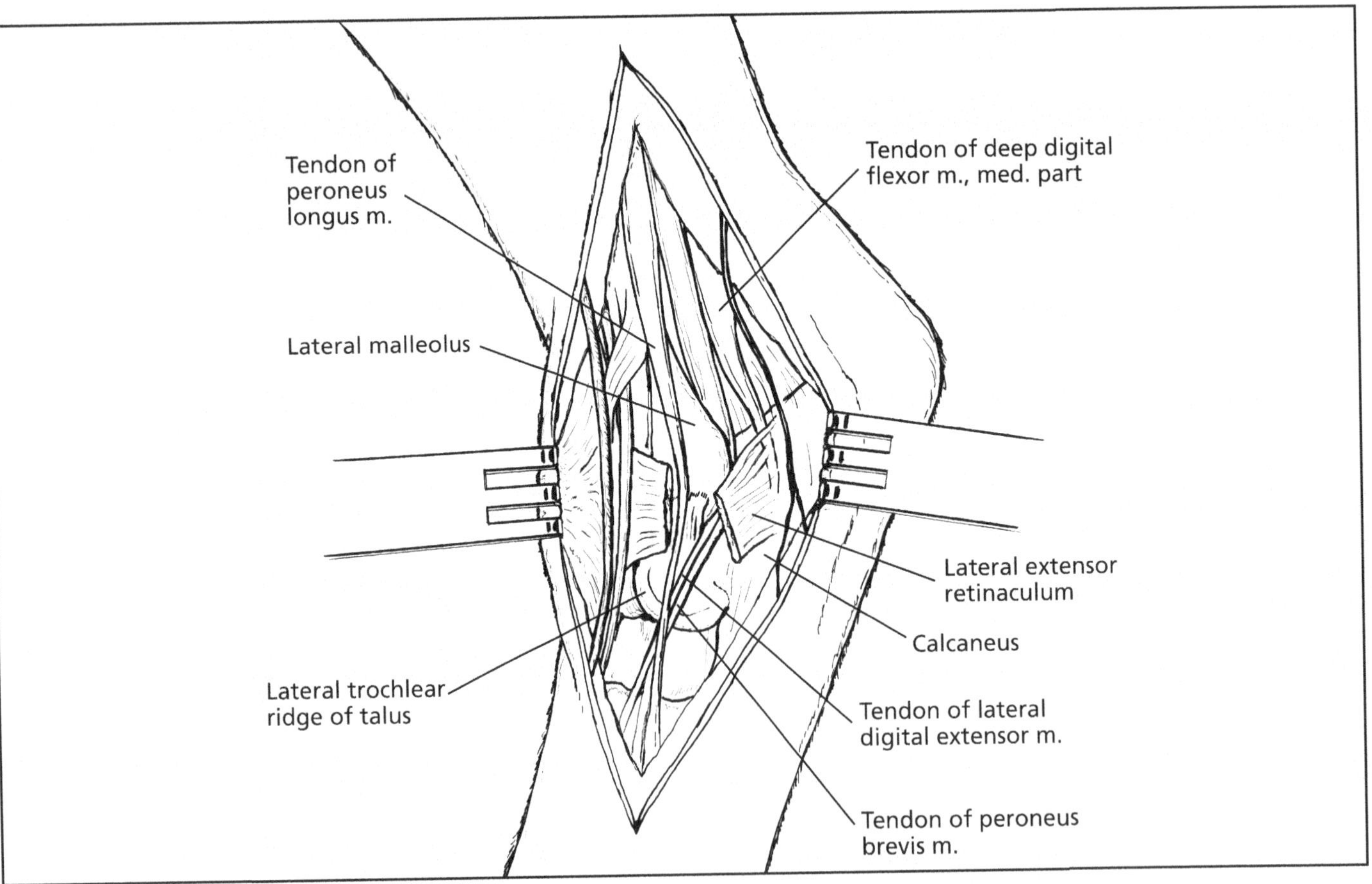


**Figure 7-14.** Approach to the lateral bones of the tarsus. The skin incision is centered over the lateral surface of the tarsocrural joint. It extends from the level of the lateral saphenous vein down to the level of the tarsometatarsal joint. The subcutaneous tissue and crural fascia are incised on the same line and are retracted with the skin. The tendon of the peroneus longus muscle is seen on the cranial aspect of the lateral malleolus and the lateral digital extensor and peroneus brevis tendons are caudal to the malleolus. The extensor retinaculum overlying the lateral malleolus is incised parallel to the peroneus longus tendon so the tendon can be retracted cranially. (After Piermattei DL, Johnson KA. An Atlas of Surgical Approaches to the Bones and Joints of the Dog and Cat 4th ed. Philadelphia: Saunders, 2004, 387).

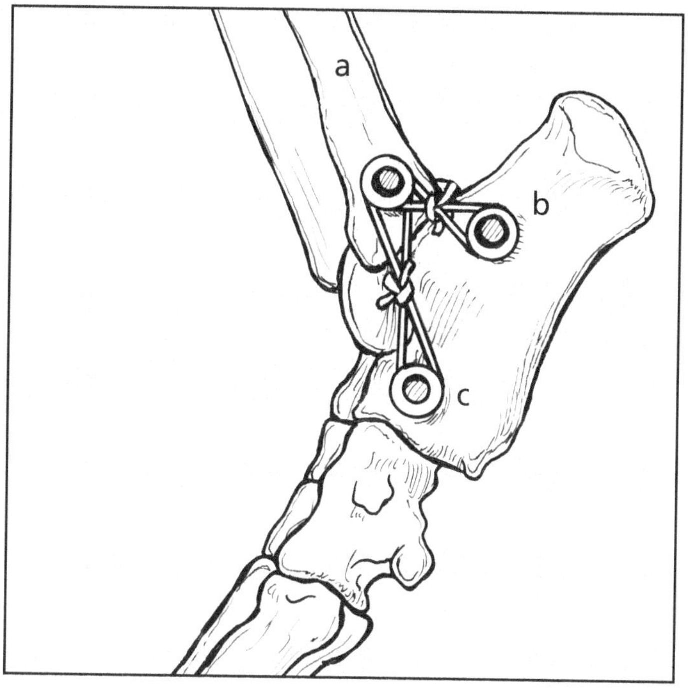


**Figure 7-15.** Prosthetic imbrication of the lateral tarsus. This procedure may be done using screws and washers or suture anchors. Suture is anchored from the origin of the lateral collateral ligament to the distal insertions of both the long and the short portions of the ligament. The origin anchor is located just proximal to the lateral malleolus. The location is more caudal than that of the corresponding anchor for medial collateral ligament imbrication *(a.)* The insertion anchor for the short portion of the ligament is placed just proximal and plantar to the articular surface of the calcaneus *(b.)* The insertion anchor for the long portion of the ligament is placed through a tubercle located at the base of the calcaneus *(c.)* The origin anchor is sutured to both insertion anchors using heavy gauge suture. (After Aron DN, Purinton PT. Replacement of the collateral ligaments of the canine tarsocrural joint: a proposed technique. Vet Surg 14:178, 1985).

The short medial collateral ligament divides into 2 parts as it passes underneath the long medial collateral ligament. One part inserts on the talus and the other inserts on the first and second metatarsal bones (See Figure 7-3).

The short lateral collateral ligaments consist of 2 horizontal components. One of the short ligaments, the fibulocalcanear, runs from the fibular malleolus, passes underneath the long ligament, and inserts on the calcaneus. The other short ligament, the fibulotalar, inserts on the lateral ridge of the talus (See Figure 7-3). Minor rotational instability can be detected if the fibulocalcanear or both ligaments are ruptured, whereas disruption of only the fibulotalar ligament causes no apparent instability. With instability, a distinct motion or "click" of the tarsocrural joint can be felt while testing in flexion.

The short fibulotalar ligament can avulse from its insertion leaving a bony fragment from the talar ridge in the joint. Although disruption of this ligament alone does not cause detectable joint instability, the fragment disrupts the talar articular surface and needs to be replaced and stabilized. Because the calcaneus overlaps the lateral talar ridge, radiographic examination for a bone fragment in this region requires more than standard dorsalplantar and lateral projections. A flexed dorsoplantar radiographic view of the tarsocrural joint can be done to visualize the lateral talar ridge.

Grade II to III sprain injuries of the medial or lateral short collateral ligaments are repaired with suture or imbrication techniques and avulsed pieces of bone are reattached if they are large enough.

## Diagnosis and Surgical Treatment of the Short Medial or Short Lateral Collateral Ligaments

### Physical Exam

Diagnosing rupture of the short collateral ligaments requires a high index of suspicion since the intact long portions of the ligaments provide varus and valgus stability. A sedated exam may be required. The injured limb is compared with the opposite side to verify the presence of laxity. While keeping the tarsocrural joint in 60° to 90° of flexion, the tibia is fixed with one hand while the foot is rotated medially and laterally with the other hand. Laxity associated with external rotation of the paw is consistent with short medial collateral ligament instability and laxity with internal rotation of the paw is consistent with short lateral collateral ligament instability.

### Flexed Dorsoplantar Radiographic View

This radiographic view is used to outline the trochlear ridges of the talus. With a standard cranial caudal view of the tarsus the calcaneus obscures the lateral trochlear ridge. If there is a suspicion of rupture of the short lateral collateral ligament it is useful to visualize the lateral trochlear ridge for an avulsed bony fragment. Sedation is needed to obtain this view.

The dog is positioned in dorsal recumbency. A box is placed on the table and will be used to support the distal hind limbs. Sand bags or a V-shaped trough can be used to support the thoracic area. The distal limbs are flexed at the stifles and tarsal joints, and the tarsal joints are placed on top of the box. Tape is used to keep both stifles close together in the flexed position. A positioning device (approximately 5 cm thick sponge or rolled cotton) is placed between the right and left tarsal joints. The tarsal joint is flexed with an angle of 10 to 15° between its long axis and the radiographic beam. The x-ray beam is collimated tightly to achieve maximal detail of 1 tarsal joint. (Figure 7-16).

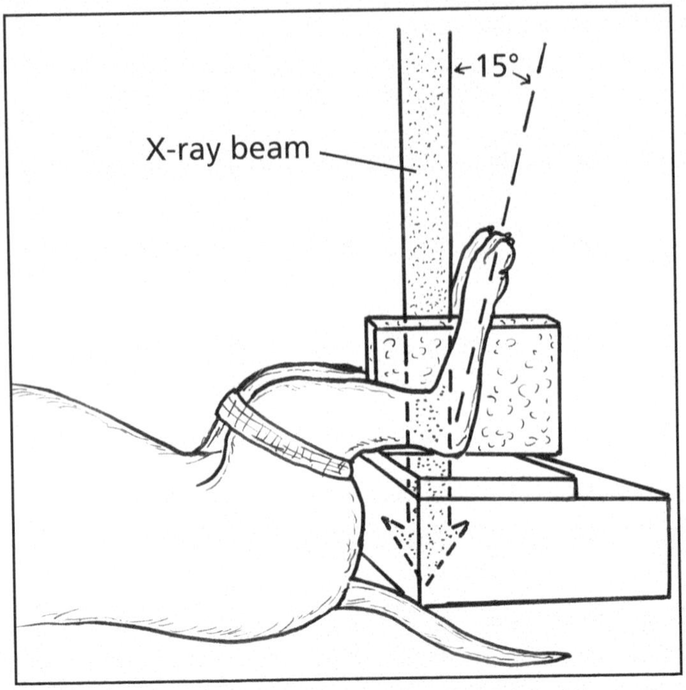


**Figure 7-16.** Flexed dorsoplantar view of the tarsus. The patient is positioned in dorsal recumbency and the distal limbs are flexed and placed on an elevated support. Tape is used to keep both stifles close together in flexed position. A positioning device (approximately 5 cm thick sponge) is placed between the right and left tarsal joints. The tarsal joint is flexed with an angle of 10 to 15° between its long axis and the radiographic beam. (After Miyabayashi T et al. Use of a flexed dorsoplantar radiographic view of the talocrural joint to evaluate lameness in two dogs. JAVMA 199(5):598, 1991).

### Surgical Stabilization - Isolated Rupture of the Short Medial or Short Lateral Collateral Ligaments

The surgical approach to the medial or lateral side is as described for medial and lateral collateral ligament rupture. Ligament damage is likely to be so extensive that a primary suture repair such as a locking loop will be unreliable. If a suture repair is performed, it is supplemented with prosthetic imbrication.

To perform prosthetic imbrication, suture is anchored to the origin and insertion sites of the short collateral ligaments. Origin anchors for medial or lateral collateral ligaments are placed in their respective malleolus using a suture anchor or screw and washer. The insertion site for the medial short collateral ligament is the proximoplantar quadrant of the medial aspect of the talus (See Figure 7-12). The insertion anchor for the short lateral portion of the collateral ligament is placed in the calcaneus, adjacent to the proximal talocalcaneal articulation (See Figure 7-15). The origin and insertion ends of the suture are tied together with the joint held in approximately 90° of flexion. Heavy gauge nonabsorbable suture, such as 50 to 80 pound test fishing line, is suitable for this repair.

### Avulsion Fracture of the Talar Insertion of the Short Lateral Collateral Ligament

The patient is positioned in lateral recumbency with the affected limb up. The proximal region of the lateral talar ridge is surgically approached by performing a lateral approach to the tarsal joint with an osteotomy of the distal fibula. The skin incision is centered over the lateral surface of the tarsocrural joint. It begins proximally at the level of the lateral saphenous vein and continues distally to the level of the tarsometatarsal joint. The subcutaneous tissue and crural fascia are incised on the same line as the skin and are retracted with the skin. The peroneus longus tendon is located along the cranial edge of the fibula. The extensor retinaculum overlying the lateral malleolus is incised parallel to the peroneus longus tendon and the tendon is retracted cranially (See Figure 7-14). The distal fibula is freed from remaining fascial tissue. An osteotomy of the distal fibula is performed, just above the lateral malleolus, using an oscillating saw or osteotome. The bone fragment is retracted distally to expose the talus. The joint capsule is incised parallel to the joint surfaces. The bone fragment is anatomically reduced using either bone reduction forceps or digital pressure. The fragment is stabilized using 1 to 2 K-wires (size 0.035 or 0.045 inch) placed in normograde fashion, through the fractured talar fragment, across the fracture site and into the talus (Figure 7-17). The K-wires should be countersunk to avoid pin contact with the opposing articular surface of the tibia. Alternatively, biodegradable polydioxanone pins can be placed (Orthosorb Resorbable Pins; Johnson and Johnson Gateway, Raynham, MA). The joint capsule is closed using absorbable suture. The fibula is stabilized by pin and tension band fixation (Figure 7-17).

## Aftercare

## Non-Surgical Treatment of Sprain Injuries

### Grade 1 Sprain

Cold therapy is applied for 1 to 2 days and is followed by heat therapy for 1 to 2 days. External support is not necessary. Animals are treated with NSAIDs for 1 week and exercise is restricted to short (5 minute) leash walks 3 to 4 times daily for 7 to 10 days, followed by another 7 to 10 days of light exercise such as leash walking or free movement in a small run. By the end of the third week, most animals can be allowed unrestricted activity.

### Grade 2 Sprain

Cases treated conservatively have the joint immobilized with a splint for 2 weeks followed by 1 to 2 weeks in a soft padded bandage. Light activity is started at

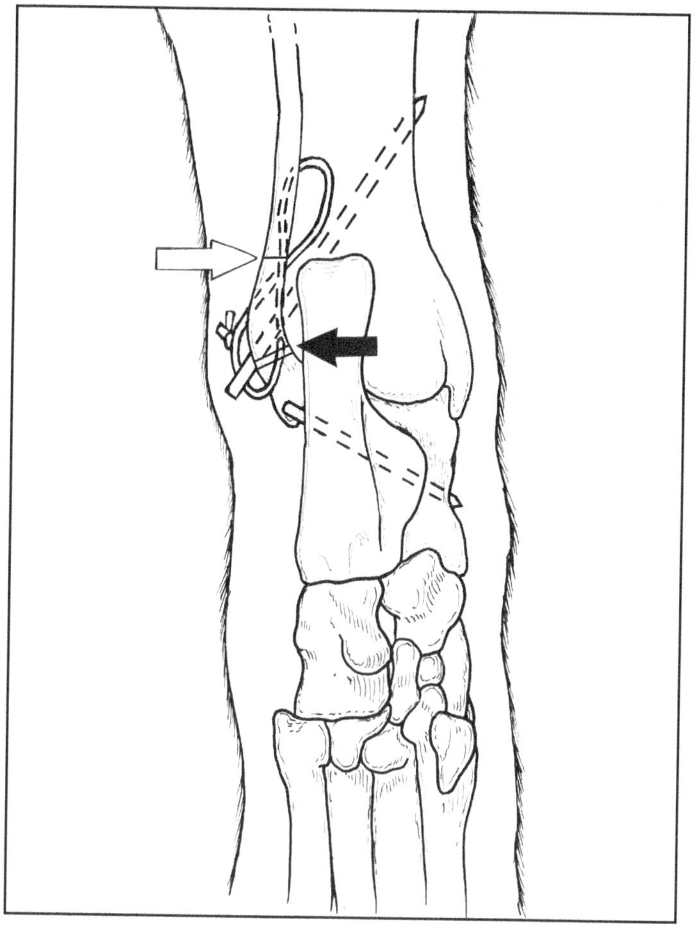

**Figure 7-17.** Stabilization of the short lateral collateral ligament insertion. An osteotomy of the distal fibula is performed just proximal to the lateral malleolus *(open arrow)*. The talar bone fragment is stabilized using 1 to 2 K-wires placed across the fracture site *(closed arrow)*. The distal fibula has been stabilized by a tension band fixation.

the removal of the splint and slowly increased toward normal between 6 and 8 weeks after injury, although there should be no exuberant off leash activity until at least 12 weeks after the injury. Nonsteroidal anti-inflammatory drugs are administered at a tapering dose as described for 2 to 4 weeks. Injectable polysuflated glycosaminoglycan is administered at a tapering frequency as described for 4 to 12 weeks.

## Suggested Readings


1. Aron DN: Prosthetic ligament replacement for severe tarsocrural joint instability. J Amer An Hosp Assoc 23:41, 1987.
2. Beale B: Surgical treatement of talus fractures. In Bojrab MJ, Ellison GW, Slocum B (eds): Current Techniques in Small Animal Surgery, 4th ed: Baltimore: Williams and Wilkins, 1998, p 1264.
3. Behrens F, Kraft EL, Oegema-TR J: Biochemical changes in articular cartilage after joint immobilization by casting or external fixation, J Orthop Res 12:335-343, 1989.
4. Burgess R, Elder S, McLaughlin R et al.: In vitro biomechanical evaluation and comparison of FiberWire, FiberTape, OrthoFiber, and nylon leader line for potential use during extraarticular stabilization of canine cruciate deficient stifles. Vet Surg 39:208-215, 2010.
5. Clark GN: Malleolar shearing injuries treated by double ligament replacement. In Bojrab MJ, Ellison GW, Slocum B: Current Techniques in Small Animal Surgery, 4th ed.: Baltimore: Williams & Wilkins, 1998, 1261.
6. Heinrichs K: Superficial Thermal Modalities. In Millis DL, Levine D, Taylor RA: Canine Rehabilitation and Physical Therapy: St Louis: Saunders, 2004, 100-285.
7. Jaeger GH, Roe SC: Isometry of potential suture attachment sites for the medial aspect of the tibiotarsal joint. Vet Comp Orthop Traumatol 18:73-76, 2005.
8. Jaeger GH, Wosar MA, Marcellin-Little DJ, et al: Use of hinged fixation for adjunctive joint stabilization in dogs and cats: Fourteen cases (1999-2003). J Am Vet Med Assoc 227: 586-591, 2005
9. Keller WG, Aron DN, Rowland GN et al: The effect of trans-stifle external fixation and hyaluronic acid therapy on articular cartilage in the dog. Vet Surg 23:119-128, 1994.
10. Mayabayashi T, Biller DS, Manley PA, et al: Use of a flexed dorsoplantar radiographic view of the talocrural joint to evaluate lameness in two dogs. J Am Vet Med Assoc 199(5):598, 1991.
11. Neil KM, Caron JP, Orth MW: The role of glucosamine and chondroitin sulfate in treatment for and prevention of osteoarthritis in animals. J Am Vet Med Assoc 226:1079-1088, 2005.
12. Piermattei DL, Flo GL: Principles of joint surgery. In Brinker, Piermattei and Flo's Handbook of Small Animal Orthopedics and Fracture Repair, 3rd ed. Philadelphia: W.B. Saunders Co., 1997, 203-212.
13. Piermattei DL, Flo GL. Fractures and other orthopedic injuries of the tarsus, metatarsus, and phalanges. In Brinker, Piermattei DL, Flo GL, eds.: Handbook of Small Animal Orthopedics and Fracture Repair, 3rd ed.: Philadelphia: WB Saunders, 1997, 610.
14. Piermattei DM, Johnson KA: An Atlas of Surgical Approaches to the Bones and Joints of the Dog and Cat 4th ed: Philadelphia: Saunders, 2000.
15. Roe S: Injury and Diseases of Tendons. In Bloomberg MS, Dee JF, Taylor RA: Canine Sports Medicine and Surgery: Philadelphia: W. B. Saunders Co., 1998, 92-99.
16. Sjöström L, Håkanson N: Traumatic injuries associated with the short lateral collateral ligaments of the talocrural joint of the dog. J Small Anim Pract 35:163, 1994.
17. Todhunter RJ, Lust G: Polysulfated glycosaminoglycan in the treatment of osteoarthritis. J Am Vet Med Assoc 204:1234-1251, 1994.


# Tarsal Shearing Wounds Treated by Open Wound Healing, Prosthetic Imbrication and External Fixation

## Definition and Indications

Shearing injuries are commonly encountered in small animal practice. With minor to moderate shearing wounds, soft tissues of the distal limbs are avulsed or abraded following vehicular trauma. There is loss of skin, subcutaneous tissues, ligaments, and often bone. Shearing wounds tend to be heavily contaminated with dirt, asphalt, hair and organic debris. The medial aspect of the distal portion of the limbs is affected most often, and tarsal injuries predominate over carpal injuries. The appearance of shearing wounds suggests that many animals are oriented in a prone position with the hind limb abducted at the time of injury. This would expose the medial aspect of the tarsus to the ground if the limb was caught under the car at the moment of contact. The collateral ligament support of the tarsus often is lost, even in smaller wounds, due to the prominent position of the malleolus.

The extent of ligamentous damage is estimated based on visual inspection of the wound, palpation under heavy sedation, and survey and stress radiographs (See Figure 7-7). Mild shearing wounds have collateral ligament injury but no loss of bone. Moderate shearing wounds have ligament injury and bone loss, which can range from loss of the malleolus only to malleolar, tarsal and metatarsal involvement. Loss of bone from the articular surface of the tarsocrural joint is a severe shearing injury. The technique indicated for stabilization of collateral ligaments depends on the degree of damage to osseous structures in the tarsus and the expected activity level of the dog. Some animals with minor to moderate shearing injury do well treated conservatively, with splint fixation alone, for 6 to10 weeks. This technique relies on periarticular scar tissue to stabilize the joint. Moderate shearing injury with damage limited to malleoli and collateral ligaments can be repaired using prosthetic imbrication techniques as previously described for collateral ligament ruptures. Further stabilization can be achieved by placing a transarticular external fixator. Surgical stabilization procedures can be initiated early in the healing process.

## Techniques

### Conservative Management of Minor to Moderate Shearing Wounds

The wound is treated with lavage, debridement, and daily bandage changes until infection and contamination are controlled. This can generally be accomplished within the first week of the injury. The tarsus is immobilized with a soft padded bandage and splint **(see Chapter 1, Initial Wound Management of Contaminated and Infected Wounds)**. The soft padded bandage and splint should extend from mid-tibia to the digits (see Figure 7-8). The average time for second intention healing is approximately 7 weeks.

The frequency of bandage changes depends on the size of the wound and degree of exudate. Daily bandage changes are usually required for the first two to three weeks. Once a healthy bed of granulation tissue is established, the frequency of bandage changes can be gradually decreased. Exam or sterile gloves are worn for bandage changes. Bandage materials to be applied to the wound are placed on a clean impermeable surface. Disposable styrofoam or paper trays are useful for this purpose. The type of contact layer used changes with progression from an exudative open wound bed to a healthy bed of granulation tissue **(see Chapter 1, Initial Wound Management of Contaminated and Infected Wounds)**.

The necessity for antibiotics in the presence of open shearing wounds is unproven. The most important protocol with shearing wounds is thorough lavage and debridement of necrotic tissue. Aseptic technique is followed during bandage changes and bandages are immediately changed if "strike through" occurs. It is reasonable to provide broad spectrum antibiotics when bone is not yet covered by granulation tissue. The wound is cultured after initial lavage with a sterile isotonic solution such as physiologic saline or lactated ringer's solution. Antibiotics can be adjusted based on culture and sensitivity results. Antibiotics can usually be discontinued when granulation tissue covers the bone.

There can be a temptation to suture the wound if there are skin edges that can be apposed. This is not recommended initially due to the risk of trapping contaminating microbes within the wound. Additionally the success of conservative treatment requires the formation of periarticular fibroplasia during the course of wound granulation and contraction.

Manipulation of the unstable tarsal joint and fragile wound bed causes patient discomfort. Appropriate analgesia and sedation are required to perform bandage changes. A combination of an opiate and alpha 2 agonist (such as morphine, fentanyl, hydromorphone, oxymorphone or buprenorphine with dexmedetomidine) provides good analgesia and sedation for most cases.

### Surgical Stabilization of Shearing Wounds

The timing of surgical stabilization must be considered. Early stabilization, between days 4 and 7 post injury, can be successful and is recommended. Tarsal shearing wounds are stabilized with prosthetic imbrication as described for collateral ligament ruptures. A significant difference is that the malleolus is absent in most shearing wounds, thus, it cannot be used as a landmark for placement of fixation devices.

The proximal suture anchor is placed in the tibia, just proximal to the tarsocrural joint. The normal anatomy of the talus or calcaneus, depending on whether the shearing wound is medial or lateral, is sometimes altered. Thus, the correct insertion sites for the short and long portions of the collateral ligaments are estimated. The short insertion site is located in the proximal portion of the talus or calcaneus and the long insertion site is in the distal portion of the talus or calcaneus (medial or lateral stabilization, respectively). Due to the contaminated nature of the wound, monofilament nonabsorbable suture such as nylon line is used. The tarsus is stabilized with either a splint or an external fixator during the granulation and epithelialization phases of wound management.

A transarticular external fixator is placed as described (see Transarticular External Fixation of the Tarsus). Some external fixator designs are static whereas some are equipped with a hinge. Hinges for transarticular external fixators (SK range of motion hinge, modified angular hinge, Imex Veterinary Inc., Longview TX; Slocum Joint Hinge, Slocum Enterprises, Eugene, OR) permit limited movement in one plane to promote joint health while providing stability (See Transarticular External Fixation of the Tarsus).

## Aftercare

Daily bandage changes are performed until a healthy granulation bed is present. Appropriate analgesia and sedation are needed for bandage changes. Dosages and types of medications are adjusted to individual needs. Protocols consisting of an opioid mixed with a tranquilizer or an alpha-2 agonist are effective. In general, patients with an external fixator in place experience less discomfort during bandage changes. As the wound bed matures, bandage changes become easier.

If a soft padded bandage and splint is used instead of an external fixator it is placed for approximately 6 weeks. The splint is changed weekly to twice weekly and if areas of pressure irritation are identified the position of the splint can be changed. For example, a lateral splint can be moved to the medial side or an area of irritation over a bony protuberance such as the tuber calcanei can be covered with a "donut" of bandage material to relieve pressure. After splint removal a soft padded bandage is placed for 2 weeks.

Broad spectrum bactericidal antibiotics, such as cephalosporins, can be administered during the initial phases of wound management when there is exposed bone that is not yet covered with a bed of granulation tissue. If antibiotics have been used they are usually discontinued when bone is resurfaced with granulation tissue. Sterile technique is maintained at all times during bandage changes. When the wound bed is covered with healthy granulation tissue, decisions can be made regarding the best means of skin reconstruction. Most cases heal completely by second intention but some will require a skin stretching/relaxation technique, skin graft or skin flap. The appropriate procedure can then be performed. Clinical judgment will be needed in selecting a reconstructive technique based on having to work around any external fixator pins that may be present.

If a hinged external connecting system is used, it can be locked down during the early phases of healing. Depending on the type of hinge, this is done by an adjustment on the hinge or by placing an added connecting rod on the cranial surface of the joint for the first 3 weeks (See External Fixation of the Tarsus). If a hinged external fixator is used, it is kept in place for 6 to 8 weeks. When the hinged external fixator is removed a soft padded bandage is placed for 2 weeks. The soft padded bandage provides some protection to the joint and promotes gradual transference to full joint motion after removing the external fixator or splint. If a static external fixator (one without a hinge) is used it is removed in approximately 4 weeks and replaced with a splint. The splint is kept on for 3 weeks and then replaced with a soft padded bandage for 2 weeks.

Exercise is restricted to short (maximum 10 minute) leash walks 3 to 5 times daily for 12 weeks after surgery. Rehabilitation is begun at 10 to 12 weeks and consists of gradually increased leash walks, controlled swimming (for example 3 ten- minute sessions per week) or both. Underwater treadmill therapy can also be started.

Animals with articular trauma can be started on glucosamine/chondroitin oral supplements (Coseqin, Dasuquin, Nutramax Laboratories, Edgewood, MD) or injectable polysulfated glycosaminoglycan (Adequan, Novartis Animal Health, Greensboro, NC) soon after injury to help protect the proteoglycan content of joint cartilage.

## Advantages and Disadvantages

Supporting the tarsus with an external fixator during wound management requires an additional surgery and expense. However, many patients require anesthesia for wound debridement and the fixator can be placed at this time. Patients with unstable joints are more comfortable during bandage changes with an external fixator in place. In the author's experience, joint stabilization using both a prosthetic imbrication technique and transarticular external fixation provides good to excellent postoperative function.

Waiting until soft tissues are healed prior to surgical intervention creates a more protracted recovery time and recently healed tissues must be incised to make a surgical approach. The potential risk with early stabilization (4 to 7 days post injury) is implant infection that would necessitate future removal of anchors and suture material. This is not a frequent problem with monofilament suture. If early surgical repair is performed, clients should be educated about the possibility of future suture removal if infection occurs.

The need to treat shearing wounds with antibiotics is unproven. Most shearing wounds are initially contaminated but not infected and there has been no difference in outcomes whether patients receive antibiotics or not. The disadvantage to their use is additional cost, possible complications such as gastrointestinal upset, and the potential for the formation of resistant bacteria. The most important aspect of wound management is to use sterile technique during bandage changes.

Conservative management is the least invasive and least costly method for treating shearing wounds. However, stabilization of tarsal shearing wounds is not difficult and patients are usually going to be anesthetized during the course of wound management. Surgical stabilization can be recommended for most patients with unstable joints unless cost dictates otherwise.

## Suggested Readings

1. Aron DN: Prosthetic ligament replacement for severe tarsocrural joint instability. J Am Anim Hosp Assoc 23:41, 1986.
2. Beardsley SL, Schrader SC: Treatment of dogs with wounds of the limbs caused by shearing forces: 98 cases (1975-1993). J Am Vet Med Assoc 208(8):1071, 1995.
3. Diamond DW, Besso J, Boudrieau RJ: Evaluation of joint stabilization for treatment of shearing injuries of the tarsus in 20 dogs. J Am Anim Hosp Assoc 35:147, 1999.
4. Swaim SF: Management and bandaging of soft tissue injuries of dog and cat feet. J Am Anim Hosp Assoc 21:329-40, 1985.
5. Swaim SF, Henderson RA: Small Animal Wound Management 2nd ed: Baltimore: Williams and Wilkins, 1997, 141.
6. Swaim SF, Pope ER: Early management of limb degloving injuries. Sem Vet Med Surg (Small Animal) 3:274, 1988).

# Severe Tarsal Shearing Wounds Treated by Early Arthrodesis Using External Fixation

### Definition and Indications

Tarsal shearing injuries that result in loss of bone from the articular surface of the tibia or talus are considered severe shearing wounds and require a salvage procedure (either arthrodesis or amputation). Arthrodesis is performed by removing articular cartilage and using a transarticular external fixator to confer rigid stabilization to the tarsus. Arthrodesis can be done within the first week after injury. The external fixator must remain in place until arthrodesis is completed so a type II frame design is applied and is supplemented with connecting rods that span the cranial surface of the joint to provide increased resistance to bending (See Transarticular External Fixation of the Tarsus).

### Technique

Dirty or contaminated wounds are initially treated using standard lavage, debridement, and bandaging. Copious lavage with a sterile isotonic solution such as saline or lactated ringers is chosen. In highly contaminated wounds a 1:40 (0.05%) solution of chlorhexidine diacetate is also useful for reducing bacterial numbers in the wound. A splint is incorporated into the soft padded bandage during this stage for patient comfort (see Chapter 1, Initial Wound Management of Contaminated and Infected Wounds, and chapter II, Bandages, Pads, Splints and Slings). The use of antibiotics is of undetermined benefit with a well-managed open wound. Most shearing wounds are initially contaminated but not infected. If antibiotics are to be used, a culture of the wound is taken after lavage with sterile saline. Broad spectrum bactericidal antibiotics such as cephalosporins are begun while waiting for culture and sensitivity results. Arthrodesis is performed once the exudative phase of wound healing is completed and the tissues appear healthy. There may still be exposed bone. It is not necessary to wait for granulation tissue to cover all bony surfaces prior to performing arthrodesis.

A dorsal approach is made that extends from the distal tibia to the proximal metatarsals. Some shearing wounds are so extensive that a surgical skin incision is not required. All articular surfaces will need to be exposed in order to remove articular cartilage. If necessary to improve exposure, the proximal extensor retinaculum is incised to mobilize the cranial tibial and long digital extensor tendons. The cranial tibial tendon can be incised as it crosses the tarsocrural joint, but the long digital extensor tendon must be left intact (Figure 7-18). The small intertarsal ligaments that connect the tarsal bones are incised as needed. Articular cartilage is removed using a high speed drill and bur. The goal is to remove as much of the articular cartilage as possible down to subchondral bone. A Freer elevator can be used to lever open joint spaces and improve visibility. When removing the cartilage from the tarsocrural joint, it is especially important to form 2 congruent surfaces. The

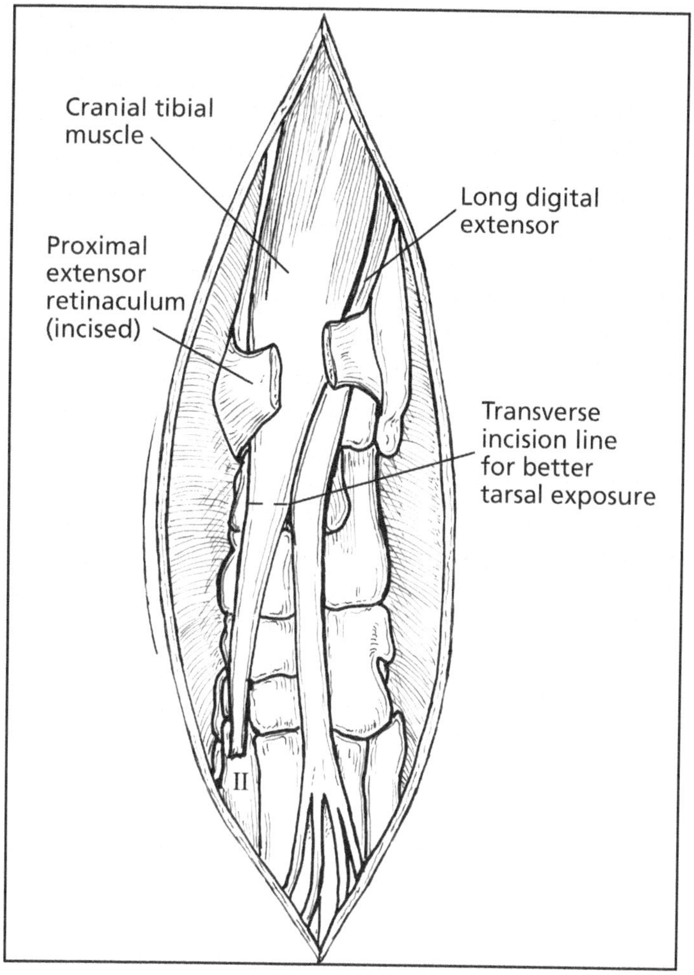


**Figure 7-18.** Dorsal approach to the tarsus. A dorsal approach is made from the distal tibia to the proximal metatarsals. The proximal extensor retinaculum that covers the dorsal tendons is incised. If necessary to improve exposure, the cranial tibial tendon is incised transversely as it crosses the tarsocrural joint, but the long digital extensor tendon must be left intact.

bur follows the normal contour of the tibial and talar articular surfaces without removing their ridges. The cartilage is removed from the proximal and distal joint surfaces of the tarsocrural, talocalcaneocentral, calcaneoquartal, centrodistal, and tarsometatarsal joints (See Figure 7-2).

The surgeon is mindful that the perforating metatarsal artery passes between metatarsals II and III just distal to the tarsometatarsal joint. This component of the blood supply may have been damaged from the shearing wound but this area is still treated carefully while removing cartilage from the tarsometatarsal joint.

A cancellous bone graft can be placed between articular surfaces to promote osteogenesis. Autogenous graft can be harvested from the ipsilateral greater tubercle of the humerus or allograft can be placed. Frozen or freeze-dried bone allograft can be purchased from a supplier (Veterinary Transplant Services; Kent, WA). This graft consists of demineralized bone matrix and cancellous chips. It is rehydrated then mixed with the patient's blood and packed between the articular surfaces.

Standard closure with absorbable suture is performed on subcutaneous tissue and skin that can be approximated without tension as long as there is healthy tissue beneath. When in doubt tissues are left open. The external fixation system is placed across the tarsocrural joint and positioned at a pre-determined angle **(see Transarticular External Fixation of the Tarsus)**. The standing angle of the tarsus varies from 130° to 150° in the average dog and 115° to 125° in the cat. To tailor the angle to the individual, the standing angle of the opposite limb is measured preoperatively with a goniometer or with a conformable template. These devices can be autoclaved and used intraoperatively to ascertain the angle.

For added stability, a normograde intramedullary pin can be placed from the plantar aspect of the tarsus into the medullary cavity of the tibia. The pin size is approximately 40% of the medullary canal diameter of the tibia. A small incision is made over the plantar aspect of the talus. Using a high speed drill and chuck, the pin is introduced in a normograde manner through the talus into the medullary cavity of the tibia. There can be a tendency to angle the pin too far cranially such that it engages the cranial cortex of the tibia rather than advancing to the proximal metaphysis. This is corrected by redirecting the pin to be parallel with the caudal cortex of the tibia. The pin is advanced until it engages the proximal metaphysis of the tibia but does not penetrate the tibial plateau (Figure 7-19). A paired pin is used to estimate the penetration depth of the intramedullary pin. The pin is cut short at the plantar aspect of the talus.

A type II external fixation device is applied (see Transarticular External Fixation of the Tarsus). The device must withstand significant bending forces for a long period of time because it requires at least 12 weeks to achieve arthrodesis. Some or all of the pins on each side of the joint should be full pins meaning they penetrate both the medial and lateral skin surface. To improve durability of the external fixator it is best to use positive profile pins. Positive profile pins have threads added to the part of the pin that will engage the bone and have superior resistance to loosening (See Transarticular External Fixation of the Tarsus).

The surgical site is bandaged using a contact layer that will promote granulation tissue formation. If cancellous bone grafts have been used, the contact layer should

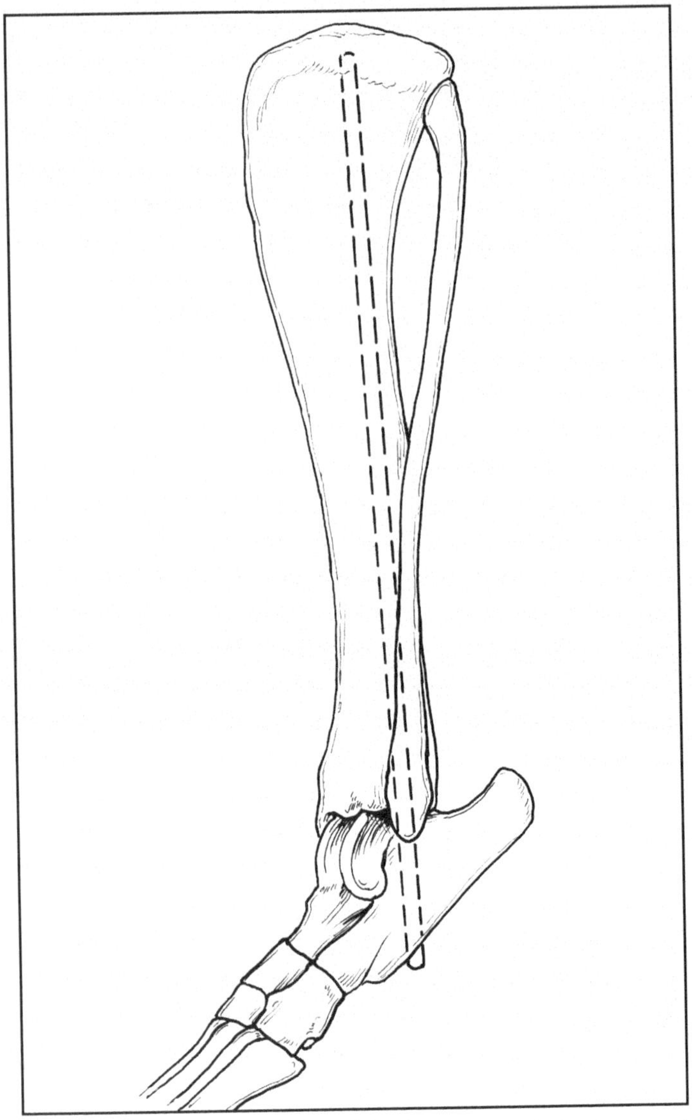

**Figure 7-19.** Transarticular pin for adjunctive stabilization of the tarsocrural joint. To add stability to tarsal arthrodesis a normograde intramedullary pin can be placed from the tarsocrural joint to the tibia. The pin size is approximately 40% of the medullary canal diameter of the tibia. The pin is introduced in a normograde manner through the talus into the medullary cavity of the tibia. The pin is advanced until it engages the proximal metaphysis of the tibia but does not penetrate the tibial plateau. The pin is cut short at the plantar aspect of the talus.

not adhere to the grafts such that they would be disturbed at bandage change. A soft padded bandage is placed over the contact layer and encompasses the external fixator. Once a healthy bed of granulation tissue has formed, a decision should be made whether the wound will heal by second intention or whether some type of reconstruction will be needed, i.e. skin stretching, graft, or flap.

## Aftercare

The open wound and external fixator are bandaged as one unit. The bandage is changed once daily initially, and then every 2 days, once a healthy minimally exudative granulation bed has formed. At this point, reconstructive skin surgery can be considered. The frequency of bandage changes may be decreased further once healing is advanced if healing by second intention is to take place. When soft tissues are healed, including any skin reconstruction, a "bumper bandage" may be applied. This bandage covers only the connecting bar and clamps of the external fixator to prevent damage from the sharp ends of cut pins. The ends of the cut pins may also be covered with caps so that if the bandage does come off the pins will not scratch the patient or owners (Imex Veterinary Inc., Longview, TX). A bumper bandage need only be changed when it becomes soiled; approximately weekly or every two weeks. Radiographs are taken every 4 to 6 weeks to evaluate healing. Arthrodesis is complete when joint spaces are replaced with healing bone. Without complications, the fixator can usually be removed by 12 to 14 weeks. If an intramedullary pin was used, it is also removed at this time. It is generally unnecessary to place a splint or soft padded bandage after removal of an external fixator. If pin tract infections have created focal skin lesions, a soft padded bandage can be placed for approximately 3 days to protect these areas.

If antibiotics were started they are generally discontinued once a healthy bed of granulation tissue is established.

Exercise restriction is continued for 4 to 6 weeks following external fixator removal as a precaution in letting pin tract sites in the bone heal. During this time, animals are outside only on a leash. The duration of leash walks may be gradually increased during this time.

## Advantages and Disadvantages

Arthrodesis in the early healing phase of shearing injuries is a viable alternative to more traditional management of allowing all soft tissues to heal prior to definitive stabilization. This technique promotes a shortened hospital stay and the stability it provides improves patient comfort. Potential complications include pin tract infections and premature pin loosening. Pin tract infections that are minor to moderate can be controlled with broad spectrum antibiotics such as amoxicillin clavulanate. If pin loosening occurs prior to the completion of arthrodesis, those pins may need to be changed or the fixation system revised. External fixation devices are ultimately removed so long term implant infection will not occur.

Placing a normograde intramedullary pin from the tarsocrural joint into the proximal tibia increases the stability of the repair for correct placement. If one is not accustomed to normograding a pin in the tibia in this direction it can take more than one attempt. There is a possibility of pin loosening that would require removal in the future.

Harvesting a cancellous autograft adds approximately 15 minutes of surgical time to the procedure and creates an additional surgical site for the patient. Freeze dried or frozen cancellous allograft is effective and avoids surgical time and morbidity. The only disadvantage is the additional cost of purchase and shipping for the allograft. Cancellous bone graft is not essential in these cases. Acceleration of arthrodesis has not been proven when cancellous graft is used for immediate arthrodesis of shearing wounds.

## Suggested Readings


1. Benson JA, Boudrieau RJ: Severe carpal and tarsal shearing injuries treated with an immediate arthrodesis in seven dogs. J Am Anim Hosp Assoc 38:370, 2002.
2. Corr S: Management of distal limb shearing injuries in cats: J Feline Med Surg 11:747-757, 2009.
3. Kirsch JA, Déjardin LM, DeCamp CD, et al: In vitro mechanical evaluation on the use of an intramedullary pin-plate combination for pantarsal arthrodesis in dogs. Am J Vet Res 66:125-131, 2005.
4. Piermattei DL, Flo GL. Handbook of Small Animal Orthopedics and Fracture Repair, 3rd ed.: Philadelphia: WB Saunders, 1997, 629.


# Severe Tarsal Shearing Wounds Treated by Delayed Arthrodesis Using Bone Plating

## Definition and Indications

Pantarsal arthrodesis with the use of a bone plate is indicated when there is no longer exposed bone. Dorsal, medial or lateral bone plates can be placed. Pantarsal arthrodesis is performed in all cases. Selective arthrodesis of the tarsocrural joint alone is associated with chronic lameness that results from excessive loading of low-motion distal joints.

## Techniques

### Pantarsal Arthrodesis with a Dorsal Bone Plate

The animal is positioned in dorsal recumbency to facilitate access to all tarsal joints. The skin is incised over the cranial medial surface of the tarsal joint and extends from the distal third of the tibia to the middle of the metatarsal bones. The subcutaneous tissues are incised and the extensor retinaculum is incised to allow separation of the cranial tibial and long digital extensor tendons. Hemostasis is achieved with the use of electrocautery. A tourniquet is not necessary in most cases. The cranial tibial tendon is retracted medially and the long digital extensor tendon is retracted laterally. All horizontal joint spaces are exposed by incising the small intertarsal ligaments if they have not been destroyed by trauma. Articular cartilage is removed from the tarsocrural, talocalcaneocentral, calcaneoquartal, centrodistal and tarsometatarsal joints (See Figure 7-2). The surgeon is mindful that the perforating metatarsal artery passes in a dorsal to plantar direction between metatarsals II and III just distal to the tarsometatarsal joint. This area is treated carefully during cartilage removal at the tarsometatarsal level. Articular cartilage is removed using a high speed drill and bur. A freer elevator can be used to lever open joint spaces and improve visibility. The goal is to remove as much of the articular cartilage as possible down to subchondral bone. Excessive subchondral bone is not removed as this can delay arthrodesis. When removing the cartilage from the tarsocrural joint, it is important to form 2 congruent surfaces. The bur follows the normal contour of the tibial and talar articular surfaces without removing their ridges.

### A Dynamic Compression Plate (DCP) or Lengthening Plate

A dynamic compression plate (DCP) or lengthening plate can be applied. The bone plate is pre-contoured to the desired angle of fusion using a table top plate bender. Torque irons can be used to grasp the plate and complete the bend. The angle is verified during surgery using a sterilized goniometer and adjusted if necessary. The acute bend is positioned in the plate over the distal aspect of the talus (the neck of the talus). The most common angle for the dog ranges from 135 to 145 degrees. The angle can be estimated more accurately by measuring the standing angle of the opposite tarsal joint with a goniometer prior to surgery. The functional standing angle of the tarsus for the cat is 115 to 125 degrees (Figure 7-20A & B).

A sample of cancellous bone can be obtained from the patient's ipsilateral humerus as described for arthrodesis of shearing wounds. Alternatively, frozen or freeze-dried bone graft can be purchased from a supplier (Veterinary Transplant Services; Kent, WA (www.vtsonline.com).

A dynamic compression plate (DCP) or lengthening plate can be applied (See Figure 7-20A & B). A lengthening plate has 4 screw holes at either end but has no holes in the middle of the plate. This type of plate is more resistant to bending in the region devoid of screw holes compared to a standard bone plate. With any plate, there must be adequate length to ensure

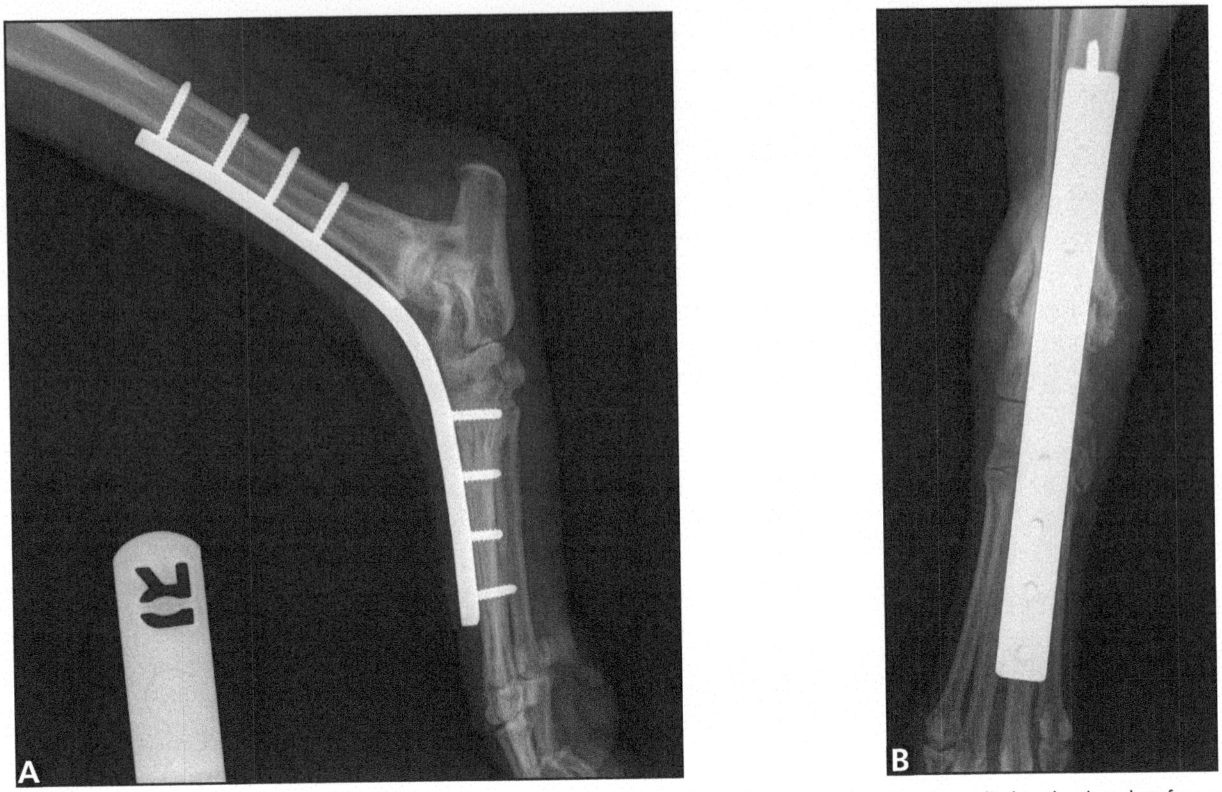


**Figure 7-20.** Tarsal arthrodesis by dorsal bone plate. A lengthening plate or dynamic compression plate is applied to the dorsal surface of the tarsocrural joint. The acute bend of the plate is positioned over the talus. There must be adequate length to ensure at least 3 screws in the distal tibia and 3 screws in the third metatarsal bone. Care is taken to position metatarsal screws in the middle of the bone. **A.** Lateral radiographic projection. **B.** Craniocaudal radiographic projection.

3 screws in the distal tibia and 3 screws in the third metatarsal bone. The plate is centralized over the metatarsal bone first by marking the position of the distal screw hole. The plate is removed and the drill is positioned in the center of the metatarsal bone to make the first hole. The plate is replaced and secured at the first screw hole. The remaining metatarsal screw holes are drilled and screws are placed. The joint is inspected to ensure that there is no varus or valgus malposition and the remaining screws in the distal tibia are placed. Lengthening plates are available in multiple sizes (Synthes, Paoli, PA; Veterinary Orthopedic Implants, S Burlington, VT).

Bone plates can be supplemented with an intramedullary pin. The intramedullary pin is inserted through the plantar aspect of the talus and advanced in normograde fashion into the proximal tibial metaphysis. The pin size should be 40 % of the diameter of the medullary canal of the tibia. The pin must not penetrate the stifle joint. A paired pin of the same size can be used to estimate the position of the intramedullary pin. The pin is cut short at the plantar aspect of the tarsocrural joint (See Figure 7-19).

The cranial tibial tendon is sutured to local soft tissues. During wound closure it is important not to create tension at the cranial (flexion) surface of the tarsocrural joint. This is the region where the cranial tibial artery becomes the dorsal pedal artery and a tight closure here can impinge the blood supply to the dorsal and plantar aspects of the paw. Subcutaneous tissues are not sutured. The intradermal layer is closed with 3-0 to 4-0 absorbable suture if desired. Skin is sutured in an interrupted or continuous (such as Ford interlocking) pattern. Approximately 2 staggered rows of multiple punctate releasing incisions can be placed to mitigate tension and postoperative swelling (See Wounds with nonapposable edges--potential for apposition and relief of tension related scars, closure--relaxing incisions, multiple punctate releasing incisions).

## Pantarsal Arthrodesis with a Medial or Lateral Plate

The patient is positioned in lateral recumbency with the affected limb down and the other pelvic limb abducted and secured with tape. A medial approach is made to the tarsal area. The skin incision extends from the distal third of the tibia to the middle of the metatarsals. The subcutaneous tissues are incised. The joint spaces are exposed from distally to proximally. The periarticular soft tissues of the tarsometatarsal, centrodistal, and talocalcaneocentral joints are incised and the joint spaces are levered open with the help of a freer elevator or small Hohman retractor. Articular cartilage is removed with the use of a high speed bur. The tarsocrural joint is exposed next. If the medial malleolus is still present the distal aspect of the malleolus is removed using an osteotome and mallet or oscillating saw (See Figure 7-11). Excision of the malleolus facilitates placement of the medial bone plate. Articular cartilage is removed from the tarsocrural space. All of the debrided joint spaces are lavaged with saline and the bone plate is applied.

The arthrodesis angle for the dog is 130 to 150 degrees and for the cat 115 to 125 degrees. A bone plate designed for this purpose is available. The pantarsal arthrodesis plate (Veterinary Orthopedic Implants, South Burlington, VT; Jorgenson Laboratories Inc., Loveland, CO) has a pre-formed angle of 135 degrees. This is a hybrid plate with larger screw holes proximally and smaller screw holes distally. The proximal screw holes are 3.5 mm in diameter and the distal screw holes are 2.7 mm in diameter. There is a left and a right plate. The selected bone plate is centered on the tibia and metatarsus and secured with a screw in the center of the talus. Screws are then placed in the following order: proximal metatarsal bone, distal metatarsal bone, remaining metatarsal bone, distal tibia and remaining tibia (Figure 7-21A & B).

The dermal layer is sutured with absorbable monofilament in a continuous pattern. If tension is present, approximately 2 staggered rows of multiple punctuate releasing incisions can be placed to mitigate tension and postoperative swelling (See Wounds with nonapposable edges--potential for apposition and relief of tension related scars, closure--relaxing incisions, multiple punctuate releasing incisions). Skin is closed routinely.

Plate application is similar for lateral positioning but the distal fibula rather than the medial malleolus is excised to permit plate application. The patient is positioned in lateral recumbency with the affected limb up. A skin incision is made over the caudolateral aspect of the distal tibia extending to the middle of the metatarsal bones (See Figure 7-14). The distal fibula is excised using an osteotomy and mallet or an oscillating saw. Joint surfaces are exposed and articular cartilage removed using a high speed bur. The lateral hybrid plate is positioned over the tibia, tarsal joint and metatarsal bone V. The selected bone plate is centered on the tibia and metatarsus and secured with a screw in the calcaneus and talus. Screws are then placed in the following order: proximal metatarsal bone, distal metatarsal bone, remaining metatarsal bone, distal

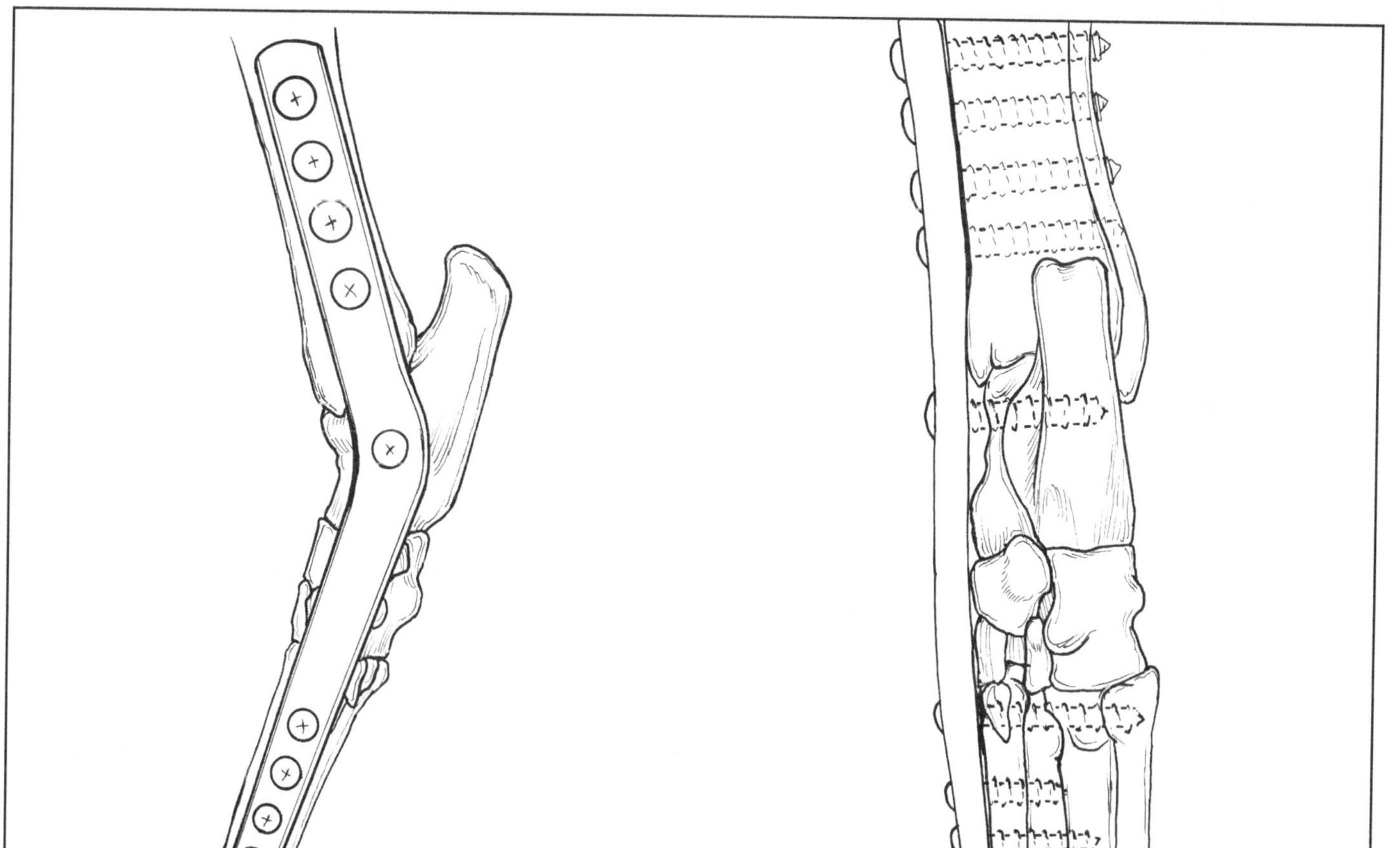


**Figure 7-21.** Medial pantarsal arthrodesis plate. This is a hybrid angled plate applied to the medial aspect of the tarsal joint after removal of the medial malleolus. There are holes for 4 screws in the tibia, one in the talus, and 4 in the metatarsal bones. Care is taken to position the metatarsal screws in the center of the bone. **A.** Medial view. **B.** Caudal view.

tibia and remaining tibia. Closure is as described for medial plate application.

## Aftercare

The operated limb is protected with a modified Robert Jones bandage for one day. This bandage is changed and replaced with a soft padded bandage and lateral splint. The splint remains in place for approximately six weeks. The splint is changed weekly and if areas of pressure irritation are identified the position of the splint can be changed. For example, a lateral splint can be moved to the medial side or an area of irritation over a bony protuberance such as the tuber calcanei can be covered with a "donut" of bandage material to relieve pressure. The splint is transitioned to a soft padded bandage which is placed for approximately 2 weeks and changed weekly or as needed. Exercise is restricted to cage confinement with short leash walks for approximately 12 weeks or until arthrodesis has progressed well. In 12 weeks, longer leash walks may be allowed but no off-leash activity is advised until the completion of arthrodesis. This is usually expected within 12 to 16 weeks. Radiographs are taken at 8 weeks postoperatively and then monthly until arthrodesis is complete. Implant removal may ultimately be required due to irritation from the implant, loosening of the implant or the development of drainage. Owners should be prepared for potential implant removal within approximately one year of surgery.

## Advantages and Disadvantages

The disadvantage of performing a delayed arthrodesis for shearing wounds is increased hospitalization and overall healing time. The advantage of a bone plate over an external fixator for arthrodesing closed wounds is that, with an external fixator, pin tracts and pin loosening can develop during the time it takes to achieve arthrodesis. The bone plate involves less attention to the implants early in the healing process. Long term, however, the bone plate may need to be removed as an additional surgical procedure.

A lengthening plate applied to the dorsal surface of the joint is more resistant to compressive bending forces than a DCP plate due to the absence of screw holes in the center. There may be an increased incidence of screw loosening with these plates compared to DCP plates. It is possible that repetitive bending imposed during weight-bearing may be translated from the lengthening plate to the screws and thus contributes to screw loosening.

A disadvantage of using lateral or medial plates for pantarsal arthrodesis is that the visualization of the tarsal joint spaces is reduced compared to the dorsal approach so it can be more challenging to remove articular cartilage. There is a theoretical advantage of medial or lateral bone plating as opposed to dorsal. The dorsal surface of the tarsocrural joint is the compression side and thus is more susceptible to bending than the medial or lateral side. Medial and lateral bone plates should be less susceptible to breaking than dorsal bone plates. This theoretical advantage has not been demonstrated in clinical trials.

Placement of a medial bone plate for tarsal arthrodesis has been associated with compromise of the vascular supply to the paw resulting in necrosis of the plantar aspect of the paw. It is speculated that the perforating metatarsal artery could be injured either by laceration during cartilage debridement of the tarsometatarsal joint or by impingement from drilling or screw penetration of metatarsal II.

Placing a normograde intramedullary pin from the tarsocrural joint into the proximal tibia increases the stability of the repair. The advantage to this is improved efficiency of arthrodesis with potentially decreased risk of implant loosening. This is most applicable when choosing a dynamic compression plate. The DCP plate is inherently less stiff than a lengthening plate because there are screw holes over the tarsocrural joint.

The placement of multiple punctate releasing incisions parallel to the major incision has the advantage of minimizing postoperative wound tension and swelling of the paw. These are placed even if the primary incision is readily closed without significant tension. These incisions must be covered with a bandage until they heal. This is not a clinically significant issue because the arthrodesis is protected with a soft padded bandage and splint regardless. The punctate incisions heal within the first week.

Harvesting a cancellous autograft adds approximately 15 minutes of surgical time to the procedure and creates an additional surgical site for the patient. Freeze dried or frozen cancellous allograft is effective and avoids surgical time and morbidity. The only disadvantage is the additional cost of purchase and shipping.

## Suggested Readings

1. DeCamp CE, Martinez SA, Johnston SA: Pantarsal arthrodesis in dogs and a cat: 11 cases (1983-1991). J Am Vet Med Assoc 213:1705-1707, 1993.
2. Gorse MJ, Earley TD, Aron DN: Tarsocrural arthrodesis: long-term functional results. J Am Anim Hosp Assoc 27:231-235, 1991.
3. Johnson AL, Dunning D: Atlas of Orthopedic Surgical Procedures of the Dog and Cat: St. Louis: Elsevier Saunders, 2005, 90-91.

4. Kirsch JA, Déjardin LM, DeCamp CD, et al.: In vitro mechanical evaluation on the use of an intramedullary pin-plate combination for pantarsal arthrodesis in dogs. Am J Vet Res 66:125-131, 2005.
5. McKee WM, May C, Macias C, Lapish JP: Pantarsal arthrodesis with a customized medial or lateral bone plate in 13 dogs. Vet Record 143:165-170, 2004.
6. Roch SP, Clements DN, Mitchell RAS et al: Complications following tarsal arthrodesis using bone plate fixation in dogs. J Small Anim Pract 49:117-126, 2008.

# Plantar Intertarsal Subluxation and Luxation

## Definition and Indications

Three distinct plantar ligaments have been described, referred to as the medial, middle, and lateral plantar ligaments (See Figure 7-4). The medial plantar ligament leaves the plantar surface of the sustentaculum tali and attaches to the central tarsal bone and distally to the tarsometatarsal joint capsule. The middle is the most commonly injured plantar ligament. The middle plantar ligament originates on the body of the calcaneus and attaches to the fourth tarsal bone before inserting on the base of the fourth and fifth metatarsals. The lateral plantar ligament leaves the caudolateral surface of the calcaneus and unites with the long lateral collateral ligament before inserting on the base of the fifth metatarsal bone. Rupture of the plantar ligaments destabilizes the proximal intertarsal joint.

The proximal intertarsal joint is comprised of calcaneoquartal and talocalcaneocentral joints. Subluxation of the proximal intertarsal joint is seen radiographically as an increased space between the calcaneus and 4th tarsal bones (the calcaneoquartal joint) with a stable talocalcaneocentral joint (Figure 7-22). Luxation, which is less common, is seen radiographically as an increased space between both the talocalcaneocentral and the calcaneoquartal joints. There is marked dorsal displacement of the distal tarsus at the proximal intertarsal joint with complete luxation (Figure 7-23).

Subluxation of the proximal intertarsal joints is a common tarsal injury in small animals and often occurs with no history of trauma. Middle-aged collies and Shetland Sheepdogs appear to be overly susceptible to plantar ligament ruptures. Clinically, the affected hock is not especially painful despite local swelling, and a moderate plantigrade stance occurs with weight bearing. Bilateral injuries are common. The diagnosis is confirmed with stress radiography. A mediolateral radiograph, with the joint stressed in flexion, will confirm the instability. Avulsed fragments of bone may be seen either from the fourth tarsal bone or the base of the calcaneus.

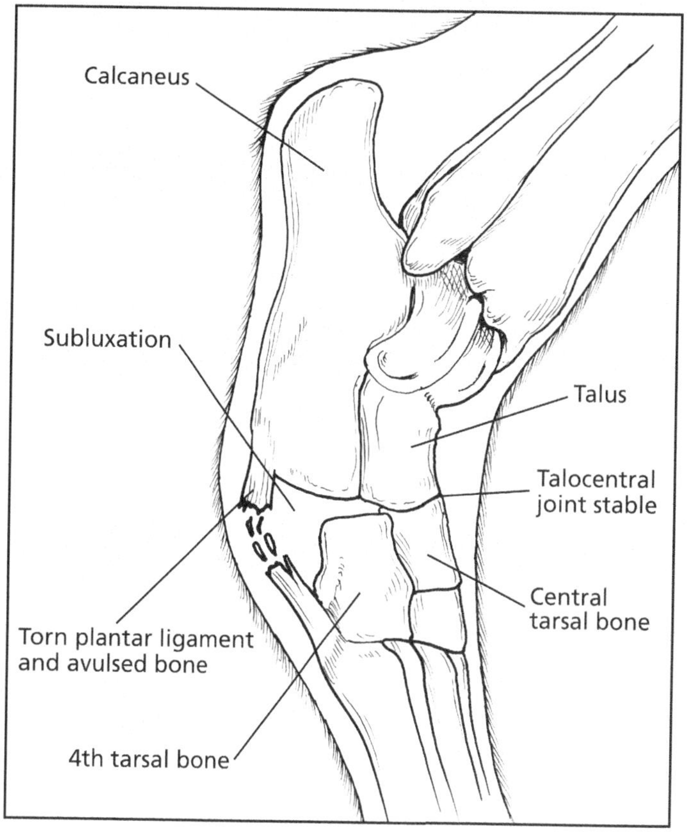


**Figure 7-22.** Proximal intertarsal subluxation. Subluxation of the proximal intertarsal joint is seen radiographically as an increased space between the calcaneus and 4th tarsal bones with a stable joint space between the talus and central tarsal bones. (After Piermattei DL, Flo GL, DeCamp CE. Brinker, Piermattei and Flo's Handbook of Small Animal Orthopedics and Fracture Repair 4th ed. St. Louis: Saunders Elsevier, 2006, 701).

Luxation of the proximal intertarsal joint is associated with severe trauma and is more likely to be associated with fractures of the tarsal bones than subluxation injuries. There is no breed predisposition for this injury. On radiographs, the talus is displaced in a plantar direction and the distal aspect of the tarsus is displaced in a dorsal direction. A luxation of the proximal intertarsal joint is distinguished from a subluxation by the marked dorsal displacement of the distal tarsus at the proximal intertarsal joint (See Figure 7-23).

## Techniques

Conservative management of plantar intertarsal subluxations and luxations with casts or splints is rarely successful. Arthrodesis of the calcaneoquartal joint is recommended and can be accomplished with a lateral bone plate or external fixator.

### Proximal Intertarsal Arthrodesis with a Lateral Bone Plate

The patient is placed in lateral recumbency with the affected limb up. A lateral approach to the calcaneus and metatarsus is made. The skin incision extends from the proximal calcaneus to the middle of the fifth

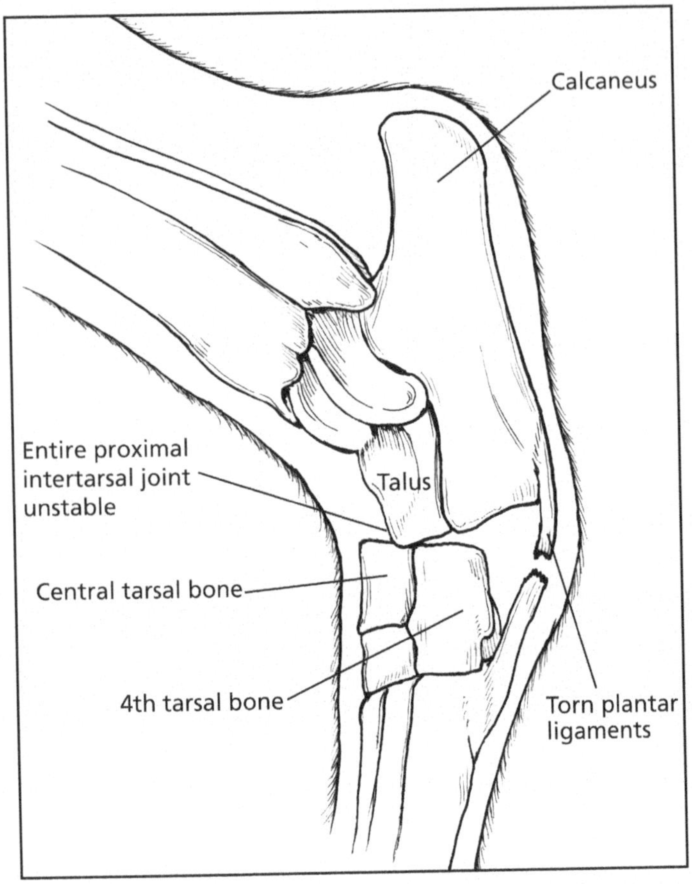


**Figure 7-23.** Proximal intertarsal luxation. Luxation of the proximal intertarsal joint is seen radiographically as increased space between the calcaneus and 4th tarsal bones in addition to marked displacement of the joint space between the talus and central tarsal bones. (After Piermattei DL, Flo GL, DeCamp CE. Brinker, Piermattei and Flo's Handbook of Small Animal Orthopedics and Fracture Repair 4th ed. St. Louis: Saunders Elsevier, 2006, 703).

metatarsal bone. The subcutaneous and deep crural fascia is incised. The superficial digital flexor tendon is retracted medially and the abductor digiti quinti muscle is elevated to expose the calcaneus, fourth tarsal bone, and base of the fifth metatarsal bone (Figure 7-24). The paw is stressed medially and articular cartilage is removed from the calcaneoquartal joint using a high speed bur. A Freer elevator can be used to lever open joint spaces and improve visibility. In preparation for plating, it may be necessary to smooth the base of the fifth metatarsal bone and a portion of the fourth tarsal bone with an oscillating saw or high speed bur to accommodate the plate. The surgical site is lavaged and bone graft is packed into the proximal intertarsal joint. A cancellous bone graft can be obtained from the patient's ipsilateral humerus as described for arthrodesis of shearing wounds. Alternatively, frozen or freeze-dried bone graft can be purchased from a supplier (Veterinary Transplant Services; Kent, WA. www.vtsonline.com ). It is not essential to use cancellous bone graft with this surgery.

A standard dynamic compression plate or locking plate (Synthes, West Chester, PA) size 2.7 mm or 3.5 mm, is chosen according to the size of the patient. At least three screws are placed in the calcaneus and three in the metatarsus. The distal screw into the calcaneus should also engage the talus. The order of screw placement is important to ensure centralization over the small metatarsal bones. The first screw is placed in the proximal hole through the calcaneus, the plate is correctly positioned over the metatarsus, and a screw is placed in the distal plate hole through metatarsal bones 5 and 4. The remaining plate holes are drilled and screws are placed (Figure 7-25). When drilling holes into the calcaneus, they should not be placed too close to the plantar cortex, as this may cause a stress riser and promote fracture of the calcaneus.

The metatarsal bone is smaller than the calcaneus and it may be desirable in some cases to use smaller screws in the metatarsus to avoid exceeding 30% of the bone diameter. A hybrid dynamic compression bone plate designed for carpal arthrodesis (Jorgensen Laboratories, Inc., Loveland, CO) can be adapted to partial tarsal arthrodesis. The hybrid bone plate is available as a 2.0/2.7-mm or a 2.7/3.5-mm size. The plate is applied as described for standard bone plate application, from the lateral calcaneus to the lateral metatarsal bones, with smaller screws engaging the distal holes. The distal plate also tapers in width and in thickness to facilitate tension-free closure over the implant.

After bone plate application, the surgical site is thoroughly lavaged with sterile saline. The calcaneoquartal joint can then be packed with cancellous bone to promote early arthrodesis although this is not essential with this surgery. A sample of cancellous bone can be obtained from the patient's ipsilateral humerus as described for arthrodesis of shearing wounds. Alternatively, frozen or freeze-dried bone graft can be purchased from a supplier (Veterinary Transplant Services; Kent, WA. www.vtsonline.com). Subcutaneous tissues are sutured with 3-0 to 4-0 absorbable suture followed by skin. There is a tendency for tension to be present over the distal incision which can promote postoperative swelling. Multiple punctuate releasing incisions can be placed to prevent significant postoperative swelling (See Chapter 3).

### Proximal Intertarsal Arthrodesis with an External Fixator

The patient is placed in lateral recumbency with the affected limb up. A craniolateral approach to the calcaneus and metatarsus is made. The skin incision is intended to be cranially located to not interfere with external fixator placement.

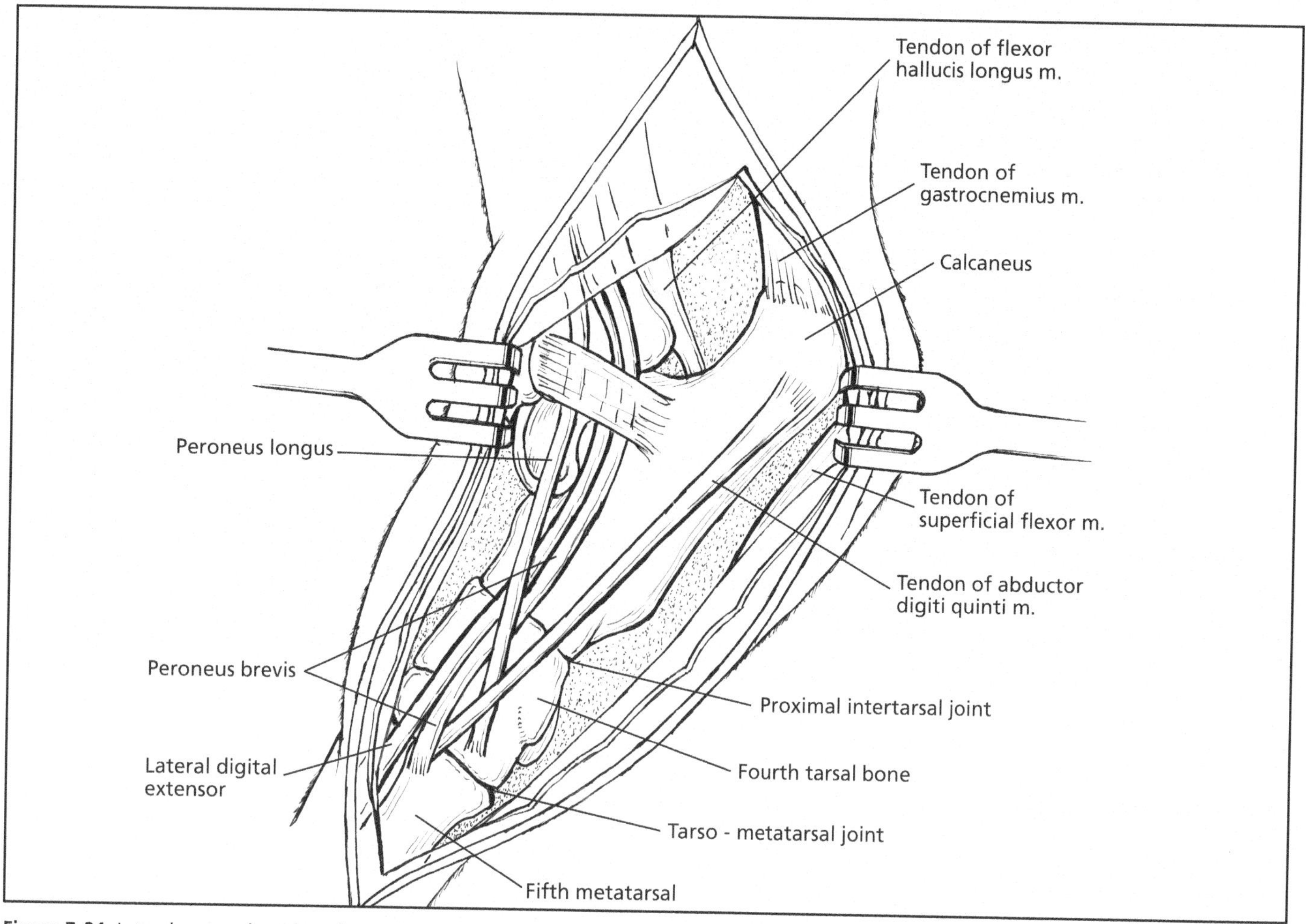


**Figure 7-24.** Lateral approach to the calcaneus and metatarsus. The skin incision extends from the proximal calcaneus to the middle of the fifth metatarsal bone. The subcutaneous and deep crural fascia are incised. The superficial digital flexor tendon is retracted and the abductor digiti quinti muscle is elevated to expose the calcaneus, fourth tarsal bone, and base of the fifth metatarsal bone. (After Piermattei DL, Johnson KA. An Atlas of Surgical Approaches to the Bones and Joints of the Dog and Cat 4th ed. Philadelphia: Saunders, 2004, 383).

The skin incision extends from the proximal calcaneus to the proximal aspect of the fifth metatarsal bone. The subcutaneous and deep crural fascia is incised. The superficial digital flexor tendon is retracted caudally and the abductor digiti quinti muscle is elevated to expose the calcaneus and fourth tarsal bone (See Figure 7-24). The paw is stressed medially and articular cartilage is removed from the calcaneoquartal joint using a high speed bur. A Freer elevator can be used to lever open joint spaces and improve visibility. The calcaneoquartal joint can then be packed with cancellous bone to promote early arthrodesis although this is not essential with this surgery. A sample of cancellous bone can be obtained from the patient's ipsilateral humerus as described for arthrodesis of shearing wounds. Alternatively, frozen or freeze-dried bone graft can be purchased from a supplier (Veterinary Transplant Services; Kent, WA. www.vtsonline.com).

The dermal tissue are closed with 3-0 to 4-0 absorbable suture followed by routine skin closure. A type II external fixator is applied to the proximal intertarsal joint. Two center-threaded positive profile fixation pins are placed transversely through the calcaneus and talus and two are placed through the fourth tarsal bone (Figure 7-26). An appropriately sized pre-drill is used prior to placing each pin. If there is not enough room to place 2 pins through the fourth tarsal bone, the distal most pin can be placed through the proximal metatarsal bones. The pins are affixed to connecting rods with clamps or with epoxy putty (Oatey epoxy putty, Oatey, Cleveland, OH). The epoxy putty is kneaded for approximately 1 minute and pressed onto the pin/rod interface. This epoxy is fully set in approximately 20 minutes.

## Aftercare

Subluxation and luxation injuries that are stabilized with a bone plate are protected with a lateral splint extending from the proximal tibia to the digits for approximately 4 weeks postoperatively. The splint is changed weekly and if areas of pressure irritation are identified the position of the splint can be changed. For example, a lateral splint can be moved to the medial side or an area of irritation over a bony protuberance such as the tuber calcanei

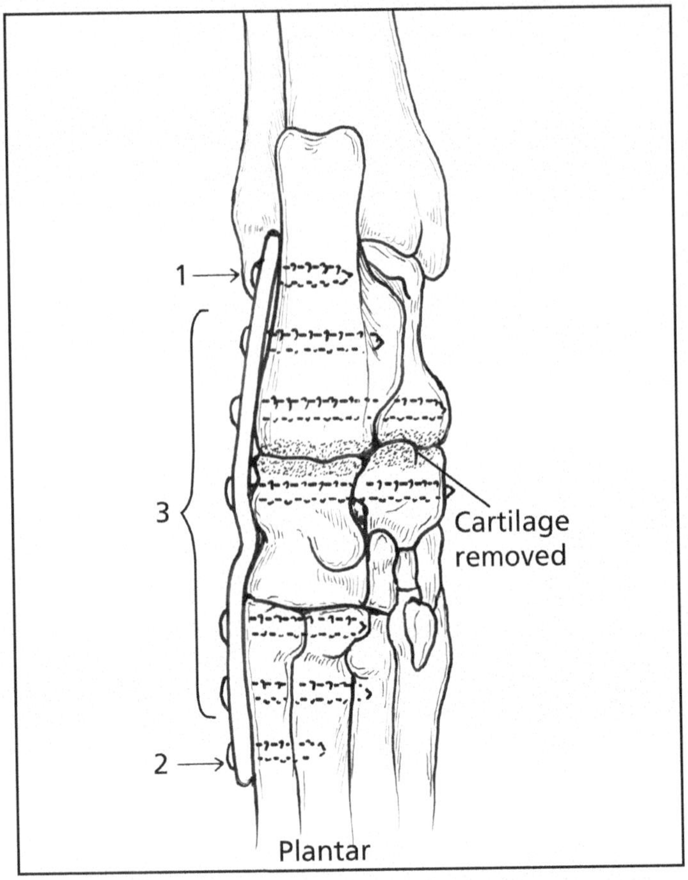


**Figure 7-25.** Lateral bone plating for partial tarsal arthrodesis. The lateral aspect of the fourth tarsal bone and the base of the fifth metatarsal bone have been flattened to accommodate the plate. The plate traverses the proximal and distal intertarsal joints and the tarsometatarsal joint. Three screws have been placed in the calcaneus and 3 in the metatarsus, with one placed in the fourth and central tarsal bones. The order of screw placement is important to ensure centralization over the small metatarsal bones. The first screw *(1)* is placed in the proximal hole through the calcaneus, the plate is correctly positioned over the metatarsus, and the second screw *(2)* is placed in the distal plate hole through metatarsal bones 5 and 4. The remaining plate holes *(3)* are filled.

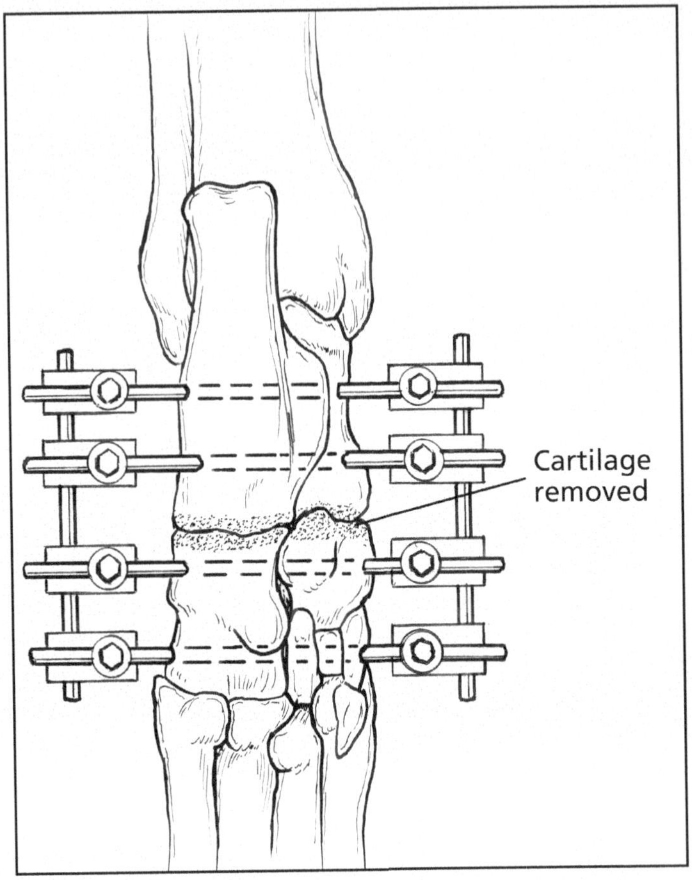


**Figure 7-26.** External fixation for partial tarsal arthrodesis. Cartilage is removed from the proximal intertarsal joint space. A type II external fixator traverses the proximal intertarsal joint. Two center-threaded positive profile fixation pins are placed through the calcaneus and talus and 2 are placed through the fourth and central and fourth and numbered tarsal bones. The pins are secured to connecting rods with clamps or with epoxy putty. (After Piermattei DL, Flo GL, DeCamp CE: Brinker, Piermattei and Flo's Handbook of Small Animal Orthopedics and Fracture Repair, 4th ed. St Louis: Saunders Elsevier, 2006, 701).

can be covered with a "donut" of bandage material to relieve pressure. Exercise is restricted to short, 5 to 10 minute leash walks, 3 to 5 times daily for 8 to 12 weeks or until fusion is verified on radiographs. Radiographs are taken 8 weeks postoperatively and then every 4 to 6 weeks as needed until arthrodesis of the proximal intertarsal joint is achieved.

Metatarsal screws may loosen over time and necessitate removal of the plate. This typically occurs after arthrodesis has been accomplished so the plate can be removed and not replaced. This is done no sooner than 4 to 6 months postoperatively. The distal screws are most apt to loosen since the tarsometatarsal joint is not arthrodesed. If the screws loosen prior to complete fusion of the calcanoquartal joint, they can be removed while leaving the remaining implants in place.

External fixators are covered with a circumferential soft padded bandage and changed weekly or as needed. After 3 to 4 weeks the circumferential bandage is removed and a "bumper" bandage placed that just covers the connecting rods. The external fixator is maintained until radiographic signs of advanced proximal intertarsal joint fusion are seen, which usually occurs by 8 to 10 weeks. Exercise is restricted to short, 5 to 10 minute leash walks, 3 to 5 times daily for 8 to 12 weeks or until fusion is verified on radiographs.

## Advantages and Disadvantages

Partial arthrodesis by means of a bone plate is straightforward and effective in achieving arthrodesis of the proximal intertarsal joint. The plate may very well loosen over time and need to be removed. The tarsometatarsal joint is not arthrodesed so micromotion exists at this site and promotes implant loosening. This is not a significant issue if arthrodesis is complete prior to the onset of implant loosening.

A hybrid dynamic compression bone plate (carpal arthrodesis plate) is designed to have smaller screws placed in the distal holes and thereby accommodates the smaller metatarsal bones. The disadvantage of hybrid plates is that they are available in limited sizes and lengths compared to standard dynamic compression plates.

An external fixator frame is less expensive than a bone plate and particularly useful if there are open wounds. There is no need for a second open surgery to remove implants as there may be with a bone plate. There is a potential for pin tract infections to develop but these are localized and respond to systemic antibiotics. Epoxy putty can be used instead of bone clamps and may be easier to place if there is limited space between pins. Epoxy putty adheres well to pins. A 25 mm segment of epoxy paste is comparable in strength to a medium KE clamp. Epoxy putty is especially useful in this external fixator because the limited space between pins can impede placement of standard clamps.

A cancellous bone graft should speed arthrodesis. However, arthrodesis usually occurs readily without a bone graft in this situation. The added surgical time or expense for a graft is not always necessary for proximal intertarsal arthrodesis. Grafting is most applicable for unstable luxation injuries.

# Suggested Readings


1. Allen MJ, Dyce J, Houlton JEF: Calcaneoquartal arthrodesis in the dog. J Small Anim Pract 34:205-210, 1993.
2. Fettig AA, McCarthy RJ, Kowaleski MP: Intertarsal and tarsometatarsal arthrodesis using 2.0/2.7-mm or 2.7/3.5-mm hybrid dynamic compression plates. J Am Anim Hosp Assoc 38:364-369, 2002.
3. Johnson AL, Dunning D: Atlas of Orthopedic Surgical Procedures of the Dog and Cat: St. Louis: Elsevier Inc., 2005, 92-95.
4. Piermattei DL, Flo GL: Fractures and other orthopedic injuries of the tarsus, metatarsus, and phalanges. In Brinker, Piermattei, and Flo's Handbook of Small Animal Orthopedics and Fracture Repair, 3rd ed.: Philadelphia: WB Saunders, 1997, 607-655.
5. Piermattei DL. An Atlas of Surgical Approaches to the Bones and Joints of the Dog and Cat, 4th ed.: Philadelphia: Saunders, 2004.
6. Roe SC, Keo T: Epoxy putty for free-form external skeletal fixators. Vet Surg 26:472-77, 1997.
7. Staudte KL, Gibson NR, Read RA et al: Evaluation of a metal acrylic repair product as a clamp for an external fixator. Vet Comp Orthop Traumatol 17:97-103, 2004.


# Dorsal Intertarsal Subluxation

## Definition and Indications

Subluxation of the calcaneoquartal, talocalcaneocentral, and centrodistal joints (proximal or distal intertarsal joints) in a dorsal direction is less common than plantar injury. Numerous short intertarsal ligaments stabilize the dorsal, medial and lateral portions of the proximal and distal intertarsal joints. The condition is not usually associated with external trauma. Dorsal instabilities may occur more often than plantar instabilities in cats. Dorsal subuxation affects the compression, versus the tension, side of the joint and thus is more stable with weight-bearing and less stable during the swing phase of the gait. Diagnosis can be challenging. The animal is able to stand with a normal joint angle because the plantar ligament is intact, but the dorsal instability produces inflammation and pain and causes a mild lameness. Physical examination will show excessive laxity of the intertarsal joints. Diagnosis is confirmed with stress radiographs demonstrating dorsal opening of the joint space. Most have a medial (talocalcaneocentral) or lateral (calcaneoquartal) component (Figure 7-27A & B).

Although the primary injury involves the dorsal supporting ligaments, injury to the medial or lateral short ligaments at the level of the intertarsal joints can induce varus or valgus positioning of the paw (See Figure 7-27B). The presence of medial or lateral instability in addition to dorsal instability warrants surgical repair of these is also indicated (See Figures 7-12 and 7-15).

Conservative treatment with splinting may be adequate for isolated dorsal injuries (without medial or lateral instability) in non-athletic animals. Surgical treatment is indicated for athletic animals with any intertarsal injury and for non-athletes that have combined dorsal and medial or lateral instability. Traditionally, partial tarsal arthrodesis to stabilize the dorsal compartment was the surgical treatment of choice. Newer surgical approaches provide internal splinting of the dorsal surface of the joint, as opposed to arthrodesis, to induce fibrous healing. These techniques appear to be as effective as arthrodesis.

## Techniques

### Stabilization with Screws and Washers

Rather than performing an arthrodesis on the unstable part of the joint, the joint space can be bridged with internal fixation.

The patient is placed in dorsal recumbency with the affected limb pulled caudally. A skin incision is centered over the dorsal aspect of the proximal intertarsal joint. The site(s) of instability are located. A dorsal approach to the tarsus is made. The incision extends from the distal tibia to the proximal metatarsal bones. The long digital extensor tendon is separated from the cranial tibial tendon and retracted laterally (See Figure 7-18).

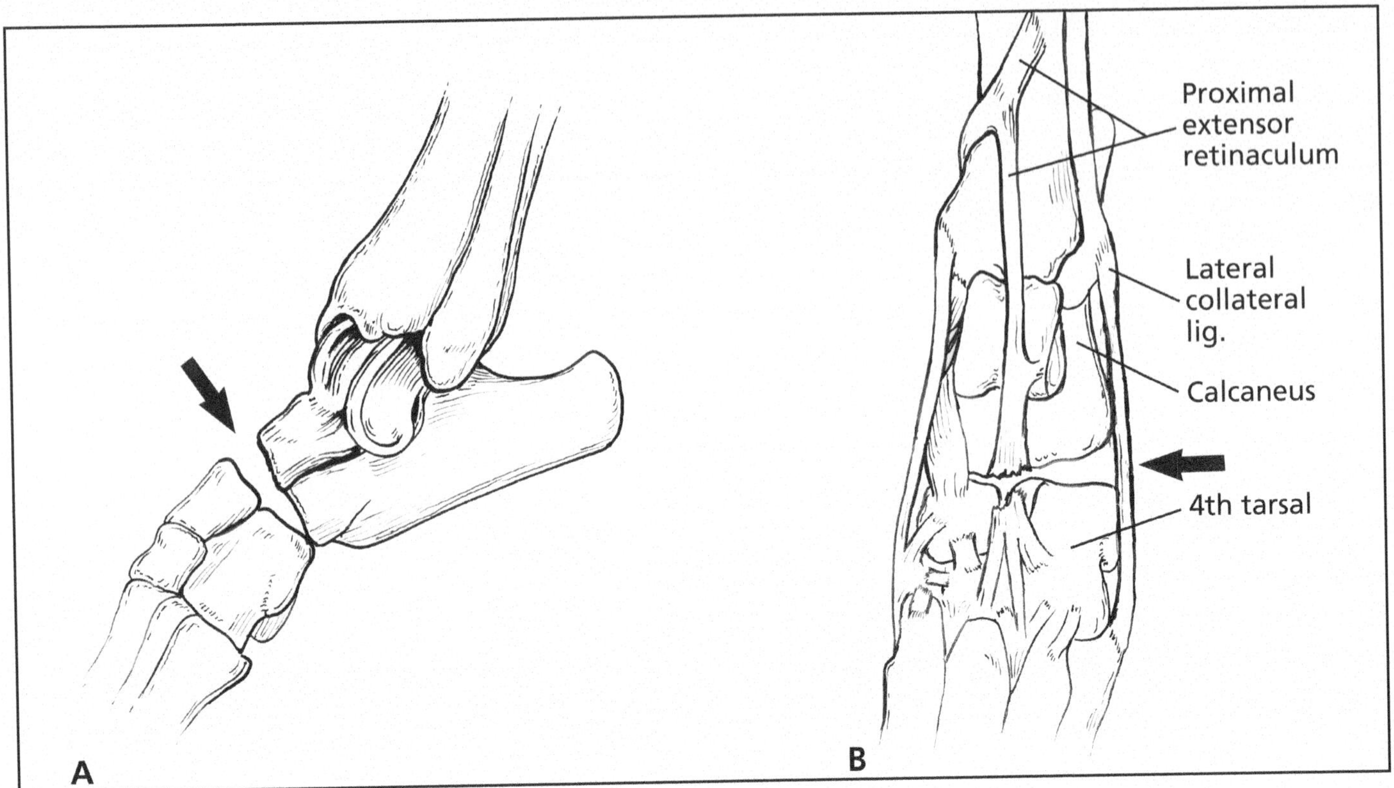


**Figure 7-27.** Dorsal intertarsal subluxation. **A.** Stress radiographs demonstrate opening of the dorsal intertarsal joint space in the lateral projection *(arrow)*. **B.** Wedging between the calcaneus and 4th tarsal bone is seen in the cranial-caudal projection *(arrow)*. (After Piermattei DL, Flo GL, DeCamp CE: Brinker, Piermattei and Flo's Handbook of Small Animal Orthopedics and Fracture Repair, 4th ed. St Louis: Saunders Elsevier, 2006, 703).

The affected joint space is located. Potential sites of instability include the proximal intertarsal (talocalcaneo-central or calcaneoquartal) joints (See Figure 7-27) or distal intertarsal (central distal) joints (See Figure 7-29).

A screw and washer are placed on either side of the affected joint. Screw size ranges from 2.0. 2.7 or 3.5 depending on the size of the dog. With instability of the calcaneoquartal joint, a screw and washer are placed on the craniolateral surface of the calcaneus and the craniolateral surface of the fourth tarsal bone. Cerclage wire (approximately 20 gauge), or heavy gauge suture is anchored beneath the washer on either side in a figure 8 pattern and tightened (Figure 7-28A, B and C).

For instability of the distal intertarsal joint one screw is placed on the cranial surface of the central tarsal bone and one on the cranial surface of the 3rd tarsal bone. Cerclage wire (approximately 20 gauge) is anchored beneath the washer on either side and tightened (Figure 7-29A, B and C).

The subcutaneous layer is closed with 3-0 to 4-0 absorbable suture in a simple continuous pattern followed by the skin.

### Stabilization with a Bone Plate

The bone plate described for this surgical procedure is a ComPact Unilock 2.0/2.4 System (Synthes, Inc., Maxillofacial, Paoli, PA.). The 2.0 mm locking plate is useful in cats and small dogs and the 2.4 mm plate in larger dogs. This system is more stable than a standard plate (See Figure 7-28B & C) and thus the use of only 1 to 2 screws on either side of the unstable joint. The screws can be placed through the near cortex of the bone. It is not necessary to penetrate both cortices with this system.

The site(s) of instability are located. For example, with instability of the calcaneoquartal joint the plate is centered over the craniolateral surface of the proximal intertarsal joint. Two screws are placed in the more proximal tarsal bone (the calcaneus) and two screws are placed in the distal tarsal bone (the fourth tarsal bone). The screws are tightened (See Figure 7-28B).

With instability of the distal intertarsal joint, a 2 hole plate is positioned over the cranial aspect of the central and 3rd tarsal bones. One screw is placed in the central and one in the 3rd tarsal bone (See Figure 7-29C).

Small standard plates (veterinary cuttable plate, 2.0 mm DCP or LC-DCP plates, Synthes Veterinary, Paoli, PA) can be used instead of the specialized plate described. Without the locking mechanism both cortices should be penetrated and additional screws placed.

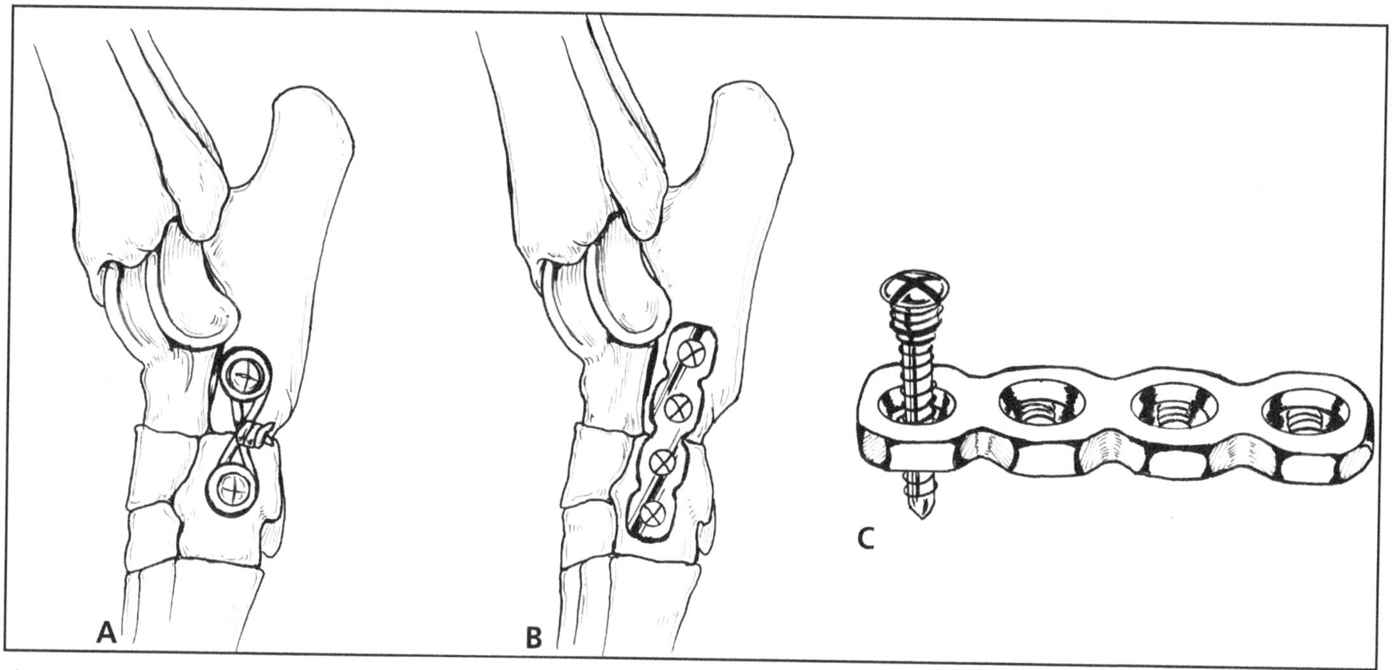


**Figure 7-28.** Fixation of dorsal intertarsal subluxation. **A.** The intertarsal joint is stabilized with a screw and washer anchored in the calcaneus and the 4th tarsal bone. Cerclage wire or heavy gauge suture is anchored to both screws and tightened. **B., C.** The affected joint space may also be bridged with a small locking bone plate.

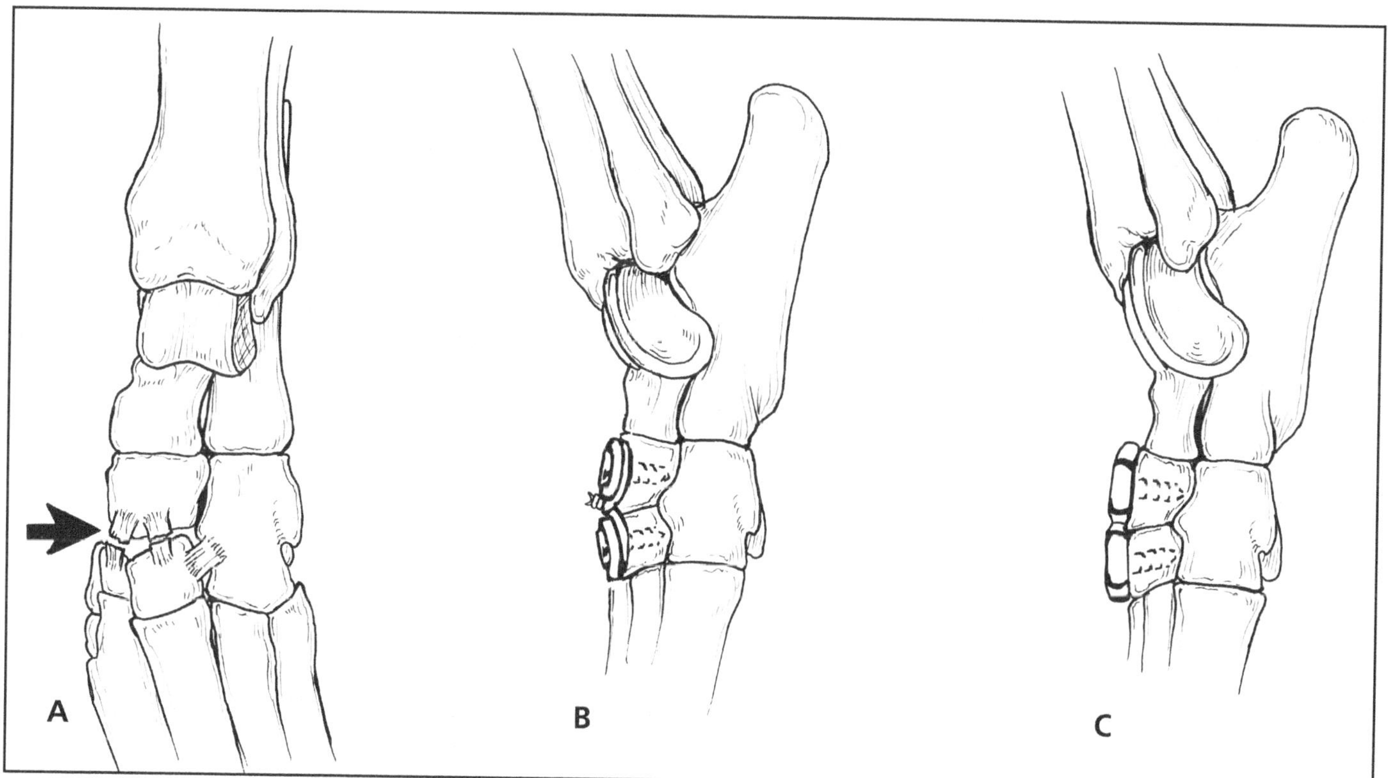


**Figure 7-29.** Dorsal subluxation of the central-distal joint space. **A.** There is instability between the central and numbered tarsal bones in the cranial-caudal radiographic projection *(arrow)*. **B.** The central-distal joint space is stabilized with screws and washers anchoring heavy gauge suture or cerclage wire. **C.** The central-distal joint may also be bridged with a small locking bone plate.

The subcutaneous layer is closed with 3-0 to 4-0 absorbable suture in a simple continuous pattern followed by the skin. In the presence of tension, multiple punctate relaxing incisions may be placed (See Chapter 3).

## Aftercare

Dorsal intertarsal subluxation injuries stabilized with locking plates do not require splinting postoperatively. Those injuries stabilized with standard bone plates or screws, washers and cerclage wire are protected with a lateral splint extending from the mid tibia to the digits for approximately 3 weeks postoperatively with weekly changes. The splint is replaced with a soft padded bandage for 1 week. Exercise is restricted to short, 5 to 10 minute leash walks, 3 to 5 times daily for 8 weeks postoperatively.

Screws and cerclage wire or bone plates should ideally be removed approximately two months postoperatively to prevent joint ankylosis from chronic absence of motion.

### Advantages and Disadvantages

Bridging the region of instability to induce fibrous healing has advantages over partial tarsal arthrodesis. Surgical time is shorter and fibroplasia occurs more quickly postoperatively than joint fusion. Screws and washers are less expensive than specialized bone plates (ComPact Unilock, Synthes, Inc, Paoli, PA) and can be effective for this purpose. However, if the suture or cerclage wire breaks prematurely an additional surgery may be required. The specialized plates are less likely to fail than suture or wire. The cost of this system is greater than a standard cuttable bone plate but the advantage is the use of fewer screws and unicortical screw placement.

If bone plates are used for this surgery, joint ankylosis can occur over time so plate removal is recommended. Despite this concern, excellent results are reported with cases whose owners chose not to have implant removal.

## Suggested Readings

1. Guillard MJ: Dorsal tarsal instability in three racing greyhounds. J Small Anim Pract 44:415-417, 2003.
2. Hurter K, Schawalder P, Schmokel HG: Talocalcaneocentral luxation combined with lateral instability of the talocrural joint in a dog and cat. Vet Comp Orthop Traumatol 17:53-56, 2004.
3. Johnson AL, Dunning D: Atlas of Orthopedic Surgical Procedures of the Dog and Cat: St. Louis: Elsevier Inc., 2005, 92-93.
4. Voss K, Keller M, Montavon PM: Internal splinting of dorsal intertarsal and tarsometatarsal instabilities in dogs and cats with the ComPact UniLock 2.0/2.4 System. Vet Comp Orthop Traumatol 17:1250130, 2004.

## Luxation of the Base of the Talus

### Definition and Indications

This is an infrequent injury involving the talocalcaneocentral joint. This injury is distinguished from hyperextension with luxation of the proximal intertarsal joint by the direction of the talus. With luxation of the base of the talus, the talus displaces dorsally (Figure 7-30A & B). This is in contrast to hyperextension with luxation of the proximal intertarsal joint, in which case the talus displaces in a plantar direction (See Figure 7-23). Animals with luxation of the base of the talus usually present with non-weightbearing lameness and significant swelling of the tarsus. The injury is diagnosed with standard radiographs of the tarsus and is most apparent in the lateral view. Surgery is indicated for this injury. Because some cases have concurrent injury of the medial collateral ligament, the tarsus should be evaluated for medial instability. If medial stability is detected, a prosthetic imbrication repair is performed as described for medial collateral ligament rupture.

### Technique

The dog is positioned in dorsal recumbency and the tarsus is immobilized so that the plantar surface is parallel with the table. A dorsomedial incision is made over the central tarsal bone and talus. The cranial branch of the medial saphenous vein is retracted laterally or ligated. The cranial tibial tendon is retracted medially and the long digital extensor tendons are retracted laterally (See Figure 7-18). The base of the talus is reduced by opening the proximal intertarsal joint. This joint is opened by applying flexion and lateral distraction on the metatarsus. A 3.5 or 4.0 mm screw is placed between the distal talus and calcaneus. The screw is placed as a positional screw rather than a lag screw (See Figure 7-30B).

The dermal layer is closed with 3-0 to 4-0 absorbable suture in a simple continuous pattern followed by the skin. In the presence of tension, multiple punctate relaxing incisions may be placed (See Chapter 3).

### Aftercare

A lateral splint is placed that extends from the digits to the proximal tibia. The splint is maintained for 4 weeks. The splint is changed weekly and if areas of pressure irritation are identified the position of the splint can be changed. For example, a lateral splint can be moved to the medial side or an area of irritation over a bony protuberance such as the tuber calcanei can be covered with a "donut" of bandage material to relieve pressure. This splint is replaced with a soft padded bandage for 2 weeks. Exercise is restricted to short leash walks only for 8 weeks followed by gradual return to normal activity. The screw is not removed unless it becomes loose.

### Advantages and Disadvantages

Surgical stabilization for this injury is advantageous. Most patients respond well to surgical repair. Closed reduction and stabilization with a cast or splint does not yield reliable results and is not recommended.

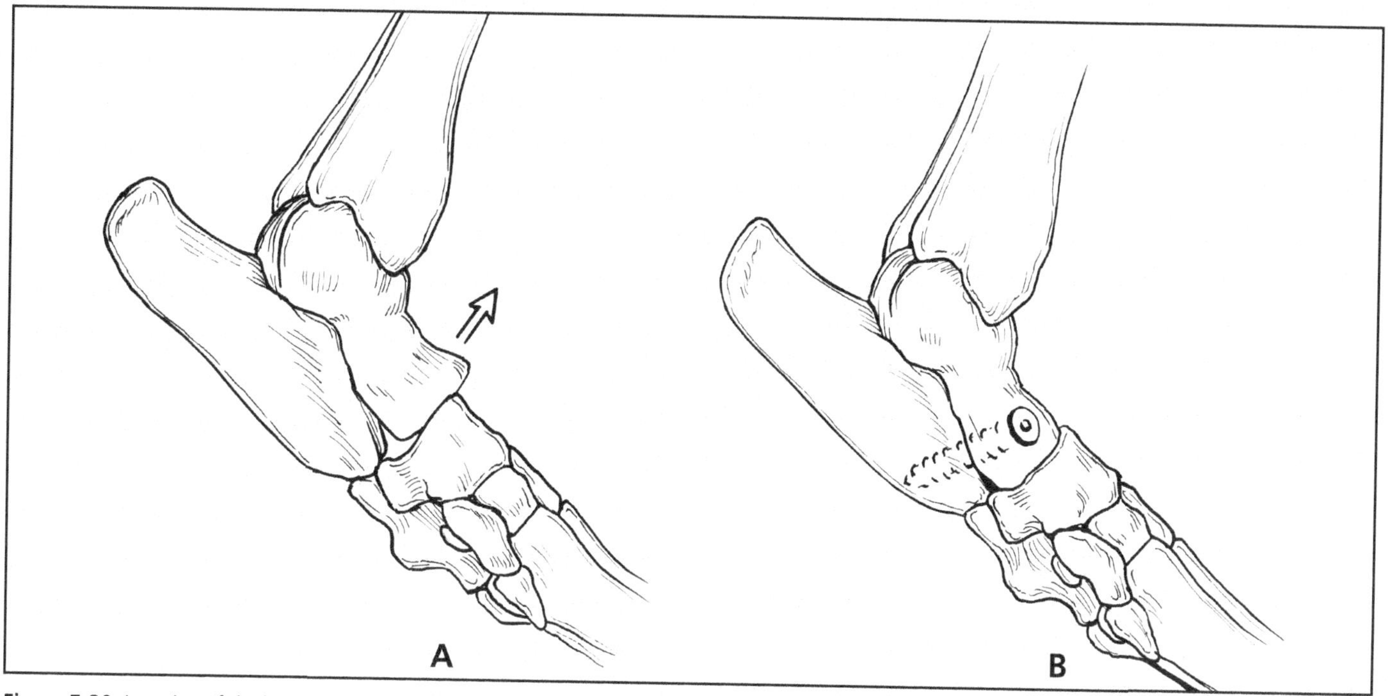


**Figure 7-30.** Luxation of the base of the talus. **A.** This injury is distinguished by dorsal displacement of the base of the talus *(arrow)*. **B.** Fixation is achieved with a positional screw from the talus to the calcaneus. (After Piermattei DL, Flo GL, DeCamp CE: Brinker, Piermattei, and Flo's Handbook of Small Animal Orthopedics and Fracture Repair 4th ed. St. Louis: Saunders Elsevier, 2006, 686).

## Suggested Readings

1. Piermattei DL, Flo GL, DeCamp CE: Brinker, Piermattei, and Flo's Handbook of Small Animal Orthopedics and Fracture Repair, 4th ed.: St. Louis: Saunders Elsevier, 2006,686.

# Tarsometatarsal Joint Subluxation

## Definition and Indications

Instability of the plantar or medial aspect of the tarsometatarsal joint produces significant lameness and often a plantigrade stance. Plantar instability results from disruption of the plantar ligament at the level of the tarsometatarsal joint. This is a hyperextension injury at the level of the proximal intertarsal joint. Whereas proximal intertarsal subluxation often occurs with no external trauma, tarsometatarsal injury is usually related to a known traumatic event. The degree of instability can be either subluxation or luxation of the tarsometatarsal joint space. Cast or splint stabilization is usually unsuccessful. Surgical stabilization by means of partial tarsal arthrodesis is indicated for both subluxation and luxation injuries of the plantar tarsometatarsal joint.

Medial or lateral instability of the tarsometatarsal joint is a result of collateral ligament injury and can occur singly or along with plantar or dorsal instability. Medial instability is a significant injury because the medial tarsus is the weightbearing side and attempted weightbearing exacerbates the valgus angulation of the paw (Figure 7-31A & B). These cases do not respond well to external coaptation. Medial or lateral instability alone can be treated with collateral ligament reconstruction. There is a concern that undetected injury to the plantar ligament could be present that would result in persistent lameness. Surgical stabilization by means of partial arthrodesis is recommended for medial-lateral and plantar instability.

Partial arthrodesis is done using a bone plate that extends from the level of the talus or calcaneus to the metatarsal bones. If there is a medial component to the instability, the bone plate may be placed medially, and laterally if there is a lateral component.

Tarsaometatarsal instability confined to the dorsal plane is rarely reported. As with dorsal instability at the proximal intertarsal level, this injury is not usually associated with an acute traumatic event. A chronic low grade lameness is reported and animals bear weight on the affected limb. The standing angle is normograde. Palpation may reveal dorsal instability and stress radiographs confirm the diagnosis. External coaptation for 4 weeks can be adequate for these cases and should be tried prior to surgical intervention. If conservative management does not resolve the lameness, the area of instability can be stabilized using a dorsal locking plate or veterinary cuttable plate as described for dorsal intertarsal instability. Chronic cases should be treated by arthrodesis of the tarsometatarsal joint as described for plantar instability.

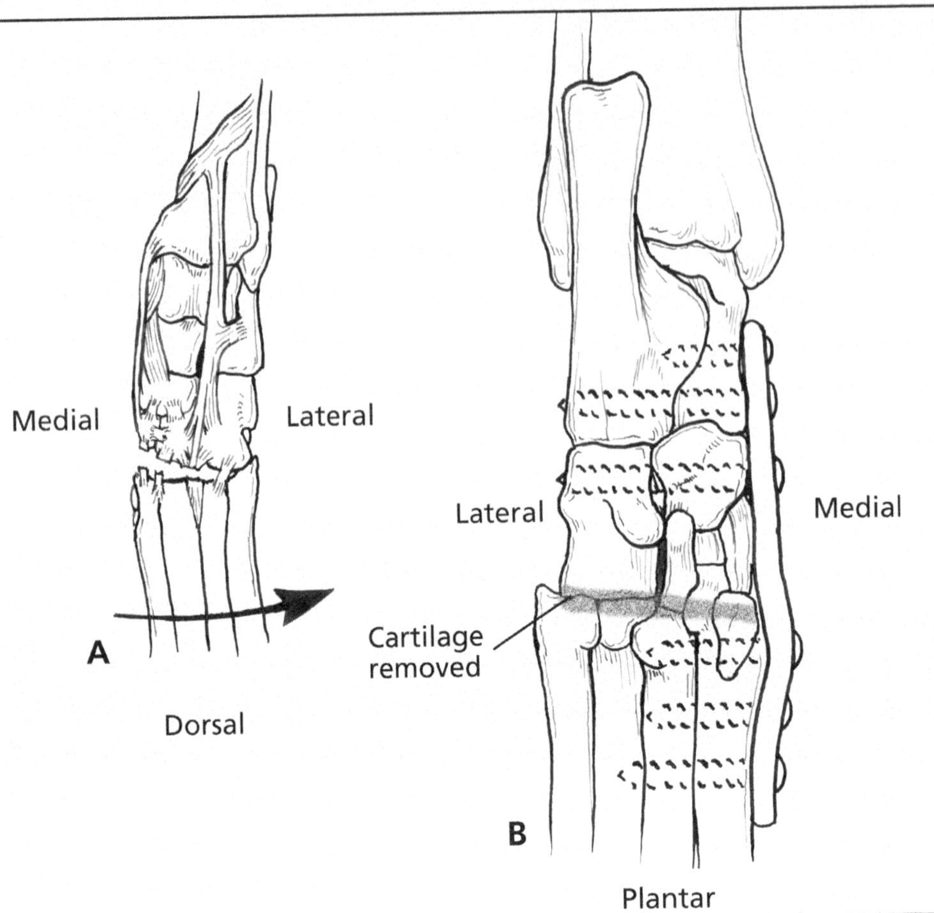


**Figure 7-31.** Dorsomedial instability of the tarsometatarsal joint. **A.** Ligament disruption between the numbered tarsal bones and the metatarsal bones can induce dorsal medial instability. There is excessive valgus deviation of the paw *(arrow)*. **B.** The tarsometatarsal joint is arthrodesed using a bone plate. Cartilage is removed from the tarsometatarsal joint but a bone graft is not essential. The bone plate may be placed medially or laterally and extends from the level of the talus or calcaneus to the metatarsal bones.

## Techniques

### Arthrodesis of the Tarsometatarsal Joint by Use of a Lateral Bone Plate

The patient is positioned in lateral recumbency with the affected limb up to approach the lateral aspect of the tarsus. The skin incision extends from the proximal calcaneus to the middle of the fifth metatarsal bone. The subcutaneous and deep crural fascia are incised. The superficial digital flexor tendon is retracted caudally and the abductor digiti quinti muscle is elevated to expose the calcaneus, fourth tarsal bone, and base of the fifth metatarsal bone (See Figure 7-25). The paw is stressed medially and articular cartilage is removed from the third, fourth and fifth tarsometatarsal joints using a high speed bur. It is not usually possible to gain access to the second tarsometatarsal joint from the lateral approach. A Freer elevator can be used to lever open joint spaces and improve visibility. In preparation for plating, it is necessary to smooth the base of the fifth metatarsal bone and a portion of the fourth tarsal bone with an oscillating saw or high speed bur. Prior to plating, the surgical site is lavaged and the tarsometatarsal joints are packed with cancellous autograft harvested from the patient's ipsilateral humerus or frozen or freeze-dried allograft (Veterinary Transplant Services; Kent, WA).

Dynamic compression plates are usually of the 2.7 mm or 3.5 mm screw size. Approximately 2 screws are placed in the base of the calcaneus, 1 to 2 through the fourth tarsal bone, and 3 in the metatarsal bones. The order of screw placement is important to ensure centralization over the small metatarsal bones. The first screw is placed in the proximal hole through the calcaneus, the plate is correctly positioned over the metatarsus, and a screw is placed in the distal plate hole through metatarsal bones 5 and 4. The remaining plate holes are drilled and screws placed. The distal screw into the calcaneus should also engage the talus. Care is taken to avoid placement of a screw through the calcaneoquartal joint.

The dermal layer is closed with 3-0 to 4-0 absorbable suture in a simple continuous pattern followed by the skin. In the presence of skin tension, multiple punctate relaxing incisions may be placed (See Chapter 3).

### Arthrodesis of the Tarsometatarsal Joint by use of a Medial Bone Plate

The patient is positioned in lateral recumbency with the affected limb down. The skin incision extends from the region of the medial malleolus to the distal second metatarsal bone. The medial collateral ligaments are identified and preserved (See Figure 7-11A). Deep fascia is incised to expose the medial surface of the talus, the proximal and distal intertarsal joints, the tarsometatarsal joint and the 2nd metatarsal bone. The medial aspect of the tarsometatarsal joint is opened by applying a valgus stress on the paw. A small high speed bur is used to remove cartilage from the second and third tarsometatarsal joints. The surgeon is careful to protect the perforating metatarsal artery as it passes between the 2nd and 3rd metatarsal bones. It is not essential to place a cancellous bone graft in the tarsometatarsal joint. A bone plate (usually 2.7 mm DCP plate) is positioned over the talus and 2nd metatarsal bone. It is contoured if needed. Two screws engage the talus, 1 screw traverses the central and fourth tarsal bones, and 3 screws engage the 2nd or 2nd and 3rd metatarsal bones (See Figure 7-31B).

The dermal layer is closed with 3-0 to 4-0 absorbable suture in a simple continuous pattern followed by the skin. In the presence of tension, multiple punctate relaxing incisions may be placed (See Chapter 3).

## Aftercare

A tarsometatarsal arthrodesis is protected with a lateral splint extending from the proximal tibia to the digits for approximately 4 weeks postoperatively with weekly splint changes. If areas of pressure irritation are identified the position of the splint can be changed. For example, a lateral splint can be moved to the medial side or an area of irritation over a bony protuberance such as the tuber calcanei can be covered with a "donut" of bandage material to relieve pressure. This splint is replaced with a soft padded bandage for 2 weeks. Exercise is restricted to short, 5 to 10 minute leash walks, 3 to 4 times daily until fusion is verified on radiographs. Radiographs are taken 8 weeks postoperatively and then every 4 weeks as needed until arthrodesis of the tarsometatarsal joint is achieved. Metatarsal screws may loosen over time and necessitate removal of the plate. This typically occurs after arthrodesis has been accomplished so the plate can be removed and not replaced. Animals that do not have screw loosening but do display a chronic mild lameness after arthrodesis should also have the bone plate removed. This is done no sooner than 4 to 6 months postoperatively.

## Advantages and Disadvantages

Stabilizing tarsometatarsal instability by means of arthrodesis is effective and associated with good long term results. Placing bone plates on either the medial or lateral sides requires less soft tissue dissection than dorsal approaches. It is logical to place a medial bone plate for medial instability however a lateral bone plate has been shown to successfully stabilize both medial and lateral instability. The advantage of the lateral plate is there is more bone for proximal screw purchase with the calcaneus than with the talus. This may be most significant in small patients. The disadvantage of bone plates is that in some cases they are associated with chronic mild lameness. The source of mild lameness is unclear. It could be referable to rigid fixation of low motion joints or to screws traversing metatarsal bones. Bridging two or more metatarsal bones with a screw results in loss of flexibility between adjacent bones and may produce lameness. Most animals with successful arthrodesis that have a continued mild lameness will become sound when the bone plate is removed.

# Suggested Readings


1. Dyce J, Whitelock RG, Robinson KV, et al: Arthrodesis of the tarsometatarsal joint using a laterally applied plate in 10 dogs. J Small Anim Pract 39:19-22, 1998.
2. Guillard MJ. Dorsal tarsal instability in three racing greyhounds. J Small Anim Pract 44:415-417, 2003.
2. Johnson AL, Dunning D: Atlas of Orthopedic Surgical Procedures of the Dog and Cat: St. Louis: Elsevier Inc., 2005, 92-93.
3. Muir P, Norris JL: Tarsometatarsal subluxation in dogs: partial arthrodesis by plate fixation. J Am Anim Hosp Assoc 35:155-162, 1999.
4. Piermattei DL, Flo GL, DeCamp CE: Brinker, Piermattei, and Flo's Handbook of Small Animal Orthopedics and Fracture Repair, 4th ed.: St. Louis: Saunders Elsevier, 2006, 710-712.
5. Piermattei DL, Johnson KA: An Atlas of Surgical Approaches to the Bones and Joints of the Dog and Cat, 4th ed.: Saunders, 2004.


# Talocalcaneal Luxation

## Definition and Indications

Talocalcaneal luxation is an uncommon injury. The talocalcaneal joint is a low motion joint. The major structures maintaining stability of the talocalcaneal joint are two strong ligaments, the proximal and distal talocalcaneal ligaments that cross the internal surfaces of the talus and calcaneus. There are no external ligaments that directly connect the talus and calcaneus. In some cases the talocalcaneal luxation is dramatic and can be seen radiographically as a wide separation between the two bones. These cases often have displacement of the proximal intertarsal joint as well (Figure 7-32A & B). Both talocalcaneocentral and calcaneoquartal joint displacement has been reported to occur with talocalcaneal luxations. More subtle cases of talocalcaneal luxation may require rotational stress views to aid in the diagnosis. Surgical stabilization of talocalcaneal luxations is recommended. Securing the talus to the calcaneus by means of a lag or positional screw has been successful in a small number of cases. Although there is a concern of screw breakage secondary to residual motion between the talus and calcaneus, this has not been a clinical problem.

### Technique

The tarsus is exposed using a dorsomedial approach. The incision extends from the distal fourth of the tibia to the base of metatarsal II. The subcutaneous and crural fasciae are incised on the same line as the skin and retracted with the skin. The tendon of the cranial tibial muscle is retracted laterally so that the joint capsule on the dorsal aspect of the tarsus may be incised and retracted (See Figure 7-18). If there is luxation of the proximal intertarsal joint (the calcaneoquartal or talocalcaneocentral joints) the luxation is reduced. This is done by flexing the tarsocrural joint and using a combination of pointed reduction forceps and digital pressure to manipulate the talus and calcaneus into place. Once the proximal intertarsal joint is reduced, the tarsocrural joint is held in slight extension and pointed reduction forceps are placed across the talus and calcaneus to stabilize and compress the talocalcaneal joint. Depending on the size of the animal, a 2.7 mm or 3.5 mm positional bone screw is placed from the distal aspect of the talus (the head or neck of the talus) to the calcaneus (Figure 7-32C & D). The stability of the talocalcaneal and proximal intertarsal joints is ascertained. Usually stabilizing the talus and calcaneus results in stabilizing the proximal intertarsal joint as well, as long as the collateral ligaments are intact.

A technique for applying additional stability to the talocalcaneocentral join has been described. A small screw with washer or a suture anchor is placed in the central tarsal bone in a medial to lateral direction. This anchor is connected to the previously placed talar screw with heavy gauge nylon.

The dermal layer is closed with 3-0 to 4-0 absorbable suture in a simple continuous pattern followed by the skin. In the presence of tension, multiple punctate relaxing incisions may be placed (See Chapter 3).

### Aftercare

The tarsus is protected with a lateral splint and soft padded bandage that extends from the proximal tibia to the digits. The splint is placed for approximately 4 weeks. The splint is changed weekly and if areas of pressure irritation are identified the position of the splint can be changed. For example, a lateral splint can be moved to the medial side or an area of irritation over a bony protuberance such as the tuber calcanei can be covered with a "donut" of bandage material to relieve pressure. This splint is replaced with a soft padded bandage for 2 weeks. Exercise is restricted to short, 5 to 10 minute leash walks, 3 to 4 times daily for 8 weeks postoperatively. Follow up radiographs are performed at 8 weeks postoperatively to evaluate joint stability and integrity of the implants.

### Advantages and Disadvantages

Traversing a low motion joint with a metal implant and not arthrodesing the joint applies cyclic loading forces to the implant. The screw that traverses the talocalcaneal joint can become loose or break over time. This complication has not yet been reported but there are low numbers of cases. If implant loosening occurs, the implant can be removed. Stabilization of the joint is expected by 3 to 6 months postoperatively.

If there is only mild displacement between the talus and calcaneus, conservative treatment with a splint can be attempted. The potential disadvantage is arthritic change resulting from a low motion joint experiencing excessive mobility over time. Placing a screw between the calcaneus and talus is relatively straightforward and could limit the risk of arthritic change.

## Suggested Readings

1. Gorse MJ, Purinton PT, Penwick RC et al: Talocalcaneal luxation. An anatomic and clinical Study. Vet Surg 19:429-434, 1990.
2. Hurter K, Schawalder P, Schmokel HG: Talocalcaneocentral luxation combined with lateral instability of the talocrural joint in a dog and a cat. Vet Comp Orthop Traumatol 17:53-56, 2004.
3. Macias C, McKee WM, May C: Talocalcaneal luxation with plantar displacement of the head of the talus in a dog and a cat. Vet Record 147:743-745, 2000.
4. Piermattei DM, Johnson KA. An Atlas of Surgical Approaches to the Bones and Joints of the Dog and Cat, 4th ed.: Philadelphia: Saunders, 2004, 312-315.376-379.

## Strain Injury

### Definition and Indications

Tendons extend from muscle bellies and insert on bone. Tendon architecture is similar to ligaments in that they are composed primarily of type I collagen arranged in parallel bundles. The individual bundles are surrounded by loose connective tissue called endotenon. Epitenon surrounds the entire group of bundles and paratenon covers and separates different tendon bellies thus providing smooth gliding function. Tendons that are encased within a synovial lining do not have a paratenon.

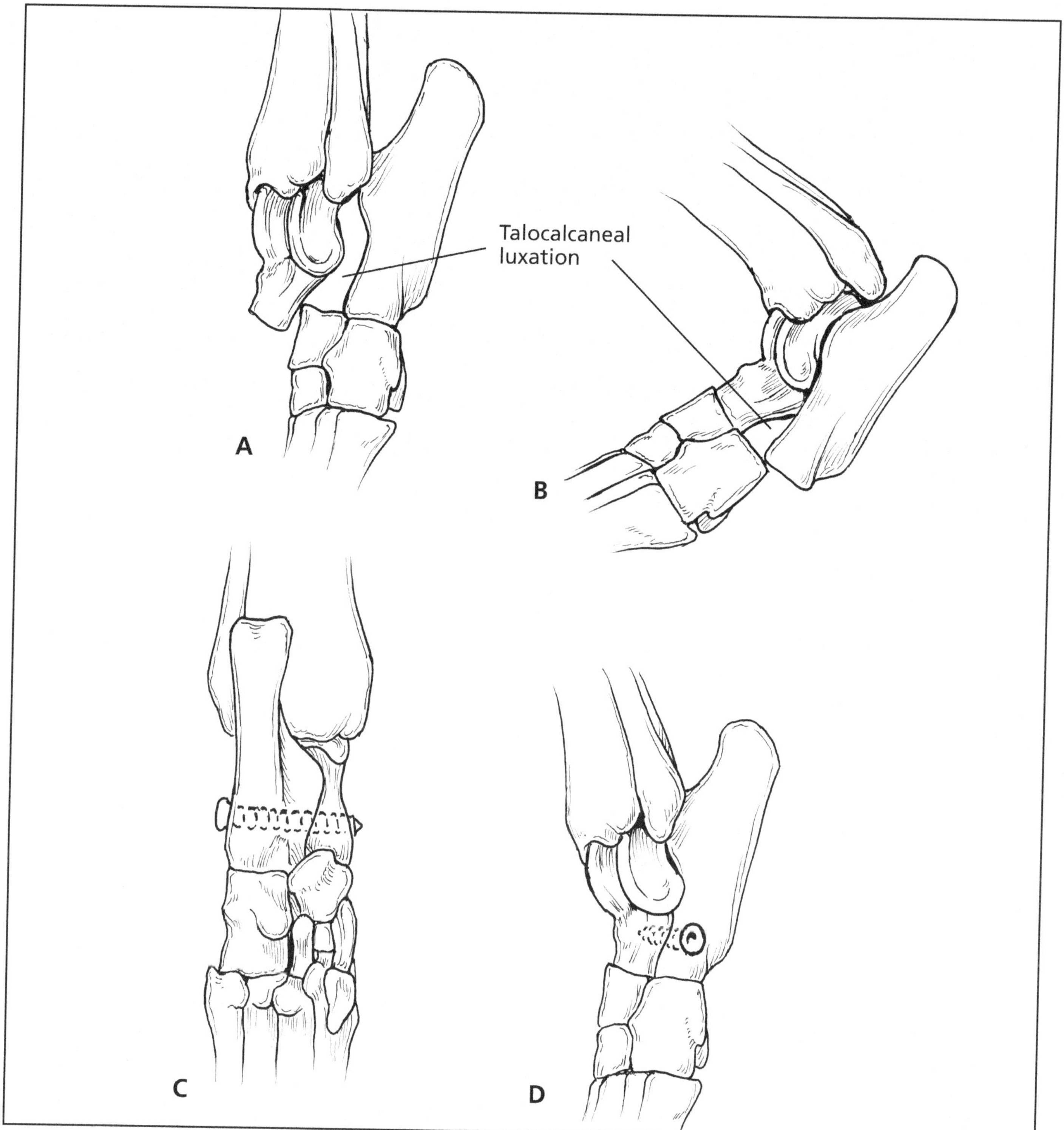


**Figure 7-32.** Talocalcaneal luxation **A.** Obliqued cranial-caudal radiographic projection and **B.** Lateral projection show medial and plantar displacement of the head of the talus. **C.** and **D.** Caudal and lateral views (respectively). The talus and calcaneus are reduced and stabilized with a lag screw.

Injury to a tendon is referred to as a strain. Strains can occur in the muscle belly, the musculotendinous junction, or in the tendon. As with other tissues tendons undergo inflammatory, reparative and remodeling (or maturation) stages of healing. The inflammatory stage occurs within the first 3 days and ends with the deposition of randomly oriented collagen by about the fifth day. The reparative stage follows and lasts for approximately 4 weeks. The reparative phase is marked by increasing collagen content and alignment of fibers parallel to lines of stress. During the remodeling phase type III collagen is gradually replaced by type I.

Evaluation of tendon healing demonstrates that a healing tendon has 56% of its original strength at 6 weeks and 79% at 1 year following injury. An approximation for tendon healing strength is "50% by 50 days". The resistance to gap formation is an essential component of tendon repair. In repaired canine tendons, gaps less than 3 mm increase in strength between 10 and 42 days postoperatively. Gaps greater than 3 mm markedly impair healing because they do not develop significant increase in strength during this time. Successful tendon repair depends on selecting suture patterns that resist gap formation and controlling motion during the first six weeks of healing. Suture patterns described for tendon anastomosis include the three-loop pulley (Figure 7-33), continuous cruciate (Figure 7-34A & B) and locking loop (See Figures 7-9 & 7-10).

Tendons take more than 12 weeks to become strong enough for unrestrained active loading. Normal forces associated with muscle contraction strain tendons to only 25% to 33% of their maximal capability. The strength obtained by 6 weeks after tenorrhaphy is adequate to withstand limited exercise.

The suture material chosen for tendon repair should be monofilament to promote smooth gliding through the tissue and should also be slowly absorbable or nonabsorbable to allow time for adequate return of tensile strength.

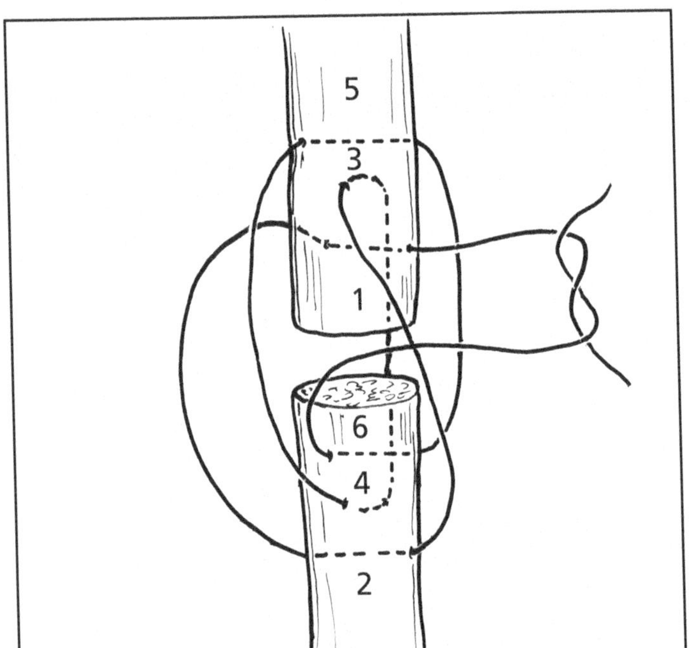


**Figure 7-33.** Three-loop pulley suture. The three-loop pulley is a 3 dimensional suture pattern created by placing suture passes approximately 60 degrees apart around a tendon. There are 3 passes of suture with 2 parts to each pass (1 and 2, 3 and 4, 5 and 6). After each pass, the needle is moved around the tendon by approximately 60 degrees before beginning the next pass of suture. The distances from the severed end of the tendon for suture passes are near-far (1 and 2), middle-middle (3 and 4), far-near (5 and 6). The "near" needle passes are approximately 0.5 cm from the cut edge of the tendon, the "middle" passes are 1.0 cm and the "far" passes are 1.5 cm. The 2 free ends of suture are tied. (After Berg RJ, Egger EL. In vitro comparison of the three loop pulley and locking loop suture patterns for repair of canine weightbearing tendons and collateral ligaments. Vet Surg 15:107, 1986.

## Techniques

### Three-Loop Pulley Pattern

The three-loop pulley is a 3 dimensional suture pattern created by placing suture passes approximately 60 degrees apart around a tendon. There are 3 passes of suture with 2 parts to each pass. After each pass, the needle is moved around the tendon by about 60 degrees before beginning the next pass of suture. The distances from the severed end of the tendon for suture passes are described as near-far, middle-middle, far-near. The "near" needle passes are 0.5 cm from the cut edge of the tendon, the "middle" passes are 1.0 cm and the "far" passes are 1.5 cm. The 2 free ends of suture are tied snugly with a double throw followed by 3 single throws (See Figure 7-33). A monofilament suture such as nylon or polypropylene in size 2-0 to 0 is chosen for a medium to large-sized dogs. When tension is applied to the tendon or ligament, the suture material glides within the tissue in a pulley fashion such that an equal amount of tension is supported by each of the three loops. This redistribution of tension is optomized if each loop is tightened prior to tying the final knot.

### Continuous Cruciate Pattern

The continuous cruciate pattern is useful for tenorrhaphy of flat tendons. The continuous cruciate pattern is started by joining the 2 cut edges of the tendon with a simple continuous pattern that proceeds in a cranial to caudal direction. The knot is left untied at the start of the pattern so the suture remains as a free end. The second row is redirected from caudal to cranial with each suture pass overlapping a passage in the first row to form "X's" or a cruciate pattern. The 2 ends of the suture are alternately tightened until the tendon ends are tightly apposed, and then the suture ends are tied with square knots (See Figure 7-34). Depending on the size of the tendon, either 2-0 or 0 monofilament suture is chosen for this pattern.

### Locking Loop Pattern

The locking loop pattern creates 4 loops of suture that grasp bundles of tendon tissue when the suture is tightened. There are transverse and longitudinal components to this pattern. To allow the loops to tighten on the tendon bundles, the transverse components must be superficial to the longitudinal ones. The first pass of the suture is transverse. This pass is begun approximately 1 cm from the torn edge of the tendon. The suture is passed in a medial to lateral direction. The second pass of the suture is longitudinal. The

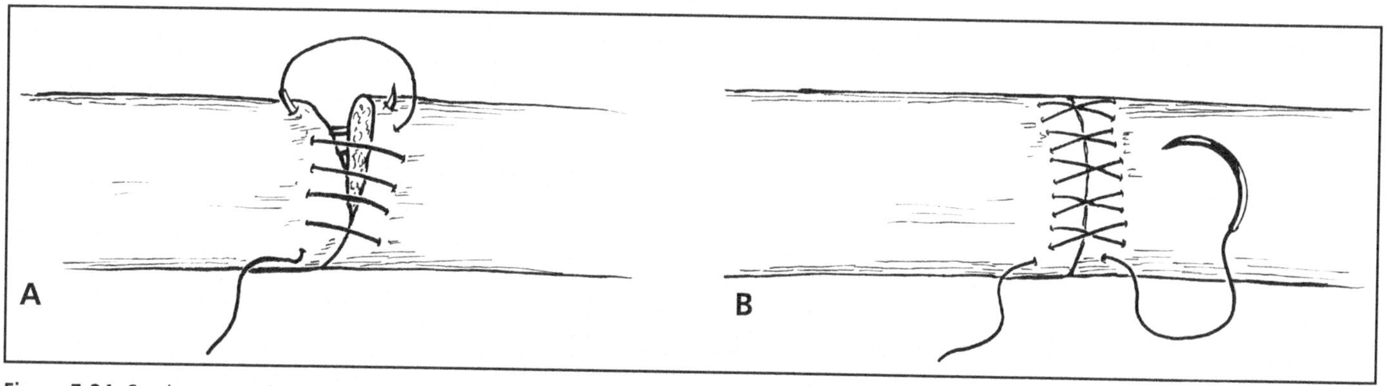


**Figure 7-34.** Continuous cruciate pattern. **A.** The continuous cruciate pattern is started by joining the 2 cut ends of the tendon with a simple continuous pattern that proceeds in a cranial to caudal direction. The knot is left untied at the start of the pattern so the suture remains as a free end. **B.** The second row is redirected from caudal to cranial such that its strands overlie those of the first row to form a series of "X's". The 2 ends of the suture are alternately tightened until the tendon ends are tightly apposed, and then the suture ends are tied.

needle re-enters the tendon directly behind the first pass of the suture. The needle is directed distally and deep to the transverse portion, parallel to the fibers of the tendon, and exits at the distal end. The needle enters the opposite side of the tendon and the pattern is repeated to form the 4 locking loops (See Figure 7-9). The 2 ends of the suture are tightly tied. The suture material is size 2-0 to 0 in a medium-to large dog. A smooth surface suture material such as nylon or polypropylene is chosen to allow free gliding through the tendon as the knot is tightened. It is possible in larger tendons to place 2 locking loop patterns side by side. This provides a stronger repair than placing a single suture (See Figure 7-10).

## Aftercare

Postoperative immobilization is for surgically repaired tendons similar to that described for a grade 3 sprain injury. The tendon repair is immobilized postoperatively with an external fixator or splint. A transarticular external fixator can be placed for 4 weeks then removed and replaced with a soft padded bandage and splint for 2 weeks then a soft padded bandage alone for 1 to 2 weeks. Alternatively a soft padded bandage and splint can be placed for 4 to 6 weeks and then changed to a soft padded bandage alone for 1 to 2 weeks. The splint is changed weekly and if areas of pressure irritation are identified the position of the splint can be changed. For example, a lateral splint can be moved to the medial side or an area of irritation over a bony protuberance such as the tuber calcanei can be covered with a "donut" of bandage material to relieve pressure.

A joint supplement is recommended for the entire period of immobilization. Polysulfated glygosaminoglycan (Adequan, Novartis Animal Health US Inc, Greesnboro, NC) may be administered at a dose of 4.4 mg/kg intramuscularly (IM) or subcutaneously (SQ) twice weekly for 4 weeks, then once every 2 to 4 weeks. The subcutaneous form is off-label but has been used by the author with better owner compliance than with IM administration. Oral glucosamine/chondroitin supplements (Cosequin, Dasuquin, Nutramax Laboratories, Edgewood, Md) may be used instead of injectable chondroitin.

## Advantages and Disadvantages

Although the locking loop suture pattern (see sprain injury) is described for use in ligament and tendon repair, it is weaker than both the three-loop pulley and the continuous cruciate pattern. The three-loop pulley suture has been shown to be more resistant to gap formation than 2 locking-loop sutures in canine Achilles tendon repair. The three-loop pulley suture is most suited to cylindrically shaped versus flat tissue because there is some tendency for this suture pattern to cause bunching up of a flat tendon.

Placing an external fixator can induce greater articular cartilage damage than a splint because it completely immobilizes the joint, which reduces the proteoglycan content of the cartilage. A splint permits some motion, which benefits cartilage health. Joint immobilization for 4 weeks reduces the proteoglycan content of articular cartilage. The proteoglycan content improves when the joint is allowed to move again but it is important to control weight-bearing forces during this phase of recovery to protect the cartilage. This is done by transitioning from an external fixator to a soft padded bandage with splint and then to a soft padded bandage alone. Having an external fixator in place for a limited time has the advantage of protecting the surgical repair during the early phases of healing when it is most vulnerable. There are usually fewer rechecks needed with an external fixator compared to a soft padded bandage and splint.

## Suggested Readings

1. Berg RJ, Egger EL: *In vitro* comparison of the three-loop pulley technique and locking loop suture patterns for repair of canine weightbearing tendons and collateral ligaments. Vet Surg 15:107-110, 1986.
2. Dueland R, Quenin J: Triceps tenotomy: biomechanical assessment of healing strength. J Am Anim Hosp Assoc 16:507-512, 1980.
3. Gelberman RH, Boyer MI, Brodt MD, et al.: The effect of gap formation at the repair site on the strength and excursion of intrasynovial flexor tendons. J Bone Joint Surg (Am) 81:975-982, 1999.
4.Keller WG, Aron DN, Rowland GN, et al.: The effect of trans-stifle external skeletal fixation and hyaluronic acid therapy on articular cartilage in the dog. Vet Surg 23:119-128, 1994.
5. Moores AP, Owen MR, Tarlton JF. The three-loop pulley suture versus two locking-loop sutures for the repair of canine Achilles tendons. Vet Surg 33:31-37, 2004.
6. Renberg WC, Radlinsky MG. In vitro comparison of the locking loop and continuous cruciate suture patterns. Vet Comp Orthop Traumatol 14:15-18, 2001.
7. Williams J: Wound Healing: Tendons, Ligaments, Bone, Muscles and Cartilage. In Millis DL, Levine D, Taylor RA: Canine Rehabilitation and Physical Therapy: St. Louis: Saunders, 2004, 100.


# Injury to the Common Calcanean Tendon

## General Information

Injury to the common calcanean, or Achilles, tendon usually occurs at the distal insertion on the calcaneus. Injury can also occur at the proximal origin of the gastrocnemius muscle or along the length of the tendon. The common calcanean tendon has 3 parts: the gastrocnemius, the combined tendon, and the superficial digital flexor tendon. The gastrocnemius muscle originates on the distal femur and its tendon provides the most significant component of the calcanean tendon. The gastrocnemius tendon inserts on the proximal lateral aspect of the tuber calcanei. The combined tendon comprises the tendons of the biceps, gracilis and semitendinosus muscles and attaches medially on the tuber calcanei. The superficial digital flexor tendon caps the tuber calcanei, attaching on either side, and continues distally to insert on the plantar aspect of the middle phalanges.

In animals with an intact calcanean tendon apparatus, there is a normal flexion angle of the tarsocrural joint while standing. This angle is approximately 140 degrees in the dog and 120 degrees in the cat. The standing angle will match the contralateral side. On physical examination, the animal is placed in lateral recumbency and the limb is held at a normal standing angle. In this position, flexing the tarsocrural joint to 90 degrees should produce tension in the calcanean tendon. Damage to the calcanean tendon creates varying degrees of a plantigrade stance, depending on the type of injury, and there may be laxity of the calcanean tendon when the joint is flexed to 90 degrees.

There is a classification system that describes 3 types of common calcanean tendon injuries. A Type 1 injury is complete rupture of all 3 components of the common calcanean tendon. Dogs with complete tendon rupture have a plantigrade stance. When the stifle joint is held at a normal standing angle, the tarsocrural joint can be completely flexed beyond 90 degrees. A gap between tendon ends may be palpable and there may be a visible laceration of the skin and underlying tissues. A Type 2 injury involves rupture of some but not all 3 major components of the common calcanean tendon. The most common presentation of this is called a type 2C injury. A type 2C injury is avulsion of the gastrocnemius tendon insertion on the tuber calcanei with an intact superficial digital flexor tendon. A unique postural change occurs when the superficial digital flexor tendon remains functional but there has been disruption at some point along the calcanean tendon. With a plantigrade stance, there is increased tension on the intact superficial digital flexor tendon. This tendon exerts more force on its attachment, the plantar aspect of the middle phalanges, and causes flexion of the digits in a characteristic "claw" appearance (Figure 7-35). A type 3 injury is inflammation of the tendon. A type 3 injury causes lameness that becomes worse with exercise but the angle of the stance is normal. On palpation, a thickening is palpable just proximal to the calcaneus.

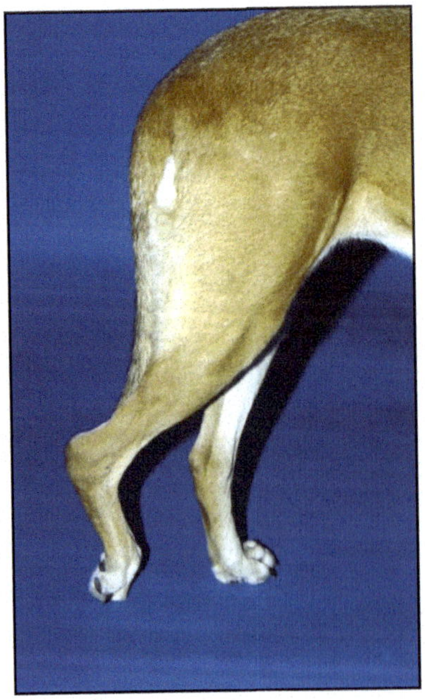

**Figure 7-35.** Stance with Achilles tendon injury. Avulsion of the gastrocnemius tendon insertion on the calcaneus causes excessive flexion of the digits due to the tension of the superficial digital flexor tendons on the middle phalanges.

Radiographs are evaluated for soft tissue swelling along the common calcanean tendon and soft tissue calcification within the tendon. With distal avulsion injuries, the proximal calcaneus may be roughened and bony fragments may be present. There may also be a "beaklike" projection of bone on the plantar aspect of the tuber calcanei (Figure 7-36). This represents chronic proliferation of bone at the retinacular attachments of the superficial digital flexor tendon. Increased stress on this tendon presumably elicits this response. Avulsion of the medial or lateral heads of the gastrocnemius muscle is associated with distal displacement of the fabella at the level of the stifle.

Ultrasonographic examination of the common calcanean tendon has been described. Because of the superficial position of the common calcanean tendon, it is accessible for ultrasonographic examination and the architecture of the tendons can be evaluated. It is possible to diagnose both complete and partial ruptures of the tendon with ultrasound.

Injuries that require treatment by tenorrhaphy (Type I or II lesions) require a period of immobilization afterwards. Tendons heal relatively slowly in that a healing tendon has been shown to have 56% of its original strength at 6 weeks. It is imperative to resist gap formation in the healing tendon and as little as a 3 mm gap can markedly impair ultimate tendon healing. Thus, the tenorrhaphy is protected with either a soft padded bandage and splint or a transarticular external fixator postoperatively. The external fixator can be a static or mobile hinged fixator. The hinged fixator is initially locked down for complete immobilization but then loosened to permit motion in a single plane (see Transarticular External Fixation of the Tarsus). It has been shown that transarticular external fixation of the tarsus does not limit strain in the mid-portion of an intact gastrocnemius tendon. This does not necessarily reflect strain forces in a sutured tendon or at the insertion of a repaired tendon on the tuber calcanei. Based on clinical experience the author currently recommends transarticular external fixation for surgical repair of Achilles tendon injuries.

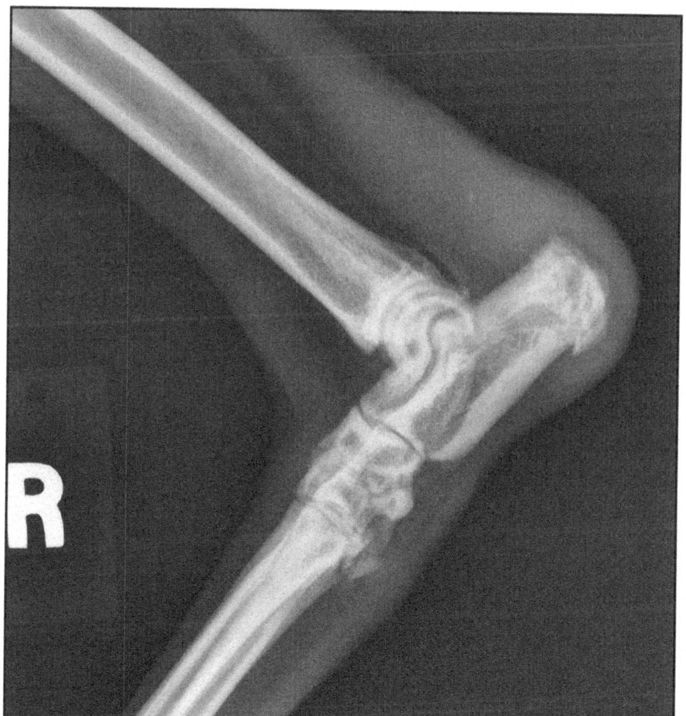


**Figure 7-36.** Lateral radiographic appearance of the proximal calcaneus with a roughened edge, bony fragments, and "beaklike" projection of bone on the plantar aspect of the tuber calcanei.

## Suggested Readings

1. Kramer M, Gerwing M, Michele U et al: Ultrasonographic examination of injuries to the Achilles tendon in dogs and cats. J Small Anim Pract 42:531-535, 2001.
2. Lister SA, Renberg WC, Roush JK: Efficacy of immobilization of the tarsal joint to alleviate strain on the common calcaneal tendon in dogs. Am J Vet Res 70:134-140, 2009.
3. Meutstege, FJ: The classification of canine Achilles' tendon lesions. Vet Comp Orthop Traumatol 6:53-55, 1993.
4. Reinke JD, Mughannam AJ, Owens JM: Avulsion of the gastrocnemius tendon in 11 dogs. J Am Anim Hosp Assoc 29:410-418, 1993.

# Rupture or Laceration of the Common Calcanean Tendon

### Definition and Indications

This is a type 1 lesion of the common calcanean tendon. Complete disruption of the common calcanean tendon can be caused by laceration, traumatic separation, or fatigue rupture. The injury can occur at any point from the musculotendinous junction to the tuber calcanei. Significant loss of tendon length can result from retraction of the tendon end and necrosis following injury. Diagnosis can be made by observing postural changes, directly palpating the tendon defect, and ultrasound examination of the tendon. Calcanean tendon rupture or laceration should be repaired as soon as possible after the injury. Moderate tendon debridement is suggested for injuries that are more than 4 hours old or that are contaminated.

### Technique

The skin is incised along the lateral border of the calcanean tendon. The incision extends approximately 6 cm proximal and distal to the defect. The superficial digital flexor tendon is repaired separately from the gastrocnemius and combined tendons. The three-loop pulley suture is recommended for repair of the gastrocnemius and combined tendons. It is not always possible to distinguish between the gastrocnemius and combined tendon intraoperatively. If this is the case, the tendons may be repaired as one unit using the three-loop pulley suture. The three-loop pulley suture is placed as described for treatment of strain injury (See Figure 7-33). Monofilament nylon or polypropylene (size 0 on a medium - large size dog) is used. Size 2-0 horizontal mattress sutures of the same materials may be placed between tendon ends for supplemental fixation. The superficial digital flexor tendon is repaired separately using a locking loop suture pattern. Size 2-0 to 0 monofilament nylon or polypropylene suture is used (See Figures 7-9 and 7-10). The soft tissues and skin are closed routinely in layers.

The joint is placed in mild extension to relieve tension on the repair. The tarsocrural joint is immobilized postoperatively with a lateral splint and soft padded bandage. Alternatively, a transarticular external fixator may be applied (See Transarticular External Fixation of the Tarsus).

## Aftercare

The tenorrhaphy is protected with a lateral splint and soft padded bandage for 6 weeks. The splint is changed weekly and if areas of pressure irritation are identified the position of the splint can be changed. For example, a lateral splint can be moved to the medial side or an area of irritation over a bony protuberance such as the tuber calcanei can be covered with a "donut" of bandage material to relieve pressure. When the splint is removed, it is replaced with a soft padded bandage for an additional 2 weeks. Alternatively, a transarticular fixator can be placed for 4 weeks. The external fixator is checked weekly to biweekly after surgery. The external fixator is removed at 4 weeks and a lateral splint with soft padded bandage is placed extending from just distal to the stifle to the digits. The splint remains on for 2 weeks with weekly changes. The splint is replaced with a soft padded bandage for 2 to 3 weeks. Another option is placement of a mobile hinged external fixator. This can be locked down to restrict all motion for the first 3 weeks then loosened to permit motion in 1 plane. The hinged external fixator is removed at 6 weeks (see Transarticular External Fixation of the Tarsus).

Restricted exercise is maintained for a total of 12 weeks after surgery. Exercise consists of short, 10 minute, leash walks 3 to 5 times daily. After this, normal exercise is gradually reintroduced over a 4 week period of time.

A joint supplement is recommended for the entire period of immobilization. Polysulfated glygosaminoglycan (Adequan, Novartis Animal Health US Inc, Greensboro, NC) may be administered at a dose of 4.4 mg/kg intramuscularly (IM) or subcutaneously (SQ) twice weekly for 4 weeks, then once every 2 to 4 weeks. The subcutaneous form is off-label but has been used by the author with better owner compliance than with IM administration. Oral glucosamine/chondroitin supplements (Cosequin, Dasuquin, Nutramax Laboratories, Edgewood, Md) may be used instead of injectable chondroitin.

## Advantages and Disadvantages

The three-loop pulley suture is well suited for cylindrically shaped tendons, such as the common calcanean tendon, and has been shown to provide more tensile strength and resistance to gap formation than the locking-loop pattern. Significant tensile forces are exerted on the calcaneal tendon and this is exacerbated by loss of tendon length due to injury or retraction of the tendon ends. Thus, a pattern providing more tensile force is desirable.

Immobilization of the tendon is needed to reduce the chance of suture failure and gap formation during walking. The advantage of an external fixator is that greater joint immobilization can be achieved than with casting or splinting. Additionally, prolonged splinting can lead to pressure wounds or dermatitis. There should be fewer rechecks with an external fixator than with a cast or splint. The disadvantage of placing an external fixator is increased surgical time, the possibility for developing pin tract infections, and potential damage to articular cartilage. With experience, surgical time to place this fixation system is minimal. Pin tract infections can be minimized by correct pin placement (see external fixation of the tarsus) and generally respond to broad spectrum antibiotics if they do occur. The external fixator is placed for approximately 4 weeks. Immobilization for this period of time decreases the proteoglycan content of joint cartilage. The proteoglycan content improves after remobilization; however there is cartilage damage from the application of full weight bearing forces. In order to protect the joint, weightbearing forces can be gradually applied by first applying a splint for 2 weeks and then a soft padded bandage for 2 weeks.

# Suggested Readings

1. Aaron DN: Tendons. In Bojrab MJ, ed.: Current Techniques in Small Animal Surgery 3rd ed.: Philadelphia: Lea and Febiger, 1990, 549.

2. Berg RJ, Egger EL: In vitro comparison of the three loop pulley and locking loop suture patterns for repair of canine weightbearing

tendon and collateral ligaments. Vet Surg 15:107, 1986.
3. Keller WG, Aron DN, Rowland GN, et al.: The effect of trans-stifle external skeletal fixation and hyaluronic acid therapy on articular cartilage in the dog. Vet Surg 23:119-128, 1994.
3. Meutstege, FJ: The classification of canine Achilles' tendon lesions. Vet Comp Orthop Traumatol 6:53-55, 1993.
4. Montgomery R, Fitch R. Muscle and tendon disorders. *In* Slatter D, ed.: Textbook of Small Animal Surgery 3rd ed. Philadelphia: Saunders, 2003, 2264.
5. Moores AP, Owen MR, Tarlton JF: The three-loop pulley suture versus two locking-loop sutures for the repair of canine Achilles tendons. Vet Surg 33:131-137, 2004.

# Avulsion of the Gastrocnemius Tendon Insertion

## Definition and Insertions

This is categorized as a type IIC injury of the common calcanean tendon. The superficial digital flexor tendon is intact but the gastrocnemius tendon is detached from its insertion on the calcaneus. The combined tendon may also be involved. Injuries of the common calcanean tendon insertion involve either a separation of the tendon from the bone or avulsion of small or large bone fragments. Avulsion with large bone fragments occurs in young animals, less than 2 years old, and is associated with incomplete maturation of bone at the site of tendon insertion. In middle aged, large breed dogs with tendinosseous junction injury the associated bony fragments are small. Based on histopathological data in the dog, it is thought that the gastrocnemius tendon finally tears after long-term subclinical trauma.

Clinically animals with a type IIC lesion of the common calcanean tendon stand with the stifle in extension and slight to moderate flexion of the tarsus or "dropped hock". These animals display a distinct flexion of the digits when standing (See Figure 7-35). This stance results from increased tension on the superficial digital flexor tendon that induces flexion of the phalanges. The increased tension on the superficial digital flexor tendon is caused by the plantigrade stance. On palpation of the distal tendon, edema is present acutely, followed by fibroplasia and muscle retraction chronically. Careful palpation just proximal to the calcaneus may reveal a gap beneath the superficial digital flexor tendon. With time, this region can become occupied with fibrous tissue and give the impression during palpation that the tendon is intact. Radiographically there may be small avulsion fragments or bony proliferation on the tuber calcanei (See Figure 7-36). This represents chronic proliferation of bone at the retinacular attachments of the superficial digital flexor tendon. Increased stress on this tendon presumably elicits this response.

Avulsion of the gastrocnemius tendon in dogs does not respond well to casting or splinting and should be surgically repaired. There is evidence that in cats, unlike dogs, external coaptation is a viable method of repair. In dogs, surgical repair with adequate postoperative immobilization is indicated and often successful. For surgical repair the distal end of the debrided tendon is affixed to the calcaneus by means of suture and a bone tunnel. In chronic cases, resection of fibrous tissue at the distal end of the common calcanean tendon creates a gap that can prohibit direct apposition of the tendon to the calcaneus. In these circumstances, the surgical options indicated include tendon lengthening procedures, tendon transposition, autograft, supplementation with mesh or combinations of these techniques. Tendon transposition involves releasing the insertion sites of the peroneus longus and brevis tendons and redirecting them proximally to suture them to the severed end of the calcanean tendon. Autograft is obtained by harvesting the patient's fascia lata tissue and suturing it over the repaired calcaneal tendon. Synthetic mesh is made of polypropylene (Premilene mesh, B. Braun Medical, Inc., Bethlehem, PA) and is capable of withstanding mechanical stress. In addition its porosity permits fibrous tissue ingrowth. Pantarsal arthrodesis is a salvage procedure if tendon repair is unsuccessful.

## Techniques

### Suturing Achilles Tendon to Calcaneus

A lateral paramedian approach is made over the distal tendon and tuber calcanei (Figure 7-37). Beginning proximally, the superficial digital flexor tendon is separated from the gastrocnemius tendon by sharply incising subcutaneous and retinacular tissues. The superficial digital flexor tendon is then retracted medially to expose the calcaneus. In acute injuries the avulsed end of the gastrocnemius tendon will be clearly visible. The tendon is debrided to create a smooth end for suturing. In chronic cases considerable debridement is necessary to resect fibrous tissue attachments from the calcaneus. Moving in a proximal direction, fibrous tissue is resected until normal appearing tendon is reached. In some chronic cases complete resection of fibrous tissue would create too large of a gap and is not possible. It may be difficult to distinguish the combined tendon from the gastrocnemius tendon and in this case they are sutured as one unit.

The gastrocnemius tendon is reattached to the tuber calcanei by means of a bone tunnel and a modified

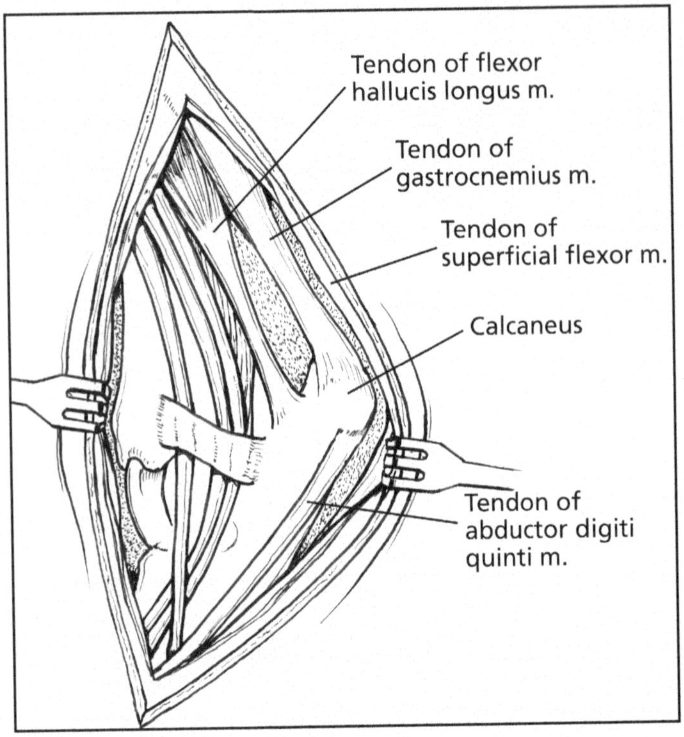


**Figure 7-37.** Approach to the lateral calcaneus. A lateral paramedian approach is made over the distal Achilles tendon and tuber calcanei. Beginning proximally, the superficial digital flexor tendon is separated from the gastrocnemius tendon by sharply incising subcutaneous and retinacular tissues. The superficial digital flexor tendon is then retracted toward the medial side to expose the calcaneus. (After Piermattei DL, Johnson KA. An Atlas of Surgical Approaches to the Bones and Joints of the Dog and Cat 4th ed. Philadelphia: Saunders, 2004, 383).

three-loop pulley suture (Figure 7-38A through H). If a stump of soft tissue is present on the calcaneal tuberosity it is not removed. Monofilament suture is used (nylon or polypropylene size 0 to 1 for a medium - large size dog). To drill a single lateral-to-medial bone tunnel, a 1.5 to 2.0 mm drill bit is used and the hole is placed just distal to the site of tendon insertion on the calcaneus. A modified three-loop pulley suture consists of 3 needle passes in different planes of the tendon and a repeating lateral to medial pass through a bone tunnel in the calcaneus. Each needle pass moves circumferentially around the tendon with each pass 60 degrees from the preceding one and penetrating at 3 different distances from the avulsed end of the tendon. The "far" needle pass is 1.5 cm from the end of the tendon, the "middle" pass is 1.0 cm, and the "near" pass is 0.5 cm from the end of the tendon. The first needle pass is from lateral-medial through the bone tunnel and then medial-lateral through the "far" position in the tendon (See Figure 7-37A & B). The second needle pass is from lateral to medial in the bone tunnel and then caudomedial-craniolateral through the "middle" position in the tendon (See Figure 7-37C & D). The third needle pass is from lateral to medial through the bone tunnel and then craniomedial-caudolateral through the "near" position in the tendon (See Figure 7-38E & F). The suture is tightened and tied to pull the avulsed tendon end against the tuber calcanei (See Figure 7-38G & H). The knot is tied with a double (surgeon's) throw followed by 3 square knots.

The tenorrhaphy is protected with either a soft padded bandage and splint or a transarticular external fixator postoperatively (See Transarticular External Fixation of the Tarsus). The external fixator can be a static or mobile hinged fixator. The hinged fixator is initially locked down for complete immobilization but then loosened to permit motion in a single plane. The joint is placed in mild extension when placing the fixator to relieve tension on the repair (see Transarticular External Fixation of the Tarsus).

## Supplemented Repair

Autograft and Mesh: Autogenous or synthetic material can be used to supplement a calcanean tendon repair. To collect autogenous tissue, a craniolateral approach to the distal femur is performed. A strip of fascia lata, approximately 10 cm x 2 cm, is harvested. The graft is placed over the medial aspect of the gastrocnemius tendon and longitudinally wrapped around the gastrocnemius tendon repair (Figure 7-39). The graft is secured proximally to the tendon with simple interrupted sutures of non absorbable or slowly absorbable suture material (2-0 polydioxanone, nylon, and polypropylene). Distally the graft is secured to the calcaneus by suturing to regional periosteum or soft tissue, if available, or by passing suture through 1 to 2 bone tunnels created in the calcaneus. The bone tunnels are created using a high speed drill and 1.5 mm drill bit (See Figure 7-39).

Polypropylene mesh can be used as the sole means of supplementation or it can be used along with a fascia lata graft. The sheet of mesh is removed from the sterile package and a section is cut that corresponds to the required length. The length of the mesh extends from the junction of the middle and distal one-third of the Achilles tendon to the tuber calcanei. The sheet of mesh is folded so that it is 3 layers thick. The folded mesh is applied to the lateral aspect of the Achilles tendon and secured with 2-0 suture (polydioxanone, nylon, polypropylene). The mesh is sutured along the tendon with simple interrupted sutures and distally to the periosteum of the calcaneus or through 1 to 2 bone tunnels created in the calcaneus (See Figure 7-39).

## Tendon Lengthening Procedures

Tendons that have undergone contracture can be lengthened using various patterns including the V to Y plasty and the sliding Z plasty (See Figures 7-40 and 7-41). The V to Y plasty is located at the muscu-

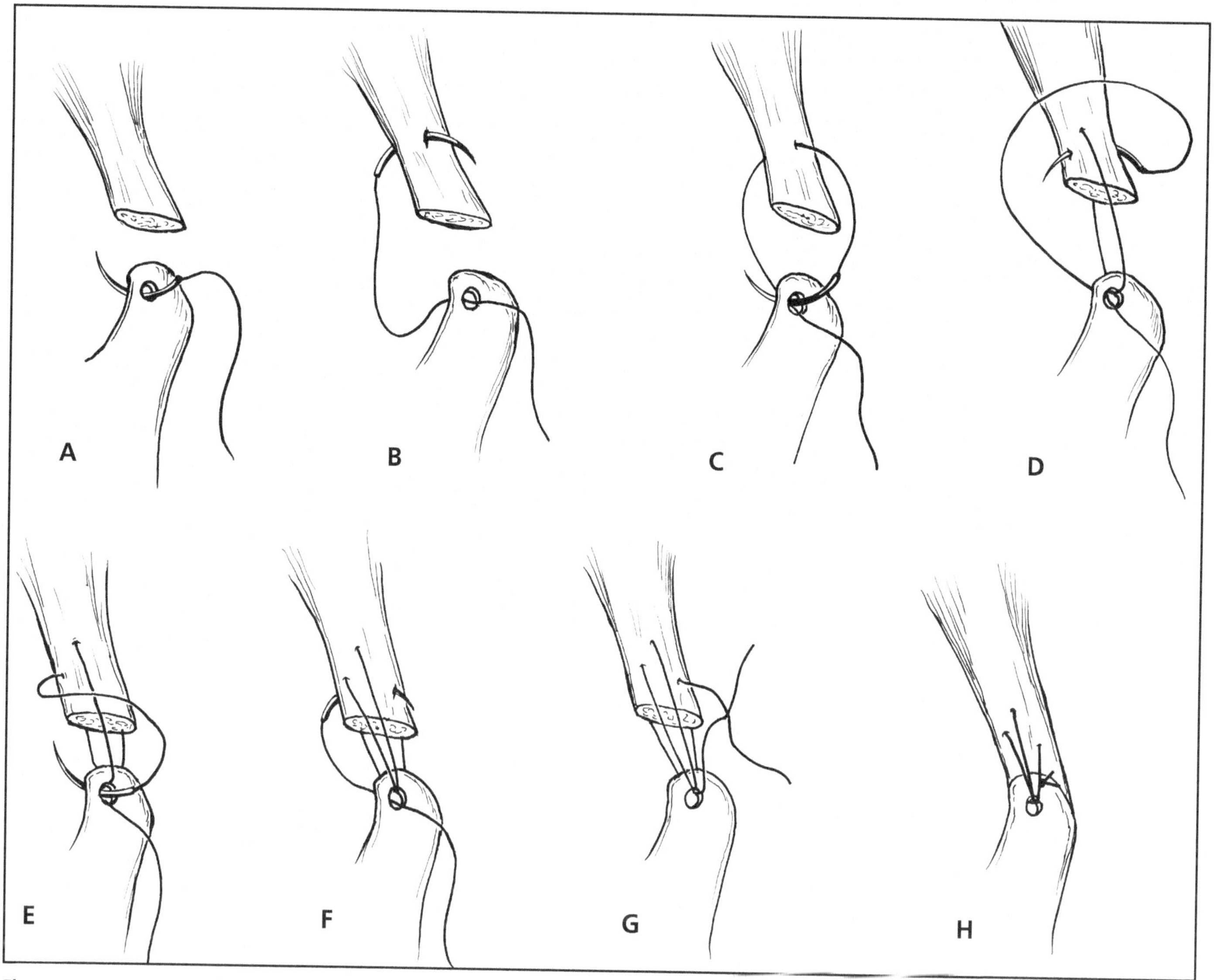


**Figure 7-38.** Modified three-loop pulley suture. A modified three-loop pulley suture consists of 3 needle passes in different planes of the tendon and a repeating lateral to medial pass through a bone tunnel in the calcaneus. Each needle pass moves circumferentially around the tendon with each pass 60 degrees from the preceding one and penetration at 3 different distances from the avulsed end of the tendon. The "far" needle pass is 1.5 cm from the end of the tendon, the "middle" pass is 1.0 cm, and the "near" pass is 0.5 cm from the end of the tendon. **A.** The drill hole in the calcaneus is placed just distal to the site of tendon insertion. **B.** The first needle pass is from lateral-medial through the bone tunnel and then medial-lateral through the "far" position in the tendon. **C., D.** The second needle pass is from lateral to medial in the bone tunnel and then caudomedial-craniolateral through the "middle" position in the tendon. **E., F.** The third needle pass is from lateral to medial through the bone tunnel and then craniomedial-caudolateral through the "near" position in the tendon. **G., H.** The suture is tightened and tied to pull the avulsed tendon end against the tuber calcanei. (After Moores AP, Comerford EJ et al. Biomechanical and clinical evaluation of a modified 3-loop pulley suture pattern for reattachment of canine tendons to bone. Vet Surg 33:391, 2004).

lotendinous portion of the gastrocnemius tendon. The point of the V points proximally. The V incision is made and the tendon is advanced distally. The tendon is secured to the distal tendon stump using a 3-loop pulley pattern as shown or using a modified 3-loop pulley pattern through bone tunnels. Proximally the tissues are closed in an inverted Y pattern using simple interrupted sutures using 2-0 slowly absorbable or non-absorbable suture (Figure 7-40A & B).

The sliding Z plasty is carried out in the tendinous portion of the gastrocnemius tendon. The proximal end of the tendon is transected transversely half way through its width then split longitudinally for the desired length. The length is estimated by the gap between the distal tendon and the calcaneus insertion site. The distal end is transversely transected the remaining width so that there are 2 free segments of tendon. The elongated segments on the tendon ends are sutured together using a three-loop pulley pattern using 2-0 to 0 non-absorbable suture (Figure 7-41A & B).

## Tendon Transposition

The tendons of the peroneus longus (PL) and peroneus brevis (PB) are transposed through drill holes in the calcaneus and anastomosed to the distal gastrocnemius or combined tendon (See Figure 7-42). The PB and PL are small diameter tendons so both should

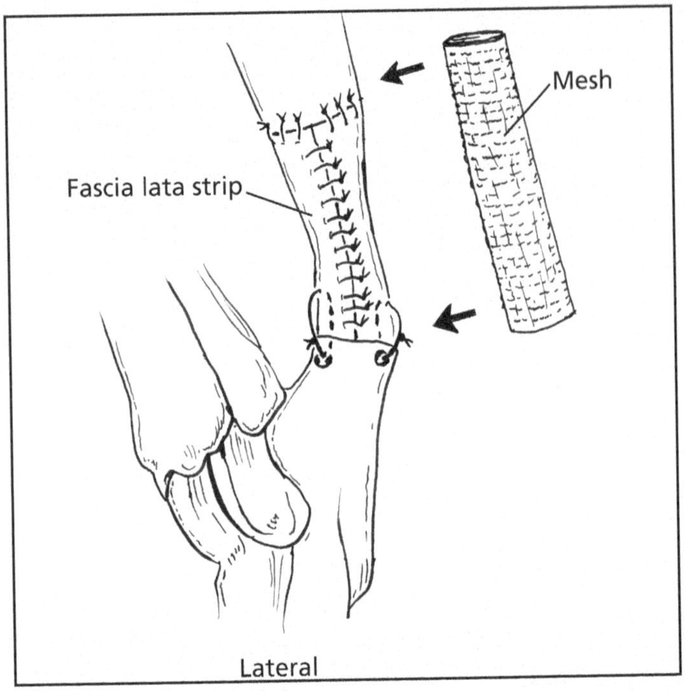


**Figure 7-39.** Supplementation of calcanean tendon repair. A strip of fascia lata has been wrapped and sutured around the lateral aspect of the gastrocnemius tendon repair site and secured proximally with simple interrupted sutures. Distally the graft is secured to the calcaneus using sutures through small bone tunnels. Mesh can be sutured to the repair for added strength.

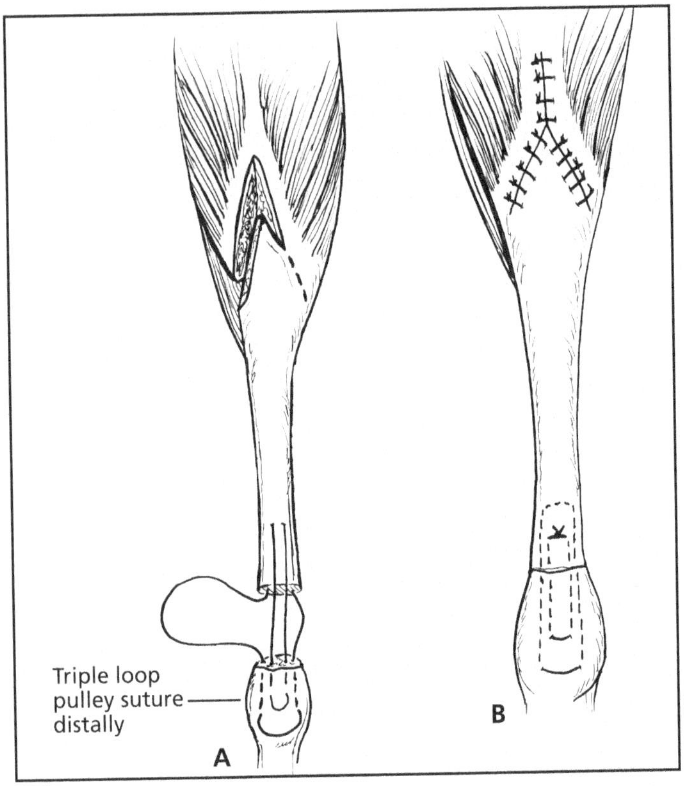


**Figure 7-40.** Tendon lengthening: V to Y. **A.** The V to Y plasty is located at the musculotendinous portion of the gastrocnemius tendon. The point of the V points proximally. The V incision is made and the tendon is advanced distally. The tendon is secured to the distal tendon stump using a 3-loop pulley pattern as shown or using a modified 3-loop pulley pattern through bone tunnels. **B.** Proximally the tissues are closed in an inverted Y pattern using simple interrupted sutures. (After Aron DA. Tendons. In Bojrab MJ: Current Techniques in Small Animal Surgery 3rd ed. Philadelphia: Lea and Febiger, 1990, 559).

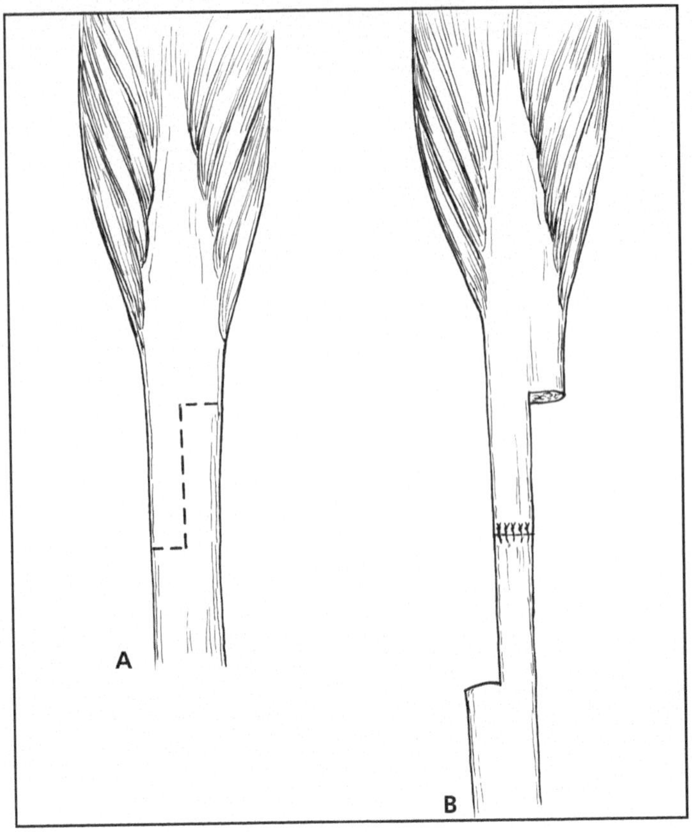


**Figure 7-41.** Tendon lengthening: sliding Z plasty. The sliding Z plasty is carried out in the tendinous portion of the gastrocnemius tendon. **A.** The proximal end of the tendon is transected half way through its width then split longitudinally for the desired length. The length is estimated by the gap between the distal tendon and the calcaneus insertion site. The distal end is transversely transected the remaining width so that there are 2 free segments of tendon. **B.** The elongated segments on the tendon ends are sutured together using an interrupted cruciate pattern or a triple loop pulley pattern. (After Fahie MA. Healing, diagnosis, repair, and rehabilitation of tendon conditions. Vet Clin No Am Small Anim 35:1195, 2005).

be used in the anastomosis. The PB muscle originates from the lateral surface of the distal 2/3 of the tibia and fibula and inserts at the proximal end of metatarsal V. The PL muscle originates from the proximolateral portion of the tibia and fibula and inserts on the fourth tarsal bone and the plantar surface of the metatarsals.

The PB tendon is sharply transected at its insertion on the proximal part of metatarsal V. The tendon is mobilized proximally to the muscle belly. The PL tendon is also sharply transected at the level of the proximal aspect of metatarsal V and mobilized proximally. Two tunnels are created in the tuber calcaneus using a 2.0 mm drill bit. One tunnel is drilled in a plantaro-lateral to dorso-medial direction and the other is drilled in a plantaro-medial to dorso-lateral direction. Using traction sutures the PB tendon is passed from distal to proximal through the lateral bone tunnel and the PL tendon is passed in the opposite direction. If it seems difficult to mobilize enough PL tendon to pass through

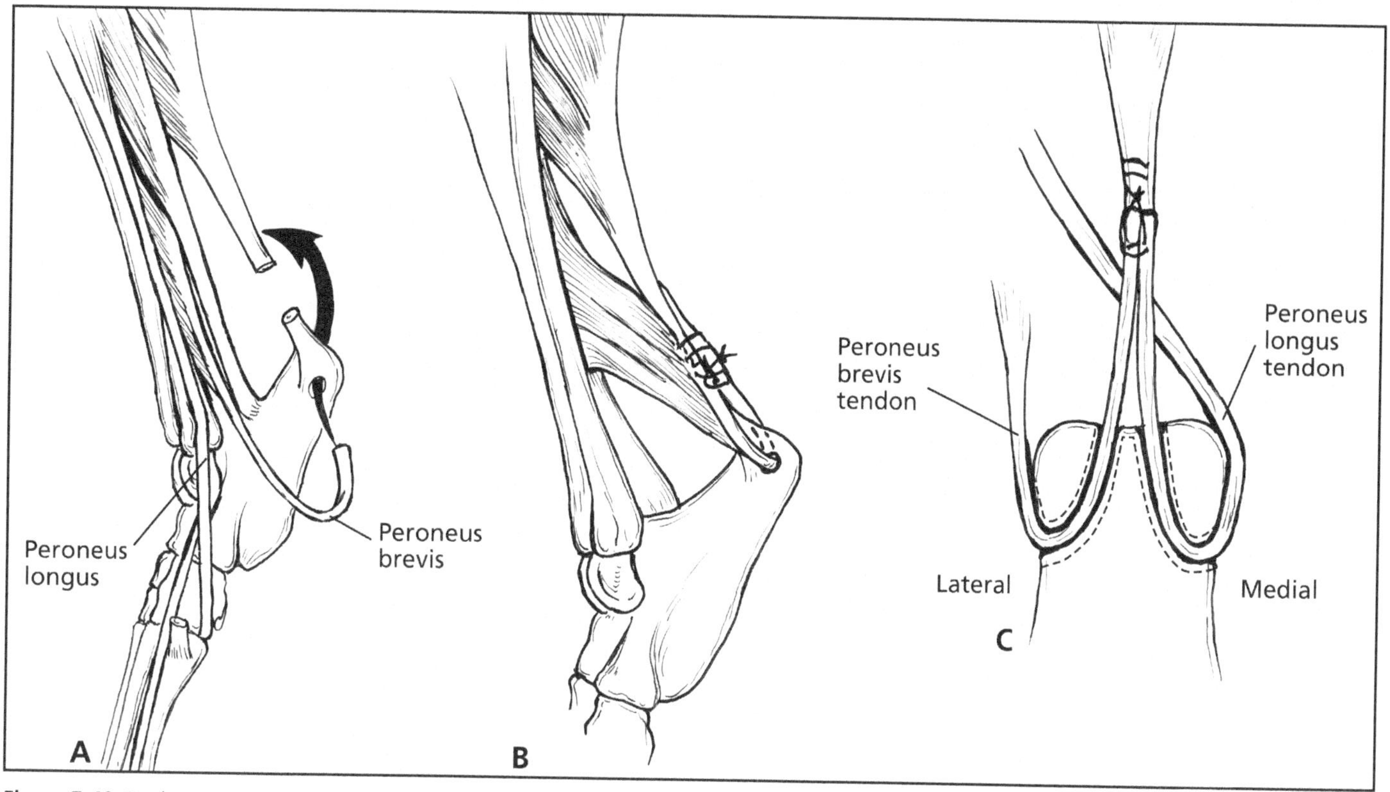


**Figure 7-42.** Tendon transposition. **A.** Severed insertional end of the peroneus brevis muscle to be threaded through a tunnel in the tuber calcaneus and sutured to the severed end of the gastrocnemius muscle *(arrow)*. **B.** The peroneus longus and peroneus brevis insertional ends have been threaded through the matching tunnels in the calcaneal tuber and sutured to the severed end of the gastrocnemius tendon. **C.** Caudal view of the calcaneal tuber with the tendons threaded through their tunnels. (After Sivacolundhu RK, Marchevsky AM, Read RA et al. Achilles mechanism reconstruction in four dogs. Vet Comp Orthop Traumatol 14:25, 2001).

a medially located bone tunnel it is possible to pass both tendons through the laterally located bone tunnel. It may be necessary to start with a larger lateral bone tunnel to do this. This decision should be made prior to drilling both bone tunnels so that the lateral may be enlarged without risking weakening of the proximal calcaneus. The ends of the PB and PL are trimmed to remove any tendon damaged by the traction sutures. The two tendons are sutured to the distal aspects of either the gastrocnemius or the combined tendon using size 2-0 nylon or polypropylene in a three loop pulley pattern (Figure 7-42A, B & C).

## Aftercare

The external fixator is kept in place for approximately 4 weeks. The fixator is checked weekly to biweekly. After removing the external fixator, a splint is placed for 2 to 3 weeks followed by a soft padded bandage for 2 to 3 weeks to transition to full weight bearing. Alternatively, a mobile hinged external fixator can be placed. This fixator can be locked down for the first 3-4 weeks of healing and then loosened to allow controlled movement in one plane (See Transarticular External Fixation of the Tarsus).

If a splint is used for immobilization rather than an external fixator, it is kept on for 6 weeks with weekly bandage changes. The splint extends from the digits to just below the stifle joint. The splint is changed weekly and if areas of pressure irritation are identified the position of the splint can be changed. For example, a lateral splint can be moved to the medial side or an area of irritation over a bony protuberance such as the tuber calcanei can be covered with a "donut" of bandage material to relieve pressure.

When the splint is removed, a soft padded bandage is placed for 2 to 3 weeks with weekly changes.

A joint supplement is recommended for the entire period of immobilization. Polysulfated glygosaminoglycan (Adequan, Novartis Animal Health US Inc, Greensboro, NC) may be administered at a dose of 4.4 mg/kg intramuscularly (IM) or subcutaneously (SQ) twice weekly for 4 weeks, then once every 2 to 4 weeks. The subcutaneous form is off-label but has been used by the author with better owner compliance than with IM administration. Oral glucosamine/chondroitin supplements (Cosequin, Dasuquin, Nutramax Laboratories, Edgewood, Md) may be used instead of injectable chondroitin.

Exercise is restricted for 12 to 16 weeks postoperatively and consists of short, maximum 10 minute, leash walks

3 to 4 times daily. Exercise is then gradually increased over the next 4 weeks.

## Advantages and Disadvantages

The modified three-loop pulley suture pattern is biomechanically superior to the locking loop pattern when reattaching calcanean tendon to bone. The modified three-loop pulley pattern resists gap formation more than the locking loop. This is particularly important in tendon healing. Repaired canine tendons with greater than a 3 mm gap do not gain significant strength between the first 10 to 42 days of healing. A lack of strength during this time would make a tendon repair vulnerable to failure.

Calcaneal tendon injuries undergo significant contraction and fibrotic change. The fibrotic disorganized portion of the tendon stump should be removed so that the remaining tissue appears grossly normal to achieve good tendon healing. This often creates a significant gap between the distal tendon and the calcaneus. Initially tendon lengthening procedures can be used to close the gap. The sliding Z plasty provides a greater increase in tendon length than the V to Y procedure but it is more invasive. In the author's experience large tendon gaps can be closed without using the sliding Z plasty if tendon transposition is employed along with V to Y lengthening. Tendon transposition removes the normal function of these tendons. The function of the peroneus longus and peroneus brevis tendons is to flex the tarsus. The peroneus longus tendon also pronates the hindpaw. Loss of these functions after tendon transposition has not caused detectable gait problems postoperatively.

It is advantageous to remove all traumatized and abnormal tendon prior to repair. However, closure of the gap must be possible given the techniques described. In very chronic cases surgeons must use their best judgement when determining how much tendon to excise. The extremely thickened portion of retracted tendon must be removed but it is sometimes necessary to leave some of the more proximal portion of tendon intact even if it does not appear completely normal by gross inspection. More tendon can always be excised as surgery progresses if that is deemed possible.

The advantage of an external fixator is that it avoids pressure wounds that can occur with long-term splinting. It is desirable to have this degree of immobilization early in healing to avoid gap formation but the tendon must also experience weightbearing forces to have appropriate alignment of collagen fibers. The external fixator is left on for approximately 3 to 4 weeks and is then removed to allow more weight-bearing forces to be applied to the tendon. The disadvantage of placing an external fixator is increased surgical time, the possibility for developing pin tract infections, and potential damage to articular cartilage from immobilization.

The disadvantages can be managed or overcome. With experience, surgical time to place this fixation system is minimal. Pin tract infections can be minimized by correct pin placement (see external fixation of the tarsus) and generally respond to broad spectrum antibiotics if they do occur. Joint immobilization for 3 to 4 weeks can decrease the proteoglycan content of cartilage. Since the external fixator is in place for approximately 4 weeks, immobilization for this period of time decreases the proteoglycan content of joint cartilage. The proteoglycan content improves after remobilization, but at the cost of cartilage damage from the application of full weight bearing forces. In order to protect the joint, weightbearing forces are gradually added by transitioning from the external fixator to a splint and then a soft padded bandage. The provision of a glucosamine/chondroitin supplement may also be protective.

The advantage of autograft and mesh supplementation is the provision of increased strength to the repair. This is especially advantageous in more chronic cases requiring large resections of disorganized tissue from the distal end of the tendon. The disadvantage of autograft collection is increased surgical dissection. A potential concern is that placing an autograft around the tendon isolates it from the blood supply provided by surrounding soft tissues. This potential concern has not been recognized clinically.

Prolene mesh is an inert material that does not engender an inflammatory reaction. It serves as bridgework for the organized ingrowth of collagen fibrils. One rare complication that the author has encountered is exposure of the mesh through the skin several months after surgery. Excising all visible exposed portions of the mesh and resuturing the skin over the area successfully managed this problem.

# Suggested Readings

1. Berg RJ, Egger EL: In vitro comparison of the three-loop pulley technique and locking loop suture patterns for repair of canine weightbearing tendons and collateral ligaments. Vet Surg 15:107, 1986.
2. Choksey A, Soonawalla D, Murray J: Repair of neglected Achilles tendon ruptures with Marlex mesh. Injury 27:215-217, 1996.
3. Gall TT, Santoni BG, Egger EL et al.: In vitro biomechanical comparison of polypropylene mesh, modified three-loop pulley

suture pattern, and a combination for repair of distal canine Achilles' tendon injuries. Vet Surg 38:845-851, 2009.
4. Jann HW, Alexander JW: Using a modified three-loop pulley tenorrhaphy to repair avulsion of the gastrocnemius tendon in dogs. Vet Med 841, 1996.
5. Meutstege, FJ. The classification of canine Achilles' tendon lesions. Vet Comp Orthop Traumatol 6:53-55, 1993.
6. Moores AP, Comerford EJ, Tarlton JF et al.: Biomechanical and clinical evaluation of a modified 3-loop pulley suture pattern for reattachment of canine tendons to bone. Vet Surg 33:391-397, 2004.
7. Mughannam A, Reinke J: Avulsion of the gastrocnemius tendon in three cats. J Am Anim Hosp Assoc 30:550-556, 1994.
8. Reinke JD, Mughannam AJ, Owens JM: Avulsion of the gastrocnemius tendon in 11 dogs. J Am Anim Hosp Assoc 29:410-418, 1993.
9. Sivacolundhu RK, Marchevsky AM, Read RA, et al.: Achilles mechanism reconstruction in four dogs. Vet Comp Orthop Traumatol 14:25-31, 2001.
10. Swiderski J, Fitch RB, Staatz A et al.: Sonographic assisted diagnosis and treatment of bilateral gastrocnemius tendon rupture in a Labrador retriever repaired repaired with fascia lata and polypropylene mesh. Vet Comp Orthop Trauamatol 18:258-63, 2005.

# Chronic Calcaneal Tendonitis

## Definition and Indications

Chronic inflammation of the common calcanean tendon just proximal to the tuber calcanei occasionally occurs in large breed dogs. This condition has been classified as a Type 3 lesion of the common calcanean tendon. There is a persistent mild lameness that is exacerbated with exercise but a normograde stance. On palpation there is thickening of the distal 2 to 4 cm of the tendon. When the stifle joint is held at a normal standing angle, the common calcanean tendon becomes taut at 90 degrees of flexion, which is normal, and there is no abnormal flexion of the digits. This disturbance may represent a chronic moderate strain injury of the gastrocnemius tendon. This condition may progress to a type IIC injury. A type IIC injury represents avulsion of the gastrocnemius tendon of insertion with an intact superficial digital flexor tendon.

## Technique

Treatment consists of resting the tendon by immobilizing the tarsocrural joint. This can be accomplished by immobilizing the tarsocrural joint with a soft padded bandage and splint or a customized orthotic brace (OrthoPets, Denver, CO) or by external fixation. The joint should be protected from usual weight bearing forces for approximately 16 weeks.

## Aftercare

The lateral splint and soft padded bandage is placed for approximately 8 weeks. The splint and bandage are changed weekly and if areas of pressure irritation are identified the position of the splint can be changed. For example, a lateral splint can be moved to the medial side or an area of irritation over a bony protuberance such as the tuber calcanei can be covered with a "donut" of bandage material to relieve pressure. After approximately 8 weeks, the splint is replaced with a soft padded bandage for 2 to 3 weeks with weekly changes.

A custom orthotic device may be ordered to fit the tarsocrural joint of the individual patient. This requires creating a negative model of the limb using fiberglass casting tape and submitting this model for fabrication of the custom device. The device can be designed as a dynamic orthotic which will allow increasing ranges of flexion during the healing period.

Either a static or dynamic tranarticular external fixator can be placed. A static fixator remains on for 4 weeks. After 4 weeks, the external fixator is removed and replaced with a splint for 4 weeks and then a soft padded bandage for 2 weeks. During the first 12 weeks of healing exercise is restricted to short, 10 minute, leash walks 3 to 4 times daily. After this, exercise is gradually reintroduced over 4 to 8 weeks. There is no outdoor off leash activity until the end of the 4 week reintroduction period.

## Advantages and Disadvantages

There is a good chance for ameliorating tendon inflammation by non-invasive means; either splinting or use of a custom orthotic device. These are a good alternatives to external fixation in most cases. The disadvantage of splinting for such a long period of time is the risk for pressure wounds or dermatitis as well as repeat visits to change the bandage and splint. There is significant cost associated with custom orthotic devices, but they are non-invasive and can provide gradually increased stress to the tendon. Furthermore the device can be re-used after initial treatment.

# Suggested Readings

1. Case JB, Palmer R, Valdes-Martinez A, et al: Gastrocnemius tendon strain in a dog treated with autologous mesenchymal stem cells and custom orthosis. Vet Surg 42: 355-360, 2013.
2. Meutstege FJ. The classification of canine Achilles' tendon lesions. Vet Comp Orthop Traumatol 6:53-55, 1993.
3. Piermattei DL, Flo GL. Brinker, Piermattei and Flo's Handbook of Small Animal Orthopedics and Fracture Repair, 3rd ed. Philadelphia: W B Saunders Co, 1997, 622.

# Gastrocnemius Tears at the Musculotendinous Junction

## Definition and Indications

Complete separation of the gastrocnemius tendon from the proximal junction with the muscle belly occasionally occurs. The musculotendinous junction is more vulnerable to rupture than the muscle itself, most likely because muscle tissue has greater elasticity and because of the change of tissue strength at this junction. Complete musculotendinous junction tears result in collapse of the tarsocrural joint. Frequently the site of damage is painful on deep palpation and there may be associated bruising. Swelling can be palpated acutely, and more chronically, the area is fibrosed and thickened. Surgical repair is indicated if the injury is significant enough to induce a plantigrade stance of the tarsus. Surgical reapposition is recommended for recent injuries. Chronic injuries or those that have had a failed attempt at surgical repair are candidates for pantarsal arthrodesis (see severe tarsal shearing wounds treated by early arthrodesis using external fixation) to restore weightbearing function to the limb.

## Technique

A lateral skin incision is made over the junction of the proximal and middle 1/3 and of the common calcanean tendon. The area of separation is located and debrided as necessary to visualize the free end of the tendon. Structures to be aware of in the caudal region of the tibia include the peroneal and tibial nerves. The peroneal nerve courses over the lateral head of the gastrocnemius muscle and then passes between the flexor hallicus longus and peroneus longus muscles. The tibial nerve passes between the 2 heads of the gastrocnemius muscle and continues distally along the lateral surface of the deep digital flexor muscle.

The junction between muscle and tendon is repaired with a tendon suture pattern such as the locking loop (See Figure 7-9). The locking loop pattern has transverse and longitudinal components that, when tightened, grasp bundles of tendinous tissue. To be effective the transverse component must be superficial to the longitudinal one. In this application the proximal suture ends are tied over a sterile button (polypropylene or titanium surgical button: Imex Vet Inc., Longview, TX) to disperse tension. The suture is tied with one surgeon's throw followed by 3 square knots. If there is room, an identical locking loop pattern is placed adjacent to the first to increase the security of the repair. Several horizontal mattress sutures are placed at the musculotendinous junction (Figure 7-43).

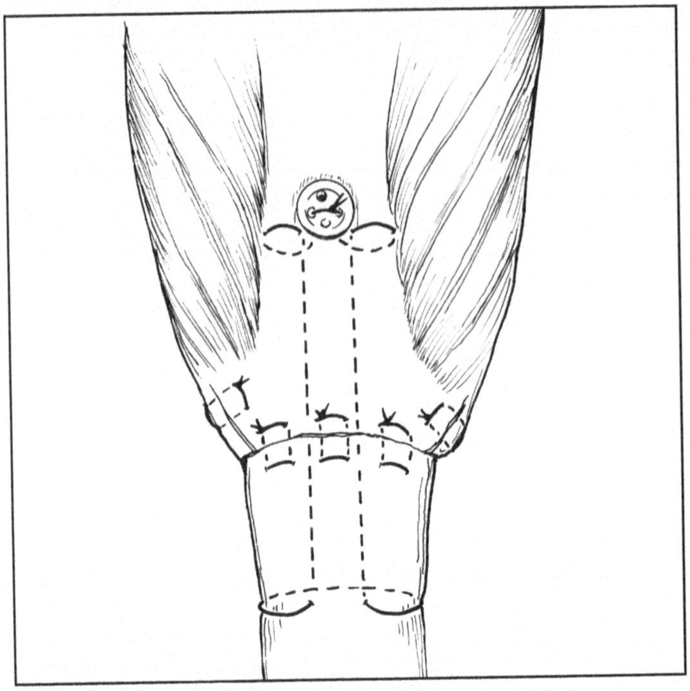

**Figure 7-43.** Locking loop repair of gastrocnemius muscle-tendon disruption. (See Figure 7-9). Proximally the suture ends are tied over a sterile button to disperse tension. The suture is tied with one surgeon's throw followed by 3 single throws. Several horizontal mattress sutures are placed at the musculotendinous junction. (After Aron DN. Tendons. In Bojrab MJ: Current Techniques in Small Animal Surgery 3rd ed. Philadelphia: Lea and Febiger, 1990, 553).

## Aftercare

The repair is protected with a full length splint that extends from the mid-femur to the digits for 4 weeks. The stifle joint is splinted at approximately 140 degrees of flexion. The splint is changed weekly and if areas of pressure irritation are identified the position of the splint can be changed. For example, a lateral splint can be moved to the medial side or an area of irritation over a bony protuberance such as the tuber calcanei can be covered with a "donut" of bandage material to relieve pressure.

Exercise is limited to short, 10 minute, leash walks 3 to 4 times daily. No off-leash activity is allowed for 12 weeks postoperatively.

## Advantages and Disadvantages

There is a chance that the repair may break down by suture pulling through the muscular tissue and owners must be made aware of this possibility. Using a stent, such as a sterile button, in the muscular tissue may help to limit tensile pull through the tissue. Immobilization is necessary to protect the repair but with increasing duration of splinting there is the risk of dermatitis and pressure wounds. Weekly bandage changes help to identify potential areas of pressure irritation.

In very chronic cases or those that have not succeeded surgically, a pantarsal arthrodesis will restore weight-bearing capacity to the limb. The advantage of pantarsal arthrodesis is the ability to achieve a functional limb. The disadvantage is surgical invasiveness, the loss of joint mobility, protracted healing time, and potential for implant loosening or infection.

## Suggested Readings


1. Aron DN. Tendons: In Bojrab MJ, ed.: Current Techniques in Small Animal Surgery, 3rd ed.: Philadelphia: Lea & Febiger, 1990, 549.
2. Reinke JD, Kus SP: Achilles mechanism injury in the dog. Comp Contin Educ 4:639-645, 1982.
4. Robinson A: Atraumatic bilateral avulsion of the origins of the gastrocnemius muscle. J Small An Prac 40:498, 1999.


# Rupture of the Gastrocnemius Muscle

### Definition and Indications

Rupture of the gastrocnemius muscle is a rare occurrence in dogs and cats. In dogs, gastrocnemius muscle rupture has been associated with trauma, corticosteroid administration, and parasitic myositis. Complete rupture of the gastrocnemius muscle belly results in changes in the tarsus similar to other calcanean mechanism injuries. Glucocorticoids can induce muscle degeneration by increasing protein catabolism, inhibiting synthesis of myofibrillar proteins, and reducing fibroblast proliferation. Certain diagnostic procedures are indicated when this injury is suspected. Physical examination may show clear evidence of this injury. On physical examination, the caudal aspect of the stifle joint may be swollen, tender or bruised. There may be palpable laxity of the calcanean tendon. To evaluate this, the limb is held at a normal standing angle and the tarsus is flexed. The calcanean tendon should become taut at approximately 90 degrees of flexion. Laxity indicates rupture. Additional diagnostics may include ultrasound examination of the muscle and electromyography. Screening tests for hyperadrenocorticism are indicated if serum chemistry or physical exam findings are suggestive of this. Muscle biopsies at the time of surgery are warranted if an underlying myopathy is suspected.

Therapy indicated for acute muscle rupture consists of cold packs for the first 1 to 2 days and nonsteroidal anti-inflammatory drugs. After this, swelling is reduced and the injured muscle can be palpated to assess the severity of injury. With complete ruptures of the gastrocnemius muscle a gap is palpable and some degree of plantigrade stance is observed. Surgical reapposition of muscle ruptures is indicated if muscle rupture is complete and a palpable gap is present or a visible gap is seen on ultrasound. Surgical repair is not always successful and a pantarsal arthrodesis may be required as a salvage procedure.

### Technique

The skin is incised over the caudolateral aspect of the ruptured portion of the gastrocnemius muscle. The surgeon must be aware of the sciatic nerve branches in this area. The peroneal nerve crosses over the lateral aspect of the proximal gastrocnemius muscle and the tibial nerve enters the crus between the two heads of the muscle at the level of the stifle. Horizontal mattress sutures using polydioxanone (size 2-0 to 0) are placed to appose the muscle. Suture ends can be tied over sterile surgical buttons (Imex Vet, Inc., Longview, TX) to redistribute pressure. The remaining tissues are closed in layers.

### Aftercare

Immediately after surgery, cold packs are placed over the surgical site every 4 to 6 hours for 24 hours. Nonsteroidal anti-inflammatory drugs are administered for 2 weeks postoperatively.

A lateral splint and soft padded bandage is placed from the femur to the digits with the stifle joint positioned at approximately 140 degrees of flexion. The splint is placed for 4 weeks. The splint is changed weekly and if areas of pressure irritation are identified the position of the splint can be changed. For example, a lateral splint can be moved to the medial side or an area of irritation over a bony protuberance such as the tuber calcanei can be covered with a "donut" of bandage material to relieve pressure.

If pantarsal arthrodesis has been performed, the tarsocrural joint is supported with a lateral splint and soft padded bandage for the first 6 weeks or until arthrodesis has begun to be radiographically visible. The splint is changed weekly. Radiographs are taken every 8 weeks and again monthly until arthrodesis is complete. The bone plate may require future removal if screw loosening or drainage develops.

### Advantages and Disadvantages

The advantage of surgical apposition of the gastrocnemius muscle is the potential to restore a normal standing angle and function of the limb with normal mobility of the tarsus. The chance of failure is high. Even with initial surgical success, re-injury of the muscle is reported. Although it is more invasive, pantarsal arthrodesis is a more reliable method of repair. The advantage of pantarsal arthrodesis is the high success rate. The disadvantage of pantarsal arthrodesis is that it is invasive and eliminates range of motion in the tarsus. It is reasonable to attempt one surgical repair of the muscle and resort to pantarsal arthrodesis if this is unsuccessful. For clients who want the best chance for only one surgery, pantarsal arthrodesis is a good initial recommendation.

# Suggested Readings


1. Braund KB: Endogenous causes of myopathies in dogs and cat. Vet Med 618-628, 1997.
2. Mitchell M: Spontaneous repair of a ruptured gastrocnemius muscle in a dog. J Am Anim Hosp Assoc 16:513, 1980.
3. Rewarts JM, Grooters AM, Payne JT, et al.: Atraumatic rupture of the gastrocnemius muscle after corticosteroid administration in a dog. J Am Vet Med Assoc 210:655, 1997.


# Luxation of the Superficial Digital Flexor Tendon

## Definition and Indications

The superficial digital flexor muscle runs deep to the lateral head of the gastrocnemius muscle and is intimately attached with this muscle at its origin. The superficial digital flexor tendon winds around the tendon of the gastrocnemius at the middle of the tibia, caps the tip of the calcaneus, and attaches medially and laterally on the tuber calcanei by means of dense retinacular fascia (Figure 7-44A). The superficial digital flexor cap is made up of fibrocartilage, and a synovial bursa exists between the tendon and the tip of the calcaneus. Displacement of the superficial digital flexor tendon can occur and is over-represented in Collies and Shetland Sheepdogs. The etiology is uncertain but is thought to relate to the anatomical structure of the calcaneus in affected dogs. Affected dogs are reported to have a shallow groove in the tip of the calcaneus. This conformational abnormality may decrease the stability of the superficial digital flexor tendon and allow it to luxate (Figure 7-44B). A congenital etiology is suspected although some cases are preceded by a traumatic event. Although lateral luxation predominates, medial luxation occurs as well.

This injury creates a variable degree of lameness. The majority of dogs bear weight on the affected leg although intermittent periods of non-weightbearing occur. Unilateral luxations are more common than bilateral. Diagnosis is established with careful palpation of the calcaneal bursa and superficial digital flexor tendon. A consistent finding is palpable distension of the calcaneal bursa. When the tarsocrural joint is extended, the tendon can be displaced manually from the calcaneal groove. Lateral radiographs show a soft tissue swelling around the tip of the calcaneus without bony changes.

## Technique

For a lateral luxation the patient is positioned in lateral recumbency with the affected limb down on the table. An incision is made over the plantaromedial aspect of the calcaneus for a lateral luxation. The incision extends proximally 4 cm from the point of the calcaneus and distally one-half the length of the calcaneus. The skin is retracted and an incision is made parallel to the superficial digital flexor tendon into the fluid distended calcaneal bursa. The bursa is flushed to remove debris. The superficial digital flexor tendon is separated from the gastrocnemius and combined tendons in order to provide enough mobility to position and suture the tendon. The tendon is centered over the intertubercular groove. The tissue on the edge of the superficial digital flexor tendon is sutured to the medial retinacular tissue using 2-0 nylon or polypropylene in a simple interrupted pattern (Figure 7-44). The tarsocrural joint is moved through a range of motion to verify proper positioning of the tendon. The remaining soft tissues are closed in layers.

Medial luxation of the superficial digital flexor tendon is approached similarly with interrupted sutures placed in the lateral retinacular tissues (Figure 7-44A through E).

## Aftercare

A lateral splint and soft padded bandage extending from the digits to the proximal tibia is applied. The splint is placed for 4 weeks with weekly changes. The splint is replaced with a soft padded bandage for 1 to 2 weeks. Exercise is restricted to short, 10 minute, leash walks for 6 weeks after surgery.

## Advantages and Disadvantages

Correcting a superficial digital flexor tendon luxation is a straightforward surgery and is associated with very good results. Failures have been reported when non-absorbable suture is used and when the bandage has been removed prior to 4 weeks postoperatively.

# Suggested Readings


1. Mauterer JV, Prata RG, Carberry CA, et al.: Displacement of the tendon of the superficial digital flexor muscle in dogs: 10 cases (1983-1991). J Am Vet Med Assoc 203(8):1162-1165, 1993.
2. Reinke JD, Mughannam AJ: Lateral luxation of the superficial digital flexor tendon in 12 dogs. J Am Anim Hosp Assoc 29:303-309, 1993.

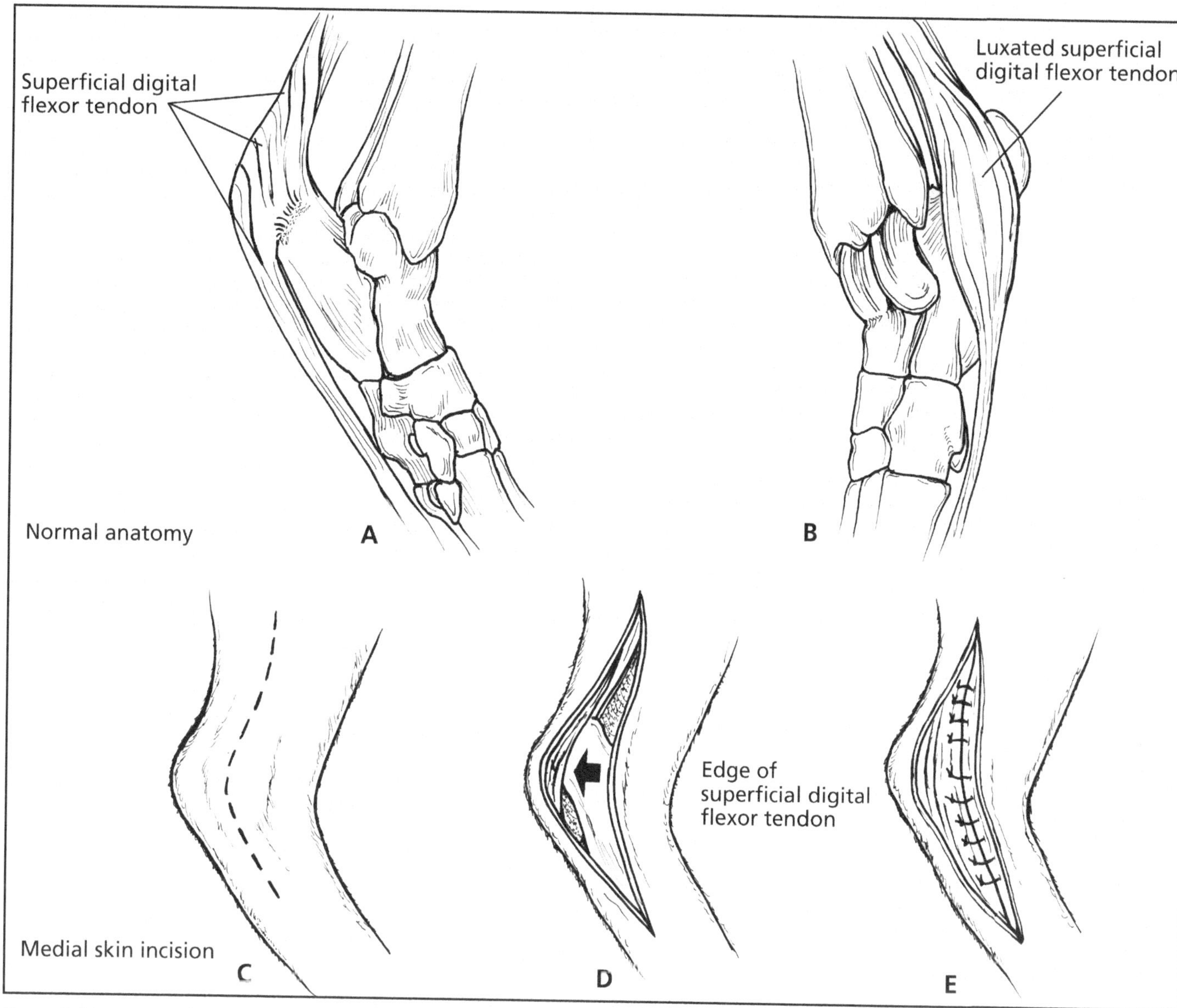


**Figure 7-44.** Luxation of the superficial digital flexor tendon. **A.** Normal anatomy of the superficial digital flexor tendon. The superficial digital flexor tendon caps the tuber calcanei and attaches medially and laterally on the tuber calcanei by means of dense retinacular fascia. **B.** Luxation of the superficial digital flexor tendon. For lateral luxation to occur medial retinacular attachments are disrupted. **C.** The luxation is corrected surgically. An incision is made over the plantaromedial aspect of the calcaneus for a lateral luxation. The incision extends proximally 4 cm from the point of the calcaneus and distally one-half the length of the calcaneus. **D.** The skin is retracted and an incision is made parallel to the superficial digital flexor tendon *(arrow)* into the fluid -distended calcaneal bursa. **E.** The tendon is centered over the intertubercular groove and the edge of the superficial digital flexor tendon is sutured to the medial retinacular tissue using non-absorbable suture in a simple interrupted pattern. (After Reinke JD, Mughannam AJ. Lateral luxation of the superficial digital flexor tendon in 12 dogs. J Amer Anim Hosp Assoc 29:303, 1993).

# Transarticular External Fixation of the Tarsus

## Definition and Indications

Several orthopedic conditions of the tarsus are treated using a transarticular external fixator to support the joint during healing. Examples include temporary stabilization of collateral ligament and calcanean tendon repairs and arthrodesis for severe shearing wounds. The two fundamental components of an external fixator are the fixation pins and the connecting rods. Fixation pins are placed percutaneously through the skin and into the bone with the use of a power drill. The pin always engages both the near and far cortex of the bone. A half-pin enters the skin and subcutaneous tissues on one side, engages both cortices of the bone, but does not exit the skin on the opposite side. An external fixator that consists of all half pins is referred to as a type I frame (See External Fixation of Radial Fractures).

A full pin penetrates the skin and subcutaneous tissues on one side, both cortices of the bone, and then proceeds through the skin on the opposite side. The pins are held on the outside of the bone by connecting rods. A full pin is supported by connecting rods on both sides. An external fixator that incorporates full pins is referred to as a type II frame (See External

Fixation of Radial Fractures). Fixation pins can be either smooth or threaded. The benefit of threaded pins is greater strength at the pin-bone interface. Modern threaded pins are a "positive profile" design meaning that the threads are not cut into the stainless steel but are raised above the core diameter of the pin. Newer versions do not have raised threads but rather have an altered design at the thread-non thread junction that confers stiffness to the pin (tapered run out feature; Imex Veterinary Inc, Longview, TX). Pins can be threaded either on the center of the pin or on the end. Centrally threaded designs are for full pin placement and end threaded designs are for half pin placement.

## Techniques

### Introduction: Principles of External Fixation

Transarticular external fixators used to support tendon or ligament repairs are kept in place for approximately 4 weeks. Systems used for arthrodesis are kept in place for approximately 12 weeks. The longevity of an external fixator is directly related to the pin-bone interface. The pin-bone interface can be threatened first by localized thermal bone injury and second by excessive local stress on individual pins. These problems can be limited by proper pin placement. Thermal bone injury is minimized by pre-drilling. This is necessary because most fixator pins are designed with a trocar point that has no spiral channels to release bone shards during placement. Bone impacts around the rotating tip of the pin and creates friction and heat. To avoid this a sharp drill bit that is slightly smaller than the diameter of the fixator is used to make the initial path through the bone.

Excessive local pin stress is avoided by placing enough pins. Generally at least 3 pins are placed on either side of the fracture. There is no significant benefit to placing greater than 4 pins on either side of the fracture. Larger pins have a greater surface area and thus lower levels of stress at the pin-bone interface. The pin must not exceed 30% of the bone diameter however or iatrogenic fracture can occur through the pin site.

The interface between the pin and the skin is created and maintained in a way that will avoid pressure on the skin and excessive motion of the skin. This promotes rapid healing of the wound and helps to prevent pin tract infections. A stab incision is made in the skin and extended down to the bone prior to introducing the bone drill. Once the fixator pin is in place, the skin is inspected for tension. Any tension at the pin site is relieved with a small releasing incision. These skin incisions are not sutured. The connecting rod and clamps must not contact the skin since this can create irritation and skin wounds. Techniques for bandaging the limb after pin placement are designed to stabilize the skin at the interface with the pin.

The normal standing angle of the tarsus is 130 to 150° in the dog and 115 to 125° in the cat. The external fixator construct must be designed to position the tarsocrural joint in an appropriate degree of flexion. A plate bender can be used to contour the connecting rods to the desired angle. It can be challenging to get enough bend in the bar this way. Alternative designs obviate the need to place a bend in the connecting rod. These designs include the use of hinges (either static or mobile), construction of a modified clamp to hold the connecting rods at an angle, the use of flexible tubing that is filled with acrylic, and the placement of a simple 3 pin frame. The 3 pin frame is intended to be used for short periods of external fixation.

There are specific considerations when placing pins in the metatarsal bones. First, the central metatarsal bones are positioned cranial to the lateral and medial bones. Due to this arrangement, it is impossible to apply a pin across all 4 metatarsal bones and an attempt is made to engage 2 metatarsal bones. Secondly, pins should only be placed in the proximal two-thirds of the metatarsal bones. Pins placed more distally may interfere with the metatarsal/metacarpal pad and could impede the animal's ability to bear full weight on the limb.

Techniques for applying transarticular external skeletal fixation are described in this section.

### Three Pin Type II Frame

This frame is used for short, 3 to 4 week, episodes of transarticular external fixation. The pin placement is as follows: one pin in the distal tibia, one through the calcaneus, and one through the proximal metatarsal bones. Because so few pins are used, this system is often applied using full pins (type II external fixator) in which case the pins are centrally-threaded. The tibial and calcaneal pins are secured to one connecting rod on the medial and lateral sides using single clamps. The metatarsal pins are secured to a second connecting rod on the medial and lateral sides with single clamps and double clamps are used to attach the proximal and distal connecting rods together (Figure 7-45).

### Hinged Frame for a Dynamic External Fixator

A mobile hinge permits physiologic flexion and extension during healing while preventing medial and lateral or rotational movement. These systems provide a level of stability while maintaining more normal

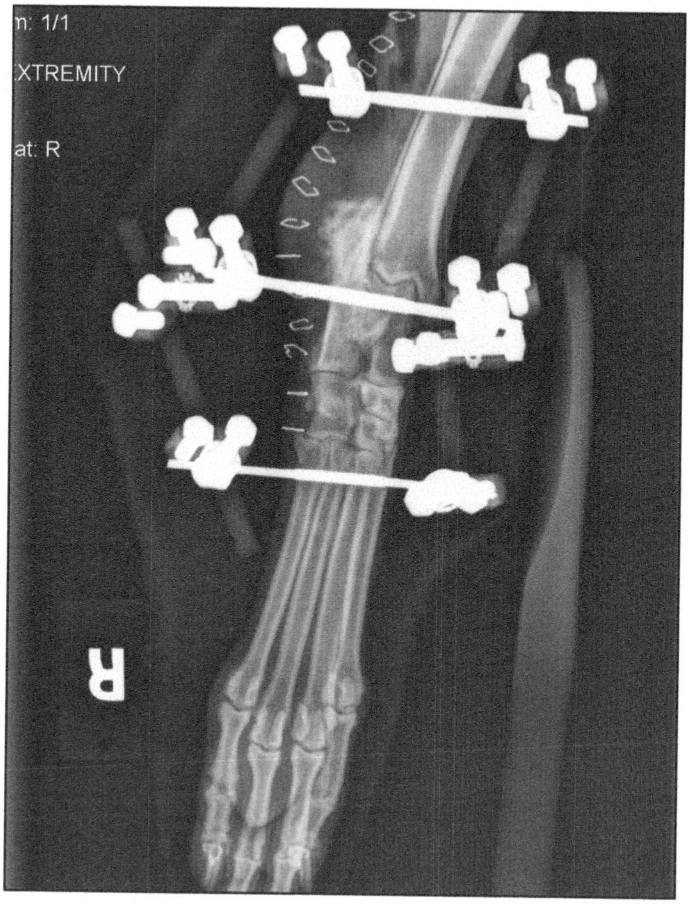


**Figure 7-45.** Three pin frame. Craniocaudal view tarsus. The tarsocrural joint is stabilized using one pin in the distal tibia, one through the calcaneus and one through the metatarsal bones. The pins are secured to connecting rods with clamps. Connecting rods are carbon fiber and thus not radiopaque.

homeostasis of cartilage than with static external fixation (Figure 7-46). There are hinges specifically designed for transarticular external fixation (Figure 7-47A) Range of Motion Hinge, Imex Veterinary Inc., Longview, TX)) and those that are created by modifying external fixator components to create a hinge (Figure 7-47B); Imex Veterinary Inc., Longview, TX). Both types of hinges use hybrid connecting rods. Hybrid connecting rods are the same width as standard connecting rods but have a threaded end. The hinge has internal threads on each side that accept the threads of a hybrid connecting rod.

A modified hinge (See Figure 7-47B) is created by converting a hinge designed for circular external fixation into a mobile hinge for transarticular external fixation (Angular hinge; Imex Veterinary Inc., Longview, TX). This requires exchanging a shorter bolt in the hinge for a longer bolt and tightening it with nuts. Hybrid connecting rods of the appropriate length are chosen for the tibia and the metatarsus. Each hybrid rod is inserted into the hinge with a nut and tightened (See Figure 7-47B).

The hinge is placed at the level of the tarsocrural joint, centered medially over the ridges of the talus. The most proximal pin is placed in the tibia and connected to the hybrid rod with a single clamp. The most distal pin is placed in the metatarsal bones and connected to the hybrid rod with a single clamp. Additional pins are added to the tibia, calcaneus and metatarsal bones and secured to the connecting rods with single clamps (See Figure 7-46).

To obtain a non-moveable frame, the tarsocrural joint can be spanned with a cranial connecting rod. This connecting rod is attached to the proximal and distal

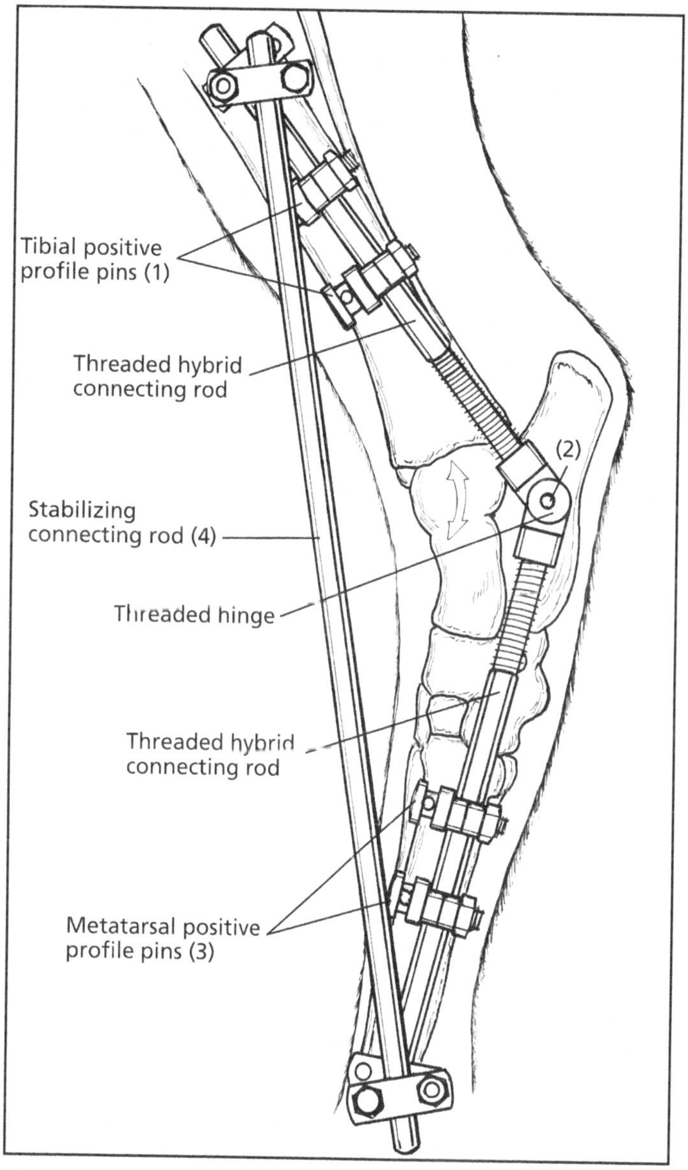


**Figure 7-46.** Hinged Frame for a Mobile External Fixator. This frame spans the tarsocrural joint and permits movement in a single plane. Two external fixation pins are placed in the tibia *(1)* one pin is placed in the calcaneus *(2)* and one pin in the proximal metatarsal bones *(3)*. Two pins may be placed in the metatarsal bones for increased stability of the fixator. Pins are secured to connecting rods with single clamps and the proximal and distal connecting rods are joined by a hinge. (4) A stabilizing connecting rod can be added to create a static fixation during initial healing.

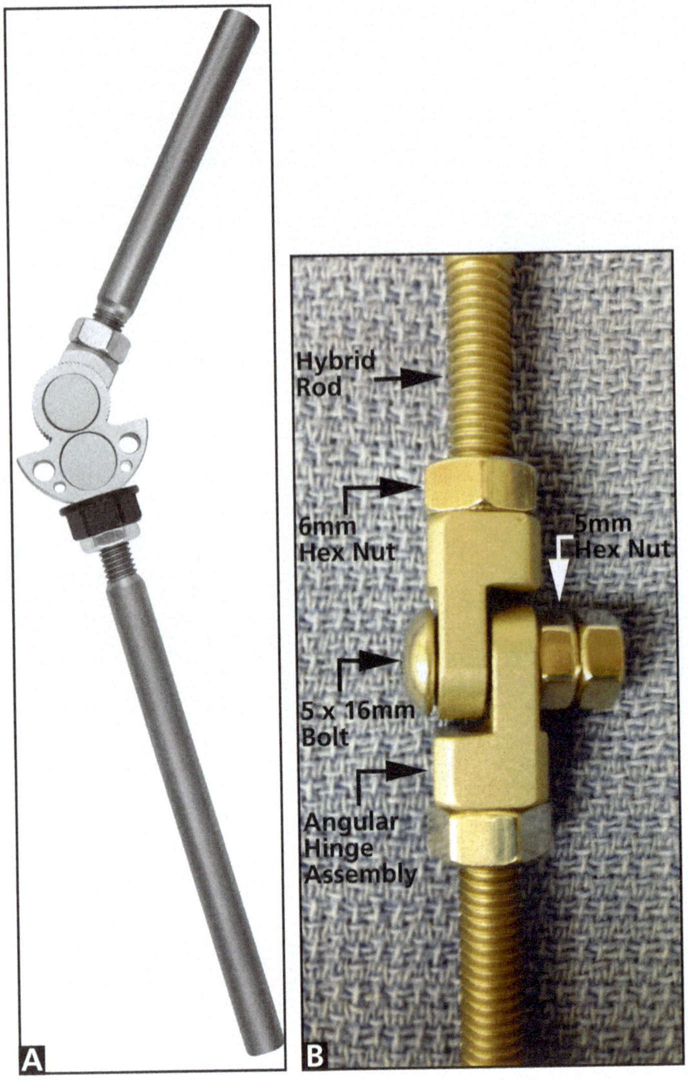


**Figure 7-47.** Mobile Hinges used for External Fixation. **A.** Range of motion hinge. This hinge joins proximal and distal connecting rods and can be adjusted to provide a desired range of motion. **B.** Modified hinge. This hinge is created using an angular hinge that is designed for circular external fixation. The short bolt of the angular hinge is exchanged for a longer bolt. The bolt is tightened with two 5 mm hex nuts. Each side of the hinge has internal threads that accept the threads of a hybrid connecting rod. (Imex Veterinary, Inc., Longview, TX).

portions of the tibia and metatarsal connecting rods using double clamps. An assistant holds the tarsocrural joint at the desired angle as the surgeon tightens the clamps of this connecting rod. The frame can be adjusted for complete stability early in the healing process, such as the first 3 weeks, and can then be transitioned to a mobile hinge for the remainder of the healing process. The frame is transitioned to a mobile hinge by removing the cranial connecting rod (See Figure 7-46).

## Modified Clamp for a Static External Fixator

Modified clamps are derived from the components of single clamps (Imex Veterinary Inc., Longview, TX) and are used to secure the connecting rods of a transarticular external fixator at an angle (Figure 7-48A). Two modified clamps are used for the articulation and are connected by two short pieces of Steinmann pins (Figure 7-48B). The angle of this articulation is adjustable but once the bolts are tightened the fixation is secure.

A fixator frame constructed from modified clamps is very stable and with a sufficient number of pins can be used for tarsocrural arthrodesis. For this purpose, 3 pins are placed in the tibia, 1 in the talus, 1 in the central and fourth tarsal bones, and 2 in the metatarsal bones (Figure 7-48C). For added stiffness cranial connecting rods can be added.

## Acrylic External Fixator System

The acrylic pin external fixator system (APEF system, Innovative Animal Products, Rochester, MN.) replaces standard connecting rods and clamps with polymethyl methacrylate columns (See Figure 7-49). The system has different sizes of flexible tubing. An acrylic column using 21 mm diameter tubing is comparable in strength to the traditional medium Kirschner-Ehmer frame (KE external skeletal fixation, Imex Veterinary Inc., Longview, TX). This system can be used to provide transarticular support to the tarsus. For a medium-sized dog, 2 to 4 size medium, positive profile, center threaded pins are placed through both cortices of the tibia and 2 to 4 small, positive profile, center threaded pins are placed in the metatarsal bones. The flexible plastic tubing is pushed over the fixator pins on both sides. The liquid and powder components of the acrylic are mixed to initiate a polymerization reaction and the liquid acrylic is poured into the tubes. An assistant holds the tarsus at the desired angle of flexion until the acrylic solidifies (Figure 7-49).

## Kirschner-Ehmer Frame

The Kirschner-Ehmer (KE) frame is the prototype veterinary external fixator. Current systems (Imex SK, Imex Veterinary Inc., Longview, TX; Securos External Fixation, Securos Inc., Fiskdale MA) have stronger components and are more convenient to place. The KE external fixator consists of small (3.2 mm) and medium (4.8 mm) stainless steel connecting rods and clamps. Unlike newer clamps, KE clamps cannot be taken apart and placed onto the connecting rod during fixator assembly. KE clamps have to be placed onto the connecting rod at the beginning of the procedure. KE clamps cannot accommodate passage of the threaded components of positive profile pins. Given the inherent weaknesses with the KE system it is best to apply it as a type II fixator (Figure 7-50).

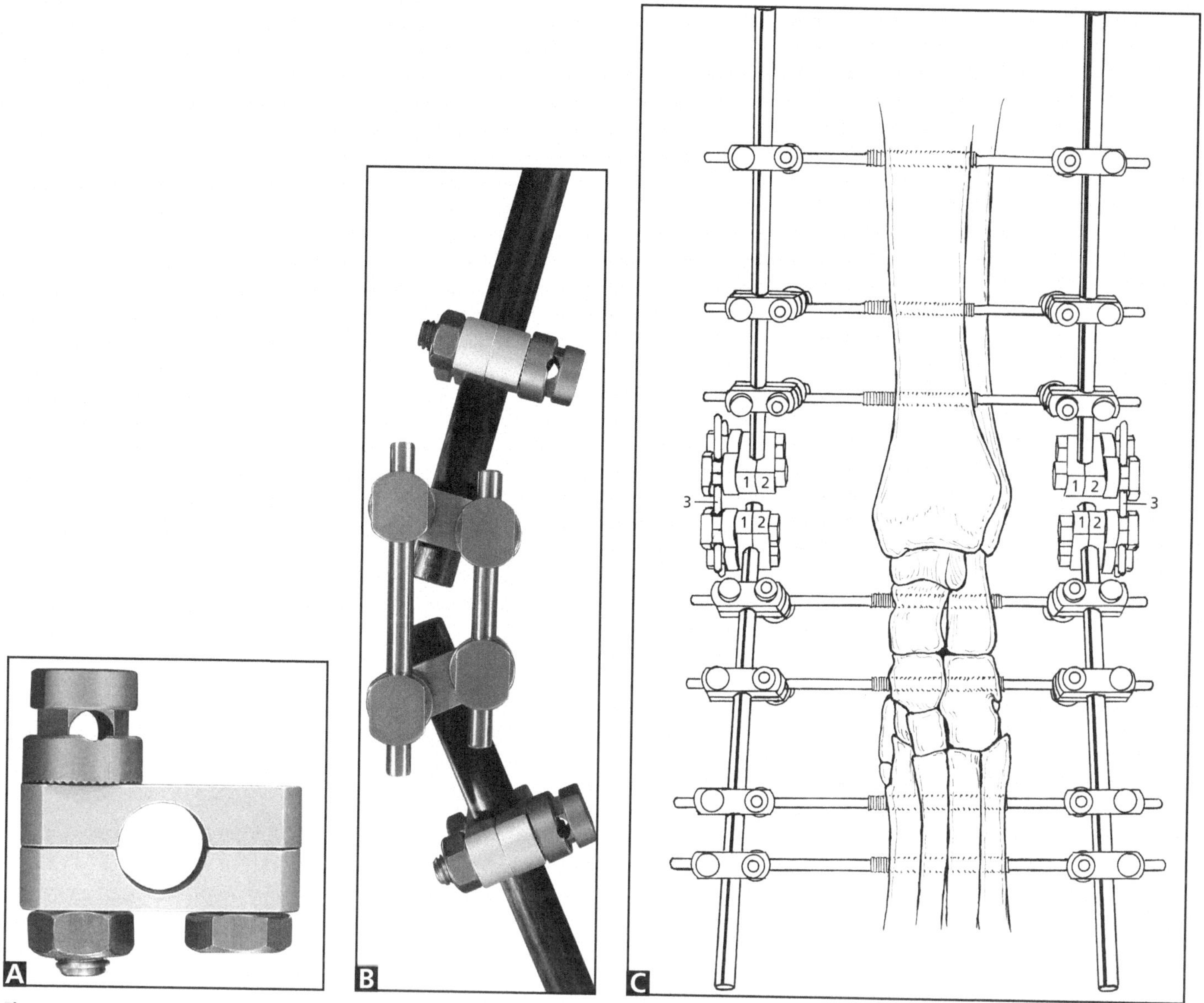


**Figure 7-48.** Modified Clamp for a Static External Fixator. **A.** Single clamps. Each clamp is composed of 2 halves. The halves are secured together by 2 bolts. The larger bolt is the primary pin gripping bolt and the smaller is the secondary bolt. Each half of the bolt is different. One half has a threaded hole and a smooth hole and the other has 2 smooth holes **B.** The modified clamp is designed by using the 2 halves of a single clamp that contain smooth (non-threaded) holes only. The 2 halves are assembled with pin gripping bolts and nuts. The two clamps are connected by Steinmann pins that are cut short and placed through the pin gripping bolts. **C.** The modified clamps can be used as part of a very stable frame design. For this purpose the fixator frame is completed by placing 2 to 3 pins in the tibia, 2 to 3 pins in the metatarsals, and if desired 1 pin through the talus and 1 through the central and fourth tarsal bones (Imex Veterinary Inc., Longview, TX).

A KE external fixator can be placed across a joint by bending the connecting rod. The connecting rods are smaller than others so are easier to bend. The connecting rods are bent to a normal standing angle, approximately 130 to 150 degrees in the dog or 115 to 125 degrees in the cat, and attached with clamps to the proximal and distal pins. Remaining clamps have been pre-placed on the connecting rod. An additional full pin is placed in the tibia and metatarsal bones, and half pins are then directed through the clamps into the distal tibia and tarsal bones. Cranial connecting rods are placed for increased resistance to bending (See Figure 7-50).

## Aftercare

A soft padded bandage is placed from just below the stifle to the distal extent of the digits. Bandaging the fixator helps prevent excessive skin movement around the fixator pins and helps to reduce swelling. Foam rubber or sponge material is placed between the connecting rods and the skin (Figure 7-51) to stabilize the skin. For the first 2 weeks postoperatively, the external fixator and paw are covered with a soft padded bandage. The bandage is changed 1 to 2 days postoperatively and then weekly.

By 2-3 weeks postoperatively, the bandage can usually be reduced to a "bumper bandage". Surgical sponges

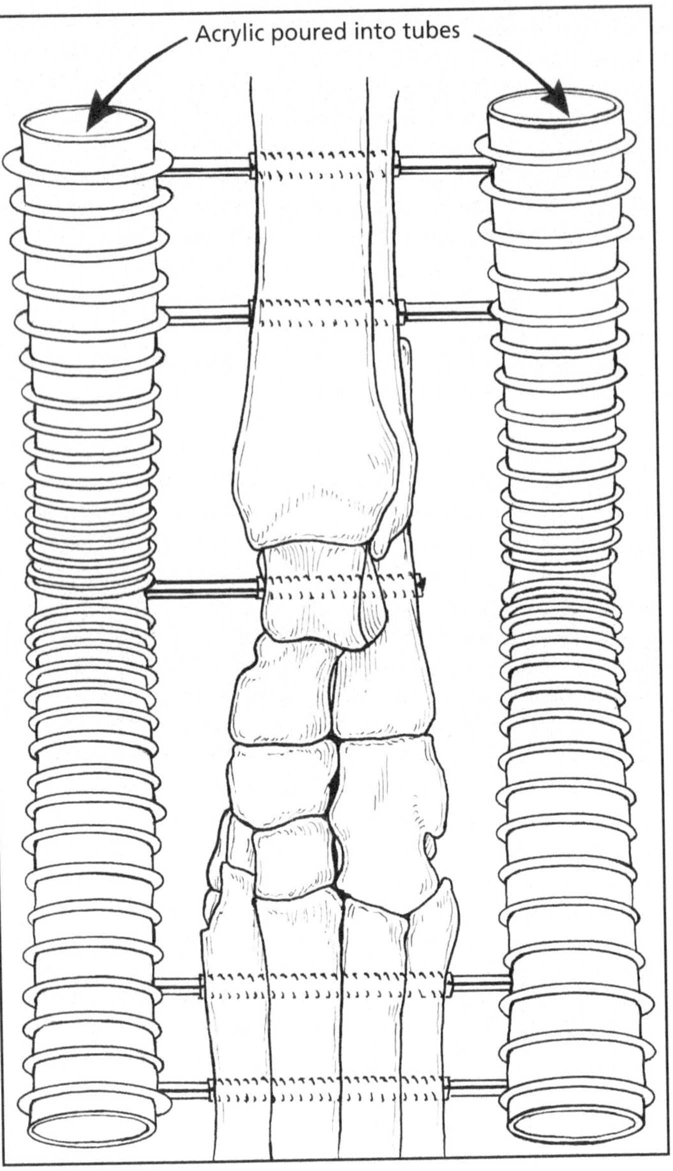


**Figure 7-49.** Transarticular external fixator: Acrylic type. Two to 4 positive profile pins are placed through both cortices of the tibia, 1 to 2 pins through the tarsal bones, and 2 to 3 pins are placed in the metatarsal bones. Flexible plastic tubing is pushed over the fixator pins on both sides. The liquid and powder components of the acrylic are mixed and the acrylic is poured into the plastic tubes. (APEF system, Innovative Animal Products, Rochester, MN.)

are still placed between the skin and the connecting rods. Elastic tape (VetWrap) is used to encircle the fixator and sponges. The purpose of the bandage is to prevent the fixator from becoming caught on things and to protect the patient and the owner. Bumper bandages are changed every 2 weeks or as needed.

The sites where the pin enters the skin are examined at the time of bandage changes. Some degree of redness, mild swelling, and scant discharge is normal within the first week. Triple antibiotic ointment is placed at the pin entrance sites during the first 2 weeks using a sterile swab or gloved finger. Enlargement of the skin wound around the pin, or the presence of a purulent discharge signifies irritation and probably infection of the pin site. This is treated with broad spectrum antibiotics. A veterinarian should examine the fixator at approximately 2 to 3 week intervals.

## Advantages and Disadvantages

Postoperative joint immobilization protects healing and inhibits gap formation in ligaments and tendons. This goal must be balanced with the overall health of the joint cartilage. Rigid fixation with an external fixator reduces the glycosaminoglycan (GAG) content of the cartilage matrix to a greater degree than splinting, which permits 8 to 15 degrees of motion. Joints that are completely immobilized for significant periods of time, such as 6 weeks, can have a decrease in GAG content by approximately 30% compared to a lesser degree with cast fixation. The advantage of rigid external fixation is that it confers stability and is generally easier to manage than a splint. The disadvantage, in terms of cartilage health, can be managed by placing the fixator for a limited period of time and then converting it to splints and bandages that permit increasing degrees of mobility. Alternatively, hinged fixators can be used. Hinged fixators confer a physiologic degree of motion when absolute stability is not necessary.

Hinged external fixator frames are advantageous for support of shearing wound cases. Disruptive rotational or varus-valgus motion is prohibited but physiologic motion around a single axis, flexion and extension, is maintained. A mobile hinge system would be a disadvantage if absolute stability were needed, such as with pantarsal arthrodesis.

The modified clamp can be readily constructed from standard components (Imex Veterinary Inc., Longview, TX) and is very stable. This clamp cannot be mobilized and is useful for very stable frames.

The KE system is familiar to many veterinarians and may be less expensive than other systems. The connecting rods are not difficult to bend. The biomechanical weakness of the connecting rods and clamps limit its use.

An advantage of most external fixator frames is the potential to modify pin placement after surgery. The acrylic external fixator system is less expensive than the others and slightly faster to construct. However it is a static system that cannot be readily modified after it is placed.

External fixators are also useful in cases that have received skin grafts over the joint surface. Limiting motion facilitates the healing of grafts and simplifies bandaging of the skin graft.

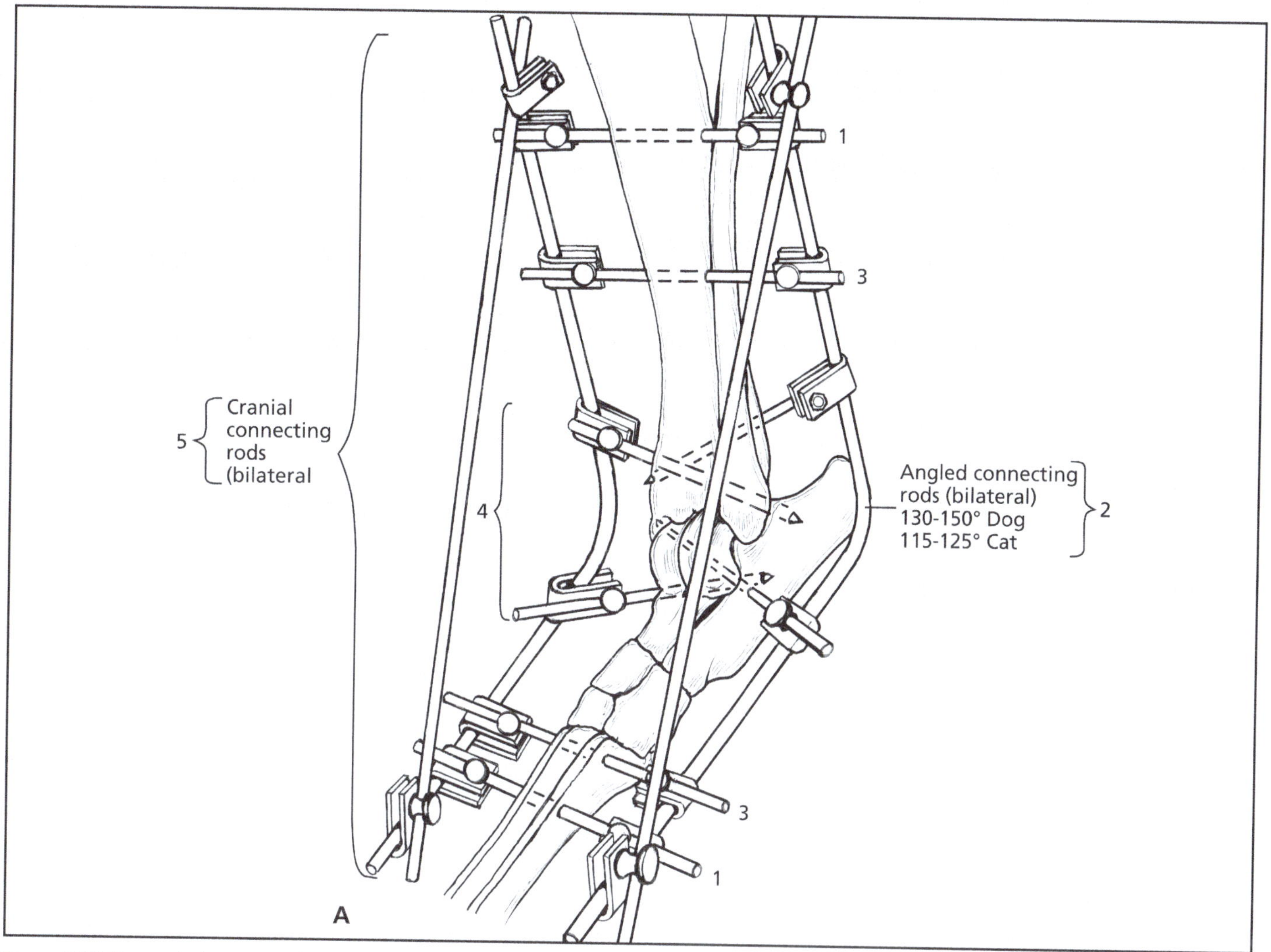


**Figure 7-50.** Transarticular external fixator: Kirschner-Ehmer (KE) type. Type II KE placed for tarsal arthrodesis. The first step is placement of a full pin proximally in the tibia and distally in the metatarsals *(1)*. Next the connecting rods are bent to a normal standing angle, approximately 140 degrees in the dog *(2)*, and attached with clamps to the proximal and distal pins. Remaining clamps have been pre-placed on the connecting rod and remaining pins are directed through the clamps and into the bone. An additional full pin is placed in the tibia and metatarsal bones *(3)* and half-pins are placed in the distal tibia and talus *(4)*. Cranial connecting rods are placed for increased resistance to bending *(5)*.

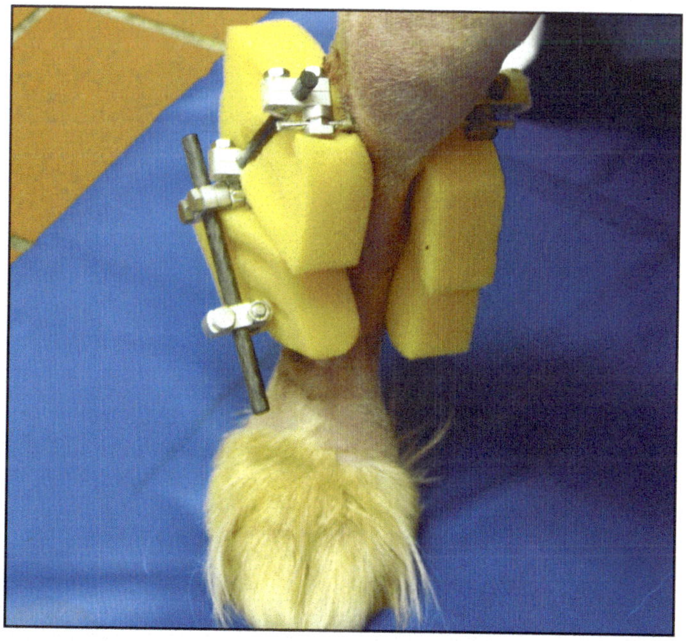

**Figure 7-51.** External fixation bandage: sponge placement between connecting rods and skin.

# Suggested Readings


1. Anderson MA: Using transarticular external skeletal fixation devices. Vet Med: 468-472, May 1998.
2. Behrens F, Kraft EL, Oegema-TR J: Biochemical changes in articular cartilage after joint immobilization by casting or external fixation, J Orthop Res 12:335-343, 1989.
3. Jaeger GH, Wosar MA, Marcellin-Little DJ et al.: Use of hinged transarticular external fixation for adjunctive joint stabilization in dogs and cats: 14 cases (1999-2003). J Am Vet Med Assoc 227:586-591,2005.
4. Kraus KH, Toombs JP, Ness MG. External Fixation in Small Animal Practice. Malden, MA: Blackwell Science Ltd: 2003, 5-78.
5. King M, Jerram R: Achilles tendon rupture in dogs. Comp Cont Educ Small Anim Pract 25:613-620, 2003.


# Malleolar Fractures

## Definition and Indications

The medial and lateral malleolus serve as the origin for the respective collateral ligaments. Fracture of either malleolus results in significant tarsal joint instability and requires surgical repair.

## Techniques

Malleolar fractures are commonly repaired using a tension band fixation. This fixation consists of 2 small pins or K-wires that traverse the fracture line and anchor in the far cortex of the tibia. A cerclage wire is placed around the pins and through a hole in the distal tibia in a figure 8 fashion. The purpose of the figure 8 wire is to counteract the tension applied on the fracture site by the pull of the collateral ligament. Special care is taken not to penetrate the tarsocrural joint with the K-wires. The malleoli extend distal to the articular surface, so the pins must be angled proximally enough to avoid the joint. An alternative to tension band fixation is lag screw fixation of the fractured malleolus.

### Medial Malleolar Fracture

The skin incision is centered over the medial surface of the tarsocrural joint. The incision begins at the distal fourth of the tibia and continues distally to the level of the tarsometatarsal joint. The subcutaneous tissue and crural fascia are incised on the same line as the skin. Soft tissues are retracted (See Figure 7-11).

The distal bone fragment is grasped with small pointed bone reduction forceps and held at the fracture site. Using a high speed drill, 2 K-wires are advanced into the malleolus and into the opposite cortex of the tibia. A small hole is drilled in the distal tibia for passage of the figure 8 cerclage wire. The cerclage wire is anchored behind the K-wires, crossed to form a figure 8, passed through the drill hole and tightened (Figure 7-52A). The K-wires are cut and bent and the cerclage wire is cut to a length of 2 to 3 twists. The subcutaneous layer is closed with absorbable suture followed by skin closure.

Alternatively the medial malleolus can be secured by means of a lag screw from the malleolus into the distal tibia (Figure 7-52B). To place a lag screw, the near cortex (the distal fragment of the medial malleolus) is over-drilled and the far cortex (the distal tibia) is drilled according to the core diameter of the screw. For a medium sized dog, a 3.5 mm screw is placed. The near cortex would be drilled with a size 3.5 mm drill bit and the far cortex would be drilled with a size 2.5 mm drill bit. The drill holes are tapped with a 3.5 mm tap (Figure 7-52C).

### Lateral Malleolar Fracture

The lateral malleolus is approached by centering the skin incision over the lateral surface of the tarsocrural joint (See Figure 7-14). The incision begins proximally at the level of the lateral saphenous vein and continues distally to the level of the tarsometatarsal joint. The subcutaneous and crural fascia is incised along the same line as the skin and is retracted with the skin.

The peroneus longus tendon overlies the lateral malleolus (See Figure 7-14). The extensor retinaculum is incised parallel to the cranial edge of the tendon so that the tendon can be retracted. The distal bone fragment is grasped with bone reduction forceps and held at the fracture site. A K-wire is directed from the lateral malleolus up the shaft of the fibula. The hole for anchoring the figure 8 wire is made in the distal tibia. Cerclage wire is anchored beneath the end of the K-wire and through the proximal hole and tightened (See Figure 7-52A). Subcutaneous tissue and skin are closed in layers.

In some animals the lateral malleolus is too small for normograde placement of K-wires. In these cases, the distal fragment is secured directly to the distal tibia by means of K-wires or a lag screw (See Figure 7-52C).

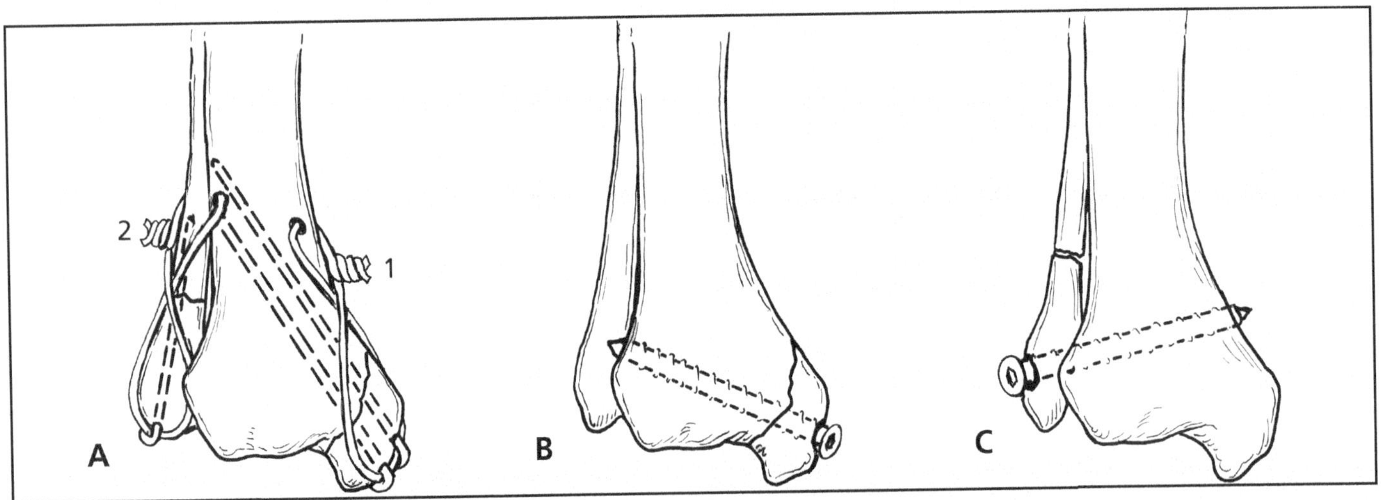


**Figure 7-52.** Malleolar fractures: tension band fixation. **A.** Two small pins traverse the medial malleolus and fracture line and far cortex of the tibia. A cerclage wire is placed around the pins and through a hole in the distal tibia in a figure 8 fashion *(1)*. A K-wire and figure 8 cerclage wire are used to repair a lateral malleolar fracture *(2)*. **B., C.** Medial and lateral malleolar fractures repaired with lag screws.

## Aftercare

A lateral splint and soft padded bandage extending from the digits to the proximal tibia is placed for 2 to 3 weeks with weekly changes. Exercise is limited to short leash walks for 8 weeks. Radiographs are taken at approximately 8 weeks postoperatively to assess healing.

## Advantages and Disadvantages

A lag screw can be placed in slightly less time than a tension band fixation and there are no sharp cerclage wire ends in the subcutaneous tissues. The disadvantage of a lag screw is that a relatively large hole must be drilled in the malleolus. The malleolus tends to be small and the large drill hole could risk fracture of the bone fragment.

# Suggested Readings


1. Boudrieau RJ: Fractures of the Tibia and Fibula. In Slatter D, ed.: Textbook of Small Animal Surgery 3rd ed: Philadelphia: Saunders, 2003, 2144.
2. Johnson AL, Dunning D: Atlas of Orthopedic Surgical Procedures of the Dog ad Cat. St. Louis: Elsevier Saunders, 2005, 200.
3. Piermattei DL, Flo GL, DeCamp CE: Brinker, Piermattei, and Flo's Handbook of Small Animal Orthopedics and Fracture Repair, 4th ed: St. Louis: Saunders Elselvier, 2006, 658.


# Distal Tibial Physeal Fractures

## Definition and Indications

Distal tibial physeal fractures occur following traumatic injury in young animals. Despite involvement of the physis, growth disturbance with this injury is rare. Surgical repair is usually accomplished with cross pins. Very occasionally, it is possible to perform a closed reduction of a physeal fracture using traction to manipulate the distal fragment into position in an anesthetized animal. Reduction is maintained with external coaptation. However, most cases require surgical repair.

## Technique

The skin is incised on the cranial medial aspect of the tibia from the distal diaphysis of the tibia to the middle of the tarsal joint. The origin of the medial collateral ligament can be seen at the distal medial malleolus and the tendon of the tibialis caudalis muscle can be seen caudal to the malleolus (See Figure 7-11). The fracture is carefully reduced to minimize trauma to the physeal cartilage. Reduction is maintained with a pointed reduction forceps or with manual pressure. A K wire is advanced from the medial malleolus up into the lateral tibial metaphysis to penetrate the lateral tibial cortex. Next a K-wire is advanced from the lateral aspect of the distal fragment to the medial aspect of the proximal fragment (Figure 7-53). Each pin is bent and cut. The intradermal layer is closed with absorbable suture followed by skin.

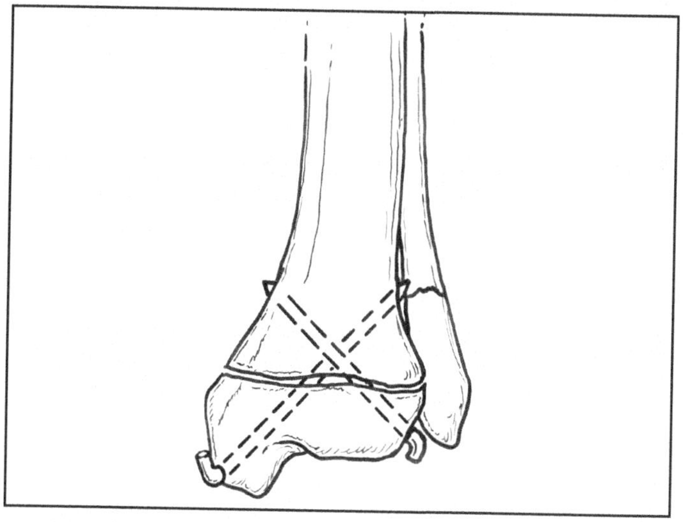

**Figure 7-53.** Distal tibial physeal fractures: cross pin repair. A Kirschner wire is advanced from the medial malleolus up to the tibial diaphysis. A second Kirschner wire is placed from the lateral aspect of the distal fragment to the medial aspect of the proximal fragment. The pins are bent and cut short.

## Aftercare

A lateral splint and soft padded bandage that extends from the proximal tibia to the digits is placed for 2 to 3 weeks with weekly changes. Exercise is limited to short 10 minute leash walks 3 to 4 times daily with indoor crate rest for 4 weeks. Radiographs are taken at 4 weeks postoperatively to evaluate healing. Implant removal may be required if the pins cause soft tissue irritation or become loose.

## Advantages and Disadvantages

The advantage to surgical repair of distal physeal fractures is that it is relatively straightforward and results in stable fixation. The disadvantage to closed reduction is that anatomic reduction may not be achieved or maintained by external coaptation. Imperfect reduction close to a joint can result in significant rotational or angular deformity.

# Suggested Readings


1. Johnson AL, Dunning D. Atlas of Orthopedic Surgical Procedures of the Dog and Cat. St. Louis: Elsevier Saunders, 2005, 198-199.


# Fractures of the Tarsal Bones

## General Information

Fractures of the tarsal bones can be single or can involve multiple bones. Some fracture patterns are seen most commonly in racing Greyhounds whereas others occur in all breeds. Most tarsal bone fractures are repaired with the use of lag screws. To do this, the near cortex is overdrilled using a drill bit that is the same size as the thread diameter of the screw. The far cortex is drilled with a smaller size that equals the core diameter of the screw. Comminuted tarsal bone fractures with small bone fragments are often repaired by placing a bone plate to buttress that portion of the tarsus.

# Fractures of the Calcaneus

## Definition and Indications

A calcaneal fracture completely disrupts the common calcanean tendon apparatus. The result is a plantigrade stance and marked displacement of the proximal bony fragment due to the tensile force of the calcanean tendon. The proximal half of the calcaneus is referred to as the tuber calcanei and the middle portion is the shaft. The distal portion is the base of the calcaneus. Fractures occur most commonly at the tuber or in the shaft and less commonly near the base. Fractures at the base of the calcaneus disrupt the origin of the plantar ligament and therefore cause subluxation and hyperextension of the calcaneoquartal joint.

Calcaneal fractures are common in racing greyhounds and, in this breed, often occur in conjunction with central tarsal bone fractures. Chronologically, the central tarsal bone fails, and next the head of the talus is displaced distally into the fracture gap of the central tarsal bone. Tension from the common calcaneal tendon and loss of dorsomedial support place abnormal stress on the calcaneus and plantar ligaments. Relief of the accumulated forces on the lateral and plantar aspect of the tarsus occurs by fracture of the calcaneus. If the calcaneus remains intact as the central tarsal bone collapses, the brunt of the remaining fracture forces are conferred to the fourth tarsal bone and cause it to fracture.

Tension band wire fixation can be an effective repair for non-comminuted calcaneal fractures. Simple or comminuted calcaneal fractures can be repaired using a bone plate or a bone plate supplemented with an intramedullary pin. Fractures of the distal calcaneus (the base of the calcaneus) that do not have a large enough piece of bone to accommodate a plate can be stabilized with tension band fixation anchored to the fourth tarsal bone. Avulsion fractures from the base of the calcaneus that involve only a small piece of bone are treated with partial tarsal arthrodesis to restore plantar support.

## Techniques

### Tension Band Fixation for Proximal Fractures of the Calcaneus

Tension band fixation is often used for proximal avulsion fragments. The patient is placed in lateral recumbency with the affected leg up. The skin incision begins on the lateral side of the common calcanean tendon just proximal to the tuber calcanei and extends to the level of the fourth tarsal bone (See Figure 7-24). The skin and subcutaneous tissues are reflected to expose the deep fascia. The lateral border of the tendon of the superficial digital flexor muscle is located. An incision is made parallel to the lateral border of the tendon. To free the tendon, the incision is made through deep fascia and the lateral retinacular attachment of the tendon to the calcaneus, and is continued proximally. The tendon is separated from the gastrocnemius tendon and retracted medially.

The proximal bone fragment is grasped with pointed reduction forceps and manually held in correct position for normograde pin insertion. Two intramedullary pins are inserted down the shaft of the calcaneus and cerclage wire is anchored around the proximal pins and through a distal transverse hole in the bone (Figure 7-54A, B & C). It is not necessary to pre-drill for pin placement in the calcaneus of young dogs. In older animals a pre-drill may be necessary because the bone of the calcaneus is so dense. If a pre-drill is required, the drill size is slightly smaller than the intramedullary pin. The 2 pins are placed in a slightly lateral and slightly medial orientation to minimize postoperative irritation of the overlying superficial digital flexor tendon. A transverse hole is drilled in the shaft of the calcaneus with a small drill bit (size 2.0 mm in a medium dog). The size of cerclage wire must be large enough to resist fatigue. The following sizes are recommended: up to 15 to 20 pounds, 22 gauge (0.635 mm); 20 to 40 pounds, 20 gauge (0.812 mm); and over 40 pounds, 18 gauge (1.02 mm). The cerclage wire is placed in figure eight fashion and the proximal pins are bent over to the side and cut short. The cerclage wire is cut between the first and second twist.

If there is a larger fragment of proximal bone, the tension band is placed in a different manner. A single larger intramedullary pin is selected for normograde placement. Prior to placing the pin, a transverse hole is drilled through the proximal fragment and through the distal shaft of the bone using a drill bit. Next a bone tunnel slightly smaller than the pin is pre-drilled down the shaft of the calcaneus using a drill bit. The pin is normograded into the calcaneus, cut short, and then countersunk using a pin punch and mallet (Securos Inc., Fiskdale, MA). The appropriate size wire is passed through the 2 transverse holes in a figure eight pattern and tightened. The cerclage wire is cut short (Figure 7-55A-C).

The superficial digital flexor tendon is sutured to the retinacular fascia using interrupted non-absorbable sutures. The dermal layer is closed with absorbable suture followed by skin closure.

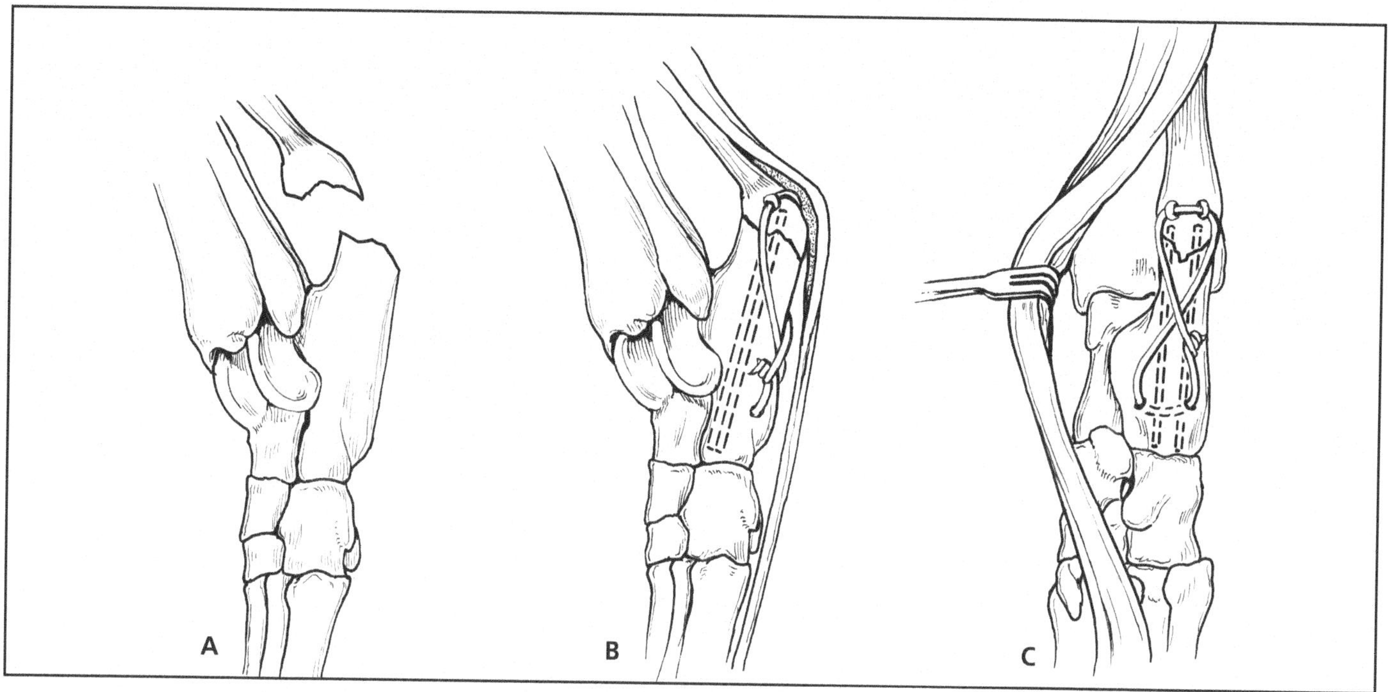


**Figure 7-54.** Proximal calcaneal avulsion fractures: tension band fixation. **A.** Calcaneal avulsion fracture. **B., C.** Lateral and plantar views (respectively) with a small proximal avulsion fragment, the tension band fixation is placed using 2 K-wires or small pins and a figure 8 cerclage wire. Two Kirschner wires or small pins are placed in a slightly lateral and slightly medial orientation through the fracture segment and into the shaft of the calcaneus. (After Piermattei DL, Flo GL, DeCamp CE: Brinker, Piermattei and Flo's Handbook of Small Animal Orthopedics and Fracture Repair, 4th ed. St Louis: Saunders Elsevier, 2006, 671).

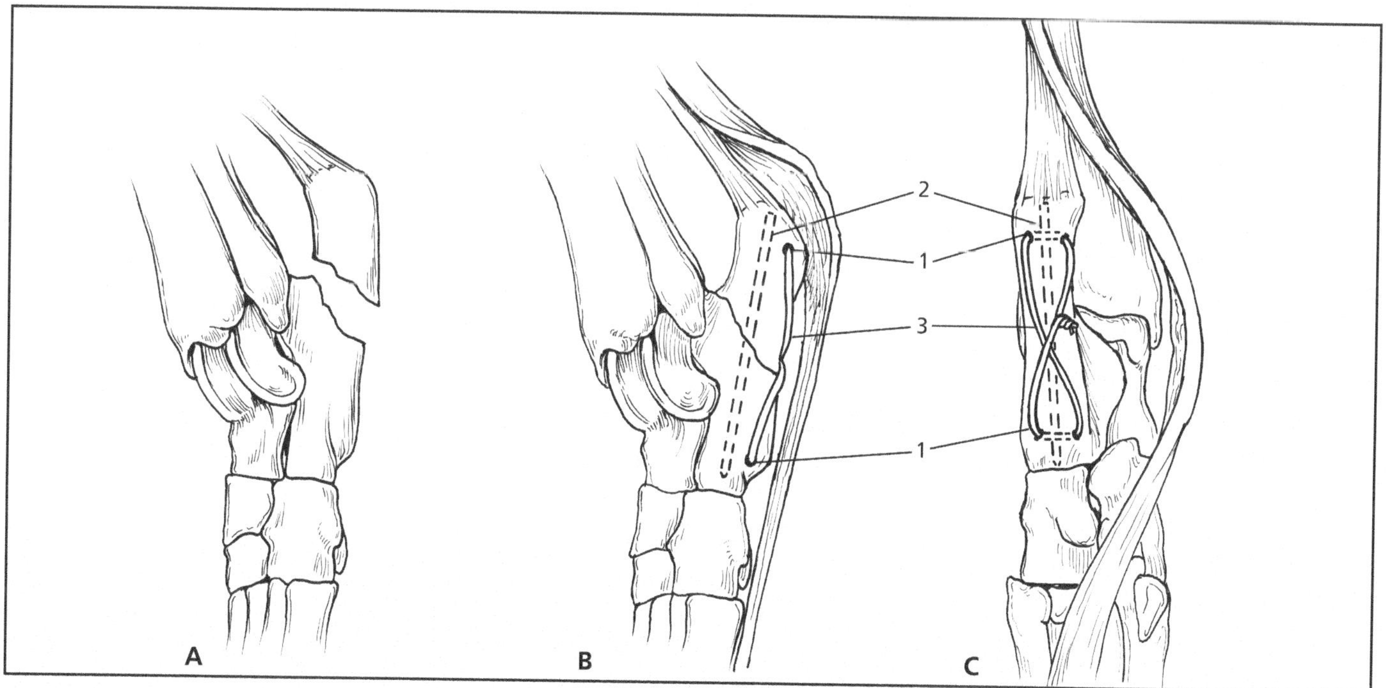


**Figure 7-55.** Mid-shaft calcaneal fractures: tension band fixation. **A.** Mid-shaft calcaneal fracture. **B., C.** Lateral and plantar views (respectively). Prior to placing the pin, one transverse hole is drilled through the proximal fragment and another through the distal fragment *(1)*. A single intramedullary pin is placed in normograde fashion down the shaft of the calcaneus after a pre-drilled tunnel of slightly smaller diameter has been made *(2)*. The pin is cut as short as possible and then countersunk. Cerclage wire is passed through the 2 transverse holes in a figure eight pattern and tightened *(3)*. (After Piermattei DL, Flo GL, DeCamp CE: Brinker, Piermattei and Flo's Handbook of Small Animal Orthopedics and Fracture Repair, 4th ed. St Louis: Saunders Elsevier, 2006, 672).

## Tension Band Fixation for Distal Fractures of the Calcaneus

This injury usually involves a slab fracture of bone from the base of the calcaneus with attached plantar ligament. The small fragment of bone is secured to its origin with a lag screw and the calcaneus is further stabilized with a pin and tension band fixation. A lateral approach to the calcaneus is made as described for tension band fixation for proximal fractures of the calcaneus (See Figure 7-24). The superficial digital flexor tendon is freed from its retinacular attachment and displaced medially. The small distal fragment of bone is grasped with bone reduction forceps. A 2.0 mm or 2.7 mm screw is placed in lag fashion by using a standard drill size in the far cortex and an over drill for the glide hole in the near cortex. An intramedullary pin is placed from the proximal calcaneus into the 4th tarsal bone. A pilot hole is placed first using a drill bit that is slightly smaller than the intramedullary pin. The pin is countersunk below the level of the proximal calcaneus using a pin punch and mallet (Securos Inc., Fiskdale, MA). Two transverse holes are drilled next: one through the proximal aspect of the calcaneus and the other through the plantar tubercle of the fourth tarsal bone (Figure 7-56A through D). The appropriate size wire is passed through the 2 transverse holes in a figure eight pattern and tightened. The cerclage wire is cut short.

The superficial digital flexor tendon is sutured to the retinacular fascia using interrupted non-absorbable

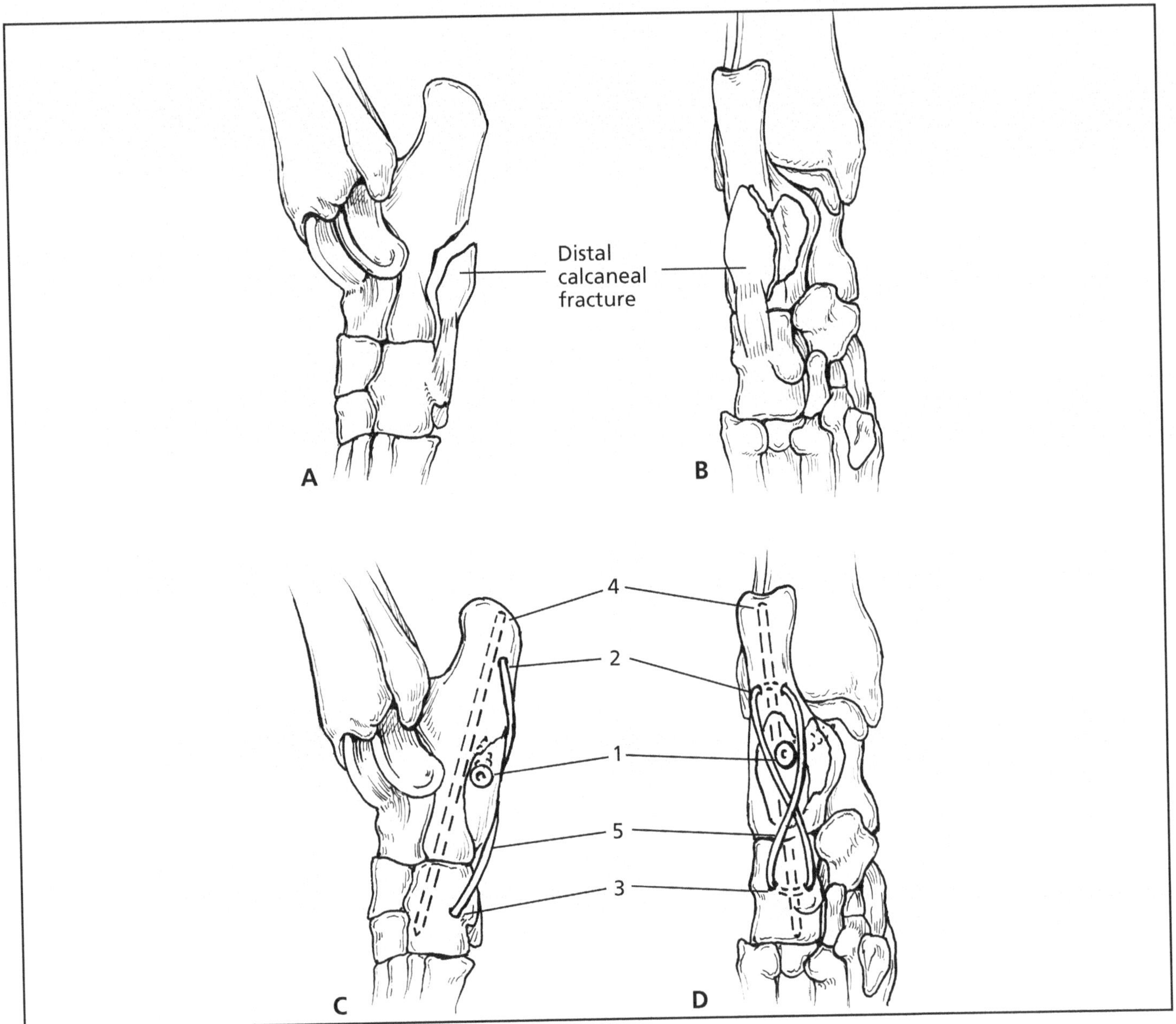


**Figure 7-56.** Distal fractures of the calcaneus: tension band fixation. **A., B.** Lateral and plantar views (respectively). Distal calcaneal fracture. **C., D.** Lateral and plantar views (respectively). The small fragment of bone is secured to its origin with a lag screw *(1)*. Prior to pin placement one transverse hole is drilled proximally in the calcaneus *(2)* and another distally through the plantar tubercle of the fourth tarsal bone *(3)*. The intramedullary pin is placed in normograde fashion and countersunk *(4)*. Cerclage wire is passed through the 2 transverse holes in a figure eight pattern and tightened *(5)*. (After Piermattei DL, Flo GL, DeCamp CE: Brinker, Piermattei and Flo's Handbook of Small Animal Orthopedics and Fracture Repair, 4th ed. St Louis: Saunders Elsevier, 2006, 672).

sutures. The dermal layer is closed with absorbable suture followed by skin closure.

### Bone Plate Fixation of the Calcaneus

Fractures of the mid-portion of the calcaneus are most amenable to bone plating because there is room for screw placement proximally and distally. The calcaneus must be large enough to permit the placement of 5 to 6 screws along the length of the bone. A size 2.7 mm bone plate will fit most medium sized dogs whereas a veterinary cuttable plate (Synthes Veterinary, Paoli, PA) is useful for smaller animals. For added stiffness, an intramedullary pin can be placed as well as a bone plate. This is particularly useful with comminuted calcaneal fractures to improve resistance to bending (Figure 7-57).

The patient is positioned in lateral recumbency with the affected limb up. A lateral approach is made to the calcaneus (See Figure 7-24). An intramedullary pin is placed in normograde fashion, using a slightly smaller pre-drilled tunnel, and anchored in the distal calcaneus. The bone plate is placed along the lateral or caudolateral aspect of the calcaneus. Screws are placed bicortically when possible and through one cortex if impeded by the pin.

The superficial digital flexor tendon is sutured to the retinacular fascia using interrupted non-absorbable

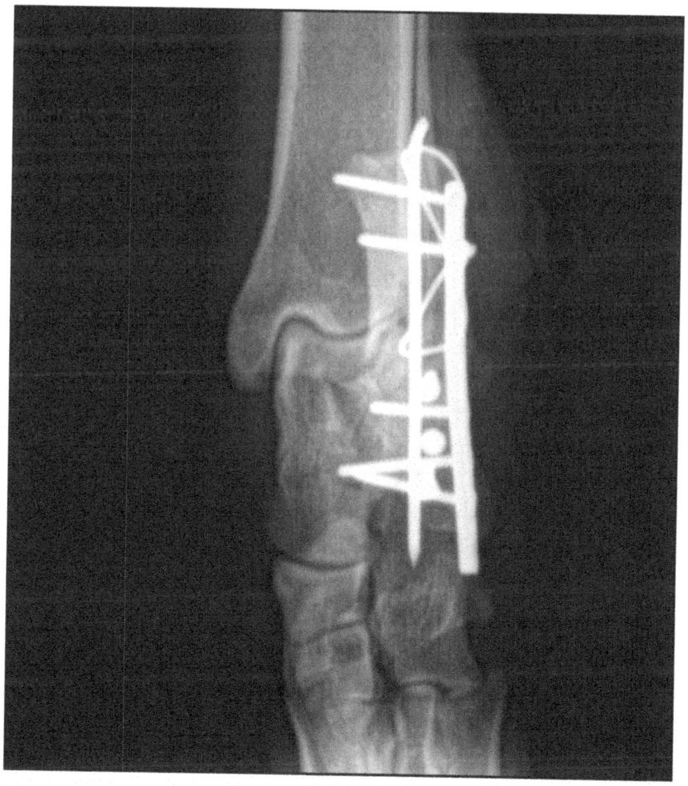

**Figure 7-57.** Bone plate fixation of the calcaneus craniocaudal projection. Fracture is stabilized with a 2.7 mm bone plate and screws. Due to comminution, the fracture was also stabilized with an IM pin and cerclage wire tension band and lag screws.

sutures. The dermal layer is closed with absorbable suture followed by skin closure. Two rows of staggered multiple punctate releasing incisions are placed on either side of the skin incision to ease tension on the skin closure over the bone plate.

### Proximal Intertarsal Arthrodesis for Small Distal Avulsion Fractures of the Calcaneus

This injury causes a loss of plantar support. The avulsed piece of distal bone is not substantial enough to permit lag screw fixation and therefore plantar stability is restored with a partial tarsal arthrodesis. A laterally-placed bone plate is used to stabilize the calcaneoquartal joint following debridement of articular cartilage from this joint. This technique is performed as described for hyperextension with luxation of the proximal intertarsal joint (See Figure 7-25)

## Aftercare

The tarsocrural joint is supported with a soft padded bandage that extends from the proximal tibia to the digits for the first week postoperatively. A short lateral splint and soft padded bandage is indicated for comminuted calcaneal fractures and for partial tarsal arthrodesis. This splint remains in place for approximately 4 weeks with weekly changes. Exercise is limited to short, 10 minute, leash walks 3 to 4 times daily until fracture healing or arthrodesis is documented on radiographs.

## Advantages and Disadvantages

Proximal calcaneal fractures are readily repaired with pins and tension band fixation. The proximal fragment is not large enough to permit bone plating. Mid body calcaneal fractures can be repaired with either a pin and tension band wire or with a bone plate. The advantages of pin and tension band wire are reduced cost compared with bone plating. The disadvantage of pin and tension band wire fixation is that the calcaneus is a very dense bone and pin placement is difficult without pre-drilling. Furthermore, the proximal part of the pin can interfere with the superficial digital flexor tendon if it is not adequately countersunk. A bone plate occupies more space under the skin compared to pin and tension band wire. This can create tension of the skin incision that results in dehiscence. This problem can be avoided by placing approximately 2 staggered rows of multiple punctate releasing incisions on either side of the skin incision. The punctate incisions must be bandaged but heal within one week postoperatively.

The advantage of a combined intramedullary pin and bone plate for a comminuted fracture is improved stabilization by reducing stress on the bone plate. The area of comminution does not need to be reconstructed but rather is supported proximally and distally by screws through the bone plate with axial support provided by the intramedullary pin.

# Suggested Readings

1. Bloomberg MS, Taylor RA, Dee JF: Canine Sports Medicine and Surgery. Philadelphia: W.B. Saunders Co.: 1998, 124-129.
2. Hulse D, Hyman W, Nori M, et al: Reduction in plate strain by addition of an intramedullary pin. Vet Surg 26:451-459, 1997.
3. Piermattei DL, Flo GL, DeCamp CE: Brinder, Piermattei, and Flo's Handbook of Small Animal Orthopedics and Fracture Repair 4th ed.: St. Louis: Saunders Elsevier, 2006, 661.

# Talus Fractures

## Definition and Indications

The talus consists of a body, neck, and head. The body is the enlarged proximal portion that articulates with the distal tibia and fibula. The neck is the middle portion of the talus and the head is the distal portion that articulates with the central tarsal bone. Fractures of the talus may be intra-articular or extra-articular. Intra-articular fractures include those involving the medial or lateral trochlear ridges proximally or the head of the talus distally. Extra-articular fractures may involve the neck, body, or head of the talus. Regardless of whether the fracture is intra-articular or extra-articular, all talus fractures should be repaired surgically for optimal function with the least degree of osteoarthritis. Simple fractures are repaired with lag screws or K-wires. Highly comminuted fractures, especially those affecting intra-articular surfaces, may require pantarsal arthrodesis.

Because the calcaneus overlaps the lateral talar ridge, radiographic examination for a fracture in this region may require more than standard dorsoplantar and lateral projections. A flexed dorsoplantar radiographic view of the tarsocrural joint can be done to visualize the lateral talar ridge (See Figure 7-16).

## Techniques

### Talar Ridge Fractures

Medial talar ridge fractures are approached by performing an osteotomy of the medial malleolus. Lateral talar ridge fractures require an osteotomy of the distal fibula. To perform an osteotomy of the medial malleolus, the skin incision is centered over the medial surface of the tarsocrural joint. The incision starts over the distal fourth of the tibia and continues distally to the level of the tarsometatarsal joint. The subcutaneous and crural fascia are incised and retracted with the skin. The joint capsule is incised on either side of the medial collateral ligament parallel to the long axis of the ligament. These incisions should completely penetrate the joint capsule to permit visualization of the interior joint surfaces. This helps to judge the angle of the osteotomy.

The osteotomy of the medial malleolus is performed with an osteotome and mallet. The osteotomy angle should remove most of the origin of the medial collateral ligament but must not be large enough to invade the weightbearing articular surface of the distal tibia (Figure 7-58A ,B & C). While performing the osteotomy, the surgeon should periodically check the depth of the cut to avoid cutting into the medial ridge of the talus. It may be necessary to incise part of the proximal extensor retinaculum to obtain the proper angle of the osteotome. Distal retraction of the malleolus and attached ligaments and pronation of the tarsus provides visualization of the articular surface of the talus.

The fracture site is visualized by evacuating the fracture hematoma from the articular surface. The fracture fragment is anatomically reduced. Digital pressure or pointed reduction forceps are used to keep the fragment in place while implanting either a lag screw or Kirschner wires (Figure 7-59). If the fragment is large enough, a lag screw is placed. The size of the screw selected depends on the fracture fragment but is usually 1.5 to 3.5 mm in diameter. One or two lag screws are placed or one lag screw can be supplemented with K-wires. To place the lag screw, the near cortex is over-drilled, the far cortex is drilled according to the core diameter of the screw, and the screw head is countersunk. The head of the screw must rest below the articular surface of the talus. If the fragment is so small that placement of a lag screw would risk fissuring the fragment, the entire repair can be done with K-wires. Most fractures can be adequately repaired with 0.035 or 0.045-inch K-wires. The wires must also be countersunk so that they are below the articular surface. As an alternative to stainless steel K-wires, biodegradable polydioxanone pins can be placed (Orthosorb Pins; DePuy Orthopaedics; Johnson and Johnson, Warsaw, IN). Lag screws or pins are advanced until they firmly engage the opposite cortex.

The medial malleolus is replaced by means of a tension band fixation as described for repair of medial malleolar fractures (See Figure 7-52). The joint capsule is reapposed to the edges of the collateral ligament using absorbable interrupted sutures. The dermal layer is closed with absorbable suture followed by skin closure.

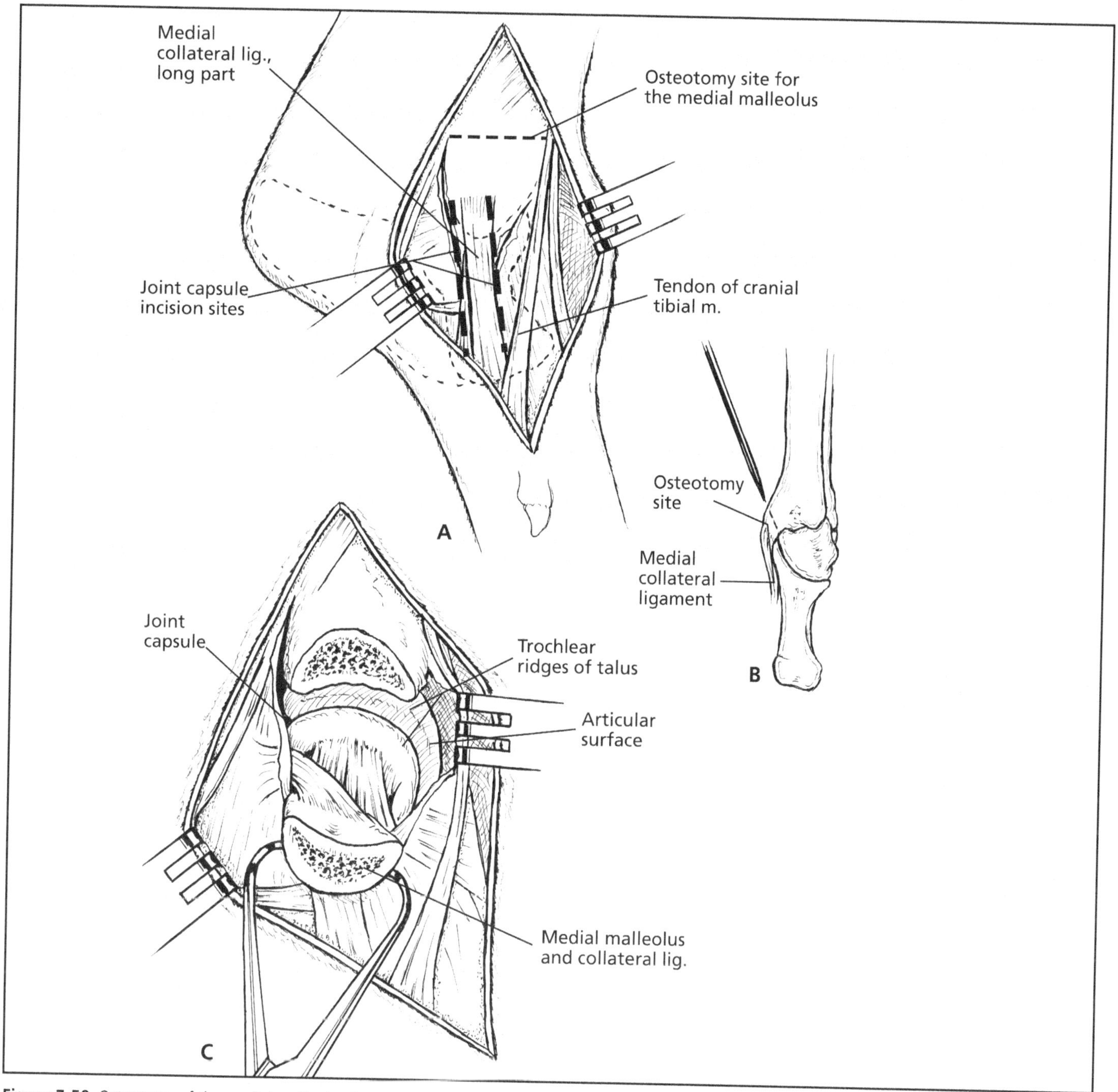


**Figure 7-58.** Osteotomy of the medial malleolus for approach to the trochlear ridge of the talus. **A.** The joint capsule is incised on either side of the collateral ligament. **B.** The osteotomy angle should remove most of the origin of the medial collateral ligament but must not be large enough to invade the weightbearing articular surface of the distal tibia. **C.** Distal retraction of the malleolus and attached ligaments and pronation of the tarsus provides visualization of the articular surface of the talus. (After Piermattei DL, Johnson KA. An Atlas of Surgical Approaches to the Bones and Joints of the Dog and Cat 4th ed. Philadelphia: Saunders, 2004).

The lateral ridge of the talus is exposed by performing an osteotomy of the distal fibula. The skin incision is centered over the lateral tarsocrural joint. The incision starts at the level of the lateral saphenous vein proximally and extends to the level of the tarsometatarsal joint distally. The subcutaneous and crural fascia are incised and retracted with the skin. The extensor retinaculum overlying the fibula is incised parallel to the dorsal edge of the peroneus longus tendon. The peroneus longus tendon can then be retracted cranially. The peroneus brevis and lateral digital extensor tendons are retracted caudally and the joint capsule is incised cranial and caudal to the lateral collateral ligament (See Figure 7-14). The angle of the osteotomy is transverse to the long axis of the tibia and fibula. The distal segment of the fibula should be long enough to accommodate 2 lag screws or a tension band fixation repair. Fracture fragments are stabilized as described for fractures of the medial ridge of the talus. The osteotomy of the fibula is repaired as described for distal fibula fractures (See Figure 7-52).

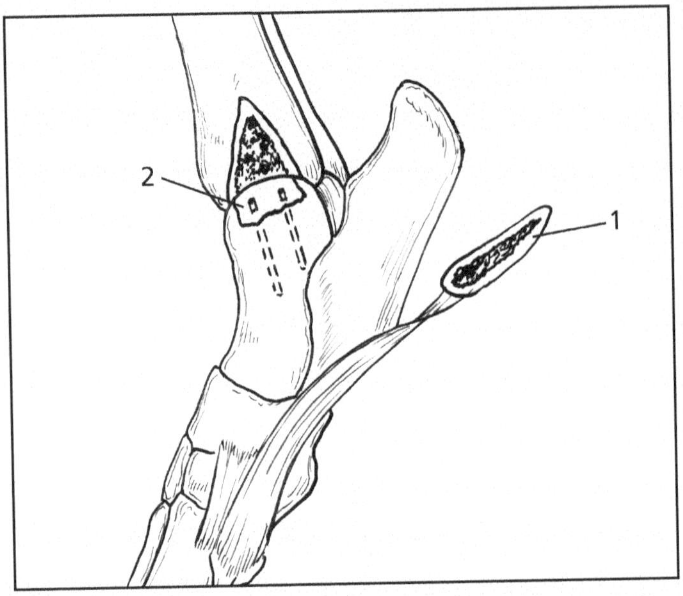


**Figure 7-59.** Repair of medial talar ridge fracture. Medial malleolus with attached medial collateral ligament is reflected *(1)*. Medial talar ridge fracture repaired with 2 countersunk k-wires *(2)*. (See Figure 7-52 for replacement of medial malleolus). (After Piermattei DL, Flo GL, DeCamp CE: Brinker, Piermattei and Flo's Handbook of Small Animal Orthopedics and Fracture Repair 4th ed. St Louis: Saunders Elsevier, 2006, 683).

The joint capsule is reapposed to the edges of the collateral ligament using absorbable interrupted sutures. The dermal layer is closed with absorbable suture followed by skin closure.

## Talar Neck Fractures

Fractures of the neck of the talus are often accompanied by luxation of the distal fracture fragment. The fracture surface rotates distally (Figure 7-60A, B & C).

The fracture is surgically repaired by repositioning the fragment and securing it with a lag screw. The patient is positioned in lateral recumbency with the affected limb down. The talus is approached medially. The skin incision extends from the medial malleolus to the base of the 2nd metatarsal bone. The subcutaneous tissues and skin are retracted. The deep fascia is incised between the tendon of the cranial tibial muscle and medial collateral ligament (See Figure 7-11). A metatarsal vein branches from the saphenous vein and overlies the cranial tibial tendon. This vein may be cauterized. The cranial tibial tendon is retracted in a dorsal or plantar direction as needed to visualize the fracture. Fascia lying on the surface of the talus is incised and elevated to improve exposure. The fracture fragment is anatomically reduced and kept in position with pointed reduction forceps. Reduction may be facilitated by flexing the tarsus while applying pressure to the lateral surface of the joint. This opens the medial aspect of the joint. The fracture is stabilized by placing a screw from the neck of the talus into the calcaneus. The size of the screw is chosen according to the size of the fragment. A 3.5 mm diameter screw is usually appropriate for a medium to large sized dog. It is not necessary to place a lag screw in this case. The hole is drilled from the distal talar fragment, in a caudolateral direction, into the body of the calcaneus (See Figure 7-60B & C).

The subcutaneous layer is closed with absorbable suture followed by skin closure.

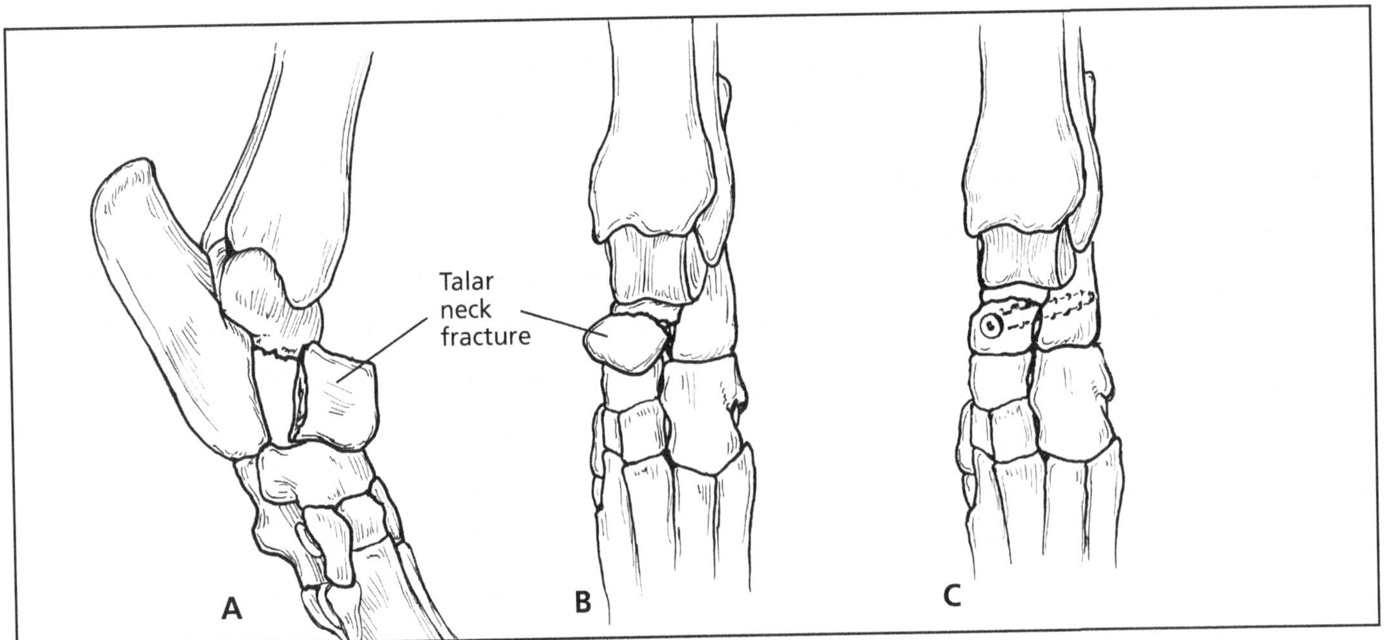


**Figure 7-60.** Talar neck fracture: Lag screw stabilization. **A., B.** Medial and dorsal views (respectively). Talar neck fracture with cranial displacement of the fracture fragment. **C.** Dorsal view, the fracture is stabilized by placing a screw from the neck of the talus into the calcaneus. The hole is drilled from the distal talar fragment, in a caudolateral direction, into the body of the calcaneus. (After Piermattei DL, Flo GL, DeCamp CE: Brinker, Piermattei and Flo's Handbook of Small Animal Orthopedics and Fracture Repair 4th ed. St Louis: Saunders Elsevier, 2006, 684).

## Talar Head Fractures

Fractures of the head, or distal portion, of the talus are accessed by a medial approach as described for talar neck fractures (See Figure 7-11). To visualize the head of the talus it is helpful to retract the cranial tibial tendon in a plantar direction. The fracture is reduced and stabilized with digital pressure or with pointed reduction forceps. Placing the joint in extension may facilitate reduction. The fracture is stabilized with crossing K-wires or with a T plate (Synthes Veterinary, Paoli PA) To place K-wires, one wire is placed from the caudomedial aspect of the distal fragment, in a proximal direction, into the craniolateral aspect of the trochlea of the talus. The articular surface of the trochlea is not penetrated with the pin. A second K-wire is placed from the proximal, caudomedial aspect of the talus, in a distal direction, into the craniolateral aspect of the distal fragment (Figure 7-61A & B).

In medium-sized to larger dogs, talar head fractures may be stabilized with a modified T-plate. A standard 1.5, 2.0, or 2.7 mm T-plate is modified by cutting the long arm of the plate to a workable length. Usually it is only possible to have one hole proximal to the fracture line. The plate is applied over the dorsal aspect of the head and neck of the talus with 2 holes distally and one hole proximally (See Figure 7-61B). Each screw penetrates both the near and far cortex of the talus. The dermal layer is closed with absorbable suture followed by skin closure.

## Aftercare

Surgical repairs of the talus are protected with a lateral splint and soft padded bandage that extends from the proximal tibia to the digits. The splint is kept on for 4 weeks with weekly changes. Exercise is limited to short, 10 minute, leash walks 3 to 4 times daily during this time. Exercise is gradually increased when fracture healing is documented radiographically. Radiographs are taken 6 to 8 weeks postoperatively to evaluate healing.

## Advantages and Disadvantages

The most significant disadvantage to the surgical correction of fractures of the trochlea of the talus is the need for osteotomy of the medial or lateral malleolus. It is necessary to approach the joint in this way in order to have adequate visualization of the fracture. Careful osteotomy and secure stabilization of the osteotomy are essential. The disadvantage to using stainless steel K-wires and screws for intra-articular fractures is the potential for interfering with the articular surface. It is important to completely countersink implants to avoid articular damage. Small absorbable pins are available and are advantageous for use in joints. The disadvantage of absorbable pins is their moderate expense.

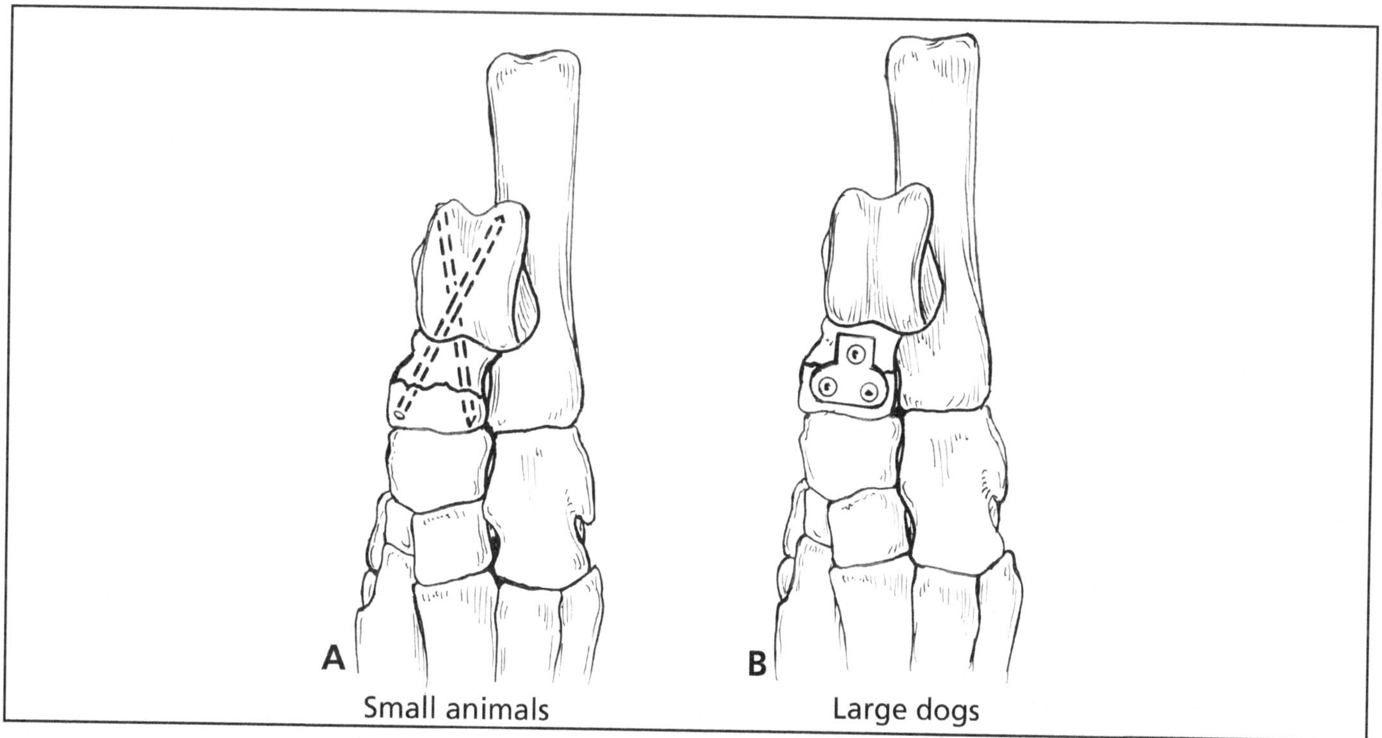


**Figure 7-61.** Talar head fracture repair: K -wire and modified T-plate. **A.** K-wires repair: One wire is directed from the caudomedial aspect of the distal fragment, in a proximal direction, into the craniolateral aspect of the trochlea of the talus. The articular surface of the trochlea is not penetrated with the pin. A second K-wire is placed from the proximal, caudomedial aspect of the talus, in a distal direction, into the craniolateral aspect of the distal fragment **B.** Modified T-plate: The plate is applied over the dorsal aspect of the head and neck of the talus with 2 holes distally and one hole proximally. (After Beale B. Surgical treatment of talus fractures. In Bojrab MJ: Current Techniques in Small Animal Surgery 4th ed. Baltimore: Williams and Wilkins, 1998, 1236).

## Suggested Readings

1. Beale B: Surgical treatment of talus fractures. In Bojrab MJ, Ellison GW, Slocum B. Current Techniques in Small Animal Surgery 4th ed.: Baltimore: Williams and Wilkins: 1998, 1264-1267.
2. McCartney WT, Carmichael S: Talar neck fractures in five cats. J Small Anim Pract 41:204-206, 2000.
3. Nixon AJ, Fortier LA, Goodrich LR, Ducharme NG: Arthroscopic reattachment of osteochondritis dissecans lesions using resorbable polydioxanone pins. Equine Vet J 36:376-383, 2004.
4. Piermattei DL, Flo GL, DeCamp CE: Brinker, Piermattei, and Flo's Handbook of Small Animal Orthopedics and Fracture Repair, 4th ed.: Philadelphia: W B Saunders, 2006, 661.
5. Piermattei DL, Johnson KA. An Atlas of Surgical Approaches to the Bones and Joints of the Dog and Cat 4th ed. Philadelphia: Saunders, 2004, 380, 388.

## Central Tarsal Fractures

### Definition and Indications

Central tarsal fractures are most commonly reported in racing greyhounds but do occur in other breeds. The central tarsal bone touches all other bones in the tarsal joint and acts as a medial support or buttress for the tarsus. In racing dogs, stresses are greater on the outside limb. In dogs racing counterclockwise, intense compressive forces are concentrated in the medial aspect of the right tarsus. Once the buttress action of the central tarsal bone is lost, the talocalcaneocentral joint collapses. Joint collapse leads to varus deformity and loss of limb function. Central tarsal fractures may induce secondary fractures. Among racing greyhounds with central tarsal bone fractures, secondary fractures occur 64% of the time. The most common secondary fracture involves the fourth tarsal bone. A triad of fractures occurs in some cases and involves the fourth tarsal bone, calcaneus, and base of the lateral aspect of metatarsal V. There are 5 types of central tarsal bone fractures (Figure 7-62A, B & C). Type I is a dorsal slab fracture that is not displaced. A Type II is the same fracture but with displacement. Type III is a medial fracture of the central tarsal bone (Figure 7-63A, B, C & D). The fracture fragment is usually displaced medially and dorsally. Type IV is fractured in 2 planes: medial and dorsal (Figure 7-64A, B, C & D). Type IV is the most frequent type of central tarsal bone fracture in racing dogs and occurs 5 times more often than types I or II. Type V is a severely comminuted fracture (Figure 7-65A, B & C).

Types I and II fractures are suspected when point pain is produced over the central tarsal area with digital palpation. Type I fractures require a high index of suspicion for diagnosis. Different types of screw fixation are indicated for the different types of fractures. Types I, II, and III fractures are repaired with solitary screws. Type I and II fractures are repaired with a lag screw placed in a dorsal to plantar direction (See Figure 7-62C). The type III fracture is repaired with a single medial to lateral screw (See Figure 7-63C, D). Some surgeons recommend repairing a type III fracture with 2 screws: one from medial to lateral and one from dorsal to plantar. The thinking behind the additional screw is that some type III fractures actually are type IV fractures with a poorly visible dorsal slab fracture line. Type IV fractures are repaired with 2 lag screws at approximately 90 degrees from each other (See Figure 7-64C, D). All screws are placed as lag screws. Type V fractures have been reconstructed successfully using internal

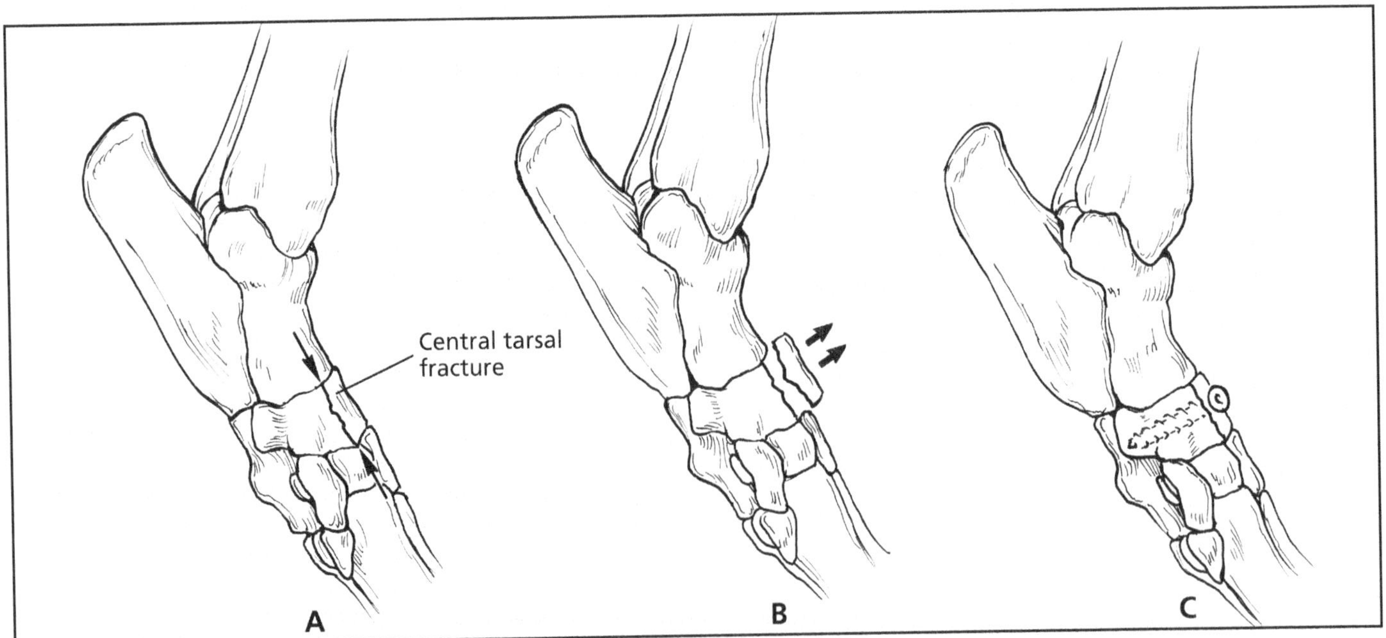


**Figure 7-62.** Central tarsal fracture Types I and II. **A.** Type I central tarsal bone fracture *(fracture line between arrows)*. **B.** Type II is the same fracture but with displacement *(arrows)* **C.** Type I and II fractures are repaired with a lag screw placed in a dorsal to plantar direction. (After Boemo CM. Specific tests for tarsal injury. In Bojrab JM, Ellison GW, Slocum B: Current Techniques in Small Animal Surgery 4th ed. Baltimore: Williams and Wilkins, 1998, 1253).

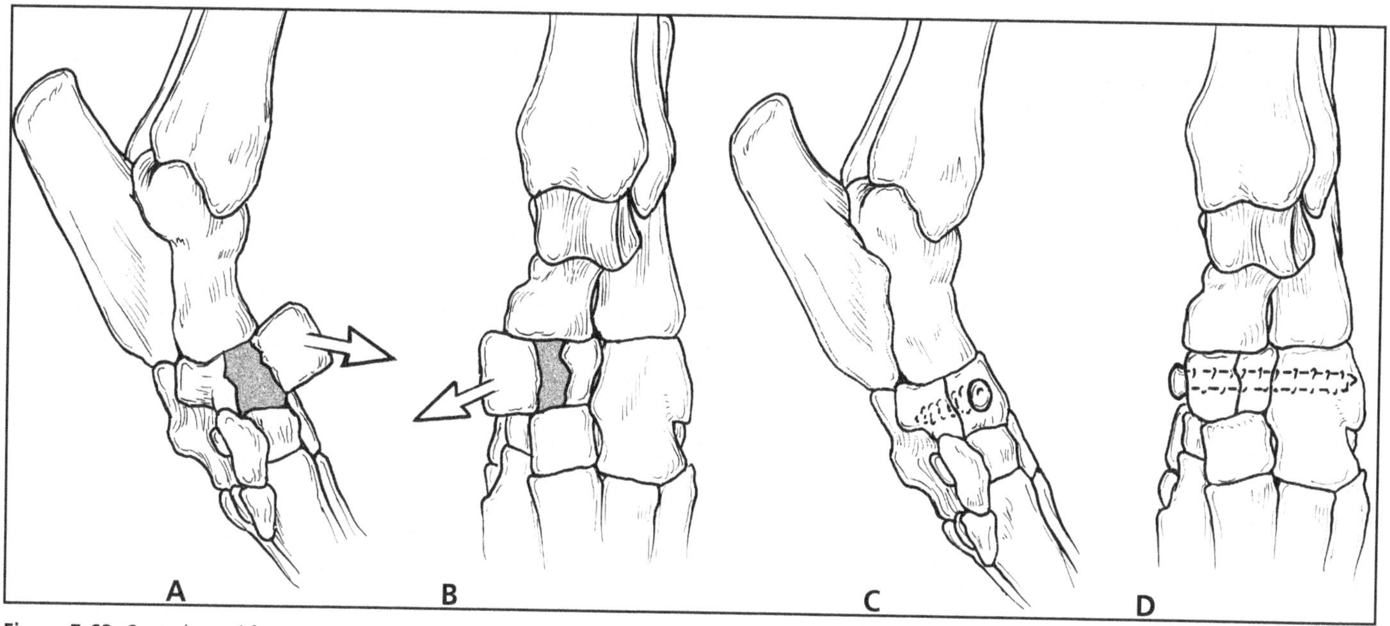


**Figure 7-63.** Central tarsal fracture Type III. Type III central tarsal bone fracture with **A.** cranial and **B.** medial displacement *(arrows)*. **C., D.** Medial and dorsal views (respectively). The type III fracture is repaired with a single medial to lateral screw. (After Boemo CM. Specific tests for tarsal injury. In Bojrab JM, Ellison GW, Slocum B: Current Techniques in Small Animal Surgery 4th ed. Baltimore: Williams and Wilkins, 1998, 1253).

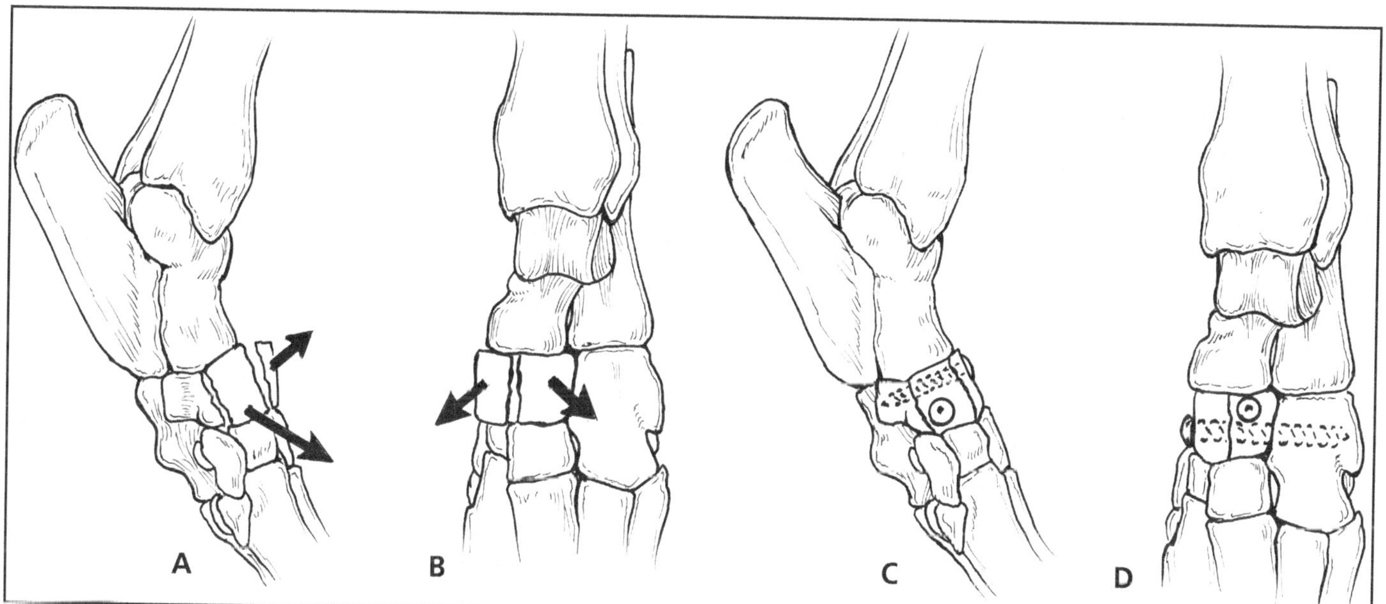


**Figure 7-64.** Central tarsal fracture Type IV. **A., B.** Type IV central tarsal bone fracture occurs in 2 planes: medial and dorsal *(arrows)*. **C., D.** Medial and dorsal views (respectively). Type IV fractures are repaired with 2 screws: one medial to lateral and one dorsal to plantar. The mediolateral screw is placed at the junction of the middle and distal third of the bone, and the dorsoplantar screw is placed at the junction of the proximal and middle third of the bone. (After Boemo CM. Specific tests for tarsal injury. In Bojrab JM, Ellison GW, Slocum B: Current Techniques in Small Animal Surgery 4th ed. Baltimore: Williams and Wilkins, 1998, 1254).

fixation by surgeons experienced with this injury. Central tarsal fractures that cannot be reconstructed can be managed with a medial buttress plate or dorsal T plate and cancellous bone graft (See Figure 7-65C, D). The objective is to restore and maintain the normal joint space and thereby prevent deformity of the foot. The prognosis after central tarsal bone fractures is related to the fracture type. Good healing and return to competitive racing is reported in 88% of greyhounds with surgical stabilization of central tarsal fractures.

Secondary fractures occur most frequently with types IV and V central tarsal bone fractures. The higher grades of central tarsal fractures induce medial collapse of the joint and thereby transfer more stresses to other tarsal bones. The most common bone to be fractured along with the central tarsal bone is the fourth tarsal bone. Specific repair is not needed in most cases of fourth tarsal bone and fifth metatarsal bone fractures. Restoration of medial support of the tarsus by repairing the central tarsal bone indirectly stabilizes the fourth tarsal bone, and screws are anchored into the fourth tarsal

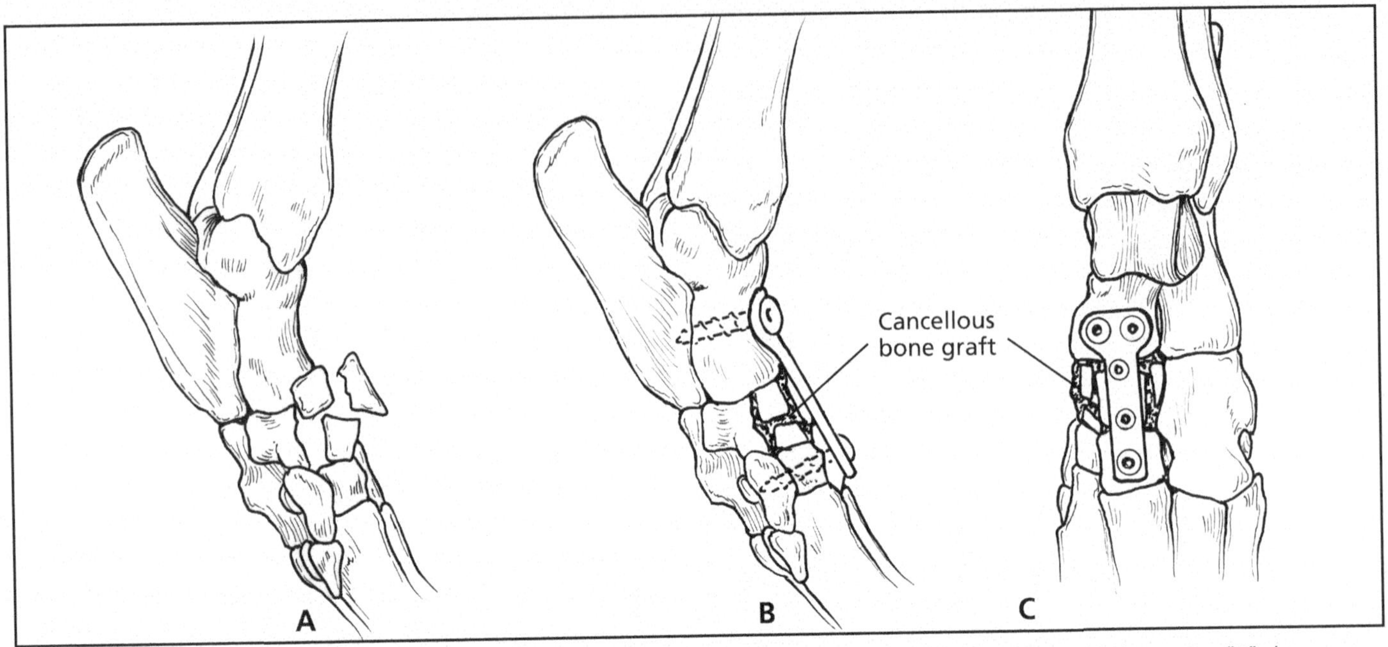


**Figure 7-65.** Central tarsal fracture type V. **A.** Type V is a highly comminuted fracture of the central tarsal bone. **B.** A straight plate or **C.** a "T" plate in conjunction with a bone graft can be used for repair. (After Boemo CM. Specific tests for tarsal injury. In Bojrab JM, Ellison GW, Slocum B: Current Techniques in Small Animal Surgery 4th ed. Baltimore: Williams and Wilkins, 1998, 1255).

bone routinely for repair of type III and IV fractures. Fractures of the fourth tarsal bone and base of the fifth metatarsus do not influence the outcome of surgical repair and do not impede return to racing.

Fracture of the calcaneus can negatively influence the outcome of central tarsal fracture repair. The types of calcaneal fractures reported include slab fracture of the calcaneal base, transverse calcaneal fracture, comminuted calcaneal fracture, and avulsion fracture of the base of the calcaneus. Comminuted calcaneal fractures and avulsion fractures of the base of the calcaneus can be surgically repaired but carry a poor prognosis for return to full athletic function.

## Techniques

The dog is positioned on its back and the hock is immobilized so that the plantar surface of the tarsus is parallel with the table. The central tarsal bone is approached with a dorsal incision. The incision is centered directly over the fracture on the dorsomedial aspect of the tarsus, at the junction of the dorsal branches of the medial and lateral saphenous veins (Figure 7-66). Soft tissues are bluntly dissected with a periosteal elevator to the level of the central tarsal bone, just distal to the cranial tibial tendon. The long digital extensor tendon is elevated and retracted laterally, and the cranial tibial tendon is retracted medially.

### Central Tarsal Bone-Types I – IV Fractures

Central tarsal fractures I through IV are stabilized with single lag screws. Lag screws are placed by overdrilling the near cortex and drilling the far cortex according to the smaller, or core, diameter of the screw. If a partially threaded screw is used, both cortices are drilled according to the core diameter of the screw. In fracture types I and II, the fracture is reduced and stabilized with pointed reduction forceps. A screw hole for either a 2.0 mm or 2.7 mm cortical screw is placed into the center of the dorsal fracture fragment in lag fashion and directed in a dorsoplantar direction. The screw engages the plantar process of the central tarsal bone (See Figure 7-62C).

In fracture types III and IV, reduction is obtained by hyperextending and externally rotating the tarsus. The fracture is held in reduction using pointed reduction forceps. Type III fractures are stabilized with a mediolateral lag screw placed at the junction of the middle and distal third of the bone (See Figure 7-63C & D). Alternatively, a type III fracture can be repaired as a type IV fracture on the assumption that a non-visible dorsal slab fracture may be present. Exact placement of these screws is critical to ensure that they will both fit. The mediolateral screw is placed at the junction of the middle and distal third of the bone, and the dorsoplantar screw is placed at the junction of the proximal and middle third of the bone. The medial fragment is repaired first. The mediolateral screw hole is begun just proximal to the origin of the intertarsal ligament that connects the central tarsal bone to the second tarsal bone. A 3.5 or 4.0 mm cancellous screw is lagged in a mediolateral direction and seats into the fourth tarsal bone. Using a partially threaded 4.0 mm screw for this gives an extra millimeter of clearance for the second screw. The second screw, size 2.0 or 2.7 mm, is placed in a dorsoplantar direction. The drill bit is angled so that it will miss the mediolateral screw and also avoid entering the joint space above (See Figure 7-65C & D).

If secondary fractures are present in the fourth tarsal bone they may reduce spontaneously during reduction of the central tarsal bone. The mediolateral screw in the central tarsal bone engages the fourth tarsal bone and thus provides stability. If additional stability is needed, a second screw can be placed from the second tarsal bone, in a mediolateral direction, through the third tarsal bone and into the fourth tarsal bone (see Figure 7-1 for anatomy). Fractures of the base of the fifth metatarsal bone do not need to be surgically repaired. Calcaneal fractures, if present, are repaired as described.

The subcutaneous and intradermal tissues are closed in layers with absorbable suture followed by skin closure.

### Central Tarsal Bone-Type V Fracture

A type V fracture can be repaired with multiple lag screws but is most often bridged with cancellous bone grafting and a medial butress bone plate to prevent medial collapse of the joint and varus deformity of the paw. The surgical approach is dorsal to the central tarsal bone, as described for fracture types I through IV (See Figure 7-66), with proximal and distal extension of the incision as needed to visualize the talus and proximal metatarsal bones. Fragments of the bone are left in place, and a cancellous autograft or allograft (Freeze dried cancellous bone, Veterinary Transplant Services, Kent, WA) is placed. The central tarsal bone region is bridged with a 2.7 mm T-plate (Synthes, Paoli, PA). The proximal "T- shaped"cross portion of the plate is fixed to the head of the talus. On the vertical part of the "T" the middle screw holes are unfilled, and the distal screw hole is fixed to the third tarsal bone (See Figure 7-65C). Cartilage may be removed from the talocalcaneocentral and centrodistal joints to promote arthrodesis versus ankylosis of the joint. Cartilage is removed using a small high speed bur.

The subcutaneous layer is closed with absorbable suture followed by skin closure. Multiple punctate releasing incisions may be placed on either side of the incision to minimize postoperative swelling (See Chapter 3).

## Aftercare

The operated limb is placed in a short lateral splint and soft padded bandage. The splint extends from the digits to the proximal tibia. The splint is maintained for 4 weeks, with changes once to twice weekly. Exercise is restricted to short leash walks for 8 weeks followed by a gradual return to normal activity. Implants need only be removed if they become loose or if a screw has been placed into the talocalcaneocentral joint. For central tarsal fractures repaired with a bridging bone plate, the limb is splinted for 6 weeks and exercise limited to leash walks for approximately 16 weeks.

## Advantages and Disadvantages

Surgical repair of central tarsal bone fracture types I through IV yields an excellent chance for return to full function. Dogs with type V fractures can occasionally have excellent recoveries but more commonly do not return to prior athleticism. Type I fractures can heal with external coaptation instead of surgery. The disadvantage to this approach is that dorsal migration of the slab fracture often occurs during healing. This can create arthritic change and chronic lameness in the joint. The advantage to surgery is immediate security of fracture fragments and the best chance for full recovery. The advantage to repairing a type V fracture primarily, with lag screws, is restoration of joint anatomy and medial support. However, many of the fragments are extremely small and are not incorporated into the fracture repair. Ultimately, ankylosis of the talocalcaneocentral and other intertarsal joints is common with comminuted central tarsal bone fractures repaired in this way. Ankylosis in not necessarily a negative result and is compatible with return to athleticism. The potential disadvantage to lag screw reconstruction is implant failure and destabilization of the medial tarsal joint. Buttressing the fracture with a bone plate carries a lower risk of failure. If this technique is chosen, there is an advantage to treating it as an arthrodesis and removing cartilage from the proximal and distal intertarsal joints. This should promote more rapid bony bridging.

# Suggested Readings

1. Boemo CM. Specific Tests for Tarsal Injury: In Bojrab JM: Current Techniques in Small Animal Surgery 4th ed. Baltimore: Williams and Wilkins, 1998, 1252-1254.
2. Boudrieau RJ, Dee JF, Dee LG: Central tarsal bone fractures in the racing Greyhound: A review of 114 cases. J Am Vet Med Assoc 184:1486-1491, 1984.
3. Boudrieau RJ, Dee JF, Dee LG: Treatment of central tarsal bone fractures in the racing Greyhound. J Am Vet Med Assoc 184:1492-1500.
4. Guilliard MJ: Fractures of the central tarsal bone in eight racing Greyhounds. Vet Rec 147:512-515, 2000.

# Central Tarsal Bone Fracture - Luxation

## Definition and Indications

Luxation of the central tarsal bone occurs sporadically in all breeds. The injury has been reported following vigorous exercise. The central tarsal bone luxates in a dorsomedial direction and often accompanies a fracture of the plantar tubercle of the central tarsal bone (Figure 7-67A, B & C). The fractured fragment remains attached to the plantar ligaments. Clinically, the protruded central tarsal bone may be palpable below the subcutaneous tissues. If the luxation is complete, medial tarsal support is lost and a mild varus deformity may be observed. Diagnosis is made with standard lateral and craniocaudal radiographs of the tarsocrural joint. Surgical stabilization is indicated.

## Technique

The surgical approach is carried out as described for central tarsal bone fractures. The animal is positioned on its back and the hock is immobilized so that the plantar surface of the tarsus is parallel with the table. The central tarsal bone is approached with a dorsal incision. The incision is centered over the dorsomedial aspect of the tarsus, at the junction of the dorsal branches of the medial and lateral saphenous veins (See Figure 7-66). Soft tissues are bluntly dissected with a periosteal elevator to the level of the central tarsal bone, just distal to the cranial tibial tendon. The long digital extensor tendon is elevated and retracted laterally, and the cranial tibial tendon is retracted medially.

The central tarsal bone is reduced and then stabilized. To facilitate reduction of the central tarsal bone, a spreading device (Wallace knee retractor, Securos Inc., Fiskdale, MA) can be used to open the joint space. The central tarsal bone is held in place digitally or with pointed reduction forceps. The bone is stabilized with a 3.5 mm lag screw. The screw is directed in a medial to lateral direction from the central tarsal bone into the fourth tarsal bone (See Figure 7-67C).

The dermal layer is closed with absorbable suture followed by skin closure. Multiple punctate releasing incisions may be placed on either side of the incision to minimize postoperative swelling (See Chapter 3).

## Aftercare

A short lateral splint and soft padded bandage is placed from the digits to the middle of the tibia. The splint is maintained for 3 to 4 weeks with changes once to twice weekly. Exercise is restricted to short leash walks for 8 weeks followed by gradual resumption of activity. Radiographs are obtained 4 to 6 weeks postoperatively to assess positioning of the central tarsal bone and implant. The stabilizing screw is only removed if it becomes loose.

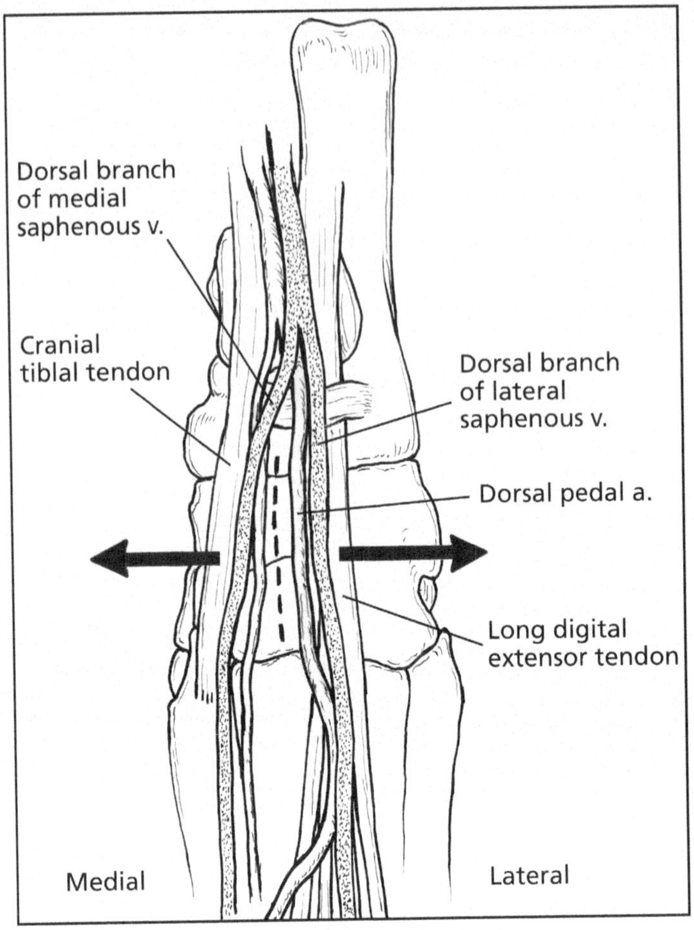


**Figure 7-66.** Surgical approach to the central tarsal bone. The central tarsal bone is approached with a dorsal incision. The incision is centered directly over the fracture on the dorsomedial aspect of the tarsus, at the junction of the dorsal branches of the medial and lateral saphenous veins (broken line). Soft tissues are bluntly dissected with a periosteal elevator to the level of the central tarsal bone, just distal to the cranial tibial tendon. The long digital extensor tendon is elevated and retracted laterally, and the cranial tibial tendon is retracted medially *(arrows)*. (After Boudrieau, RJ, Dee JF, Dee LG. Treatment of central tarsal bone fractures in the racing Greyhound. J Am Vet Med Assoc 184:1492, 1984).

## Advantages and Disadvantages

Surgical correction of this injury is advantageous. Most patients respond very well to surgery. The central tarsal bone must be anatomically positioned prior to stabilization with a lag screw. Fracture of the plantar tubercle of the central tarsal bone has not negatively influenced clinical outcome. Closed reduction and splint or cast fixation is rarely successful and is not recommended.

# Suggested Readings


1. Lorinson D, Grösslinger K: Central tarsal bone luxation in three non-racing dogs. Vet Comp Orthop Traumatol 14:229-31, 2001.
2. Piermattei DL. Flo GL, DeCamp CE: Brinker, Piermattei, and Flo's Handbook of Small Animal Orthopedics and Fracture Repair, 4th ed: St. Louis: Saunders Elsevier, 2006, 661-713.

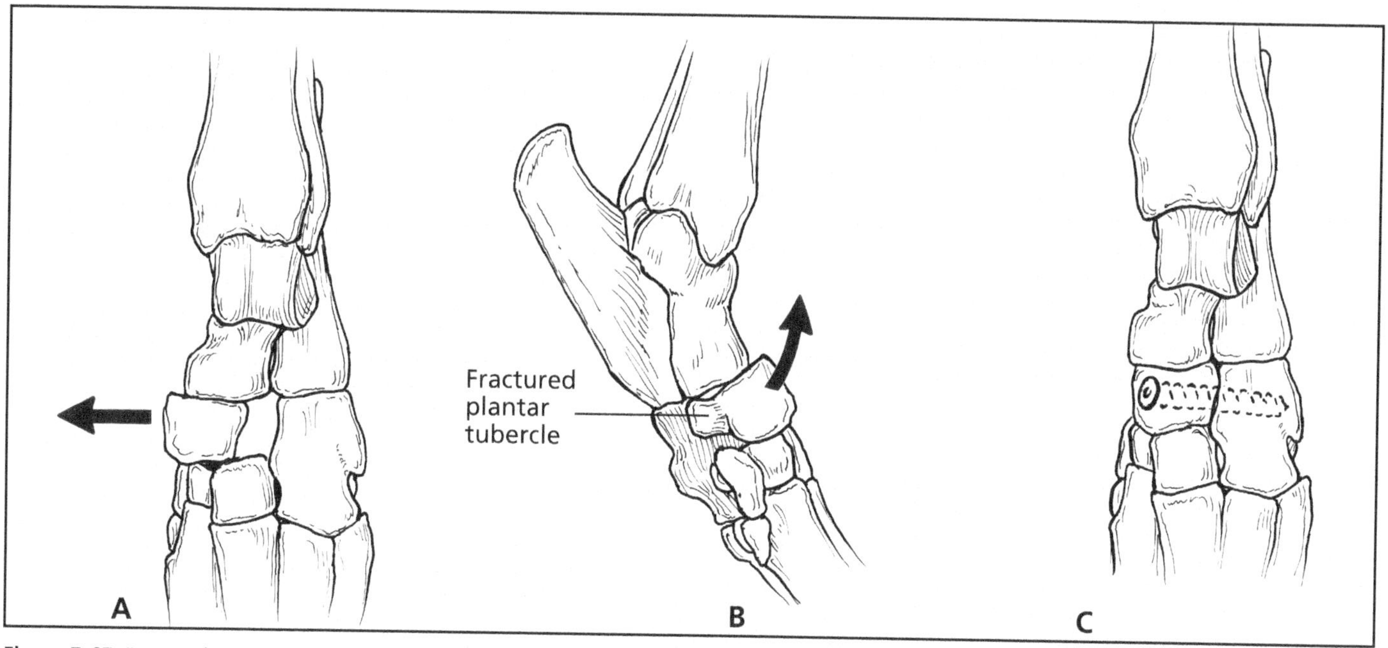


**Figure 7-67.** Fracture-luxation of the central tarsal bone. **A., B.** Dorsal and medial views (respectively). The central tarsal bone luxates in **A.** a medial *(arrow)* **B.** dorsal direction *(arrow)*. **C.** The fracture is stabilized with a countersunk lag screw placed in a medial to lateral direction from the central tarsal bone into the fourth tarsal bone. (After Piermattei DL, Flo GL, DeCamp CE. Brinker, Piermattei, and Flo's Handbook of Small Animal Orthopedics and Fracture Repair 4th ed. St. Louis: Saunders Elsevier, 2006, 699).

# Fractures of the Numbered Tarsal Bones

## Definition and Indications

### Third Tarsal Bone

Fractures of the first and second tarsal bones are extremely rare. Fracture of the third tarsal bone occasionally occurs. Third tarsal bones may be fractured on the dorsal surface similar to types I and II central tarsal bone fractures (Figure 7-68A, B & C). This fracture is treated with lag screw fixation.

### Fourth Tarsal Bone

Most fourth tarsal bone fractures occur in conjunction with central tarsal bone fractures. Approximately 40 per cent of greyhounds with central tarsal bone fractures have a compression fracture of the fourth tarsal bone. Repair of fourth tarsal bone fractures is indirectly achieved by repairing the central tarsal bone fracture. A medial to lateral screw through the central tarsal bone engages the 4th tarsal bone (See Figure 7-64D). If required an additional screw can be placed from the second and third tarsal bones into the fourth tarsal bone screw.

## Techniques

### Third Tarsal Bone

The skin incision is made over the dorsal-medial aspect of the tarsal bones as described for repair of central tarsal bone fractures (See Figure 7-66). The incision is centered between the two branches of the saphenous vein. The cranial tibial tendon is retracted medially and the long digital extensor tendons are retracted laterally. The dorsal pedal artery is avoided. The fracture fragment is held in reduction with digital pressure or pointed reduction forceps. A lag screw, size 1.5mm to 4.0 mm, is placed from the dorsal to the plantar aspect of the third tarsal bone (See Figure 7-68B & C).

### Fourth Tarsal Bone

The surgical approach is as described for repair of a central tarsal fracture (See Figure 7-66). A medial to lateral lag screw is placed from the central to the fourth tarsal bone (See Figures 7-63D and 7-64D).

The subcutaneous layer is closed with absorbable suture followed by skin closure.

## Aftercare

The tarsocrural joint is immobilized with a lateral splint and soft padded bandage that extends from the digits to the mid-tibia. The splint is maintained for 4 weeks. Exercise is restricted to crate rest and short leash walks for 8 weeks followed by a gradual return to normal activity. Radiographs are taken at approximately 6 weeks postoperatively to evaluate healing and implant position. Implants are only removed if they become loose.

## Advantages and Disadvantages

The potential disadvantage of surgical stabilization of a third tarsal bone fracture is inadvertent placement of

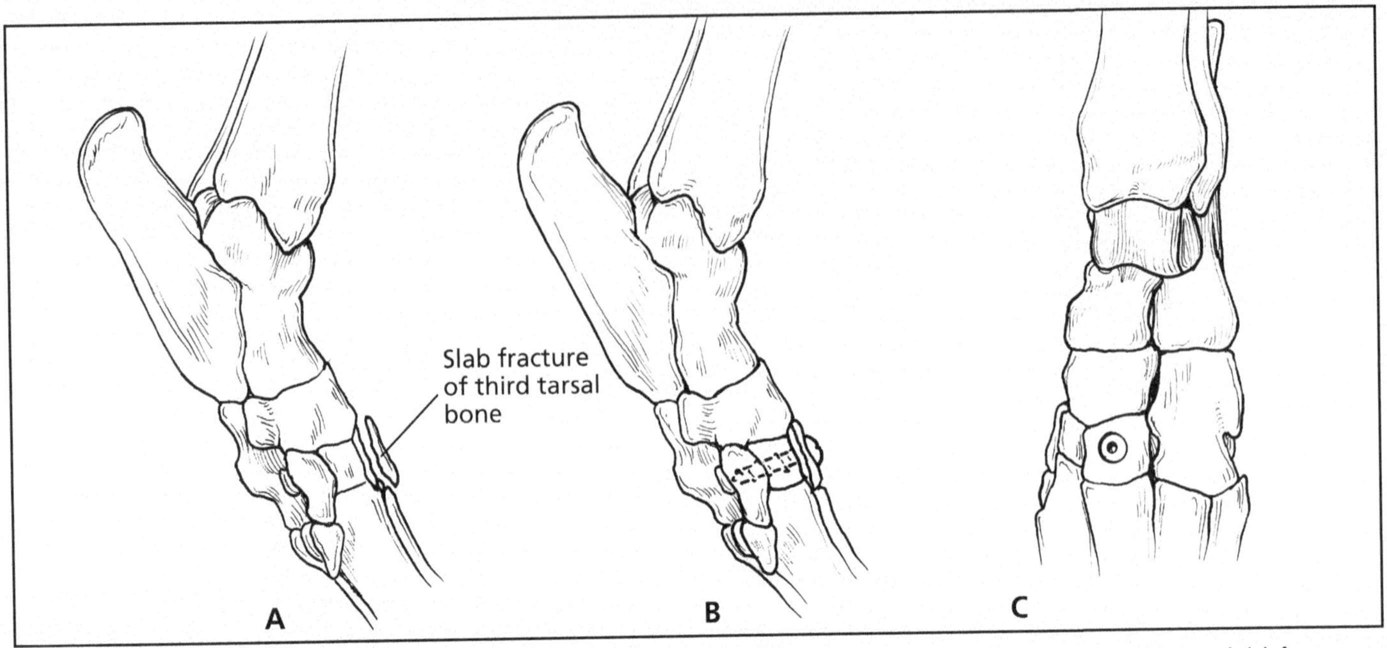


**Figure 7-68.** Fracture of the third tarsal bone. **A.** Third tarsal bone dorsal slab fracture. **B., C.** Medial and dorsal views (respectively). Dorsal slab fracture of the third tarsal bone repaired with a lag screw directed in a cranial to caudal direction. (After Piermattei DL, Flo GL, DeCamp CE. Brinker, Piermattei, and Flo's Handbook of Small Animal Orthopedics and Fracture Repair 4th ed. St Louis: Saunders Elsevier, 2006, 699).

a screw within a proximal joint space. A craniocaudal screw placed in the third tarsal bone, for example, could invade the centrodistal joint. This could promote loosening of the screw or induce discomfort. Careful screw placement should avoid this problem. If a screw is seen to enter the centrodistal or tarsometatarsal joint space on radiographs, it is replaced or scheduled for removal when the fracture has healed.

## Suggested Readings

1. Dee JF: Tarsal Injuries. In Bloomberg MS, Dee JF, Taylor RA: Canine Sports Medicine and Surgery. Philadelphia: W.B. Saunders Co., 1998, 120-137.
2. Boudrieau RJ, Dee JF, Dee LG: Treatment of central tarsal bone fractures in the racing Greyhound. J Am Vet Med Assoc 12:1492-1500, 1984.

# Chapter 8

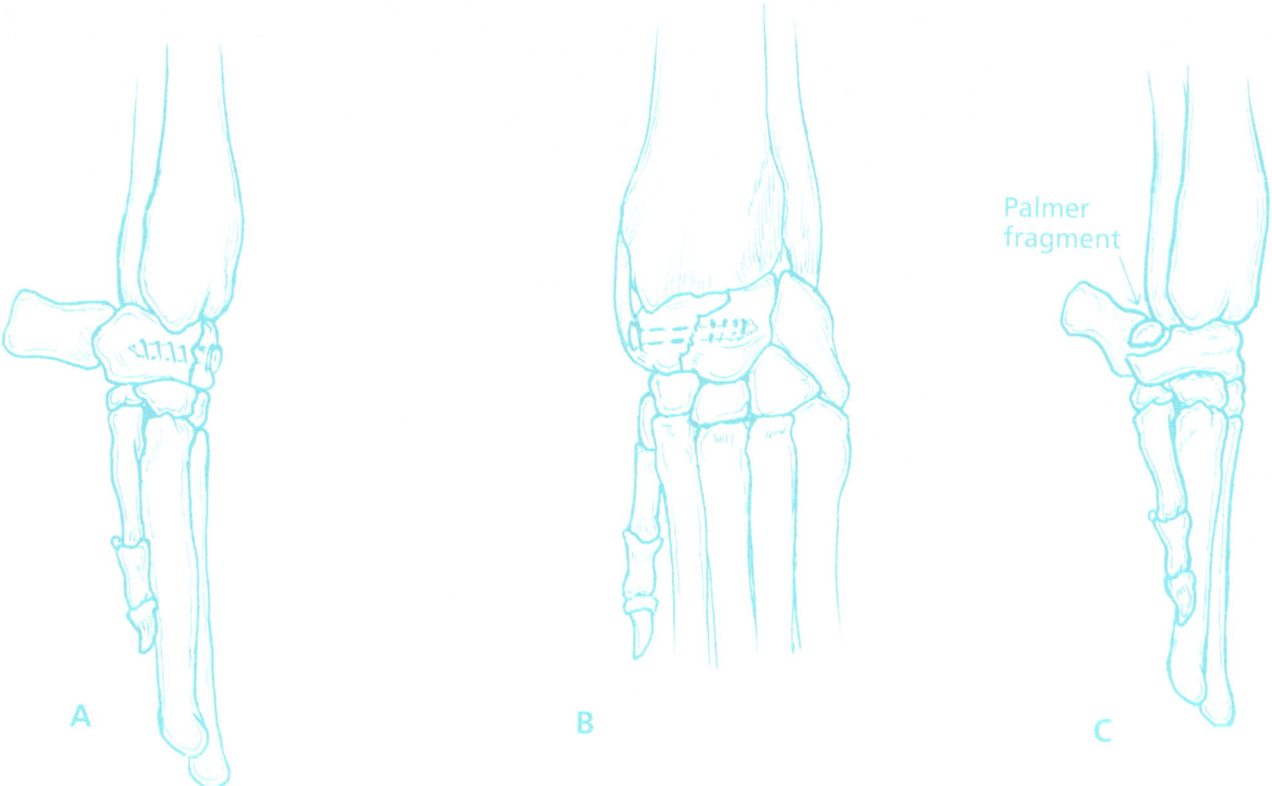


## Orthopedic Injuries of the Carpal Area

Janet Welch, D.V.M., D.A.C.V.S.

# Anatomy of the Distal Forelimb

## Osseous Structures

The radius and ulna are the long bones of the antebrachium. At the elbow joint the radius is positioned laterally to the ulna and at the carpal joint the radius is medial to the ulna. The distal aspect of the radius is the radial styloid process and the distal aspect of the ulna is the ulnar styloid process (Figure 8-1). On the cranial aspect of the radius there are 3 grooves for extensor tendons. The tendons, from medial to lateral, are the abductor pollicus longus, the extensor carpi radialis, and the common digital extensor.

The osseous components of the carpus include seven small bones arranged into two rows. The proximal row contains the radial, ulnar, and accessory carpal bones. The radial and ulnar carpal bones are arranged side by side in the proximal row. The accessory carpal bone is located in a proximal and palmar position with relation to the ulnar carpal bone. The radial carpal bone is the largest and articulates with the radius. The ulnar and accessory carpal bones articulate with the styloid process of the ulna. The accessory carpal bone serves as a lever arm for some of the flexor muscles of the carpus. The distal row of carpal bones consists of four bones numbered from the medial to the lateral side. These increase in size from medial to lateral and are the first, second, third and fourth carpal bones (See Figure 8-1).

## Nomenclature of the Carpal Joints

The antebrachiocarpal joint is located between the distal part of the radius and ulna and the proximal

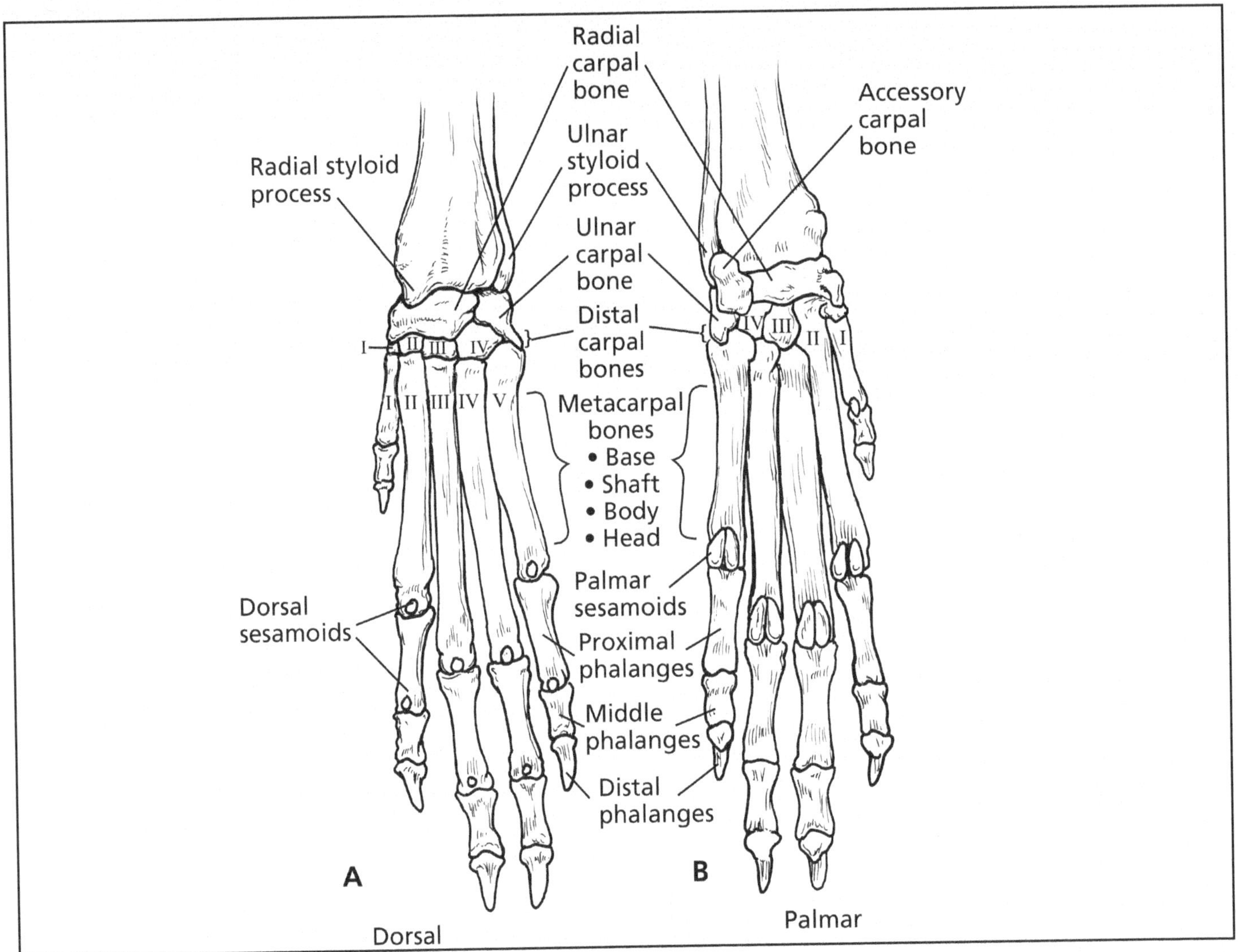


**Figure 8-1.** Osseous structures of the left distal forelimb. Carpal bones–seven carpal bones arranged in two rows. Proximal row–radial carpal bone medially; ulnar carpal bone laterally; accessory carpal bone proximal and palmar to ulnar carpal bone. Distal row–first *(I)* to fourth *(IV)* from medial to lateral. Metacarpal bones–first *(I)* to fifth *(V)* from medial to lateral. Each bone consists of base, shaft or, body, and head from proximal to distal. First metacarpal bone is vestigial. Digits–first *(I)* to fifth *(V)* from medial to lateral. Phalanges of digits–proximal, middle, distal. Sesamoid bones–dorsal sesamoids: one in extensor tendons of digits II-V at metacarpophalangeal joint. Palmar sesamoids–two on palmar surface of metacarpophalangeal joint (After Piermattei DL, Flo GL, DeCamp CE: Brinker, Piermattei and Flo's Handbook of Small Animal Orthopedics and Fracture Repair 4th ed. St Louis: Saunders Elsevier, 2006, 383).

row of carpal bones. The middle carpal joint is located between the two rows of carpal bones. The carpometacarpal joints are located between the carpus and metacarpus. Joints between the individual carpal bones of each row are the intercarpal joints. The motion of the carpal joint as a whole is primarily flexion and extension in a craniocaudal plane with some lateral movement. Greatest movement occurs in the antebrachiocarpal and middle carpal joints.

## Ligaments

In the carpus there are no long collateral ligaments that span all three of the carpal joint spaces. Medial and lateral support is provided by short radial and ulnar collateral ligaments. Cranial and caudal support is provided by dorsal and palmar radiocarpal ligaments and a palmar ulnocarpal ligament. Additional small intercarpal ligaments are present on the dorsal and palmar surfaces. The distal radius and styloid process of the ulna are connected by the radioulnar ligament (Figure 8-2A, B & C).

The short radial collateral ligament consists of a straight and an oblique part. The straight part runs from the proximal aspect of the styloid process of the radius to the medial part of the radial carpal

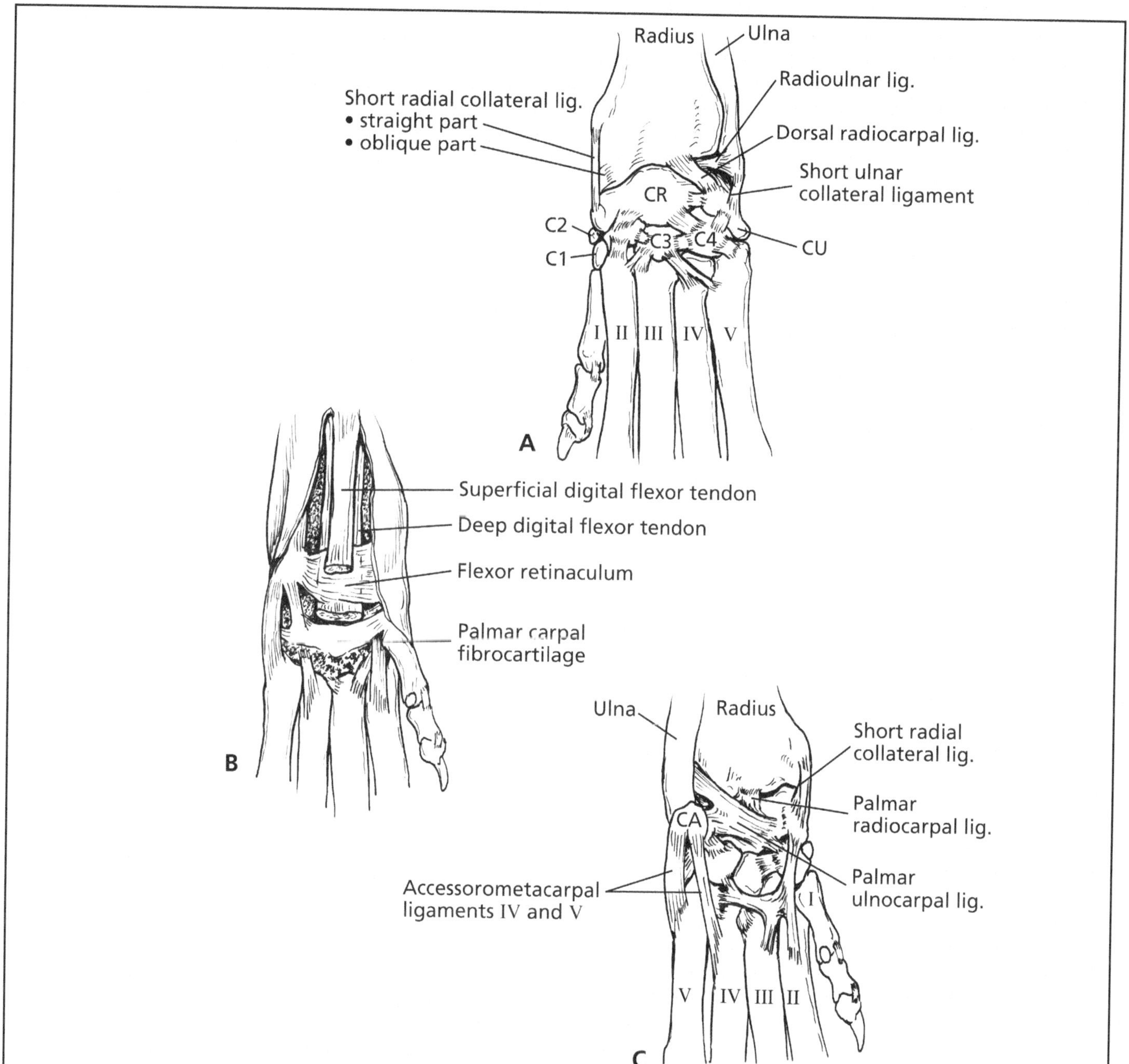


**Figure 8-2.** Ligamentous structures of the carpus. **A.** Dorsal aspect. *CR* = Radial carpal. *CU* = ulnar carpal. *C1* to *C4* = first, second, third, fourth carpals. I to *V* = metacarpals. **B.** Superficial ligaments of left carpus, palmar aspect. **C.** Deep ligaments of left forepaw, palmar aspect. *CA* = accessory carpal. *I* to *V* = metacarpals. (After Evans HE, Miller's Anatomy of the dog, 3rd ed.: Philadelphia: W B Saunders, 1993).

bone. The oblique part leaves the styloid process and runs obliquely to the palmaromedial surface of the radial carpal bone. The short ulnar collateral ligament extends from the styloid process of the ulna to the ulnar carpal bone (See Figure 8-2). The accessory carpal bone is stabilized distally by two ligaments which originate near its proximal free end. Distally one attaches to metacarpal V and one to metacarpal IV.

The flexor retinaculum is a fascial tissue that attaches laterally to the medial aspect of the accessory carpal bone, medially to the styloid process of the radius, and distally to the palmar projections of the radial and first carpal bones. One part of the flexor retinaculum overlies the superficial digital flexor tendon and the other part is between the superficial digital flexor tendon and the deep digital flexor tendon (See Figure 8-2).

The palmar carpal fibrocartilage is a thick band of fascial tissue that is located just distal to the flexor retinaculum. It crosses the palmar surfaces of the carpal bones and attaches to all except the accessory carpal bone. This tissue becomes thickest distally where it attaches to the palmar surfaces of the distal row of carpal bones and the adjacent surfaces of the proximal parts of metacarpals III, IV, and V. The palmar carpal fibrocartilage flattens the palmar irregularities of the carpometacarpal joint and provides a smooth, deep surface for the flexor tendons (See Figure 8-2).

## Tendons

The dorsolateral antebrachial muscles and their tendons function as the extensors of the carpal and digital joints. These are the extensor carpi radialis, common digital extensor, lateral digital extensor, extensor pollicis longus and abductor pollicis longus. The majority of these muscles arise from the lateral epicondyle of the humerus. Distally the extensor retinaculum covers the tendons of the extensor carpi radialis, common digital extensor and lateral digital extensor tendons. The extensor carpi radialis runs underneath the abductor pollicis longus tendon to insert on the proximal and dorsal surfaces of metacarpals II and III. The common digital extensor tendon has four divisions that insert on the distal phalanges of digits II, III, IV and V. The lateral digital extensor tendon lies between the common digital extensor and the ulnaris lateralis. It inserts on the distal phalanges of digits III, IV and V. The ulnaris lateralis is the only flexor tendon originating from the lateral epicondyle. It inserts on the lateral aspect of the proximal end of metacarpal V and the accessory carpal bone. The abductor pollicis longus muscle inserts on the proximal end of metacarpal I (Figure 8-3).

The tendons inserting on the caudal aspect of the carpal joint include the superficial and deep digital flexors, the flexor carpi radialis and the flexor carpi ulnaris. The superficial digital flexor tendon covers the deep digital flexor and inserts on the proximal palmar surfaces of the middle phalanges of digits II, III, IV and V. The deep digital flexor tendon has three bellies of origin that arise from the humerus, radius and ulna. The three muscle bellies fuse at the carpus to form a single tendon. At the metacarpophalangeal joint, the

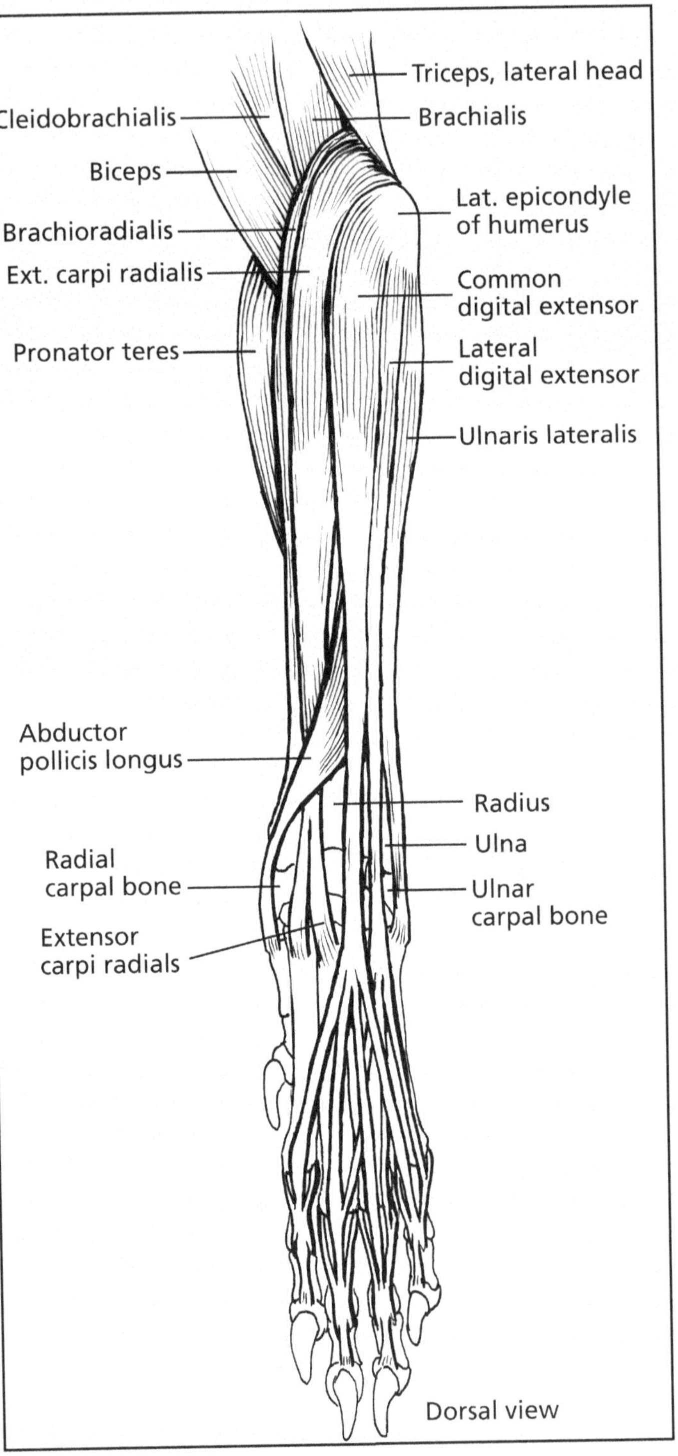


**Figure 8-3.** Dorsal tendons of the carpus. (After Evans HE, DeLahunta A, Miller ME. Guide to the Dissection of the Dog 5th ed. Philadelphia:W. B. Saunders Co., 2000).

deep digital flexor tendon passes through the superficial digital flexor tendon. The deep digital flexor tendon inserts on the palmar surface of the proximal end of the distal phalanx of each digit. The flexor carpi radialis lies between the pronator teres muscle and superficial digital flexor muscles proximally. It inserts on the palmar side of the proximal ends of metacarpals II and III. The flexor carpi ulnaris consists of an ulnar head and a humeral head. Both components insert on the accessory carpal bone (Figure 8-4).

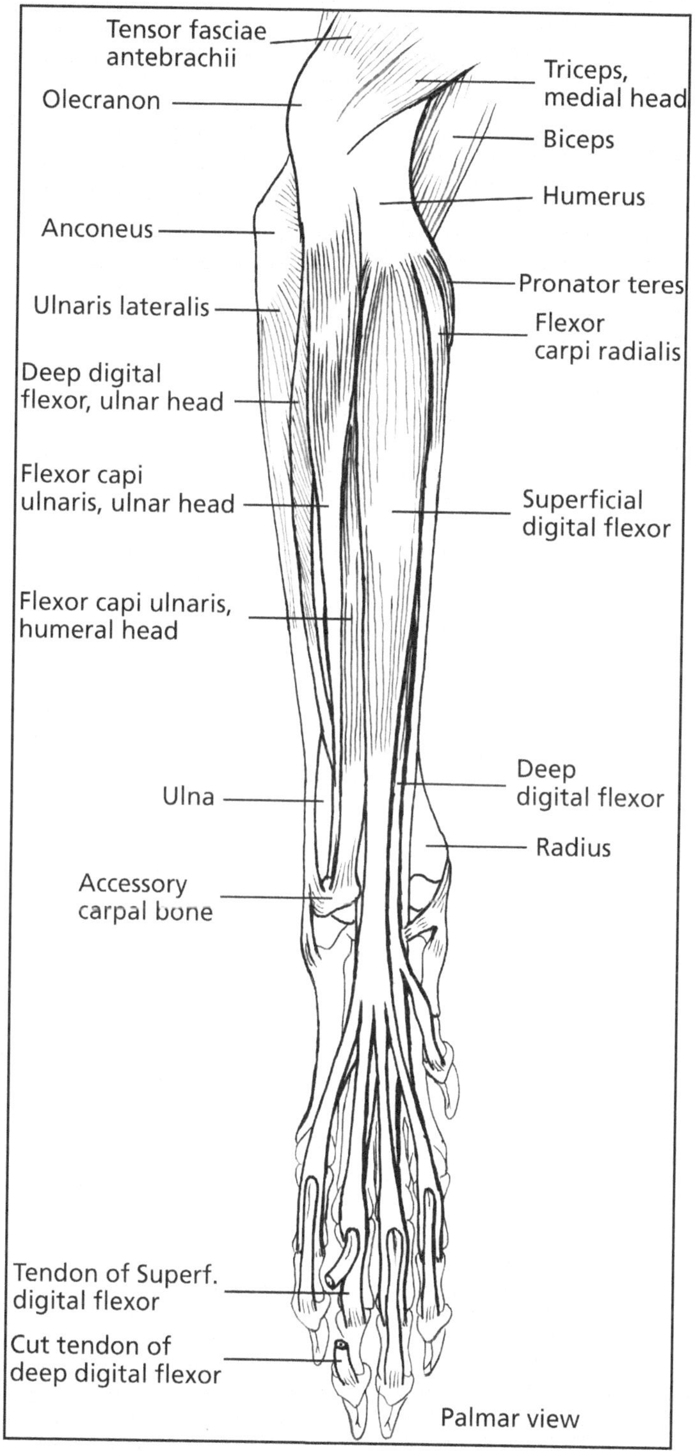


**Figure 8-4.** Palmar tendons of the carpus. (After Evans HE, DeLahunta A, Miller ME. Guide to the Dissection of the Dog 5th ed. Philadelphia:W. B. Saunders Co., 2000).

### Blood Supply

The major arterial supply to the forepaw is provided by the median artery. The brachial artery in the proximal forelimb gives rise to the interosseous artery just distal to the elbow joint and continues as the median artery. Distally the palmar aspect of the paw is supplied by branches of the median artery. The dorsum of the paw is supplied by the cranial superficial antebrachial artery which is a branch from the brachial artery.

## Suggested Readings

1. Evans HE, Miller ME: Miller's Anatomy of the Dog 3rd ed. Philadelphia: W.B. Saunders, 2003.
2. Piermattei DL, Flo GL, DeCamp CE. Fractures and Other Orthopedic Conditions of the Carpus, Metacarpus, and Phalanges. In Brinker, Piermattei, and Flo's Handbook of Small Animal Orthopedics and Fracture Repair, 4th ed. St. Louis: Saunders Elsevier, 2006, 382-385.

## Hyperextension Injury

### Definition and Indications

The carpal joint is normally held at 10 to -12° of extension. Hyperextension of the carpus usually results from a jumping or falling injury in midsize to large breeds of dogs. Other less common modes of hyperextension include vehicular trauma and injury while running. Affected animals have swelling in the limb, and although they may not bear weight initially after the event, they become weightbearing within 5 to 7 days. There is a variable degree of extension in the paw ranging from 20 degrees to completely palmigrade. There is discomfort with palpation and range of motion which significantly declines in the first week. The pathology of hyperextension injury is rupture of the fibrous tissues supporting the flexor surface, namely, the flexor retinaculum and palmar carpal fibrocartilage. The flexor tendons are not torn in this injury. The only tendon that provides stability to the radiocarpal joint in extension is the flexor carpi ulnaris and sectioning of this tendon causes only slight hyperextension.

Standard 2 view radiographs will ordinarily show soft tissue swelling but no clear hyperextension. It is essential to obtain stress views to diagnose and categorize the injury. Stress views are obtained in lateral position. The radius is stabilized with a protected hand or encircling tape or gauze. A wooden spoon or dowel is used to put upward pressure on the palmar aspect of the paw to apply a force to the carpus.

The three articular levels of the joint, the antebrachiocarpal, middle carpal, and carpometacarpal, are evaluated radiographically. It is helpful to obtain a stress view of the unaffected side for comparison.

When stressed, the uninjured carpus will maintain a normal angle (10 to 12 degrees of extension) and the carpal bones maintain normal positioning. With hyperextension injury at the antebrachiocarpal joint, the only change is an increased angle of extension. With middle carpal instability, there is a gap between the palmar process of the ulnar carpal bone and the base of metacarpal V. With carpometacarpal instability, the numbered carpal bones seem to disappear because the metacarpal bones overlap them (Figure 8-5A through D).

When interpreting radiographs it is possible to miss antebrachiocarpal instability when distal instability is also present. Hyperextension injury of the antebrachiocarpal joint can induce an intraarticular fracture of the palmar aspect of the radius. The presence of this fracture is clear evidence of antebrachiocarpal instability.

In most hyperextension cases the only viable treatment for the injury is arthrodesis. Splinting or casting may be tried in smaller dogs or cats. The antebrachiocarpal joint is responsible for most of the normal motion of the carpus. Hyperextension injury here requires arthrodesis at all joint levels and thus the joint is permanently held at a normal standing angle. Hyperextension at the level of the middle carpal or carpometacarpal level can be treated with partial carpal arthrodesis and thus maintain significant range of motion. Partial carpal arthrodesis can be accomplished with a cross-pinning technique or with the use of a T-plate. Standard straight plates are not recommended for partial carpal arthrodesis. The presence of antebrachiocarpal instability mandates arthrodesis of all 3 joint levels. It is not acceptable to single out the antebrachiocarpal joint for arthrodesis because the distal low-motion joints will develop degenerative change when subjected to greater motion.

## Techniques

### Partial Carpal Arthrodesis Using T-plate Fixation

Partial carpal arthrodesis may be performed with a bone plate or with cross-pins. T-plates are useful for this purpose and come in a range of sizes. The patient is positioned in lateral recumbency with the affected limb up. A dorsal midline approach is made from the level of the distal radius to the midmetacarpal level. Bleeding is controlled with electrocautery. The extensor carpi radialis and common digital extensor tendons are retracted medially and laterally (Figure 8-6A & B). Articular cartilage of the middle carpal and carpometacarpal joints is removed using a high speed bur and

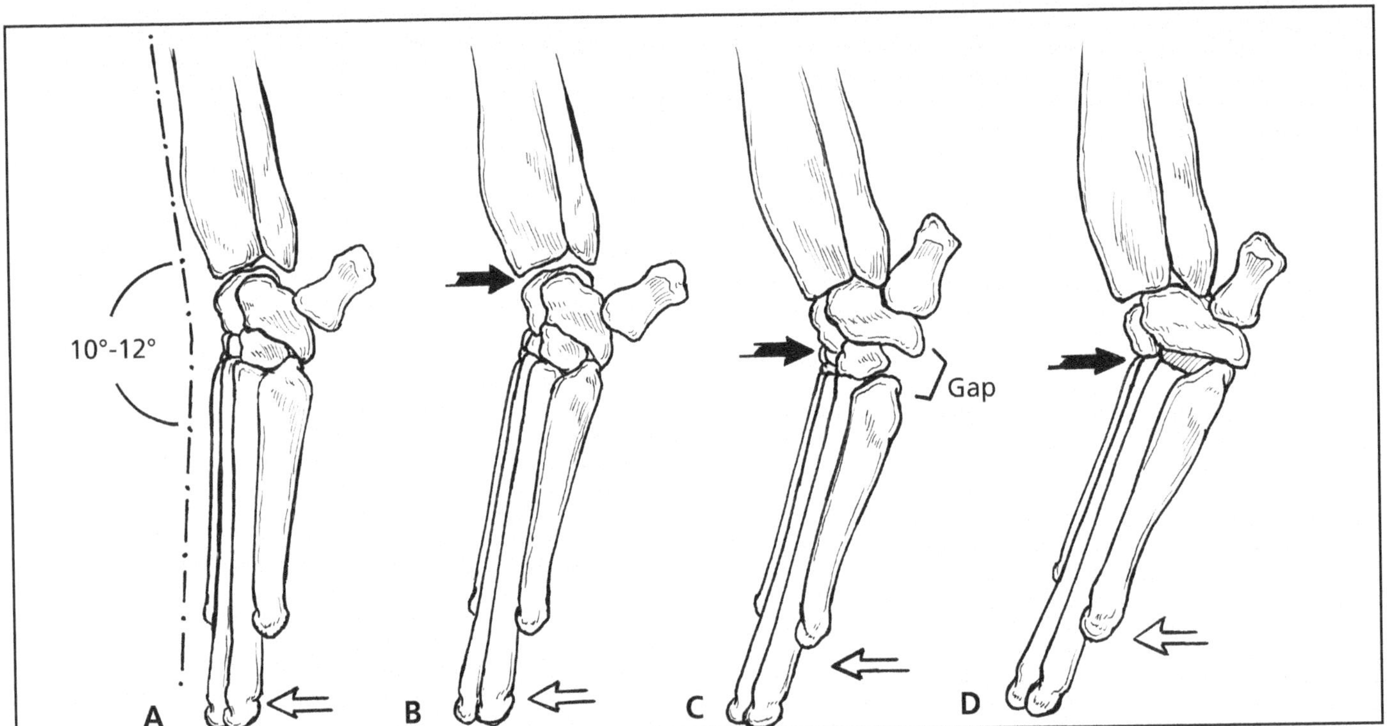


**Figure 8-5.** Stress radiographs for diagnosis of carpal hyperextension injury. Open arrows indicate stress application. **A.** The carpal joint is normally held at 10-12 ° of extension. Stress lateral radiograph of normal radial carpal joint shows maximal extension of 10 to 12 degrees. **B.-D.** Hyperextension injury may affect the carpus at the antebrachiocarpal, middle carpal, or carpometacarpal levels and may affect more than one level (closed arrows indicate level of instability). **B.** With hyperextension injury at the antebrachiocarpal joint, the only change is an increased angle of extension. **C.** With middle carpal instability, there is a gap between the palmar process of the ulnar carpal bone and the base of metacarpal V (bracket). **D.** With carpometacarpal instability, the numbered carpal bones seem to disappear because the metacarpal bones overlap them. (From Piermattei DL, Flo GL, DeCamp CE. Brinker, Piermattei, and Flo's Handbook of Small Animal Orthopedics and Fracture Repair 4th ed. St. Louis: Saunders Elsevier, 2006, 399).

saline lavage. A freer elevator is useful for opening up joint spaces. Cartilage is removed without excessive removal of subchondral bone. It is more important to remove cartilage from horizontal than from vertical joint spaces. The insertions of the extensor carpi radialis tendon on proximal metacarpals II and III are preserved. The tendon insertion on metacarpal III can be transected and sutured to the adjacent tendon to improve exposure for bone plate application. A cancellous bone graft is placed between articular surfaces to promote osteogenesis. Autogenous graft can be harvested from the ipsilateral greater tubercle or allograft can be used. Frozen or freeze-dried bone allograft can be purchased from a supplier (Osteo-allograft Orthomix; Veterinary Transplant Services; Kent, WA). A veterinary T-plate (sizes 1.5/2.0 mm or 2.7/3.5 mm Synthes, West Chester, PA) is positioned over the distal most aspect of the radial carpal bone (Figure 8-7). The plate must be small enough to avoid impinging on the distal radius. The two screws in the radial carpal bone are angled proximally to gain adequate purchase in the bone. The articular surface must not be penetrated and the screw length must not be excessive as this could irritate the palmar soft tissues. The distal portion of the plate is positioned over metacarpal III with holes drilled and screws placed in the distal 2 holes. The remaining middle screw hole is either placed in the 3rd carpal bone or in the base of metacarpal III with holes drilled and screws placed in the distal holes. The surgeon should assess stability of the antebrachiocarpal joint intraoperatively after performing a partial carpal arthrodesis. If the

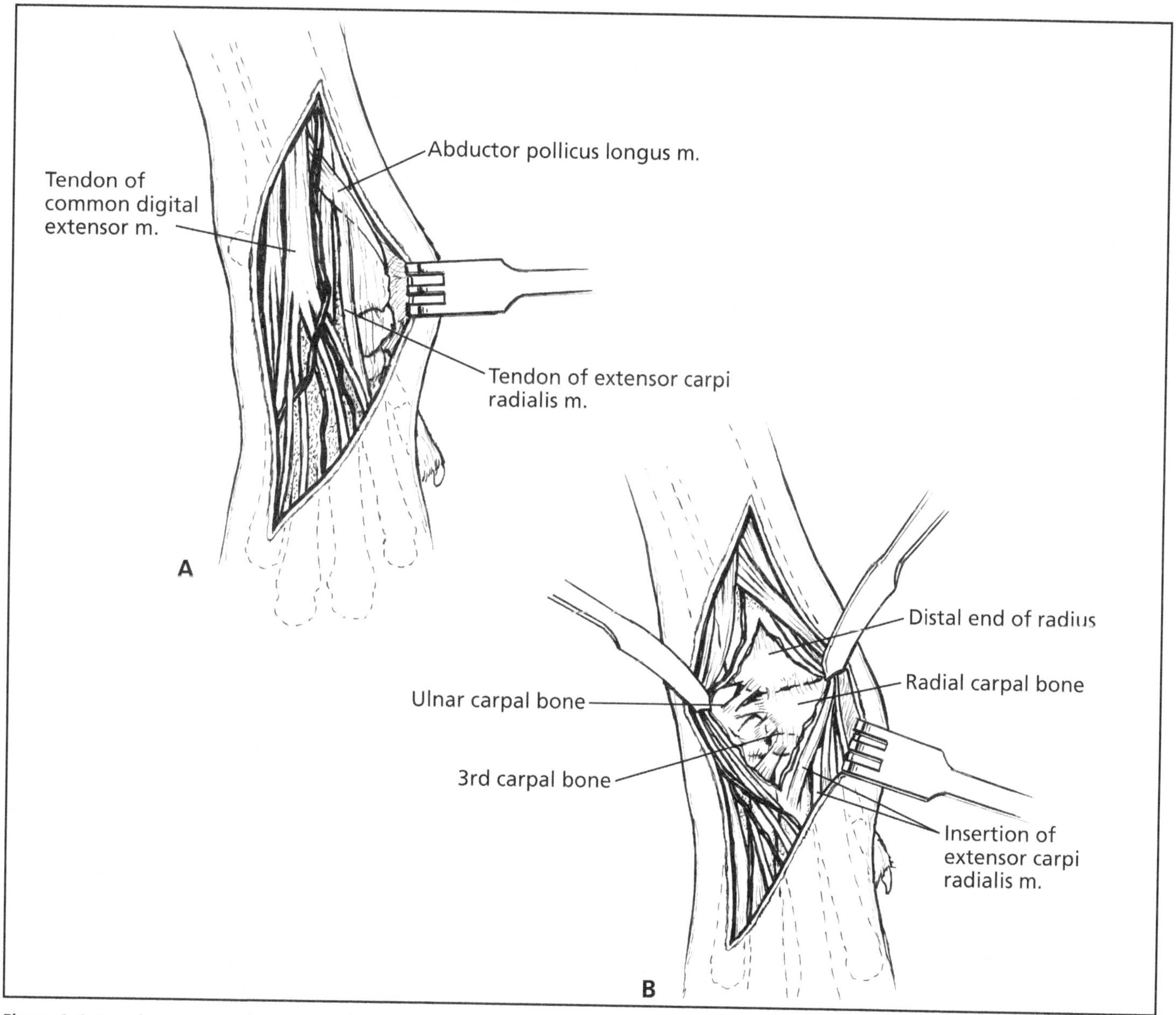


**Figure 8-6.** Dorsal approach to the radiocarpal joint. **A.** A dorsal midline approach is made from the level of the distal radius to the midmetacarpal level. Subcutaneous tissues are incised to expose the extensor carpi radialis and common digital extensor tendons. **B.** The tendons are retracted medially and laterally and the carpal joints are exposed. (After Piermattei DL, Johnson KA. An Atlas of Surgical Approaches to the Bones and Joints of the Dog and Cat 4th ed. Philadelphia: Saunders, 2004, 255).

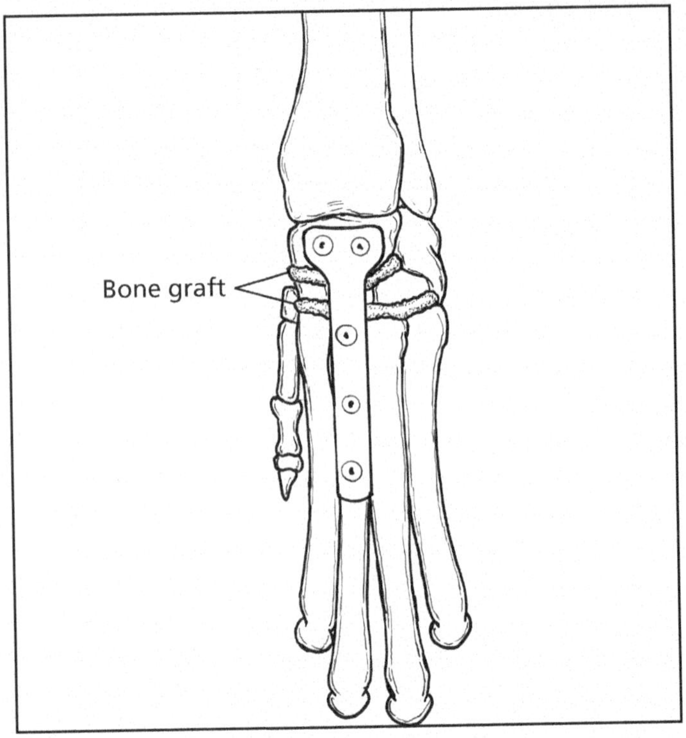


**Figure 8-7.** Partial carpal arthrodesis with a T-plate. Articular cartilage of the middle carpal and carpometacarpal joints is removed, and a cancellous bone graft is placed in the joint spaces. The proximal part of a veterinary T-plate is affixed to the distal most aspect of the radial carpal bone. The distal portion of the plate is affixed to metacarpal III.

degree of extension remains excessive, the procedure is converted to a pancarpal arthrodesis as described below.

Subcutaneous tissue and skin are closed in layers. In the presence of tension, multiple punctate relaxing incisions may be placed (See Chapter 3).

### Pancarpal Arthrodesis

A dorsal bone plate is commonly used for this procedure. The patient is positioned in lateral recumbency with the affected limb up. The skin and subcutaneous tissues are incised over the dorsal surface of the joint from the distal third of the radius to the distal third of the metacarpus. Bleeding is controlled with electrocautery. The extensor carpi radialis and common digital extensor tendons are isolated (See Figure 8-7). The common digital extensor tendon is retracted laterally and the extensor carpi radialis tendons are incised at their insertions on the metacarpal bones with retraction of the muscle medially. The joint capsule is incised to enter the joint spaces. A high speed bur and saline lavage are used to remove articular cartilage from all three levels of joint spaces. A freer elevator can be used to wedge open joint spaces for more complete access. Cartilage is removed without excessive removal of subchondral bone. It is more important to remove cartilage from horizontal than from vertical joint spaces. The surgical wound is lavaged and a cancellous bone graft is packed into the prepared joint spaces (see partial carpal arthrodesis).

The joint is stabilized with a carpal arthrodesis plate (Veterinary Orthopedic Implants, Inc., South Burlington, VT) (Figure 8-8A & B). This plate has useful design features. There are larger screw holes for the radius (3.5 mm) and smaller screw holes for metacarpal III (2.7 mm). A center hole is provided that can accept either size screw. The center hole is positioned over the radial carpal bone. The plate is available in smaller sizes to accommodate smaller bones. The width of the distal aspect of the plate is tapered and the distal plate is thinner to minimize tension on overlying soft tissues at wound closure. The plate produces approximately a 5 to 10° angle of extension when applied to the joint without contouring. The plate is secured to the radiocarpal bone first and then to metacarpal III. Drill holes in metacarpal III should be positioned in the middle of the bone as much as possible. Eccentric screw positioning can increase the risk of iatrogenic fracture through the bone. The remaining plate holes are filled. (See Figure 8-8).

Dermal tissue and skin are closed in layers. In the presence of tension, multiple punctate relaxing incisions may be placed (See Chapter 3).

## Aftercare

A soft padded bandage and splint that extends from the proximal radius to the digits is placed for partial and pancarpal arthrodesis. The splint is made from

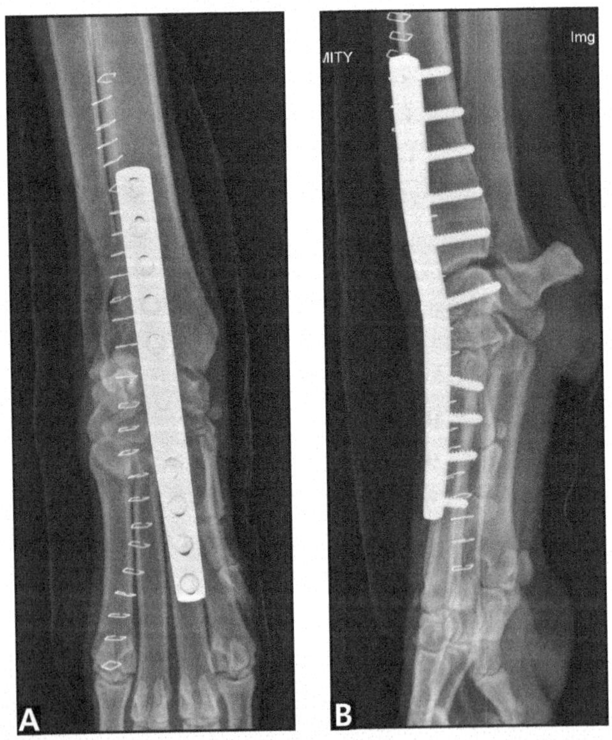


**Figure 8-8.** Pancarpal arthrodesis with a bone plate.

molded fiberglass and is contoured to the palmar aspect of the antebrachium. A donut pad can be placed around the carpal foot pad to help prevent pressure injury (see Chapter 2). The splint is maintained for 6 weeks postoperatively or until there is evidence of bone bridging. Patients are confined in a small indoor area and leash walked only until fusion is obtained. Radiographs are repeated at 6 week intervals until fusion is completed. Radiographic fusion is progressing well when there is bony bridging of joint spaces. Fusion is considered to be complete when there is no visible joint space. With pancarpal arthrodesis bony bridging is anticipated to occur in the distal joints (intercarpal and carpometacarpal) by 12 weeks after surgery. Bony bridging of the antebrachiocarpal joint takes longer and has been shown to take up to 30 weeks. Implants may need to be removed if persistent lameness is present after fusion. Implant removal is delayed until at least 6 to 12 months after surgery.

### Advantages and Disadvantages

The disadvantage of a pancarpal arthrodesis is permanent loss of joint motion and circumduction of the limb during the swing phase of the gait. Despite this owner satisfaction with pancarpal arthrodesis is high. A potential risk with pancarpal arthrodesis is metacarpal fracture at the distal region of the bone plate. Covering slightly more than 50% of the length of the metacarpal bone with the bone plate was found to be protective. A potential disadvantage has been raised with carpal arthrodesis in cats. The elimination of the ability to pronate and supinate could be more problematic in this species than in dogs. Despite this concern, cats tolerate pancarpal arthrodesis very well with many cats just showing a reduced height of jumping or a reduction in their willingness to jump and climb.

The advantage of partial carpal arthrodesis is preservation of joint motion and the potential for return to athleticism. Although range of motion is still present in the antebrachiocarpal joint, it is reduced by approximately 50% of normal. The disadvantage is the potential for degenerative joint disease to develop at the antebrachiocarpal joint. Degenerative change could result from unidentified injury at the antebrachiocarpal joint or from surgical technique.

Specific surgical technique complications with partial carpal arthrodesis are excessive subchondral bone removal and implant interference with the distal radius. Excessive subchondral bone removal from the middle carpal joint space can cause collapse of the radial carpal bone and widening of the antebrachiocarpal joint space. This complication can lead to degenerative joint disease at the antebrachiocarpal level. Implant interference with the distal radius is a concern when using bone plates for pancarpal arthrodesis. The size of the T-plate must allow full joint extension without interference with the distal radius. The plate is placed as distally as possible on the radial carpal bone and screws are angled proximally for adequate bone purchase. Straight bone plates are contraindicated for partial carpal arthrodesis. With these plates, it is virtually impossible to obtain adequate stabilization without impinging on the distal radius.

## Suggested Readings

1. Calvo I, Farrell M, Chase D et al. Carpal arthrodesis in cats. Long-term functional outcome. Vet Comp Orthop Traumatol 22:498-504, 2009.
2. Clarke SP, Ferguson JF, Miller A et al. Clinical evaluation of pancarpal arthrodesis using a CastLess Plate in 11 dogs. Vet Surg 38:852-860, 2009.
3. Denny HR, Barr RS. Partial carpal and pancarpal arthrodesis in the dog: a review of 50 cases. J Small Anim Pract 32:329-34, 1991.
4. Haburjak JJ, Lenehan TM, Davidson CD, et al. Treatment of carpometacarpal and middle carpal joint hyperextension injuries with partial carpal arthrodesis using a cross pin technique: 21 cases. Vet Comp Orthop Traumatol 16:105-11, 2003.
5. Li A, Gibson N, Carmichael S et al. Thirteen pancarpal arthrodesis using 2.7/3.5 mm hybrid dynamic compression plates. Vet Comp Orthop Traumatol 12:102-7, 1999.
6. Piermattei DL, Flo GL, DeCamp CE: Brinker, Piermattei, and Flo's Handbook of Small Animal Orthopedics and Fracture Repair 4th ed. St. Louis: Saunders Elsevier, 2006, 399-409.
7. Michal U, Flückiger M, Schmökel H. Healing of dorsal pancarpal arthrodesis in the dog. J Small Anim Pract 44:109-112, 2003.
8. Willer RL, Johnson KA, Turner TM et al. Partial carpal arthrodesis for 3rd degree carpal sprains: a review of 45 carpi. Vet Surg 19:334-40, 1990.

# Collateral Ligament Instability of the Antebrachiocarpal Joint

### Definition and Indications

#### Rupture of the short radial collateral ligament

Joint subluxation occurs when there is a grade 3 injury of the radial collateral ligament and may result from an acute athletic event or vehicular trauma. Vehicular trauma can induce isolated ligament rupture or shearing injury. Shearing injury produces extensive soft tissue loss and often loss of the medial portions of the radial styloid process and radial carpal bones. Lesser grades of sprain injury in the anetebrachiocarpal joint (Grades 1 or 2 sprain) may produce discomfort, loss of strength in the ligament, and if chronic, the formation of enthesophytes at the origin or insertion of the ligament.

Antebrachiocarpal subluxation resulting from injury to

the short radial collateral ligament is more common than injury to the short ulnar collateral ligament. The short radial collateral ligament extends from the medial distal radius to the radial carpal bone and is composed of a straight and an oblique part (See Figure 8-2C). Because the paw is normally in 10 to 15° of valgus, weight bearing on the limb tends to further destabilize the medial side if there is instability of the short radial collateral ligament.

Grade 3 sprains of the short radial collateral ligament require surgical stabilization. This is carried out by suturing the ligament if it is still identifiable and supporting the repair with a prosthetic imbrication technique. This is done by anchoring heavy gauge suture at the origin and insertion sites of the ligament. The suture may be secured with bone anchors or through drill tunnels.

### Carpal shearing injury with damage to articular structures

Shearing injury of the carpus results from vehicular trauma. The medial surface of the carpus is affected more often than the lateral surface. Contact with pavement erodes skin and underlying soft tissues and can shear away the medial surfaces of the radius, carpal bones and their attached collateral ligaments. This is a highly contaminated injury. Treatment of shearing wounds involves wound lavage, debridement, bandaging techniques to stimulate granulation tissue, and collateral ligament stabilization. Damage to articular surfaces of the anetbrachiocarpal joint is best treated by pancarpal arthrodesis.

## Techniques

### Rupture of the short radial collateral ligament

The patient is positioned in lateral recumbency with the affected paw down to expose its medial surface. A skin incision is made directly over the distal 1/3 of the radius to the proximal 1/3 of the second metacarpal bone. The remnants of the collateral ligament are located immediately deep to the antebrachial fascia and the tendon of the abductor pollicus longus (See Figure 8-6A). If the ligament ends are intact enough to hold sutures they are apposed using a locking loop pattern (See Figure 7-9). The suture repair is supplemented with prosthetic imbrication. This is accomplished with bone tunnels or suture anchors. Bone tunnels are made with a relatively small drill bit (1.5 to 2.0 mm). There are 2 sites of origin for the ligament in the distal radius and therefore 2 drill tunnels are created. One is located in the tubercle proximal to the styloid process for the straight portion of the ligament and the other is more distal for the oblique portion. The third drill hole for one insertion is made through the medial prominence of the radial carpal bone using caution to avoid the articular surfaces of the bone. A single suture is placed to connect the proximal, middle and distal fixation sites in a figure 8 style. The suture is tightened to the point where the joint is stable but still able to move, and is tied (Figure 8-9A, B & C).

Dermal tissue and skin are closed in layers. In the presence of tension, multiple punctate relaxing incisions may be placed (See Chapter 3).

### Reconstruction of carpal shearing injury

Once the patient is hemodynamically stabilized general anesthesia is used to lavage and debride the wound. The patient is positioned in lateral recumbency with the affected limb down to expose the medial surface. Wound treatment is carried out as described for shearing wounds (see Chapters 1 and 2). Ligament stabilization can be carried out early in the healing process while the wound is still being managed as an open wound with sterile bandage changes. Once gross contamination is resolved and wound exudation is minimal, surgical stabilization is performed. Short radial collateral ligament stabilization can be performed as described for closed collateral ligament rupture (See Figure 8-9) using drill tunnels. If there is enough loss of bone from the medial distal radius and radiocarpal bone to preclude the creation of drill tunnels, suture anchors are used. The distal medial radius is visualized and the prior location of the styloid process is estimated. An appropriately-sized drill hole is placed at this location and a suture anchor is placed (Imex Veterinary Inc., Longview, TX; Securos Veterinary Orthopedics, Charlton, MA; or Arthrex Vet Systems Bonita Springs, FL). The proximal to distal midpoint of the radial carpal bone is located and a suture anchor is placed here for the insertion site of the ligament (Figure 8-10). Heavy gauge suture, such as 40 to 60 pound test leader line or braided material (Fiberwire, Arthrex Vet Systems, Bonita Springs, FL) is used to connect the proximal distal fixation sites in a figure 8 style. The suture is tightened to the point where the joint is stable but still able to move, and is tied.

The carpal joint is stabilized with a soft padded bandage or splint or a type II external fixator (see external fixation of distal radial fractures). A type II external fixator is placed with the carpal joint held in a straight position. Two to 3 pins are placed in the radius and 2 to 3 pins in the metacarpal bones (See Figure 8-10). It is not necessary to use modified clamps or hinges as described for temporary external fixation of

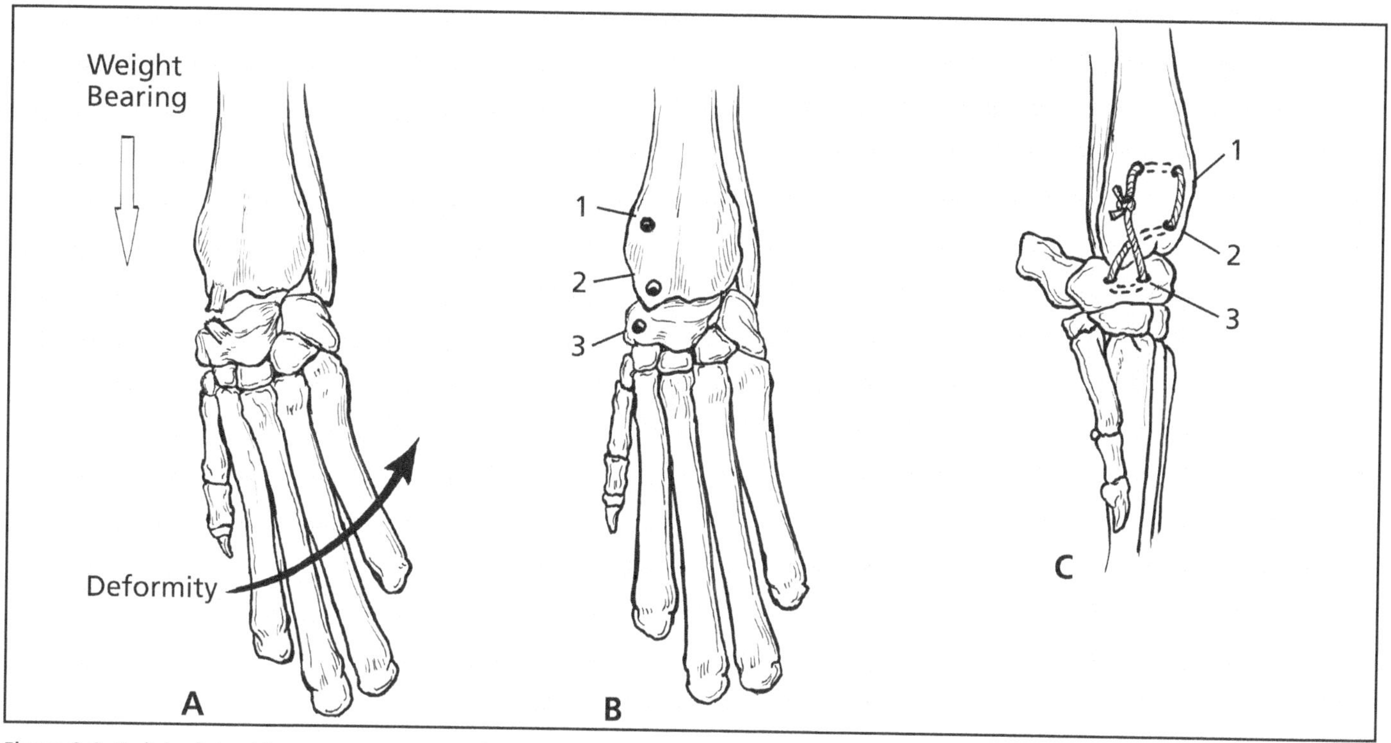


**Figure 8-9.** Radial collateral ligament rupture. **A.** Medial collateral ligament rupture. Valgus deformity *(closed arrow)* with weightbearing *(open arrow)*. **B.** Tunnels drilled at the origin and insertion sites to accommodate stabilizing suture. There are 2 sites of origin in the distal radius. One is located in the tubercule proximal to the styloid process to simulate the straight portion of the ligament *(1)* and the other is more distal to simulate the oblique portion *(2)*. The third tunnel is made through the medial prominence of the radial carpal bone *(3)* using caution to avoid the articular surfaces of the bone **C.** A single suture is placed to connect the *(1)* proximal *(2)* middle and *(3)* distal fixation sites. (After Boemo CM. Diagnostic tests for fractures, luxations, and radial carpal injuries. In Bojrab JM, Ellison GW, Slocum B: Current Techniques in Small Animal Surgery 4th ed. Baltimore: Williams and Wilkins, 1998, 1103).

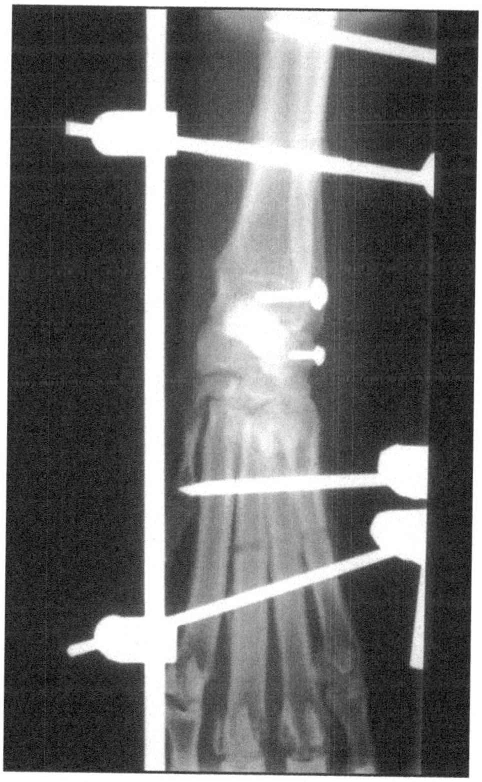

**Figure 8-10.** External fixation of the antebrachiocarpal joint to stabilize a shearing injury.

the carpus because angulation is not required between the proximal and distal pins.

## Arthrodesis of Shearing Injury with Damage to Articular Structures

Damage to articular surfaces of the distal radius or carpal bones is treated by arthrodesis. Arthrodesis can be done immediately, within the first week of injury, through the open wound bed. Gross contamination is treated initially with wound lavage and sterile dressing application (see Chapters 1 & 2). Once visible contamination has been resolved arthrodesis may be performed. Articular cartilage is removed and the carpal joint is stabilized with external fixation. This procedure can be coordinated with surgical wound debridement.

The patient is placed in sternal recumbency with the limb pulled forward or in lateral recumbency with the open wound bed facing up. The cartilaginous surfaces of the antebrachiocarpal, middle carpal and carpometacarpal joints are exposed through the shearing wound itself. If needed the wound may be enlarged to access these surfaces. A small round bur is used to remove cartilage in conjunction with saline lavage. Excessive subchondral bone removal is avoided. A type II external fixator is applied as described for support of collateral ligament injuries (See Figure 8-10). For the purpose of arthrodesis more pins are used. Four pins are placed in the radius and 3 pins in the metacarpal bones. An autogenous cancellous bone graft can be harvested from the ipsilateral humerus or an allograft can be placed (Osteoallograft Orthomix; Veterinary Transplant Services; Kent, WA). Cancellous bone is packed deeply into joint spaces prior to applying the external fixator. The radiocarpal joint is placed at approximately 10 degrees of extension. A modified clamp (See Figure 7-48) or acrylic external fixator (See Figure 7-49) can be used to achieve angulation of the joint.

Pancarpal arthrodesis can be carried out with a bone plate but bacterial contamination must be well under control. Surgery is delayed until wound exudation and visible contamination are resolved and granulation tissue covers the bone. The granulation tissue is incised directly over the bone and the cartilaginous surfaces are prepared for arthrodesis as usual. The joint is stabilized with a carpal arthrodesis plate (Veterinary Orthopedic Implants, Inc., South Burlington, VT) (See Figure 8-8).

## Aftercare

### Rupture of the Short Radial Collateral Ligament

The carpus is immobilized in a straight position using a soft padded bandage and caudal splint for 4 to 6 weeks. The splint is changed every 1 to 2 days perioperatively and then as needed. The splint is removed and the joint is stabilized with a soft padded bandage at a normal standing angle for an additional 2 weeks. Exercise is strictly controlled for the first 8 weeks and then progressively increased over a period of another 4 to 6 weeks.

### Reconstruction of Carpal Shearing Injury

Wounds are managed open with daily sterile bandage changes (See Chapter 3). A non-adherent dressing is placed as a contact layer over the wound bed once the exudative phase is completed. Wound stimulating agents may be used on the wound bed. The skin underneath the connecting rod is stabilized with gauze sponges or foam pads to help prevent pin tract irritation. A soft padded bandage encircles the entire external fixator and limb. Bandage changes are done daily to every other day initially and then decreased in frequency according to wound healing. Once a healthy bed of granulation tissue completely covers all bone surfaces bandage changes can usually be decreased to twice weekly. Broad-spectrum antibiotics such as cephalosporins may be prescribed. Once a viable bed of granulation tissue is present systemic antibiotics are withdrawn.

Exercise is strictly controlled for the first 8 weeks and then progressively increased over a period of another 4 to 6 weeks.

### Arthrodesis of Shearing Wounds with Damage to Articular Surfaces

Wound management is conducted as described for reconstruction of carpal shearing injury. Arthrodesis is expected to occur within 3 to 4 months following surgery. Wound closure by epithelialization and contraction is expected to occur within 6 to 10 weeks following injury. A minority of cases require skin grafts for wound closure. Grafting can be done while the external fixator is in place or after the external fixator has been removed (see Chapter 3). Postoperative radiographs to assess arthrodesis are taken at 8 weeks after surgery and then monthly until arthrodesis is complete. The external fixator should be checked for clamp tightness and pin loosening every 2 to 4 weeks. Pin tract sites are evaluated for purulent discharge indicating pin tract infection. Patients developing pin tract infection are treated with broad spectrum antibiotics such as cephalosporins or clavulanic potentiated amoxicillin for 10 to 14 days.

## Advantages and Disadvantages

### Rupture of the Short Radial Collateral Ligament

The advantage of surgical stabilization of the collateral ligament is adequate resistance to valgus deviation of the paw. Splinting only without surgical stabilization is unlikely to provide sufficient stability to medial collateral ligament injuries due to intrinsic medial stresses present in the antebrachiocarpal joint.

### Reconstruction of Carpal Shearing Injuries

Shearing wounds that are reconstructed rather than arthrodesed can have good to excellent long term results with maintenance of joint motion. The disadvantage is the potential for degenerative joint disease. The presence of degenerative joint disease is commonly seen with long term follow up of shearing wounds but many of these patients still experience good clinical function. Owners are advised of the potential for degenerative joint disease before performing this surgery.

The advantage of placing an external fixator to support ligament reconstruction of shearing wounds is assurance of adequate immobilization postoperatively. A splint allows some degree of mobility but can slip or be removed by the patient. Destabilization in the early phases of healing will disrupt the fibroplastic response and can lead to joint laxity and progressive degenerative change. Furthermore prolonged splinting can cause pressure sores over bony protuberances. The disadvantage of external fixators is increased surgical time and the potential for skin tract infections. If these do occur they are localized and resolve with pin removal. External fixators are kept on for a relatively short time for shearing wound reconstruction to minimize cartilage damage due to immobilization.

### Arthrodesis of Shearing Wounds with damage to Articular Surfaces

The advantage of immediate arthrodesis for severe shearing wounds with articular damage is improved patient comfort and shorter hospital stays. Surgical stabilization can be carried out at the time of surgical debridement thus limiting the number of times the patient must be anesthetized. The potential disadvantage is increased risk of implant infection but this has not been a long term problem with external fixation since implants are removed. The disadvantage is a change in gait. Most patients have comfortable use of their limb following arthrodesis but there can be noticeable circumduction to the gait.

The potential disadvantage of performing pancarpal arthrodesis with a bone plate is long term infection requiring future plate removal. Waiting until exudation and visible contamination are resolved and the bone is covered with granulation tissue decreases this risk. Sterile procedure is followed during bandage changes and granulation and re-epithelialization occur directly over the implant. Owners are informed that bone plate removal may be required in the future.

The disadvantage to placing a cancellous graft in an early shearing wound is that some of the graft can be lost to the external environment. Graft placement can be delayed until there is a healthy granulation bed that completely covers the bone but a second anesthetic procedure would be required.

# Suggested Readings


1. Benson JA, Boudrieau RJ. Severe carpal and tarsal shearing injuries treated with an immediate arthrodesis in seven dogs. J Amer Anim Hosp Assoc 38:370-380, 2002.
2. Corr S. Intensive, extensive, expensive. Management of distal limb shearing injuries in cats. J Fel Med and Surg 11:747-757, 2009.
3. Diamond DD, Besso J, Boudrieau RJ. Evaluation of joint stabilization for treatment of shearing injuries of the tarsus in 20 dogs. J Amer Anim Hosp Assoc 35:147-153, 1999.
4. Johnson KA. Carpal Injuries. In Bloomberg MS, Dee JF, Taylor RA: Canine Sports Medicine and Surgery. Philadelphia: WB Saunders Co., 1998, 100-119.
5. Piermattei DL, Flo GL, DeCamp CE. Brinker, Piermattei, and Flo's Handbook of Small Animal Orthopedics and Fracture Repair 4th ed. St. Louis: Saunders Elsevier, 2006, 399-409.


# Luxation of the Antebrachiocarpal Joint

## Definition and Indications

Luxation of the antebrachiocarpal joint in dogs is a highly disruptive injury associated with ruptures of multiple ligaments including the short radial collateral and ulnar collateral ligaments, the dorsal and palmar radiocarpal ligaments and the palmar ulnocarpal ligaments. On physical exam, in addition to varus-valgus instability, the radius is dorsally displaced from the carpal bones and can be moved in a dorsal to palmar direction (Figure 8-11A & B). Repair of individual structures is not feasible and the joint must be salvaged with a pancarpal arthrodesis.

Antebrachiocarpal luxation in cats can be caused by rupture of the short radial collateral ligament alone. The short radial collateral ligament is anatomically different in the cat compared to the dog. In dogs, the short radial collateral ligament of the carpus consists of straight and oblique portions. Both portions originate on the distal radius. The straight portion inserts on the radial carpal bone and the oblique portion inserts on the palmarodistal portion of the radial carpal bone. In cats, the straight part of the ligament is absent. The medial collateral ligament consists only of a single broad portion that extends from the dorsal aspect of the radius to the palmar aspect of the radial carpal bone. The ligament acts to oppose palmar dislocation of the radial carpal bone rather than medial opening of

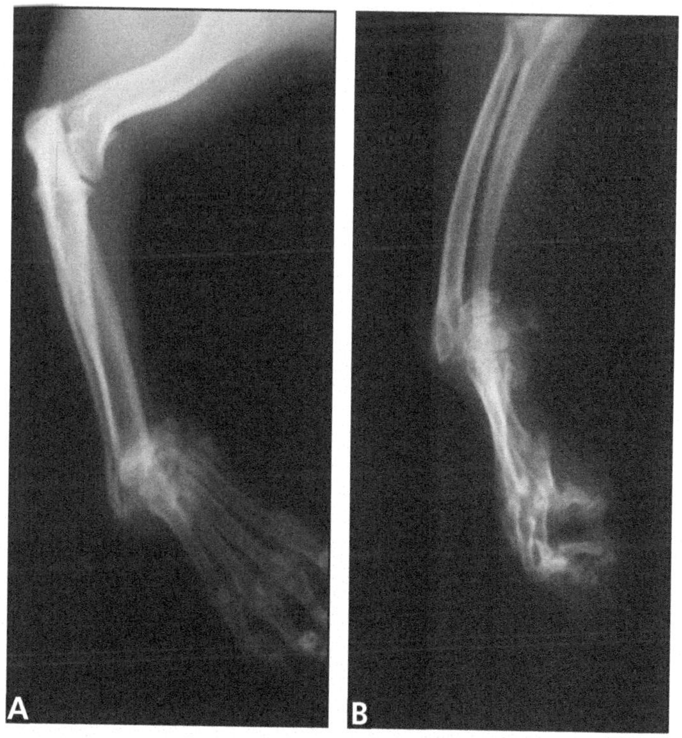


**Figure 8-11.** Luxation of the radiocarpal joint. All ligaments are ruptured and instability is seen in **A.** medial-lateral and **B.** dorsal planes.

the joint. Rupture of the short radial collateral ligament in combination with rupture of the dorsomedial joint capsule can result in complete antebrachiocarpal luxation in cats. Although pancarpal arthrodesis can be successfully performed in cats, it may be unnecessary. Open reduction and internal fixation of the medial collateral ligament can stabilize the joint.

## Techniques

### Antebrachiocarpal Joint Luxation in Dogs

In dogs pancarpal arthrodesis is performed as described for carpal hyperextension injuries (See Figure 8-8).

### Antebrachiocarpal Joint Luxation in Cats

Cats are treated with prosthetic ligament stabilization rather than pancarpal arthrodesis. The patient is positioned in lateral recumbency with the affected limb down to expose the medial surface. A medial skin incision is performed extending from the distal 1/3 of the radius to the proximal 1/3 of the second metacarpus. The abductor pollicus longus muscle can be seen superficial to the medial collateral ligament (See Figure 8-3). The antebrachiocarpal joint is manually reduced. The ruptured ends of the medial collateral ligament are visualized and if the ligament is capable of holding sutures the ends are apposed with a locking loop pattern (See Figure 7-9). A prosthetic imbrication technique is used to bridge the origin and insertion sites of the ligament. These sites are located similarly to the origin and insertion of the oblique portion of the short radial collateral ligament in the dog (See Figure 8-9B). A small (1.5 mm) screw is placed in the dorsomedial aspect of the distal radius and a second screw (1.5 mm or 1.0 mm, Synthes Maxillofacial, Paoli, PA) is placed in the palmar aspect of the radial carpal bone. The joint capsule is sutured with absorbable material in an interrupted pattern. Size 2-0 to 0 non-absorbable suture (polypropylene or nylon) is placed around the two screws and washers in a figure 8 pattern and tightened, taking care not to restrict the normal range of motion.

Dermis and skin are closed in layers. In the presence of tension, multiple punctate relaxing incisions may be placed (See Chapter 3).

## Aftercare

### Pancarpal arthrodesis (dog)

A soft padded bandage and splint is placed that extends from the proximal radius to the digits. The splint is made from molded fiberglass and is contoured to the palmar aspect of the antebrachium. A donut pad can be placed around the carpal foot pad to help prevent pressure injury (See Chapter 2). The splint is maintained for 6 weeks postoperatively. Patients are confined in a small indoor area and leash walked only until fusion is obtained. Radiographs are taken at 8 weeks postoperatively and repeated at 4 to 6 week intervals until fusion is completed.

### Collateral ligament stabilization (cats)

For cats treated with collateral ligament stabilization, a padded bandage with palmar fiberglass splint is placed from the proximal radius to the digits with the paw held in a straight position. The soft padded bandage and splint are maintained for 3 weeks then changed to a soft padded bandage for 2 weeks. Exercise is restricted to a confined indoor area with no jumping at all for 12 weeks. Radiographs are taken 8 weeks postoperatively to evaluate the position of the screws and the alignment of the joint.

## Advantages and Disadvantages

Pancarpal arthrodesis is the only viable option for total antebrachiocarpal joint luxation in the dog and generally produces a very functional and comfortable gait. Implant loosening or chronic low grade infection may necessitate implant removal after completion of arthrodesis.

The advantage of ligament reconstruction versus arthrodesis in cats is that it preserves joint motion and, in particular, supination and pronation which are important for normal gaiting, playing and grooming. A technical challenge with this technique is the small size of the radial carpal bone which limits screw size and positioning. A smaller implant (a size 1.0 mm screw) may be more suitable than the standard 1.5 mm screw size.

## Suggested Readings

1. Voss K, Geyer H, Montavon PM. Antebrachiocarpal luxation in a cat. Vet Comp Orthop Trauamtol 16:266-270, 2003.

# Middle Carpal Subluxation

## Definition and Indications

Subluxation at the level of the middle carpal joint is induced by ligamentous instability between the radial carpal and second carpal bones (Figure 8-12A, B & C. Instability may also occur between the second carpal and metacarpal II and, in both situations, causes valgus positioning of the paw. Medial instability is palpable and is detected using standard or stress radiographs.

## Technique

The patient is positioned in lateral recumbency with the affected limb down to expose the medial surface. A dorsomedial skin incision is made extending from the distal 1/3 of the radius to the proximal 1/3 of

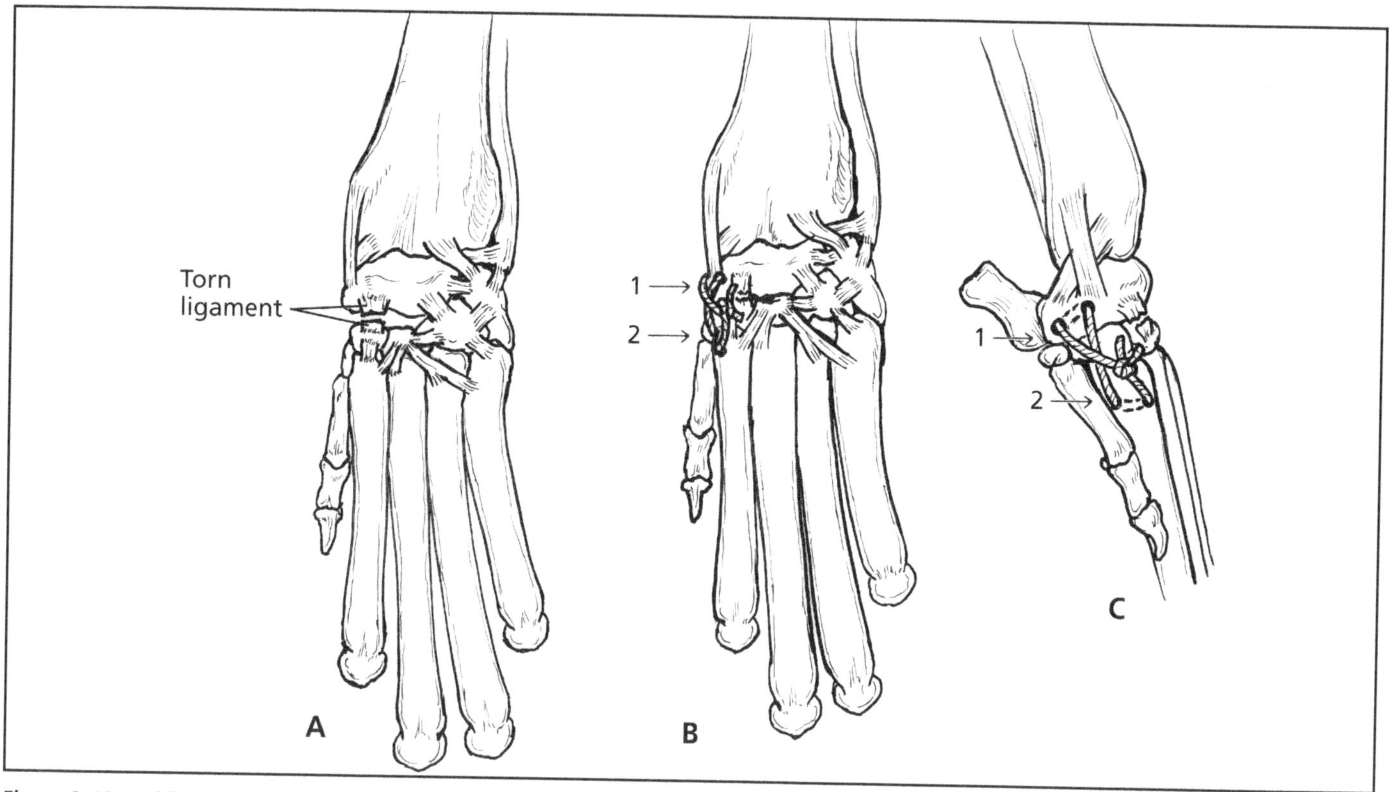


**Figure 8-12.** Middle carpal subluxation. **A.** Subluxation of the middle carpal joint by ligamentous instability between the radial carpal and second carpal bones. **B., C.** Dorsal and medial views respectively). Stabilization is achieved using bone tunnels and suture. The proximal tunnel is in the palmarmedial process of the radiocarpal bone *(1)* and the distal tunnel is in the base of metacarpal II. The bone tunnels are threaded with heavy gauge suture in a figure 8 fashion and tightened to eliminate valgus instability. (After Piermattei DL, Flo GL, DeCamp CE. Brinker, Piermattei, and Flo's Handbook of Small Animal Orthopedics and Fracture Repair 4th ed. St Louis: Saunders Elsevier, 2006, 398).

the second metacarpus. The incision is medial to the accessory cephalic vein. Subcutaneous tissue and deep antebrachial fascia are incised medial to the tendon of the extensor carpi radialis. The abductor pollicus longus muscle is located at the proximal aspect of the incision (See Figure 8-3). Using a small drill bit (1.5 to 2.0 mm) bone tunnels are drilled in the palmaro-medial process of the radial carpal bone and in the base of metacarpal II. The bone tunnels are threaded with monofilament fishing line or braided material (FiberWire; Arthrex Vet Systems, Bonita Springs, FL) in a figure 8 fashion and tightened to eliminate valgus instability (See Figure 8-12).

## Aftercare

A soft padded bandage with palmar splint that extends from the proximal radius to the digits is applied and maintained for 4 weeks with changes as needed. The splint is removed and changed to a soft padded bandage for 2 weeks. Exercise is restricted to a confined indoor area with controlled leash walks for 8 weeks postoperatively.

## Advantages and Disadvantages

Non-surgical treatment using splinting and confinement for smaller breeds with minimal laxity can be attempted. The potential disadvantage of conservative treatment is chronic instability and osteoarthritis.

## Suggested Readings

1. Piermattei DL, Flo GL, DeCamp CE. Fractures and orthopedic conditions of the forelimb. In Brinker, Piermattei, and Flo's Handbook of Small Animal Orthopedics and Fracture Repair 4th ed. St. Louis: Saunders Elsevier, 2006, 397-398.

# Distal Fractures of the Radius and Ulna

## General Information

### External Fixation for Distal Limb Fractures

External fixation devices, either linear, ring or hybrid fixators, are effective for stabilizing radius/ulna and tibia/fibula fractures. In general, bone plating is a straightforward way to treat simple long bone fractures and external fixation is well-suited for comminuted or open fractures. Ring and hybrid external fixation systems are useful for metaphyseal fractures that are close to the joint (juxta-articular) and therefore have limited space for implants.

### Linear External Fixation

Linear fixation systems consist of pins, clamps and

connecting rods. A type Ia or unilateral system employs half-pins and a connecting rod placed on one side of the limb (Figure 8-13A, B & C). A type Ib or biplanar system has half-pins placed from two different orientations on the limb, such as cranial-lateral and cranial-medial, with 2 connecting rods. There can be a linkage rod joining the 2 connecting rods. A type Ib system provides more resistance to bending than a type Ia. A type II or bilateral frame has full pins that penetrate both sides of the limb and 2 connecting rods. Half-pins may be used in addition to complete the type II frame (Figure 8-14). A type IIb frame is composed of a proximal and distal full pin and the remaining pins are half pins. Current fixation systems (Imex SK ESF System, Imex Veterinary, Inc., Longview, TX; Securos External Fixation System, Securos Veterinary

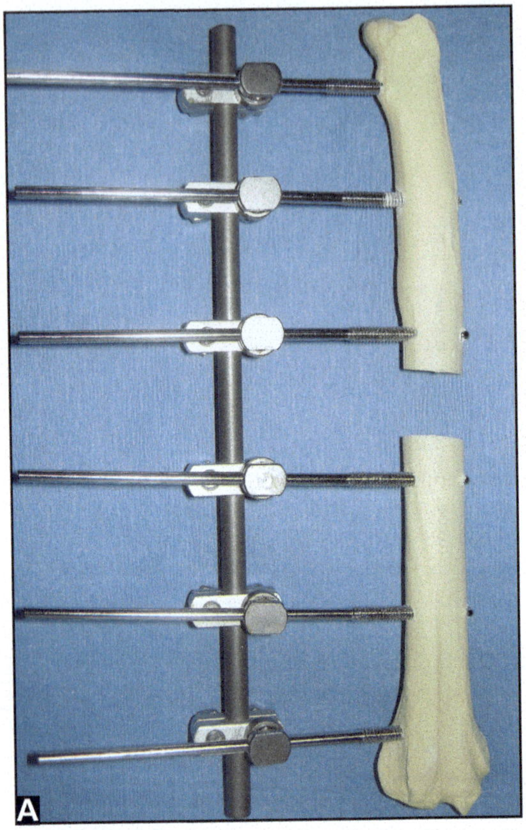


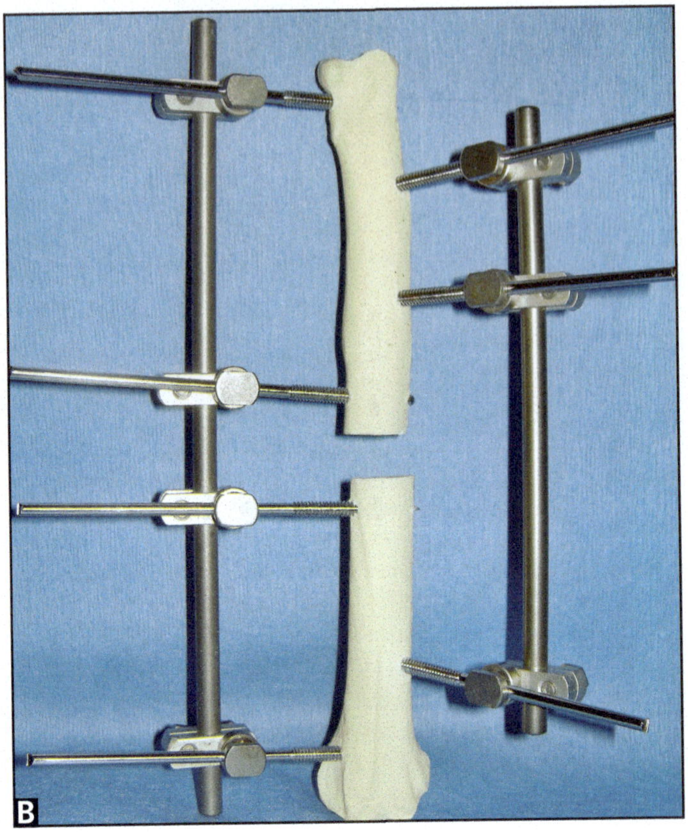


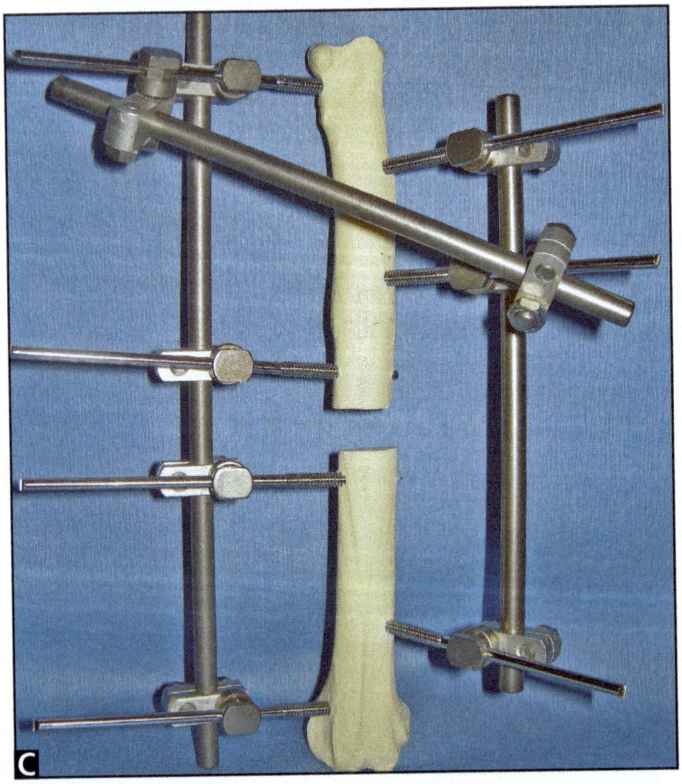


**Figure 8-13. A.** Type Ia external fixator. This unilateral system consists of half-pins and a connecting bar placed on one side of the limb. **B.** Type Ib external fixator. This fixator is biplanar and has half-pins placed from two different orientations on the limb, cranial-lateral and cranial-medial, with 2 connecting rods. **C.** A type of Ib external fixator with an articulation joining the 2 connecting rods.

Orthopedics, Charlton, MA) have stronger connecting rod and clamp components that enable the use of simpler frames, such as types Ia and Ib, compared to the more complex frames required with the Kirschner-Ehmer fixation system (KE External Skeletal Fixation System, Imex Veterinary Inc., Longview, TX). The type I frame built with the large Imex SK components is comparable in strength to the type II KE system. An additional connecting rod can also be added to type I fixation systems by attaching it right next to the primary connecting rod. Using 2 connecting rods on a type I fixation system nearly doubles the resistance to axial loading. A type Ib system can be supplemented with articulations to enhance the frame stiffness. Articulations are added connecting rods that join the two main connecting rods together (See Figure 8-13).

External fixation is usually applied using a closed or semi-closed technique. With a closed technique there is no surgical exposure of the fracture fragments and with a semi-closed technique there is a minimal incision directly over the main fracture to visualize and manipulate the proximal and distal fragments into apposition. Pins are placed through the skin and through both cortices of the bone through stab incisions. A stab incision is made through the skin down to the bone prior to pin placement. Positive profile pins are used whenever possible and are pre-drilled with a slightly smaller size drill bit. For example, a 3.2 mm pin is pre-drilled with a size 3.1 mm drill bit. Half pins are threaded on the far end of the pin and full pins are threaded in the center. A newer version of external skeletal fixation pin has a negative profile thread design but with an increased shaft diameter and decreased stress riser at the thread/non-thread junction. This design has shown improved pin strength and stiffness compared and thus can be substituted for a positive profile pin. The pin must not exceed 25% of the bone diameter to avoid iatrogenic fracture through a pin site (sizes suitable for most radial fractures range from 3/32 inch = 2.4 mm, 7/64 inch = 2.8 mm, and 1/8 inch = 3.2 mm).

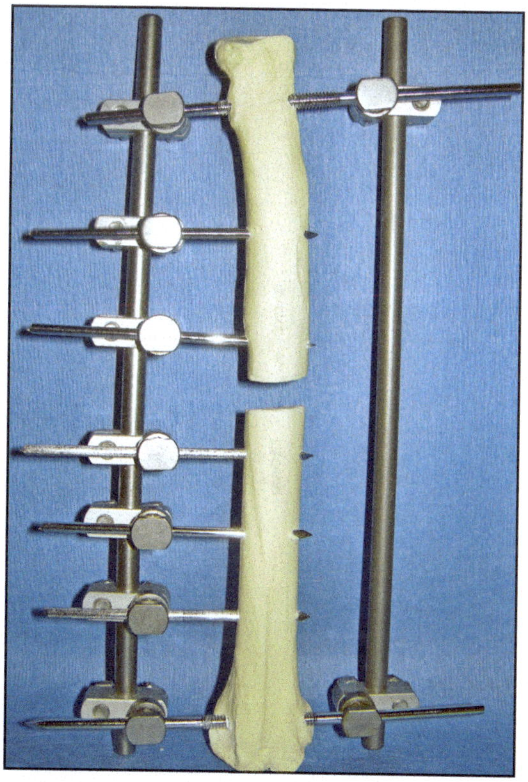

**Figure 8-14.** Type IIb external fixator. The bilateral frame has full pins that penetrate both sides of the limb, half pins, and 2 connecting rods.

The proximal and distal pins are placed first and these are attached to the connecting rods with single clamps. It is ideal to have 3 to 4 pins on either side of the fracture line. The pins should be distributed across the proximal to distal length of the bone in a far-near-near-far pattern. This means that a pin is located close to the proximal joint, close to each side of the fracture line, and close to the distal joint (See Figures 8-13 and 8-14). This configuration maximizes the resistance to bending and torsional forces. This configuration does not depict the order of pin placement but rather the ultimate spacing of the pins.

Supplementing the strength of an external fixation system becomes more important with increasing body weight and degree of comminution. Mechanisms for maximizing the strength of fixation frames for use in distal limb fractures include:

1. Placing 3 to 4 pins on either side of the fracture site whenever possible.
2. Using the largest components possible. Pins must not exceed 25 % of the diameter of the bone. The largest clamps and connecting rods that fit the pins are chosen.
3. Supplementing a type Ia frame with an additional connecting rod.
4. Constructing a type Ib frame and joining both connecting rods with articulations.
5. Placing a type II fixation frame instead of a type Ia or Ib.

## Ring and Hybrid External Fixation

It is desirable to have at least 2 to 3 pins on each side of the fracture and this may be difficult with small distal fracture fragments. In this situation, a ring fixation system or hybrid external fixator is a good choice (Figures 8-15 and 8-16A & B). Ring and hybrid fixation systems employ tensioned wires rather than fixation pins. The smaller size of the wires makes them adaptable to small bones and small fracture fragments.

A hybrid external fixator consists of ring and linear components. The aluminum ring (Imex Veterinary, Longview, TX) is secured to the distal fragment with 2 wires. Tension is applied to the wires prior to tightening the bolt using a calibrated wire tensioner. A hybrid connecting rod is attached to the ring distally and is used to anchor half pins along the length of the radius proximal to the fracture line. A hybrid connecting rod is similar to a standard connecting rod but is threaded distally so it can be anchored to the ring with hex nuts. The use of paired spherical nuts and washers permits slight angulation of the connecting rod (See Figure 8-16A & B). In this system, there are 2 kinds of clamps. A wire fixation clamp (called a cannulated/slotted wire fixation bolt) is used to anchor fixation wires to the ring and is secured to the ring with a hex nut. Standard single external fixation clamps are used to secure pins to the hybrid connecting rod. There are two types of fixation wire that can be used with the ring. The smooth wire is similar to a small Steinmann pin but with a different type of cutting point. The stopper or olive wire has a rounded deposit of stainless steel in the middle that presses against the cortex of the bone to enhance stability.

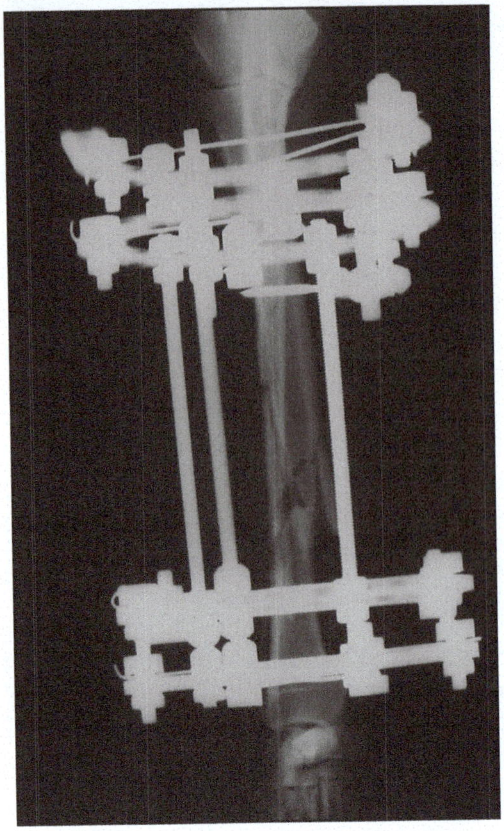

**Figure 8-15.** Ring fixation of distal radial fracture. This apparatus utilizes tension wires and is useful for small bone segments.

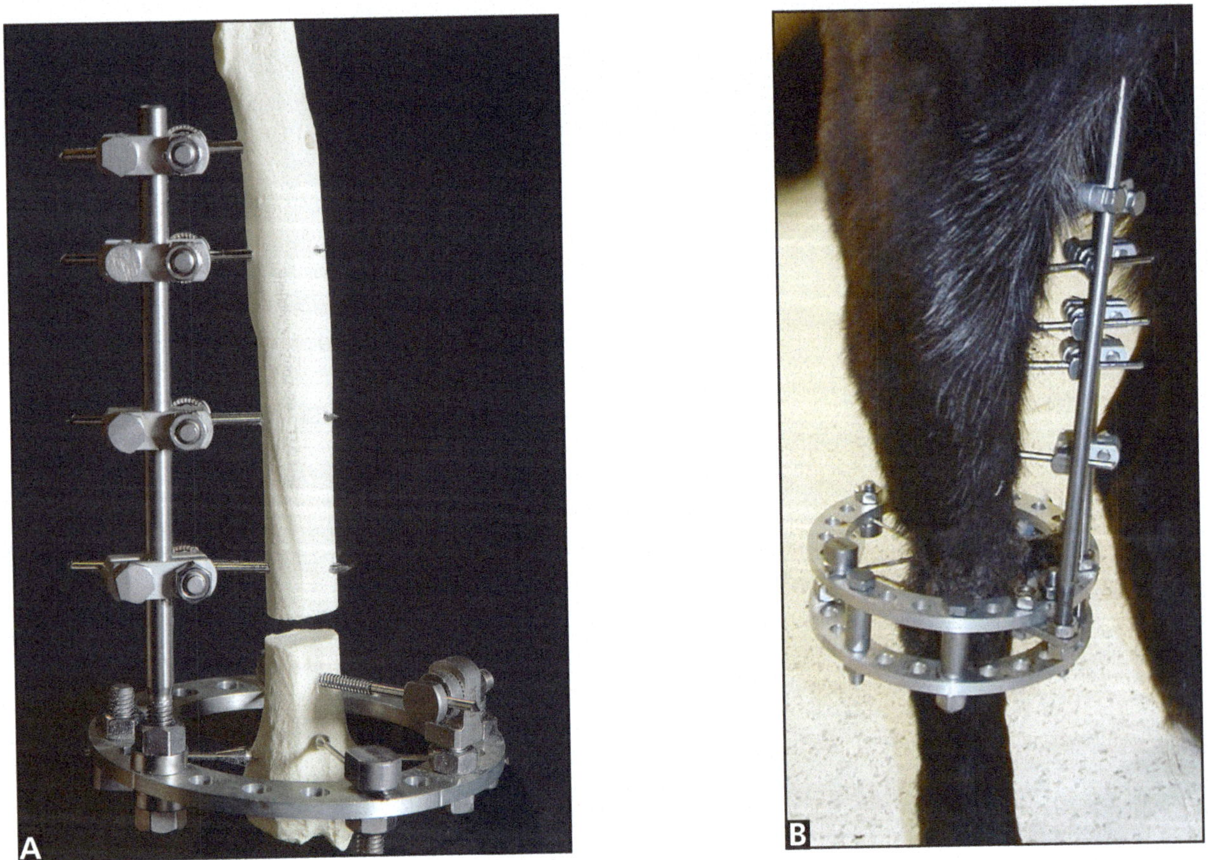


**Figure 8-16. A.** Hybrid external fixator. The small distal fracture fragment is supported with a ring and tensioned stopper wires. There is a one-hole post added to the ring to support a half-pin in the distal fragment. A hybrid connecting rod is secured to the ring with spherical nuts and washers. Half pins are added to the hybrid connecting rod using single clamps. **B.** A patient approximately 2 months postoperatively for stabilization of a juxta-articular tibial fracture. There are 2 distal rings in this frame connected with 40 mm bolts and 20 mm spacers. Half pins are secured to a hybrid connecting rod. A secondary connecting rod is secured to the distal ring with a two-hole plate and hex nuts and to the primary connecting rod with a double clamp.

A secondary connecting rod provides further stability. The secondary rod consists of a hybrid rod secured to the distal ring with hex nuts and then to the primary connecting rod with a double clamp. If a degree of angulation is desired in the secondary rod, spherical washers can be placed between the ring and the hex nut. Spherical washers are always used in pairs with one on either side of the ring. (See Figure 84 B).

## Suggested Readings


1. Farese JP, Lewis DD, Cross AR et al. Use of IMEX SK-circular external fixator hybrid constructs for fracture stabilization in dogs and cats. J Am Anim Hosp Assoc 38:279-289, 2002.
2. Griffin H, Toombs JP, Bronson DG et al. Mechanical evaluation of a tapered thread-run-out half-pin designed for external skeletal fixation in small animals. Vet Comp Orthop Traumatol 24:257-61, 2011.
3. Kraus KH, Toombs JP, Ness MG. External Fixation in Small Animal Practice. Malden, MA: Blackwell Science Ltd, 2003.
4. Lewis DD, Bronson DG, Samchukov ML et al. Biomechanics of circular external skeletal fixation. Vet Surg 27:454-464, 1998.


# Distal Radial and Ulnar Fractures: Noncomminuted and Closed

### Definition and Indications

Fractures of the distal radius and ulna are the most common fractures of the antebrachium in dogs. These fractures usually involve the junction of the distal metaphysis and diaphysis so the distal fragment is small. External coaptation with a cast or splint is not indicated for repair of most distal radial fractures. The ideal fracture to repair with external coaptation is a transverse diaphyseal fracture with at least 50% contact between the fracture ends. However, many radius and ulna fractures are close to the joint and have an oblique conformation. The obliquity of the fracture and the distraction from extension and flexor tendons promotes over-riding of the fracture ends. There is often inadequate biomechanical stability to have successful healing without surgery. The risk of treating distal radial and ulna fractures with external coaptation is magnified in toy and small breeds of dogs. Non-union of the distal radius and ulna in small breeds is a frequently reported complication. External coaptation and intramedullary pinning were found to be unacceptable methods of fixation for small dogs. The etiology of fracture non-union with external coaptation in small breeds is thought to involve poor bone apposition and stability and a more tenuous regional blood supply compared to larger dogs. Bone plate fixation has been shown to promote good to excellent fracture healing in toy and small breed dogs. Specialized plates such as stainless steel "T-plates" are applicable to this fracture. The T-shape affords greater screw placement in the distal fragment compared to a straight plate. Veterinary T-plates are available in a range of sizes that will accommodate 1.5 mm to 3.5 mm screws (Synthes, West Chester, PA; New Generation Devices, Glen Rock, NJ).

There is concern about the long-term effect of a bone plate on the bone density of the distal radius especially in small dogs. This concern has not been clearly documented. Plate removal has been advocated by some to avoid stress shielding and subsequent osteopenia. There are biodegradable bone plates (Biodegradable self-reinforced polylactide plates, Boehringher Ingelheim, Ingelheim, Germany) that can be used for radial fractures. They will resorb thus preventing stress shielding. These plates were found to be biomechanically weak unless two are stacked together to provide a more rigid plate.

Less common fractures include those involving the styloid process of the radius or ulna and the articular surface of the distal radius. Fractures of the styloid processes are generally repaired using tension band fixation. The ulnar and radial styloid processes serve as the origin of the ulnar and short radial collateral ligaments, respectively, and require surgical stabilization if fractured. Fractures of the articular surface of the radius are repaired with lag screws or bone plating. Highly comminuted articular fractures are best treated by a pancarpal arthrodesis (see pancarpal arthrodesis for carpal hyperextension injury).

## Techniques

### Bone Plate Fixation

Bone plates are usually placed on the cranial surface of the distal radius to stabilize transverse or oblique fractures. The patient is placed in a lateral position with the affected limb uppermost. To provide better access to the cranial aspect of the distal limb, sandbags or a positioning mat may be used to prop the patient into a semi sternal position. The skin incision is made on the dorsal surface of the radius and extends from the juncture of the cephalic and accessory cephalic veins to the middle of the metacarpus. The incision is lateral to the accessory cephalic vein (See Figure 8-6).

The deep fascial tissue is incised between the tendons of the extensor carpi radialis and the common digital extensor tendons. The abductor pollicis longus muscle and tendon cross over the extensor carpi radialis. It is usually necessary to transect the abductor pollicis longus tendon for adequate access to the distal radius. The fascial and periosteal tissue adjacent to the extensor tendons is incised so the extensor carpi radialis tendon is retracted medially and the common digital extensor tendon is retracted laterally. An arthrotomy incision can be made to visualize the radio-carpal joint and thus identify the distal limit for the bone plate (See Figure 8-6).

Pointed reduction forceps are used to grasp the proximal and distal fracture fragments and obtain anatomical reduction. Additional pointed reduction forceps can be used to cross an oblique fracture line and maintain reduction for plate application. Stainless steel "T" plates are available in small and larger sizes (1.5/2.0 mm and 2.7/3.5). The smaller plate is used for toy and small breed dogs and the larger plate for medium to larger dogs. The distal aspect of the plate is secured first to allow optimal positioning on the small fragment of bone followed by the proximal placement of the plate (Figure 8-17A & B).

The transected abductor pollicus longus tendon is sutured to adjacent tissues. The fascia, subcutaneous tissue and skin layers are closed. In the presence of tension, multiple punctate relaxing incisions may be placed (See Chapter 3).

### Tension Band Fixation of Styloid Process Fractures

A fracture of the ulnar styloid process is repaired with a tension band fixation using a Kirschner wire and figure eight cerclage wire. The patient is placed in lateral recumbency with the affected limb uppermost. The skin and subcutaneous tissues are incised directly over the lateral surface of the ulna, from the midshaft to the styloid process. The deep fascia is incised and surrounding tissue is elevated as needed to visualize the fracture and collateral ligament (Figure 8-18A, B & C). The fracture is held in position with pointed reduction forceps and a Kirschner wire is placed from the distal to the proximal fracture fragment. A small drill bit is used to place a hole in the proximal portion of the ulna or adjacent radius. A figure-8 cerclage wire is placed between the distal end of the Kirschner wire and through the hole in the proximal bone (See Figure 8-18B). The wire is tightened and cut.

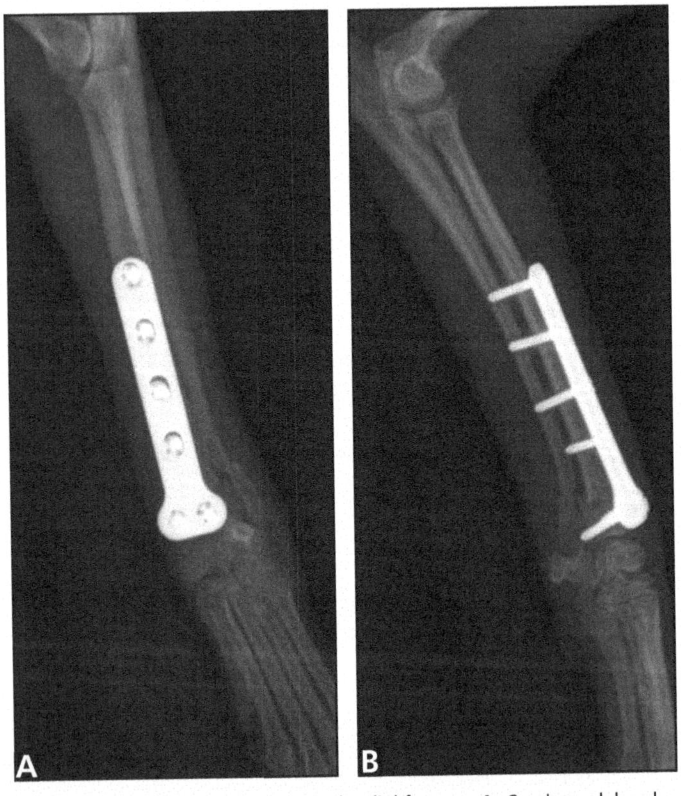


**Figure 8-17.** T plate fixation of distal radial fracture. **A.** Craniocaudal and **B.** lateral projections.

The fascia, subcutaneous tissue and skin are closed in layers.

A fracture of the radial styloid process is repaired with a tension band fixation or with a lag screw. To approach the styloid process of the radius, the patient is placed in dorsal recumbency for draping. The affected limb is abducted to expose the medial surface. The skin, subcutaneous, and deep fascial tissues are incised from the distal one-third of the radius to the proximal metacarpal bone. Surrounding tissue is elevated as needed to visualize the fracture and collateral ligaments. Small radial styloid fracture fragments can be stabilized with tension band fixation as described for ulnar styloid process fractures. Radial styloid fractures with a larger fragment can be stabilized with lag screw fixation. The screw size is usually 3.5 or 4.0 mm for a medium to large sized patient. The near cortex is drilled according to the diameter of the threads of the screw and the far cortex to the core diameter of the screw. The near cortex is slightly countersunk to seat the head of the screw. The screw is tightened. A Kirschner wire may also be placed adjacent to the lag screw for added stability (See Figure 8-18C).

The dermis and skin are closed in layers.

### Lag Screw Fixation of Distal Articular Fractures of the Radius

Distal articular fractures of the radius can be simple two piece fractures or multifragmentary. Simple two piece articular fractures are radial styloid fractures involving varying degrees of the articular surface. Larger fragments can be stabilized with 2 lag screws (Figure 8-19A). Multifragmentary fractures may be stabilized with a medially applied bone plate and screws (Figure 8-10B). Highly comminuted distal radial

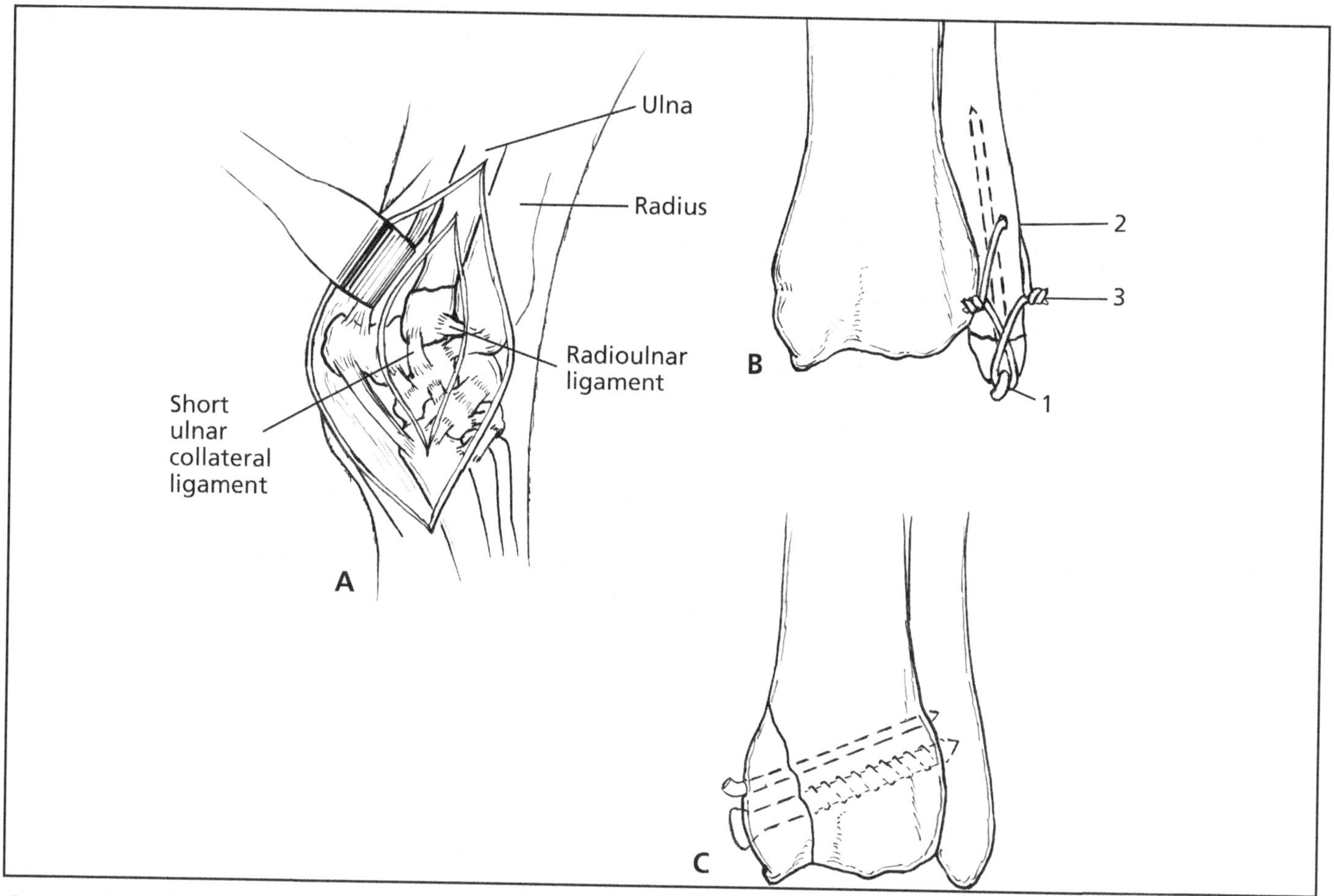


**Figure 8-18.** Styloid fracture: tension band fixation. **A.** Approach to the ulnar styloid process. Skin and subcutaneous tissues directly over the distal ulna are incised and retracted. The radioulnar and short ulnar collateral ligaments are visualized and preserved. **B.** Fractured ulnar styloid process is repaired with a tension band fixation using a K-wire and figure eight cerclage wire. The K-wire is placed from the distal to the proximal fracture fragment *(1)*. A small drill bit is used to place a hole in the proximal portion of the ulna or adjacent radius *(2)*. A figure-8 cerclage wire is placed between the distal end of the K-wire and through the hole in the proximal bone *(3)*. **C.** Fixation of radial styloid fracture with a lag screw and adjacent Kirschner wire. (After Johnson AL, Dunning D. Atlas of Orthopedic Surgical Procedure of the Dog and Cat. St. Louis: Elsevier Saunders, 2005, 31).

fractures are best treated with pancarpal arthrodesis. For fracture repair, the patient is placed in dorsal recumbency for draping. The affected limb is abducted to expose the medial surface. The skin, subcutaneous, and deep fascial tissues are incised from the mid-radius to the proximal metacarpal bone. Exposure may be improved by incising the abductor pollicus longus tendon (See Figure 8-3). To visualize the articular surface of the distal radius, the skin is retracted cranially and the joint capsule incised. The fracture fragments are reduced and held in place with pointed reduction forceps. Stabilization is achieved with lag screws or a medially applied bone plate (Figure 8-19A & B). Lag screw fixation is similar to that for radial styloid process fracture described previously. For bone plate fixation, the size of the plate is 2.7 mm for a small to medium size dog and 3.5 mm for a larger dog. The distal lag screw is placed through the plate first. The near cortex is drilled according to the diameter of the threads of the screw and the far cortex to the core diameter of the screw. The proximal screws are placed (See Figure 8-19).

The dermis and skin are closed in layers. In the presence of tension, multiple punctate relaxing incisions may be placed (See Chapter 3).

## Aftercare

Ulnar styloid fracture repairs are stabilized with a soft padded bandage and splint for approximately 2 weeks. Radial styloid and intra-articular radial fracture repairs are stabilized with a soft padded bandage and splint for approximately 4 weeks. Distal radial fractures repaired with a bone plate are stabilized with a soft padded bandage and splint for approximately 2 weeks after surgery. The splint extends from the digits to the proximal radius. The splint is changed 1 to 2 days after surgery and then weekly. Patients are confined to an indoor space or crate for 8 weeks after surgery and exercise is restricted to short (5 to 10 minute) leash walks 4 times daily. Radiographs are obtained 8 weeks postoperatively. If progression of healing is apparent and implants are stable, the length of leash walks are increased. Off-leash activity is allowed by 12 weeks postoperatively.

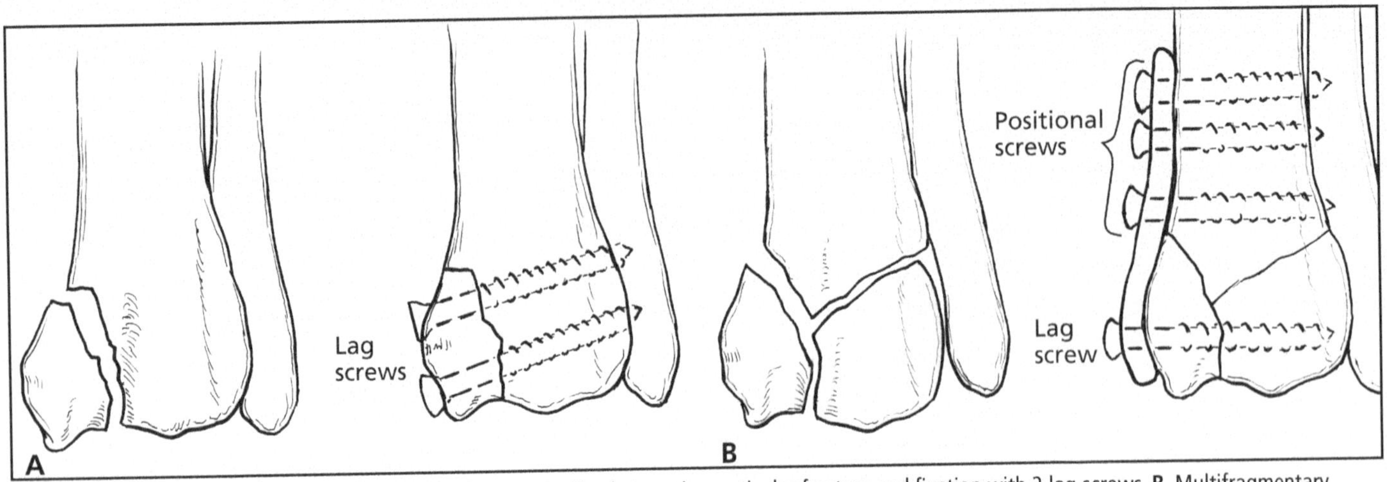


**Figure 8-19.** Distal articular radial fractures: screw fixation. **A.** Simple two piece articular fracture and fixation with 2 lag screws. **B.** Multifragmentary fracture stabilized with a medially applied bone plate using a lag screw at the articular portion and positional screws proximally.

### Advantages and Disadvantages

Veterinary T-plates are available in a range of sizes that will accommodate 1.5 mm to 3.5 mm screws. These plates are very suitable for distal radius and ulna fractures in toy breed to large breed dogs and result in successful healing for most patients. The disadvantage of placing a bone plate on the cranial surface of the distal radius is decreased carpal flexion. This is likely a consequence of the plate interfering with extensor tendons or postoperative fibrosis. This does not cause a clinical problem with function or appearance. Range of motion can be improved with physical therapy.

The advantage of surgically stabilizing radial and ulnar styloid fractures is securing the origin of the short radial and ulnar collateral ligaments. Casting or splinting will not promote reliable ligament function and could lead to long term degenerative change.

## Suggested Readings

1. Glennon JC, Flanders JA, Beck KA et al. The effect of long-term bone plate application for fixation of radial fractures in dogs. Vet Surg 23:40-47, 1994.
2. Hamilton MH, Langley Hobbs SJ. Use of veterinary mini 'T'-plate for stabilization of distal radius and ulna fractures in toy breed dogs. Vet Comp Orthop Traumatol 18:18-25, 2005.
3. Larsen LJ, Roush JK, McLaughlin RM. Bone plate fixation of distal radius and ulna fractures in small- and miniature-breed dogs. J Am Anim Hosp Assoc 35:243-250, 1999.
4. Saikku-Backstrom A, Raiha JE, Valimaa T et al. Repair of radial fractures in toy breed dogs with self-reinforced biodegradable bone plates, metal screws, and light-weight external coaptation. Vet Surg 34:11-17, 2005.

## Distal Radial and Ulnar Fractures: Comminuted or Open

### Definition and Indications

Type Ia or Ib external fixator systems are applicable to radial fractures in both small and large breeds of dogs. Although any radial fracture can be repaired with an external fixator, external fixation is particularly useful for comminuted or open fractures. External fixator frames can usually be applied to the distal limb using a closed or semi-closed surgical approach. Hybrid external fixators are useful for metaphyseal radial fractures that have a small fragment of bone distally.

### Technique

#### Linear External Fixation for Radial Fractures

The limb is surgically prepared and suspended from a ceiling hook. The limb should be positioned directly under the ceiling anchor so it is as straight as possible. The fracture site is palpated to ascertain alignment. If needed, an incision can be made directly over the fracture site in order to manipulate fragments into alignment. The landmark for the proximal radial pin is the head of the radius which can be palpated on the lateral aspect of the limb. The proximal pin is placed at least 3 to 4 cm distal to the head of the radius. Distally the radiocarpal joint is palpated or identified with a small needle and the most distal pin is placed 3 to 4 cm proximal to this site. To place a type Ia system pins are placed in a medial-lateral or cranial-medial to caudal-lateral direction. To place a type Ib system one plane of pins is cranial-medial to caudal-lateral and the second plane of pins is cranial-lateral to caudal-medial (See Figure 8-13).

After placing the proximal and distal pins, the

connecting rod is secured with single clamps. Selecting the largest connecting rod and clamps that will fit the pins improves stability. The remaining pins are distributed along the bone and secured to the connecting bar with single clamps.

### Hybrid External Fixation for Distal Radial Fractures

The patient is placed in sternal-lateral recumbency with the limb pulled cranially. Towels or sandbags placed underneath the patient help to attain a sternal-lateral position. The patient may also be positioned in dorsal recumbency with the limb abducted and pulled caudally (positioning depends on surgeon's preference). The distal ring of the fixator is placed first. A ring size is chosen that leaves ample space between the ring and skin to allow for postoperative swelling. A small stab incision is made in the skin at the proposed site for the first wire—usually starting at the cranio-medial or craniolateral aspect of the distal radius. Using a high speed drill, a stopper wire is placed from one side of the ring to the other on the lower (more distal) side of the ring. The wire is secured to the fixation bolts (cannulated/slotted bolts) on each side of the ring. The wire is placed either through the hole in the bolt or through the slot located abaxially. A second stopper wire is placed on the upper surface of the ring at a 45 to 90 degree angle to the first wire. This wire is similarly secured to the ring (See Figure 8-16). Fixation wires are tensioned using a wire tensioner device.

A hybrid rod is secured to the lateral or medial aspect of the ring with hex nuts or paired spherical nuts and washers. A single clamp is placed proximally on the hybrid connecting rod. A stab incision approximately 1 cm long is made in the skin and an appropriately sized drill bit is used to make a guide hole prior to pin insertion. The positive profile end-threaded pin (half pin) is advanced through the clamp and through both cortices of bone. The clamp is tightened to secure the pin. Two to 3 additional half pins are added to the hybrid connecting rod. If there is room in the distal fragment, an additional wire or half pin can be added by mounting it to 1- or 2-holed post that is secured to the ring (Figure 8-16).

### Aftercare

Pin tract sites must be kept clean and shifting of the skin adjacent to the pin tract should be minimized. The pin tracts are swabbed with sterile betadine or coated with triple antibiotic ointment when the bandage is changed during the first one to two weeks of surgery. The skin is stabilized by placing foam pads or gauze sponges between the skin and connecting rods of the fixator. The entire fixator is then covered with a soft padded bandage and changed weekly. By 3 weeks after surgery, the pin tract sites should be stabilized and the fixator is simply covered with soft padded bandage material. The fixator components should be checked for loosening 2 to 4 weeks postoperatively and tightened if necessary. Radiographs are performed approximately 8 weeks after surgery to assess healing and again in 4 weeks if necessary until fixator removal.

### Advantages and Disadvantages

A closed or semi-closed approach is advantageous for promoting biologic fracture healing which is especially meaningful in a comminuted fracture. The benefit of a hybrid fixator is the ability to obtain multiple points of fixation in a small distal fragment using tensioned wires. The disadvantage of external fixation is the potential for pin tract infections and the need for more frequent rechecks than are usually required for bone plates. Pin tract infections respond to antibiotic therapy and resolve with pin removal.

## Suggested Readings

1. Farese JP, Lewis DD, Cross AR et al. Use of IMEX SK-circular external fixator hybrid constructs for fracture stabilization in dogs and cats. J Am Anim Hosp Assoc 38:279-289, 2002.
2. Lewis DD, Bronson DG, Samchukov ML et al. Biomechanics of circular external skeletal fixation. Vet Surg 27:454-464, 1998.

## Angular Limb Deformity

### Definition and Indications

In a young animal, any forelimb trauma has the potential to induce an angular limb deformity. The distal ulnar physis is especially vulnerable to traumatic injury due to its conical shape. This shape, unique to dogs, has a physiologic purpose. The distal ulnar physis provides 100% of the long bone growth to the ulna distal to the elbow joint whereas radial growth is shared by the distal and proximal physes (60% distal and 40% proximal). The conical shape of the distal ulnar physis increases the growth surface area by 1.5 times over a flat area of the same diameter. This shape also carries a greater risk of crushing injury (Salter Harris V) because a shearing force that otherwise could spare the germinal cells translates into a crushing force on at least one side of the ulna. Crushing injury damages the vascular supply to germinal cells in the physis and leads to premature closure. Because the radius and ulna are connected by the interosseous and the radioulnar ligaments, stagnated growth of the ulna interferes with radial growth. Typical angular changes of the radius are: valgus deformity, craniocaudal bending (procurvatum), rotational deformity, and distal ulnar subluxation in the elbow joint. The potential for traumatic injury to the distal radial or ulnar physis should be considered in any forelimb trauma case in a young dog. Cellular injury at the level of the physis has been shown to precede the onset of carpal valgus by 2 to 4 weeks. The earliest radiographic sign of physeal closure of the distal ulna is an area of closure at the apex (pointed) area of the physis followed in 3 to 4 weeks by growth plate ossification. Young dogs with seemingly mild injuries, such as a history of jumping or a greenstick fracture of the radius, are at risk for angular limb deformity. Owners should be cautioned to observe for angular changes in these cases. Besides Salter Harris crushing injury, other causes of physeal closure include breed proclivities, synostosis between the radius and ulna, and inflammatory conditions such as hypertrophic osteodystrophy. Chondrodystrophic dogs are predisposed to angular deformities. Giant breed dogs may have retained cartilaginous cores that disrupt growth. Synostosis between the radius and ulna develops from diaphyseal fractures of the bones that heal with a common callus or from surgical stabilization that bridges the 2 bones in a growing animal.

Surgical correction of forelimb deformities requires assessment of which growth plate(s) are closed, the degree of angulation, and whether there is reduced range of motion or discomfort in the elbow or carpal joints. The goal of surgery is to achieve varus-valgus, rotational and procurvatum angles that are normal or close to normal. Correction in the cranial-caudal plane is prioritized compared to the sagittal plane. Animals tolerate excessive procurvatum better than varus-valgus or rotational deformity. The choice for which surgical technique to use depends on the degree of angulation and the growth potential remaining in that patient. The least invasive and least technically demanding technique is partial distal ulnar ostectomy for premature closure of the distal ulnar physis. As the sole method of treatment, this procedure is most effective in young dogs (median age 5 months) with less than 25 degrees of carpal valgus deformity. Partial ulnar ostectomy must be combined with corrective radial osteotomy or ostectomy in mature patients or with immature patients having more pronounced angulation. Partial ulnar ostectomy will not be successful as the sole method if there is partial closure of the distal radial physis as well as ulnar physeal closure. Partial closure of the radial physis usually affects the lateral portion of the physis. As the medial portion of the radius continues to grow, valgus angulation of the distal radius continues despite release from the ulna. This may account for some of the failures of ulnar ostectomy alone to correct radial deformities. Preoperative radiographs are carefully evaluated to fully assess physeal involvement.

Correction of the radius can be performed as an oblique osteotomy, a closed wedge ostectomy or dome-shaped osteotomy. For all of these procedures, it is also necessary to perform an ulnar ostectomy as described to permit movement of the radius. An ostectomy, versus an ulnar osteotomy, minimizes visible protrusion of the ulna that can occur after angular correction. Radial osteotomy or ostectomy is designed to correct rotational, varus-valgus, and procurvatum deformity. Patients that have significant loss of limb length, greater than 20% compared to the normal side, are considered for distraction osteogenesis with a ring or hybrid external fixator.

Stabilization of radial osteotomies or ostectomies is achieved using either bone plates or external fixation. A T-plate is useful for maximizing screw purchase in the small fragment of the distal radius (See Distal Radial and Ulnar Fractures: Non-comminuted and Closed (See Figure 8-17). External fixation options include linear, circular or hybrid frames (See Fractures of the Radius and Ulna, Introduction: External Fixation for Distal Limb Fractures (See Figure 8-16). Linear frames consist of threaded pins secured to connecting rods with clamps. Circular frames are constructed with tensioned wires anchored to aluminum rings. The rings are connected to each other by means of threaded connecting rods. Hybrid frames combine both ring and linear connecting rod components. A hybrid connecting rod is threaded at one end so it can be anchored to a distal ring using paired hex nuts. The remainder of the rod is smooth to accommodate standard linear fixation pins.

Timing of surgical correction is most urgent when joint subluxation is present. Patients are evaluated for elbow or radiocarpal joint pain by putting these joints through a range of motion. A painful response suggests joint subluxation. Radiographs are useful for confirming the presence of subluxation of the elbow joint but less so for the radiocarpal joint. Subluxation of the radiocarpal joint is difficult to appreciate radiographically because craniocaudal deformities obscure the appearance of the joint. Suspicion of radiocarpal joint subluxation is therefore based on clinical signs. The presence of advanced osteoarthritic change or deformed bony structures in the radiocarpal joint is an indication for angular correction and joint arthrodesis.

## Techniques

### Preoperative Assessment

Surgical correction begins by accurate preoperative

assessment of the degree of deformity. An accurate method of measurement, the center of rotation of angulation or CORA, has been described. This technique involves determining the angle formed by the joint surfaces of the elbow and radiocarpal joints (the joint orientation lines) with the anatomic line of the long axis of the radius (the anatomic axis). In the craniocaudal view, the joint orientation line for the elbow is drawn from the lateral-most aspect of the radial head to the medial-most aspect of the medial coronoid process. The joint orientation line for the carpus is drawn along the articular surface of the distal radius (Figure 8-20A). In the craniocaudal view, the anatomic axis of the radius is drawn by connecting points in the middle of the bone 25%, 50%, and 75% along its length. In the craniocaudal view of a normal dog, the radial anatomic axis intersects with the joint orientation line to form an angle that is close to perpendicular (85° at the medial aspect of the elbow joint and 87° at the lateral aspect of the radiocarpal joint). These angles are called the joint orientation angles. The vertical line corresponding to the joint orientation angle is the joint orientation axis.

The anatomic axis and the joint orientation axis should overlap. In angular limb cases, these lines do not overlap. The angle formed by the intersection of the joint orientation axis and the anatomic axis is the degree of deformity. If the deformity involves just one joint—usually the radiocarpal joint—it is a uniapical deformity (Figure 8-20B). If both the radiocarpal and elbow joint reference axes do not overlap the anatomic axis, there is a biapical deformity (Figure 8-20C). Corrective osteotomies may be required at both sites to realign the elbow and carpal joints. Biapical deformities that are on opposite sides of the anatomic axis are called partially compensated. A proximal varus deformity with a distal valgus deformity is a common example of a partially compensated deformity.

There is normally curvature present in the canine radius in the sagittal plane. The angle of natural procurvatum is approximately 25 degrees (Figure 8-20D).

## Partial Ulnar Ostectomy

Partial ulnar ostectomy involves excising a portion of distal ulna to release the "bowstring" effect of a shortened ulna on the radius. The patient is placed

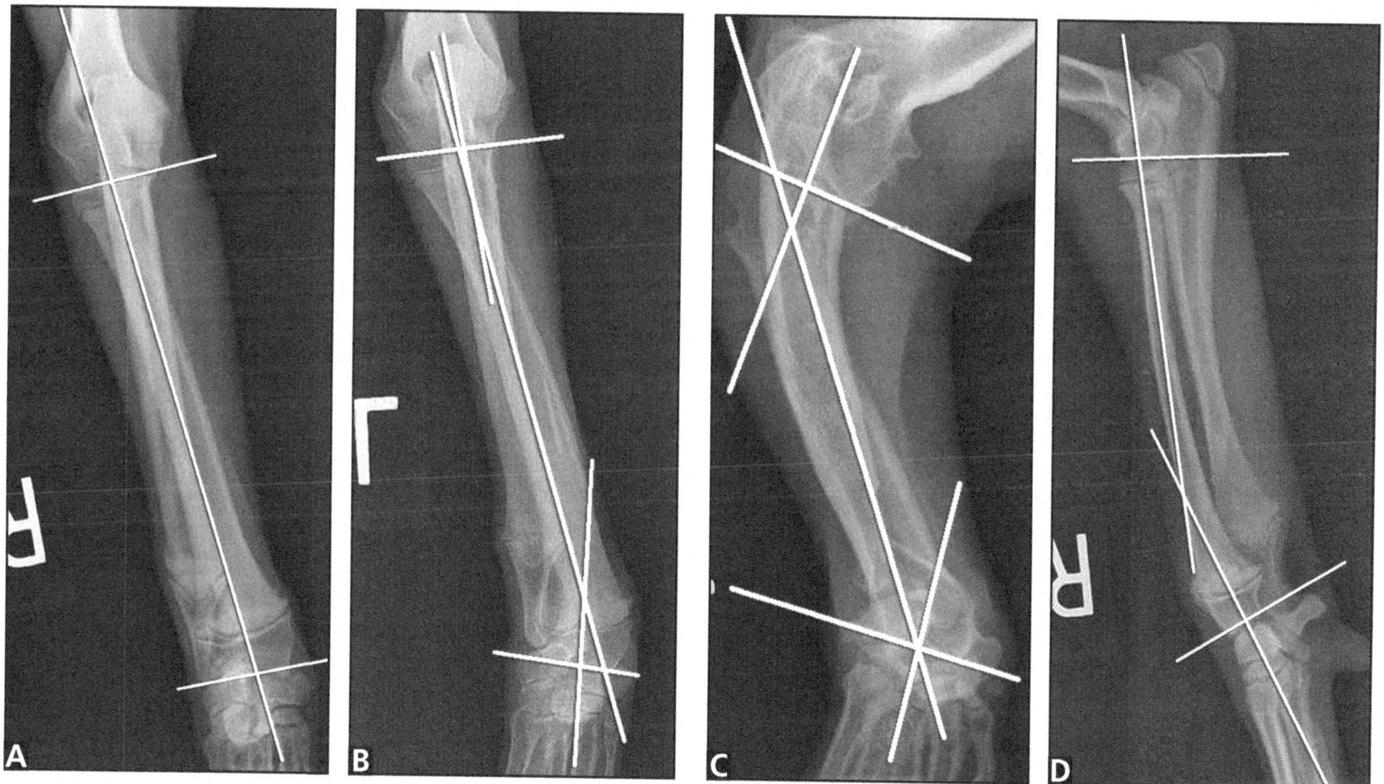


**Figure 8-20.** Angular limb deformities: Normal, uniapical and biapical. **A.** Normal radius: In the craniocaudal view of a normal dog, the radial anatomic axis intersects with the joint orientation line to form an angle that is close to perpendicular (85° at the medial aspect of the elbow joint and 87° at the lateral aspect of the radiocarpal joint). These angles are called the joint orientation angles. The vertical line corresponding to the joint orientation angle is the joint orientation axis. The anatomic axis and the joint orientation axis should overlap. In angular limb cases, these lines do not overlap. **B.** Uniapical deformity: The angle formed by the intersection of the joint orientation axis and the anatomic axis is the degree of valgus deformity. The point of intersection of the joint orientation axis and the anatomic axis is called the center of rotation of angulation or CORA. **C.** Biapical deformity: If both the elbow joint and the carpal joint orientation axes do not overlap the anatomic axis, there is a biapical deformity. This is a partially compensated deformity because the direction of the CORAs are on opposite sides of the anatomic axis. **D.** Normal canine radius in the sagittal plane. There is normal curvature in this plane.

in lateral recumbency and the abdomen is prepped and draped in as well as the forelimb. The abdomen is also prepared and draped in preparation to collect a fat graft from the umbilical region. On the forelimb, the skin incision is made directly over the ulna from the mid-diaphysis to the styloid process. The fascial layer is incised between the ulnaris lateralis and the lateral digital extensor tendons to expose the ulna. A periosteal elevator is used to elevate the surrounding musculature and Hohmann retractors are placed between the radius and ulna at the intended ostectomy site. A power oscillating saw is used to excise a portion of the distal ulna. The segment of excised bone should at least equal 1.5 times the width of the ulna or approximately 2 cm (Figure 8-21). Periosteum is removed from this site along with the bone to prevent rapid callus formation. A fat graft is harvested by incising skin and subcutaneous tissues over the umbilical region and sharply penetrating the linea to exteriorize falciform fat. A segment of fat is collected as a single block of tissue and placed at the ostectomy site. Subcutaneous tissues and skin are closed over the ulna and abdominal closure is performed routinely.

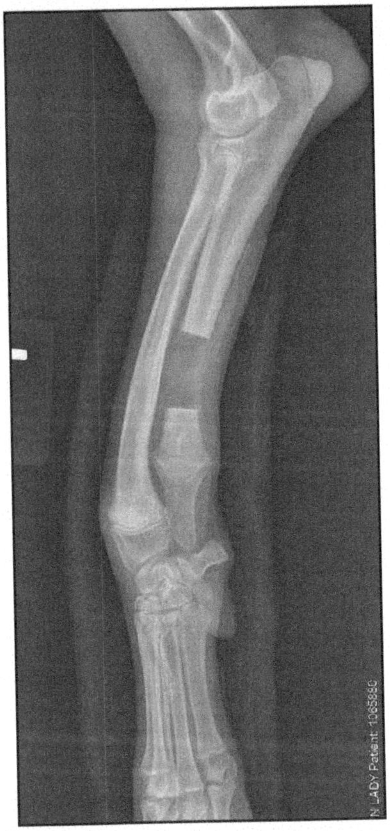

**Figure 8-21.** Partial ulnar ostectomy. A portion of the distal ulna approximately 1.5 times the width of the ulna has been removed to release the "bowstring" effect of a shortened ulna on the radius.

## Corrective Radial Ostectomy: Closed Wedge with Bone Plate Fixation

The patient is placed in sternal-lateral recumbency with the limb pulled cranially. Towels or sandbags placed underneath the patient help to attain a sternal-lateral position. A lateral approach directly over the distal ulna is made and a partial ulnar ostectomy is performed as described. The ulna must be released in order to be able to move the radius after radial ostectomy. A segment of ulna is removed rather than making a single cut so that the ulna will not protrude noticeably beneath the skin after repositioning the radius. A dorsal approach to the radius is performed by incising skin and subcutaneous layers and retracting the extensor carpi and common digital extensor tendons (See Figure 8-6). The abductor pollicus longus tendon is transected. An assistant holds the limb so that the paw is flat on the table and the entire dorsal surface of the radius is facing up. Two K-wires (.062 size) are placed prior to performing the osteotomy. Each wire is placed in a medial to lateral direction. The proximal K-wire is placed parallel to the elbow joint, and the distal one is placed parallel to the radio-carpal joint (Figure 8-22A-D). The distal K-wire is also oriented to reflect the degree of external rotation by tilting the pin to be parallel with the dorsum of the paw (Figure 8-22A inset). Using a power oscillating saw, proximal and distal cuts are made parallel with the proximal and distal K-wires. The widest portion of the wedge is medial. Excessive procurvatum (cranial-caudal) deformity is corrected by angling the blade dorsally while making the proximal cut for the wedge ostectomy. The wedge is removed. The pins are aligned parallel to one another as the ostectomy site is closed. The resulting transverse osteotomy is temporarily stabilized with two crossed K-wires. The osteotomy is then stabilized with a T-plate. A size 1.5/2.0 T-plate is placed in small dogs and a 2.7/3.5 mm in large dogs (Synthes, Paoli, PA; New Generation Devices, Glen Rock, NJ). The distal screw holes of the plate are placed first to obtain optimal positioning in the small fragment and then the remaining holes are filled. Open screw holes should be avoided directly over the osteotomy. All K-wires are removed.

Dermis and skin are closed in layers. In the presence of tension, multiple punctate relaxing incisions may be placed (See Chapter 3).

## Corrective Radial Osteotomy: Dome Osteotomy with Bone Plate Fixation

Corrective radial osteotomy can be performed using a circular saw blade (TPLO saw blades; New Generation Devices Glen Rock, NJ). The patient is placed in sternal-

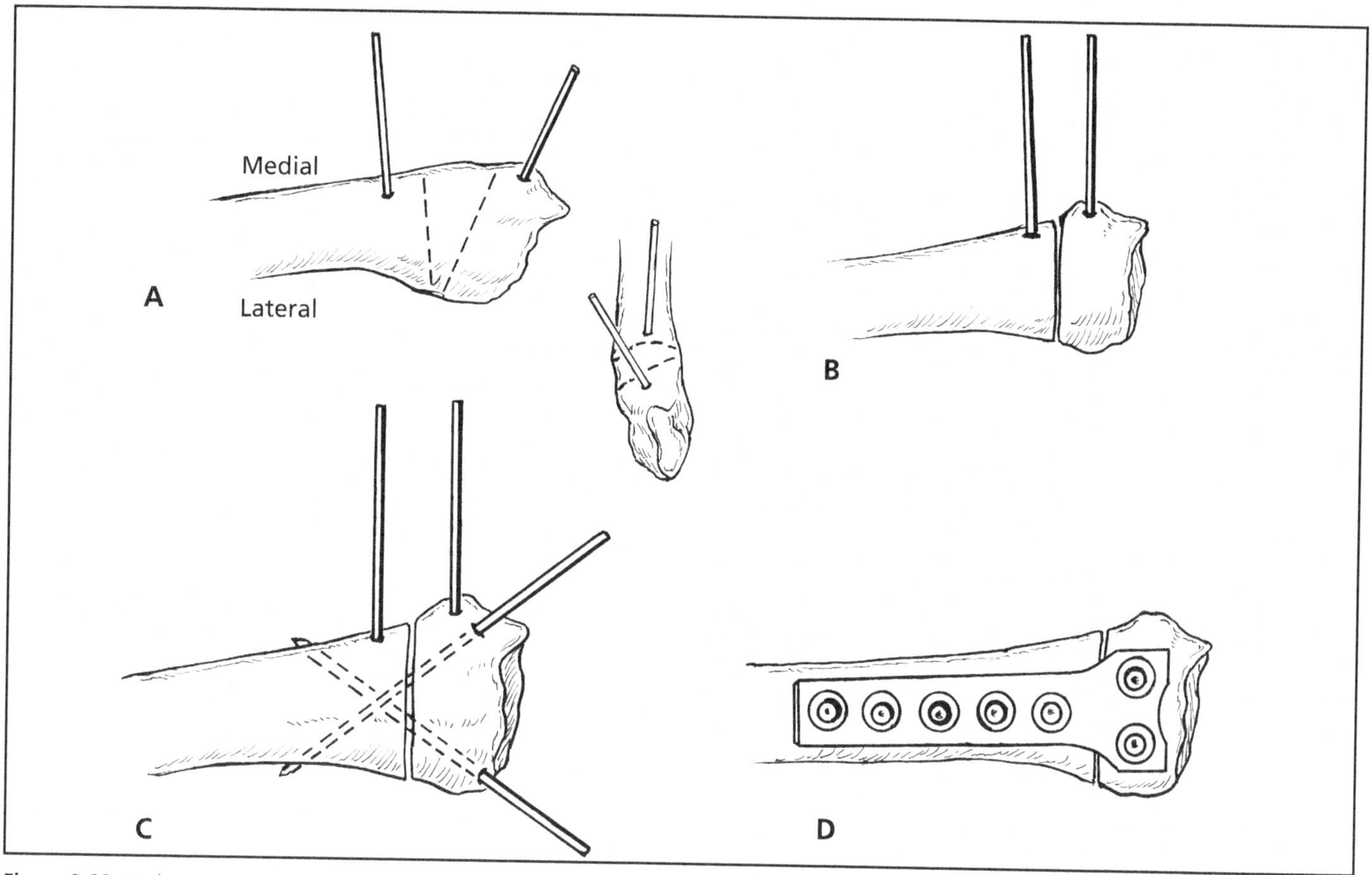


**Figure 8-22.** Wedge ostectomy and T plate fixation for angular deformity of the radius. **A.** Two K-wires are placed, in a medial to lateral direction, on either side of the proposed ostectomy. The proximal K-wire is placed parallel to the elbow joint, and the distal K-wire is placed parallel to the radiocarpal joint. The distal K-wire is oriented to reflect the degree of external rotation by tilting the wire parallel with the dorsal aspect of the paw *(inset)*. **B.** Using a power oscillating saw, proximal and distal cuts are made parallel with the proximal and distal K-wires and the wedge is removed. The widest portion of the wedge is medial. The pins are aligned parallel to one another. **C.** Additional K-wires may be placed as temporary cross pins through the osteotomy line to prepare for placing the bone plate. **D.** The resulting transverse osteotomy is stabilized with a T-plate. (After Balfour RJ, Boudrieau RJ, Gores BR. T-plate fixation of distal radial closing wedge osteotomies for treatment of angular limb deformities in 18 dogs. Vet Surg 29:207, 2000).

lateral recumbency with the limb pulled cranially. Towels or sandbags placed underneath the patient help to attain a sternal-lateral position. A lateral approach to the distal ulna is made and a partial ulnar ostectomy is performed as described. The ulna must be released in order to be able to move the radius after radial ostectomy. A segment of ulna is removed rather than making a single cut so that the ulna will not protrude noticeably beneath the skin after repositioning the radius. A dorsal approach to the radius is performed by incising skin and subcutaneous layers and retracting the extensor carpi and common digital extensor tendons (See Figure 8-6). Prior to performing the osteotomy, an assistant holds the limb so that the paw is flat on the table and the entire dorsal surface of the radius is facing up. The size of saw blade that is chosen should have a diameter that closely matches the diameter of the radius to be cut. The medial-lateral center of the blade is aligned with the center of the radius. The saw blade is offset from the CORA location by the radius of the saw blade (Figure 8-23A & B). The distal fragment is rotated until the valgus deformity is corrected. Once the desired position is established, it is helpful to place a temporary pin or cross pins across the osteotomy site during bone plate application as described for wedge ostectomy of the radius. A size 1.5/2.0 T-plate is placed in small dogs and a 2.7/3.5 mm in large dogs (Synthes, Paoli, PA; New Generation Devices, Glen Rock, NJ). The distal screw holes of the plate are placed first to obtain optimal positioning in the small fragment and then the remaining holes are filled. Open screw holes should be avoided directly over the osteotomy. All K-wires are removed.

### Corrective Radial Osteotomy: Open Wedge Stabilized with Type II External Fixator

The patient is placed in sternal-lateral recumbency with the limb pulled cranially. Towels or sandbags placed underneath the patient help to attain a sternal-lateral position. A lateral approach to the distal ulna is made and a partial ulnar ostectomy is performed as described. The ulna must be released in order to be able to move the radius after radial ostectomy. A segment of ulna is removed rather than making a single cut so that the ulna will not protrude noticeably beneath the skin after repositioning the radius. A

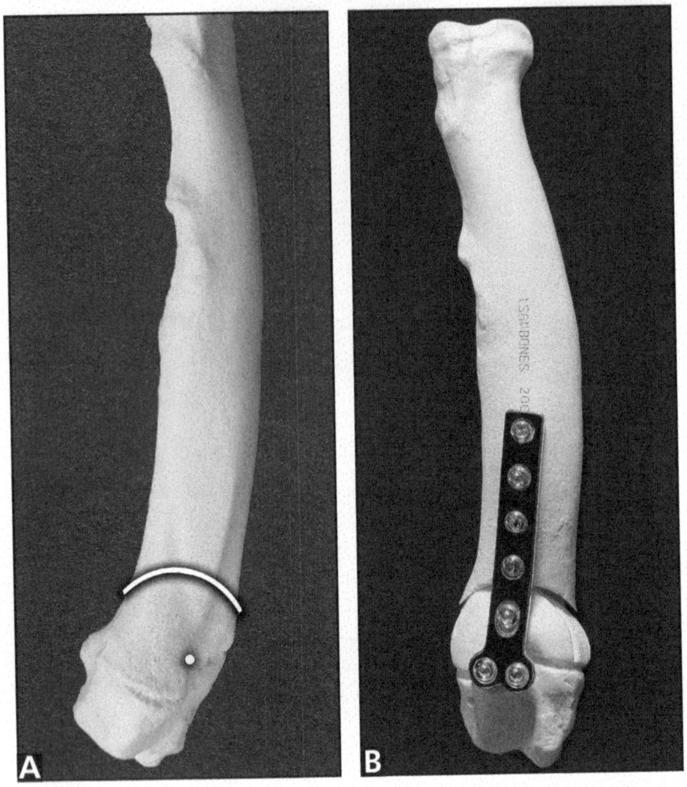


**Figure 8-23.** Circular radial osteotomy to correct angular limb deformity. Radial osteotomy can be performed using a circular saw blade. The size of saw blade that is chosen should have a diameter that closely matches the diameter of the radius to be cut. **A.** Location of the cut to be made in the distal radius using a circular saw blade. The cut is offset from the CORA location by the radius of the saw blade. **B.** The distal segment of bone is rotated into straight alignment with the proximal segment and stabilized with a T plate.

dorsal approach to the radius is performed by incising skin and subcutaneous layers and retracting the extensor carpi and common digital extensor tendons (See Figure 8-6). Prior to performing the osteotomy, an assistant holds the limb so that the paw is flat on the table and the entire dorsal surface of the radius is facing up. Centrally-threaded external fixation pins are placed transversely through stab incisions in the skin at the most proximal and distal extent of the radius (Figure 8-24A-D). Each pin is parallel to its respective joint orientation line. An oblique osteotomy is made parallel to the distal radial pin at the site of maximal deformity of the bone (the CORA) using an oscillating saw). The proximal and distal pins are then aligned so that they are parallel with one another and may be adjusted if needed so that the limb is visibly straight. The proximal and distal pins are attached to a connecting rod using single clamps. Medial and lateral connecting rods are used; thus creating a type II external fixator. A type Ib or hybrid external fixator are also well-suited for this type of osteotomy (See Figures 8-13 & 8-16).

## Aftercare

### Partial Ulnar Ostectomy

A soft padded bandage and splint are placed for approximately 1 week to protect the fat graft from motion. Follow up exam and radiographs are taken at approximately 4 weeks postoperatively. If the angular deformity has visibly progressed by evaluation of the limb and of the angles on radiographs, corrective osteotomy of the radius is required for a successful outcome. If the deformity is unchanged or improved, recheck again at 8 weeks to assess progress.

### Corrective Radial Osteotomy or Ostectomy

Exercise is restricted to a confined indoor area and short leash walks for 8 weeks postoperatively. If the radius has been stabilized with a bone plate and there are just two screws in the distal fragment, a soft padded bandage and splint may be placed for 2 to 3 weeks after surgery for supplementary stabilization. Splinting is not necessary if 3 screws are in place in the distal fragment. If the radius has been stabilized by an external fixator, the pin tract sites must be kept clean and shifting of the skin adjacent to the pin tracts should be minimized. The pin tracts are swabbed with sterile betadine or coated with triple antibiotic ointment during the first 10 to 14 days after surgery. The skin is stabilized by placing foam pads or gauze sponges between the skin and connecting rods of the fixator (See Figure 8-21). The entire fixator is then covered with a soft padded bandage and changed weekly. By 3 weeks after surgery, the pin tract sites should be stabilized and the fixator is simply covered with soft padded bandage material. The fixator components should be checked for loosening 2 to 4 weeks postoperatively and tightened if necessary.

Postoperative physical therapy is recommended to minimize the tendency for reduced range of motion of the radiocarpal joint after angular correction and bone plating. The radiocarpal joint is slowly flexed and extended 5 to 10 repetitions twice daily. If a postoperative splint has been placed, range of motion exercises are delayed until splint removal.

Radiographs are obtained 6 to 8 weeks after surgery and if needed again at 4 to 6 weeks to assess healing. Once significant bone healing is documented radiographically exercises may be gradually increased over a 4 week period of time.

## Advantages and Disadvantages

### Partial Ulnar Ostectomy

Partial ulnar ostectomy is a technically simple procedure and is less invasive than corrective radial osteotomy or

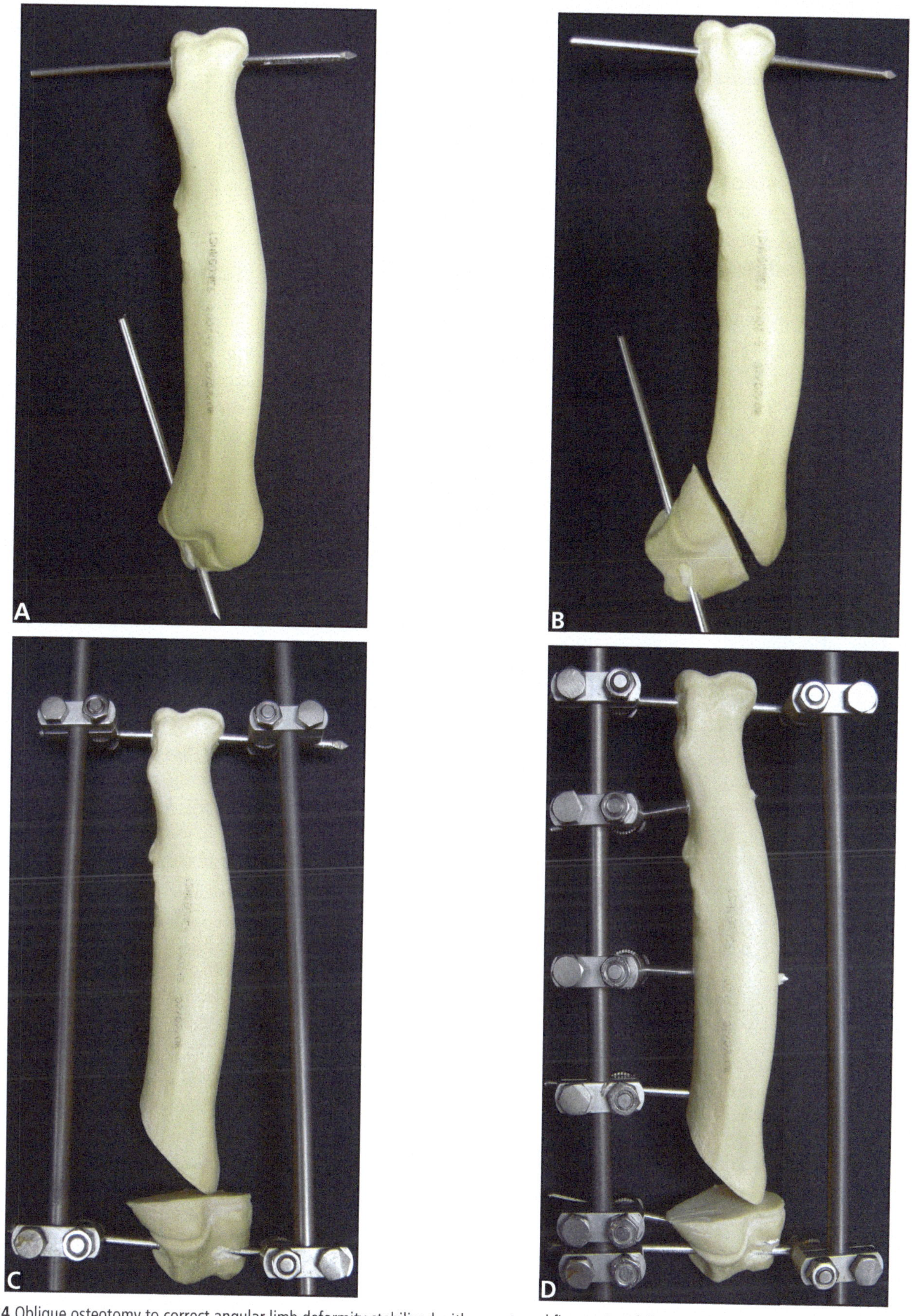


**Figure 8-24.** Oblique osteotomy to correct angular limb deformity stabilized with an external fixator. **A.** A full external fixation pin is placed parallel to the proximal joint and parallel to the distal joint. **B.** The osteotomy is made with an oscillating saw parallel to the distal pin. **C.** The pins are aligned so that they are parallel and medial and lateral connecting rods are secured to each pin with clamps. **D.** The remaining fixator frame is constructed with ½ pins.

ostectomy. If a patient's age and degree of angulation are such that partial ulnar ostectomy can be curative it is advantageous to do the procedure. If angular correction does not occur or is insufficient, a second anesthetic episode is required to correct the deformity.

### Corrective Radial Osteotomy or Ostectomy: Closed Wedge Ostectomy with Bone Plate Fixation, Dome Osteotomy with Bone Plate Fixation, Open Wedge Osteotomy with External Fixation

There are advantages to creating an osteotomy with a circular saw blade rather than a closing wedge ostectomy. By virtue of offsetting the cut by the radius of the blade, there is more room for placement of implants distally. Furthermore, the angular correction can be fine-tuned by pivoting bone segments until final alignment is achieved rather than having to create additional cuts as required with a wedge ostectomy. The disadvantage is a limited ability to correct large rotational defects with the circular osteotomy. The maximum rotational correction possible is approximately 10°.

The advantage of external fixation versus bone plating is a less invasive approach. Additionally, hybrid fixation can simplify stabilization of small distal radial fragments. It is possible to secure 2 to 3 wires to a single ring when it would not be possible to place 3 screws in a small juxta-articular fragment of bone. The disadvantage to external fixation is postoperative management of pin tract sites and the necessity for more frequent postoperative rechecks for bandage changes compared to a bone plate.

## Suggested Readings

1. Balfour RJ, Boudrieau RJ, Gores BR. T-plate fixation of distal radial closing wedge osteotomies for treatment of angular limb deformities in 18 dogs. Vet Surg 29:207-217, 2000.
2. Farese JP, Lewis DD, Cross AR et al. Use of IMEX SK-circular external fixator hybrid constructs for fracture stabilization in dogs and cats. J Amer Anim Hosp Assoc 38:279-289, 2002.
3. Fox DB, Tomlison JL, Cook JL et al. Principles of uniapical and biapical radial deformity correction using dome osteotomies and the center of rotation of angulation methodology in dogs. Vet Surg 35:67-77, 2006.
4. Henney LH, Gambardella PC. Premature closure of the ulnar physis in the dog: a retrospective clinical study. J Am Anim Hosp Assoc 25:573-581, 1989.
5. Lewis DD, Radasch RM, Beale BS et al. Initial experience with the IMEX circular external skeletal fixation system. Vet Comp Orthop Traumatol 12:118-27, 1999.
6. Quinn MK, Ehrhart N, Johnson AL et al. Realignment of the radius in canine antebrachial growth deformities treated with corrective osteotomy and bilateral (type II) external fixation. Vet Surg 29:558-563, 2000.
7. Vandewater A, Olmstead ML, Stenvenson S. Partial ulnar ostectomy with free autogenous fat grafting for treatment of radius curvus in the dog. Vet Surg 11:92-99, 1982.

# Radial Carpal Bone Fractures

## Definition and Indications

Radial carpal bone fractures are rare. They tend to occur in active sporting dogs and in dogs that are allowed ample amounts of free off-leash activity. Affected dogs are usually young to middle aged adult males and the injury is frequently bilateral. A history of a traumatic event is only rarely reported and the lameness is usually chronic, intermittent and progressive. The length of time between the onset of the problem and presentation to a veterinarian has been shown to range from months to years. Clinical signs include mild to moderate lameness, reduced range of motion, soft tissue swelling and pain on joint manipulation. Definitive diagnosis is made by radiographs. The most common appearance is a dorsal slab fracture visible in the lateral view or an oblique midbody fracture visible in the cranial caudal view (Figure 8-25A, B & C). The two fracture patterns can be present simultaneously.

The fractures may occur as a result the application of repetitive stress, an inherent weakness of the structure of the radial carpal bone, or a combination of these factors. The radial carpal bone has 3 ossification centers that should fuse by 3 to 4 months of age: the radial, central and intermediate. The plane of fusion of these ossification centers corresponds to the two main fracture lines that are seen clinically. It is possible that incomplete fusion of these ossification centers could predispose some dogs to this injury.

Optimal treatment recommendations are unclear. Clinically there has been little difference between lag screw fixation, small fragment removal or conservative therapy. Pancarpal arthrodesis has shown the most satisfactory long term results. A reasonable approach would be to recommend lag screw fixation for the cases that are diagnosed early and do not have degenerative joint disease on initial radiographs. If degenerative change is already present, pancarpal arthrodesis is recommended as a first choice procedure.

## Technique

### Lag screw fixation

The patient is placed in sternal-lateral recumbency with the limb pulled cranially. Towels or sandbags placed underneath the patient help to attain a sternal-lateral position. The skin and subcutaneous tissues are incised dorsally, beginning 3 to 4 cm proximal to the radial carpal joint and extending distally to the middle of the metacarpus (See Figure 8-6). Deep dissection is continued between the extensor carpi radialis and common digital extensor tendons and the tendons are

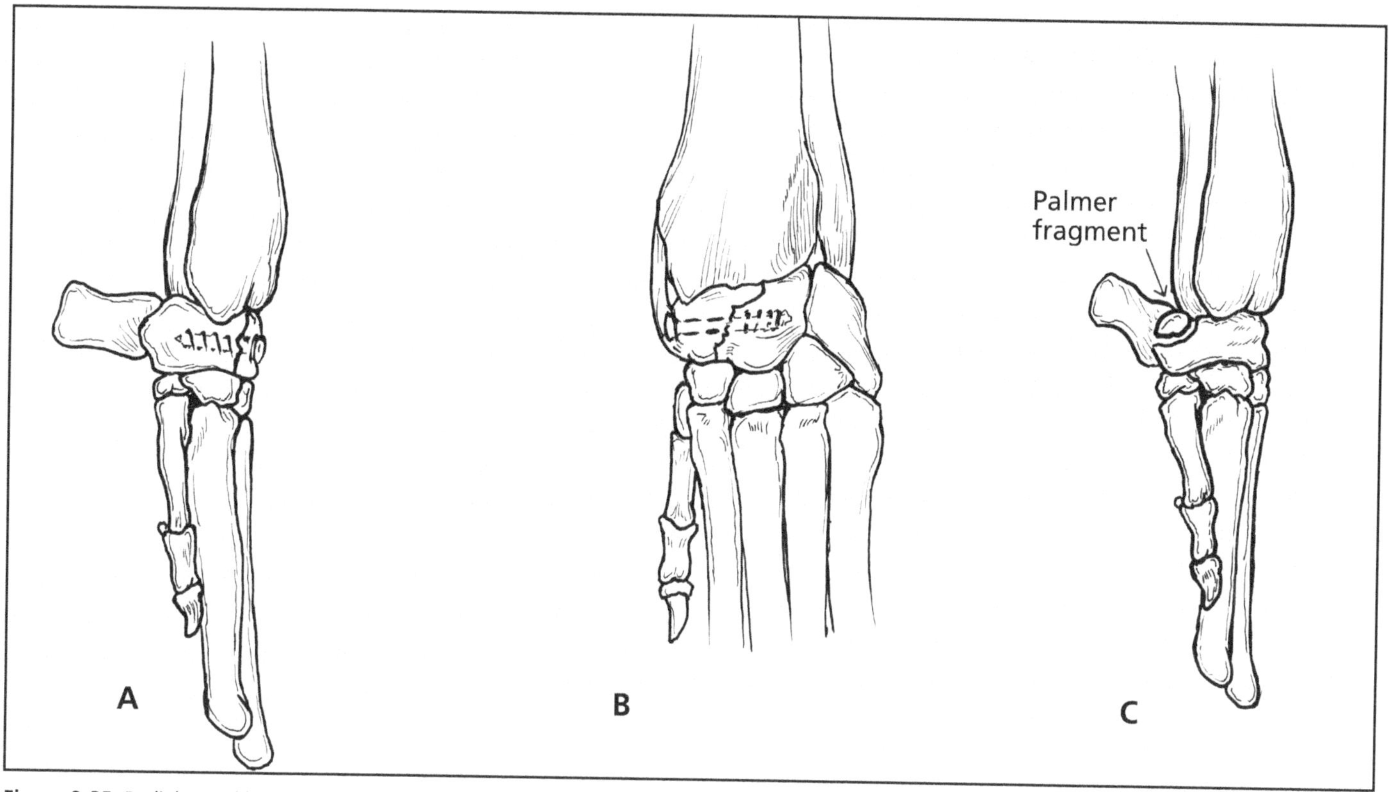


**Figure 8-25.** Radial carpal bone fracture. **A.** lag screw is placed distally on the dorsal surface of the radial carpal bone and advanced in a dorsopalmar direction. **B.** Medial-lateral oblique fractures are stabilized by introducing a lag screw through the body of the radial carpal bone in a medial to lateral direction. The head of the screw is placed through the insertion of the short radial collateral ligament **C.** Fragments involving the palmar portion of the radial carpal bone are excised. (Figs A, B after Johnson AL, Dunning D. Atlas of Orthopedic Surgical Procedures of the Dog and Cat. St Louis: Elsevier Saunders, 2005, 210-211; Fig C after Piermattei DL, Flo GL, DeCamp CE. Brinker, Piermattei, and Flo's Handbook of Small Animal Orthopedics and Fracture Repair 4th ed. St. Louis: Saunders Elsevier, 2006, 391).

retracted. The joint capsule is incised to expose the radial carpal bone.

Dorsal fragments that are too small to be stabilized are excised. Larger fragments are reduced and held in place with pointed reduction forceps. A small (1.5 to 2.0 mm) lag screw is placed in a dorsopalmar direction and angled slightly proximally. The screw hole in the dorsal fragment is countersunk. The screw is started quite distal on the dorsal margin of the radial carpal bone to avoid the screw head from interfering with the distal end of the radius.

Medial-lateral oblique fractures are stabilized by introducing a small (2.0, 2.7 or 3.5 mm) screw in lag fashion through the body of the radial carpal bone in a medial to lateral direction. The screw should not enter the joint space between the radial and ulnar carpal bones. The head of the screw is placed through the insertion of the short radial collateral ligament.

Fragments involving the palmar portion of the radial carpal bone may be treated by excising the fragment. The fragment does not involve the primary weight-bearing surface of the bone.

Dermis and skin are closed routinely. In the presence of tension, multiple punctate relaxing incisions may be placed (See Chapter 3).

## Aftercare

Activity is restricted to confined indoor rest with short (10 minute) leash walks for 8 weeks postoperatively. For cases treated with lag screw fixation, a soft padded bandage and splint is placed for 3 weeks postoperatively and changed weekly. For cases treated with fragment excision, a soft padded bandage and splint is placed for 10 days after surgery. Cases treated with fragment excision should have exercise restricted to leash walks for 4 weeks after surgery.

## Advantages and Disadvantages

The advantage of lag screw fixation of radial carpal fractures is the potential for interfragmentary compression and healing. Satisfactory outcomes have been reported in racing greyhounds. Patients with a chronic insidious lameness may respond more poorly to lag screw fixation due to remodeling of bone fragments or pre-existent degenerative joint disease. A pancarpal arthrodesis, although more invasive, will likely produce better results in chronic cases.

## Suggested Readings

1. Gnudi G, Mortellaro CM, Bertoni G et al. Radial carpal bone fracture in 13 dogs. Vet Comp Orthop Traumatol 16:178-183, 2003.
2. Johnson AL, Dunning D. Atlas of Orthopedic Surgical Procedures of the Dog and Cat. St Louis: Elsevier Saunders, 2005, 210-211.
3. Johnson KA. Carpal injuries. Bloomberg, Dee, Taylor. Canine Sports Medicine and Surgery. Philadelphia: W. B. Saunders Co., 1998, 106-107.
4. Li A, Bennett D, Gibbs C et al. Radial carpal bone fractures in 15 dogs. J Small Anim Pract 41:74-79, 2000.
5. Tomlin JL, Pead MJ, Langley-Hobbs SJ et al. Radial carpal bone fracture in dogs. J Am Anim Hosp Assoc 37:173-178, 2001.


# Radial Carpal Bone Luxation

## Definition and Indications

Radial carpal bone luxation in the dog is rare. The injury occurs in large and small breed dogs with no history of major trauma. The radial carpal bone is displaced in a palmar direction. The mechanism for luxation is reported to be simultaneous hyperextension and pronation of the paw followed by immediate supination. The short radial collateral ligament and dorsal joint capsule rupture, but the palmar ligament that connects the radial carpal bone to the second and third metacarpals remains intact (See Figure 8-2C). The radial carpal bone luxates caudally then rotates 90 degrees in a medial direction around the intact palmar ligament (Figure 8-26A, B & C).

There is a case report of dorso-medial luxation of the radial carpal bone in a dog. The suspected mechanism of injury is similar to that for palmar luxation but with an intact or partially intact radial collateral ligament. The intact ligament limits displacement of the radial carpal bone to the dorso-medial position.

Surgical stabilization of radial carpal bone luxation consists of replacing the radial carpal bone, securing it to the ulnar carpal bone, and stabilizing the short radial collateral ligament.

## Technique

The patient is placed in sternal-lateral recumbency with the limb pulled cranially. Towels or sandbags placed underneath the patient help to attain a sternal-lateral position. The skin and subcutaneous tissues are incised dorsally, beginning 3 to 4 cm proximal to the radial carpal joint and extending distally to the middle of the metacarpus (See Figure 8-6). Deep dissection is continued between the extensor carpi radialis and common digital extensor tendons and the tendons are retracted. The joint capsule is incised to expose the area of the radial carpal bone.

The radial carpal bone is located and the lateromedial rotation is corrected first. Next, the bone is reduced dorsally into the joint space and secured with a K-wire introduced from the medial non-articulating surface of the radial carpal bone into the ulnar carpal bone. If possible, proximal and distal remnants of the short

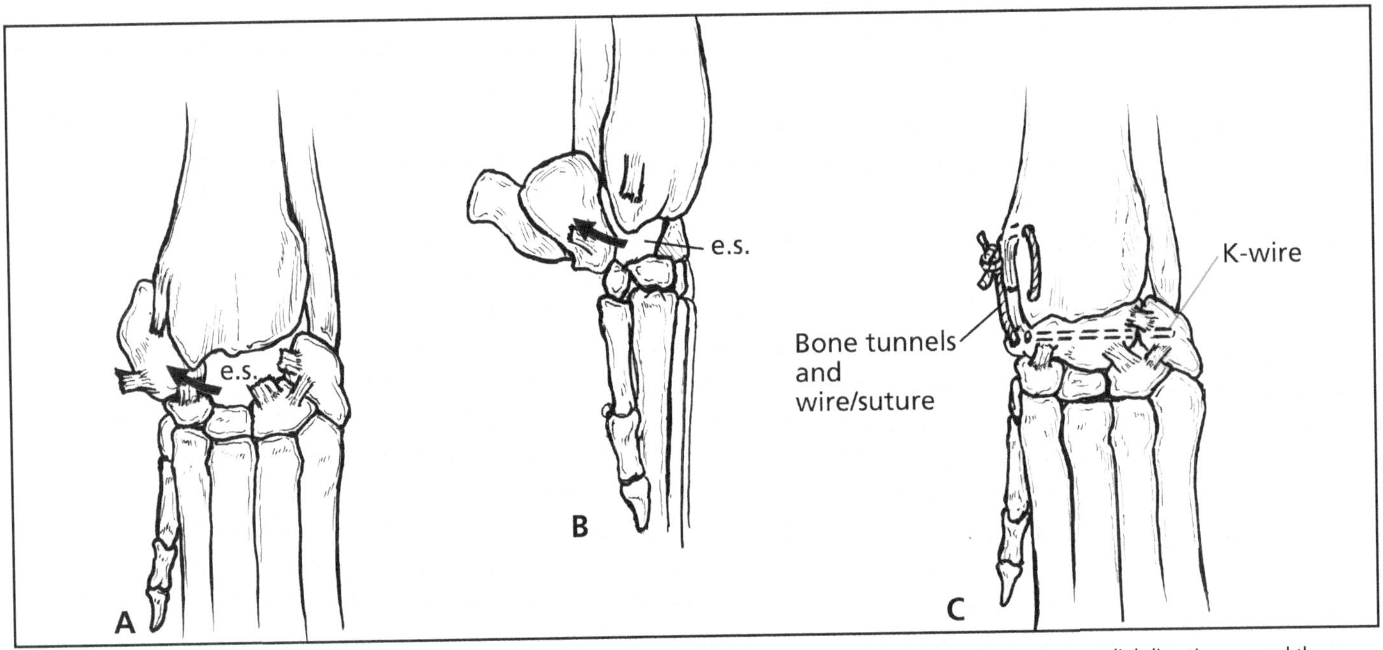


**Figure 8-26.** Luxation of the radiocarpal bone. **A., B.** The radial carpal bone luxates caudally then rotates 90 degrees in a medial direction around the palmar radiocarpal ligament *(arrows)*. **C.** The radial carpal bone is reduced dorsally into the joint space and secured with a K-wire introduced from the medial non-articulating surface of the radial carpal bone into the ulnar carpal bone. The radial collateral ligament is stabilized using bone tunnels and heavy gauge suture. One bone tunnel is in the medial prominence of the radial carpal bone and two are in the distal radius. (After Boemo CM. Diagnostic test for fractures, luxations, and radial carpal injuries. In Bojrab MJ, Ellison GW, Slocum B: Current Techniques in Small Animal Surgery 4th ed. Baltimore: Williams and Wilkins, 1998, 1108).

radial collateral ligament are sutured together (See Figures 7-9 and 7-10). A prosthetic imbrication of the short radial collateral ligament is always performed whether or not the ligament has been primarily repaired. Drill tunnels are placed in the distal radius to simulate the origin of the straight and oblique portions of the short radial collateral ligament as described for radial collateral ligament rupture (See Figure 8-9). Alternatively, a screw and washer or suture anchor may be placed just proximal to the styloid process of the radius to serve as the origin site for the ligament. Heavy gauge nylon suture (40 to 80 pound test fishing line or cerclage wire) is anchored at the origin of the collateral ligament and then underneath the K-wire that is securing the radial carpal bone to the ulnar carpal bone. The K-wire is bent over and cut.

Dermis and skin are closed. In the presence of tension, multiple punctate relaxing incisions may be placed (See Chapter 3).

### Aftercare

The carpus is immobilized using a soft padded bandage and caudal splint for 4 weeks after surgery followed by 2 weeks in a soft padded bandage alone. The bandage is changed weekly. Exercise is restricted to indoor confinement with short 10 minutes leash walks for 8 weeks after surgery. Exercise is gradually reintroduced over a 4 week period of time.

### Advantages and Disadvantages

Surgical stabilization of radial carpal bone is considered successful in returning dogs to sound function.

## Suggested Readings

1. Piermattei DL, Flo GL, DeCamp CE: Brinker, Piermattei, and Flo's Handbook of Small Animal Orthopedics and Fracture Repair 4th ed. St. Louis: Saunders Elsevier, 2006, 388-389.
2. Miller A, Carmichael S, Anderson TJ et al. Luxation of the radial carpal bone in four dogs. J Small Anim Pract 31:148-154, 1990.
3. Palierne S, Delbeke C, Asimus E eta l. A case of dorso-medial luxation of the radial carpal bone in a dog. Vet Comp Orthop Trauamatol 21:171-176, 2008.

## Accessory Carpal Bone Fractures

### Definition and Indications

Accessory carpal bone fractures occur in racing greyhounds but can be seen sporadically in other large breed dogs. The injury mechanism is avulsion of tendon or ligament attachment sites on the accessory carpal bone as a result of strenuous activity. In racing greyhounds the injury occurs predominantly on the right forelimb consistent with the counterclockwise direction of track racing. Clinical signs are an acute to subacute mild lameness after running. On physical examination there is swelling of the carpus, pain with pressure in the region of the accessory carpal bone, and pain on carpal flexion.

A classification system identifies 5 types of accessory carpal bone fractures (Figure 8-27A-D):
Type I Avulsion fracture of the distal margin of the accessory carpal bone at the origin of the accessori-oulnar ligaments. This is an articular fracture.
Type II Avulsion fracture of the proximal margin at the insertions of the palmar, radiocarpal, and ulnocarpal ligaments. This is an articular fracture.
Type III Avulsion fracture of the distal palmar (non-articular) margin of the accessory carpal bone at the origin of the accessoriometacarpal IV and V ligaments.
Type IV Avulsion fracture at the proximal palmar (non-articular) margin of the accessory carpal bone at the insertion of the flexor carpi ulnaris muscle. Type V Comminuted fracture of the body of the accessory carpal bone. This may extend into the articular surface.

Type I fractures comprise 67% of the accessory carpal bone fractures in racing greyhounds and type III injuries are the least common. Type II injuries are usually seen concurrently with type I fractures. In other breeds types IV and V fractures predominate.

Fracture types I and II are articular and there is potential for significant arthritis to develop in the acccessorioulnar carpal joint without intervention. Surgical therapy for fracture types I to III is required for good function and consists of screw stabilization of avulsed bone fragments. Simply excising fragments is not advised because the ligament attachment is lost and joint instability results. Screws are not placed in lag fashion because over-drilling the near cortex runs the risk of splitting the small piece of bone. Screw fixation of fracture types I to III yields excellent results and return to athleticism in most cases.

Fracture type IV is an avulsion of the flexor carpi ulnaris muscle insertion and occurs most often in breeds other than the racing greyhound. This injury causes mild but persistent lameness without surgery. If the fragment is large enough it is secured with a screw, but if not, fragment excision with this type of fracture can be satisfactory. Fracture type V is comminuted and although stabilization with multiple small screws is feasible, most cases respond well to cast fixation.

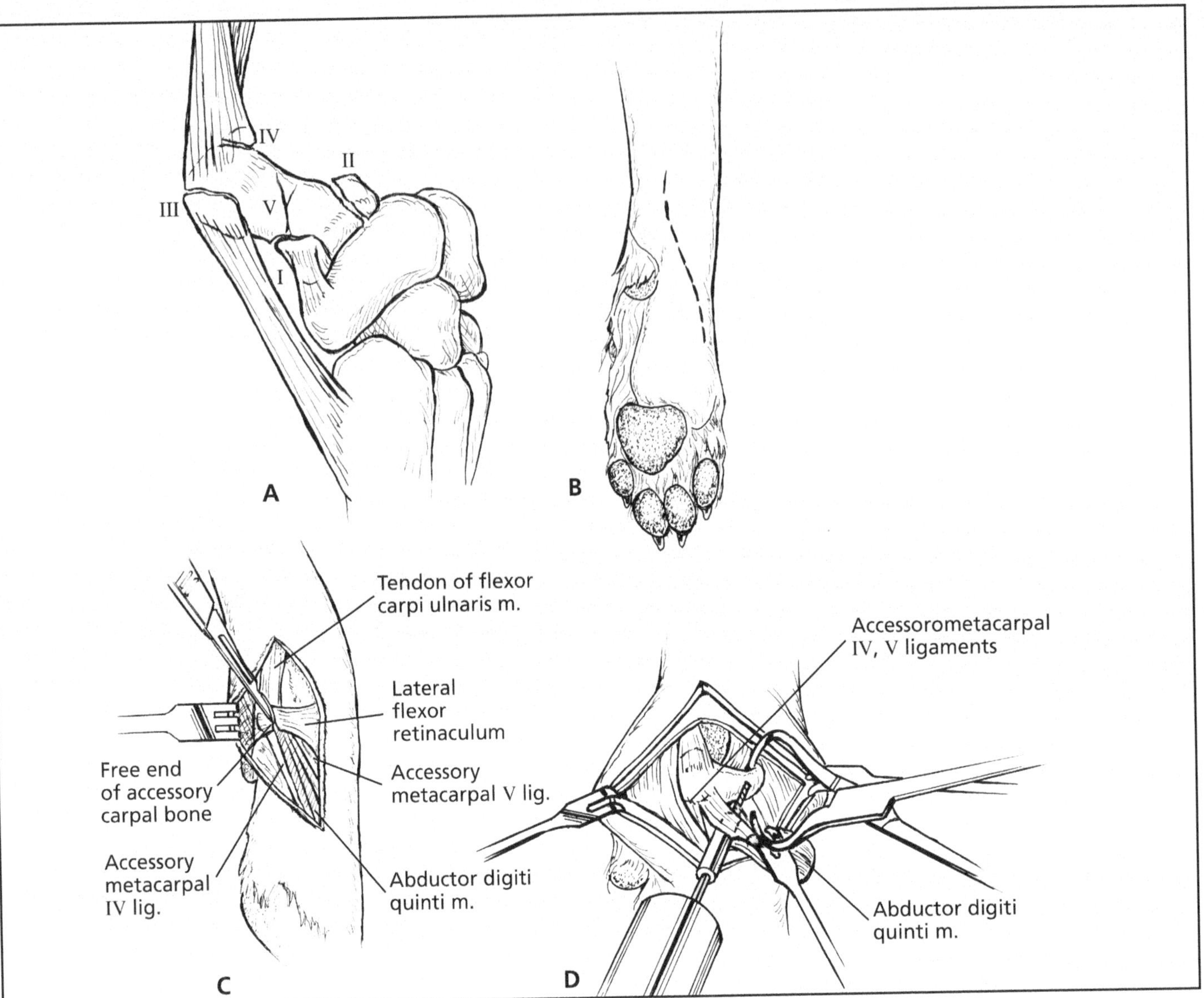


**Figure 8-27.** Accessory carpal bone fractures: Types, approach and repair. **A.** A classification system identifies 5 types of accessory carpal bone fractures. Type I is an avulsion fracture of the distal margin of the accessory carpal bone at the origin of the accessoroulnar ligaments. Type II is an avulsion fracture of the proximal margin at the insertions of the palmar, radiocarpal, and ulnocarpal ligaments. Type III is an avulsion fracture of the distal palmar (non-articular) margin of the accessory carpal bone at the origin of the accessorometacarpal IV and V ligaments. Type IV is an avulsion fracture at the proximal palmar (non-articular) margin of the accessory carpal bone at the insertion of the flexor carpi ulnaris muscle. Type V is a comminuted fracture of the body of the accessory carpal bone **B.** A 5 cm long incision is made on the palmarolateral aspect of the carpus and continued through the subcutaneous tissues to expose the palmar carpal fascia. **C.** The palmar carpal fascia is incised over the lateral aspect of the accessory carpal bone. The fascia is reflected to expose the accessory carpal bone and its associated ligaments. The abductor digiti quinti muscle is bluntly separated from the accessorometacarpal IV and V ligaments, transected at its origin, and reflected distally. **D.** Reduction is achieved and maintained with small pointed reduction forceps. Type I fracture being stabilized with a small screw placed in a distal to proximal direction. (After Johnson KA, Dee JF, Piermattei DL. Screw fixation of accessory carpal bone fractures in racing Greyhounds: 12 cases (1981-1986). J Am Vet Med Assoc 194:1618, 1989).

# Techniques

## Fracture Types I – III

The patient is positioned in lateral recumbency. A 5 cm long incision is made on the palmarolateral aspect of the carpus and continued through the subcutaneous tissues to expose the palmar carpal fascia. This fascia is incised over the lateral aspect of the accessory carpal bone. The fascia is reflected to expose the accessory carpal bone and its associated ligaments. The abductor digiti quinti muscle is bluntly separated from the accessoriometacarpal IV and V ligaments, transected at its origin on the accessory carpal bone, and reflected distally. In cases with fracture types I and II a lateral arthrotomy of the accessorioulnar joint is performed to evaluate the articular surfaces and visualize the fracture fragments. Reduction is achieved and maintained with small pointed reduction forces. The ulnar nerve and palmar interosseous artery are located medial to the accessory carpal bone and are avoided. All 3 fracture types are stabilized with a small (1.5 or 2.0 mm screw) placed in a distal to proximal direction. An appropriate drill hole (1.1or 1.5 mm) is placed through both sides of the fracture. Screws are not placed in lag fashion and screw heads are not countersunk. Smaller secondary chip fragments are excised. The origin of the abductor digit quinti muscle and palmar carpal retinacular fascia are sutured with 3-0 absorbable material and subcutaneous tissues and skin are closed in layers.

### Fracture Type IV

This avulsion injury tends to involve only part of the insertion of the flexor carpi ulnaris tendon (See Figure 8-27A). The patient is positioned in lateral recumbency. A palmarolateral incision is made over the accessory carpal bone (See Figure 8-27B). Subcutaneous and fascial tissues are incised. A longitudinal incision is made through the distal insertion site of the flexor carpi ulnaris tendon to expose the dorsal surface of the bone. The bony fragment is usually small and is therefore excised. If the fragment is large enough it is reduced with pointed reduction forceps and stabilized with a positional screw (1.5 to 2.0 mm) placed in a proximal to distal direction. The tendon incision is closed with 3-0 absorbable suture and fascial, subcutaneous and skin layers are closed in layers.

### Fracture Type V

Comminuted accessory carpal bone fractures tend to heal well with external coaptation. If there is an intra-articular fragment that appears to be large enough for screw fixation, surgical stabilization of that component is attempted. The positioning and surgical approach are as described for fracture types I to III.

## Aftercare

Stabilization with a soft padded bandage and splint is required for variable periods of time with accessory carpal bone fractures. The splint is made from fiberglass casting tape molded to the palmar aspect of the paw in 20 degrees of flexion. The paw is placed in slight flexion to relieve stress on the accessory carpal bone. The splint is changed weekly.

After screw fixation of accessory carpal bone fractures the soft padded bandage and splint is maintained for 4 weeks. Strict confinement and exercise control is required until 8 weeks postoperatively, followed by gradually increasing activity over the next 4 weeks.

After excision of fragments only, usually fracture type IV injuries, the soft padded bandage and splint are maintained for 2 weeks followed by a soft padded bandage for 2 weeks.

Type V fractures are stabilized with a soft padded bandage and splint until radiographic signs of advanced healing are seen which usually occurs by 6 weeks. The splint is changed weekly or as needed. Exercise is restricted to relatively short and controlled leash walks for an additional 3 to 4 weeks after splint removal.

## Advantages and Disadvantages

The clear advantage to open reduction and internal fixation of intra-articular accessory carpal bone fractures is to avoid or minimize degenerative change. The additional benefit is to stabilize ligament and tendon attachment sites. The disadvantage to attempting to stabilize a type V fracture is the potential for an ineffective surgical procedure. A surgical exploration is recommended for type V fractures that have an articular component. Splint stabilization will still be required for healing of the remaining fragments.

# Suggested Readings

1. Piermattei DL, Flo GL, DeCamp CE: Brinker, Piermattei, and Flo's Handbook of Small Animal Orthopedics and Fracture Repair 4th Edition. St Louis: Saunders Elsevier, 2006, 392-396.
2. Johnson KA, Dee JF, Piermattei DL. Screw fixation of accessory carpal bone fractures in racing Greyhounds: 12 cases (1981-1986). J Amer Vet Med Assoc 194:1618-1625, 1989.

# Soft Tissue Injury Related to the Accessory Carpal Bone

## Definition and Indications

The flexor carpi ulnaris muscle inserts on the accessory carpal bone via tendons from the humeral and ulnar heads. Strain injury of the flexor carpi ulnaris tendon and tearing of the palmar retinacular fascia directly over the accessory carpal bone have been reported.

Flexor carpi ulnaris tendonopathy presents as weight-bearing lameness with visible swelling and thickening over the tendon and accessory carpal bone. There is no palpable joint laxity. There is a painful response to palpation of the swelling. Weimeraners may be over-represented for flexor carpi ulnaris tendonopathy. Radiographs show soft tissue swelling around the tendon and accessory carpal bone and possibly osteophyte formation on the accessory carpal bone (Figure 8-28). Ultrasound examination of the tendon may show disruption of normal tendon architecture compared to the unaffected side.

Tears of the palmar superficial fascia are distinguished from flexor carpi ulnaris tendonopathy by deep palpation just below the accessory carpal bone. Palpation of a horizontal dimple in this location corresponds to a tear in the palmar fascia. Dogs with this injury are reported to respond very well to surgical exploration and closure of the defect.

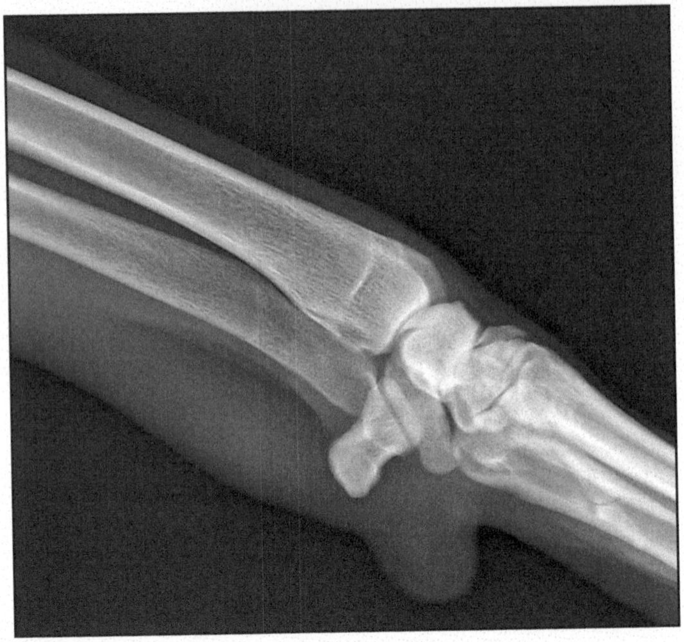

**Figure 8-28.** Radiograph of a Weimaraner with tendonopathy of the flexor carpi ulnaris. There is soft tissue thickening of the distal tendon at the palmar aspect of the carpus.

## Technique

### Flexor Carpi Ulnaris Tendonopathy

This condition is treated conservatively by rest, external coaptation and anti-inflammatory medication. One report states successful resolution with external coaptation followed by topical flumethasone (Flucort, Fort Dodge Animal Health, Fort Dodge, Iowa) and dimethyl sulfoxide (DMSO; Domoso gel, Wyeth Animal Health, Guelph, Ontario, Canada) applied twice daily. Coaptation consists of a soft padded bandage and palmar flexion splint that is made using fiberglass casting tape molded to the palmar aspect of the paw in 20 degrees of flexion.

### Tears of the Palmar Superficial Fascia

The patient is placed in lateral recumbency. An incision is made over the palmarolateral aspect of the accessory carpal bone as described for the surgical approach to accessory carpal bone fractures (See Figure 8-27). The incision deviates laterally around the accessory carpal pad. Subcutaneous tissues are incised. The injury is visible as a horizontal tear in the superficial fascia along the palmar border of the accessory carpal bone. In chronic cases overlying fibrous tissue must be carefully incised and partially removed to locate the horizontal tear. The tear is sutured using 2-0 polydioxanone in an interrupted cruciate pattern. Subcutaneous tissues and skin are closed in layers.

## Aftercare

Flexor carpi ulnaris tendonopathy is treated by immobilization with a soft padded bandage and splint for 3 weeks with weekly changes. The splint is then changed to a soft padded bandage for 1 to 2 weeks. Non-steroidal anti-inflammatory drugs may be given for approximately 2 weeks during immobilization. When all dressings are removed topical medication with flumethasone and dimethyl sulfoxide twice daily for 1 to 2 weeks can be used if lameness is still present.

After repair of a palmar superficial fascia tear, the paw is stabilized in a soft padded bandage and palmar flexion splint as described for flexor carpi ulnaris tendonopathy. The splint is maintained for 3 weeks then is changed to a soft padded bandage for 2 weeks.

For both types of injury exercise is restricted to indoor rest with short (10 min) leash walks for 6 weeks. After 6 weeks exercise is gradually increased over 2 to 4 weeks.

## Advantages and Disadvantages

There are anecdotal reports of palmar fascial tears responding well to conservative management. However, there have been dogs with chronic injuries that did not recover with rest, but returned to normal function after surgery. The disadvantage of conservative therapy is the potential for chronic lameness.

# Suggested Readings


1. Kuan SY, Smith BA, Fearnside SM et al. Flexor carpi ulnaris tendonopathy in a Weimaraner. Aust Vet J 85:401-404, 2007.
2. Guilliard MJ, Mayo AK. Tears of the palmar superficial fascia in five racing Greyhounds and a Labrador retriever. J Small Anim Pract 41:218-220, 2000.
3. Roe SC. Injury and Diseases of Tendons. In Bloomberg MS, Dee JF, Taylor RA: Canine Sports Medicine and Surgery. Philadelphia: W. B. Saunders Co., 1998, 98.

# Chapter 9

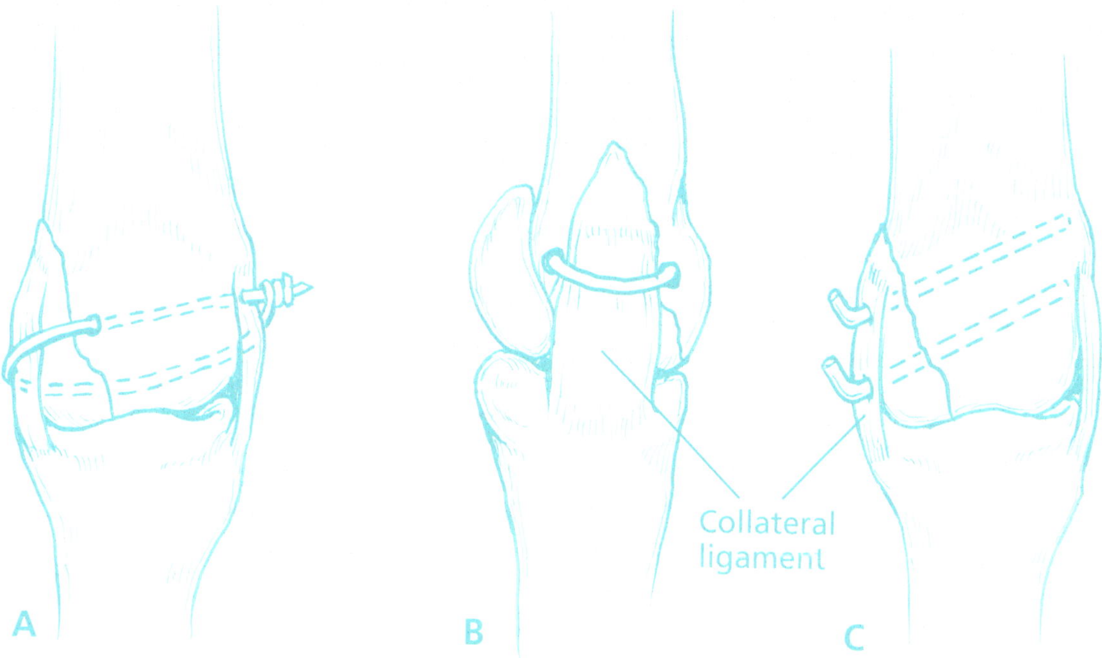


## Orthopedic Injuries of the Metatarsal, Metacarpal and Phalangeal Areas

Janet Welch, D.V.M., D.A.C.V.S.

# Anatomy

## Osseous Structures

Metacarpal bones have three anatomical regions. The proximal end of the bone is the base, the mid portion is the shaft or body, and the distal end is the head. The primary weight-bearing bones are the third and fourth digits. The metacarpal and metatarsal bones are numbered from the medial to the lateral side. The first metacarpal bone of the forepaw is usually present, although it is a vestigial structure and is much shorter than the others. Proximally the first metacarpal bone articulates with the first carpal bone and distally it articulates with the proximal phalanx of the first digit and a single palmar sesamoid bone. To be correct, the term dewclaw is used only in the hindlimb. Distally, metacarpal and metatarsal bones II through V articulate with the corresponding digits. Each of the four main digits (II through V) contains 3 phalanges, referred to as proximal, middle and distal. Each individual phalanx consists of a base proximally and a head distally. The base of the proximal phalanx articulates with the head of its corresponding metacarpal or metatarsal bone at an angle of approximately 110 degrees. In this position the proximal phalanx is nearly parallel to the ground. The middle phalanx articulates with the proximal phalanx at a palmar/plantar angle of approximately 135 degrees. The middle phalanx articulates with the distal phalanx at nearly a right angle. Each distal phalanx has a projection of bone from the palmar border of the base which serves as the insertion of the deep digital flexor tendon. The rounded dorsal part of the base is the extensor process on which the common digital extensor tendon is inserted. A thin shelf of bone, the ungual crest, overlaps the claw on the distal phalanx. Two sesamoid bones are located on the palmar/plantar surface of each metacarpo- or metatarsophalangeal joint (digits II to V). A single small sesamoid bone is located dorsally in the extensor tendons of digits II to V at the level of the metacarpo- or metatarsophalangeal joint and a small cartilaginous nodule is located on each of the distal interphalangeal joints (See Figure 8-1).

## Muscles and Tendons

Four interosseous muscles arise from the palmar or plantar sides of the metacarpal and metatarsal bones. These muscles cover most of the palmar or plantar surfaces of the bones. Each interosseous muscle divides into two branches, which attach by tendons to the proximal phalanges. Each tendinous insertion of this muscle has a palmar sesamoid embedded in it (Figure 9-1).

Extensor tendons traverse the dorsal surfaces of the paw to insert on either the metacarpal and metatarsal bones or on the digits. In the forelimb, the common digital extensor tendon has four branches that insert on digit. The lateral digital extensor tendon inserts on digits III, IV and V. Proximally, the extensor carpi radialis inserts on the dorsal bases of metacarpals II and III. The ulnaris lateralis inserts on the base of metacarpal V. The abductor pollicis longus inserts on the proximal medial part of metacarpal I (See Figure 8-3).

Flexor tendons traverse the palmar or plantar surface of the paw. On the palmar surface the flexor carpi radialis tendon inserts on the proximal ends of metacarpals II and III. The superficial digital flexor tendon inserts on the proximal palmar surfaces of the

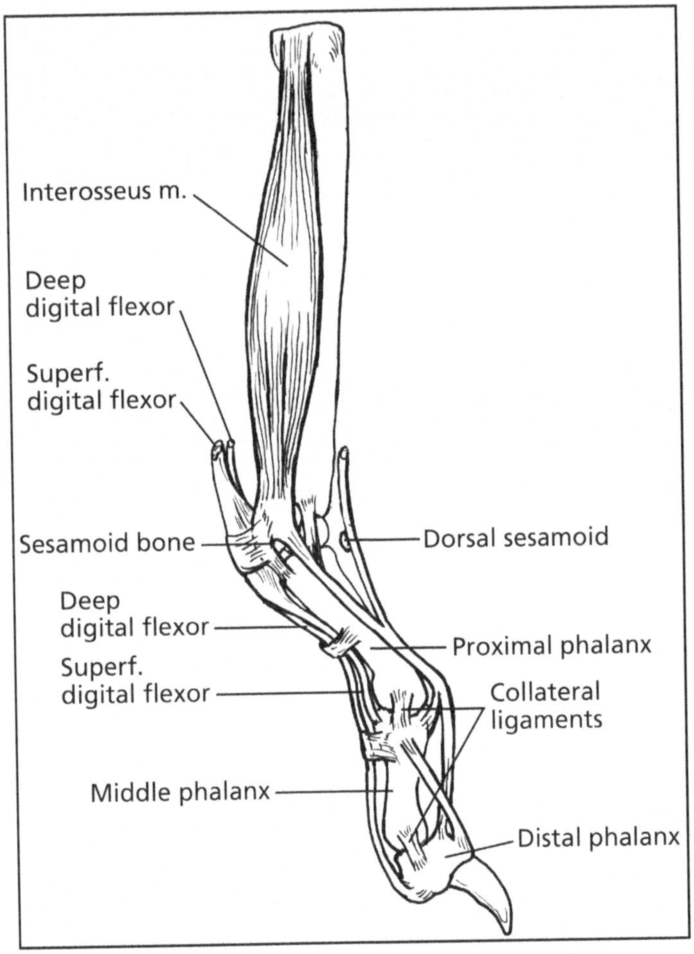


**Figure 9-1.** Anatomy of the digits. Each digit has a proximal, middle and distal phalanx. The superficial digital flexor tendon inserts on the proximal palmar/plantar aspect of the middle phalanx. The deep digital flexor tendon inserts on the palmar/plantar tubercle of the distal phalanx. Four interosseous muscles arise from the palmar or plantar sides of the metacarpal and metatarsal bones. These muscles cover most of the palmar or plantar surfaces of the bones. Each interosseous muscle divides into two branches, which attach by tendons to the proximal phalanges. Each tendinous insertion of this muscle has a sesamoid embedded in it. A smaller sesamoid is located at the dorsal aspect of the metacarpo- or metatarsophalangeal joint. (After Evans HE, DeLahunta A, Miller ME. Guide to the Dissection of the Dog 5th ed. Philadelphia:W. B. Saunders Co., 2000).

middle phalanges of the digits II through V. At the metacarpophalangeal joint, each forms a collar around the deep digital flexor tendon that passes through it. The deep digital flexor tendon inserts on the proximal end of the distal phalanx of each digit (See Figure 8-4).

In the hindlimb, the long digital extensor tendon has four branches that insert on each digit. The short digital extensor muscle is located underneath the long digital extensor tendons. This muscle has three tendons that insert on digits II, III and IV. The cranial tibial tendon inserts on the proximal surface of metatarsals I and II. The peroneus longus tendon inserts on the fourth tarsal bone and the plantar aspect of the proximal ends of metatarsals I, II and V. The peroneus brevis tendon inserts on the base of metatarsal V. The lateral digital extensor tendon inserts on digit V (See Figure 7-6).

## Ligaments

The metacarpo- and metatarsophalangeal joints have a joint capsule and medial and lateral collateral ligaments which unite the metarcarpal and metarsal bones with the corresponding proximal phalanx. Each phalangeal joint also has a joint capsule and medial and lateral collateral ligaments (See Figure 9-1).

## Blood Supply

The dorsal blood supply to the forepaw is formed from the cranial superficial antebrachial artery. This artery branches into the dorsal common digital arteries

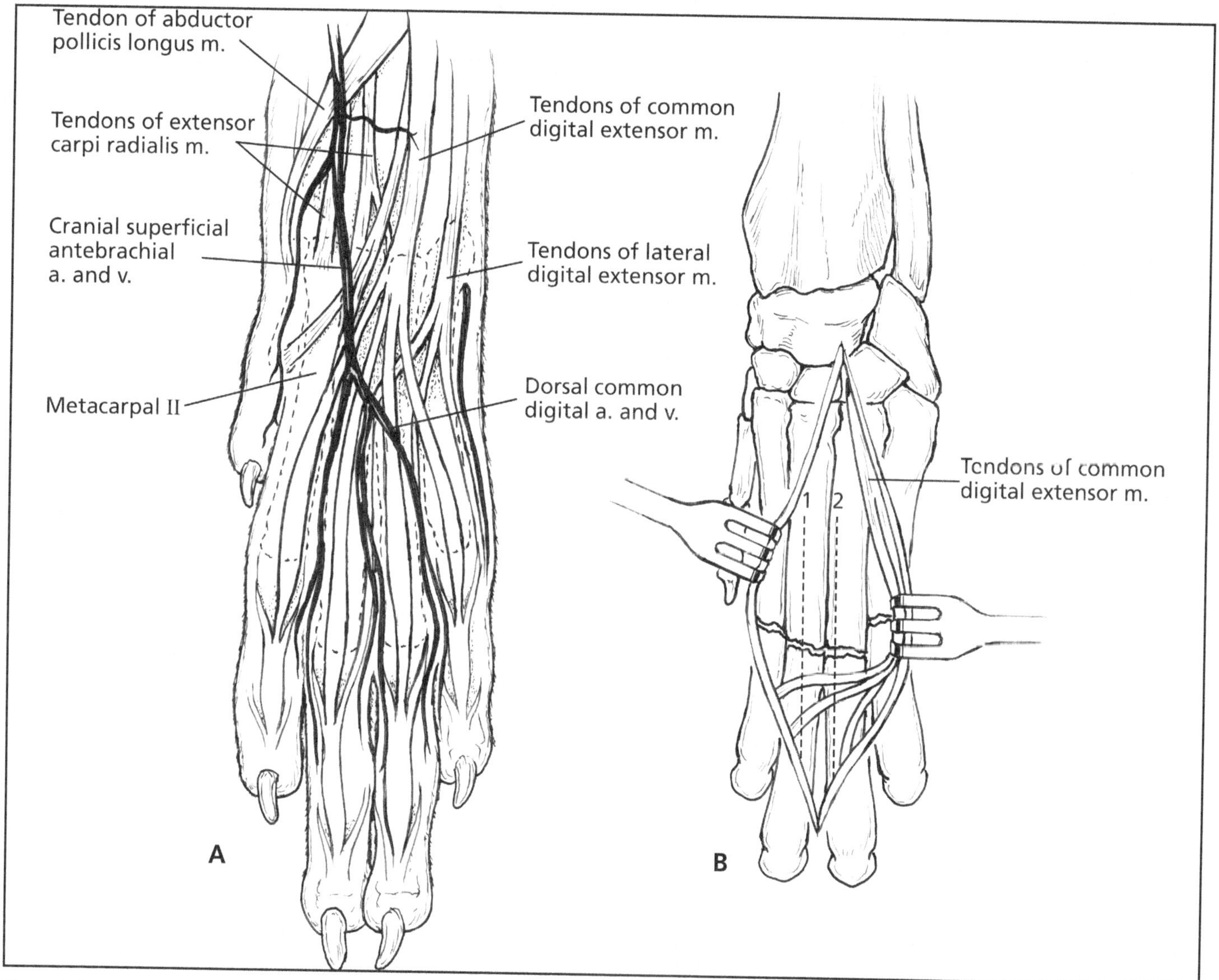


**Figure 9-2.** Metacarpal bone anatomy and surgical approach. **A.** In the forelimb, the common digital extensor tendon has four branches that insert on their respective digits. The lateral digital extensor tendon inserts on digit III, IV and V. Proximally, the extensor carpi radialis inserts on the dorsal bases of metacarpals II and III. The abductor pollicis longus tendon inserts on the proximal medial part of metacarpal I. The dorsal blood supply to the forepaw is formed from the cranial superficial antebrachial artery. This artery branches into the dorsal common digital arteries which run between the common digital extensor tendons in the area of the metacarpals. The location of the skin incision varies according to the bones that need to be exposed. **B.** If a single metacarpal or metatarsal bone is fractured, the incision is located directly over the bone *(1)*. Two adjoining bones are approached by an incision between them *(2)*. (After Piermattei DL, Johnson KA: An Atlas of Surgical Approaches to the Bones and Joints of the Dog and Cat 4th ed. Philadelphia:Saunders, 2004, 267).

which run between the common digital extensor tendons in the area of the metacarpals (Figure 9-2A & B). The palmar blood supply is formed from the median artery. This artery branches into the palmar common digital arteries.

The blood supply to the hindpaw is similar. The metatarsals and digits are supplied by dorsal common digital arteries. These arteries are formed by a branch of the cranial tibial artery and a branch of the saphenous artery. The cranial tibial artery terminates as the dorsal pedal artery which becomes the perforating metatarsal artery. This artery passes from the dorsal to the plantar aspect of the hindpaw between proximal metatarsals II and III.

# Metacarpal and Metatarsal Fractures

## Definition and Indications

Metacarpal and metatarsal fractures are usually caused by motor vehicle trauma or other direct injury to the foot. Single metatarsal or metacarpal bone fractures are seen less often than multiple. The treatment choices for fractures of the metacarpal and metatarsal bones include external coaptation or surgical stabilization. External coaptation with a soft padded bandage and splint can be recommended for stabilization if one or two metacarpal or metatarsal bones are fractured. Surgical stabilization is indicated when greater than 2 bones are fractured or if the 2 main weightbearing bones (metacarpal or metatarsal III or IV) are fractured and displaced. Fractures of the proximal region of the metacarpal or metatarsal bones tend to be less displaced than mid-shaft or distal fractures. In this situation of proximal fractures with minimal displacement, external coaptation of greater than two fractured bones can be suitable.

Displaced fractures of the proximal portion (base) of metacarpal/metatarsal II or V benefit from surgical stabilization. These bones are sites of ligamentous insertion, and instability here leads to varying degrees of valgus displacement with metacarpal/metatarsal II or varus displacement with metacarpal/metatarsal V. With metacarpal II and metatarsal V, fractures of the distal end (head) can result in instability of the metacarpo- or metatarsophalangeal joint due to disruption of the collateral ligaments at this site. These fractures also benefit from surgical stabilization. Persistent joint instability and degenerative joint disease are likely without surgical fixation.

Reported surgical techniques for shaft fractures include intramedullary pin placement, bone plating or external fixation. Intramedullary pins do not provide any improvement in fracture alignment compared with external coaptation. Intramedullary pin placement is hampered by the anatomy of the metacarpal and metatarsal bones. Pins cannot be normograded directly up the bone without damaging the metacarpo- or metatarsophalangeal joints. The pin must be introduced through the dorsal surface of the distal fracture fragment and advanced into the proximal piece. This requires choosing small pins so that the pin can bend during placement. The stability provided by IM pins is weak due to small pin size and frequent lack of ancillary fixation such as cerclage wires because fractures are short oblique. There is a newer method of pin fixation referred to as dowel pin fixation that has been effective in cats and small dogs. This method involves introducing the pin at the fracture site rather than through the distal fracture fragment. This method allows larger pins to be placed and has yielded good results.

Bone plates are available in a range of sizes appropriate for metacarpal and metatarsal bone fractures. Veterinary cuttable plates for 1.5 and 2.0 mm screws (Synthes, Paoli, PA, Veterinary Orthopedic Implants, South Burlington, VT) are well suited for repair of these fractures, as they allow the placement of more screws per unit length than conventional plates and their low profile minimizes soft tissue coverage problems.

External fixation stabilization for metacarpal and metatarsal fractures can be very effective and particularly useful for comminuted or open fractures. Most external fixators used for metacarpal or metatarsal fractures employ epoxy putty rather than standard connecting rods. External fixation using small pins (K-wires) and epoxy putty permits a free-form external fixation frame with pins placed in different planes. This type of frame is very useful when multiple metacarpal or metatarsal bones are fractured and in patients with open wounds.

Fractures of the base (proximal) aspect of the metacarpal or metatarsal bones can be stabilized with lag screws or tension band fixation using K-wires and cerclage wire. Fractures of the head (distal) aspect of the bones can be stabilized with hemicerclage wire, K-wires or small lag screws.

## Techniques

### External Coaptation: Soft Padded Bandage and Splint

A soft padded bandage and splint are applied from the digits to the mid-radius or tibia (See Figure 7-8). Fiberglass casting tape is used to make a molded splint for the palmar or plantar aspect of the paw.

### Surgical Stabilization of Metacarpal and Metatarsal Fractures

For metacarpal fractures the patient is placed in sternal recumbency with the palmar surface of the paw on the table. For metatarsal fractures the patient is in dorsal recumbency with the plantar surface of the paw on the table.

### Bone Plate Application

The surgical approach is the same for metacarpal and metatarsal fractures. The location of the skin incision varies according to the bones that need to be exposed. If a single metacarpal or metatarsal bone is fractured, the incision is located directly over the dorsal surface of the bone. Two adjoining bones are approached by an incision between them (See Figure 9-2B). Bleeding is managed using electrocautery. It is not usually necessary to apply a tourniquet, but if a tourniquet is used, it is placed for a maximum of 30 to 60 minutes. When approaching the metatarsal bones, the perforating branch of the dorsal pedal artery, located between bones II and III, should be protected.

Once the skin is incised, subcutaneous tissues are undermined as needed to access the fractured bones. Next deep fascia is incised. Deep fascia is incised over bone II to expose metacarpals II and III, and over bone V to expose bones IV and V. Extensor tendons are elevated and retracted. The fracture ends are levered into position using a Freer elevator. If the fracture is oblique, reduction can be maintained using pointed reduction forceps. Bone plates are contoured with a small plate bender if needed and applied to the dorsal surface of the bone (Figure 9-3A & B). Veterinary cuttable plates are available in size 1.5/2.0 and 2.0/2.7. Alternatively, size 2.0 dynamic compression plates (DCP) may be used as well as smaller plates if necessary (Synthes, Paoli, PA, Veterinary Orthopedic Implants, Burlington, VT).

Skin is closed with 3-0 to 4-0 suture in a simple interrupted pattern. Subcutaneous and intradermal sutures are avoided in metacarpal or metatarsal fracture repair due to the risk of snug closure of the deeper layers interrupting blood supply to the paw. Multiple punctate releasing incisions may be placed on both sides of the primary incision. The limb is covered with a soft padded bandage.

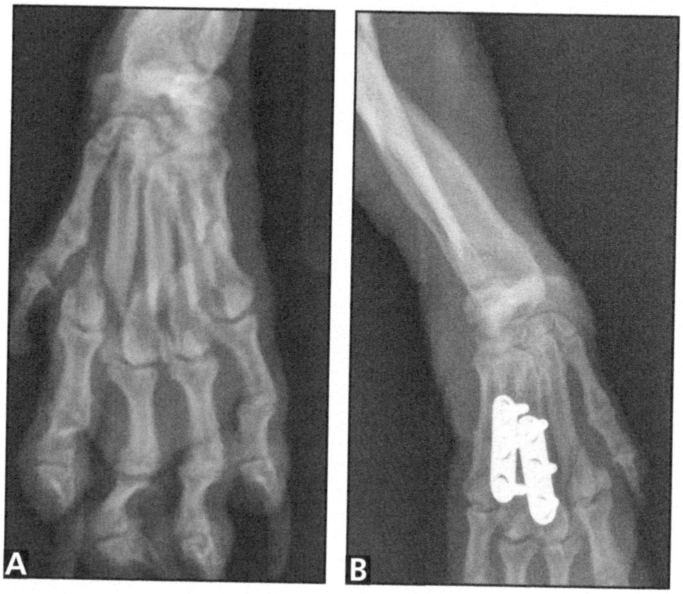


**Figure 9-3.** Metacarpal fractures stabilized using small bone plates and screws. Bone plates are placed on the two major weightbearing bones metacarpals III and IV. **A.** Preoperative craniocaudal view. **B.** Postoperative craniocaudal view.

### Dowel Pin Fixation

This technique is applicable to cats and small dogs. A short longitudinal incision is made over the dorsal surface of the metacarpus/metatarsus centered over the fracture site. If there are fractures involving more than one bone the incision is extended by 3 to 4 cm for exposure. The fracture fragments are grasped with mosquito hemostats or Brown Adson forceps. A K-wire is chosen that almost completely fills the medullary canal. This pin is retrograded into the medullary canal of the longer bone fragment. The pin is cut so that approximately 1 to 2 cm protrudes from the fracture end. The two fracture fragments are distracted to insert the protruding pin into the medullary canal of the opposite fracture fragment. The fracture is reduced using gentle twisting motions. If needed, the end of the K- wire being inserted into the opposite fracture fragment can be shortened to facilitate insertion (Figure 9-4A & B).

Skin is closed with 3-0 to 4-0 suture in a simple interrupted pattern. Subcutaneous and intradermal sutures are avoided in metacarpal or metatarsal fracture repair due to the risk of snug closure of the deeper layers interrupting blood supply to the paw. Multiple punctate releasing incisions may be placed on both sides of the primary incision. The limb is covered with a soft padded bandage.

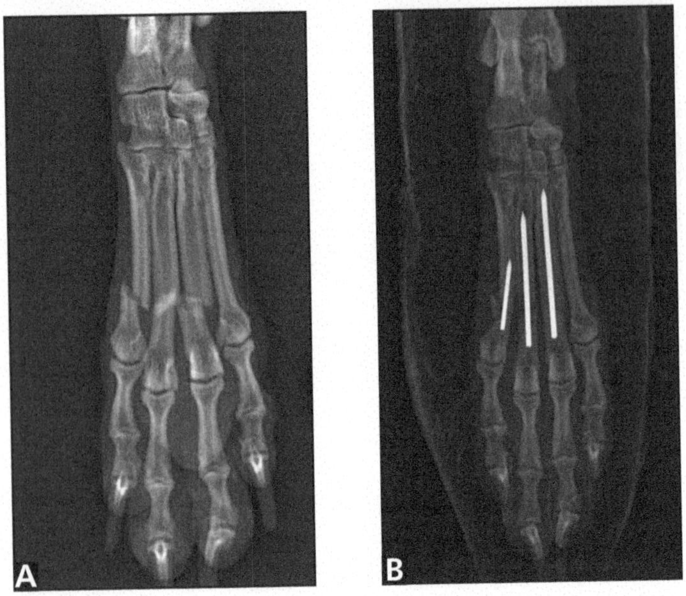


**Figure 9-4.** Dowel pin fixation of metacarpal and metatarsal fractures. **A.** Preoperative craniocaudal radiographic projection of fractured metatarsal bones 3, 4 and 5 in a small breed dog. **B.** Postoperative radiographic projection of dowel pin fixation. For each metatarsal fracture, a pin was retrograded into the medullary canal of the longer bone fragment. The pin was cut short so that 1 to 2 cm protruded from the fracture end. The two fracture fragments were distracted to insert the protruding pin into the opposite fragment and the fracture was reduced.

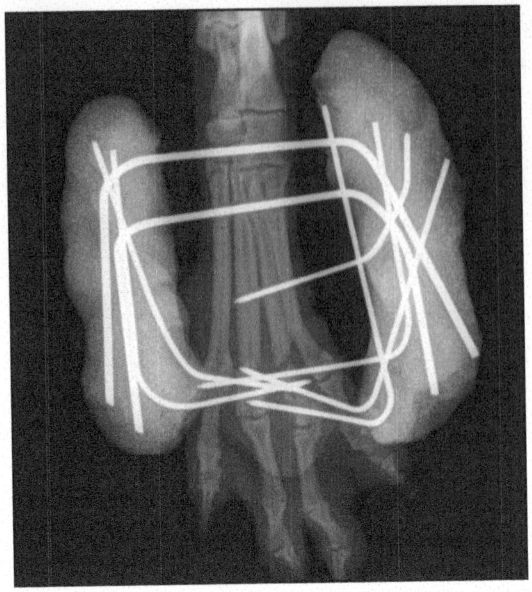

**Figure 9-5.** External fixation of metacarpal and metatarsal fractures: Closed external fixation. Postoperative craniocaudal radiographic projection of metatarsal fracture repair. The first pin was placed proximally in a medial-lateral plane through the distal row of tarsal bones and a second transverse pin was placed through the proximal metatarsal bones. The remainder of the pins were half pins that each engaged one to two metacarpal or metatarsal bones. Each pin was bent to bring the free ends of the pins into line with each other parallel to the axis of the limb. A bolus of rapid-set epoxy putty was pressed onto the ends of the pins.

## External Fixation of Metacarpal and Metatarsal Fractures: Closed Technique

Small pins (K-wires, small Steinmann pins or mini to small positive profile external fixation pins) are placed into the metacarpal or metatarsal bones through stab incisions in the skin. The first pins are placed in a transverse direction through the proximal base of the four main metacarpal or metatarsal bones (Figure 9-5). Alternatively, the pin may also be placed through the distal row of the carpal or tarsal bones. If possible, two transverse proximal pins are placed. The remainder of the pins, including all pins in the distal section, are half pins. Pins are not necessarily placed in the same plane and pins may engage more than one metacarpal or metatarsal bone each to maximize bone purchase. Distal pins tend not to engage more than 2 bones because of the arched configuration of the distal metacarpal and metatarsal bones.

Each pin is bent 1 to 2 cm from the skin surface to bring the free ends of the pins into a line that is parallel with the axis of the limb. The pins will act as a scaffold for the epoxy putty. Pins are bent either to the medial or lateral side to create a type II external fixator. Postoperative radiographs can be taken prior to application of the epoxy putty to ensure that pins do not invade the metacarpal or metatarsophalangeal joints and to check for gross malalignment of the fracture fragments. The paw is then aligned and held in position while the epoxy putty is pressed onto the bent pins. There should be a gap of 1 to 2 cm between the epoxy and the skin to accommodate postoperative swelling without having the epoxy impinge on the skin.

The pin tract sites are coated with triple antibiotic ointment and the skin is stabilized by placing foam sponges or gauze pads between the epoxy connecting rod and the skin. The entire paw and external fixator are then covered with a soft padded bandage.

## External Fixation of Metacarpal and Metatarsal Fractures: Open Technique

Proximal full pins are placed as described for closed external fixation. One to two proximal full pins are placed. For distal pin placement a small incision is made directly over the fracture site. A K-wire is retrograded through the fracture site and exits proximal to the distal articular surface of the head of the metacarpal or metatarsal bone. The drill is attached to the distal end of the pin. The fracture is reduced and the pins are driven into the proximal metacarpal or metatarsal bones. The free ends of the pins are bent 1 to 2 cm from the skin surface and directed to converge at the dorsum of the paw. A bolus of rapid-set epoxy putty (Oatey epoxy putty, Oatey, Cleveland, OH) is pressed onto the ends of the pins. (Figure 9-6A & B).

Surgical incisions are closed with 3-0 to 4-0 skin

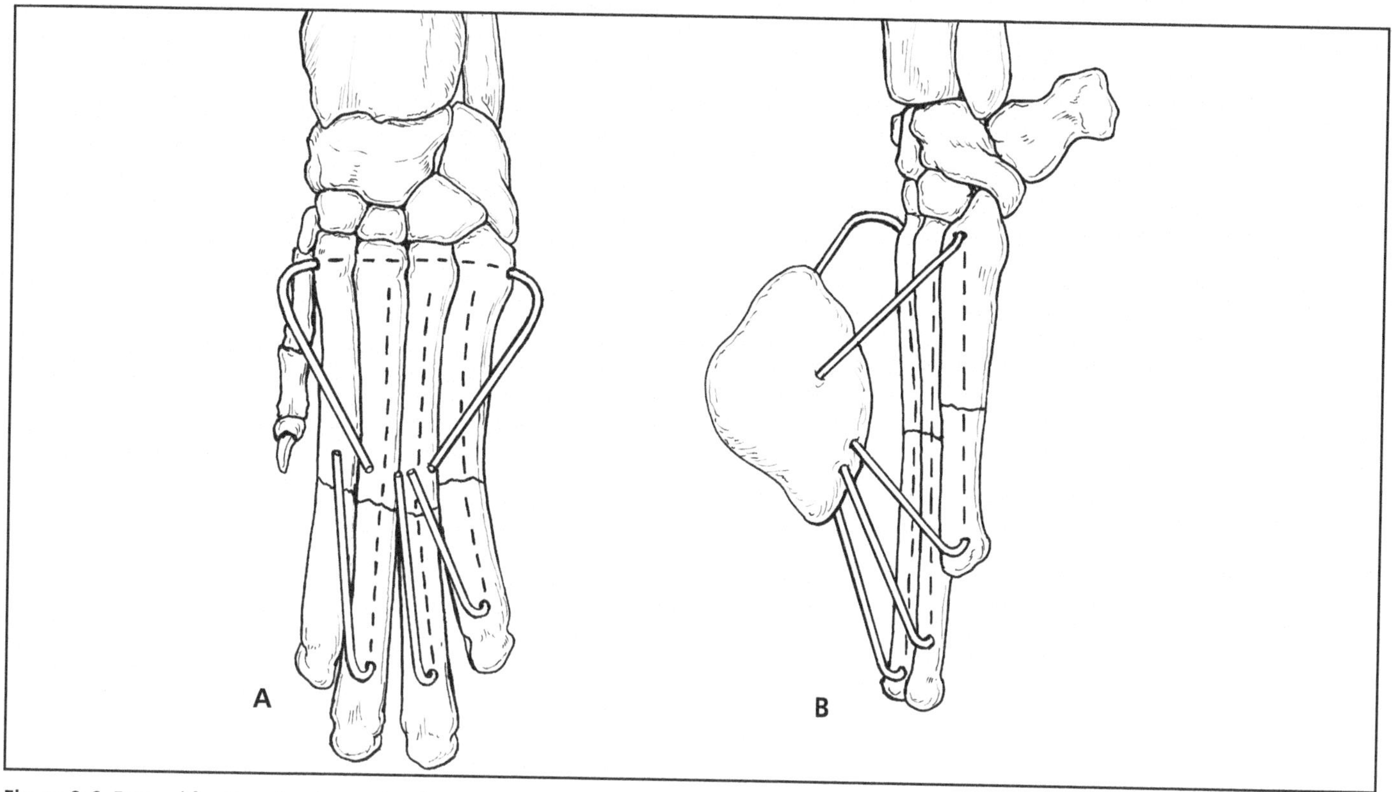


**Figure 9-6.** External fixation of metacarpal and metatarsal fractures: Open external fixation. **A.** The first pin is placed proximally in a medial-lateral plane through the base of the metacarpal or metatarsal bones. Distally K-wires are normograded through the fracture site and lodged in the proximal fracture fragment. It is most important to stabilize the major weightbearing bones (3rd and 4th metacarpal/metatarsal bones). The 3rd, 4th, and 5th metacarpal bones are stabilized in this fracture. The free ends of all 4 pins are bent and directed to converge at the dorsum of the paw. **B.** A bolus of rapid-set epoxy putty is pressed onto the ends of the pins.

sutures in a simple interrupted pattern. The pin tract sites are coated with triple antibiotic ointment and the skin is stabilized by placing foam sponges or gauze pads between the epoxy connecting rod and the skin. The entire paw and external fixator are then covered with a soft padded bandage.

## Fractures of the Base of the Metacarpal and Metatarsal Bones: Lag Screw and Tension Band Fixation

A skin incision is made directly over the base of the fractured metacarpal or metatarsal bone. Subcutaneous tissues are incised and extensor tendons are retracted. If the fracture is oblique it can be stabilized with screw fixation (Figure 9-7). Smaller sized lag screws, such as 1.5 or 2.0 mm, are appropriate for most cases. The lag screws are placed in standard fashion, by overdrilling the near cortex according to the thread diameter, and drilling the far cortex according to the core diameter of the screw. The lag screws are placed perpendicular to the fracture line. One to 2 screws are used.

If the fracture fragment is small, it is best to place a positional screw. With a positional screw, both cortices are drilled according to the smaller or core diameter of the screw. Compared to a lag screw, this technique has less risk of fissuring the fragment.

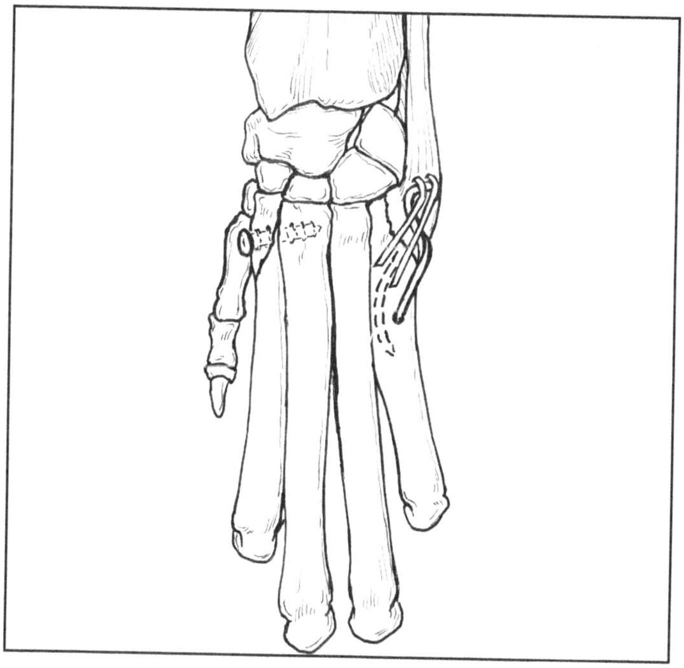

**Figure 9-7.** Stabilization for fractures of the base of metacarpal bones II and V. Oblique fracture of the base of metacarpal 2 is repaired with a lag screw engaging the fracture fragment and the adjacent metacarpal bone. Fracture of the base of metacarpal V is repaired with a tension band fixation: the proximal fracture fragment is stabilized with 1 to 2 K-wires advanced into the distal fragment and a figure 8 cerclage wire is anchored at the proximal aspect of the pins and through a small drill tunnel in the distal fragment. The pins are bent and cut short. (After Piermattei DL, Flo GL, DeCamp CE: Brinker, Piermattei and Flo's Handbook of Small Animal Orthopedics and Fracture Repair 4th ed. St. Louis: Saunders Elsevier, 2006, 413).

Tension band fixation can also be used to stabilize the fracture fragment. This technique is useful for smaller fracture fragments. One to two K-wires are directed from the fracture fragment into the medullary cavity of the metacarpal or metatarsal bone. The pins are advanced until resistance is felt. A drill hole is created in the distal bone. Cerclage wire (sized 22 gauge for a medium to large sized dog) is anchored in the drill tunnel and behind the pins in a figure 8 pattern and tightened. The pins are bent and cut (See Figure 9-7).

Skin incisions are closed with 3-0 to 4-0 suture in a simple interrupted pattern.

### Fracture Fixation of the Head of the Metacarpal Bone

Fracture of the head, or distal end, of the metacarpal or metatarsal bone produces instability of the metacarpophalangeal joint because the collateral ligaments originate here. The fragment may be quite small. Surgical stabilization is recommended for best results especially in the athletic animal and particularly if it involves the primary weightbearing digits 3 and 4.

A skin incision is made directly over the affected metacarpal or metatarsal bone. If the fragment is small drilling of the fragment is avoided because it could readily fissure. Instead two small holes (1.1 to 2.0 mm drill bit) are drilled in the dorsal and palmar or plantar aspect of the metacarpal or metatarsal bone (Figure 9-8A, B & C). Cerclage wire (size 22 gauge for a medium to large-sized dog) is introduced through the drill holes and around the fragment. The wire is tightened to secure the fragment to the bone.

If the fragment is larger it can be secured with K-wires or a small positional screw. One to two K-wires (size .045 for a medium dog) is inserted through the fragment to engage the opposite cortex of the bone. The ends are gently bent and cut (See Figure 9-5C).

The skin is closed with 3-0 to 4-0 suture in an interrupted pattern. A soft padded bandage with palmar splint is placed for 4 weeks and changed as needed.

## Aftercare

For fractures repaired with external coaptation, the soft padded bandage and splint are kept on for approximately 6 weeks with weekly changes. Radiographs are obtained at 6 to 8 weeks, and if callus formation is seen the splint may be removed. It is not necessary to wait for disappearance of the fracture line prior to splint removal. Exercise is restricted to leash walks only for 8 weeks and gradually increased over an additional 4 weeks.

Metacarpal or metatarsal fractures repaired with internal fixation should be protected with a soft padded bandage and splint for approximately 4 weeks postoperatively. The splint extends from the radius or tibia to the digits. The splint is changed weekly. External fixators are bandaged using sterile gauze pads or foam sponges between the skin and epoxy putty bar to limit swelling and stabilize the pin-skin interface. The entire paw and external fixator are covered with a soft padded bandage for the first 3 to 7 days after surgery to help minimize swelling of the paw. After this, the digits do not need to be completely covered by the bandage. The external fixator is covered with

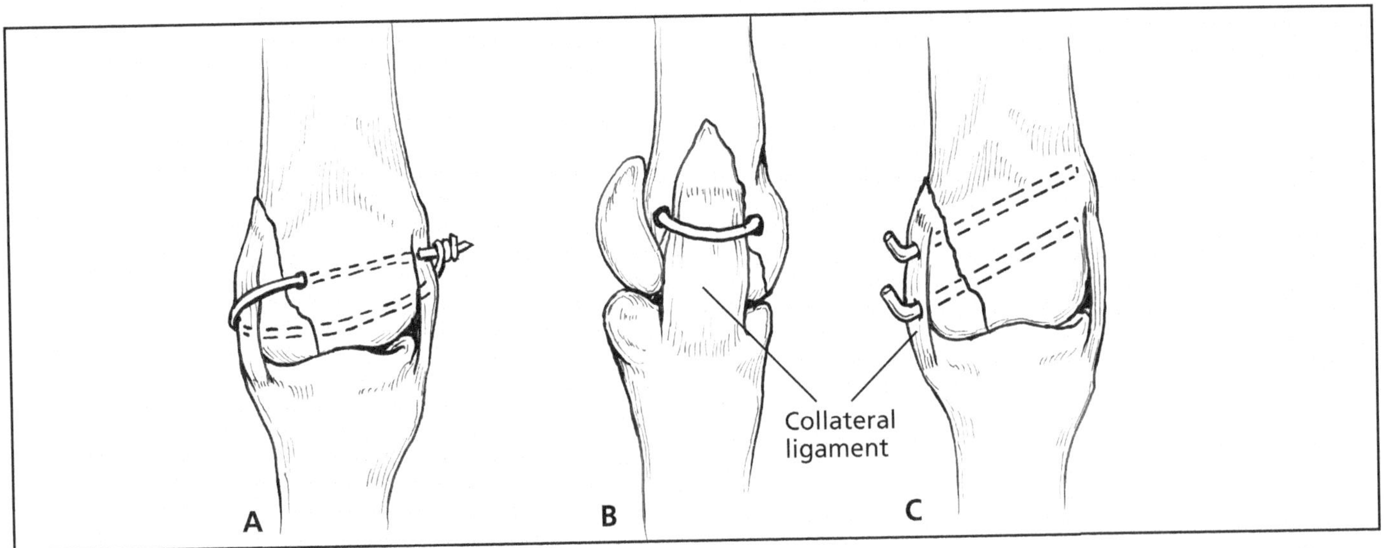


**Figure 9-8.** Fracture fixation of the head of the metacarpal bone. **A.** craniocaudal view and **B.** lateral view of the head of the metacarpus. Two small holes are drilled in the dorsal and palmar/ plantar aspects of the bone. Cerclage wire is introduced through the drill holes and around the fragment. The wire is tightened to secure the fragment to the bone. **C.** Craniocaudal view of a larger fragment secured with K-wires. The K-wires penetrate the collateral ligament. (After Piermattei DL, Flo GL, DeCamp CE: Brinker, Piermattei and Flo's Handbook of Small Animal Orthopedics and Fracture Repair 4th ed. St. Louis: Saunders Elsevier, 2006, 419).

a bandage during the entire time that it is in place to prevent trauma to the fixator. With all patients, exercise is restricted to short 10 minute leash walks 3 to 4 times daily for approximately 8 weeks until progressive fracture healing is seen radiographically. Normal activity is then gradually reintroduced over 4 weeks.

### Advantages and Disadvantages

The advantage of external coaptation is that it is non-invasive. This option is ideally limited to treatment of minimally displaced fractures in one or two metacarpal or metatarsal bones because it will not consistently improve bone alignment. There is no clear advantage to normograde intramedullary pin placement. This technique does not offer any improvement over external coaptation alone in terms of fracture alignment and involves a surgical approach. For displaced fractures, bone plating or external fixation provides improved alignment compared to intramedullary pins.

Dowel pin fixation, a form of intramedullary pin placement, can be effective in cats and small dogs and has been shown to improve fracture alignment and decrease the incidence of malunion compared to external coaptation with a splint. The surgical approach for this technique is less extensive than with bone plate fixation.

The disadvantage of bone plating is that it involves a surgical approach over the length of the metacarpal or metatarsal bone and may require more than one incision if all metacarpal or metatarsal bones are fractured. Patients with damage to the paw can have compromised circulation or open wounds and a large skin incision could be detrimental to the soft tissues. In these circumstances, either multiple fractured bones or open fractures, external fixation is an excellent option. This technique is versatile and pin size can be tailored to the size of the bone fragments. It can be done completely closed or through a minimal incision over the fracture line. Closed external fixation is preferable as this does not compromise the extraosseous blood supply and therefore provides the greatest potential for biologic fracture healing. Closed external fixation will not create the anatomic reduction that can be obtained with bone plating but precise anatomic reduction is not mandatory to achieve a good functional outcome with metacarpal or metatarsal fractures.

A potential risk with surgical fixation of metacarpal or metatarsal fractures, particularly when multiple bones are stabilized, is postoperative swelling and in rare cases devitalization of skin over the paw. The cranial superficial antebrachial artery of the forepaw, dorsal pedal artery of the hindpaw, and their branches can be compromised by the initial trauma and further with a surgical approach. Incision closure can be accomplished with skin sutures alone to avoid the risk of deeper suture layers constricting blood supply to the paw. During surgery every attempt is made to preserve the perforating metatarsal artery that passes between metatarsals II and III. Multiple punctuate releasing incisions help to reduce postoperative swelling. Bandages must not be placed too tightly, should be adequately padded and should extend to the distal aspect of the digits.

## Suggested Readings


1. Degasperi B, Gradner G, Dupre G. Intramedullary pinning of metacarpal and metatarsal fractures in cats using a simple distraction technique. Vet Surg 36:382-388, 2007.
2. De La Puerta BD, Emmerson T, Moores AP et al. Epoxy putty external skeletal fixation for fractures of the four main metacarpal and metatarsal bones in cats and dogs. Vet Comp Orthop Traumatol 21:451-458, 2008.
3. Evans HE, Christensen GC. Miller's Anatomy of the Dog 2nd ed. Philadelphia: WB Saunders Co., 1979, 192-222; 365-373, 398-407, 706-708; 740-746.
4. Faulkner Besancon M, Conzemius MG, Evans RB et al. Distribution of vertical forces in the pads of Greyhounds and Labrador Retrievers during walking. Am J Vet Res 65:1497-1501, 2004.
5. Kapatkin A, Howe-Smith R, Shofer F. Conservative versus surgical treatment of metacarpal and metatarsal fractures in dogs. Vet Comp Orthop Traumatol 13:123-127, 2000.
6. Muir P, Norris JL. Metacarpal and metatarsal fractures in dogs. J Small Anim Pract 38:344-348, 1997.
7. Okumura M, Watanabe K, Kadosawa T et al. Surgical salvage from comminuted metatarsal fracture using a weight-bearing pin-putty apparatus in a dog. Aust Vet J 78:95-98, 2000.
8. Piermattei DL, Flo GL, DeCamp CE. Fractures and orthopedic conditions of the forelimb. Brinker, Piermattei, and Flo's Handbook of Small Animal Orthopedics and Fracture Repair, 4th ed. St. Louis: Saunders Elsevier,2006, 412-428.
9. Van Ee RT, Blass CE. Arthrodesis of the metatarsophalangeal joints in a dog. J Am Vet Med Assoc 194:82-84, 1989.
10. Zahn K, Kornmayer M, Matis U. Dowel pinning for feline metacarpal and metatarsal fractures. Vet Comp Orthop Traumatol 20:256-263, 2007.


## Phalangeal Fractures

### Definition and Indications

#### Diagnosis and Guidelines for Treatment

Phalangeal fractures are associated with a variable degree of lameness. Palpation of the affected bone elicits discomfort and crepitus or instability is often detected. Diagnosis is made with radiographs.

Shaft fractures of the proximal or middle phalanx can heal well with external coaptation. Surgical stabilization for shaft fractures of the proximal and middle phalanges is considered if the fragments are completely overriding or if the patient is a performance animal.

Surgical implants consist of lag screws, cerclage wire, and mini plates.

Fractures of the base or head of the phalanx are articular and usually involve the insertion of the collateral ligaments. These fractures should be treated surgically. Surgical treatment consists of stabilization of the fragment or digit amputation. If the fragments are too small or comminuted to be repaired, amputation can be performed. If possible, the fracture fragments are surgically stabilized using a small positional screw. If the fracture is open and comminuted, amputation is the best option.

In rare cases of proximal or middle phalangeal fractures, healing results in a protrusion of bone that puts pressure on adjacent soft tissues and induces lameness. This complication has been reported with fracture of the middle phalanx and can be successfully treated with surgical excision of the protruding piece of bone.

Digit amputation is indicated for open comminuted proximal or middle phalangeal fractures and for most distal phalangeal fractures especially if they are articular. Open phalangeal fractures are frequently comminuted and highly contaminated. These fractures have a poor prognosis for healing due to fracture severity and vascular compromise. Fractures of the distal phalanx have such small fragments that attempts at internal fixation are unlikely to be successful.

Amputation of the second and fifth digits at any level is well-tolerated in most dogs. Amputation at the metacarpo- or metatarsophalangeal joints of the middle digits, 3 and 4, can have more impact on a patient's athleticism because they are the major weightbearing digits. With these digits, more distal amputations are preferred.

# Technique

## Diagnosis

For radiographic examination, a standard dorso-palmar/plantar projection is taken along with a lateral. The lateral projection is most helpful if the toes are spread with the aid of tape applied to the nail of the second and fifth digits. This is referred to as a "fan lateral". Oblique projections can be added if needed.

### External Coaptation for Shaft Fractures of the Proximal and Middle Phalanx

A fractured digit can be stabilized by taping it to an adjacent intact digit. An elasticized form of tape is used (Elastoplast, Beiersdorf-Jobst Inc., Charlotte, NC). The fractured and intact digits are encompassed with 1 inch wide elasticized tape. This is referred to as "phalangeal stripping". Care should be taken not to place the tape too tightly to prevent circulatory compromise. Only one piece of tape is necessary and two pieces of tape could cause excessive pressure on the digits. A short soft padded bandage may also be applied. A splint is not required since primary stability comes from the intact digit taped to the fractured digit. The bandage extends from the distal radius or distal tibia and covers the digits.

### Surgical Fixation for Shaft Fractures of the Proximal and Middle Phalanx

The patient is positioned in sternal recumbency for the forelimb and in dorsal recumbency for the hindlimb. The approach is made directly over the affected phalanx. The main blood supply from the dorsal common digital arteries and the palmar/plantar common digital arteries is preserved. A Freer elevator is used to reflect fascial tissues and vessels away from the phalanx. The fracture fragments are handled carefully using Brown-Adson forceps and digital manipulation. Oblique and spiral fractures can be immobilized with small pointed reduction forceps and then stabilized with screws. Small implants (screw size 1.3, 1.5; Synthes, Paoli, PA) are used. Screws are often placed in a positional manner instead of lag screws. Lag screws risk fissuring small pieces of bone because the near cortex is overdrilled according to the thread diameter of the screw. Positional screws are drilled according to the core diameter in both far and near cortices. Short oblique, transverse or comminuted fractures can be stabilized or bridged with a mini cuttable plate and screws (1.0 and 1.3 mm titanium adaption plates, Maxillofacial Division, Synthes Inc., Paoli, PA).

The skin is closed with interrupted 3-0 to 4-0 sutures.

### Surgical Fixation for Base or Head Fractures of the Proximal and Middle Phalanx

To surgically stabilize fractures of the base or head of the proximal and middle phalanx, a dorsal approach is performed as described for shaft fractures of the phalanx. The fracture fragment is held in place with digital pressure or gently-placed small pointed reduction forceps. A small screw (size 1.0, 1.3, or 1.5) is placed in a positional fashion. The near cortex is not overdrilled as it would be with lag screw placement. Care is taken not to penetrate the articular surface with the screw.

The skin is closed with interrupted 3-0 to 4-0 sutures.

### Digit Amputation

Amputation of the middle or distal phalanges requires preservation of the digital pad. The skin incision begins dorsally over the most proximal phalanx to be amputated and continues distally to encircle the nail. The digital pad is spared. Soft tissue is sharply dissected away from the bone and disarticulation is performed between the proximal and middle or middle and distal phalanges. Using rongeurs, the condylar portion of the remaining phalangeal head is removed. (See Chapter 4).

The soft tissues are sutured to create a Y-shaped incision. Subcutaneous tissues are closed with 3-0 to 4-0 absorbable suture in an interrupted pattern and skin sutures are placed in an interrupted pattern.

Amputation at the metarcarpo- or metatarsophalangeal joint requires excision of the digital pad. A dorsal skin incision is begun at the level of the distal metacarpus or metatarsus. The skin incision curves around to the palmar or plantar aspect of the digit. The metacarpo- or metatarsophalangeal joint is disarticulated. Soft tissues are sharply incised and blood vessels are cauterized or ligated. The palmar sesamoids should be excised. The distal condylar area of the metacarpal or metatarsal head is removed using rongeurs. Alternatively, the distal end of the bone is amputated with an oscillating saw or gigli wire. On the medial and lateral digits, 2nd and 5th, the distal end of the metacarpal/metatarsal bone can be amputated using a beveled cut to improve the cosmetic appearance. The medial and lateral sides of the incision are sutured together using 3-0 to 4-0 absorbable suture for the subcutaneous tissues and 3-0 to 4-0 suture for the skin.

## Aftercare

All fractures of the phalanges that are surgically repaired are stabilized with a soft padded bandage and splint for 3-4 weeks and then a soft padded bandage for 2 weeks. Splints or bandages are changed weekly. Shaft fractures that are stabilized by coaptation only are kept bandaged for approximately 6 weeks. For the first 2 to 3 weeks, an elasticized tape bandage "phalangeal stripping" and soft padded bandage are applied. For the following 3 to 4 weeks, just "phalangeal stripping" is used. All patients have exercise restricted to short controlled leash walks only for the first 6 to 8 weeks after injury. Radiographs are taken at 8 weeks to assess healing. When significant healing is evident, exercise is gradually reintroduced over a 4 week period of time.

## Advantages and Disadvantages

The advantage to surgically stabilizing shaft fractures of the proximal or middle phalanx is improved fracture alignment and potentially a more rapid and complete return to function. This is most significant in performance animals. Many shaft fractures can be treated with external coaptation alone and thereby avoid a surgery. The potential disadvantage is malunion or production of healing bone that induces pressure-related discomfort and/or wounds of the surrounding soft tissues.

There is a distinct advantage to surgical treatment of base or head fractures of the proximal or middle phalanx. These are articular fractures that often involve the collateral ligament insertion. Malunion or persistent instability here can result in arthritis and chronic discomfort. Any digit fracture that is open or comminuted and any articular fracture of the distal phalanx are best treated with amputation. Surgical intervention in these cases carries a high risk of failure. Amputation at the metacarpal or metatarsal region of the main weightbearing digits (3 and 4) can result in some degree of disability in that foot, particularly in a performance animal. High amputation of the 2nd or 5th digits is better tolerated.

# Suggested Readings


1. Anderson MA, Muhlbauer MC. Radiographic diagnosis—aberrant bone growth following a phalangeal fracture. Vet Radiol Ultrasound 38:48049, 1997.
2. Evans HE, Miller ME: Miller's Anatomy of the Dog 3rd ed. Philadelphia: W.B. Saunders, 2003.
3. Piermattei DL, Flo GL, DeCamp CE. Fractures and Other Orthopedic Conditions of the Carpus, Metacarpus, and Phalanges. In Brinker, Piermattei, and Flo's Handbook of Small Animal Orthopedics and Fracture Repair, 4th ed. St. Louis: Saunders Elsevier, 2006, 420-426.
4. Piras A. Phalangeal Fractures. Proceedings of the 2005 ACVS Veterinary Symposium, San Diego, CA, 220-222, 2005.


# Ligamentous Injuries of the Phalanges (Toe Dislocations)

## Definition and Indications

Injury to the collateral ligaments of the digits is categorized as first, second or third degree sprains as with other ligament injuries. (See Chapter 7). First and second degree sprain injuries do not require surgical intervention whereas a third degree sprain is a complete ligament rupture. This level of injury is best treated with surgical stabilization. Chronic third degree sprains that are accompanied by arthritic change or acute sprains accompanied by a comminuted articular fracture are best treated by amputation.

Phalangeal subluxations and luxations are rare injuries in the pet population but relatively common in sporting dogs. Predisposing conditions are thought to be uneven running or racing surfaces and potentially the animal's digit conformation. A "spread toe" conformation of the digits or excessively long nails may make an animal more vulnerable to this injury. At times this injury is simply associated with an abrupt change in direction at a high speed. In the racing greyhound, the distal interphalangeal joint is commonly involved.

Clinical signs vary with the extent of the sprain injury. Animals with first or second degree sprains have minimal or absent lameness. There may be palpable swelling of the affected digit and manipulation may elicit a pain response. First degree injuries are stable whereas second degree sprains often have mild instability. The stability of the phalangeal joints is ascertained by holding the digit in extension and applying a varus and valgus force to the digit.

In the case of a third degree sprain, there is usually some lameness apparent at the walk. Animals with a completely dislocated joint have significant lameness and are reactive to palpation. There is palpable swelling of the joint along with instability and possibly rotation of the phalanx. Radiographs are taken as described for fractures of the phalanx. A standard dorsopalmar or -plantar projection is done along with a "fan lateral" to separate the individual digits. With third degree sprains the subluxation or luxation can be visualized. Small avulsed fragments of bone are sometimes seen.

Luxation or subluxation of the digits is a serious injury in the performance dog, and early treatment is indicated. Surgical repair has yielded better results than external splinting. Results of surgical treatment are best when performed within the first 10 days after the injury. Fibroplasia of the joint capsule and collateral ligament structures makes accurate suturing difficult after this time.

## Techniques

### First and Second Degree Sprains

Treatment for these injuries is conservative. Cold therapy is applied for five minutes 3 to 6 times daily for the first 1-2 days and NSAID therapy is administered for 5 to 7 days. If mild joint laxity is detected, the affected digit may be stabilized using phalangeal stripping, by encircling the unstable digit and the adjacent digit with elastic tape (Elastoplast, Beiersdorf-Jobst Inc., Charlotte, NC). Shortening the nail is helpful to decrease the leverage on the affected joint. The tape bandage is used for approximately 2 weeks. Local treatment with dimtheyl sulfoxide (DMSO; Domoso gel, Wyeth Animal Health, Guelph, Ontario, Canada) can be applied twice daily for 2 weeks.

Occasionally second degree sprains with notable laxity do not improve after conservative management. These injuries require surgical stabilization in performance or working animals.

### Third Degree Sprains

Primary surgical repair of a luxated or subluxated phalanx consists of suturing the joint capsule and collateral ligament(s). The patient is placed in lateral recumbency with the side of the digit to be operated up. With bilateral collateral ligament ruptures, the patient is placed in sternal/oblique recumbency for the forepaw and dorsal recumbency for the hindpaw, so that both sides of the joint are accessible. A dorsal surgical incision is made directly over the affected phalangeal joint. The fascia adjacent to the extensor tendons is incised and the extensor tendon is retracted to expose the joint. The joint capsule and collateral ligaments are inspected. The joint capsule and collateral ligaments are sutured as one layer using 3-0 to 4-0 synthetic absorbable or non-absorbable suture in a horizontal mattress pattern. Two to three interrupted mattress sutures are placed. Lastly the fascia in the area is encompassed with a single large purse-string mattress suture (Figure 9-9). This procedure is repeated on the other side in the case of bilateral ligament ruptures.

The extensor tendon is replaced dorsally and if necessary a few sutures are placed in the edge of the tendon and joint capsule to stabilize it. The subcutaneous tissue and skin are closed in layers.

## Aftercare

Subluxation or luxation injuries stabilized with suture repair are protected with a splint and soft padded bandage for 2 weeks and transitioned to a soft padded bandage for an additional 2 weeks. The bandages or splints extend from the distal radius or tibia and over the digits. Bandages are changed weekly. Exercise is limited to short 10 minute leash walks for 6 weeks.

Second degree sprain injuries with instability are stabilized with phalangeal stripping for 2 weeks. Exercise is limited to short leash walks for approximately 3 weeks.

## Advantages and Disadvantages

The advantage of surgical stabilization of luxated phalangeal joints is patient comfort and the potential to return to prior athleticism with performance

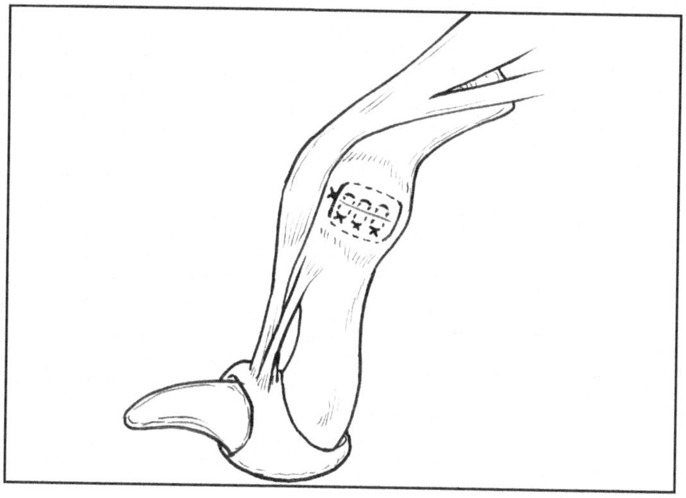

**Figure 9-9.** Surgical repair of phalangeal sprain injury. Primary surgical repair of a luxated or subluxated phalanx consists of suturing the joint capsule and collateral ligament(s). The joint capsule and collateral ligaments are sutured as one layer in a horizontal mattress pattern. Two to three interrupted mattress sutures are placed (After Piermattei DL, Flo GL, DeCamp CE: Brinker, Piermattei and Flo's Handbook of Small Animal Orthopedics and Fracture Repair 4th ed. St. Louis: Saunders Elsevier, 2006, 424).

animals. Even in companion animals complete luxation of a digit is uncomfortable and can create chronic lameness if not surgically repaired.

# Suggested Readings

1. Piermattei DL, Flo G. Brinker, Piermattei, and Flo's Handbook of Small Animal Orthopedics and Fracture Repair, 3rd ed. Philadelphia: W B Saunders, 1997, 381-389.
2. Piras A. Ligamentous injuries of the digits. Proceedings of the 2005 ACVS Veterinary Symposium, San Diego, CA, 218-219, 2005.

# Sesamoid Fragmentation

## Definition and Indications

In the four major digits there are 2 paired sesamoids on the palmar/plantar surface of the metacarpo- and metatarsophalangeal joints. There is a single small dorsal sesamoid in the extensor tendon of each of the four major digits. The anatomy of the metacarpo- and metatarsophalangeal sesamoids is the same. The palmar/plantar sesamoids of the four main digits (II to V) are numbered from 1 to 8 in a medial to lateral direction starting with the second digit. The joint capsule envelops the distal metacarpus/metatarsus, proximal phalanx and 2 palmar/plantar sesamoids of each digit (Figure 9-10).

The palmar/plantar sesamoids are firmly supported by several ligaments. The proximal ends of the sesamoid bones are embedded in the interosseous muscles of the second to fifth digits rather than being supported by ligaments. The inter-sesmoidean ligament joins the 2 sesamoids, the medial and lateral sesmoidean ligaments support the sides of the sesamoids, and the distal aspects of the sesamoids are supported by the distal sesmoidean ligaments and the cruciate ligaments. In summary, each pair of sesamoids is stabilized by 8 ligaments, by the joint capsule and by the interosseous muscles (See Figure 9-10).

The sesamoids function as a pulley for the flexor tendons on the palmar/plantar surface of the paw. The flexor tendons follow the direction of the metacarpal/metatarsal bones. The metacarpal/metatarsal bones diverge distally. Because of this diverging alignment, the flexor tendons of the middle digits (3 and 4) lie centrally in the groove between the palmar/plantar sesamoids, whereas the tendons to digits 2 and 5 are eccentrically located. Here, the tendons overlay the second and seventh sesamoids. The second and seventh sesamoids have higher rates of fragmentation which likely reflects an increase in force from their respective flexor tendons.

Fracture of the palmar/plantar sesamoid bones occurs primarily in greyhounds, but has also been reported in rottweilers and other breeds. The 2nd and 7th sesamoids are most commonly affected in all breeds. In greyhounds, the sesamoids of the right fore and right hindlimbs are most commonly involved.

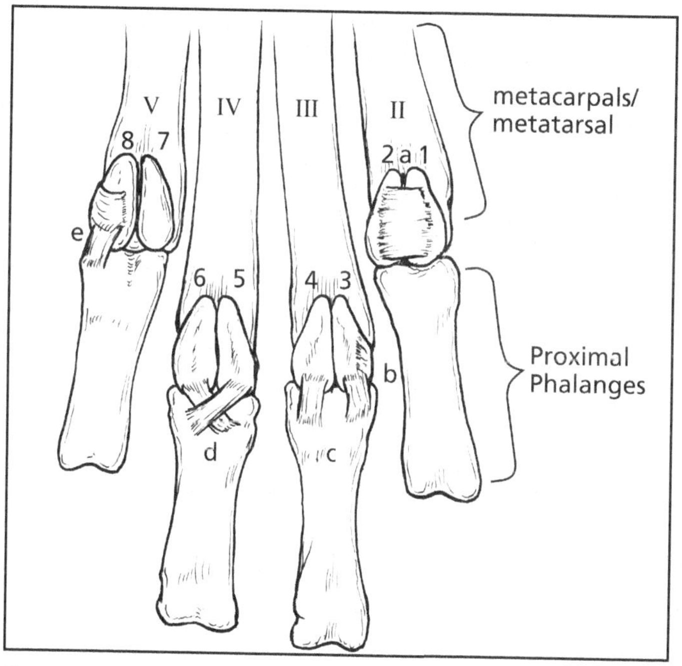


**Figure 9-10.** Anatomy of the sesamoid bones and ligaments. In the four major digits there are 2 paired sesamoids on the palmar/plantar surface of the metacarpo- and metatarsophalangeal joints. The anatomy of the metacarpo- and metatarsophalangeal sesamoids is the same. The palmar/plantar sesamoids of the four main digits (II to V) are numbered from 1 to 8 in a medial to lateral direction starting with the second digit. Ligamentous attachments of the palmar/plantar sesamoids include the inter-sesmoidean ligament *(a)*, medial sesmoidean ligament *(b)*, distal sesmoidean ligament *(c)*, cruciate ligaments *(d)*, and the lateral sesmoidean ligaments *(e)*. (After Mathews KG, Koblik PD, Whitehair JG et al. Fragmented palmar metacarpophalangeal sesamoids in dogs: a long term evaluation. Vet Comp Orthop Traumatol 14:7, 2001).

On radiographs there is a well-defined transverse fracture of the mid to distal third of the sesamoid. The injury is traumatic in origin. In other breeds, the etiology is not so definitive. The sesamoid may have multiple areas of fragmentation and proposed etiologies include congenital, traumatic, and degenerative. A congenital condition of bipartite sesamoids is described whereby the 2 fragments have rounded edges and there is no lameness attributable to the sesamoids. Some authors propose that degenerative fragmentation could be caused by disordered ossification or vascular compromise. Although rottweilers are over-represented, other breeds are reported. The metacarpophalangeal sesamoids are more commonly afflicted than the hindlimb sesamoids.

Clinical signs of sesamoid fracture and degeneration are similar, especially in chronic cases. The presenting history may be one of sudden lameness which subsides and then returns only after exercise. On physical exam, distinct pain is elicited by flexing the metacarpo- or metatarsophalangeal joints. The normal metacarpo- or metatarsophalangeal joint should flex to a 90 degree angle. A dog with sesamoid pain will significantly react to full flexion and may only have a 45 degree angle or less. Standard 2 view radiographs are obtained for diagnosis. Not all dogs with radiographic fragmentation of the sesamoids have associated clinical signs.

The recommended treatment for sesamoid fragmentation is conservative. Surgical excision of fragments is recommended only for unremitting discomfort and lameness.

## Techniques

### Conservative Treatment

In the acute stage treatment consists of NSAIDs and stabilization with a soft padded bandage and splint. Nonsteroidal anti-inflammatory drugs are administered for 1 to 2 weeks. The paw is bandaged with a "clamshell" splint that extends past the end of the digits. The splint remains in place for 1 week. At this time, passive range of motion exercises are begun and continued for 1 week.

Chronic sesamoid fragmentation or degeneration is also treated with NSAIDs and splinting. A depot steroid injection can be administered instead of treating with NSAIDs. Methyprednisolone (Depomedrol, Pfizer, New York, NY) at a dose of 0.5 mls is injected around the sesamoid.

### Surgical Treatment

The patient is placed in sternal recumbency for the forelimb and dorsal recumbency for the hindlimb. The surgical approach to the sesamoids is simplified if the injury involves the second or fifth digits. The sesamoid can be approached without invading the major metacarpal or metatarsal pad. This is usually possible because the 2nd and 7th sesamoids are most commonly affected. To approach the sesamoids of the second or fifth digits (the 1st, 2nd, 7th, 8th sesamoids), a skin incision is made on the palmar or plantar surface of the paw, just medial or lateral to the large central pad, respectively. The incision is directly over the sesamoid at the metacarpo- or metatarsophalangeal joint. The superficial flexor tendon is located and the annular ligament that attaches it to the sesamoids is incised on the side nearest to the affected bone. The flexor tendons are retracted and fragments of the sesamoid are sharply dissected away from their ligamentous attachments. Care is taken not to incise the collateral ligaments of the metacarpophalangeal joint. If a piece less than one third of the total bone is fractured, it is conventional to leave the larger fragment and remove the smaller. When the fracture is in the center portion, both fragments are removed.

Dermis and skin are closed in layers.

## Aftercare

For conservative treatment, a splint is maintained for one week. After the splint is removed, flexion exercises of the metacarpophalangeal joint are begun. The joints are gently flexed and extended as a group for 10 to 15 repetitions twice daily. Exercise is restricted to leash walks only for 4 to 8 weeks. For chronic cases treated with steroid injection, this can be repeated if needed in 4 to 6 weeks.

For surgical treatment, the paw is supported by a soft padded bandage that extends from the distal radius or distal tibia and covers the digits. The bandage is maintained for 7 to 10 days after surgery.

## Advantages and Disadvantages

There is an advantage to avoiding surgery in these cases. Lameness attributable to sesamoid disease may resolve satisfactorily with conservative treatment alone. In cases that undergo sesamoid excision, lameness often improves initially but may recur over time. There is a possibility that sesamoid excision may be associated with significant progression of degenerative joint disease radiographically. The sesamoids have numerous ligamentous attachments and disrupting these attachments could destabilize the metacarpo- or metatarsophalangeal joint. Surgery should be reserved for cases that have continued lameness that does not resolve with at least 8 weeks of conservative management.

## Suggested Readings


1. Mathews KG, Koblik PD, Whiteair JG et al. Fragmented palmar metacarpophalangeal sesamoids in dogs: a long-term evaluation. Vet Comp Orthop Traumatol 14:7-14, 2001.
2. Piermattei DL, Flo G. Brinker, Piermattei, and Flo's Handbook of Small Animal Orthopedics and Fracture Repair, 3rd ed. Philadelphia: W B Saunders, 1997, 382-384.
3. Read RA, Black AP, Armstrong SJ et al. Incidence and clinical significance of sesamoid disease in Rottweilers. Vet Rec 130:533-5, 1992.
4. Robins GM, Read RA. Diseases of the Sesamoid Bones. Bloomberg MS, Dee JF, Taylor RA. Canine Sports Medicine and Surgery. Philadelphia: W.B. Saunders Co., 1998, 255-264.

# Part Three: Athletic and Working Dog Injuries

# Chapter 10

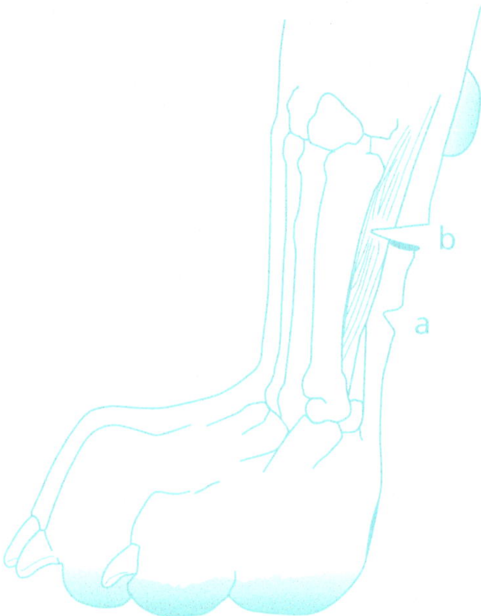


## Athletic and Working Dog Injuries

Robert L. Gillette, D.V.M., M.S.E

# General Information

The veterinary profession is currently witnessing an increased demand from clientele for information concerning performance of the canine athlete or working dog. The canine athlete can present uncommon challenges to the general practitioner. Some examples of these types of dogs include the sprint athlete, the endurance athlete and the workout companion. Some of the sprint activities include Greyhound racing, lure and field coursing, flyball, and agility. Some of the endurance activities include sled dog racing, upland bird hunting, game hunting, herding and the detection dogs. Recently there have been an increasing number of dogs participating with their owners during workouts. Workout companions accompany their owners while they jog, skate, hike, bike or perform many other exercise activities.

These dogs perform daily activities at a higher level than the normal pet or companion dog. If trained properly their body is stronger and can handle the extremes of their normal workload. In some instances, this higher level of activity combined with extended working periods predisposes these dogs to distal limb injuries. The paw is the part of body that makes the most contact with the surface and the factors surrounding this interaction create the potential for injury. The environment in which they work can affect the incidence of injury. Some dogs have to work in areas where the surface is rough or inconsistent. A rough surface will create injuries to the pads or webbing. An inconsistent surface will create injuries to the digits, metacarpus, tarsus and carpus.

In general the body condition of the canine athlete or working dog is much higher than that of the normal pet dog. Their training and conditioning programs are designed to prepare their bodies for the extremes of their work. If they are taken out of this training regimen their overall body condition will decline. The overall body condition of the dog should be taken into consideration when developing a treatment plan. Any amount of time away from their work will require at least that amount of time to recondition the body. For example, if they are rested for two weeks it will take at least two more weeks for their body to return to its previous condition level. This means that an injury will keep this dog out of work for at least four weeks. Therefore, it is very important that any injury be diagnosed properly at the initial examination. This is not as important in the pet dog as it is in the athletic or working dog. A misdiagnosis could lead to unnecessary downtime for the athletic dog.

In every lameness diagnostic work-up, it is important to palpate the entire musculoskeletal system. The athletic or working dog may not exhibit any lameness because the perceived pain is not great enough to produce a visual lameness. The dog may be too stoic. Although the dog does not feel the pain the structural fault will still alter the movement of the body's musculoskeletal structure. The altered forces related to this abnormal movement predisposes the rest of the musculoskeletal system to potential secondary injury. The secondary injury results in a visual lameness in the dog that warrants a veterinary consultation. The veterinarian should avoid the temptation to develop a treatment plan based upon the client's lameness description. If the described lameness is related to the secondary injury and not the primary injury, that was the underlying injury cause, the therapeutic regimen may result in failure or injury reoccurrence. For this reason, palpation of the entire musculoskeletal system should be included in every diagnostic work up of an athletic or working dog.

The initial treatment selection can also play a role in the amount of time away from work. The dog may not exhibit any reaction to the initial injury out in the field or while performing its specific activity. The drive and excitement to perform is so great that it often over-rides any perception of pain. If an injury is suspected or observed, injury management should begin immediately. First, stop the dogs activity and apply ice or any form of hypothermic application to the site of the suspected injury. Apply ice for at least 15 minutes to the injured site. Repeat this every hour for at least 6 hours post injury.

The initial injury treatment plan should allow for the injury to heal but require the least amount of time for rehabilitation. This starts with correctly identifying the tissue that is injured. It includes selecting the treatment that addresses the injured tissue yet requires the least amount of time to heal. For instance, the plan might utilize a splint to minimize tissue movement during the initial healing process. Lastly, the mental issues associated with the athletic or working dog and the management program of the dog's handler must be addressed. A lot of athletic dogs are considered "high drive dogs". They have a great need to perform their work. This can lead to management problems because their high energy level and related activity can disrupt the healing process.

# Skin Injuries

## Cracked Nails

### Definition and Indications

Cracked nails can be distal or proximal (Figure 10-1) They can be a painful condition that can cause gait abnormalities depending on the depth of the crack. The cause of the crack should be determined. The crack can be painful; however, if unnoticed or untreated, bacterial invasion can lead to infection of the nail or nail bed causing further pain. Treatment of any infection, sealing the crack and support of the injured area are indicated.

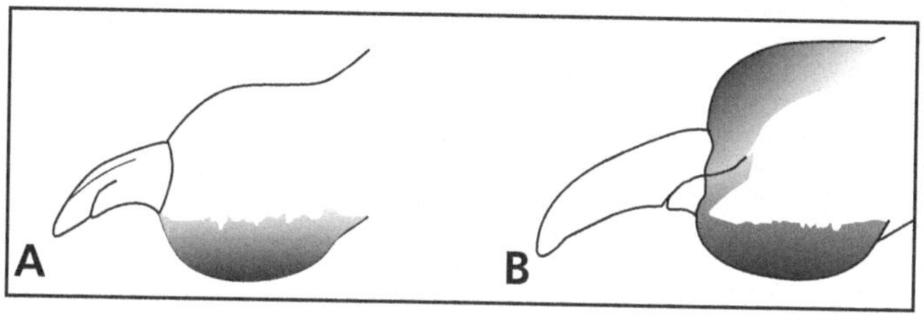


**Figure 10-1.** Toenail cracks **A.** Distal nail crack. **B.** Proximal nail crack into the nail bed.

Cracked nails can result from poor conditioning of the nails, which may be related to poor hair and skin condition. This is reflected by hard brittle nails. A thorough physical examination is indicated for these dogs.

Some owners believe long nails are an advantage for their dogs based on the "cleat theory". The belief is that longer nails provide maximum grip and better traction, similar to cleats on human athletic shoes. However, since the nail is attached to the digital bony structure, a long nail will act as a lever and put undo forces on digital bones and joint, predisposing to digital injuries. Thus, short nails are indicated for canine athletes to prevent cracked nails and other digital orthopedic injuries.

The length of the toenail can be related to the occurrence of toe dislocations. A long nail predisposes the toe to dislocation. Proponents of long nails suggest that longer nails help to provide surface traction however, the toenail plays a very minor role in surface traction. The paw pads provide almost all of the traction that occurs at impact. With soft surfaces like a racetrack, the webbing helps to provide traction. The disadvantages of long nails far outweigh any potential benefit. The longer nail acts like a fulcrum, which increases detrimental forces placed upon the bone and ligamentous structures of the paw (Figure 10-2).

Longer nails predispose the digits to fractures, dislocations and nail injuries. Toe nails should be maintained so that when the dog is standing on a hard surface the nail does not touch the ground. A sheet of paper should be able to slide easily between the surface and the end of the nail.

Nail trauma can result in a cracked nail with pain from the initial trauma and pain from hematoma development within the nail. Radiographic examination to evaluate potential fracture of the distal phalanx, the result of any hematoma pressure, and support of the injured area are indicated.

### Techniques

If a cracked nail is long and presented immediately after it occurs, it should be clipped. The area should be cleaned with an antibiotic/antiseptic solution and dried. The crack is then repaired with cyanoacrylate/super glue to seal out contamination and hold the nail segment together. A bandage can be applied for 2 to 3 days.

If the nail and/or nail bed are infected, the dog may need sedation prior to treatment. The digit and nail should be clipped and cleansed and an antibiotic/antiseptic soak performed. In some cases it may be necessary to remove the nail or entire distal phalanx (onychectomy) to eliminate the infection and pain. (See Chapter 6) The paw should be bandaged for seven days with periodic bandage changes.

If the cracked nail is due to poor conditioning of

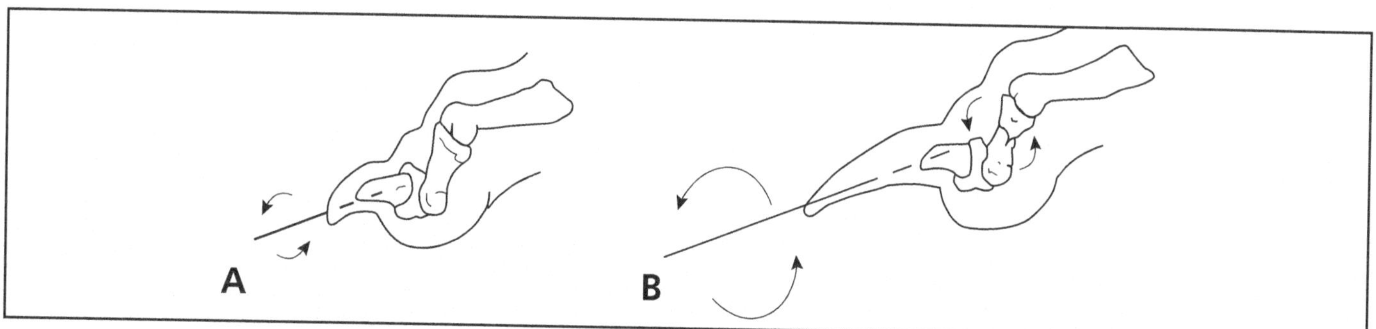


**Figure 10-2.** Nail length and predisposition to injury. **A.** Short nail-less leverage to cause digital injury *(short arrows)*. **B.** Long nail-more leverage to cause digital injury *(long arrows)*.

the dog, a thorough physical examination should be performed. Adjustments should be made in the nutrition and conditioning of the dog as needed, or any underlying disease conditions should be treated.

If nails are cracked because the owner is leaving them long to conform with the "cleat theory", the dangers of long nails should be discussed with the owner. The nails should be cut to an acceptable length.

A radiograph should be taken of digits that have nail injuries due to trauma to check for possible fracture of the distal phalanx. If trauma has caused a hematoma of the nail, a hole should be drilled in the nail to relieve pressure. This is followed by application of a bandage and a flex splint that extends beyond the digits. (See Chapter 2). If the nail is injured without a fracture of the distal phalanx, the splint is left on for 1 week. With a fracture of the distal phalanx, the splint should remain in place for at least 2 weeks followed by another radiograph to assess the status of the fracture.

### Aftercare

When the cracked nail is infected, the dog should be placed on systemic antibiotics. Exercise should be restricted for a period of 7 to 10 days.

If the cracked nail is associated with trauma and a fracture of the distal phalanx, radiographs 2 weeks post trauma will determine whether the fracture is healing. If the fracture is not healed further splinting is needed and exercise should be restricted for another 7 to 10 days.

### Advantages and Disadvantages

A problem with severely cracked nails or infected cracked nails is that treatment requires restricted exercise. This interferes with the dogs work, athletic performance or training for a period of time.

Conditioning with these underlying nail problems predisposes the dog to multiple nail involvement, which could complicate (i.e. involve more) treatment.

## Suggested Readings

1. Blythe, LL, Gannon, JR, Craig, AM: Care of the Racing Greyhound: A Guide for Trainers, Breeders, and Veterinarians. American Greyhound Council, Inc. Abilene, KS 1994.
2. Gillette, RL, Nails: Long or Short, The Athletic and Working Dog Newsletter, 1:2, 2002.
3. Swaim SF, Henderson RA: Small Animal Wound Management, 2nd ed.: Baltimore: Williams and Wilkins, 1997, 13, 53, and 295.

## Bruised Nails

### Definition and Indications

Sometimes trauma can cause a build-up of blood between the nail and distal phalanx. The nail is painful on palpation. If it is a light colored nail, the blood can be visualized. Sometimes bruised nails can be associated with blood dyscrasias. Check the other nails and the gingiva for petechia to rule out a hematological abnormality. Perform blood tests if warranted. If the bruise is not associated with blood dyscrasias, trauma can be assumed to be the cause. Radiographs are indicated to rule out a distal phalangeal fracture, especially in a dark-nailed dog.

### Techniques

Treatment can be addressed in two ways, either leave it on or remove the nail.

#### Leaving the Nail

Epsom salt soaks can help relieve the pain and heal a bruised nail. Soak the paw twice daily for 5 days.

#### Nail Removal

Remove the nail by cutting it back to the point of the bruise using nail clippers. Sedation is required for this procedure.

#### Aftercare

Rest the dog for 5 to 10 days. After nail removal, bandage the paw for 1 to 2 weeks with periodic changes. (See Chapter 2). Place the dog on systemic antibiotics to help prevent infection of the exposed nail.

### Advantages and Disadvantages

Leaving the nail on can be advantageous because it saves the nail. However, it may not be possible to resolve the problem by just soaking the paw. Removing the nail increases the chance of resolving the issue. It does, however, increase the therapy and recovery time.

## Suggested Readings

1. Blythe, LL, Gannon, JR, Craig, AM: Care of the Racing Greyhound: A Guide for Trainers, Breeders, and Veterinarians. American Greyhound Council, Inc. Abilene, KS 1994.
2. Gillette, RL, Nails: Long or Short, The Athletic and Working Dog Newsletter, 1:2, 2002.
3. Swaim SF, Henderson RA: Small Animal Wound Management, 2nd ed.: Baltimore: Williams and Wilkins, 1997, 13, 53, and 295.

## Avulsed Nails

### Definitions and Indications

In some instances the nail will come off and leave the distal phalanx exposed. Examine the paw for any dermatological causes. If the nail has fallen off due to an underlying dermatological issue, the treatment plan should address that problem. Causes of nail avulsion include a cracked nail getting caught on something or blunt trauma.

### Techniques

If the avulsion is related to trauma, radiographs are needed to check for any other trauma related injuries that might be present. Treat the avulsed nail as an open wound until a new nail grows. Onychectomy is an alternative treatment. (See Chapters 1 and 5).

### Aftercare

See aftercare of removed bruised nails.

### Advantages and Disadvantages

If the avulsed nail is treated as an open wound, the nail bed can produce new nail material. This can, however, result in a distorted nail that can cause further problems. These chronic problems diminish the performance level of the active and working dog. Performing an onychectomy, removes the distal phalanx and eliminates any potential follow-up nail problems.

## Suggested Readings


1. Blythe, LL, Gannon, JR, Craig, AM: Care of the Racing Greyhound: A Guide for Trainers, Breeders, and Veterinarians. American Greyhound Council, Inc. Abilene, KS 1994.
2. Gillette, RL, Nails: Long or Short, The Athletic and Working Dog Newsletter, 1:2, 2002.
3. Swaim SF, Henderson RA: Small Animal Wound Management, 2nd ed.: Baltimore: Williams and Wilkins, 1997, 13, 53, and 295.


## Pads Injuries

### General Information

Visually examine the pads for any problems or abnormalities. Pad condition can be related to overall body health and condition. Check for prior disease history or health changes by taking a thorough patient history. Poorly conditioned pads are prone to damage. Check for hard, cracked, brittle or dry pads. First, check for any growths or abnormal looking pads. If any are seen, biopsies should be performed to determine the nature of the lesion. The growths should be removed or the problem disease addressed appropriately.

Pad lesions are common in athletic and working dogs. In general, treatments for these lesions are the same as those described in Chapter 4.

### Corns

### Definitions and Indications

Corns are a cause of pad pain primarily in greyhounds (Figure 10-3). This pathological condition can cause a leg carrying lameness in greyhounds. The digital pads are most commonly affected. There are three theories as to the cause of the condition. One theory is that cuts or punctures result in scar tissue accumulation. Related to this is the theory that the presence of a small foreign body in the pad produces an accumulation of scar tissue at the lesion site. This results in a thickened hard "corn" as the body attempts to isolate the foreign body. Another theory is that a papilloma viral infection causes the lesion. With the pressure and abrasion of walking, the papilloma is pressed into deeper pad layers forming a painful "corn". A third theory is that chronic low grade pressure on the digital pad skin by the distal interphalangeal joint in the presence of relatively sparse fibroadipose tissue results in a callus/"corn-like" lesion.[8]

Greyhounds affected with "corns"/warts usually have a history of being racing dogs at sometime in their life. The condition can affect one or more paws and one or more pads on a paw. Pads of the third and fourth digits (weight-bearing digits) are the most commonly affected digits.[2,5,8] Corns can be managed medically or surgically.

### Techniques

Softening the pads using a pad softening solution and slicing off the corn's surface every month to two months is a non-surgical option for treating corns. Soaking the paw and applying manual pressure to the pad to express the corn has been described. Other

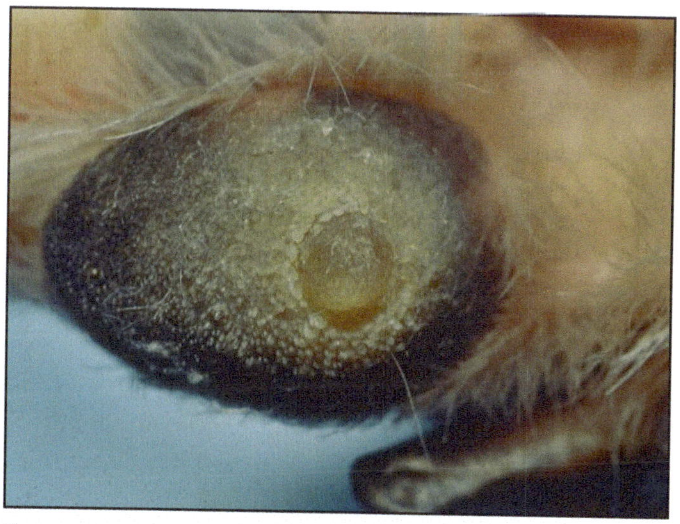

**Figure 10-3.** Corn on the pad of a racing greyhound. (From Swaim SF, Bohling MW, Wright JC, et al: Paw pad pain: A review of corns in dogs. Vet Med 109: 61, 2014.)

treatments and "home remedies" have been reported.[8]

The corn can be surgically removed by excising it from the pad. A number 15 scalpel blade is used to create a full thickness eliptical incision around the corn. The corn is removed leaving any subcutaneous fibroadipose tissue that may be present. A 3-0 monofilament nylon or polypropylene suture is used in a simple interrupted or far-near-near-far pattern to close the incision. A technique that may help delay the return of the corn is to cauterize the underlying tissue and allowing it to heal as an open wound.

The definitive technique for eliminating the corn and associated problems is to surgically remove the digit with the affected pad (See Chapter 6).

### Aftercare

When the corn has been surgically removed with suturing, bandaging with padding under the metacarpal/metatarsal pad or use of "clam shell" splints for 2 weeks should be considered to keep pressure off of the digital pads as they heal. If the tissue is cauterized and the lesion is left open, bandages should be applied for a period of two weeks. Again, padding under the metacarpal/metatarsal pad or "clam shell" splints should be considered to keep pressure off of digital pads at they heal. The bandages should be changed and the lesion cleansed every three to four days. Systemic antibiotics and analgesics should be given while the lesion is open. (See Chapters 2 and 6).

Based on clinical findings and preliminary research, prevention of the return of corns is based on relieving pressure on the involved pads. Padded booties of some sort could be helpful. The subdermal injection of silicone block gel particles under the involved pads has shown promise.

### Advantages and Disadvantages

The nonsurgical option is time intensive and does not eliminate the problem.

If the corn is excised and the pad has been sutured, pain is relieved, but the corn will return in 2 to 9 months. The client should be informed of this before the procedure is performed. Cauterizing the underlying tissue helps to delay the return of the corn. The recovery from this procedure can be painful and requires two to four weeks of bandaging.

The advantage of toe removal is that the affected tissues are removed. The disadvantage is that this procedure can only be used on 1 to 2 digits per paw. This technique is not an option on paws that have multiple toes affected. There is also the possibility that a corn will develop on an adjacent digit after removing an affected digit. Cutting out the corn, removes the source of the pain, but return of the corn is inevitable.

## Suggested Readings


1. Andelman NC: Dermatology, *In* Bloomberg MS, Dee JF, Taylor RA, eds.: Canine Sports Medicine and Surgery, Philadelphia, WB Saunders, 1998, 35.
2. Balara JM, McCarthy RJ, Kivpal M, et al: Clinical, histologic and immunohistochemical characterization of wart-like lesions on the paw pads of dogs: 24 cases (2000-2007) J Am Vet Med Assoc. 234: 1555-1558, 2009
3. Blythe, LL, Gannon, JR, Craig, AM: Care of the Racing Greyhound: A Guide for Trainers, Breeders, and Veterinarians. American Greyhound Council, Inc. Abilene, KS 1994.
4. Borghese IF: Corns and warts: Definitions, causes, and treatments. Celebrating Greyhounds. 8:48, 2003.
5. Guilliard MJ, Segboer I, Shearer DH: Corns in dogs: Signalment, possible aetiology and response to surgical treatment. J Small Animal Pract. 51: 162, 2010.
6. Kapatkin AS, Garcia-Nolan T, Hayashi K: Carpus, metacarpuys, and digits. In Tobia KM, Johnston SA, eds.: Veterinary Surgery, Small Animal, Vol 2.: St. Louis, Elsevier-Saunders, 2012, 785.
7. Swaim SF, Amalsadvala T, Marghitu DB, et.al: Pressure reduction effects of subdermal silicone block gel particle implantation: A preliminary study. WOUNDS 16:299-312, 2004.
8. Swaim SF, Bohling MW, Wright JC, et al: Paw pad pain: A review of corns in dogs. Vet Med 109: 61, 2014.


# Muscle Injuries Associated with the Distal Extremities

### General Information

The interosseous muscles are the main muscle group of the distal appendage. Injuries to these muscles in the back legs are rare, but the muscles of the front paw are predisposed to injury. The carpus is hyperextended on impact and the metacarpal bones are spread apart. This occurs at the same time that the muscles are contracting. These combined actions predispose the interosseous muscles to injury.

# Interosseous Myositis or Muscle Strain

### Definition and Indications

The muscles of the distal extremity can be strained just like any other muscle of the body. Point pain on the caudal aspect of the metacarpal region can be indicative of myositis or muscle strain. Radiographs should be taken to rule out any problems associated with the bones in that area. Palpation can help to rule out tendon problems. A tendon injury will have pain associated with toe extension whereas interosseous muscles do not exhibit pain on slight toe extension.

### Techniques
Treatment involves application of a flexion splint to minimize the distractive forces on the injured muscles. (See Chapter 2).

### Aftercare
The splint is left on for 3 to 5 days and the dog is cage or crate rested for 10 days. Nonsteroidal anti-inflammatory drugs such as Metacam (The oral dose is 0.2 mg/kg as a single dose on the first day followed by 0.1 mg/kg given once every 24 hours thereafter) are given for 3 to 5 days to help reduce inflammation.

### Advantages and Disadvantages
A flexion splint reduces the healing time. If proper diagnostic techniques are not used, the condition may be misdiagnosed as a tendon problem. This results in improper treatment and increased recovery time. Application of a flexion splint reduces the forces that act to impede tissue healing.

## Suggested Readings

1. Blythe LL, Gannon, JR, Craig, AM: Care of the Racing Greyhound: A guide for Trainers, Breeders, and Veterinarians. American Greyhound Council, Inc. Abilene, KS 1994.
2. Dee JF, Dee LG, Eaton-Wells RD: Injuries of high performance dogs. In Whittick WG, ed.: Canine Orthopedics, 2nd ed.: Philadelphia: Lea and Febiger, 1990.
3. Ferguson RG: Treatment of soft tissue musculoskeletal injuries. The TG Hungerford Refresher Course for Veterinarians. Proceedings 122, Postgraduate in Veterinary Science, University of Sydney, Australia, 1989.


## Interosseous Muscle Tears or Ruptures

### Definitions and Indications
These usually present as an acute swelling on the caudal aspect of the metacarpal region. If not recognized initially, they can later present as point pain over the torn muscle. Swelling will be dependent upon which muscle is injured and the location of the injury. Muscle tears can also result from external lesions. If the lesion is deep enough the muscles can also be lacerated when the skin is cut. Radiographs should be taken to rule out any bony lesions.

### Techniques
Initial treatment is cold therapy. An ice pack or other cold medium is applied for 10 to 15 minutes at a time. Repeat every hour for up to 12 hours. Treatment is dependent upon the damage to other tissues. Assess the injury initially for skin damage and tendon status, as well as ascertaining if innervation has been affected. Treatment of these problems is discussed in other areas of the book. Once the status of the lesion has been established and the tendon and neuronal status have been determined to be intact the muscle or skin and muscle damage can be addressed. Muscle tears or lacerations in the area of the caudal metacarpal region are usually treated conservatively. If the skin has been cut the wound is debrided and cleaned. Simple-interrupted sutures and tension sutures of non-absorbable material are used to hold the skin edges together. The muscle tissue does not usually need to be sutured.

### Aftercare
Once the initial therapy is concluded a flexion splint is applied and left on for 5 days in cases where only the muscle tissue has been affected. (See Chapter 2). In cases where the skin and muscle have been cut, the paw is placed in a flexion splint for a total of 14 days. Check and replace the splint after 7 days to make sure the site has not become infected. Oral antibiotics are indicated if the clinician feels the lesion warrants antibiotic therapy. Nonsteroidal anti-inflammatory drugs are given to help reduce swelling and inflammation. The dog should be cage or crate rested for 10 to 14 days.

Return to activity starts after the rest period. Both the 5 days of rest associated with injury of the muscle alone or the 14 days of rest associated with a laceration that includes both the skin and the muscle is followed by a time of limited activity. For muscle rehabilitation therapy, controlled leash walks are used for the next 5 to 7 days. Activities are introduced by having the dog do uphill runs for front leg injuries. The dog starts at the bottom of the hill and runs uphill, where he is caught and led downhill on a lead. Usually 50 to 100 yards is sufficient. Four to 5 repetitions are performed once a day. Level ground running is best for reconditioning rear leg injuries. Conditioning activity is performed for 7 days after which the dog can return to normal activity.

### Advantages and Disadvantages
Conservative treatment without any splinting or rest will prolong the recovery time. This is detrimental to the conditioning level of the canine athlete or working dog.

Splinting the paw in a flexion splint initially enhances healing of the injured tissues. Progressively increasing the physical stresses on the palmar tissues, lines up and strengthens the collagen tissue associated with healing. It decreases the chance of reoccurrence.

## Suggested Readings

1. Blythe LL, Gannon, JR, Craig, AM: Care of the Racing Greyhound: A guide for Trainers, Breeders, and Veterinarians. American Greyhound Council, Inc. Abilene, KS 1994.
2. Dee JF, Dee LG, Eaton-Wells RD: Injuries of high performance dogs. In Whittick WG, ed.: Canine Orthopedics, 2nd ed.: Philadelphia: Lea and Febiger, 1990.
3. Ferguson RG: Treatment of soft tissue musculoskeletal injuries. The TG Hungerford Refresher Course for Veterinarians. Proceedings 122, Postgraduate in Veterinary Science, University of Sydney, Australia, 1989.

# Synovial Injuries

### General Information

The synovial joints of the distal extremities are held together by ligaments and are encased by a synovial sheath. Each synovial joint has a sheath that covers it like a sleeve. The synovial sheath is a strong, fibrous (collagen) tissue that encloses the joint space and serves to help support the joint. It produces synovial fluid that lubricates and protects the hyaline cartilage and inner lining of the joint. Synovial fluid is a transparent, viscid fluid secreted by the synovial membrane and found in joint cavities, bursa, and tendon sheaths. Ligaments are fibrous structures designed to prevent abnormal motion of a joint and connect bones to bones.

# Acute Carpal Synovitis

### Defintions and Indications

Synovitis is the inflammation of a synovial (joint-lining) membrane. It is usually painful and characterized by swelling, due to effusion in the synovial space. It differs from a sprain in that ligament tissues are usually associated with sprains. In a joint with synovitis, the ligamentous structures are intact but the synovial structures and membrane are involved. The high forces related to activity that affects a joint can lead to acute synovitis. Acute swelling of the joint after activity should be taken seriously. Radiographs should be taken to rule out any bone or ligamentous disruption. If these structures are intact then the inflammation may be associated with the synovial structures. If synovial inflammation is not addressed in a timely fashion it can lead to a weakened and inflamed synovial structure.

### Techniques

If there is no fracture or sprain and synovitis is diagnosed, a conservative management program can be developed to treat the injury. Joint immobilization reduces stress on the inflamed tissues. A flexion splint is placed over the joint as described in Chapter 2. A non-steroidal anti-inflammatory drug (NSAID) therapy regimen is initiated. To help reduce joint inflammation and enhance the production of healthy synovial fluid, a polysulfated glycosaminoglycan (PSGAG) (Adequan®) is given intramuscularly at a dose of 0.02 mg per pound body weight.

### Aftercare

The splint is kept on for 5 to 7 days. A non-steroidal anti-inflammatory drug can be given for the duration of the management program to help minimize pain associated with the injury. It is usually not needed for longer than 10 to 14 days. The PSGAG's are given twice weekly for 2 weeks post diagnosis. Exercise and activity should be restricted for 14 to 21 days. Activities are introduced by having the dog do uphill runs. The dog starts at the bottom of the hill and runs uphill, where he is caught and led downhill on a lead. This activity is performed for 7 days before returning the dog to normal activity.

### Advantages and Disadvantages

Splinting the injury reduces stress on the synovial tissues and helps to stop the inflammatory cycle. The PSGAG treatments enhance the healing process and minimize healing disruptions.

The patient should be monitored for any deleterious affects of a long term regimen that includes NSAID's and PSGAG's. There are reports that long term use of NSAID's can be harmful to the gastrointestinal tract. The molecule of the PSGAG is somewhat similar to the heparin molecule. Because of these similarities, the occurrence of blood dyscrasia's should be monitored in patients that have had previous blood problems.

## Suggested Readings

1. Blythe LL, Gannon, JR, Craig, AM: Care of the Racing Greyhound: A guide for Trainers, Breeders, and Veterinarians. American Greyhound Council, Inc. Abilene, KS 1994.
2. Dee JF, Dee LG, Eaton-Wells RD: Injuries of high performance dogs. In Whittick WG, ed.: Canine Orthopedics, 2nd ed.: Philadelphia: Lea and Febiger, 1990.
3. Ferguson RG: Treatment of soft tissue musculoskeletal injuries. The TG Hungerford Refresher Course for Veterinarians. Proceedings 122, Postgraduate in Veterinary Science, University of Sydney, Australia, 1989.

# Chronic Carpal Synovitis

### Defintions and Indications

Joints with synovitis do not ususally present immediately nor is synovitis suspected in a lameness that has been present for a period of time. In cases of delayed diagnosis the carpal joint will be swollen. Ligaments will be intact upon examination and there will be no boney alteration in the radiograph.

### Techniques

The treatment plan for chronic carpal synovitis is the same as that described for the acute injury.

### Aftercare

Activity and exercise are limited for 21 days. A flexion splint is placed over the joint to restrict movement for 7 days. Epsom salt soaks may help to enhance healing of chronic synovitis. These soaks are initiated after the splint is removed and can be continued for up to 4 days. Pour enough Epsom salt into a bowl to supersaturate the water. A hand towel or wash cloth is placed in the bowl until it is soaked. The towel is placed on a plate and then set in a microwave oven for 15 to 30 seconds depending on the strength of the microwave. It is then tested to make sure it is not too hot to be placed on the leg. The soaked towel or wash cloth can then be wrapped around or placed on the injured area. It is left in place for 10 to 15 minutes twice daily. After the initial Epsom salt soaks, hot water soaks can be used for another 5 to 7 days. Each soaking treatment is followed by applying passive range of motion (PROM) to the affected joint. This involves flexing and extending the joint 15 times twice a day. Light exercise is allowed after 21 days and regular activity can be initiated in 28 days.

### Advantages and Disadvantages

There is usually a lot of fibrous tissue accumulation associated with chronic synovitis of the carpus. Epsom salt soaks and hot water soaks combined with the PROM exercises help to increase the range of motion in the joint.

It is important to rinse off the Epsom salt after each soak. Ingestion of Epsom salt can cause diarrhea. It is common for the injury to return in highly active dogs and in these patients an ongoing management program may be required for the duration of their career.

## Suggested Readings


1. Blythe LL, Gannon, JR, Craig, AM: Care of the Racing Greyhound: A guide for Trainers, Breeders, and Veterinarians. American Greyhound Council, Inc. Abilene, KS 1994.
2. Dee, JF, Dee, LG and Eaton-Wells, RD. Injuries of high-performance dogs. In Canine Orthopedics, Second Edition. Whittick, WG, ed. Lea and Febiger, Philadelphia 1990.
3. Ferguson, RG. Treatment of soft tissue musculoskelatal injuries. Greyhound Medicine and Surgery, The T G Hungerford Refresher Course for Veterinarians: Proceedings 122, Post Graduate in Veterinary Science, University of Sydney, Australia, 1989.


## Acute Sesamoidal Synovitis

### Definitions and Indications

This is a very common issue in the athletic or working dog and it is very important to determine the significance of the problem. This can occur in any of the 4 paws, on both the front and back legs. It is most commonly found in the sesamoids of the second and fifth digit. The dog might exhibit a toe-touching lameness on the affected paw. On presentation, the affected joint will appear swollen. The normal metacarpo/tarsophalangeal joint should flex to a 90 degree angle. A dog with sesamoidal synovitis will have pain when the joint is flexed and it is very common for flexion of the joint to be restricted to a 45 degree angle or less.

### Techniques

Treatment begins with oral or systemic NSAID's for 5 to 7 days. It is important to minimize surface impact and activity of the joint. A flexion splint can be applied for 7 days to the front leg to stabilize the affected joint. In the back leg a splint that extends past the end of the toes, e.g. "clam shell" splint, (See Chapter 2) can help reduce stress on the sesamoid tissues. More aggressive therapy includes using an anti-inflammatory paint of methylprednisilone mixed in Dimethyl Sulfoxide (DMSO). The paint is applied to the inflamed sesamoid twice daily for 5 days. Another method of applying the methylprednisilone is by injecting 10 mg (0.5 milliliters) around the sesmoid.

### Aftercare

The paw should be rested for 7 days. Then flexion exercises are initiated and continued for 7 days. These involve flexing the joint 15 times twice daily. Hot packs or soaks should be applied 10 to 15 minutes prior to the exercises to help loosen the tissue. After 14 days the dog can return to normal activity. If this does not work retirement from the activity that is affected by the problem should be discussed with the handler.

### Advantages and Disadvantages

Sesamoid problems are often insignificant and frequently overlooked. The key to management is recognizing them as a potential problem. Once they are recognized treating them aggressively is very beneficial to the patient.

DSMO and methylprednisone can affect owners or handlers physically. Gloves should be worn whenever handling this drug.

## Suggested Readings

1. Blythe LL, Gannon, JR, Craig, AM: Care of the Racing Greyhound: A guide for Trainers, Breeders, and Veterinarians. American Greyhound Council, Inc. Abilene, KS 1994.
2. Dee, JF, Dee, LG and Eaton-Wells, RD. Injuries of high-performance dogs. In Canine Orthopedics, Second Edition. Whittick, WG, ed. Lea and Febiger, Philadelphia 1990.
3. Ferguson, RG. Treatment of soft tissue musculoskelatal injuries. Greyhound Medicine and Surgery, The T G Hungerford Refresher Course for Veterinarians: Proceedings 122, Post Graduate in Veterinary Science, University of Sydney, Australia, 1989.

# Chronic Sesamoidal Synovitis

### Definitions and Indications

This problem usually presents as a slight lameness that has been undiagnosed for a long period of time. The dog might exhibit a toe-touching lameness on the affected paw. The joint can appear very swollen and it usually has minimal flexibility. Pain will be present on flexion of the metacarpo/tarsophalangeal joint. It usually occurs in older dogs that show evidence of multiple musculoskeletal problems. There will be no ligament instability or any boney alterations. After the entire musculoskeletal system has been evaluated, and if no other problems have been found related to the lameness or the drop in performance, then consider chronic sesmoidal synovitis as the significant issue.

### Technique

Treatment is similar to that for acute cases but recovery is less likely. Treatment begins with oral or systemic NSAID's for 5 to 7 days. Methylprednisilone 10 mg (0.5 milliliters) is injected around the sesmoid. A flex splint is applied for 7 days to the front leg to stabilize the affected joint. In the back leg, a splint that extends past the end of the toes, e.g. "clam shell" splint, (See Chapter 2) is used to reduce stress on the sesmoid tissues.

### Aftercare

The splint should be left in place for 10 to 14 days. Flexion exercises are initiated and continued for 7 days after the splint is removed. These exercises involve flexing the joint 15 times twice daily. Hot packs or soaks should be applied 10 to 15 minutes prior to the exercises to help loosen the tissue. At this point the dog can return to normal activity. If this does not work retirement from the activity that is affected by the problem should be discussed with the handler.

### Advantages and Disadvantages

Identifying or correctly diagnosing chronic sesamoidal synovitis is a key component in resolving the related lameness. The treatment plan increases the chances of returning to normal. Unfortunately, the chronicity of the problem results in a low chance of recovery.

## Suggested Readings

1. Blythe LL, Gannon, JR, Craig, AM: Care of the Racing Greyhound: A guide for Trainers, Breeders, and Veterinarians. American Greyhound Council, Inc. Abilene, KS 1994.
2. Dee JF, Dee LG, Eaton-Wells RD: Injuries to high-performance dogs. In Whittick WG, ed.: Canine Orthopedics, Philadelphia: Lea and Febiger, 1990.
3. Ferguson RG: Treatment of soft tissue musculoskeletal injuries. Greyhound Medicine and Surgery, The TG Hungerford Refresher Course for Veterinarians: Proceedings 122, Postgraduate in Veterinary Science. University of Sydney, Australia, 1989.

# Toe Dislocations (Ligamentous Injuries of the Phalanges)

### General Information

The toe is made up of 3 phalangeal bones (1 proximal, 2 middle & 3 distal) and 2 interphalangeal joints. Toe dislocation is a common injury in the athletic and working dog, especially those that work in the field environment. There are three degrees of toe dislocation (See Chapter 9, Ligamentous Injuries of the Phalanges).

### First Degree Dislocations

### Definitions and Indications

A first degree dislocation involves a stretching of the ligament and synovial structure but the ligament does not rupture. This can occur in any digit. It usually occurs to the proximal interphalangeal joint, but it can occur in the distal interphalangeal joint also. It rarely occurs in the metacarpo/metatarsophalangeal joint. This will often go unnoticed in the working or athletic dog. The dog will exhibit an acute transient lameness post workout. This will be followed by a return to observable soundness. Because the dog appears sound and does not show any further lameness, the normal working routine is maintained. In reality the dog has altered its gait to compensate for the pain. At a later date there will be a breakdown of one of the other joints related to the altered gait. This will result in a recurring lameness because the primary gait abnormality has not been addressed.

### Techniques

The dog should be stopped from participating in the activity or work. An NSAID regimen can be initiated.

### Aftercare

Treatment is followed by 3 to 5 days of rest and the dog is placed on nonsteroidal anti-inflammatory drugs for pain.

### Advantages and Disadvantages

To minimize future problems, it is important to recognize this problem early. It is important to initiate the return to function gradually over a 2-week period to prevent re-injury.

## Suggested Readings


1. Blythe LL, Gannon, JR, Craig, AM: Care of the Racing Greyhound: A guide for Trainers, Breeders, and Veterinarians. American Greyhound Council, Inc. Abilene, KS 1994.
2. Dee, JF, Dee, LG and Eaton-Wells, RD. Injuries of high-performance dogs. In Canine Orthopedics, Second Edition. Whittick, WG, ed. Lea and Febiger, Philadelphia.
3. Early TD, Dee JF. Trauma to the carpus, tarsus and phalanges of dogs and cats. Vet Clin North Am 10:717, 1980.
4. Ferguson, RG. Treatment of soft tissue musculoskelatal injuries. Greyhound Medicine and Surgery, The T G Hungerford Refresher Course for Veterinarians: Proceedings 122, Post Graduate in Veterinary Science, University of Sydney, Australia, 1989.


### Second Degree Dislocation
### Definitions and Indications

A level 2 dislocation involves a rupture of one of the joint ligaments but not the synovial sheath. The toe will present with a swelling around the joint but the toe will appear to be in place. Manipulation of the toe will show that the joint will come out of place. Radiographs should be taken to confirm that the bony structures are intact.

### Technique

If the injury is acute, ice packs (cryotherapy or hypothermic therapy) should be applied to the joint for 15 minutes every hour for 6 hours. A splint should be applied to the paw to eliminate further trauma to the joint. In the author's experience it is best to allow 12 to 24 hours of crate rest with the splint to let the injury subside. Surgery can be performed to reattach the two ends of the ligaments.

### Aftercare

The splint should remain in place for at least 14 days. The dog should be crate rested for 7 days following removal of the splint. The dog can begin light activity for 7 days. Hot packs or soaks should be applied 10 to 15 minutes prior to the exercises to help loosen the tissue and cryotherapy should be applied to the joint post work for 15 minutes. The dog can return to normal work 28 days post-surgery.

### Advantages and Disadvantages

Early diagnosis of the problem and immediate initiation of the treatment regimen allows for a more successful prognosis and an early return to function. It is important to repair the joint structure as soon as possible. Don't wait a week or 2.

If the joint is not stabilized in some manner, this will turn into an ongoing lameness.

## Suggested Readings


1. Blythe LL, Gannon, JR, Craig, AM: Care of the Racing Greyhound: A guide for Trainers, Breeders, and Veterinarians. American Greyhound Council, Inc. Abilene, KS 1994.
2. Dee, JF, Dee, LG and Eaton-Wells, RD. Injuries of high-performance dogs. In Canine Orthopedics, Second Edition. Whittick, WG, ed. Lea and Febiger, Philadelphia, 1990.
3. Early TD, Dee JF. Trauma to the carpus, tarsus and phalanges of dogs and cats. Vet Clin North Am 10:717, 1980.
4. Ferguson, RG. Treatment of soft tissue musculoskelatal injuries. Greyhound Medicine and Surgery, The T G Hungerford Refresher Course for Veterinarians: Proceedings 122, Post Graduate in Veterinary Science, University of Sydney, Australia, 1989.


### Third Degree Toe Dislocation
### Definitions and Indications

In a third degree dislocation the entire support structure for the joint is disrupted. The ligaments and synovial structure have been ruptured and do not support the joint. The joint is out of place and manipulation cannot return it to its normal alignment.

### Techniques

Surgery is required to restructure the joint. The ligaments and surrounding soft tissue are sutured using 4 to 6 horizontal mattress sutures of 4-0 polydioxanone (PDS) suture.

### Aftercare

The paw is then splinted for 6 weeks. If this procedure fails, a toe amputation may be required.

### Advantages and Disadvantages

Repairing the ligament and soft tissues of the third degree toe dislocation allows the dog to keep the toe.

If this procedure fails there is a lot of rehabilitation time lost. Most dogs can perform very well after a toe amputation. To save the potential time lost due to surgical repair, some veterinarians elect to perform a toe amputation first.

# Suggested Readings

1. Blythe LL, Gannon, JR, Craig, AM: Care of the Racing Greyhound: A guide for Trainers, Breeders, and Veterinarians. American Greyhound Council, Inc. Abilene, KS 1994.
2. Dee, JF, Dee, LG and Eaton-Wells, RD. Injuries of high-performance dogs. In Canine Orthopedics, Second Edition. Whittick, WG, ed. Lea and Febiger, Philadelphia 1990.
3. Early TD, Dee JF. Trauma to the carpus, tarsus and phalanges of dogs and cats. Vet Clin North Am 10:717, 1980.
4. Ferguson, RG. Treatment of soft tissue musculoskelatal injuries. Greyhound Medicine and Surgery, The T G Hungerford Refresher Course for Veterinarians: Proceedings 122, Post Graduate in Veterinary Science, University of Sydney, Australia, 1989.


# Tendon Injuries

# Sprains

## General Information

The athletic and working dog places a greater amount of physical stress on the musculoskeletal structure than the typical pet dog. Tendons are flexible tissues with no blood vessels within them. There are three levels of tendon injury in relation to strain injuries. In a first degree tendon injury there is a strain of the tendonous structure but no tissue separation. In a second degree tendon injury there is a partial disruption of the tendon structure. In a third degree tendon injury there is total disruption of the tendon structure. Tendons can also be lacerated traumatically. The palmar and plantar digital flexors are common sites of injury. In these areas the tendons are contained within tendonous sheaths. Sometimes the sheath becomes irritated (tenosynovitis) in addition to the tendon injury.

## First Degree Superficial and Deep Digital Flexor Tendon Injury

## Definitions and Indications

(See Chapter 7, Ligament and Tendon Injuries)
This is usually a mild injury. The history will usually include a description of the dog working and suddenly becoming lame. They appear to recover from the injury and usually are sound or have improved greatly the next day. This type of injury may result in an inflamed tendon sheath without any apparent tendon damage. Flexion and extension of the metacarpo/metatarsophalangeal joints of the paw will elicit a pain response or have restricted movement. Point pressure placed directly over the digital flexor tendons may also illicit a pain response. Swelling will be evident in this area depending on the severity of the injury. In old chronic injuries the tendons will feel thickened and enlarged. Radiographs should be taken to confirm that there is no bony involvement.

## Techniques

The dog's performance abilities and expectations dictate the therapy regimen. No treatment is needed if there are no problems in performance and no apparent lameness. The problem should be noted in the record and the dog should be watched for any performance changes in subsequent activities or work. If a drop in performance or lameness occurs, the dog should be reevaluated by the veterinarian for any significant trauma in this area.

If a lameness is evident or the dog's performance has been affected and it is related to a first degree tendon injury, then treatment is warranted. Conservative management should begin with an oral systemic NSAID regimen and a PSGAG regimen.

If this approach does not work, methylprednisilone can be injected along the line of the tendons and the dog rested for 7 to 10 days. If this regimen does not improve the damaged structure it is best to discuss, with the handler, reducing activity or retiring the dog from the activity that creates the ongoing or reoccurring lameness (See Chapter 7, Ligament and Tendon Injuries).

## Aftercare

The NSAID regimen is continued for 5 to 7 days. The intramuscular polysulfated glucosaminoglycans (Adequan) is given twice weekly for two weeks.

Moist, wet hot packs should be applied twice daily to the injured region for 5 to 7 days. A flexed splint can be placed on the paw for 5 to 7 days to minimize physical stress on the tendonous structures. Rest is indicated for 2 weeks. The return to activity should be gradual over a 2 to 4 week period.

## Advantages and Disadvantages

Identifying this injury early and treating it aggressively will minimize any decline in performance and reduce healing time.


# Suggested Readings

1. Dee, JF, Dee, LG and Eaton-Wells, RD. Injuries of high-performance dogs. In Canine Orthopedics, Second Edition. Whittick, WG, ed. Lea and Febiger, Philadelphia 1990.
2. Ferguson, RG. Treatment of soft tissue musculoskelatal injuries. Greyhound Medicine and Surgery, The T G Hungerford Refresher Course for Veterinarians: Proceedings 122, Post Graduate in Veterinary Science, University of Sydney, Australia, 1989.

## Second Degree Supericial and Deep Flexor Tendon Injury

### Definition and indications

(See Chapter 7, Ligament and Tendon Injuries)
The history will usually include a description of the dog working and suddenly becoming lame. Dogs do not appear to recover quickly from this kind of injury. There will be a lameness and swelling in the area of the damaged tissue. This type of injury may result in an inflamed tendon sheath without any apparent tendon damage. Flexion and extension of the metacarpo/tarso-phalangeal joints of the paw will elicit a pain response or cause restricted movement. Point pressure placed directly over the digital flexor tendons may also illicit a pain response. Radiographs should be taken to confirm that there is no bony involvement.

### Techniques

The athletic activity or work should be stopped and the paw should be supported to minimize further damage to the tendon. Cryotherapy should be initiated by the handler. At clinical presentation a flex splint should be applied. Surgery is usually not indicated in a second degree injury.

### Aftercare

An oral systemic NSAID regimen and a PSGAG regimen should be initiated. The NSAID regimen is continued for 5 to 7 days. The intramuscular polysulfated glucos-aminoglycans (Adequan) is given twice weekly for 2 weeks. A flexed splint is placed on the paw for 10 to 14 days to minimize physical stress on the tendinous structures. Crate rest is indicated for the next 10 to 14 days. Moist, wet hot packs should be applied twice daily to the injured region for 5 to 7 days following splint removal. The crate rest is followed by limited activity for the next 10 to 14 days. The return to activity should be gradual over a 2 to 4 week period.

### Advantages and Disadvantages

Identifying this injury early and treating it aggressively will minimize any decline in performance and reduce healing time.

The rest needed for the healing process in this therapy regimen will sometimes affect the mentality of the high-drive athletic and working dog. At any point in their rest period their pent-up energy will cause them to try to get out and run. This will usually result in a set-back and disruption of the healing process.

## Suggested Readings

1. Dee, JF, Dee, LG and Eaton-Wells, RD. Injuries of high-performance dogs. In Canine Orthopedics, Second Edition. Whittick, WG, ed. Lea and Febiger, Philadelphia 1990.
2. Ferguson, RG. Treatment of soft tissue musculoskelatal injuries. Greyhound Medicine and Surgery, The T G Hungerford Refresher Course for Veterinarians: Proceedings 122, Post Graduate in Veterinary Science, University of Sydney, Australia, 1989.

## Third Degree Superficial and Deep Digital Flexor Tendon Injury

### Definition and indications

(See Chapter 7, Ligament and Tendon Injuries)
As with the other levels of digital tendon injury, the history will often include a description of the dog working and suddenly becoming lame. Usually the lameness is apparent the next day. The dog sometimes appears to recover from the injury and is sound or has improved greatly by the next day. Because of this scenario many of these injuries present as chronic injuries. A few days to weeks later the structure of the paw will be altered and the handler will see that the dog is lame. These structural alterations have been described as a "dropped toe" (superficial digital tendon rupture) or a "sprung toe" (deep digital tendon rupture) depending on which tendon is affected. In these injuries there is complete fiber disruption or an avulsion at the insertion of the tendon. Rupture of both tendons results in a flat, flaccid toe.

Healing of a ruptured tendon is affected by capillaries and fibroblasts which grow in from the adjacent tendon sheath and connective tissue, and which can lead to scar tissue formation. Scar tissue does not have the same elasticity as the normal tendon. It is important to minimize adhesion formation during the healing process. Adhesions can result in restricted movement. Collagen fiber alignment is dependent on the distance between the ends of the damaged tendon and the amount of tension placed on the healing tissue. It is important to know that the digital tendons in the paw run within sheaths. If possible, it is important to preserve the gliding function of the extensors and flexors of the carpus and tarsus. Excessive tension and activity delays healing, but allowing a slight amount of tension helps orient the collagen fibers along normal planes of force. A slight amount of tension is needed to enhance the strength of the healing tissue and will help reduce adhesion formation.

### Techniques

Treatment of a third degree tendon injury involves repairing the tendon structure. The tendon ends are secured in apposition by the placement of one or two locking loop sutures using PDS. Simple interrupted sutures of fine PDS or Vicryl are used to suture the tendon ends together. The skin incision is closed using simple interrupted sutures to appose the skin edges and tension sutures to minimize stress on the skin edges.

In front leg injuries, a flexion splint is placed on the leg to help support tissue healing. In rear leg injuries a padded splint is placed on the paw that extends past the end of the toes, e.g. a "clam shell" splint. (See Chapter 2).

### Aftercare

The splint is left in place for 7 to 10 days. The skin sutures are removed in 7 to 10 days. A splint is then repositioned on the distal limb and left on for another 7 to 10 days. This is followed by limited activity for the next 10 to 14 days. The return to activity should be gradual over a 2 to 4 week period.

### Advantages and Disadvantages

Identifying this injury early and treating it aggressively will minimize any decline in performance and reduce healing time.

The rest needed for the healing process in this therapy regimen will sometimes affect the mentality of the highly-driven athletic and working dog. At any point in their rest period their pent-up energy will cause them to try to get out and run. This will usually result in a set-back and disruption of the healing process.

## Suggested Readings

1. Blythe, LL, Gannon, JR, & Craig, AM: Care of the Racing Greyhound: A Guide for Trainers, Breeders, and Veterinarians. American Greyhound Council, Inc. Abilene, KS, 1994.
2. Dee, JF, Dee, LG and Eaton-Wells, RD. Injuries of high-performance dogs. In Canine Orthopedics, Second Edition. Whittick, WG, ed. Lea and Febiger, Philadelphia 1990.
3. Ferguson, RG. Treatment of soft tissue musculoskelatal injuries. Greyhound Medicine and Surgery, The T G Hungerford Refresher Course for Veterinarians: Proceedings 122, Post Graduate in Veterinary Science, University of Sydney, Australia, 1989.

## Palmar or Plantar Lacerations

### Definitions and Indications

Traumatic lacerations are common in the athletic and working dogs (Figure 10-4). The surfaces can be rough or the presence of sharp debris can predispose the soft tissue proximal to the accessory pad to injury. These lacerations can be skin only (superficial) or can involve the digital flexor tendons (deep).

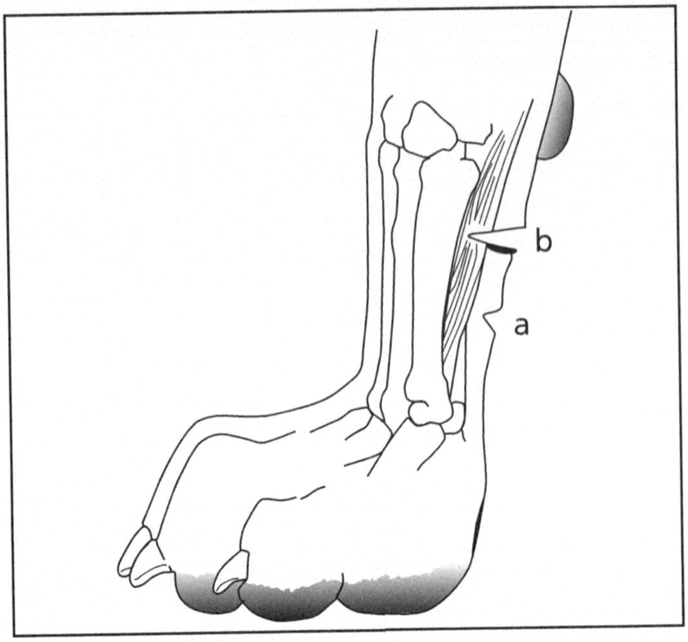


**Figure 10-4.** Depth of the palmar or plantar lacerations. Superficial, *(a)* Deep, *(b)* transecting underlying tendons and muscles.

The superficial lacerations are common injury in field dogs or dogs that work in an urban environment. Depending upon the cause, they can be clean lacerations or they can be related to blunt trauma. This area is very vascular and, because of its proximity to the ground, it is exposed to contamination. It is important to clean and debride the area extensively. Foreign material is also quite commonly found in these lacerations.

### Techniques

The first step is to clean the wound and stop any bleeding. A radiograph should be taken to help identify any foreign material or bony involvement. Manipulation of the digits will indicate if any tendons have been severed. Healing of this area can involve a lot of scar tissue. Scar tissue complicates healing by causing contracture. Any bleeding vessels are ligated. Closing the skin with a nonabsorbable monofilament suture material in a simple interrupted or mattress pattern has been successful in the author's experience. There are no subcuticular sutures used and none of the underlying tissue is sutured. The paw is then placed in a flexion splint or cast for 14 days. The flexion splint reduces the strain on the sutured skin and underlying structures, which promotes healing.

### Aftercare

The splint should be removed and the lesion checked after one week. The splint is replaced and left on for another week. The dog is rested for 2 weeks with no activity except for that during urination and defecation on a leash. The splint is removed after 14 days. The dog is then crate rested for 7 days. This is followed by 5 to 10 minute leash walks twice a day for 7 days. After 28 days the dog can return to normal activity.

### Advantages and Disadvantages

Subcuticular sutures in lacerations of the palmar and plantar regions tend to create a lot of fibrous and or scar tissue. This reactive tissue, and/or the adhesions associated with healing, often interferes with the ability of the tendons to move and function smoothly. Using only skin sutures and applying a flexion splint appears to decrease the amount of reactive tissue. This results in a reduced rehabilitation period and more flexible joint.

## Suggested Readings

1. Early, TD, Dee, JF. Trauma to the carpus, tarsus and phalanges of dogs and cats. Vet Clin North Am 10:717, 1980.
2. Swaim SF, Henderson RA: Small Animal Wound Management, 2nd ed.: Baltimore: Williams and Wilkins, 1997, 13.

# Index

A
Abrasions
deep palmar/plantar pad, 171-173
superficial palmar/plantar pad, 169-171
Acaricidal therapy, for acral lick dermatitis, 220
Acemannan, 29
Achilles tendon suturing, 289-290, 291
Acral lick dermatitis, 212
definition and indications for, 216-217
diagnosis of, 217, 218
therapy for, 217-224
advantages and disadvantages of, 225-226
aftercare for, 224-225
Activated bovine collagen, 34-35
Acupuncture, for acral lick dermatitis, 221
Adequan® (PSGAG), 254, 384, 388, 389
Adhesive tape
porous, 50-52
advantages and disadvantages of, 52
aftercare for, 51-52
application of, 51
definition and indications for, 50-51
waterproof, 52-53
Adhesive tape-pressure bandage, elastic, 53-55
Adhesive tape stirrups, 46-48
with carpal flexion splint, 63
Allergy treatment, for acral lick dermatitis, 219-220
advantages and disadvantages of, 225
aftercare for, 225
Aminoglycosides, 3, 4
Amitriptyline, 222
Amoxicillin, 3
Amoxicillin-trihydrate, 3, 178
Ampicillin, 4
Amputation
dewclaw, 234-235
digit, 236-241
Analgesia, 6-9
regional, 7-8
Anesthesia, 6-9
Antebrachial muscles, dorsolateral, 326
Antebrachiocarpal joint, 324-325
collateral ligament instability of, 331-335
luxation of, 335-336
Antibiotics
for acral lick dermatitis, 219, 224-225
for contaminated and infected wound treatment, 3-4
for tarsal shearing injuries, 262, 263, 264
Antidepressants, for acral lick dermatitis, 222
Antimicrobials, 3
Antirobe (clindamycin), 4
Antivenin, 213-215
Anxiolytics, for acral lick dermatitis, 222
Arthrodesis
advantages and disadvantages of, 266-267
of carpal joint shearing wounds, 333-334, 335
delayed
advantages and disadvantages of, 270
for tarsal shearing injuries, 267-270
for gastrocnemius muscle rupture, 297-298
for gastrocnemius tears, 297
pancarpal, 330, 331, 336
pantarsal
with dorsal bone plate, 267
for gastrocnemius muscle rupture, 297-298
for gastrocnemius tears, 297
with medial or lateral bone plate, 268-269
partial carpal, 328-330, 331
for plantar intertarsal subluxation/luxation, 271-272, 274-275
proximal intertarsal
of calcaneus, 311
for plantar intertarsal subluxation/luxation, 271-272, 274-275
for severe tarsal shearing injuries, 264-267
of tarsometatarsal joint, 279
by lateral bone plate, 280-281
by medial bone plate, 281
Athletic dogs, 378
avulsed nails in, 380-381
bruised nails in, 380
cracked nails in, 379-380
muscle injuries in, 382-384
pad injuries in, 381-382
palmar/plantar lacerations in, 390-391
synovial injuries in, 384-386
tendon injuries in, 388-390
toe dislocations in, 386-387
Autografts, for gastrocnemius tendon insertion avulsion, 290, 294
Avulsions
nail, 380-381
palmar/plantar pad, 171-173
Azithromycin (Zythromax), 4

B
Bacitracin, 24-25
Bactoderm (mupirocin ointment), 220
Bandages
adherent, 38-39
after carpal/tarsal flexion surface wound repair, 144-146
after onychectomy, 230-231
for carpal-metacarpal/tarsal-metatarsal wounds, 73
for carpal/tarsal extension surface wounds, 115
for chronic calcaneal tendonitis, 295
for deep pad ulcerations, 179-180
for deep palmar/plantar pad abrasions, partial avulsions, and deep burns, 171-173
for digital flexor tendon luxation, 298
donut-type, 55-57, 174, 178
elastic
adhesive tape-pressure, 53-55
for paw surgery, 168
for phalangeal sprains, 370
for pad puncture wounds, 174-175
padded
for metacarpal/metatarsal fractures, 363, 366-367
for peripheral nerve repair, 79
for sesamoid fragmentation, 372
primary layer, 38-48
secondary layer, 48-50, 55-58
sterile, 2
for superficial palmar/plantar pad abrasions and burns, 169-171
for tarsal joint sprains, 252-253
for tarsal shearing injuries, 262, 263
tertiary layer, 50-55
for wounds over carpal/tarsal flexion surfaces, 118
Baytril, 3
Behavior alteration, for acral lick dermatitis, 222-224
Betamethasone valerate, 220
Bone
drilling, 164-165
exposed, wound closure with, 163-165
granulation tissue coverage of, 164-165
Bone grafts, cancellous
advantages and disadvantages of, 267
for plantar intertarsal subluxation/luxation, 272

for severe tarsal shearing injuries, 265
Bone plate fixation
advantages and disadvantages of, 270
of calcaneus, 311-312
closed wedge with, 348, 352
for distal radial and ulnar fractures, 341-342, 344
dome osteotomy with, 348-349, 352
for dorsal intertarsal subluxation, 276-278
with intramedullary pin, 268
lateral
for plantar intertarsal subluxation/luxation, 271-272, 274-275
for tarsometatarsal joint instability, 280
for metacarpal/metatarsal fractures, 362, 363, 367
for tarsal shearing injuries, 267-270
for tarsometatarsal joint instability, 280-281
Bowstring scar, Z-plasty to release, 128-130, 131
Brachial artery, 327
Brachial plexus block, 8, 10
Bupivacaine, toxic effects of, 10
Burns, deep palmar/plantar pad, 169-173

C
Calcaneal tendonitis, chronic, 295
Calcanean tendon, common, 249
injuries to, 286-287
radiographs of, 287
tenorrhaphy for, 287
ultrasound examination of, 287
rupture or laceration of, 287-288
Calcaneoquartal joint, 247
Calcaneus, 246
fractures of, 308
aftercare of, 311
treatment of, 308-312
Camphor, for acral lick dermatitis, 220-221
Capsaicin, for acral lick dermatitis, 220-221
Carpal area orthopedic injuries
anatomy of, 324-327
angular limb deformity, 345-352
antebrachiocarpal joint, 331-336
fracture, 337-345, 352-353, 355-357
hyperextension, 327-331
luxation, 354-355
middle subluxation, 336-337
soft tissue, 357-358
Carpal bones
accessory, 324
soft tissue injury related to, 357-358
fractures of
accessory, 355-357
type IV, 357
type V, 357
types I-III, 356-357
Carpal extension surface wounds, closure for, 113-116
Carpal flexion slings, 63-64
Carpal flexion surface wounds, closure for, 116-118
Carpal joints, 324-325
middle-level subluxation of, 336-337
Carpal-metacarpal wounds
with apposable edges
extension surface, 113-116
flexion surface, 116-118
no tension, 86-88
simple interrupted skin sutures for, 89-92
staples for, 92-94
X-mattress sutures for, 92
tension, 95-96
intradermal closure of, 99-104
undermining, 96-98
delayed primary closure for, 73
with exposed bones and joints, 163-165
with nonapposable edges, 118-136
extension surface, 136-139
no potential for apposition, 139-163
open drainage of, 79-80
passive drainage of, 80-85
peripheral nerve injury and repair of, 76-79
primary wound closure for, 72
secondary wound closure for, 74-76
various shaped, 105-113
Carpal shearing injury
arthrodesis of, 333-334, 335
reconstruction of, 332-333, 334-335
Carpal sling, 65-66
Carpal synovitis
acute, 384
chronic, 384-385
Cast padding, 48, 55-57, 252
with 90/90 sling, 67
Castile soap, in lavage of exposed bone, 12, 14, 16
Casts, 252-253, 271, 278-279, 288-289, 304, 320, 328, 355
Cats
antebrachiocarpal joint luxation in, 336
deep digital flexor tenectomy for, 233-234
onychectomy for, 228-231
pad replacement in, 186-188, 193-194
Cefa-Drops/Cefa-Tabs (cefadroxil), 3
Cefadroxil (Cefa-Drops; Cefa-Tabs), 3
Cellerate RX
for contaminated and infected wounds, 34-35
with open drainage, 79
Centrodistal joint, 247
Cephadroxil, 178
Cephalexin (Keflex), 3, 178
Cephalosporins, 3, 178
Chemical deterrents, for acral lick dermatitis, 220-221, 225
ChlorhexiDerm Disinfectant (gluconate), 21, 196
Chlorhexidine diacetate (Nolvasan Solution) lavage, 12, 21, 196
Chondroitin, for tarsal joint sprains, 254
Chondroprotective agents, 254
Chronic nonhealing wound, 18
Circumferential constriction, release of, 130-132, 133
Clavamox, 3
Clavulanate potassium, 3, 178
Clavulanic acid, 3
Clindamycin (Antirobe), 4
Clomipramine, for acral lick dermatitis, 222
Clotrimazole, for acral lick dermatitis, 220
Cold therapy
for gastrocnemius muscle rupture, 297
for interosseous muscle tears or ruptures, 383
for phalangeal sprains, 370
for tarsal joint sprains, 252, 260
Collagen products, 34-35
Collateral ligaments
antebrachiocarpal joint, instability of, 331-335
avulsion of, 254
carpal, 325-326
injuries to, 369-371
medial and lateral, 247
short, 258-261
metatarsal/metacarpal, 361
rupture of, 254, 258-259, 370
diagnosis and surgical treatment of, 255-260

short radial, 331-332, 334
stabilization of, 336
Combined-V closure, 110-111
Comfor™ Foam, 57
Compression plating, 272
Contaminated/infected wounds
aftercare for, 9
closure assessment of, 17-19
debridement and lavage for, 11-15
definition of, 2
enzymatic agents for, 28-29
foreign debris in, 11
gentamicin sulfate for, 27-28
healing stimulants for, 29-35
nitrofurazone medication for, 26-27
preliminary procedures for
advantages and disadvantages of, 9-10
indications for, 2
techniques for, 2-9
silver sulfadiazine dressings for, 25-26
topical lavage agents for, 19-24
triple antibiotic medication for, 24-25
Contractions
with hydrogel dressings, 41
inhibition of, 25, 26, 32, 50
in wound healing, 18-19, 21, 30, 41, 95-96, 118-119, 121, 122, 160-163, 165, 171-173, 180, 186, 190-191, 262
Corns, 381-382
Cosequin, 254
Cranial superficial antebrachial artery, 327, 361-362
Cranial tibial artery, 250
Cryotherapy
for acral lick dermatitis, 221, 225
for toe dislocations, 387
Culture, of contaminated/infected wound, 10
Cyclooxygenase 2 (COX 2), 254

**D**

D-glucose polysaccharide
for contaminated and infected wounds, 31
with open drainage, 79
Debridement
adherent bandage, 38-39
advantages and disadvantages of, 15-16
aftercare for, 15
of blood vessels, 13
of bone, 14
for contaminated and infected wounds, 3
enzymatic, 28-29
of fascia, 13
indications for, 11
of joints, 14
of muscle, 13-14
of nerves, 13
nonsurgical, 12, 16
sharp, 15-16
of skin, 13
staged, 12, 74
techniques for, 11-15
of tendons, 14
Declawing. *See* Deep digital flexor tenectomy; Onychectomy
Deep digital flexor tenectomy, 233-234
Depomedrol (methylprednisolone), 372
Dewclaw amputation
advantages and disadvantages of, 235
aftercare for, 235
definition and indication for, 234
techniques for
in neonates, 234
in older dogs, 234-235
Dexamethasone, 220
Digit space filling, 209
Digital extensor tendons, 249, 326
Digital flexor tendons, 326, 327
deep, 249
severed, 205-206
superficial, 249
luxation of, 298, 299
Digital nerve block, 8
Digits
amputation of
advantages and disadvantages of, 240-241
aftercare for, 239
definition and indications for, 236
distal interphalangeal, 236, 237
pandigital metacarpal/metatarsal-phalangeal, 237-239
proximal interphalangeal and metacarpal/metatarsal-phalangeal, 236-237, 238-240
anatomy of, 360-362
dorsal wounds of, 168-169
luxation or subluxation of, 370
orthopedic wounds of with soft tissue salvage, 206-208
resurfacing, 206-208
Dimethyl sulfoxide
for acral lick dermatitis, 220
for phalangeal sprains, 370
for sesamoidal synovitis, 385
Distal tibial physeal fractures, 307
"Dog ear" skin
closure techniques for, 86
in combined-V closure, 110
in linear closure, 110
linear closure with, 112-113
Dogs
antebrachiocarpal joint luxation in, 336
dewclaw amputation for, 234-235
distal interphalangeal amputation for, 236, 237
onychectomy for, 228
Dolorac (capsaicin), for acral lick dermatitis, 220
Dorsal intertarsal subluxation
definition of, 275
treatment of
advantages and disadvantages of, 278
aftercare for, 277-278
indications for, 275
techniques for, 275-277
Dowel pin fixation, 363, 367
Doxepin (Sinequan®), 222
Drainage
of carpal-metacarpal/tarsal-metatarsal wounds, 72
open, 79-80
passive, 80-85
indications for, 80
medications and dressings with, 79-80
Drains
advantages and disadvantages of, 85
aftercare with, 84-85
double-exit, 84
placement of, 84
single-exit, 80-83
Dressings, 25-26, 40, 44-46
dry-to-dry, 38
gauze, 38-39, 48-50
hydrogel, 41-42

with open drainage, 79-80
roll, 48-50
Dynamic compression plates, 267-268, 280

**E**

Electronic stimulation (electroshock), for acral lick dermatitis, 224
Endorphin blockers/substitutes, for acral lick dermatitis, 222-223
Enrofloxacin, 4
Environmental modification, for acral lick dermatitis, 221-222
Enzymatic agents, 28-29
Epidural block, 8, 9, 10
Epsom salt soaks
for carpal synovitis, 385
for interdigital pododermatitis, 196
External coaptation, for metacarpal/metatarsal fractures, 363, 367
External fixation
acrylic, 302
for chronic calcaneal tendonitis, 295
for distal limb fractures, 337-339
dynamic, hinged frame for, 300-302
for gastrocnemius tendon insertion avulsion, 293, 294
hinged frame for, 304
hybrid, 339-341
for radial fractures, 345
Kirschner-Ehmer frame for, 302-303
linear, 337-339
for radial fractures, 344-345
for metacarpal/metatarsal fractures, 362, 367
closed technique, 364, 367
open technique, 364-365, 367
for plantar intertarsal subluxation/luxation, 272-274
advantages and disadvantages of, 275
principles of, 300
ring, 339-341
for severe tarsal shearing injuries, 264-267
static, modified clamp for, 302
for talar strain injuries, 285
for tarsal shearing injuries, 262-264
transarticular of tarsus, 299-305
type II
open wedge stabilized with, 349-350, 351, 352
three pin, 300
Extracellular matrix scaffolds, 43-44
Exudate, absorption of, 48, 50

**F**

Fentanyl, for snakebite, 215
Ferrage, 164-165
Fibulotalar ligament, avulsion of, 259
Flaps
bipedicle advancement, 189-190
carpal pad-single, 188-190
for carpus/tarsus extension surface wounds, 136-139
closure of in secondary wound repair, 76
hinge
advantages and disadvantages of, 146-147
for pad replacement in cats, 186-188
for wounds over carpus/tarsus flexion surfaces, 144-147
pouch, 186-188
advantages and disadvantages of, 146-147
for pad replacement, 186-188
for wounds over carpus/tarsus flexion surfaces, 142-147
reverse saphenous conduit
advantages and disadvantages of, 154
aftercare for, 154
definition and indications for, 152
technique for, 152-154
skin
advantages and disadvantages of, 146
for wounds over carpus/tarsus flexion surfaces, 139-142, 144-147
tubed pedicle
advantages and disadvantages of, 151-152
aftercare for, 151
definition and indications for, 147-148
"pancake" and, 150-151
simple, 148-150
Flexor carpi radialis tendon, 327
Flexor carpi ulnaris tendon, 327
Flexor carpi ulnaris tendonopathy, 358
Flexor retinaculum, 326
Flexor tendons
metatarsal/metacarpal, 360-361
repairs of, with carpal flexion splint, 64
sprains of
first degree, 388
second degree, 389
third degree, 389-390
Flucinolone acetonide, 220
Flucort (flumethasone), 358
Flumethasone (Flucort), 358
Fluoroquinolones, 3
Fluoxetine (Prozac), 222
Foreign debris removal, 11
Forelimb, distal
anatomy of, 324-327
angular deformities of, 345-352
blood supply of, 327
joints of, 324-325
ligaments of, 325-326
osseous structures of, 324
tendons of, 326-327
Fracture-luxation, central tarsal, 320
Fractures
calcaneal, 308-312
central tarsal, 316-319
distal tibial physeal, 307
with ferrage, 165
lavage of, 12-15
malleolar, 305-307
metatarsal and metacarpal, 362-367
of numbered tarsal bones, 321-322
phalangeal, 367-369
talar, 312-315
of tarsal bones, 307-308
Fusion podoplasty, 198-202, 203

**G**

Gastrocnemius muscle rupture, 297-298
Gastrocnemius tears, at musculotendinous junction, 296-297
Gastrocnemius tendon, 249
avulsion at insertion of, 289-294
Gauze pad dressings
advantages and disadvantages of, 39
aftercare for, 38-39
definition and indications for, 38
dry-to-dry, 38
nonadherent semiocclusive, 44-46
removing, 38
wet-to-dry, 38
Gauze roll dressing, 48-50
Gentamicin sulfate
for acral lick dermatitis, 220
for contaminated/infected wounds, 27-28

Glucocorticoids, for acral lick dermatitis, 219, 224-225
Gluconate (ChlorhexiDerm), 21, 196
Glycosaminoglycan (Adequan®), 254, 384, 388, 389
Grafts
  cancellous bone
    advantages and disadvantages of, 267
    for plantar intertarsal subluxation/luxation, 272
    for severe tarsal shearing injuries, 265
  digital pad, 241
  for gastrocnemius tendon insertion avulsion, 290, 292, 294
  mesh, 154-161,193-194, 290, 292, 294
  for pad replacement, 190-194
  in secondary wound repair, 76
  skin, 113-114, 154-160
  strip
    advantages and disadvantages of, 163
    aftercare for, 163
    definition and indications for, 161
    technique for, 162-163
  for wounds over carpus/tarsus extension surfaces, 136-139
Granulation tissue
  covering bone, 164-165
  with EMS dressing, 44
  with hydrogel dressings, 41
  in secondary wound repair, 75-76
  in undermining, 97
Granulex-V, 28-29

H
Heat therapy
  for flexor tendon sprains, 388
  for tarsal joint sprains, 252
HEET, for acral lick dermatitis, 220-221
Hemostasis, in paw wounds, 168
Hemostatic devices, 168
Hexamethyldisiloxane acrylate, with adhesive tape application, 51, 53
Hind limb
  blood supply of, 250
  ligament and tendon injuries of, 250-261
  osseous structures of, 246-247
  tendons and ligaments of, 247-250
Honey, topical
  advantages and disadvantages of, 34
  antimicrobial properties of, 33
  application technique for, 33-34
  for contaminated and infected wounds, 33-34
  definition and indications for, 33
Hybrid external fixation, radial fracture, 345
Hydrasorb, with open drainage, 79
Hydrogel dressing, 41-42
Hydrogen peroxide lavage, 23-24
Hyperextension injuries, carpal joint, 327-328
  aftercare for, 330-331
  fixation of, 328-330, 331
Hypothermic therapy, for toe dislocations, 387

I
Iamin Hydrating Gel Wound Dressing, 30
Immobilization
  for chronic calcaneal tendonitis, 295
  for common calcanean tendon rupture or lacerations, 288
  for gastrocnemius tendon insertion avulsion, 293, 294
  for tarsal joint sprains, 260-261
  for wounds over carpal/tarsal extension surfaces, 115-116
  for wounds over carpal/tarsal flexion surfaces, 118
Infection-potentiating fractions (IPFs), 11
Infections. *See* Contaminated/infected wounds



Insorb staples, 93
Interdigital lacerations
  deep, 205-206
  superficial, 204-205
Interdigital pododermatitis
  conservative incisional or excisional therapy for, 196-197
    advantages and disadvantages of, 202
    aftercare for, 201
  conservative medical therapy for, 196
    advantages and disadvantages of, 202
    aftercare for, 201
  definition of, 194-195
  diagnosis of, 195-196
  moderate excisional therapy for, 197-198
    advantages and disadvantages of, 202-203
    aftercare for, 201
  radical excisional therapy for, 198-201
    advantages and disadvantages of, 203
    aftercare for, 201-202
Interdigital wounds, 194-203
  padding for, 55, 56-57
Internal fixation
  for dorsal intertarsal subluxation, 275-278
  for metacarpal/metatarsal fractures, 363, 366-367
Interosseous muscles, 360
  strains of, 382-383
  tears or ruptures of, 383-384
Interosseous myositis, 382-383
Intracell, with open drainage, 79
Intradermal closure, 87-88
Intramedullary pinning
  for calcaneal fractures, 311-312
  for metacarpal/metatarsal fractures, 362
  with tarsal bone plating, 268
Iodine, antimicrobial activity of, 22
Isotonic saline lavage, 20-21

J
Joints, exposed, wound closure with, 163-165

K
K-wiring
  for collateral ligament rupture, 260
  for distal tibial physeal fractures, 307
  for malleolar fractures, 306-307
  for metacarpal/metatarsal fractures, 362, 363
  for radial carpal bone luxation, 354-355
  for talar head fractures, 315
  for talar ridge fractures, 312
Keflex (cephalexin), 3, 178
Kerlix® AMD Roll, 48, 50
Kerlix Roll, 48
Kirschner-Ehmer frame fixator, 302-305

L
Lacerations
  calcanean tendon, 287-288
  of common calcanean tendon, 287-288
  interdigital
    deep, 205-206
    superficial, 204-205
  of pad, 175-178
  palmar or plantar, 390-391
  of web, 204-205
Lactated Ringer's solution, 20-21
Lag screw fixation
  for central tarsal bone fracture-luxation, 320

for central tarsal fractures, 316-319
for distal radial and ulnar fractures, 342-344
for malleolar fractures, 306-307
for metacarpal/metatarsal fractures, 362, 365-366
for radial carpal bone fractures, 352-353
Lameness
after digit amputation, 240
after onychectomy, 231
with digital flexor tendon luxation, 298
with sesamoid fracture, 372
Laser therapy, for acral lick dermatitis, 221
advantages and disadvantages of, 225
aftercare for, 225
Lavage
advantages and disadvantages of, 15-16, 85
aftercare for, 15
apparatus for, 15
with exposed bone, 16
high and low pressure, 16
indications for, 11
technique in, 12-15
Lavage agents, topical, 19-24
Lavage pressure, 16
Lengthening bone plate, 267-268
Lidocaine, toxic effects of, 10
Ligament injuries
of collateral ligament, 255-260
of phalanges, 369-371
repair of with tarsal joint sprains, 254
Limb deformity, angular, 345-346
aftercare for, 350
corrective radial ostectomy for, 346-350
corrective radial osteotomy for, 348-352
partial ulnar ostectomy for, 347-348
advantages and disadvantages of, 350-352
aftercare for, 350
preoperative assessment of, 346-347
Linear closure, 109-110
for crescent-shaped wounds, 111-113

M
Magnesium sulfate soaks, 196
Malleolar fractures, 305-306
lateral, 306
medial, 306
treatment of, 306-307
Maltodextrin N.F. (D-glucose polysaccharide)
for contaminated and infected wounds, 31
with open drainage, 79
Mason metasplints, 60
Median artery, 327, 362
Mesh grafts
advantages and disadvantages of, 160
aftercare for, 159-160
contraction of holes in, 161
definition and indications for, 154
for gastrocnemius tendon insertion avulsion, 290, 292, 294
for pad replacement, 193-194
technique for, 155-158
Metacarpal area
blood supply to, 361-362
ligaments of, 361
muscles and tendons of, 360-361
Metacarpal bones
anatomy of, 360
fractures of, 362-367
head, 366
Metacarpal/metatarsal pad loss
carpal pad-single and bipedicle advancement flaps for, 188-190
with deep pad ulceration, 179-180
mesh grafts for, 193-194
pad grafts for, 190-192
phalangeal fillet for, 181-185
pouch flap for, 186-188
Metal splints
advantages and disadvantages of, 63
aftercare for, 62-63
application of, 61-62
definition and indications for, 60
full, 60, 61
types of, 60-63
Metatarsal area
blood supply to, 361-362
ligaments of, 361
muscles and tendons of, 360-361
Metatarsal bones, 246, 360
fractures of, 362-367
Metatarsal/metacarpal extensor tendons, 360, 361
Methylprednisolone (Depomedrol), 372, 385, 386
Methylsalicylate, for acral lick dermatitis, 220-221
Metronidazole, 4
Microbial evaluation/therapy, 3-4
Multiple punctate relaxing incision, 124-125
Mupirocin ointment (Bactoderm), 220
Muscle strains, in working and athletic dogs, 382-383

N
Nails
avulsed, 380-381
bruised, 380
cracks, 379-380
length of, 379
removal of, 380
Naltrexone (Trexane), for acral lick dermatitis, 222-223
Necrosis, avascular, 106-108
Neomycin, 24-25
Neomycin sulfate solution, 220
Neuroleptanalgesia
advantages of, 10
for contaminated and infected wounds, 6-7
Neuropathic pain management, 221
Nitrofurazone dressing, 26-27
Nitrofurazone/polyethylene glycol gauzes, 44, 46
Nolvasan solution, 21, 196
Nonsteroidal anti-inflammatory drugs (NSAIDs)
for carpal synovitis, 384
for digital flexor tendon sprains, 388, 389, 390
for sesamoid fragmentation, 372
for sesamoidal synovitis, 385, 386
for tarsal joint sprains, 254, 260, 261
for toe dislocations, 386-387

O
Onychectomy
advantages and disadvantages of, 231-232
aftercare for, 230-231
alternative to, 233-234
anesthetic considerations for, 229
$CO_2$ laser, 230
definition and indications for, 228
dissection, 228
nail clipper, 228-230
Open reduction and internal fixation, 336, 355-357
Ostectomy

partial ulnar, 346, 347-348, 350-352
radial, 346
Osteotomy
corrective radial, 348-352
for digit amputation, 236
for sprain injuries, 260-261
for talar ridge fractures, 312, 313
Otomax, for acral lick dermatitis, 220

**P**
Pad
deep ulceration of, 179-180
injuries to
lacerations, 175-178
palmar/plantar deep abrasions, avulsions, and burns, 171-173
palmar/plantar superficial abrasions and burns, 169-171
punctures, 173-175
in working and athletic dogs, 381-382
Pad grafts, 190-192
Pad replacement
with carpal pad-single and bipedicle advancement flaps, 188-190
with mesh grafts, 193-194
with pad grafts, 190-192
with phalangeal fillet, 181-185
with pouch flap, 186-188
Padding, 48, 55
foam sponge, 57-58
with open drainage, 79
interdigital, 55, 56-57
nonadherent semiocclusive
advantages and disadvantages of, 46
aftercare for, 45
application technique for, 44-45
definition and indications for, 44
Padding materials
cast padding, 55-57
foam sponge, 57-58
stockinette, 59-60
Palmar carpal fibrocartilage, 326
Palmar superficial fascia tears, 358
Patient evaluation, for infected wounds, 2-3
Paw bandages, pressure relief, 57-58
Paw cup, 60
advantages and disadvantages of, 63
aftercare for, 62
application of, 61
Paw wounds
carpal pad-single and bipedicle advancement flaps for, 188-190
deep abrasive, partial avulsion and deep burn, 171-173
digit orthopedic with soft tissue salvage, 206-208
digit space filling, 209
dorsal digital, 168-169
interdigital
deep lacerations in, 205-206
pododermatitis, 194-203
superficial lacerations in, 204-205
laceration, 175-178
mesh grafts for, 193-194
metacarpal/metatarsal pad loss, with deep pad ulceration, 179-180
pad grafts for, 190-192
palmar/plantar pad, 169-171
phalangeal fillet for, 181-185
pouch flap for, 186-188
puncture, 173-175
Penrose drains, 80-82, 84, 85
Peripheral nerve injury, 76-77
repair of, 77

delayed, 77, 78-79
primary, 77-78, 79
Periwound preparation, 4-6
Petrolatum-based antibiotic ointment gauzes, 44, 46
Phalangeal fillet, 181
advantages and disadvantages of, 183-185
aftercare for, 183
for digit space filling, 209
dorsal, 183, 184, 185
palmar/plantar, 181-183
to resurface digits, 206-208
Phalanges, 246-247, 360
fractures of
aftercare for, 369
diagnosis and treatment guidelines for, 367-368
treatment of, 368-369, 369
ligamentous injuries of, 369-371
Physical restraints, for acral lick dermatitis, 223-224
Pit viper envenomation, 215
indications of, 212
monitoring, 213
progression of, 213
therapy for, 213-215
Pit vipers, 212
Plantar intertarsal subluxation/luxation
definition of, 271
treatment of
advantages and disadvantages of, 274-275
aftercare for, 273-274
indications for, 271
techniques for, 271-273
Plantar ligaments, 247
Polyhexamethylene biguanide impregnated dressing, 48, 50
Polymixin, 24-25
Polysulfated glycosaminoglycans (PSGAG; Adequan®), 254, 384, 388, 389
Polyurethane foam dressing/sponge, 40
with open drainage, 79
Povidone iodine
antimicrobial activity of, 22
detergent form of, 23
lavage with, 22-23
Pressure relief, 57-58
Presutures, 103-104, 118, 121, 137
Prosthetic imbrication
for collateral ligament rupture, 256-258, 259, 260
for radial carpal bone luxation, 355
for tarsal shearing injuries, 262-264
Prozac, for acral lick dermatitis, 222
*Pseudomonas aeruginosa* infection, irrigation of, 16
*Pseudomonas* infection
nitrofurazone for, 26-27
silver sulfadiazine for, 25
Psychogenic-behavior modification, for acral lick dermatitis, 221-222
advantages and disadvantages of, 226
aftercare for, 225
Puncture wounds
open wound management for, 173-175
pseudohealing of, 175

**R**
Radial carpal bone
fractures of, 352-353
luxation of, 354-355
Radial collateral ligament, 325-326
Radiation therapy, for acral lick dermatitis, 219, 221, 225
Radical excisional therapy, for interdigital pododermatitis, 198-202,

203
Radiographs
flexed dorsoplantar, of collateral ligaments, 259-260
stress, 262, 271-272, 274-277, 279
for collateral ligament rupture, 255
for tarsal joint sprains, 251-252
Radius, 324
distal fractures of, 337-341
comminuted or open, 344-345
noncomminuted and closed, 341-344
Relaxing incisions
multiple punctate, 124-125
simple, 121-123
for wounds over carpus/tarsus extension surfaces, 136-139
Z-plasty, 127, 128, 129
Ring and hybrid fixation, 339-341
Ringer's solution lavage, 20-21
Roll dressings
advantages and disadvantages of, 50
aftercare for, 50
application technique for, 48-49
definition and indications for, 48

**S**
Saphenous artery, 362
Screw and washer fixation
for dorsal intertarsal subluxation, 275-278
for talocalcaneal luxation, 282
Screw fixation
for talus base luxation, 278-279
for tarsal bone fractures, 321-322
Second intention healing, 17, 18-19, 32, 79, 96, 123, 164, 165, 175, 221, 262-263, 266
Sensitivity test, of infected wound, 10
Sequential 7-day therapy regimen, 32
tripeptide copper complex in, 30
Serum sickness, delayed, 215
Sesamoid bones, 360
fragmentation of, 371-373
conservative treatment of, 372-373
surgical treatment of, 372-373
Sesamoidal synovitis
acute, 385
chronic, 386
Shearing injuries
carpal, 332-335
tarsal
early arthrodesis for, 264-267
open wound healing, prosthetic imbrication and external fixation for, 261-264
Silver sulfadiazine dressings, 25-26
Sinequan®, for acral lick dermatitis, 222
Single advancement flaps, 188-190
Skin flaps
advantages and disadvantages of, 146
for wounds over carpus/tarsus flexion surfaces, 139-142, 144-147
Skin grafts
advantages and disadvantages of, 160
aftercare for, 159-160
definition and indications for, 154
technique for, 155-158
for wounds over tarsal extension surfaces, 113-114
Skin injuries, 379-381
Slings
90/90, 67-69
carpal, 65-66
Velpeau, 66
Snakebite wounds
aftercare for, 215
antivenin for, 213-215
definition of, 212-213
delayed serum sickness with, 215
indications for treatment of, 212-213
initial management of, 213
monitoring for, 213
severity of, 212-214
Soft tissue injury, 357-358
Soft tissue salvage, with digit orthopedic wounds, 206-208
Specialist Cast Padding, 48, 55
Splints
after delayed tarsal arthrodesis, 270
carpal flexion, 63-64
for carpal joint hyperextension, 330-331
for carpal synovitis, 384
for carpal/tarsal extension surface wounds, 115
for chronic calcaneal tendonitis, 295
clam shell, 60
advantages and disadvantages of, 63
aftercare for, 62-63
application of, 61-62
one-half, 61, 63
for pad laceration, 178
for common calcanean tendon rupture or lacerations, 288
for deep palmar/plantar pad abrasions, partial avulsions, and deep burns, 171-173
for digital flexor tendon luxation, 298
for digital flexor tendon sprains, 390
for dorsal intertarsal subluxation, 275
full, 60-62
advantages and disadvantages of, 63
for gastrocnemius tears, 296
for gastrocnemius tendon insertion avulsion, 293
for interosseous muscle tears or ruptures, 383-384
for interosseous myositis or sprain, 383
for metacarpal/metatarsal fractures, 363, 366-367
metal, 60-63
for middle carpal subluxation, 337
for pad laceration, 178
for palmar/plantar lacerations, 390-391
for plantar intertarsal subluxation/luxation, 271, 273-274
for sesamoid fragmentation, 372
for sesamoidal synovitis, 385, 386
for talus base luxation, 278
for tarsal joint sprains, 260-261
for toe dislocations, 387
for wounds over carpal/tarsal flexion surfaces, 118
Sprains
phalangeal, 369-371
tarsal, 251, 258
aftercare for, 260-261
diagnosis and nonsurgical treatment of, 251-254
grades of, 251
surgical treatment of, 254-255
*Staphylococcus* infections, 3, 24-25
Staples, skin, 92-94
Stockinette padding, 59-60
Strain injuries, talar, 282-285
*Streptococcus* infection, 3
*Streptococcus pyogenes,* 24
Sugar, granulated, topical application of, 32-33
Surgical stabilization
for metacarpal/metatarsal fractures, 362, 363
of phalangeal sprains, 370-371
for talus base luxation, 278-279

for tarsal shearing injuries, 262-264, 263-264
Sutures
adjustable horizontal mattress, 118-121
for collateral ligament rupture, 255-256, 258
combination tension and apposition, 102
for common calcanean tendon rupture or lacerations, 287-288
continuous absorbable monofilament, 88
continuous cruciate, for talus strains, 284, 285
continuous intradermal, 118-121
continuous monofilament nonabsorbable, 87-88
for crescent-shaped wounds
central, 111-113
"fudging," 111-113
far-far-near-near, 101-102
far-near-near-far, 101-102
for gastrocnemius tears, 296
for gastrocnemius tendon insertion avulsion, 289-290, 291, 294
interrupted vertical mattress, 100, 101
intradermal, 87-89
Lembert, 103-104
locking loop
for collateral ligament rupture, 255-256
for gastrocnemius tears, 296
for talus strains, 284-285
for tarsal joint sprains, 254-255
for pad lacerations, 175-178
for palmar/plantar lacerations, 390
for palmar superficial fascia tears, 358
simple interrupted skin, 89-92
for talus strains, 284-285
for tarsal joint sprains, 254-255
tension
simple interrupted, 99-100
for wounds over carpus/tarsus extension surfaces, 136-139
three-loop pulley
for common calcanean tendon rupture or lacerations, 287-288
for gastrocnemius tendon insertion avulsion, 289-290, 291, 294
for talus strains, 284
in wound closure, 18
X-mattress (cruciate), 92, 93
Synovial injuries, 384-386
Synovial membrane inflammation, 21

T
Talocalcaneal ligament, 247
Talocalcaneal luxation, 283
definition of, 281-282
treatment of, 281-282
Talocalcaneocentral joint, 247
Talus, 246
factures of
aftercare for, 315
definition of, 312
neck, 314
ridge, 312-314
treatment of, 312-315
head fractures of, 315
luxation of base, 278-279
strain injuries of, 282-284
aftercare for, 285
treatment of, 284-285
Tap water lavage, 19-20
Tape stirrups, adhesive, 46-48, 61, 63-64, 252-253
Tarsal bones
central fracture-luxation of, 320-321
fractures of, 307-308
calcaneal fractures and, 308-312, 318
central, 316-319
fourth, 321
numbered bone, 321-322
talar, 312-315
third, 321
type V, 316, 319
types I-IV, 316-317, 318-319
Tarsal extension surface wounds, 113-116
Tarsal flexion surface wounds, 116-118
Tarsal joints
blood supply of, 250
injuries of, 250-261
collateral ligament, 255-260
sprain, 260-261
diagnosis and nonsurgical treatment for, 251-254
surgical treatment of, 254-255
ligaments of, 247-248
ruptured, 255-259
osseous structures of, 246-247
tendons of, 249
Tarsal-metatarsal wounds
with apposable edges
extension surface, 113-116
flexion surface, 116-118
no tension, 86-94
tension, 85-104
delayed primary closure for, 73
with exposed bones and joints, 163-165
with nonapposable edges, 118-136
extension surface, 136-139
with no potential for apposition, 139-163
open drainage of, 79-80
passive drainage of, 80-85
peripheral nerve injury and repair of, 76-79
primary wound closure for, 72
secondary wound closure for, 74-76
various shaped, 105-113
Tarsal shearing injuries
aftercare for, 263
definition of, 261-262
delayed arthrodesis with bone plating for, 267-270
early arthrodesis using external fixation for, 264-267
open wound healing, prosthetic imbrication and external fixation for, 261-264
treatment of, 262-264
Tarsometatarsal joint, 247
instability of, 279-280
subluxation of, 279-281
Tarsus
muscles of, 249
tendons of, 249-250
transarticular external fixation of, 299-305
Tendon transposition, 291-293
Tendonitis, chronic calcaneal, 295
Tendonopathy, flexor carpi ulnaris, 358
Tendons
lengthening of, for gastrocnemius tendon insertion avulsion, 290-291, 292
sprains of
first degree, 388
second degree, 389
third degree, 389-390
strain injuries of
healing of, 283-284
talar, 282-285
Tenectomy, deep digital flexor tendon, 233-234
Tenorrhaphy

for calcanean tendon injuries, 287
for common calcanean tendon rupture or lacerations, 288
Tension band fixation
for distal calcaneal fractures, 310-311
for malleolar fractures, 306-307
for metacarpal/metatarsal fractures, 365-366
for proximal calcaneal fractures, 308-310
for styloid process fractures, 342, 344
for talar ridge fractures, 312-314
Tension-related scars, relief of, 118
Tension relief
types of, 126
Z-plasty for, 127-133
Tension sutures
simple interrupted, 99-100
for wounds over carpus/tarsus extension surfaces, 136-139
Thiabendazole, for acral lick dermatitis, 220
Tibia, distal physeal fractures of, 307
Tissue viability, indicators of, 11-12
Toe dislocations, 369-371
first degree, 386-387
second degree, 387
third degree, 387
Tourniquets
biologic
with multiple punctate relaxing incisions, 125
with simple relaxing incision, 122
with tight closure, 120-121
with tight wound closure, 73
for paw surgery, 168
for snakebite, 213
Transport preparation, 2
Tresaderm, for acral lick dermatitis, 220
Trexane (naltrexone), for acral lick dermatitis, 222-223
Tripeptide copper complex, 30
Triple antibiotic medication, 24-25
Trypsin-balsam of Peru-castor oil, 28-29

**U**

Ulcerations, deep pad, 179-180
Ulna, 324
distal fractures of, 337-341
comminuted or open, 344-345
noncomminuted and closed, 341-344
Undermining
advantages and disadvantages of, 98
aftercare for, 97-98
definition and indications for, 96
techniques for, 96-97

**V**

V-to-Y-plasty, 134-136
Velpeau sling, 66

**W**

Web excision, for interdigital pododermatitis, 197-198, 201, 202-203
Web lacerations, 204-205
Weight-bearing, slings to prevent, 65-67
Wet-to-dry dressing, 38
Working dogs
avulsed nails in, 380-381
bruised nails in, 380
cracked nails in, 379-380
injuries of, 378
muscle injuries in, 382-384
pad injuries in, 381-382
palmar/plantar lacerations in, 390-391
synovial injuries in, 384-386
tendon injuries in, 388-390
toe dislocations in, 386-387
Wound closure
with apposable edges
extension surface, 113-116
flexion surface, 116-118
assessment of, 17-19
for carpal-metacarpal/tarsal-metatarsal wounds
with apposable edges, 86-104, 113-118
with exposed bones and joints, 163-165
with nonapposable edges, 118-163
primary, 72-73
secondary, 74-76
for chevron, crescent and triangular-shaped wounds, 105-108
for circular wounds, 109-110
for crescent-shaped wounds, 111-113
with exposed bones and joints, 163-165
with nonapposable edges, 118-136
extension surface, 136-139
no potential for apposition, 139-163
puncture, 173-175
tissue present for, 17
Wound healing stimulants, 29-35
Wound tension, 95-96
undermining to relieve, 96-98
Wounds. *See also* Contaminated/infected wounds
chevron shaped
dynamics of, 106
Y-closure of, 105-108
circular
combined-V closure of, 110-111
linear closure of, 109-110
crescent shaped
dynamics of, 106
"fudging" suture, central suture, and linear closure of, 111-113
Y-closure of, 105-108
packing of, 9-10
progression from contaminated to infected, 2
protection of during periwound preparation, 4
triangular-shaped, Y-closure of, 105-108

**Y**

Y-closure, 105-108

**Z**

Z-plasty
advantages and disadvantages of, 133
aftercare for, 132-133
definition and indications for, 126-127
dynamics of, 126
for gastrocnemius tendon insertion avulsion, 291-292, 294
relaxing incision, 127, 128, 129
to release bowstring scar, 128-130, 131
to release circumferential constriction, 130-132, 133
sliding, 291-292
techniques for, 127-132
for wounds over carpal extension surfaces, 113, 116
Zonas Porous Tape, 50
Zostrix (capsaicin), 220
Zythromax (azithromycin), 4

For Product Safety Concerns and Information please contact our EU representative GPSR@taylorandfrancis.com Taylor & Francis Verlag GmbH, Kaufingerstraße 24, 80331 München, Germany

Printed and bound by CPI Group (UK) Ltd, Croydon, CR0 4YY
22/09/2026
02220488-0001